NEW GUIDE TO
MEDICINES & DRUGS

NEW GUIDE TO
MEDICINES & DRUGS

Chief Medical Editor

Dr Kevin M O'Shaughnessy MA BM BCh DPhil FRCP FBPhS

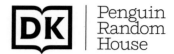

CONTRIBUTORS AND CONSULTANTS

Chief Medical Editor: Dr Kevin M O'Shaughnessy MA BM BCh DPhil FRCP FBPhS
Contributors Sanju Arianayagam MA BMBCh MRCP; Alex Azizi BA MA MRes MB BChir MRCP (UK); Timothy J Burton MA MRCP PhD; Jemima Dunne; Marie Fisk PhD MRCP; James Goodman BSc (Hons) MBChB MRCP (UK); Johann Graggaber MD MRCP; Joanna Gray MBBS MRCP (UK); Emma Hodson MA BM BCh FRCA DPhil; Bernadette Jenner MBBS BSc MRCP; Spoorthy Kulkarni MBBS MD; Ing Lu MBCHb MRCP (UK); Fraz Mir BSc MB BS FRCP; Michaela Watts RGN IP/SP

DK LONDON
Consulting Editor Martyn Page
Senior Editor Katie John
Managing Editor Angeles Gavira
Managing Art Editor Michael Duffy
Jacket Design Development Manager Sophia MTT
Jacket Designer Stephanie Cheng Hui Tan

Production Editor Gillian Reid
Senior Production Controller Meskerem Berhane
Illustrations Jo Cameron; Karen Cochrane; Tony Graham; Mike Johnson; Coral Mula; Lynda Payne
Art Director Karen Self
Associate Publishing Director Liz Wheeler
Publishing Director Jonathan Metcalf

DK DELHI
Project Art Editor Anjali Sachar
CTS Designer Umesh Singh Rawat
Senior Managing Editor Rohan Sinha
Managing Art Editor Sudakshina Basu

Pre-production Manager Sunil Sharma
Editorial Head Glenda Fernandes
Design Head Malavika Talukder

This edition published in 2021
First published in Great Britain in 1988 by
Dorling Kindersley Limited, DK, One Embassy Gardens, 8 Viaduct Gardens, London, SW11 7BW

The authorised representative in the EEA is Dorling Kindersley Verlag GmbH. Arnulfstr.
124, 80636 Munich, Germany

READER NOTICE

The *New Guide to Medicines and Drugs* provides information on a wide range of medicines, drugs, and related subjects. The book is not a substitute for expert medical advice, however, and you are advised always to consult your doctor for specific information on personal health matters. Never disregard expert medical advice or delay in seeking medical advice due to information obtained from this book. The naming of any product, treatment, or organization in this book does not imply endorsement by the Chief Medical Editor, Consulting Medical Editor, or publisher, nor does the omission of any such names indicate disapproval. The Chief Medical Editor, Consulting Medical Editor, and publisher do not accept any legal responsibility for any personal injury or other damage or loss arising from any use or misuse of the information and advice in this book.

A CIP catalogue record for this book is available from the British Library.
ISBN: 978-0-2414-7102-9

Printed in China

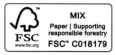

MIX
Paper | Supporting responsible forestry
FSC™ C018179

This book was made with Forest Stewardship Council™ certified paper – one small step in DK's commitment to a sustainable future.
Learn more at
www.dk.com/uk/information/sustainability

PREFACE

Modern medicines and drugs underpin our healthcare systems. Medicines are available not only on prescription, but sometimes over the counter at pharmacies or in supermarkets. Their manufacture and supply are tightly regulated. However, these medications may also be taken alongside unregulated substances such as herbal products or complementary medications. In addition, many people take more than one type of medication, and the prospect for complicated, harmful, or potentially fatal interactions between medications is increasing.

Some medicines are available over the internet, where quality and supply are increasingly difficult to control. The quality of the information is also often poor and unregulated, making deception and "fake news" a dangerous reality. Mistrust of large commercial corporations has put the pharmaceutical industry and the medicines it produces increasingly in a critical spotlight on the internet. Never has it been more important, then, that we understand the nature and risks of any medications that we take.

Before taking any medication, you should discuss it with the healthcare professional prescribing it, or if it is non-prescription, ensure that it will be safe for you. Make sure any prescriber knows about all other medications you are taking, including non-prescription and complementary treatments. Find out what the side effects of the medication may be and what treatments you should avoid taking with it. This book is not designed to replace advice from a healthcare professional, but to supplement, contextualize, and support it. Our goal is to enable the reader to make informed and safe decisions about the medications they elect to take.

This latest edition of the *New Guide to Medicines and Drugs* has detailed profiles of 285 drugs. These profiles have been updated and revised to include important changes to dosage, drug warnings, and formulations. They include nine new profiles, to reflect changes to prescribing practice. You can look up a particular drug in the profiles to find in-depth information about it, or consult parts 1 and 2 of the guide to see the classes of drugs that work in a specific condition or affect a particular part of the body. The sections on travel medicine, vitamins and minerals, drugs of abuse, and complementary and alternative medicines have all been revised where necessary. The Drug Finder now includes more than 3,000 entries, reflecting the enormous range of drugs available.

As in any area of medicine, information and opinion changes rapidly, so this guide cannot replace current advice and information from healthcare prescribers. We hope, however, that it will help you take medicines in a more informed way and improve your health and safety in the process.

Dr. Kevin O'Shaughnessy
Consulting Medical Editor

CONTENTS

3 A–Z OF DRUGS

4 INFORMATION AND INDEX

DRUG POISONING EMERGENCY GUIDE 518

INTRODUCTION

The *New Guide to Medicines and Drugs* has been planned and written to provide clear information and practical advice on drugs and medicines in a way that can be readily understood by a non-medical reader. The text reflects current medical knowledge and standard medical practice in this country. It is intended to complement and reinforce the advice given by your doctor, pharmacist, or other prescriber.

How the book is structured

The book is divided into four parts. The first part, Understanding and Using Drugs, provides a general introduction to the effects of drugs and gives advice on practical questions, such as administration and storage of drugs. Part 2, Major Drug Groups, will help you to understand the uses and mechanisms of action of the principal classes of drugs. Part 3, the A–Z of Drugs, consists of 285 detailed profiles of commonly prescribed generic drugs, profiles of vitamins, minerals, and drugs of abuse, and information on complementary and alternative medicines, and medicines and travel. Part 4 contains useful resources; a glossary of drug-related terms; the drug finder, which helps readers locate information on specific drugs through an index to over 3,000 generic and brand-name drugs; and a general index.

Finding your way into the book

The information you require, whether on the specific characteristics of an individual drug or on the general effects and uses of a group of drugs, can be easily obtained without prior knowledge of the medical names of drugs or drug classification through one of the two indexes: the drug finder or the general index. The diagram on the facing page shows how you can obtain information throughout the book on the subject concerning you from each of these starting points.

1 UNDERSTANDING AND USING DRUGS

The introductory part of the book, Understanding and Using Drugs, gives a grounding in the fundamental principles underlying the medical use of drugs. Covering such topics as classifications of drugs, mechanisms of action, and the proper use of medicines, it provides valuable background information that backs up the more detailed descriptions and advice given in Parts 2 and 3. You should read this section before seeking further specific information.

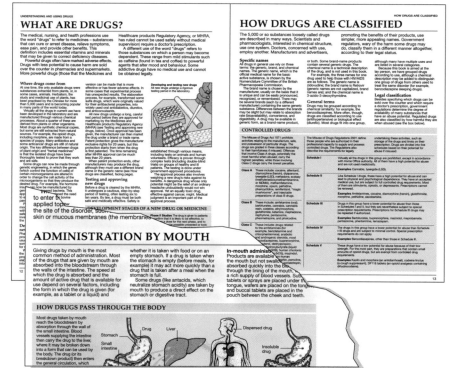

2 MAJOR DRUG GROUPS

Subdivided into sections dealing with each body system (for example, heart and circulation) or major disease grouping (for example, malignant and immune disease), this part of the book contains descriptions of the principal classes of drugs. Information is given on the uses, actions, effects, and risks associated with each group of drugs and is backed up by helpful illustrations and diagrams. Individual drugs in each group are listed to allow cross-reference to Part 3.

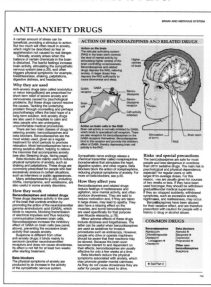

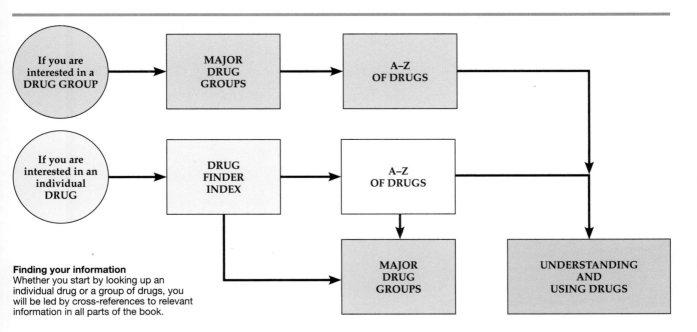

Finding your information
Whether you start by looking up an individual drug or a group of drugs, you will be led by cross-references to relevant information in all parts of the book.

3 A–Z OF DRUGS

In this part of the book, standard-format profiles of 285 generic drugs help you to find specific information quickly and easily; cross-references to relevant major drug groups are also provided. Supplementary sections give information about vitamins and minerals, drugs of abuse, complementary and alternative medicine, and medicines and travel.

4 INFORMATION AND INDEX

Useful resources, including websites, direct you to further information; the glossary explains technical words; the drug finder helps you to find information about specific brand-name drugs and generic substances; and the index enables you to look up references throughout the book.

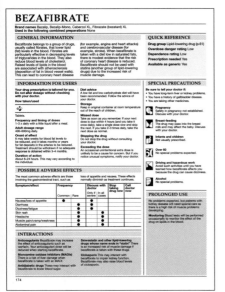

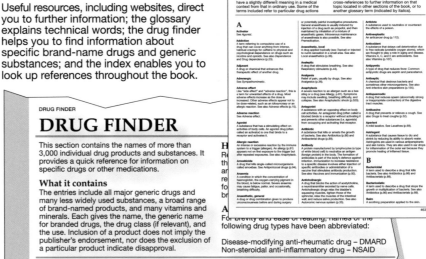

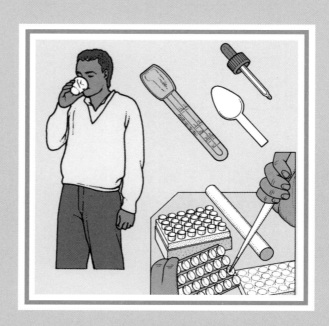

UNDERSTANDING AND USING DRUGS

WHAT ARE DRUGS?

The medical, nursing, and health professions use the word "drugs" to refer to medicines – substances that can cure or arrest disease, relieve symptoms, ease pain, and provide other benefits. This definition includes essential vitamins and minerals that may be given to correct deficiency diseases.

Powerful drugs often have marked adverse effects. Drugs with less potential to cause harm are sold over the counter in pharmacies and supermarkets. More powerful drugs (those that the Medicines and Healthcare products Regulatory Agency, or MHRA, has ruled cannot be used safely without medical supervision) require a doctor's prescription.

A different use of the word "drugs" refers to those substances on which a person may become dependent. These range from mild stimulants such as caffeine (found in tea and coffee) to powerful agents that alter mood and behaviour. Some addictive drugs have no medical use and cannot be obtained legally.

Where drugs come from

At one time, the only available drugs were substances extracted from plants, or, in some cases, animals. Herbalism, the study and medicinal use of plants, has been practised by the Chinese for more than 5,000 years and is becoming popular in many parts of the world today.

Virtually all the drugs in current use have been developed in the laboratory and are manufactured through various chemical processes. About a quarter of these are derived from plants or other organisms. Most drugs are synthetic chemical copies, but some are still extracted from natural sources. For example, the opioid drugs, including morphine, are made from a species of poppy. Many antibiotics and some anticancer drugs are still of natural origin. The key difference between drugs of plant origin and "herbal medicines" is that the isolated drugs have been thoroughly tested to prove that they work and are safe.

Some drugs can now be made through genetic engineering, in which the genes (which control the function of cells) of certain microorganisms are altered in order to change the cell activity of the microorganisms so that they produce the desired drug. For example, the hormone insulin can now be manufactured by genetically engineered bacteria. This approach has largely replaced the need to extract insulin from pig or bovine pancreas glands.

Purely synthetic drugs are either modifications of naturally occurring ones, with the aim of increasing effectiveness or safety, or drugs developed after scientific investigation of a disease process with the intention of changing it biochemically.

Developing and marketing new drugs

Pharmaceutical manufacturers find new products in various ways. New drugs are usually developed for one purpose but sometimes a variant is found to be useful for something different.

When a new drug is discovered, the manufacturer often undertakes a programme of molecular tinkering, or elaboration. This refers to investigations into variants of the drug to see if a version can be made that is more effective or has fewer adverse effects. In some cases that experimental process has unexpected results. The elaboration process, for example, transformed some sulfa drugs, which were originally valued for their antibacterial properties, into widely used oral antidiabetics, diuretics, and anticonvulsants.

All new drugs undergo a long, careful test period before they are approved for marketing by the Medicines and Healthcare products Regulatory Agency (MHRA) (see Testing and approving new drugs, below). Once approval has been given, the manufacturer can then market the drug under a brand or trade name. Patent protection gives the manufacturer exclusive rights for 20 years, but this protection starts from when the drug is first patented. The time remaining after MHRA approval can be much less than 20 years.

When patent protection ends, other manufacturers may produce the drug, although they must use a different brand name or the generic name (see How drugs are classified, facing page).

Testing and approving new drugs

Before a drug is cleared by the MHRA, it undergoes a cautious, step-by-step period of testing, often lasting six to ten years. By law, a drug must be both safe and medically effective. Safety is

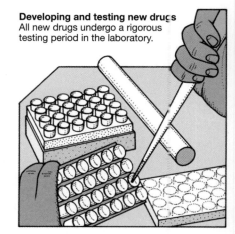

Developing and testing new drugs
All new drugs undergo a rigorous testing period in the laboratory.

established through various means, including tests on animals and human volunteers. Efficacy is proven through complex tests (including double-blind trials) on groups of healthy and ill patients. The testing is done under government-approved procedures.

The approval process also involves weighing a new drug's risks against its benefits. A dangerous drug whose only potential might be the relief of an ordinary headache undoubtedly would not win approval. Yet an equally toxic drug, effective against cancer, might. Medical judgment is an important part of the approval process.

DEVELOPMENT STAGES OF A NEW DRUG OR MEDICINE

Discovery Stage A new chemical undergoes thorough chemical and biological study. If these tests suggest it has promise as a new drug, the process of drug development starts.

Preclinical Studies The first stage of research on a new chemical includes testing on isolated organs and tissues and animal studies. These tests are required before permission can be granted for human clinical trials.

Phase I Studies This is the first stage of testing on human subjects, which usually consist of small groups of healthy volunteers, or sometimes patients. The aim is to assess both the safety of the chemical and how the body deals with it.

Phase II Studies The drug is given to patients to confirm that it is likely to be effective, to decide on a dose for the next phase, and to monitor further for possible unwanted or toxic effects. These studies are short-term (single doses or regular dosing for several weeks).

Phase III Studies Large-scale human studies are carried out to gather sufficient evidence of the drug's efficacy and safety to gain marketing approval. They must be long-term (about a year) double-blind, multi-centre, controlled trials.

Phase IV Studies Once the drug is on the market, further monitoring studies are needed to provide ongoing evidence of its overall effectiveness, safety, and usefulness.

HOW DRUGS ARE CLASSIFIED

The 5,000 or so substances loosely called drugs are described in many ways. Scientists and pharmacologists, interested in chemical structure, use one system. Doctors, concerned with use, employ another. Manufacturers and advertisers, promoting the benefits of their products, use simpler, more appealing names. Government regulators, wary of the harm some drugs may do, classify them in a different manner altogether, according to their legal status.

Specific names

All drugs in general use rely on three terms: the generic, brand, and chemical names. The generic name, which is the official medical name for the basic active substance, is chosen by the Nomenclature Committee of the British Pharmacopoeia Commission.

The brand name is chosen by the manufacturer, usually on the basis that it is unique and can be easily pronounced, recognized, or remembered. There may be several brands (each by a different manufacturer) containing the same generic substance. Differences between the brands may be slight but may relate to absorption rate (bioavailability), convenience, and digestibility. A drug may be available in generic form, as a brand-name product, or both. Some brand-name products contain several generic drugs. The chemical name is a technical description of the drug, and is not used in this book.

For example, the three names for one drug used to help those with HIV/AIDS are as follows. The generic name is zidovudine; the brand name is Retrovir (generic names are not capitalized, brand names are); and the chemical name is 3-azido-3-deoxythymidine.

General terms

Drugs may be grouped according to chemical similarity: for example, the benzodiazepines. More often, though, drugs are classified according to use (antihypertensive) or biological effect (diuretic). Most drugs fit into one group, although many have multiple uses and are listed in several categories.

Because this book is aimed at the lay person, we have grouped drugs according to use, although a chemical description may be added to distinguish one group of drugs from others used to treat the same disorder (for example, benzodiazepine sleeping drugs).

Legal classification

Besides specifying which drugs can be sold over the counter and which require a doctor's prescription, government regulations determine the degree of availability of many substances that have an abuse potential. Regulated drugs are also classified by how harmful they are when abused (see the box below).

CONTROLLED DRUGS

The Misuse of Drugs Act 1971 prohibits activities relating to the manufacture, sale, and possession of particular drugs. The drugs are graded in three classes according to their harmfulness if misused. Offences that involve Class A drugs, potentially the most harmful when abused, carry the highest penalties, while those involving Class C drugs carry the lowest penalties.

Class A	These include: cocaine, alfentanil, diamorphine (heroin), dipipanone, lysergide (LSD), methadone, ecstasy (methylenedioxymethamfetamine, or MDMA), methamfetamine, morphine, opium, pethidine, phencyclidine, remifentanil, "magic mushrooms", and injectable preparations of class B drugs.
Class B	These include: amfetamine (oral), barbiturates, cannabis, cannabis resin, codeine, ethylmorphine, glutethimide, ketamine, mephedrone, naphyrone, pentazocine, phenmetrazine, and pholcodine.
Class C	These include: drugs related to the amfetamines (for example, benzfetamine and chlorphentermine), anabolic and androgenic steroids, most benzodiazepines, buprenorphine, clenbuterol, diethylpropion, gamma hydroxybutyrate (liquid ecstasy, or GHB), human chorionic gonadotrophin (hCG), mazindol, meprobamate, non-human chorionic gonadotrophin, pemoline, phenbuterol, pipradol, somatotropin, somatrem, and somatropin.

The Misuse of Drugs Regulations 2001 define those people who are authorized in their professional capacity to supply and possess controlled drugs. The Regulations also describe the requirements for legally undertaking these activities, such as storage of the drugs and limits on their prescription. Drugs are divided into five schedules based on their potential for abuse if misused.

Schedule I	Virtually all the drugs in this group are prohibited, except in accordance with Home Office authority. All of them have a high potential for abuse and are not used medicinally. **Examples** Cannabis, lysergide (LSD).
Schedule II	Like Schedule I drugs, these have a high potential for abuse and can lead to physical and psychological dependence. They have an accepted medical use, but are subject to full controlled drug requirements. Most of them are stimulants, opioids, or depressants. Prescriptions cannot be renewed. **Examples** Amfetamines, cocaine, diamorphine (heroin), glutethimide, morphine, pethidine, secobarbital.
Schedule III	Drugs in this group have a lower potential for abuse than those in Schedules I and II, but they are nevertheless subject to special prescription requirements. Prescriptions for Schedule III drugs may be repeated if authorized. **Examples** Barbiturates, buprenorphine, mazindol, meprobamate, pentazocine, phentermine, temazepam.
Schedule IV	The drugs in this group have a lower potential for abuse than Schedule I–III drugs and are subject to minimal control. Special prescription requirements do not apply. **Examples** Benzodiazepines, other than those in Schedule III.
Schedule V	These drugs have a low potential for abuse because of their low strength. For the most part, they are preparations that contain small amounts of opioid drugs, but are exempt from controlled drug requirements. **Examples** Kaolin and morphine (an antidiarrhoeal), codeine linctus (a cough suppressant), DF118 tablets (an opioid analgesic containing dihydrocodeine).

HOW DRUGS WORK

Before the discovery of the sulfa drugs in 1935, medical knowledge of drugs was limited to possibly only a dozen or so drugs that had a clear medical value. Most of these were the extracts of plants (such as digitalis, from foxgloves), while others, such as aspirin, were chemically closely related to plant extracts (in this case, salicylic acid, from the willow tree). It was soon realized, however, that crude plant extracts had two disadvantages: they were of variable potency, and the same plant could contain a number of different substances with different actions. These might even oppose each other, or cause serious adverse effects. Now, thousands of effective drugs are available and scientific knowledge regarding drugs and their actions has virtually exploded.

Today's doctor understands the complexity of drug actions in the body, both beneficial and adverse. As a result of extensive research and clinical experience, the doctor can now also recognize that some drugs interact harmfully with others, or with certain foods and alcohol.

DRUG ACTIONS

While the exact workings of some drugs are not fully understood, medical science provides clear knowledge as to what most of them do once they enter or are applied to the human body. Drugs serve different purposes: sometimes they cure a disease, sometimes they only alleviate symptoms. Their impact occurs in various parts of the anatomy. Although different drugs act in different ways, their actions generally fall into one of three categories.

Replacing chemicals that are deficient
To function normally, the body requires sufficient levels of certain chemical substances. These include vitamins and minerals, which the body obtains from food. A balanced diet usually supplies what is needed. But when deficiencies occur, various deficiency diseases result. Lack of vitamin C causes scurvy, iron deficiency causes anaemia, and lack of vitamin D leads to rickets in children and osteomalacia in adults.

Other deficiency diseases arise from a lack of various hormones, which are the chemical substances produced by glands. Hormones act as internal messengers. Diabetes mellitus, hypothyroidism, and Addison's disease all result from deficiencies of different hormones.

Deficiency diseases are treated with drugs that replace the substances that are missing or, in the case of some hormone deficiencies, with animal or synthetic replacements.

Interfering with cell function
Many drugs can change the way cells work by increasing or reducing the normal level of activity. Inflammation, for example, is due to the action of certain natural hormones and other chemicals on blood vessels and blood cells. Anti-inflammatory drugs block the action of the hormones or slow their production. Drugs that act in a similar way are used in the treatment of a variety of conditions: hormone disorders, blood clotting problems, and heart and kidney diseases.

Many such drugs do their work by altering the transmission system by which messages are sent from one part of the body to another.

A message – to contract a muscle, say – originates in the brain and enters a nerve cell through its receiving end. The message, in the form of an electrical impulse, travels the nerve cell to the sending end. Here a chemical substance called a neurotransmitter is released, conducting the message across the tiny gap (synapse) separating it from an adjacent nerve cell. That process is repeated until the message reaches the appropriate muscle.

Many drugs can alter this process, often by their effect on receptor sites on cells (see left). Some drugs (agonists) intensify the response to cell receptor activation while other drugs (antagonists) reduce it.

Acting against invading organisms or abnormal cells
Infectious diseases are caused by viruses, bacteria, protozoa, and fungi invading the body. We now have a wide choice of drugs that destroy these microorganisms, either by halting their multiplication or by killing them directly. Other drugs treat disease by killing abnormal cells produced by the human body – cancer cells, for example.

RECEPTOR SITES

Many drugs produce their effects through their action on special sites called receptors, which may be on the surface of cells or inside them. Natural body chemicals such as neurotransmitters bind to these sites, initiating a response in the cell. A cell may have many types of receptors, each with an affinity for a different chemical. Drugs may also bind to receptors, either adding to the effect of the body's natural chemicals and enhancing cell response (agonists) or preventing such a chemical from binding to its receptor, and thereby blocking a particular cell response (antagonists).

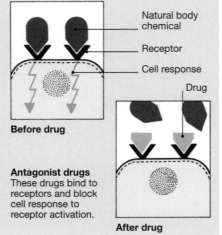

Natural body chemical

Receptor

Cell response

Drug

Before drug

Agonist drugs
These drugs bind to receptors and enhance normal cell response to receptor activation.

After drug

Natural body chemical

Receptor

Cell response

Drug

Before drug

Antagonist drugs
These drugs bind to receptors and block cell response to receptor activation.

After drug

THE EFFECTS OF DRUGS

Before a doctor selects a drug to be used in the treatment of a sick person, they carefully weigh the benefits and the risks. Obviously, the doctor expects a positive result from the drug – a cure for the condition or at least the relief of symptoms. At the same time, the doctor has to consider the risks, since all drugs are potentially harmful, some of them considerably more so than others.

Reaction time

Some drugs can produce rapid and spectacular relief from the symptoms of disease. Glyceryl trinitrate frequently provides almost immediate relief from the pain of angina; other drugs can quickly alleviate the symptoms of an asthmatic attack. Conversely, some drugs take much longer to produce a response. It may, for example, require several weeks of treatment with an antidepressant drug before a person experiences maximum benefit. This can add to anxiety unless the doctor has warned of the possibility of a delay in the onset of beneficial effects.

Adverse effects

The adverse effects of a drug (also known as side effects or adverse reactions) are its undesired effects. When drugs are taken, they are distributed throughout the body and their effects are unlikely to be restricted just to the organ or tissue we want them to affect. Other parts of the body contain receptor sites like those the drug is targeting. In addition, the drug molecule may fit other, different receptors well enough to activate or block them too.

For example, anticholinergic drugs, given to relieve spasm of the intestinal wall, may also cause blurred vision, dry mouth, and retention of urine. Such effects may gradually disappear as the body becomes used to the drug. If they persist, the dose may have to be reduced, or the time between doses may need to be increased. Reducing the dose will often reduce the severity of the adverse effect for those effects that are called "dose-related".

DOSE AND RESPONSE

People respond in different ways to a drug, and often the dose has to be adjusted to allow for a person's age, weight, or general health.

The dose of any drug should be sufficient to produce a beneficial response but not so great that it will cause excessive adverse effects. If the dose is too low, the drug may not have any effect, either beneficial or adverse; if it is too high, it will not produce any additional benefits and may produce adverse effects.

The aim of drug treatment is to achieve a concentration of drug in the blood or tissue that lies between the minimum effective level and the maximum safe concentration. This is known as the therapeutic window (or range).

For certain drugs, such as digitalis drugs, the therapeutic window is quite narrow, so the margin of safety/effectiveness is small. Other drugs, such as penicillin antibiotics, have a much wider therapeutic window.

Wide therapeutic window

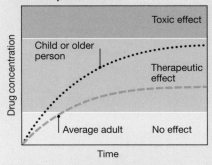

Dosage of drugs with a wide therapeutic window can vary considerably without altering the drug's effect. The effect is greater in children and older adults.

Narrow therapeutic window

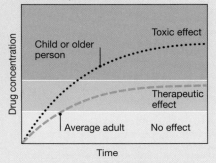

Dosage of drugs with a narrow therapeutic window must be carefully calculated to achieve the desired effect without toxicity. Children or older adults experience toxic levels earlier.

Adverse effects of some drugs can be quite serious. Such drugs are given because they may be the only treatment for an otherwise fatal disease. But all drugs are chemicals, with a potential for producing serious, toxic reactions. Some adverse effects seem not to be dose-related, and where the effect appears on first use and is unexpected, the phenomenon is called idiosyncrasy. People are genetically different and, as a result, their response to drugs differs, perhaps because they lack a particular enzyme or because it is less active than usual. For this reason, not everybody suffers even the "common" adverse effects; but, occasionally, a new adverse

effect, due to a rare and unsuspected genetic variation, will be discovered only after the drug has been taken by a large number of people.

Other adverse effects that are not dose-related are allergic reactions. These reactions do not usually appear on the first exposure to the drug but on a subsequent occasion. The symptoms are similar to those caused by other allergens and, in extreme cases, may cause anaphylactic shock (see p.520).

Beneficial vs. adverse effects

In evaluating the risk/benefit ratio of a prescribed drug, the doctor has to weigh the drug's therapeutic benefit to the sick person against the possible adverse effects. For example, such side effects as nausea, headache, and diarrhoea may result from taking an antibiotic. But the possible risks of the drug's side effects will certainly be considered acceptable if the problem is a life-threatening infection requiring immediate medical treatment. On the other hand, such side effects would be considered unacceptable for an over-the-counter drug for the relief of headaches.

Because some people are more at risk from adverse drug reactions than others (particularly those who have a history of drug allergy), the doctor normally checks whether there is any reason why a certain drug should not be prescribed (see Drug treatment in special risk groups, p.20).

PLACEBO RESPONSE

The word placebo – Latin for "I will please" – is used to describe any chemically inert substance given as a substitute for a drug. Any benefit gained from taking a placebo occurs because the person taking it believes that it will produce good results.

New drugs are almost always tested against a placebo preparation in clinical trials as a way of assessing the efficacy of a drug before it is marketed. The placebo is made to look identical to the active preparation, and the volunteers are not told whether they have been given the active drug or the placebo (so called "blinding"). Sometimes the doctor is also unaware of which preparation a person

has been given. This is known as a double-blind trial. In this way, the purely placebo effect can be eliminated and the effectiveness of the drug determined more realistically.

Sometimes just taking a medicine has a psychological effect that produces a beneficial physical response. This type of placebo response can make an important contribution to the overall effectiveness of a chemically active drug. It is most commonly seen with analgesics, antidepressants, and anti-anxiety drugs. Some people, known as placebo responders, are more likely to experience this sort of effect than the rest of the population.

DRUG INTERACTIONS

When two different drugs are taken together, or when a drug is taken in combination with certain foods or with alcohol, this may produce effects different from those produced when the drug is taken alone. Often, this is beneficial and doctors frequently make use of interactions to increase the effectiveness of a treatment. Very often, more than one drug may be prescribed to treat cancer or high blood pressure (hypertension).

Other interactions, however, are unwanted and may be harmful. They may occur not only between prescription drugs, but also between prescription and over-the-counter drugs. It is important to read warnings on drug labels and tell your doctor if you are taking any preparations – both prescription and over-the-counter, and even herbal or homeopathic remedies.

A drug may interact with another drug or with food or alcohol for a number of reasons (see below).

Altered absorption

Alcohol and some drugs (particularly opioids and drugs with an anticholinergic effect) slow the digestive process that empties the stomach contents into the intestine. This may delay the absorption, and therefore the effect, of another drug. Other drugs (for example, metoclopramide, an anti-emetic drug) may speed the rate at which the stomach empties and may, therefore, increase the rate at which another drug is absorbed and takes effect.

Some drugs also combine with another drug or food in the intestine to form a compound that is not absorbed as readily. This occurs when tetracycline and iron tablets or antacids are taken together. Milk and dairy products also reduce the

Drug absorption in the intestine

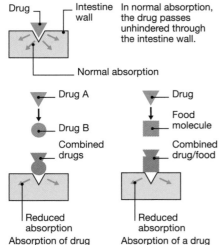

Drug — Intestine wall

In normal absorption, the drug passes unhindered through the intestine wall.

Normal absorption

Drug A
Drug B
Combined drugs

Drug
Food molecule
Combined drug/food

Reduced absorption
Absorption of drug (A) may be reduced if it combines with another drug (B).

Reduced absorption
Absorption of a drug may be reduced if it combines with a food molecule.

EXAMPLES OF IMPORTANT INTERACTIONS

Adverse interactions between drugs may vary from a simple blocking of a drug's beneficial effect to a serious reaction between two drugs that may be life-threatening. Some of the more serious adverse interactions occur between the following:

Drugs that depress the central nervous system (opioids, most antihistamines, sleeping drugs, and alcohol). The effects of two or more of these drugs together may be additive, causing dangerous oversedation.

Drugs that lower blood sugar levels and such drugs as sulfonamides and alcohol. The drug interaction increases the effect of blood-sugar-lowering drugs, thus further depressing blood sugar levels.

Oral anticoagulants and other drugs, particularly aspirin and antibiotics. As these drugs may increase the tendency to bleed, it is essential to check the effects in every case.

Monoamine oxidase inhibitors (MAOIs). Many drugs and foods can produce a severe increase in blood pressure when taken with MAOIs. Such drugs include amfetamines and decongestants; foods include cheese, herring, chocolate, red wine, and beer. Some of the newer MAOIs, however, are much less likely to interact with food and drugs.

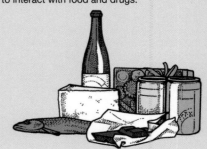

absorption of tetracycline and some other drugs, such as ciprofloxacin, by combining with the drugs in this manner.

Enzyme effects

Some drugs increase the production of enzymes in the liver that break down drugs, while others inhibit or reduce enzyme production. Thus they affect the rate at which other drugs are activated or inactivated.

Excretion in the urine

A drug may reduce the kidneys' ability to excrete another drug, raising the drug level in the blood and increasing its effect.

Receptor effects

Drugs that act on the same receptor sites (see p.14) sometimes add to each other's effect on the body, or compete with each other in occupying certain receptor sites. For example, naloxone blocks receptors used by opioid drugs, thereby helping to reverse the effects of opioid poisoning.

Similar or opposite effects

Drugs that produce similar effects (but act on different receptors) add to each other's actions. Often, lower doses are possible as a result, with fewer adverse effects. This is common practice in the treatment of high blood pressure and cancer. Antibiotics are given together as the infecting organisms are less likely to develop resistance to the drugs. Drugs with antagonistic effects reduce the useful activity of one or both drugs. For example, some antidepressants oppose the effects of anticonvulsants.

Reduced protein binding

Some drugs circulate around the body in the bloodstream with a proportion of the drug attached to the proteins of the blood

plasma. The amount of drug attached to the plasma proteins is inactive. If another drug is taken, some of the second drug may also bind to the plasma proteins and displace the first drug; more of the first drug is then active in the body.

Interaction between protein-bound drugs

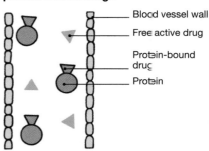

Blood vessel wall
Free active drug
Protein-bound drug
Protein

Protein-bound drug taken alone
Drug molecules that are bound to proteins in the blood are unable to pass into body tissues. Only free drug molecules are active.

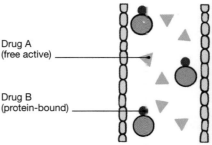

Drug A (free active)
Drug B (protein-bound)

Taken with another protein-bound drug
If a drug (B) with a greater ability to bind with proteins is also taken, drug (A) is displaced, increasing the amount of active drug.

METHODS OF ADMINISTRATION

The majority of drugs must be absorbed into the bloodstream in order for them to reach the site where their effects are needed. The method of administering a drug determines the route it takes to get into the bloodstream and the speed at which it is absorbed into the blood.

When a drug is meant to enter the bloodstream it is usually administered in one of the following ways: through the mouth or rectum, by injection, or by inhalation. Drugs that are implanted under the skin or enclosed in a skin patch also enter the bloodstream. These types are discussed under Slow-release preparations (see p.18).

When it is unnecessary or undesirable for a drug to enter the bloodstream in large amounts, it may be applied topically so that its effect is limited mainly to the site of the disorder, such as the surface of the skin or mucous membranes (the membranes of the nose, eyes, ears, vagina, or rectum). Drugs are administered topically in a variety of preparations, including creams, gels, lotions, sprays, drops, and suppositories. Most inhaled drugs also have a local effect on the respiratory tract.

Very often, a particular drug may be available in different forms. Many drugs are available both as tablets and as injectable fluid. The choice between a tablet and an injection depends on a number of factors, including the severity of the illness, the urgency with which the drug effect is needed, the part of the body requiring treatment, and the patient's general state of health, in particular their ability to swallow.

The various administration routes are discussed in greater detail below. For a description of the different forms in which drugs are given, see Drug forms (p.19).

ADMINISTRATION BY MOUTH

Giving drugs by mouth is the most common method of administration. Most of the drugs that are given by mouth are absorbed into the bloodstream through the walls of the intestine. The speed at which the drug is absorbed and the amount of active drug that is available for use depend on several factors, including the form in which the drug is given (for example, as a tablet or a liquid) and whether it is taken with food or on an empty stomach. If a drug is taken when the stomach is empty (before meals, for example) it may act more quickly than a drug that is taken after a meal when the stomach is full.

Some drugs (like antacids, which neutralize stomach acidity) are taken by mouth to produce a direct effect on the stomach or digestive tract.

In-mouth administration
Products are available that are placed in the mouth but not swallowed. They are absorbed quickly into the bloodstream through the lining of the mouth, which has a rich supply of blood vessels. Sublingual tablets or sprays are placed under the tongue, wafers are placed on the tongue, and buccal tablets are placed in the pouch between the cheek and teeth.

HOW DRUGS PASS THROUGH THE BODY

Most drugs taken by mouth reach the bloodstream by absorption through the wall of the small intestine. Blood vessels supplying the intestine then carry the drug to the liver, where it may be broken down into a form that can be used by the body. The drug (or its breakdown product) then enters the general circulation, which carries it around the body. It may pass back into the intestine before being reabsorbed into the bloodstream. Some drugs are rapidly excreted via the kidneys; others may build up in fatty tissues in the body.

Certain insoluble drugs cannot be absorbed through the intestinal wall and pass through the digestive tract unchanged. These drugs are useful for treating bowel disorders, but if they are intended to have systemic effects elsewhere they must be given by intravenous injection.

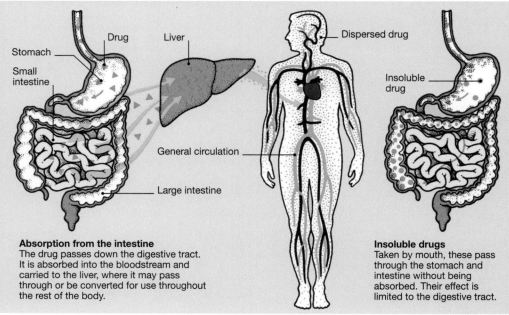

Absorption from the intestine
The drug passes down the digestive tract. It is absorbed into the bloodstream and carried to the liver, where it may pass through or be converted for use throughout the rest of the body.

Insoluble drugs
Taken by mouth, these pass through the stomach and intestine without being absorbed. Their effect is limited to the digestive tract.

RECTAL ADMINISTRATION

Drugs intended to have a systemic effect may be given in the form of suppositories inserted into the rectum, from where they are absorbed into the bloodstream. This method may be used to give drugs that might be destroyed by the stomach's digestive juices. It is also sometimes used to administer drugs to people who cannot take medication by mouth, such as those who are suffering from nausea and vomiting.

Drugs may also be given rectally for local effect, either as suppositories (to relieve haemorrhoids) or as enemas (for ulcerative colitis).

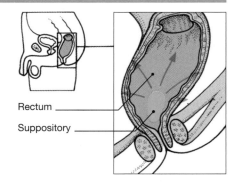

Rectum

Suppository

INHALATION

Drugs may be inhaled to produce a systemic effect or a direct local effect on the respiratory tract. Insufflation into the nose ("snorting") is a variation of this delivery method. Gases to produce general anaesthesia are administered by inhalation and are absorbed into the bloodstream through the lungs, producing a general effect on the body, particularly the brain. Bronchodilators (for certain types of emphysema, bronchitis, and asthma) are taken by inhalation for their direct effect on the respiratory tract, but some of the active drug also reaches the bloodstream. (See also p.48.)

ADMINISTRATION BY INJECTION

Drugs may be injected into the body to produce a systemic effect. One reason for injecting drugs is the rapid response that follows. Other circumstances that call for injection are when: a person is intolerant to the drug when taken by mouth; the drug would be destroyed by the stomach's digestive juices (insulin, for example); or the drug cannot pass through the intestinal walls into the bloodstream. Drug injections may also be given to produce a local effect, as is often done to relieve the pain of arthritis.

The three most common methods of injection – intramuscular, intravenous, and subcutaneous – are described in the illustration (see right). The type of injection depends both on the nature of the drug and the condition being treated.

Muscle   Vein   Skin   Fatty tissue

Intramuscular (IM) injection
The drug is injected into a muscle, usually of the thigh, the upper arm, or the buttock.

Subcutaneous (SC) injection
The drug is injected directly under the surface of the skin.

Intravenous (IV) injection
The drug is injected directly into a vein and therefore directly into the bloodstream. Drugs given by this route act more quickly than drugs given by other types of injection.

TOPICAL APPLICATION

In treating localized disorders such as skin infections and nasal congestion, it is often preferable when a choice is available to prescribe drugs in a form that has a topical, or localized, rather than a systemic effect. The reason is that it is much easier to control the effects of drugs administered locally and to ensure that they produce the maximum benefit with minimum adverse effects.

Topical preparations are available in a variety of forms, from skin creams, gels, ointments, and lotions to nasal sprays, ear and eye drops, bladder irrigations, and vaginal pessaries. It is important when using topical preparations to follow instructions carefully, avoiding a higher dose than recommended or application for longer than necessary. This will help to avoid adverse systemic effects caused by the absorption of larger amounts into the bloodstream.

SLOW-RELEASE AND MODIFIED-RELEASE PREPARATIONS

Some disorders can be treated with specially formulated preparations that can release the active drug slowly. Such preparations may be beneficial when it is inconvenient for a person to visit the doctor regularly, or when only small amounts of the drug need to be released into the body. Slow release of drugs can be achieved by depot injections, transdermal patches, capsules and tablets, and implants. Modified-release tablets and capsules are a more advanced version in which release of the active ingredient is related to time.

Slow-release capsule
Contains pellets of drug in a specially formulated coating.

Outer coating

Drug

Capsule

Transdermal patch
An adhesive, drug-impregnated pad is placed on the skin. The drug passes slowly through the skin.

Transdermal patch

Skin

Drug

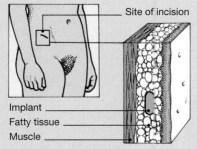

Site of incision

Implant

Fatty tissue

Muscle

Implants
A pellet containing the drug is implanted under the skin. By this rarely used method, a drug (usually a hormone) is slowly released into the bloodstream over a period of months.

DRUG FORMS

Most drugs are specially prepared in a form designed for convenience of administration. This helps to ensure that dosages are accurate and that taking the medication is as easy as possible. Inactive ingredients (those with no therapeutic effect) are sometimes added to flavour or colour the medicine, or to improve its chemical stability, extending the period during which it is effective. The more common drug forms are described below.

Tablets
These contain the drug compressed with other ingredients (see right) into a solid plug. Tablets can be either coated with a membrane that allows the drug to be released slowly for sustained effect or made up of individually layered granules for slow release; they can also be soluble in water.

Capsules
The drug is contained in a cylindrically shaped gelatin shell that breaks open after the capsule has been swallowed, releasing the drug. Slow-release capsules contain pellets that dissolve in the gastrointestinal tract, releasing the drug slowly (facing page).

Wafers/melts, pastilles, lozenges, or lollipops
The drug is contained in a small wafer (or melt) placed on the tongue and allowed to dissolve. A pastille is a medicated "sweet" that is chewed; a lozenge or lollipop is sucked.

Liquids (oral)
Some drugs are available as liquid; the active substance is combined in a solution, suspension, or emulsion with preservatives, solvents, and flavouring or colouring agents. Many liquid preparations should be shaken before use, to ensure even distribution of the active drug, or inaccurate dosages may result.

Mixture
A mixture is one or more drugs, either dissolved to form a solution or suspended in a liquid (often water).

Elixir
An elixir is a solution of a drug in a sweetened mixture of alcohol and water. It is often highly flavoured.

Emulsion
An emulsion is a drug dispersed in oil and water. An emulsifying agent is often included to stabilize the product.

Syrup
A syrup is a concentrated solution of sugar containing the active drug, with flavouring and stabilizing agents added.

Topical skin preparations
These are designed for application to the skin and other surface body tissues.

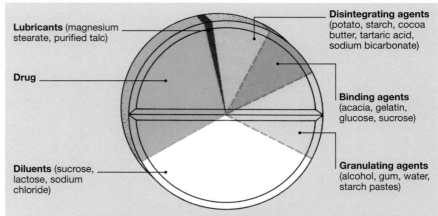

WHAT A TABLET CONTAINS

Lubricants (magnesium stearate, purified talc)

Drug

Diluents (sucrose, lactose, sodium chloride)

Disintegrating agents (potato, starch, cocoa butter, tartaric acid, sodium bicarbonate)

Binding agents (acacia, gelatin, glucose, sucrose)

Granulating agents (alcohol, gum, water, starch pastes)

Diluents add bulk. Binders and granulating agents bind the ingredients. Lubricants ensure a smooth surface by allowing the ingredients to flow during the manufacturing process.

Disintegrating agents help the tablet dissolve. A sugar coating or a transparent film protects the surface or modifies the drug's release rate. Dyes and imprints make it recognizable.

Preservatives are usually included to reduce bacterial growth. The most commonly used skin preparations are described below. (See also Bases for skin preparations, p.135.)

Creams, ointments, and gels
A cream is a non-greasy preparation that is used to apply drugs to an area of the body or to cool or moisten the skin. It is less noticeable than an ointment.

An ointment is a greasy preparation used to apply drugs to an area of the body, or as a protective or lubricant layer for the relief of dry skin conditions.

A gel is a jellylike suspension consisting of small, insoluble particles dispersed through a liquid. Most gels are non-greasy. They are most commonly used for face and scalp preparations.

Lotion
A lotion is a solution or suspension applied to unbroken skin to cool and dry the affected area. Some are more suitable for use in hairy areas because they are not as sticky as creams or ointments.

Injection solutions
Solutions for injections are sterile (germ-free) preparations of a drug dissolved or suspended in a liquid. Other chemicals (e.g., anti-oxidants and buffers) are often added to preserve the stability of the drug or to regulate the acidity or alkalinity of the solution. Most injectable drugs are packaged in sterile, disposable syringes. For details on different types, see Administration by injection, facing page.

Suppositories and pessaries
These are solid, bullet-shaped dosage forms designed for easy insertion into the rectum (suppository) or vagina (pessary). They contain a drug and an inert (chemically and pharmacologically inactive) substance often derived from vegetable oil or cocoa butter. The drug is gradually released in the rectum or vagina as the suppository or pessary dissolves at body temperature.

Eye drops
A sterile drug solution (or suspension) dropped behind the eyelid.

Ear drops
A solution (or suspension) containing a drug introduced into the ear by dropper. Ear drops are usually given to produce an effect on the outer ear canal.

Nasal drops/spray
A solution of a drug for introduction into the nose to produce a local effect.

Inhalers
Aerosol inhalers contain a solution or suspension of a drug under pressure. Dry-powder devices contain the drug in an inhalable powder form. A valve ensures delivery of a recommended dosage when the inhaler is activated. A mouthpiece facilitates inhalation as the drug is released from the canister. It is important to use the correct technique; you should follow the printed instructions carefully or ask your doctor, pharmacist, or nurse to show you what to do. Aerosol and dry-powder inhalers are widely used for asthma. (See also p.49.)

Transdermal patches
These adhesive pads are impregnated with a drug and placed on the skin. The drug is released slowly through the skin (see facing page).

DRUG TREATMENT IN SPECIAL RISK GROUPS

Different people tend to respond in different ways to drug treatment. Taking the same drug, one person may suffer adverse effects while another does not. However, doctors know that certain people are always more at risk from adverse effects when they take drugs; the reason is that in those people the body handles drugs differently, or the drug has an atypical effect. Those people at special risk include infants and children, women who are pregnant or breast-feeding, older people, and those who have long-term medical conditions, especially people with impaired liver or kidney function.

The reasons that such people may be more likely to suffer adverse effects are discussed in detail on the following pages. Others who may need special attention include those already taking regular medication who may risk complications when they take another drug. Drug interactions are discussed more fully on p.16.

When doctors prescribe drugs for people at special risk, they take extra care to select appropriate medication, adjust dosages, and closely monitor the effects of treatment. If you think you may be at special risk, be sure to tell your doctor in case they are not fully aware of your particular circumstances. Similarly, if you are buying over-the-counter drugs, you should ask your doctor or pharmacist if you think you may be at risk of experiencing any possible adverse effects or hazardous drug interactions.

INFANTS AND CHILDREN

Infants and children need a lower dosage of drugs than adults because children have a relatively low body weight. In addition, because of differences in body composition and the distribution and amount of body fat, as well as differences in the state of development and function of organs such as the liver and kidneys at different ages, children cannot simply be given a proportion of an adult dose as if they were small adults. Dosages need to be calculated in a more complex way, taking into account the child's age and weight. While newborn babies often have to be given very small doses of drugs, older children may need relatively large doses of some drugs compared to the adult dosage.

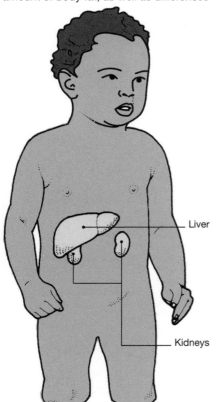

The liver
The liver's enzyme systems are not fully developed when a baby is born. This means that drugs are not broken down as rapidly as in an adult, and may reach dangerously high concentrations in the baby's body. For this reason, many drugs are not prescribed for babies or are given in very reduced doses. In older children, because the liver is relatively large compared to the rest of the body, some drugs may need to be given in proportionately higher doses.

— Liver

— Kidneys

The kidneys
During the first six months, a baby's kidneys are unable to excrete drugs as efficiently as an adult's kidneys. This may lead to a dangerously high concentration of a drug in the blood. The dose of certain drugs may therefore need to be reduced. Between one and two years of age, kidney function improves, and higher doses of some drugs may then be needed.

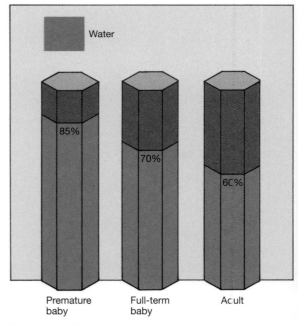

Water

85%

70%

60%

Premature baby

Full-term baby

Adult

Body composition
The proportion of water in the body of a premature baby is about 85 per cent of its body weight, that of a full-term baby is 70 per cent, and that of an adult is only 60 per cent. This means that drugs that stay in the body water will not be as concentrated in an infant's body as in an adult's, unless a higher dose relative to body weight is given.

PREGNANT WOMEN

Great care is needed during pregnancy to protect the fetus so that it develops into a healthy baby. Drugs taken by the mother can cross the placenta and enter the baby's bloodstream. With certain drugs, and at certain stages of pregnancy, there is a risk of developmental abnormalities, retarded growth, or post-delivery problems affecting the newborn baby. In addition, some drugs may affect the health of the mother during pregnancy.

Many drugs are known to have adverse effects during pregnancy; others are known to be safe, but in a large number of cases there is no firm evidence to decide on risk or safety. Therefore, the most important rule if you are pregnant or trying to conceive is to consult your doctor before taking any prescribed or over-the-counter medication.

Drugs such as cannabis, nicotine, and alcohol should also be avoided during pregnancy. A high daily intake of caffeine should be reduced if possible. Your doctor will assess the potential benefits of drug treatment against any possible risks to decide whether or not a drug should be taken. This is particularly important if you need to take medication regularly for a chronic condition such as epilepsy, high blood pressure, or diabetes.

Drugs and the stages of pregnancy

Pregnancy is divided into three three-month stages called trimesters. Depending on the trimester in which they are taken, drugs can have different effects on the mother, the fetus, or both. Some drugs may be considered safe during one trimester, but not during another. Doctors, therefore, often need to substitute one medication for another given during the course of pregnancy and/or labour.

The trimesters of pregnancy

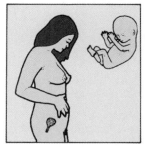

First trimester
During the first three months of pregnancy – the most critical period – drugs may affect the development of fetal organs, leading to congenital defects. Very severe defects may result in miscarriage.

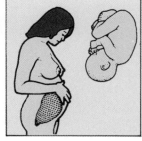

Second trimester
From the fourth to the sixth month some drugs may retard the growth of the fetus. This may also result in a low birth weight. Other drugs may affect the development of the nervous system.

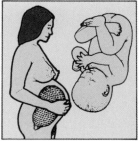

Third trimester
During the last three months of pregnancy, major risks include breathing difficulties in the newborn baby. Some drugs may also affect labour, causing it to be premature, delayed, or prolonged.

How drugs cross the placenta

The placenta acts as a filter between the mother's bloodstream and that of the baby. It allows small molecules of nutrients to pass into the baby's blood, while preventing larger particles such as blood cells from doing so. Most drug molecules are comparatively small and pass easily through the placental barrier.

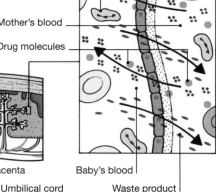

Nutrients
Blood cell
Mother's blood
Drug molecules
Wall of uterus
Placenta
Placenta
Umbilical cord
Baby's blood
Waste product

BREAST-FEEDING

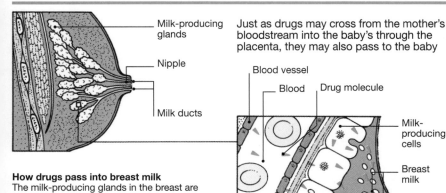

Milk-producing glands
Nipple
Milk ducts
Blood vessel
Blood
Drug molecule
Milk-producing cells
Breast milk

How drugs pass into breast milk
The milk-producing glands in the breast are surrounded by a network of fine blood vessels. Small molecules of substances such as drugs pass from the blood into the milk. Drugs that dissolve easily in fat may pass across in greater concentrations than other drugs.

Just as drugs may cross from the mother's bloodstream into the baby's through the placenta, they may also pass to the baby from the mother's milk. This means that a breast-fed baby will receive small doses of whatever drugs the mother is taking. In many cases this is not a problem, because the amount of drug that passes into the milk is too small to have any significant effect on the baby. However, some drugs can produce unwanted effects on the baby. Antibiotics may sensitize the infant and consequently prevent their use later in life. Sedative drugs may make the baby drowsy and cause feeding problems. Moreover, some drugs may reduce the amount of milk produced by the mother.

Doctors usually advise breast-feeding women to take only essential drugs. When a mother needs to take regular medication while breast-feeding, her baby may also need to be closely monitored for possible adverse effects.

OLDER PEOPLE

Older people are particularly at risk when taking drugs. This is partly due to the physical changes associated with ageing, and partly because many older people need to take several different drugs at the same time. They may also be at risk because they may be unable to manage their treatment properly, or they may lack the information to do so.

Physical changes

Older people have a greater risk of accumulating drugs in their body tissues because the liver is less efficient at breaking drugs down and the kidneys are less efficient at excreting them. Because of this, in some cases the normal adult dose will produce side effects, and a smaller dose may be needed to produce a therapeutic effect without the side effects. (See also Liver and kidney disease, below.)

Older people tend to take more drugs than younger people – many take three or more drugs at the same time. Apart from increasing the number of drugs in their systems, adverse drug interactions (see p.16) are more likely.

As people grow older, some parts of the body, such as the brain and nervous system, may become more sensitive to drugs, thus increasing the likelihood of adverse reactions from drugs acting on those sites (see right). A similar problem may occur due to changes in the percentage of body fat. Although allergic reactions (see Allergy, p.81) do not become more common due to increasing age, they are more likely because more drugs are prescribed. Accordingly, doctors prescribe more carefully for older people, especially those with disorders that are likely to correct themselves in time.

Incorrect use of drugs

Older people often suffer harmful effects from their drug treatment because they fail to take their medication regularly or correctly. This may happen because they have been misinformed about how to take it or receive vague instructions. Problems arise sometimes because the older person cannot remember whether they have taken the drug and take a double dose (see Exceeding the dose, p.30). Problems may also occur because the person is confused; this is not necessarily due to age or illness, but can arise as a result of drug treatment, especially if an older person is taking a number of different drugs or a sedative.

Prescriptions for older people should be clearly and fully labelled, and/or information about the drug and its use should be provided either for the individual or for the person taking care of them. When appropriate, containers with memory aids, such as a dosette box, should be used to dispense the medication in single doses.

Older people often find it difficult to swallow medicine in capsule or tablet form; they should always take capsules or tablets with a full glass or cup of liquid. A liquid medicine may be prescribed instead.

Effect of drugs that act on the brain

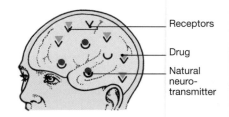

Receptors

Drug

Natural neuro-transmitter

In young people
There are plenty of receptors to take up the drug as well as natural neurotransmitters.

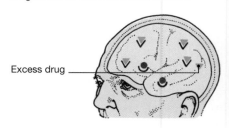

Excess drug

In older people
There may be fewer receptors so that even a reduced drug dose may be excessive.

LIVER AND KIDNEY DISEASE

Long-term illness affects the way in which people respond to drugs. This is especially true of liver and kidney problems. The liver alters the chemical structure of many drugs in the body (see How drugs pass through the body, p.17) by breaking them down into simpler substances, while the kidneys excrete drugs in the urine. If the effectiveness of the liver or kidneys is reduced, the action of drugs on the individual can be significantly altered. In most cases, people with liver or kidney disease will be prescribed fewer drugs and lower doses. In addition, certain drugs may, in rare cases, damage the liver or kidneys. For example, tetracycline can cause kidney failure in those with poor kidney function. A doctor may be reluctant to prescribe such a drug to someone with already reduced liver or kidney function in order to avoid the risk of further damage.

Drugs and liver disease

Severe liver diseases, such as cirrhosis and hepatitis, affect the way the body breaks down drugs. This can lead to a dangerous accumulation of certain drugs in the body. People suffering from these diseases should consult their doctor before taking any medication (including over-the-counter drugs and complementary or alternative remedies) or alcohol. Many drugs must be avoided completely, since they could cause coma in someone with liver damage.

Drugs and kidney disease

People with poor kidney function are at risk from drug side effects. There are two reasons for this. First, drugs build up in the system because smaller amounts are excreted in urine. Second, kidney disease can cause protein loss through the urine, which lowers the level of protein in the blood. Some drugs bind to blood proteins, and if there are fewer protein molecules, a greater proportion of the drug becomes free and active in the body.

Drug passing through body

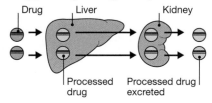

Drug   Liver   Kidney

Processed drug   Processed drug excreted

Normal liver and kidneys
Drugs are processed in the liver before being excreted by the kidneys.

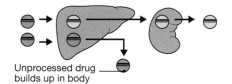

Unprocessed drug builds up in body

In liver damage
The liver cannot process enough of the drug and this builds up in the body tissues.

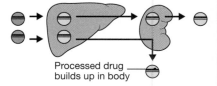

Processed drug builds up in body

In kidney damage
The kidneys cannot excrete the processed drug in the urine and drug levels in the body rise.

DRUG TOLERANCE AND DEPENDENCE

In the course of treatment with some common drugs, the body acquires the ability to adapt to the drug's effect. This response is known as tolerance. As a result, the drug dose has to be increased to achieve the same effect as before. Tolerance is not always associated with dependence (often called addiction), which is the compulsion to continue taking a drug in order to experience a desired effect, or in order to avoid the unpleasant effects that occur when it is not taken. Dependence is almost always confined to drugs that act on the brain and nervous system, such as opiates, tobacco, and alcohol.

TOLERANCE

Drug tolerance occurs as the body adapts to a drug's actions. A person taking the drug needs larger and larger doses to achieve the original effect and as the dose increases, so too do the risks of toxic effects and dependence. Although people can develop a tolerance to some drugs, it is an important characteristic of virtually all the drugs of dependence.

How tolerance develops
Drug tolerance can develop through a variety of different mechanisms, many of which are not fully understood. In some cases, the liver becomes more efficient at breaking the drug down to an inactive form. In other cases, the drug receptors adapt to the presence of the drug. In yet other cases, the drug exhausts the body's supply of chemicals necessary to produce a response.

Tolerance to one particular drug may result in the reduced effect of a drug that has similar properties or is processed in the body in the same way. This is known as cross-tolerance. For example, a regular drinker, who can tolerate high levels of alcohol (a depressant), can have a dangerous tolerance to other depressants such as sleeping drugs and anti-anxiety drugs. While cross-tolerance can often cause problems, it sometimes has a beneficial effect in allowing a substance with a less addictive potential to replace the original drug. For example, the symptoms of alcohol withdrawal can be controlled by the anti-anxiety drug diazepam, which is also a depressant.

Tolerance to some drugs has its benefits. A person can develop tolerance to the side effects of a drug while still benefiting from its useful effects. For example, many people taking antidepressants find that side effects such as dry mouth slowly disappear, with the primary action of the drug continuing (see below).

Increasing drug tolerance also has dangers. A person who has developed tolerance to a drug may keep raising the dose to sometimes toxic levels in order to achieve the desired effect.

Effects of tolerance

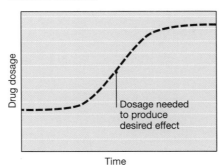

Development of tolerance
A gradually increasing dose of the drug is needed to produce the desired effect as tolerance develops over time.

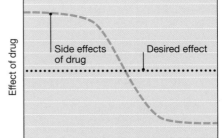

Beneficial effect of tolerance
During treatment with many drugs, the unwanted side effects decrease with time, while the desired effect of the drug is maintained.

DEPENDENCE

Drug dependence is defined as the compulsive use of a substance resulting in physical, psychological, or social harm to the user, with continued use despite the harm.

Drug dependence (now widely preferred as a term to the word addiction) applies far more widely than most people realize. It is usually thought of in association with the use of illegal drugs, such as heroin, or with excessive intake of alcohol. But millions of people are dependent on other drugs, including stimulants – such as caffeine found in coffee and tea, and nicotine in tobacco – and certain prescription medicines, such as analgesics, sleeping drugs, amfetamines, and tranquillizers.

Psychological and physical dependence
Drug dependence, implying that a person is reliant on the continued use of a substance with potential for abuse, is of two types. Psychological dependence is an emotional state of craving for a drug whose presence has a desired effect on the mind, or whose absence has an undesired effect. Physical dependence, which often accompanies psychological dependence, involves physiological adaptation to a medicine or substance that is characterized by severe physical disturbances – withdrawal symptoms – during a period of abstinence. Some drugs, such as laxatives, can produce physical dependence.

Drugs that cause dependence
Many people who need to take regular medication worry that they may become dependent on their drugs. In fact, only a few groups of drugs produce physical or psychological dependence, and most of them are substances that alter mood or behaviour. Such drugs include heroin and other opioid analgesics such as morphine and pethidine, some sleeping and anti-anxiety drugs (benzodiazepines and barbiturates), depressants (alcohol), and nervous system stimulants (cocaine, caffeine, amfetamines, and nicotine).

Antidepressant drugs do not cause psychological dependence. When a depressive illness has been treated effectively, drugs can usually be stopped

DEPENDENCE continued

without any problems, although some people may experience physical withdrawal symptoms if drugs are stopped suddenly. Consult the drug profile in Part 3 of this book to discover the dependence rating of any drug you are taking.

The use of nicotine, in the form of tobacco, and of opioid analgesics, whether controlled or uncontrolled, invariably produces physical dependence if occurring regularly over a period of time. However, it is also true that not all regular users of alcohol become dependent on it. There is debate over the definition of alcohol dependence. However, a widely used criterion is that a person is dependent on alcohol if they experience physical, psychological, social, or occupational impairment as a result of habitual, excessive alcohol consumption.

Recognizing the dangers of drug dependence

Factors that determine a person's risk of developing physical dependence include the characteristics of the drug itself, the strength and frequency of doses, and the duration of use. However, the presence of these factors does not always result in dependence. Psychological and physiological factors that are unique to each individual also enter into the equation, and there may be other, as yet unknown, factors involved. For example,

DRUG MISUSE

The term "misuse" is defined as any use of drugs that causes physical, psychological, economic, legal, or social harm to the user, or to persons who may be affected by the user's behaviour. Drug abuse commonly refers to taking drugs obtained illegally (such as heroin), but may also be used to describe the misuse of drugs generally obtainable legally (nicotine, alcohol), and to drugs obtainable through a doctor's prescription only (everything from sleeping tablets and tranquillizers to analgesics and stimulants).

The misuse of prescription drugs deserves more attention than it usually receives. The practice can include the personal use of drugs left over from a previous course of treatment, the sharing with others of drugs that have been prescribed for yourself, the deliberate deception of doctors, the forgery of prescriptions, and the theft of drugs from pharmacies. All of these practices can have dangerous consequences. Careful attention to

the advice in the section on Managing your drug treatment (p.25) will help to avoid inadvertent misuse of drugs. The dangers associated with abuse of individual drugs are discussed under Drugs of abuse (pp.446–456).

Commonly misused drugs

Alcohol	Lysergide (LSD)
Amphetamines	"Magic mushrooms"
Barbiturates	Mephedrone
Benzodiazepines	Naphyrone
Cannabis (including	Nicotine
synthetic forms	Nitrites ("poppers")
such as "Spice")	Opioids (including
Cocaine (including	heroin and
crack)	methadone)
Ecstasy (MDMA)	Phencyclidine
GHB	Volatile substances
Ketamine	(solvents)
Khat	

when the use of opioid analgesics is restricted to the short-term relief of pain in a medical setting, dependence is rare. Yet there is a high risk of physical dependence when opioid analgesics, or other drugs of abuse, are taken for non-medical reasons. There is also a risk in some cases of low-dose use when the drug is continued over a long period

(e.g. with benzodiazepines, p.39). No one can say for sure exactly what leads a person to drug-dependent behaviour. A person's psychological and physical make-up are thought to be factors, as well as the person's social environment, occupational pressures, and outlook on life.

The indiscriminate use of certain prescription drugs can also cause drug dependence. Benzodiazepine drugs can produce dependence, and this is one reason why doctors today discourage the use of any drug to induce sleep or calm anxiety for more than a few weeks. Similarly, amphetamines are no longer prescribed as appetite suppressants because of their potential for abuse.

Treating drug dependence

Treatment for drug dependence can only be effective if the person is sufficiently motivated. There are two parts to treatment. The first part, detoxification, can take different forms. In some cases, if it is possible to do so, abstinence may be abruptly imposed. Sometimes the drug may be gradually withdrawn or other safer substances substituted. For example, methadone (see p.319) is substituted for heroin. Physical or mental withdrawal symptoms may need close monitoring: for instance, withdrawal from depressants such as barbiturates or alcohol may result in seizures. Once the drug has been cleared from the body, the second part of treatment is directed towards preventing a recurrence. This can involve psychological therapies to tackle the initial cause of the dependence, such as social problems or depression. Psychotherapy, personal counselling, and the work of support organizations, such as Alcoholics Anonymous, may all play a role in overcoming dependence and preventing a recurrence.

SYMPTOMS OF WITHDRAWAL

These can range from the mild (sneezing, sweating) to the serious (vomiting, confusion) to the extremely serious (seizures, coma). Alcohol withdrawal may be associated with delirium tremens, which is very occasionally fatal. Withdrawal from benzodiazepines can sometimes involve hallucinations and seizures. But under medical guidance, withdrawal symptoms can be relieved

with doses of the original drug, or with less addictive substitutes.

Withdrawal symptoms occur because the body has adapted to the action of the drug (see Drug tolerance, p.23). When a drug is continuously present, the body may also stop the release of a natural chemical necessary for normal body function, such as endorphins (see illustrations below).

Pain and heroin withdrawal

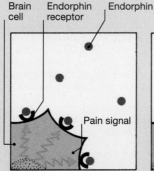

Normal brain
When no drug is present, natural substances called endorphins inhibit the transmission of pain signals.

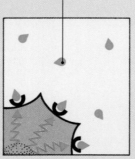

Effect of heroin
Heroin occupies the same receptors in the brain as endorphins, suppressing production of endorphins.

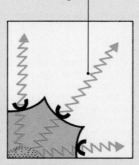

Heroin withdrawal
Abrupt withdrawal of heroin leaves the brain without a buffer to pain signals, even from minor stimuli.

MANAGING YOUR DRUG TREATMENT

A prescribed drug does not automatically produce a beneficial response. For a drug to have maximum benefit, it must be taken as directed by the doctor or manufacturer. It is estimated that four out of every six people for whom a drug is prescribed do not take it properly; one in six, not at all. The reasons include failure to understand or remember instructions, fear of adverse reactions, and lack of motivation, often arising from the disappearance of symptoms.

It is your responsibility to take a prescribed drug at the correct time, and as instructed. In order to do this, you need to know where to obtain information about the drug (see Questioning your prescriber, p.26) and to make certain that you fully understand the instructions.

The following pages describe the practical aspects of drug treatment, from obtaining a prescription and buying over-the-counter drugs to storing drugs and disposing of old medications safely. Problems caused by mismanaging drug treatment – overdosing, underdosing, or stopping the drug altogether – and long-term drug treatment are dealt with on pp.28–31. Information regarding specific drugs is given in Part 3.

OVER-THE-COUNTER DRUGS

Over-the-counter drugs are those for which a prescription is not required. All are available from pharmacies (many only from pharmacies) but some, called General Sales List (GSL) medicines, are very widely sold, even by supermarkets.

It is generally accepted that over-the-counter drugs are suitable for self-treatment and are unlikely to produce serious adverse reactions if taken as directed. But, as with all medicines, they can be harmful if misused. The ease with which they can be bought is no guarantee of their absolute safety. For this reason, the same precautions should be taken when using any over-the-counter medicine as when using a prescription drug.

Using over-the-counter drugs

A number of health problems can be treated with over-the-counter medicines; and some medicines, such as antibiotic eye drops, which were once only available with a prescription, can now be bought over the counter. However, you must follow carefully the directions on the label or patient information leaflet, particularly the advice on dosage and the circumstances in which a doctor should be consulted. Most over-the-counter drugs give clear information for users. They may warn of conditions under which the drug should not be taken, or advise you to consult a doctor if symptoms persist.

Your pharmacist is a good source of information about over-the-counter drugs and can usually tell you what is suitable for your complaint. They can also determine when an over-the-counter drug may not be effective and can warn you if self- or prolonged treatment is not advisable. When consulting the pharmacist about over-the-counter drugs, you should tell them if you are taking prescription drugs or other treatments (including complementary or alternative treatments) for any other

BUYING MEDICINES OVER THE INTERNET

There are many websites offering over-the-counter (OTC) and prescription-only medicines (POM) for sale over the internet. Buying medicines from these sites is potentially very dangerous. Many sites are operated from outside the UK, so they are not subject to UK law and the drugs they sell and the advice they give are not regulated in the same way as in the UK (through the Medicines and Healthcare products Regulatory Agency – MHRA). This means the quality of the drugs they supply cannot be guaranteed. You may even receive fake drugs, with the risk that you could suffer under- or overdosing or even toxic adverse

effects from taking the wrong drug or a toxic contaminant. You should be especially suspicious if the site will supply you with a POM medicine without a prescription or online consultation. If the site displays the logo of the Royal Pharmaceutical Society of Great Britain (a green box containing a green cross, the words "Registered Pharmacy", and a registration number) this is more reassuring, and clicking on this logo should take you to the RPS website, which will confirm the site is that of an officially UK-registered pharmacy. Also, all online drug retailers must be registered with the MHRA and display a common EU logo.

Buying over-the-counter medications
Various drugs, from cough medicine to antibiotic eye drops, are available over the counter. Your pharmacist can often help you to select the appropriate medication.

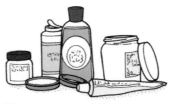
Medicated creams, lotions, and powders

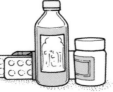
Analgesics

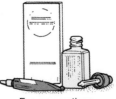
Eye preparations

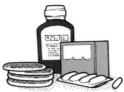
Laxatives

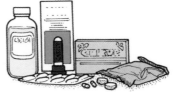
Cough and cold treatments

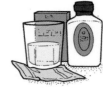
Antacids

illnesses. It is important to speak to your doctor before buying over-the-counter drugs for children. Some symptoms, such as diarrhoea in young children, should be treated only by a doctor since they may be caused by a serious condition.

PRESCRIPTION DRUGS

Prescription-only medicines (POMs) can only be prescribed by a doctor, dentist, specially qualified nurse-prescriber, or a prescribing pharmacist. Such drugs are not necessarily "stronger" or more likely to have side effects than those you can buy without prescription. Indeed, you may be given a POM that is also available over the counter. Drugs that are available only on prescription are drugs whose safe use is difficult to ensure without medical supervision.

When you are prescribed a drug, it is usually started at the normal dosage for the disorder being treated. The dosage may later be adjusted (lowered or increased) if the drug is not producing the desired effect or if there are adverse effects, or it may even be switched to an alternative drug that may be more effective.

Prescribing generic and brand-name drugs

When writing a prescription for a drug, the prescriber often has a choice between a generic and a brand-name product. Although the active ingredient is the same, two versions of the same drug may act in slightly different ways, as each manufacturer may formulate their product differently. They may also look different. In most cases, the differences are not important for the clinical effect of the drug. Generic drugs are often cheaper than brand-name products, and their use therefore provides a substantial cost-saving to the NHS.

Community pharmacists are obliged to dispense precisely what the doctor has written on the prescription form and are not allowed to substitute a generic drug when a brand-name has been specified. However, if you are prescribed a generic drug, the pharmacist is free to dispense whatever version of this drug is available. This means that your regular medication may vary in appearance each time you renew your prescription.

Hospital pharmacies often dispense generic versions of certain drugs. Therefore, if you are in hospital, the regular medication you receive may look different from the version that you are used to taking at home.

Your prescription

It is advisable for you to obtain all of your prescription drugs from the same pharmacist or at least from the same pharmacy, so that your pharmacist can advise you about any particular problems you may have, and keep supplies of any unusual drugs you may be taking.

If you need to take drugs that are prescribed by more than one doctor, or by your dentist in addition to your doctor, the pharmacist is able to call attention to possible harmful interactions. Doctors and dentists do ask if you are taking other medicines, but your regular pharmacist provides valuable additional advice.

Questioning your prescriber

Lack of information is the most common reason for drug failure. Comments like "The doctor is too busy to be bothered with a lot of questions" or "The doctor will think I'm stupid if I ask that" are common. Be certain you understand the instructions for a drug before you take it, and don't hesitate to ask if you have any questions about your drug treatment.

It is a good idea to make a list of the questions you may want to ask before your visit, and to make a few notes while you are there about what you are told. It is not uncommon to forget some of the instructions your prescriber gives you during a consultation.

Know what you are taking

Your prescriber should tell you the generic or brand name of the drug they are prescribing, and exactly what condition or symptom it has been prescribed for.

As well as telling you the name of the drug prescribed, your prescriber should explain what dose you should take, how often to take it, and whether the prescription should be repeated. Be certain you understand the instructions about how and when to take the drug (see also Taking your medication, facing page). For example, does four times a day mean four times during the time you are awake, or four times in 24 hours? Ask your prescriber how long the treatment should last; some medications cause harmful effects if you stop taking them abruptly, or do not have beneficial effects unless the course of drug treatment is completed.

To help you remember, the label on your dispensed medicine may repeat the instructions, and the pharmacist will give you a patient information leaflet that will give you detailed information about the drug. You should make sure you read this leaflet before taking your medication.

Risks and special precautions

All drugs have adverse effects (see The effects of drugs, p.15), and you should know what these are. Ask your prescriber what the possible adverse effects of the drug are and what you should do if they occur. Also ask if there are any foods, activities (such as driving), or other drugs you should avoid during treatment, and whether it is safe to drink alcohol while taking the drug.

Your prescription
Your prescription tells the pharmacist what to supply and what to put on the label. If the prescription and label differ, ask the pharmacist about it. The label may have a "do not use after" date. If it does not, ask the pharmacist to advise you. Usually, you will receive a patient information leaflet, which gives details about the drug, its adverse effects, whether it is safe for you, when not to use it, and so on. Compare this with your doctor's instructions, and ask the pharmacist about any differences.

Patient's name and address

Drug name and strength

When to take

Quantity to be dispensed

Doctor's signature

Doctor's name and address

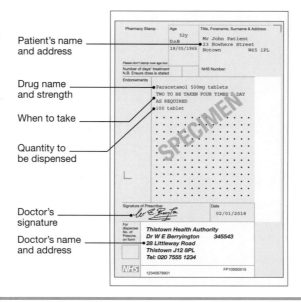

PRESCRIPTION TERMS

ac before food	**PM** evening
ad lib freely	**po** by mouth
AM morning	**pr** by rectum
bd twice a day	**prn** as needed
c with	**pv** by vagina
cap capsule	**qds** four times
cc cubic centimetre	a day
ext for external use	**s** without
gtt drops	**sr** slow release
mcg micrograms	**stat** at once
mg milligrams	**tab** tablet
ml millilitres	**tds** three times
nocte at night	a day
od each day	**top** apply topically
om each morning	**ud** use as directed
on each night	**x** times
pc after food	

TAKING YOUR MEDICATION

Among the most important aspects of managing your drug treatment is knowing how the drug is to be taken. Should it be taken on an empty stomach? With food? When? Mixed with something? Specific instructions on such points are given in the individual drug profiles in Part 3.

When to take your drugs

Certain drugs, such as analgesics and drugs for migraine, are taken only as necessary, when warning symptoms occur. Others are meant to be taken regularly at specified intervals. The prescription or label instructions can be confusing, however. For instance, does four times a day mean once every six hours out of 24 – at 8 am, 2 pm, 8 pm, and 2 am? Or does it mean take at four equal intervals during waking hours – morning, lunchtime, late afternoon, and bedtime? The latter is usually the case but you need to ask your doctor for precise directions.

The actual time of day that you take a drug is generally flexible, so you can normally schedule your doses to fit your daily routine. This has the added advantage of making it easier for you to remember to take your drugs. For example, if you are to take the drug three times during the day, it may be most convenient to take the first dose at 7 am, the second at 3 pm, and the third at 11 pm, while it may be more suitable for another person on the same regimen to take the first dose at 8 am, and so on. You must, however, establish with your doctor or pharmacist whether the drug should be taken with food, in which case you would probably need to take it with your breakfast, lunch, and dinner. Try to take your dose at the recommended intervals; if you take them too close together, the risk of side effects occurring is increased.

Four times a day?

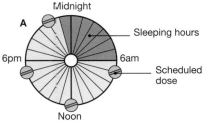

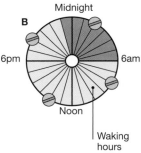

Check with your doctor whether your prescription means (A) take your drug 4 times a day during waking hours, or (B) take 4 times over a 24-hour period.

TIPS ON TAKING MEDICINES

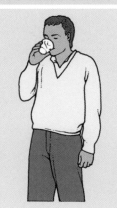

● Whenever possible, take capsules and tablets while standing up or in an upright sitting position, and take them with water. If you take them when you are lying down, or without enough water, it is possible for the capsules or tablets to become stuck in the oesophagus. This can delay the action of the drug and may damage the oesophagus.

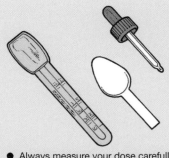

● Always measure your dose carefully, using a 5ml spoon or an accurate measure such as a dropper, children's medicine spoon, or oral syringe.

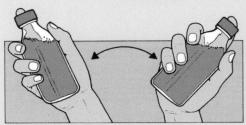

● When taking liquid medicines, make sure you shake the bottle thoroughly before measuring each dose, or you may take improper dosages if the active substance has risen to the top or settled at the bottom of the bottle.

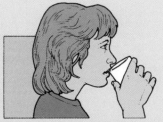

● A drink of cold water immediately after an unpleasantly flavoured medicine may hide the taste and help prevent tablets from lodging in the oesophagus.

If you are taking several different drugs, ask your doctor if they can be taken together, or if they must be taken at different times in order to avoid any adverse effects or reduced effectiveness caused by an interaction between them.

How to take your drugs

If your prescription specifies taking your drug with food, or without, it is important to follow this instruction if you are to get the maximum benefit from your treatment.

Certain drugs, such as ampicillin, should be taken on an empty stomach (usually one to two hours before eating) in order for them to be absorbed more quickly into the bloodstream; others, such as ibuprofen, should be taken with food to avoid stomach irritation. Similarly, you should comply with any instructions to avoid particular foods. Milk and dairy products may inhibit the absorption of some drugs, such as tetracycline; grapefruit juice may affect the way certain drugs are broken down in the body and significantly increase their effectiveness; alcohol is best avoided with many drugs. (See also Drug interactions, p.16.)

Inhaled corticosteroids may sometimes cause fungal infections of the mouth and/or throat. These can be avoided to some degree by rinsing the mouth and gargling with water after each inhalation.

In some cases – when taking diuretics, for example – you may be advised to eat foods rich in potassium. But do not take potassium supplements or salt substitutes unless you are advised to do so by your doctor (see potassium, p.439).

GIVING MEDICINES TO CHILDREN

A number of over-the-counter medicines are specifically prepared for children. Many other medicines have labels that give both adults' and children's dosages. For the purposes of drug labelling, anyone 12 years of age or under is considered a child.

When giving over-the-counter medicines to children, you should always follow the instructions on the label exactly and under no circumstances exceed the dosage recommended for a child. Never give a child even a small amount of a medicine intended for adult use without the advice of your doctor.

Never leave a child's medicine within reach, and remember that adults' tablets may look like sweets. Also, be aware that apparently simple adult remedies may be extremely toxic to children at an adult dose (e.g. iron tablets).

MISSED DOSES

Missing a dose of your medication can be a problem only if you are taking the drug as part of a regular course of treatment. Missing a drug dose is not uncommon and it is not a cause for concern in most cases. The missed dose may sometimes produce a recurrence of symptoms or a change in the action of the drug, so you should know what to do when you have forgotten to take your medication. For advice on individual drugs, consult the drug profile in Part 3.

Additional measures

With some drugs, the timing of doses depends on how long the actions of the drugs last. When you miss a drug dose, the amount of drug in your body is lowered, and the drug's effect may be diminished. You may therefore have to take other steps to avoid unwanted consequences. For example, if you are taking a progesterone-only oral contraceptive and you forget to take one pill at your usual time, you may need to regard it as a missed pill (see What to do if you miss a pill, p.123); you should use another form of contraception.

If you miss more than one dose of any drug you are taking regularly, you should tell your doctor. Missed doses are especially important with insulin and drugs for epilepsy.

If you frequently forget to take your medication, you should tell your doctor. They may be able to simplify your treatment schedule by prescribing a multi-ingredient preparation that contains several drugs, or a preparation that releases the drug slowly into the body over a period of time, and only needs to be taken once or twice daily.

REMEMBERING YOUR MEDICATION

If you take several different drugs, it is useful to draw up a chart to remind yourself of when each drug should be taken. This will also help anyone who looks after you, or a doctor who is unfamiliar with your treatment.

The example given here is of a dosage chart for an older woman suffering from arthritis and a heart condition who has trouble sleeping. Her doctor has prescribed the following treatment:

Bumetanide (a diuretic to counter fluid retention), one 1mg tablet in the morning.

Amiloride (another diuretic to counter the potassium loss caused by bumetanide), two 5mg tablets in the morning.

Ibuprofen (for arthritis), three 400mg tablets daily with meals.

Verapamil (to treat her heart condition), three 40mg tablets a day.

Zopiclone (a sleeping drug), one 3.75mg tablet at bedtime.

Dosage Chart

8am	1pm
1 x Bumetanide	1 x Ibuprofen
2 x Amiloride	1 x Verapamil
1 x Ibuprofen	
1 x Verapamil	

7pm	11pm
1 x Ibuprofen	1 x Verapamil
	1 x Zopiclone

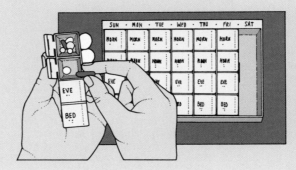

Pill, or dosette, box
Using a pill box is a handy way of making sure you take your tablets in the right order. Pill boxes are also very useful for carers of people with dementia. The boxes have a strip for each day of the week, and compartments for morning, afternoon, evening, and bedtime.

ENDING DRUG TREATMENT

As with missed doses, ending drug treatment too soon can be a problem when you are taking a regular course of drugs. With medication taken as required, you can stop as soon as you feel better.

Advice on stopping individual drugs is given in the drug profiles in Part 3. Some general guidelines for ending drug treatment are given below.

Risks of stopping too soon

Suddenly stopping drug treatment before completing your course of medication may cause the original condition to recur or lead to other complications, including withdrawal symptoms. The disappearance of the symptoms does not necessarily mean that a disorder is cured. Even if you feel better, do not stop taking the drug until the course has finished unless your doctor advises you to do so. People

taking antibiotics often stop too soon, but the full course of treatment prescribed should always be followed.

Adverse effects

Do not stop taking a medication simply because it produces unpleasant side effects. These often disappear or become bearable after a while. But if they do not, check with your doctor, who may want to reduce the dosage of the drug gradually or, alternatively, substitute another drug that does not produce the same side effects.

Gradual reduction

While many medications can be stopped abruptly, others need to be reduced gradually to prevent a reaction when treatment ends. This is the case with long-term corticosteroid therapy (see right) as well as with some antidepressants and dependence-inducing drugs.

Phased reduction of corticosteroids

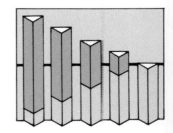

■ Corticosteroid drug

□ Natural adrenal hormone

Normal hormone level

Corticosteroid drugs suppress production in the body of natural adrenal hormones. A phased reduction of the dosage allows levels of the natural hormones to revert to normal. The last stages of withdrawal are made very slowly.

STORING DRUGS

Once you have completed a medically directed course of treatment, you should not keep any unused drugs. But most families will want to keep a supply of remedies for indigestion, headaches, colds, and so forth. Such medicines should not be used if they show any signs of deterioration, or if their period of effectiveness has expired (see When to dispose of drugs, right).

How to store drugs

All drugs, including cough medicines, iron tablets, and oral contraceptives, should be kept out of the reach of children. If you are in the habit of keeping your medicines where you will see them as a reminder to take them, leave an empty medicine container or an empty blister pack out instead, and put the drug itself safely out of reach.

Over-the-counter and prescription drugs should normally be stored in the container in which you purchased them. If it is necessary to put them into other containers, make sure you keep the original container with the label, as well as any separate instructions, for future reference.

Make certain that caps and lids are replaced and tightly closed after use; loose caps may leak and spill, or hasten deterioration of the drug.

Where to store drugs

The majority of drugs should be stored in a cool, dry place out of direct sunlight, even those in plastic containers, tinted glass, or blister packs. Room temperature, away from sources of direct heat, is suitable for most medicines. A few drugs should be stored in the refrigerator. Storage information for individual drugs is given in the drug profiles in Part 3.

Wall cabinets that can be locked are ideal for storing drugs, as long as the cabinet itself is located in a cool, dry place and not, as often happens, in the bathroom, which is frequently warm and humid.

WHEN TO DISPOSE OF DRUGS

Old drugs should be flushed down the toilet or returned to the pharmacist, but not put in the dustbin. Always dispose of:

- Any drug that is past its expiry date.
- Aspirin and paracetamol tablets that smell of vinegar.
- Tablets that are chipped, cracked, or discoloured, and capsules that have softened, cracked, or stuck together.
- Liquids that have thickened or discoloured, or that taste or smell different in any way from the original product.
- Tubes that are cracked, leaky, or hard.
- Ointments and creams that have changed odour, or changed appearance by discolouring, hardening, or separating.
- Any liquid needing refrigeration that has been kept past its expiry date.

LONG-TERM DRUG TREATMENT

Many people require regular, prolonged treatment with one or more drugs. People who suffer from chronic or recurrent disorders often need long-term or lifelong treatment with medication to help control symptoms or prevent complications. Antihypertensive drugs to manage high blood pressure and insulin or oral antidiabetic drugs for diabetes mellitus are familiar examples.

Many other disorders take a long time to cure; for example, people with tuberculosis usually need at least six months' treatment with antituberculous drugs. Long-term drug treatment may also be necessary to prevent a condition from occurring, and the drugs will need to be taken for as long as the individual remains at risk. Antimalarial drugs are a good example.

Possible adverse effects

You may be concerned that taking a drug for a long period will reduce its effectiveness or that you will become dependent on it. However, tolerance (see p.23) develops only with a few drugs; most medicines continue to have the same effect indefinitely without necessitating an increase in dosage or change in drug. Similarly, taking a drug for more than a few weeks does not normally create dependence.

Changing drug treatment

If you are taking a drug regularly, you will need to know what to do if something else occurs to affect your health. If you wish to become pregnant, for example, you should ask your doctor right away if it is preferable to continue on your regular medicine or switch to another less likely to affect your pregnancy. If you contract a new illness, for which an additional drug is prescribed, your regular treatment may be altered.

There are also a number of other reasons for changing a drug. For example, you may have had an adverse reaction to a particular drug, or an improved preparation of the drug may have become available.

Adjusting to long-term treatment

You should establish a daily routine for taking your medication in order to reduce the risk of a missed dose. Usually you should not stop taking your medication, even if there are side effects, without consulting your doctor (see Ending drug treatment, facing page). If you fear possible side effects from the drug, discuss this with your doctor.

Many people deliberately stop their drugs because they feel well or their symptoms disappear. This can be dangerous, especially with a condition like high blood pressure, which has no noticeable symptoms. Stopping treatment may lead to a recurrence or worsening of a disease. If you are uncertain about why you have to keep taking a drug, ask your doctor.

Only a few drugs require an alteration in habits. Some drugs should not be taken with alcohol; with a few drugs you should avoid certain foods. If you require a drug that makes you drowsy, you should not drive a car or operate dangerous equipment.

If you are allergic to a drug, or are taking one that should not be stopped suddenly or that may interact with other drugs, it is a good idea to carry a warning card or bracelet (MedicAlert, for example). Such information might be essential for anyone giving emergency medical treatment in an accident. More generally, a warning card or bracelet can also be helpful if you have a condition that health professionals should be aware of in an emergency, such as diabetes mellitus.

Monitoring treatment

If you are on long-term drug treatment, you will need to visit your doctor for periodic check-ups. They will check your underlying condition and monitor any adverse effects of treatment. For example, some drugs affect the levels of electrolytes (such as potassium) in the blood, and tests to measure blood electrolyte levels may be indicated. Levels of the drug in your blood may be measured. The doctor may also carry out general checks of your health, such as measuring your blood pressure and weight. People taking the anticoagulant warfarin will be given a regular blood clotting test (INR). If you are taking insulin for diabetes mellitus, in addition to regular medical checks you need to monitor the level of glucose in your blood each day.

If organ damage is a known possible risk of a drug, tests may be done to check the function of the organ. For example, blood and urine tests may be performed to check kidney and/or liver function, or a blood count to check the bone marrow function may be indicated.

EXCEEDING THE DOSE

Most people associate drug overdoses with attempts at suicide or the fatalities and near fatalities brought on by abuse of street drugs. However, drug overdoses can also occur among people who deliberately or inadvertently exceed the stated dose of a drug that has been prescribed for them by their doctor.

A single extra dose of most drugs is unlikely to be a cause for concern, although accidental overdoses can create anxiety in the individual and his or her family, and may cause overdose symptoms, which can appear in a variety of different forms.

Overdose of some drugs, however, is potentially dangerous even when the dose has been exceeded by only a small amount. Each of the drug profiles in Part 3 gives detailed information on the consequences of exceeding the dose, symptoms to look out for, and what to do. Each drug has an overdose danger rating of low, medium, or high, which are described fully on p.146.

Taking an extra dose

People sometimes exceed the stated dose in the mistaken belief that by increasing dosage they will obtain more immediate action or a more effective

Effects of repeated overdose
Too high a dose of a drug over an extended period may lead to a build-up of high levels of the drug in the body, especially if liver or kidney function is reduced.

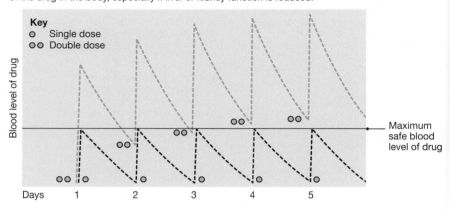

cure. This action is a particular risk with tolerance-inducing drugs (see Drug tolerance and dependence, p.23). Others exceed their dose accidentally, by miscalculating the amount or forgetting that the dose has already been taken.

Taking extra doses is often a problem in older people, who may repeat their dose through forgetfulness or confusion.

This is a special risk with medicines that cause drowsiness (see also p.22).

In some cases, especially when liver or kidney function deteriorates, the drug builds up in the blood because the body cannot break down and excrete the extra dose quickly enough, so that symptoms of poisoning may result. Symptoms of excessive intake may not be apparent for many days.

When and how to get help

If you are not sure whether or not you have taken your medicine, think back and check again. If you honestly cannot remember, assume that you have missed the dose and follow the advice given in the individual drug profiles in Part 3 of this book. If you cannot find your drug, consult your doctor. Make a note to use some system in the future which will help you remember to take your medicine.

If you are looking after an older person on regular drug treatment who suddenly develops unusual symptoms such as confusion, drowsiness, or unsteadiness, consider the possibility of an inadvertent drug overdose and consult the doctor as soon as possible.

Deliberate overdose

While many cases of drug overdose are accidental or the result of a mistaken belief that increasing the dose will enhance the benefits of drug treatment, sometimes an excessive amount of a drug is taken with the intention of causing harm or even as a suicide attempt. Whether or not you think a dangerous amount of a drug has been taken, deliberate overdoses of this kind should always be brought to the attention of your doctor. Not only is it necessary to ensure that no physical harm has occurred as a result of the overdose, but the psychological condition of a person who takes such action may indicate the need for additional medical help, especially if they are older, have a physical illness, or suffer from depression.

THE EFFECT OF DRUG OVERDOSE ON THE BODY

The effect of drug overdose on the body depends on the type of drug involved. Some drugs produce an exaggeration of the desired effect: for instance, overdose of tranquillizers leads to unconsciousness. With many drugs, the toxic overdose effects are unrelated to the action or side effects of the drug when it is taken in normal doses.

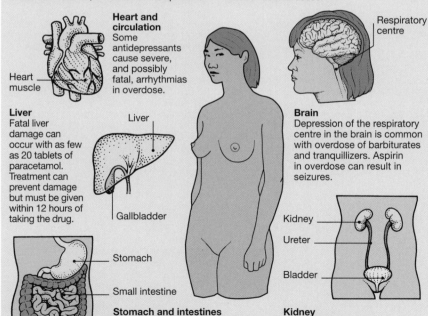

Heart and circulation
Some antidepressants cause severe, and possibly fatal, arrhythmias in overdose.

Liver
Fatal liver damage can occur with as few as 20 tablets of paracetamol. Treatment can prevent damage but must be given within 12 hours of taking the drug.

Stomach and intestines
Iron overdose causes bleeding in the digestive tract. An overdose of NSAIDs may cause ulceration of the stomach and intestines.

Brain
Depression of the respiratory centre in the brain is common with overdose of barbiturates and tranquillizers. Aspirin in overdose can result in seizures.

Kidney
An overdose of NSAIDs, particularly in people who have impaired kidney function, can result in kidney failure.

DOs AND DON'Ts

On this page you will find a summary of the most important practical points concerning the management of your drug treatment. The advice is arranged under general headings, explaining the safest methods of storing drugs and following treatment, whether it is a prescribed medicine or an over-the-counter drug. This information is equally applicable whether you are taking medicine yourself or supervising the drug treatment of someone in your care.

At the surgery or in hospital

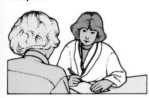

DO

✓ Tell the person prescribing your drugs about all drugs you are already taking, including prescription or over-the-counter drugs, complementary or alternative medicine, and street drugs.

✓ Tell them if you are pregnant, intending to become pregnant, or breast-feeding.

✓ Tell them about any allergic reactions you have experienced to past drug treatments.

✓ Tell them if you have a current health problem, such as liver disease, or if you think you might be at risk from drug treatment for any other reason.

✓ Discuss your drug treatment with the person prescribing your drugs and make sure you understand why you have been given a particular drug and what benefits you can expect. Often, people who do not understand the reasons for their treatment fail to take their drug correctly. Take your medicines with you when you go into hospital to ensure that the doctors know what you are taking.

DON'T

✗ Leave the surgery or hospital before you understand clearly how and when to take the drug.

At the pharmacy

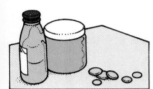

DO

✓ Ask your pharmacist's advice about over-the-counter drugs if you are not sure what you should buy, or if you think you may react adversely to a drug.

✓ Try to see the same pharmacist or use the same pharmacy to obtain your regular prescriptions.

✓ Be sure you know the name of the drug you have been prescribed. If you are getting a repeat prescription and your doctor has specified that you should always use the same brand, make sure the brand is correct.

✓ Make sure you understand what is on the drug label.

✓ Ask the pharmacist to put your drug in a container with an easy-to-remove cap if you have difficulty using child-resistant containers.

DON'T

✗ Send children to the pharmacy to get your medicine for you.

Giving medicines to children

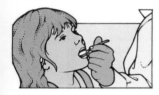

DO

✓ Check the dose on the label carefully before giving medicines to children.

✓ Make sure over-the-counter preparations you give to children under 16 years old do not contain aspirin.

✓ Make sure you use the special measuring spoon or oral syringe to administer doses from a liquid preparation more accurately and easily.

DON'T

✗ Pretend to children that medicines are sweets or soft drinks.

✗ Give any medicines to children under the age of five, except on the advice of your doctor.

Taking your drug

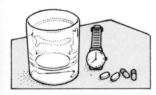

DO

✓ Make sure that your drug will not make you drowsy or otherwise affect your ability before you drive or perform difficult or dangerous tasks.

✓ Read the label carefully and do what it says. This is equally important with all types of drugs, including creams and lotions as well as drugs taken by mouth.

✓ Finish the drug treatment prescribed for you.

✓ Consult your doctor for advice if you experience side effects.

DON'T

✗ Take any prescribed or over-the-counter drugs without first consulting your doctor if you are pregnant or trying to conceive.

✗ Take any drugs after the expiry date has passed.

✗ Miss any doses; if you have trouble remembering to take your medicine, tell your doctor or pharmacist.

✗ Offer your medicine to other people or take medicine that has been prescribed for someone else (even if the symptoms are the same).

Food, drink, and drugs of abuse

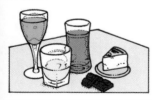

DO

✓ Check whether it is safe to take alcohol with the drugs you have been prescribed.

✓ Check that there are no foods you should avoid.

✓ Follow the timing of your drugs with respect to meals, when instructed to do so by your doctor or pharmacist.

DON'T

✗ Take drugs (except those prescribed by your doctor or other qualified prescriber) or alcohol if you are pregnant or trying to conceive. They may adversely affect the unborn baby.

✗ Take drugs of abuse under any circumstances.

Storing drugs

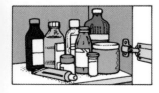

DO

✓ Take care to store drugs in a cool, dry place and protect them from light or refrigerate them, if advised to do so.

✓ Keep all drugs, including seemingly harmless ones such as cough preparations, locked away out of the reach of children.

✓ Check your medicine chest regularly in case other members of the family have left their unwanted drugs in it, and to make sure that none of the normal supplies are out of date.

✓ Keep drugs in their original containers with the original instructions to avoid confusion.

DON'T

✗ Hoard drugs at home. When you have stopped taking a prescribed drug, dispose of it unless it is part of your family first aid kit. Alternatively, take it to a pharmacist, who will dispose of it for you.

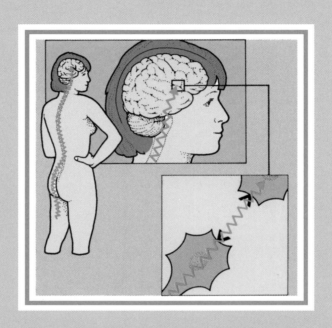

PART

2

MAJOR DRUG GROUPS

BRAIN AND NERVOUS SYSTEM
RESPIRATORY SYSTEM
HEART AND CIRCULATION
GASTROINTESTINAL TRACT
MUSCLES, BONES, AND JOINTS
ALLERGY
INFECTIONS AND INFESTATIONS
HORMONES AND ENDOCRINE SYSTEM
NUTRITION
MALIGNANT AND IMMUNE DISEASE
REPRODUCTIVE AND URINARY TRACTS
EYES AND EARS
SKIN

BRAIN AND NERVOUS SYSTEM

The human brain contains more than 100 billion nerve cells (neurons). These nerve cells receive electrochemical impulses from everywhere in the body. They interpret these impulses and send responsive signals back to various glands and muscles. The brain functions continuously as a switchboard for the human communications system. At the same time, it serves as the seat of emotions and mood, of memory, personality, and thought. Extending from the brain is an additional, large rod-shaped cluster of nerve cells that forms the spinal cord. Together, these two elements comprise the central nervous system.

Radiating from the central nervous system is the peripheral nervous system, which has three parts. One branches off the spinal cord and extends to skin and muscles throughout the body. Another, in the head, links the brain to the eyes, ears, nose, and taste buds. The third is a semi-independent network called the autonomic, or involuntary, nervous system. This is the part of the nervous system that controls unconscious body functions such as breathing, digestion, and glandular activity (see facing page).

Signals traverse the nervous system by electrical and chemical means. Electrical impulses carry signals from one end of a neuron to the other. To cross the gap between neurons, chemical neurotransmitters are released from one cell to bind on to the receptor sites of nearby cells. Excitatory transmitters stimulate action; inhibitory transmitters reduce it.

What can go wrong

Disorders of the brain and nervous system may manifest as illnesses that show themselves as physical impairments, such as epilepsy or strokes, or as mental and emotional impairments (for example, schizophrenia or depression).

Illnesses causing physical impairments can result from different types of disorder of the brain and nervous system. Death of nerve cells resulting from poor circulation can result in paralysis, while electrical disturbances of certain nerve cells cause the seizures of epilepsy. Temporary changes in blood circulation within and around the brain are associated with migraine. Parkinson's disease is caused by a lack of dopamine, a neurotransmitter that is produced by specialized brain cells.

The causes of disorders that trigger mental and emotional impairment are not known, but these illnesses are thought to result from the defective functioning of nerve cells and neurotransmitters. The nerve cells may be underactive, overactive,

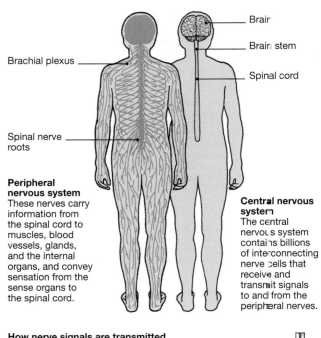

Brachial plexus

Spinal nerve roots

Brain

Brain stem

Spinal cord

Peripheral nervous system
These nerves carry information from the spinal cord to muscles, blood vessels, glands, and the internal organs, and convey sensation from the sense organs to the spinal cord.

Central nervous system
The central nervous system contains billions of interconnecting nerve cells that receive and transmit signals to and from the peripheral nerves.

How nerve signals are transmitted
A nerve signal is an electrical impulse produced by chemical reactions on the surface of the cell body of a neuron (nerve cell). The signal is transmitted by a neurotransmitter, released from the ends of a nerve fibre, that binds to a receptor on the neighbouring cell body. This, in turn, transmits the signal to another neuron or triggers a response in a muscle or organ.

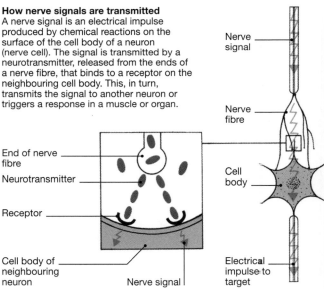

End of nerve fibre

Neurotransmitter

Receptor

Cell body of neighbouring neuron

Nerve signal

Nerve signal

Nerve fibre

Cell body

Electrical impulse to target

or poorly coordinated. Alternatively, mental and emotional impairment may be due to too much or too little neurotransmitter in one area of the brain.

Why drugs are used

By and large, the drugs described in this section do not eliminate nervous system disorders. Their function is to correct or modify the communication of the signals that traverse the nervous system. By doing so they can relieve symptoms or restore normal functioning and behaviour. In some cases,

AUTONOMIC NERVOUS SYSTEM

The autonomic, or involuntary, nervous system governs the actions of the muscles of the organs and glands. Such vital functions as heart beat, salivation, and digestion continue without conscious direction, whether we are awake or asleep.

The autonomic system is divided into two parts, the effects of one generally balancing those of the other. The sympathetic nervous system has an excitatory effect. For example, it widens the airways to the lungs, increases the heart rate, and increases the flow of blood to the arms and legs. The parasympathetic system, by contrast, has an opposing effect. It slows the heart rate, narrows the large airways, and redirects blood from the limbs to the gut.

Although the functional pace of most organs results from the interplay between the two systems, the muscles surrounding the blood vessels respond only to the signals of the sympathetic system. Whether a vessel is dilated or constricted is determined by the relative stimulation of two sets of receptor sites: alpha sites and beta sites.

Neurotransmitters
The parasympathetic system depends on the neurotransmitter acetylcholine to transmit signals from one cell to another. The sympathetic nervous system relies on epinephrine (adrenaline) and norepinephrine (noradrenaline), substances that act as both hormones and neurotransmitters.

Drugs that act on the sympathetic nervous system
The drugs that stimulate the sympathetic nervous system (see chart) are called adrenergics (or sympathomimetics). They either promote the release of epinephrine and norepinephrine or mimic their effects. Drugs that interfere with the action of the sympathetic nervous system are called sympatholytics. Alpha blockers act on alpha receptors; beta blockers act on beta receptors (see also Beta blockers, p.55).

Drugs that act on the parasympathetic nervous system
Drugs that stimulate the parasympathetic nervous system are called cholinergics (or parasympathomimetics), and drugs that oppose its action are called anticholinergics. Many prescribed drugs have anticholinergic properties (see chart, right).

Effects of stimulation of the autonomic nervous system

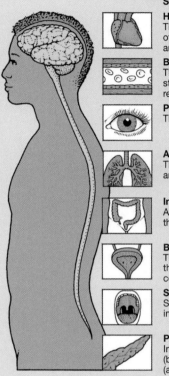

	Sympathetic	Parasympathetic
Heart	The rate and strength of the heart beat are increased.	The rate and strength of the heart beat are reduced.
Blood vessels in skin	These are constricted by stimulation of alpha receptors.	No effect.
Pupils	The pupils are dilated.	The pupils are constricted.
Airways	The bronchial muscles relax and widen the airways.	The bronchial muscles contract and narrow the airways.
Intestines	Activity of the muscles of the intestinal wall is reduced.	Activity of the muscles of the intestinal wall is increased.
Bladder	The bladder wall relaxes and the sphincter muscle contracts.	The bladder wall contracts and the sphincter muscle relaxes.
Salivary glands	Secretion of thick saliva increases.	Secretion of watery saliva increases.
Pancreas	Insulin secretion is increased (beta receptors) or reduced (alpha receptors).	Insulin secretion is increased.

Drugs that act on the autonomic nervous system

		Sympathetic	Parasympathetic
Stimulated by	Natural neurotransmitters	Epinephrine (adrenaline) Norepinephrine (noradrenaline)	Acetylcholine
	Drugs	Adrenergic (sympathomimetic) drugs (including alpha agonists, beta agonists)	Cholinergic drugs Parasympathomimetics
Blocked by	Drugs	Alpha blockers (antagonists) Beta blockers (antagonists)	Anticholinergic drugs

such as anxiety and insomnia, drugs are used to lower the level of activity in the brain. In other disorders – depression, for example – drugs are given to encourage the opposite effect, increasing the level of activity.

Drugs that act on the nervous system are also used for conditions that outwardly have nothing to do with nervous system disorders. Vomiting, for example, may be treated with drugs that directly affect the vomiting centre in the brain or block stimulatory nerve signals to the vomiting centre.

MAJOR DRUG GROUPS

Analgesics
Sleeping drugs
Anti-anxiety drugs
Antidepressant drugs
Antipsychotic drugs
Anticonvulsant drugs
Drugs for parkinsonism

Drugs for dementia
Nervous system stimulants
Drugs for migraine
Anti-emetics

ANALGESICS

Analgesics (painkillers) are drugs that relieve pain. Since pain is not a disease but a symptom, long-term relief depends on treatment of the underlying cause. For example, the pain of toothache can be relieved by drugs but can be cured only by appropriate dental treatment. If the underlying disorder is irreversible, such as some rheumatic conditions, long-term analgesic treatment may be necessary.

Damage to body tissues as a result of disease or injury is detected by nerve endings that transmit signals to the brain. The interpretation of these sensations can be affected by the psychological state of the individual, so that pain is worsened by anxiety and fear, for example. Often, a reassuring explanation of the cause of discomfort can make pain easier to bear and may even relieve it altogether. Anti-anxiety drugs (see p.39) are helpful when pain is accompanied by anxiety, and some of these drugs are also used to reduce painful muscle spasms. Some antidepressant drugs (see p.40) act to block the transmission of impulses signalling pain and are particularly useful for nerve pains (neuralgia), which do not always respond to analgesics.

Types of analgesic

Analgesics are divided into the opioids (with similar properties to drugs derived from opium, such as morphine) and non-opioids. Non-opioids include all the other analgesics, including paracetamol, nefopam, and also the non-steroidal anti-inflammatory drugs (NSAIDs), the most well known of which is aspirin. The non-opioids are all less powerful as painkillers than the opioids. Local anaesthetics are also used to relieve pain (see below).

Opioid drugs and paracetamol act directly on the brain and spinal cord to alter the perception of pain. Opioids act like the endorphins, hormones naturally produced in the brain that stop the cell-to-cell transmission of pain sensation. NSAIDs block the formation of pain-modulating substances (e.g. prostaglandins) at nerve endings at the site of pain.

When pain is treated under medical supervision, it is common to start with paracetamol or an NSAID; if neither provides adequate pain relief, they may be combined. A mild opioid (for example, codeine) may also be used. If the less powerful drugs are ineffective, a strong opioid such as morphine may be given. As there is now a wide variety of oral analgesic formulations, injections are seldom necessary to control even the most severe pain.

When treating pain with an over-the-counter preparation – for example, taking paracetamol for a headache – you should seek medical advice if pain persists for longer than 48 hours, recurs, or is worse or different from previous pain.

Non-opioid analgesics

Paracetamol

This analgesic is believed to act by reducing the production of chemicals called prostaglandins in the brain. However, paracetamol does not affect prostaglandin production in the rest of the body, so it does not reduce inflammation, although it can reduce fever. Paracetamol can be used for everyday aches and pains, such as headaches, toothache, and joint pains.

As well as being the most widely used analgesic, it is one of the safest when taken correctly. It does not usually irritate the stomach and allergic reactions are

SITES OF ACTION

Paracetamol and the opioid drugs act on the brain and spinal cord to reduce pain perception. Non-steroidal anti-inflammatory drugs (NSAIDs) act at the site of pain to prevent the stimulation of nerve endings.

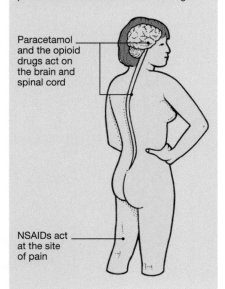

Paracetamol and the opioid drugs act on the brain and spinal cord

NSAIDs act at the site of pain

NSAIDs AND DIGESTIVE TRACT IRRITATION

NSAIDs can cause irritation, even ulceration and bleeding, of the stomach and duodenum, so they are best taken after a meal. NSAIDs are not usually given to people with stomach ulcers. An NSAID may be combined with an anti-ulcer drug (see p.67). In certain cases, a COX-2 inhibitor may be used. However, NSAIDs are usually only given in the lowest effective dose for the shortest duration.

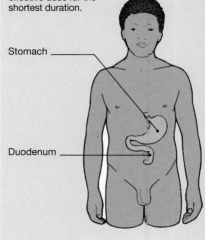

Stomach

Duodenum

rare. However, an overdose can cause severe and possibly fatal liver or kidney damage. Its toxic potential may be increased in heavy drinkers.

Non-steroidal anti-inflammatory drugs (NSAIDs): aspirin

Used for many years to relieve pain and reduce fever, aspirin also acts to reduce inflammation by blocking the production of prostaglandins, which contribute to the swelling and pain in inflamed tissue (see Action of analgesics, facing page). Aspirin is useful for headaches, toothache, mild rheumatic pain, sore throat, and discomfort caused by feverish illnesses. Given regularly, it can also relieve the

LOCAL ANAESTHETICS

These drugs are used to prevent pain, usually in minor surgical procedures: for example, dental treatment and stitching cuts. They can also be injected into the space around the spinal cord to numb the lower half of the body. This is called spinal or epidural anaesthesia and can be used for some major operations in people who are not fit for a general anaesthetic. Epidural anaesthesia is also used during childbirth.

Local anaesthetics block the passage of nerve impulses at the site of administration, deadening all feeling conveyed by the nerves they come into contact with. They do not, however, interfere with consciousness. Local anaesthetics are usually given by injection, but they can also be applied to the skin, the mouth and other areas lined with mucous membrane (such as the vagina), or the eye to relieve pain. Some local anaesthetics are formulated for injection together with epinephrine (adrenaline). Epinephrine constricts the blood vessels and prevents the local anaesthetic from being removed. This action prolongs the anaesthetic's effect.

Local anaesthetic creams are often used to numb the skin before injections in children and people with a fear of needles.

pain and inflammation of chronic rheumatoid arthritis (see Antirheumatic drugs, p.75).

Aspirin is found in combination with other substances in a variety of medicines (see Cold cures, p.52). It is also used in the treatment of some blood disorders, since aspirin helps to prevent abnormal clotting of blood by preventing platelets from sticking together (see Drugs that affect blood clotting, p.62).

Aspirin in the form of soluble tablets, dissolved in water before being taken, is absorbed into the bloodstream more quickly, thereby relieving pain faster than tablets. Soluble aspirin is not, however, less irritating to the stomach lining.

Aspirin is available in many forms, all of which have a similar effect, but because the amount of aspirin in a tablet of each type varies, it is important to read the packet for the correct dosage. Aspirin is not recommended for children aged under 16 years because its use has been linked to Reye's syndrome, a rare but potentially fatal liver and brain disorder.

Other non-steroidal anti-inflammatory drugs (NSAIDs)

These drugs can relieve both pain and inflammation. NSAIDs are related to aspirin and also work by blocking the production of prostaglandins. They are most commonly used to treat muscle and joint pain and may also be prescribed for other types of pain including period pain. For further information on these drugs, see p.74.

Combined analgesics

Mild opioids, such as codeine, are often found in combination preparations with non-opioids, such as paracetamol. The prefix "co-" is used to denote a drug combination. Although both opioids and paracetamol act centrally, these mixtures have the advantage of combining different mechanisms of action. Another advantage of combining analgesics is that the reductions in dose of the components may reduce the side effects of the preparation. Combinations can be helpful in reducing the number of tablets taken during long-term treatment.

Opioid analgesics

These drugs are related to opium, an extract of poppy seeds. They act directly on several sites in the central nervous system to block the transmission of pain signals (see Action of analgesics, above). Because they act directly on the parts of the brain where pain is perceived, opioids are the strongest analgesics and are therefore used to treat the pain arising from surgery, serious injury, and cancer. These drugs are particularly valuable for relieving severe pain during terminal illnesses. In addition, their ability to produce a state of relaxation and euphoria

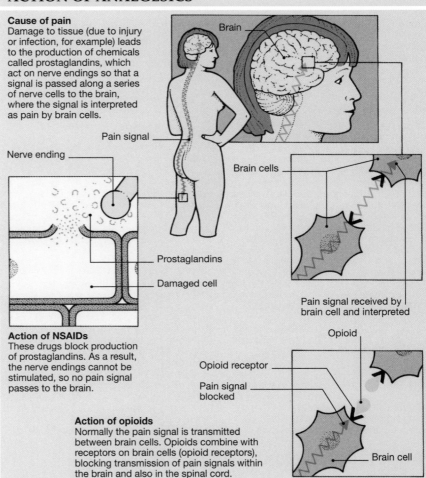

Cause of pain
Damage to tissue (due to injury or infection, for example) leads to the production of chemicals called prostaglandins, which act on nerve endings so that a signal is passed along a series of nerve cells to the brain, where the signal is interpreted as pain by brain cells.

Brain

Pain signal

Nerve ending

Brain cells

Prostaglandins

Damaged cell

Pain signal received by brain cell and interpreted

Action of NSAIDs
These drugs block production of prostaglandins. As a result, the nerve endings cannot be stimulated, so no pain signal passes to the brain.

Opioid

Opioid receptor

Pain signal blocked

Action of opioids
Normally the pain signal is transmitted between brain cells. Opioids combine with receptors on brain cells (opioid receptors), blocking transmission of pain signals within the brain and also in the spinal cord.

Brain cell

is often of help in relieving the stress that accompanies severe pain. Morphine is the best known opioid analgesic. Others include diamorphine (heroin) and pethidine. The use of these powerful opioids is strictly controlled because the euphoria produced can lead to misuse and addiction. When they are given under medical supervision to treat severe pain, though, the risk of addiction is negligible.

Opioid analgesics may prevent clear thought and cloud consciousness. Other possible adverse effects include nausea, vomiting, constipation, drowsiness, and depressed breathing. When they are taken in overdose, these drugs may induce a deep coma and lead to fatal breathing difficulties.

In addition to the powerful opioids, there are some less powerful drugs in this group that are used to relieve mild to moderate pain. They include codeine and tramadol. The opioids' normally unwanted side effects of depressing

respiration and causing constipation make them useful as cough suppressants (p.52) and as antidiarrhoeal drugs (p.68).

COMMON DRUGS

Opioids	NSAIDs (see p.74)
Buprenorphine	Aspirin *
Co-codamol	Diclofenac *
Codeine *	Etodolac
Co-dydramol	Fenbufen
Diamorphine	Fenoprofen
(heroin)	Ibuprofen *
Dihydrocodeine *	Indometacin
Dipipanone	Ketoprofen *
Fentanyl	Mefenamic acid *
Meptazinol	Naproxen *
Methadone *	Piroxicam *
Morphine *	
Oxycodone	**Other non-opioids**
Pethidine	Nefopam
Tramadol *	Paracetamol *

* See Part 3

SLEEPING DRUGS

Difficulty in getting to sleep or staying asleep (insomnia) has many causes. Most people suffer from sleepless nights from time to time, usually as a result of a temporary worry or discomfort from a minor illness. Persistent sleeplessness can be caused by psychological problems, including anxiety or depression, or by pain and discomfort arising from a physical disorder.

Why they are used

For occasional bouts of sleeplessness, simple, common remedies to promote relaxation – for example, taking a warm bath or a hot milk drink before bedtime – are usually the best form of treatment. Sleeping drugs (also known as hypnotics) are normally prescribed only when these self-help remedies have failed, and when lack of sleep is beginning to affect your general health. These drugs are used to re-establish the habit of sleeping. They should be used in the smallest dose and for the shortest possible time (not more than three weeks). It is best not to use sleeping tablets every night (see Risks and special precautions, right). Do not use alcohol to get to sleep as it can cause disturbed sleep and insomnia.

Long-term treatment of sleeplessness depends on resolving the underlying cause of the problem.

How they work

Most sleeping drugs promote sleep by depressing brain function. The drugs interfere with chemical activity in the brain and nervous system by reducing communication between nerve cells.

TYPES OF SLEEPING DRUG

Benzodiazepines These are the most commonly used class of sleeping drugs as they have comparatively few adverse effects and are relatively safe in overdose. They are also used to treat anxiety (see facing page).

Barbiturates These are now almost never used because of the risks of abuse, dependence, and toxicity in overdose. There is also a risk of prolonged sedation ("hangover").

Chloral derivatives These drugs effectively promote sleep but are little used now. If prescribed, triclofos causes fewer gastro-intestinal side effects than chloral hydrate.

Other non-benzodiazepine sleeping drugs Zopiclone, zaleplon, and zolpidem work in a similar way to benzodiazepines. They are not intended for long-term use, and withdrawal symptoms have been reported.

Antihistamines Widely used to treat allergic symptoms (see p.82), antihistamines also cause drowsiness. They are sometimes used to promote sleep.

Antidepressant drugs Some of these drugs may be used to promote sleep in depressed people (see p.40), as well as being effective in treating underlying depressive illness.

This leads to reduced brain activity, allowing you to fall asleep more easily, but the nature of the sleep is affected by the drug. The main class of sleeping drugs, the benzodiazepines, is described on the facing page.

How they affect you

A sleeping drug rapidly produces drowsiness and slowed reactions. Some people find that the drug makes them appear to be drunk, their speech slurred, especially if they delay going to bed after taking their dose. Most people find they usually fall asleep within about an hour of taking the drug.

Because the sleep induced by drugs is not the same as normal sleep, many people find they do not feel as well rested by it as by a night of natural sleep. This is the result of suppressed brain activity. Sleeping drugs also suppress the sleep

during which dreams occur; both dream sleep and non-dream sleep are essential for a good night's sleep (see The effects of drugs on sleep patterns, below).

Some people experience a variety of hangover effects the following day. Some benzodiazepines may produce minor side effects, such as daytime drowsiness, dizziness, and unsteadiness, that can impair the ability to drive or operate machinery. Older people are likely to become confused, and selection of an appropriate drug is important for them.

Risks and special precautions

Sleeping drugs become less effective after the first few nights and there may be a temptation to increase the dose. Apart from the antihistamines, most sleeping drugs can produce psychological and physical dependence (see p.23) when taken regularly for more than a few weeks, especially if they are taken in larger-than-normal doses.

When sleeping drugs are suddenly withdrawn, anxiety, seizures, and hallucinations sometimes occur. Nightmares and vivid dreams may be a problem because the time spent in dream sleep increases. Sleeplessness will recur and may lead to a temptation to use sleeping drugs again. Anyone who wishes to stop taking sleeping drugs, particularly after prolonged use, should seek their doctor's advice to prevent these withdrawal symptoms from occurring.

COMMON DRUGS

Benzodiazepines	Other non-
Flurazepam	benzodiazepine
Loprazolam	sleeping drugs
Lormetazepam	Clomethiazole
Nitrazepam ✳	Promethazine ✳
Temazepam ✳	Zaleplon
	Zolpidem
	Zopiclone ✳

✳ See Part 3

THE EFFECTS OF DRUGS ON SLEEP PATTERNS

Normal sleep can be divided into three types: light sleep, deep sleep, and dream sleep. The proportion of time spent in each type of sleep changes with age and is altered by sleeping drugs. Dramatic changes in sleep patterns also occur in the first few days following abrupt withdrawal of sleeping drugs after regular, prolonged use.

Normal sleep Young adults spend most sleep time in light sleep with roughly equal proportions of dream and deep sleep.

Drug-induced sleep has less dream sleep and less deep sleep with relatively more light sleep.

Sleep following drug withdrawal There is a marked increase in dream sleep, causing nightmares, following withdrawal of drugs used regularly for a long time.

○ Dream sleep
● Deep sleep
● Light sleep

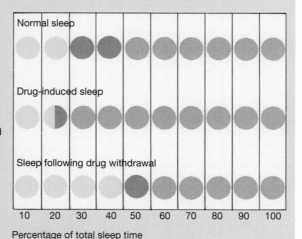

Percentage of total sleep time

ANTI-ANXIETY DRUGS

A certain amount of stress can be beneficial, providing a stimulus to action. But too much will often result in anxiety, which might be described as fear or apprehension not caused by real danger.

Clinically, anxiety arises when the balance of certain chemicals in the brain is disturbed. The fearful feelings increase brain activity, stimulating the sympathetic nervous system (see p.35), and often triggers physical symptoms: for example, breathlessness, shaking, palpitations, digestive distress, and headaches.

Why they are used

Anti-anxiety drugs (also called anxiolytics or minor tranquillizers) are prescribed for short-term relief of severe anxiety and nervousness caused by psychological problems. But these drugs cannot resolve the causes. Tackling the underlying problem through counselling and perhaps psychotherapy offers the best hope of a long-term solution. Anti-anxiety drugs are also used in hospitals to calm and relax people who are undergoing uncomfortable medical procedures.

There are two main classes of drugs for relieving anxiety: benzodiazepines and beta blockers. Benzodiazepines are the most widely used, given as a regular treatment for short periods to promote relaxation. Most benzodiazepines have a strong sedative effect, helping to relieve the insomnia that accompanies anxiety (see also Sleeping drugs, facing page).

Beta blockers are mainly used to reduce physical symptoms of anxiety, such as shaking and palpitations. These drugs are commonly prescribed for people who feel excessively anxious in certain situations, such as interviews or public appearances.

Many antidepressants (p.40), including SSRIs, clomipramine, and venlafaxine, are also useful in some anxiety disorders.

How they work

Benzodiazepines and related drugs

These drugs depress activity in the part of the brain that controls emotion by promoting the action of the neurotransmitter gamma-aminobutyric acid (GABA), which binds to neurons, blocking transmission of electrical impulses and thus reducing communication between brain cells. Benzodiazepines increase the inhibitory effect of GABA on brain cells (see panel, above), preventing the excessive brain activity that causes anxiety.

Buspirone is different from other anti-anxiety drugs; it binds mainly to serotonin (another neurotransmitter) receptors and does not cause drowsiness. Its effect is not felt for at least two weeks after starting treatment.

Beta blockers

The physical symptoms of anxiety are produced by an increase in the activity of the sympathetic nervous system.

ACTION OF BENZODIAZEPINES AND RELATED DRUGS

Action on the brain
The reticular activating system (RAS) in the brain stem controls the level of mental activity by stimulating higher centres of the brain controlling consciousness. Benzodiazepines and related drugs depress the RAS, relieving anxiety. In larger doses they depress the RAS sufficiently to cause drowsiness and sleep.

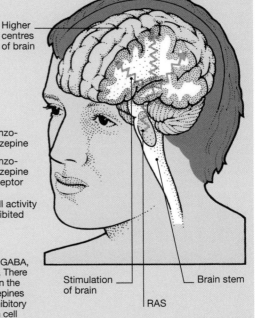

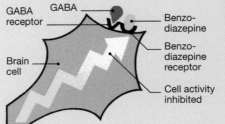

Action on brain cells in the RAS
Brain cell activity is normally inhibited by GABA, which binds to specialized cell receptors. There are also receptors for benzodiazepines on the GABA receptors themselves. Benzodiazepines bind to this receptor and promote the inhibitory effect of GABA, thereby depressing brain cell activity in the RAS.

Sympathetic nerve endings release a chemical transmitter called norepinephrine (noradrenaline) that stimulates the heart, digestive system, and other organs. Beta blockers block the action of norepinephrine, reducing physical symptoms of anxiety. For more on beta blockers, see p.55.

How they affect you

Benzodiazepines and related drugs reduce feelings of restlessness and agitation, slow mental activity, and often produce drowsiness. They are said to reduce motivation and, if they are taken in large doses, may lead to apathy. They also have a relaxing effect on the muscles, and some benzodiazepines are used specifically for that purpose (see Muscle relaxants, p.78).

Minor adverse effects of these drugs include dizziness and forgetfulness. The latter can be useful when benzodiazepines are used as sedatives for invasive procedures such as endoscopy. However, people who drive or operate machinery should be aware that their reactions may be slowed. Because the brain soon becomes tolerant to and dependent on their effects, benzodiazepines are usually effective for only a few weeks at a time.

Beta blockers reduce the physical symptoms associated with anxiety, which may promote greater mental calmness. As they do not cause drowsiness they are safer for people who need to drive.

Risks and special precautions

The benzodiazepines are safe for most people and less dangerous in overdose than other sedative drugs. The main risk is psychological and physical dependence, especially for regular users or with larger-than-average doses. For this reason, they are usually given for courses of two weeks or less. If they have been used for longer, they should be withdrawn gradually under medical supervision. If they are stopped suddenly, withdrawal symptoms, such as excessive anxiety, nightmares, and restlessness, may occur.

Benzodiazepines have been abused for their sedative effect, and are therefore prescribed with caution for people with a history of drug or alcohol abuse.

COMMON DRUGS

Benzodiazepines
Alprazolam
Chlordiazepoxide
Diazepam/
 Lorazepam ✳
Oxazepam

Beta blockers
Atenolol ✳
Bisoprolol ✳
Oxprenolol
Propranolol ✳

Other non-benzodiazepines
Buspirone

✳ See Part 3

ANTIDEPRESSANT DRUGS

Occasional moods of discouragement or sadness are normal and usually pass quickly. But more severe depression, accompanied by despair, lethargy, loss of sex drive, and often poor appetite, may call for medical attention. Such depression can arise from life stresses such as the death of someone close, an illness, or sometimes from no apparent cause.

There are three main types of drug for depression: tricyclic antidepressants (TCAs), selective serotonin re-uptake inhibitors (SSRIs), and monoamine oxidase inhibitors (MAOIs) (see Types of antidepressant, below). Lithium, a metallic element, is used to treat bipolar disorder (see Antimanic drugs, facing page). In some cases, it is used with an antidepressant for treating resistant depression. Several other antidepressants may be prescribed, including venlafaxine, mirtazepine, mianserin, and trazodone.

Why they are used

Minor depression does not usually require drug treatment; support and help in coming to terms with the cause is often all that is needed. Moderate or severe depression usually requires drug treatment, which is effective in most cases. Antidepressants may have to be taken for many months. Treatment should not be stopped too soon because symptoms are likely to reappear. When treatment is stopped, the dose should be gradually reduced over several weeks because withdrawal symptoms may occur if they are stopped suddenly.

How they work

Depression is thought to be caused by a reduction in the level of certain chemicals in the brain called neurotransmitters, which affect mood by stimulating brain cells. Antidepressants increase the level of these excitatory neurotransmitters. See Action of antidepressants (right).

Tricyclics (TCAs)

TCAs and venlafaxine block the re-uptake of the neurotransmitters serotonin and norepinephrine (noradrenaline), thereby increasing the neurotransmitter levels at receptors.

Selective serotonin re-uptake inhibitors (SSRIs)

SSRIs act by blocking the re-uptake of only one neurotransmitter, serotonin.

Monoamine oxidase inhibitors (MAOIs)

MAOIs act by blocking the breakdown of neurotransmitters, mainly serotonin and norepinephrine (noradrenaline).

How they affect you

The antidepressant effect of these drugs starts after 10 to 14 days' treatment and it may be six to eight weeks before the full effect is seen. However, side effects may happen at once. Tolerance to these side effects usually occurs and treatment should be continued.

Risks and special precautions

Overdose can be dangerous: tricyclics can produce coma, seizures, and disturbed heart rhythm, which may be fatal; monoamine oxidase inhibitors can also cause muscle spasms and even death. Both are prescribed with caution for people with heart problems or epilepsy.

MAOIs taken with certain drugs or foods rich in tyramine (for example, cheese, meat, yeast extracts, and red wine) can produce a dramatic rise in blood pressure, with headache or vomiting. People taking MAOIs are given a card that lists prohibited drugs and foods. Because of this adverse interaction, MAOIs are used much less frequently today and SSRIs or tricyclics are prescribed in preference to them, but SSRIs are not generally prescribed to anyone under the age of 18.

ACTION OF ANTIDEPRESSANTS

Normally, the brain cells release sufficient quantities of excitatory chemicals (known as neurotransmitters) to stimulate neighbouring cells. The neurotransmitters are constantly reabsorbed into the brain cells, where they are broken down by an enzyme called monoamine oxidase. In depression, fewer neurotransmitters are released. The levels of neurotransmitters in the brain are raised by antidepressant drugs.

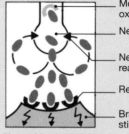

- Monoamine oxidase
- Nerve ending
- Neurotransmitters reabsorbed
- Receptor
- Brain cell stimulated

Normal brain activity
In a normal brain neurotransmitters are constantly being released, reabsorbed, and broken down.

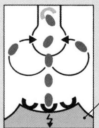

Brain activity in depression
The brain cells release fewer neurotransmitters than normal, leading to reduced stimulation.

- Brain cell poorly stimulated

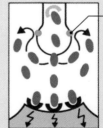

- Drug blocks reabsorption of neurotransmitter

Action of TCAs and SSRIs
TCA and SSRI drugs increase the levels of neurotransmitters by blocking their reabsorption.

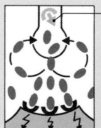

- Drug blocks enzyme

Action of MAOIs
MAOIs increase the neurotransmitter levels by blocking the action of the enzyme (monoamine oxidase) that breaks them down.

TYPES OF ANTIDEPRESSANT

Treatment usually begins with either a TCA or an SSRI.

Tricyclic antidepressants (TCAs)
Some TCAs, such as amitriptyline, cause drowsiness, which is useful for sleep problems in depression. TCAs also cause anticholinergic effects, including blurred vision, a dry mouth, and difficulty urinating.

Selective serotonin re-uptake inhibitors (SSRIs)
The SSRIs generally have fewer side effects than TCAs. The main unwanted effects of the SSRIs are nausea and vomiting. Anxiety, headache, and restlessness may also occur at the beginning of treatment.

Monoamine oxidase inhibitors (MAOIs)
These are especially effective in people who are anxious as well as depressed, or who suffer from phobias.

COMMON DRUGS

Tricyclics
Amitriptyline ✻
Clomipramine ✻
Dosulepin ✻
Doxepin
Imipramine ✻
Lofepramine ✻
Nortriptyline
Trimipramine

SSRIs
Citalopram/
 Escitalopram ✻
Fluoxetine ✻
Fluvoxamine
Paroxetine ✻
Sertraline ✻

MAOIs
Isocarboxazid
Moclobemide
Phenelzine ✻
Tranylcypromine

Other drugs
Duloxetine
Flupentixol ✻
Mianserin
Mirtazepine ✻
Reboxetine
Trazodone
Tryptophan
Venlafaxine ✻

✻ See Part 3

ANTIPSYCHOTIC DRUGS

Psychosis is a term used to describe mental disorders that prevent a person from thinking clearly, recognizing reality, and acting rationally. These disorders include schizophrenia and bipolar disorder (manic-depressive illness). The precise causes of these disorders are unknown, although a number of factors, including stress, heredity, and brain injury, may be involved. Temporary psychosis can also result from alcohol withdrawal or the misuse of mind-altering drugs (see Drugs of abuse, p.446). Various drugs are used to treat psychotic disorders (see Common drugs, below), most of which have similar actions and effects. One exception is lithium, which is particularly useful for bipolar disorder (see Antimanic drugs, right).

Why they are used

A person with a psychotic illness may recover spontaneously, and so a drug will not always be prescribed. Long-term treatment is started only when normal life is seriously disrupted. Antipsychotic drugs (also called major tranquillizers or neuroleptics) do not cure the disorder, but they do help to control symptoms.

By controlling the symptoms of psychosis, antipsychotic drugs make it possible for many affected people to live in the community and only be admitted to hospital for acute episodes.

The drug given to a particular individual depends on the nature of their illness and the expected adverse effects of that drug. Drugs differ in the amount of sedation produced; the need for sedation also influences the choice of drug.

Antipsychotics may also be given to calm or sedate a highly agitated or aggressive person, whatever the cause. Some antipsychotic drugs also have a powerful action against nausea and vomiting (see p.46), and are therefore sometimes used as premedication before a person has surgery.

How they work

It is thought that some forms of mental illness are caused by an increase in communication between brain cells due to overactivity of an excitatory chemical called dopamine. This may disturb normal thought processes and produce abnormal behaviour. Dopamine combines with receptors on the brain cells. Antipsychotic drugs reduce the transmission of nerve signals by binding to these receptors, thereby making the brain cells less sensitive to dopamine (see Action of antipsychotics, below). Some newer antipsychotic drugs, such as clozapine, risperidone, and sertindole, also bind to receptors for the chemical serotonin.

How they affect you

Because antipsychotics depress the action of dopamine, they can disturb its balance with another chemical in the brain, acetylcholine. If an imbalance occurs, extrapyramidal side effects (EPSE) may appear. These include restlessness, disorders of movement, and parkinsonism (see Drugs for parkinsonism, p.43).

In these circumstances, a change in medication to a different type of antipsychotic may be necessary. If this is not possible, an anticholinergic drug (see p.43) may be prescribed.

Antipsychotics may block the action of the neurotransmitter norepinephrine (noradrenaline). This lowers blood pressure, especially when you stand up, causing dizziness. It may also prevent ejaculation.

Risks and special precautions

It is important to continue taking these drugs even if all symptoms have gone, because the symptoms are controlled only by taking the prescribed dose.

Because antipsychotic drugs can have permanent as well as temporary side effects, the minimum necessary dosage is used. This minimum dose is found by

ANTIMANIC DRUGS

Changes in mood are normal, but when mood swings become grossly exaggerated, with peaks of elation or mania alternating with troughs of depression, it becomes an illness known as bipolar disorder, or manic-depressive illness. It is usually treated with lithium, a drug that reduces the intensity of the mania, lifts the depression, and lessens the frequency of mood swings. Because it may take weeks or even months before the lithium starts to work, an antipsychotic may be prescribed with lithium at first to give immediate relief of symptoms.

Lithium can be toxic if levels of the drug in the blood rise too high. Regular checks on the blood concentration of lithium should therefore be carried out during treatment. Symptoms of lithium poisoning include blurred vision, tremor, vomiting, and diarrhoea (see p.303).

starting with a low dose and increasing it until the symptoms are controlled. Sudden withdrawal after more than a few weeks can cause nausea, sweating, headache, and restlessness. Therefore, the dose is reduced gradually when treatment needs to be stopped.

The most serious long-term risk of antipsychotic treatment is a disorder known as tardive dyskinesia, which may develop after one to five years. This consists of repeated jerking movements of the mouth, tongue, and face, and sometimes of the hands and feet.

The condition is less common with the newer antipsychotics (atypical antipsychotics) than the older drugs (typical antipsychotics).

How they are administered

Antipsychotics may be given by mouth as tablets, capsules, or syrup, or by injection. They can also be given in the form of an intramuscular depot injection, which releases the drug slowly over several weeks.

ACTION OF ANTIPSYCHOTICS

Brain activity is partly governed by the action of a chemical called dopamine, which transmits signals between brain cells. In psychotic illness the brain cells release too much dopamine, resulting in excessive stimulation. The antipsychotic drugs help to reduce the adverse effects of excess dopamine.

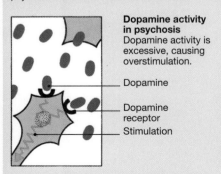

Dopamine activity in psychosis
Dopamine activity is excessive, causing overstimulation.

— Dopamine

— Dopamine receptor

— Stimulation

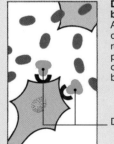

Dopamine activity blocked by drugs
Antipsychotic drugs occupy dopamine receptors and prevent the effects of excess dopamine being felt.

— Drugs

COMMON DRUGS

Typical antipsychotics
Benperidol
Chlorpromazine *
Flupentixol *
Fluphenazine
Haloperidol *
Levomepromazine
Pericyazine
Perphenazine
Pimozide
Pipotiazine
Prochlorperazine *
Promazine *
Trifluoperazine
Zuclopenthixol

Atypical antipsychotics
Amisulpride *
Aripiprazole
Clozapine *
Olanzapine *
Quetiapine *
Risperidone *
Sertindole
Zotepine

Antimanic drugs
Carbamazepine *
Lithium *
Sodium valproate *

* See Part 3

ANTICONVULSANT DRUGS

Electrical signals from nerve cells in the brain are normally finely coordinated to produce smooth movements of arms and legs, but these signals can become irregular and chaotic, and trigger the disorderly muscular activity and mental changes that are characteristic of a seizure (also called a fit or convulsion). The most common cause of seizures is the disorder known as epilepsy, which occurs as a result of brain disease or injury. In epilepsy, a seizure may be triggered by an outside stimulus such as a flashing light. Seizures can also result from the toxic effects of certain drugs and, in young children, a high temperature.

Anticonvulsant drugs are used both to reduce the risk of an epileptic seizure and to stop one that is in progress.

Why they are used

Isolated seizures seldom require drug treatment, but anticonvulsant drugs are the usual treatment for controlling seizures that are caused by epilepsy. In most cases, these drugs permit a person with epilepsy to lead a normal life.

ACTION OF ANTICONVULSANTS

Normally, the electrical activity of the brain is under good control. If an area of the brain is electrically unstable and there is an uncontrolled discharge of electrical impulses, epilepsy may occur (see Types of epilepsy, right). Anticonvulsants stabilize the electrical activity of brain cells, thus reducing the likelihood of a seizure.

Normal brain activity

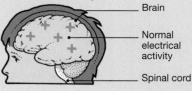

Brain

Normal electrical activity

Spinal cord

Brain activity in a seizure

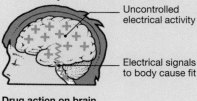

Uncontrolled electrical activity

Electrical signals to body cause fit

Drug action on brain activity

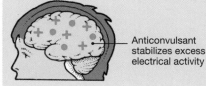

Anticonvulsant stabilizes excess electrical activity

Most people with epilepsy need to take anticonvulsants on a regular basis to prevent seizures. Usually a single drug is used, and treatment continues until there have been no attacks for at least two years. The drug prescribed depends on the type of epilepsy (see Types of epilepsy, right).

If one drug is not effective, a different one will be tried. Occasionally, it is necessary to take a combination of drugs. Even when receiving treatment, a person can suffer seizures. Repeated seizures or status epilepticus can be halted by injection of diazepam or a similar drug.

How they work

Brain cells bring about body movement by electrical activity that passes through the nerves to the muscles. In an epileptic seizure, uncontrolled electrical activity starts in one part of the brain and spreads to other parts, causing uncontrolled stimulation of brain cells. Most of the anticonvulsants have an inhibitory effect on brain cells and damp down electrical activity, preventing the excessive build-up that causes epileptic seizures (see Action of anticonvulsants, left).

How they affect you

Ideally, the only effect an anticonvulsant should have is to reduce or prevent epileptic seizures. Unfortunately, no drug prevents seizures without potentially affecting normal brain function, often leading to poor memory, inability to concentrate, lack of coordination, and lethargy. It is important, therefore, to find a drug and dosage sufficient to prevent seizures without causing unacceptable side effects. The dose has to be carefully tailored to the individual. It is usual to start with a low dose of a selected drug and to increase it gradually until a balance is achieved between the control of seizures and the occurrence of side effects, many of which wear off after the first weeks of treatment.

Blood tests are used to monitor levels of some anticonvulsants in the body as an aid to dose adjustment.

Risks and special precautions

Each anticonvulsant has its own specific adverse effects and risks; and some affect the liver's ability to break down other drugs (see Drug interactions, p.16) and may influence the action of other drugs you are taking. Doctors try to prescribe the minimum number of anticonvulsants needed to control the seizures, to reduce the risk of such interactions.

Some anticonvulsants pose risks to a developing baby – if you are hoping to become pregnant, you should discuss the risks, and whether your medication should be changed, with your doctor. People taking anticonvulsants need to take them regularly as prescribed. If levels of anticonvulsant in the body fall suddenly, seizures are very

TYPES OF EPILEPSY

The selection of anticonvulsant (anti-epileptic) drugs depends on the type of epilepsy, the age of the patient, and their particular response to individual drug treatment.

Generalized epilepsy In these forms of epilepsy, there is a widespread disturbance of the electrical activity in the brain and loss of consciousness occurs at the outset. In its simplest form, a momentary loss of consciousness occurs during which the person may stare into space. This is called an absence seizure, and mainly affects children. Seizures do not occur.

Another form of generalized epilepsy causes a brief jerk of a limb (myoclonus).

The most severe type is a tonic-clonic (grand mal) seizure, which is characterized by loss of consciousness, and seizures that may last for a few minutes.

Affected people may have one or more of these types of generalized epilepsy. Sodium valproate, lamotrigine, topiramate, levetiracetam, or the benzodiazepines are normally used for these types of epilepsy.

Partial (focal) epilepsy These types are caused by an electrical disturbance in only one part of the brain. The result is a disturbance of function, such as an abnormal sensation or movement of a limb, without loss of consciousness. In a simple partial seizure, this may precede a more serious attack associated with loss of consciousness (complex partial seizure), which may in turn progress to a generalized convulsive seizure.

Carbamazepine, lamotrigine, or phenytoin may be prescribed for this type of epilepsy.

Status epilepticus Repeated epileptic attacks without full recovery between them, or a single attack lasting more than 10 minutes, is called status epilepticus and it requires emergency treatment.

likely to occur. The dose should not be reduced or treatment stopped, except on a doctor's advice. Certain driving restrictions may apply if you have had a seizure; you need to report this to the Driver and Vehicle Licensing Agency (DVLA).

If, for any reason, anticonvulsant drug treatment needs to be stopped, the dose should be reduced gradually. People on anticonvulsant therapy are advised to carry an identification tag giving full details of their condition and treatment (see p.29).

COMMON DRUGS

Carbamazepine ✳	Lorazepam ✳
Clobazam	Midazolam
Clonazepam ✳	Oxcarbazepine
Diazepam ✳	Phenobarbital ✳
Ethosuximide	Phenytoin ✳
Gabapentin ✳	Primidone
Lamotrigine ✳	Sodium valproate ✳
Levetiracetam ✳	Tiagabine
	Topiramate
✳ See Part 3	Vigabatrin

DRUGS FOR PARKINSONISM

Parkinsonism is a general term used to describe shaking of the head and limbs, muscular stiffness, an expressionless face, and inability to control or initiate movement. It is caused by an imbalance of chemicals in the brain; the effect of acetylcholine is increased by a reduction in the action of dopamine.

The most common cause of Parkinsonism is Parkinson's disease, degeneration of the dopamine-producing cells in the brain. Other causes include the side effects of certain drugs, notably antipsychotics (see p.41), and narrowing of the blood vessels in the brain.

Why they are used
Drugs can relieve the symptoms of parkinsonism but, unfortunately, the degeneration of brain cells in Parkinson's disease cannot be halted, although drugs can minimize symptoms for many years.

How they work
Drugs to treat parkinsonism restore the balance between the chemicals dopamine and acetylcholine. They fall into two main groups: those that reduce the effect of acetylcholine (anticholinergic drugs) and those that boost the effect of dopamine.

Anticholinergics combine with receptors on brain cells, preventing acetylcholine from binding to them. This action reduces acetylcholine's relative overactivity and restores the balance with dopamine.

Dopamine cannot pass from the blood to the brain, and therefore cannot be given to boost its levels in the brain. Instead, levodopa (L-dopa), the chemical from which it is naturally produced in the brain, is combined with carbidopa (as co-careldopa) or benserazide (as co-beneldopa) to prevent it from being converted to dopamine before it reaches the brain. Amantadine (also used as an antiviral, see p.91) boosts dopamine levels in the brain by stimulating its release. Dopamine's action can also be boosted by

ACTION OF DRUGS FOR PARKINSONISM

Normal movement depends on a balance in the brain between dopamine and acetylcholine, which combine with receptors on brain cells. In parkinsonism, there is less dopamine present, with the result that acetylcholine is relatively overactive. The balance between acetylcholine and dopamine may be restored by anticholinergic drugs, which combine with the receptor for acetylcholine to block the action of acetylcholine on the brain cell, or by dopamine-boosting drugs, which increase the level of dopamine activity in the brain.

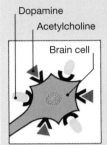

Normal chemical balance
Normally dopamine and acetylcholine are balanced.

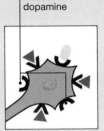

Chemical imbalance in parkinsonism
If dopamine activity is low, acetylcholine is overactive.

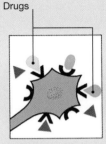

Action of anticholinergic drugs
Anticholinergic drugs displace acetylcholine and restore balance.

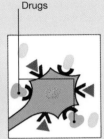

Action of dopamine-boosting drugs
These drugs increase dopamine activity and restore balance.

other drugs, including bromocriptine, pergolide, or apomorphine (injection only), which mimic the action of dopamine.

Choice of drug
Anticholinergics are used to treat parkinsonism due to antipsychotic drugs, which have dopamine-blocking properties. They are not generally used to treat parkinsonism of unknown cause because they are less effective and may increase cognitive impairment. L-dopa is usually given when the disease impairs walking; its effectiveness usually wanes after two to five years, in which case other dopamine-boosting drugs may also be prescribed.

COMMON DRUGS

Dopamine-boosting drugs	
Amantadine	Pergolide
Apomorphine	Pramipexole
Bromocriptine *	Rasagiline
Cabergoline	Ropinirole *
Entacapone	Selegiline
Levodopa * (as co-beneldopa/ co-careldopa)	**Anticholinergic drugs**
	Orphenadrine *
	Procyclidine *
	Trihexyphenidyl/ benzhexol

* See Part 3

DRUGS FOR DEMENTIA

Dementia is a decline in mental function that is severe enough to affect normal social or occupational activities. It can be sudden and irreversible, for example due to a stroke or a head injury. It can also develop gradually and may be a feature of a number of disorders, including poor circulation in the brain, multiple sclerosis, and Alzheimer's disease. Much research is in progress on the cause of Alzheimer's disease, which is the single most common cause of dementia.

Why they are used
Drugs called acetylcholinesterase inhibitors have been found to improve the symptoms of dementia in Alzheimer's disease, although they do not prevent its long-term progression.

How they work
In healthy people, acetylcholinesterase (an enzyme in the brain) breaks down the neurotransmitter acetylcholine, balancing its levels and limiting its effects. In Alzheimer's disease, there is a deficiency of acetylcholine. Acetylcholinesterase inhibitors block the action of the enzyme acetylcholinesterase, raising brain levels of acetylcholine, thus increasing alertness and slowing the rate of deterioration.

How they affect you
Drug treatment is started at a low dose following an assessment by a specialist of mental function. The dosage is increased gradually to minimize side effects. Any improvements should begin to appear in about 3 weeks. Assessment

is repeated at six-monthly intervals to decide if the treatment is beneficial.

Risks and special precautions
It is important to continue taking these drugs if they prove effective because there is a gradual loss of improvement after treatment is stopped. Side effects include urinary difficulties, nausea, vomiting, and diarrhoea. These drugs may increase the risk of seizures in some people.

COMMON DRUGS

Acetylcholinesterase inhibitors	
Donepezil *	Memantine
Galantamine	Rivastigmine *
	* See Part 3

NERVOUS SYSTEM STIMULANTS

A person's state of mental alertness varies throughout the day and is under the control of chemicals in the brain, some of which are depressant, causing drowsiness, and others that are stimulant, heightening awareness.

It is thought that an increase in the activity of the depressant chemicals may be responsible for a condition called narcolepsy, which is a tendency to fall asleep during the day for no obvious reason. In this case, the nervous system stimulants are administered to increase wakefulness. These drugs include the amfetamines (usually dexamfetamine), the related drug methylphenidate, and modafinil. Amfetamines are used less often these days because of the risk of dependence. A common home remedy for increasing alertness is caffeine, a mild stimulant that is present in coffee, tea, and cola. Respiratory stimulants related to caffeine are used to improve breathing (see right).

Why they are used

In adults who suffer from narcolepsy, some of these drugs prevent excessive drowsiness during the day. Stimulants do not cure narcolepsy and, since the disorder usually lasts throughout the person's lifetime, may have to be taken indefinitely. Methylphenidate or dexamfetamine are sometimes given to people suffering from attention deficit hyperactivity disorder (ADHD). Stimulants were once used as part of the treatment for obesity because reduced appetite is a side effect of amfetamines, but they are no longer thought appropriate for weight reduction. Diet is now the main treatment, together with orlistat if necessary.

Caffeine is added to some analgesics to counteract the effects of caffeine withdrawal, which can cause headaches, but no clear medical justification exists for this.

Apart from their use in narcolepsy, nervous system stimulants are not useful in the long term because the brain soon develops tolerance to them.

How they work

The level of wakefulness is controlled by a part of the brain stem called the reticular activating system (RAS). Activity in this area depends on the balance between chemicals, some of which are excitatory (including norepinephrine (noradrenaline)) and some inhibitory, such as gamma aminobutyric acid (GABA). Stimulants promote release of noradrenaline, increasing activity in the RAS and other parts of the brain and so raising alertness.

How they affect you

In adults, the central nervous system stimulants taken in the prescribed dose for narcolepsy increase wakefulness, thereby allowing normal concentration and thought processes to occur. They may

also reduce appetite and cause tremors. In hyperactive children, they reduce the general level of activity to a more normal level and increase the attention span.

Risks and special precautions

Some people, especially older people or those with previous psychiatric problems, are particularly sensitive to stimulants and may experience adverse effects, even when the drugs are given in comparatively low doses. They need to be used with caution in children because they can retard growth if taken for prolonged periods. An excess of these drugs given to a child may depress the nervous system, producing drowsiness or even loss of consciousness. Palpitations may also occur.

These drugs reduce the level of natural stimulants in the brain, so after regular use for a few weeks a person may become physically dependent on them for normal function. If they are abruptly withdrawn, the excess of natural inhibitory chemicals in the brain depresses central nervous system activity, producing withdrawal symptoms. These may include lethargy, depression, increased appetite, and difficulty staying awake.

Stimulants can produce overactivity in the brain if used inappropriately or in excess, resulting in extreme restlessness, sleeplessness, nervousness, or anxiety. They also stimulate the sympathetic branch of the autonomic nervous system (see p.35), causing shaking, sweating, and palpitations. More serious risks of exceeding the prescribed dose are seizures and a major disturbance in mental functioning that may result in delusions and hallucinations. Because these drugs have been abused, amfetamines and methylphenidate are classified as controlled drugs (see p.13).

ACTION OF NERVOUS SYSTEM STIMULANTS

Wakefulness is controlled by a part of the brain stem called the reticular activating system (RAS).

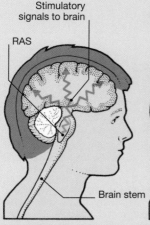

Stimulatory signals to brain

RAS

Brain stem

Normal brain activity
When the brain is functioning normally, signals from the RAS stimulate the upper parts of the brain, which control thought processes and alertness.

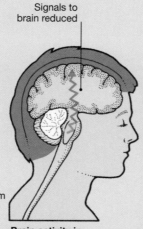

Signals to brain reduced

Brain activity in narcolepsy
In narcolepsy, the level of signals from the RAS is greatly reduced.

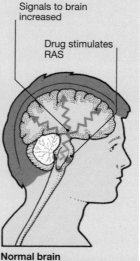

Signals to brain increased

Drug stimulates RAS

Normal brain activity restored
Central nervous system stimulants act on the RAS to increase the level of stimulatory signals to the brain.

DRUGS FOR MIGRAINE

Migraine is a term applied to recurrent severe headaches affecting only one side of the head and caused by changes in the blood vessels around the brain and scalp. They may be accompanied by nausea and vomiting and preceded by warning signs, usually an impression of flashing lights or numbness and tingling in the arms. Occasionally, speech may be impaired, or the attack may be disabling. The underlying cause of migraine is uncertain, but an attack may be triggered by a blow to the head, physical exertion, certain foods and drugs, or emotional factors such as excitement, tension, or shock. A family history of migraine also increases the chance of an individual developing it.

Why they are used

Drugs are used either to relieve symptoms or to prevent attacks. Different drugs are used in each approach, but none cures the underlying disorder. However, a susceptibility to migraine headaches can clear up spontaneously, and if you are taking drugs regularly, your doctor may recommend that you stop them after a few months to see if this has happened.

In most people, migraine headaches can be relieved by a mild analgesic (painkiller), such as paracetamol or a non-steroidal anti-inflammatory drug (NSAID), or a stronger one like codeine (see Analgesics, p.36). If nausea and vomiting accompany the migraine, tablets may not be absorbed sufficiently from the gut. Absorption can be increased if drugs are taken as soluble tablets in water or with an anti-emetic.

Some drugs used to relieve attacks can be given by injection, inhaler, nasal spray, or suppository. Preparations that contain caffeine should be avoided since headaches may be caused by excessive use or on stopping treatment. 5HT$_1$ agonist drugs (such as sumatriptan) are used if analgesics are not effective. Ergotamine is used much less often now.

The factors that trigger an individual's attacks should be identified and avoided. Anti-anxiety drugs are not usually prescribed if stress is a precipitating factor because of the potential for dependence. If the attacks occur more often than once a month and significantly disrupt daily life, drugs to prevent migraine may be taken every day. Drugs used to prevent migraine are beta blockers (see p.55), such as metoprolol or propranolol, and pizotifen (an antihistamine and serotonin blocker). Other drugs that have been used include amitriptyline (an antidepressant, see p.40), verapamil, and cyproheptadine.

How they work

The symptoms of a migraine attack begin when blood vessels surrounding the brain constrict (become narrower), producing the typical migraine warning signs. The constriction is thought to be caused by certain chemicals found in food or produced by the body. The neurotransmitter serotonin causes large blood vessels in the brain to constrict. Pizotifen and propranolol block the effect of chemicals on blood vessels and thereby prevent attacks (see Action of drugs used for migraine, above).

The next stage of a migraine attack occurs when blood vessels in the scalp and around the eyes dilate (widen). As a result, chemicals called prostaglandins are released, producing pain. Aspirin and paracetamol relieve this pain by blocking prostaglandins. Codeine acts directly on the brain, altering pain perception (see Action of analgesics, p.36). Ergotamine and 5HT$_1$ agonists relieve pain by narrowing dilated blood vessels in the scalp.

How they affect you

Each drug has its own adverse effects. 5HT$_1$ agonists may cause chest tightness and drowsiness. Ergotamine may cause drowsiness, tingling sensations in the skin, cramps, and weakness in the legs, and vomiting may be made worse. Pizotifen may cause drowsiness and weight gain. For effects of propranolol, see p.55, and for analgesics, see p.36.

Risks and special precautions

5HT$_1$ agonists should not usually be used by those with high blood pressure, angina, or coronary heart disease. Ergotamine can damage blood vessels by prolonged overconstriction so it should be used with caution by those with poor circulation. Excessive use can lead to dependence and many adverse effects, including headache. You should not take more than your doctor advises in any one week.

How they are administered

These drugs are usually taken by mouth as tablets or capsules. Sumatriptan can also be taken as an injection or a nasal spray. Ergotamine can be taken as suppositories, or as tablets that dissolve under the tongue.

ACTION OF DRUGS USED FOR MIGRAINE

The underlying cause of migraine is uncertain but symptoms occur when chemicals in the bloodstream affect blood vessels around the brain and in the scalp. In the first stage of a migraine attack, the blood vessels surrounding the brain constrict, causing warning signs (below left). In the second stage, the blood vessels in the scalp dilate, causing a severe headache (below right).

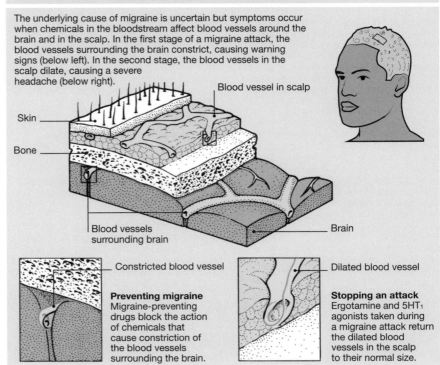

Skin

Bone

Blood vessel in scalp

Blood vessels surrounding brain

Brain

Constricted blood vessel

Preventing migraine
Migraine-preventing drugs block the action of chemicals that cause constriction of the blood vessels surrounding the brain.

Dilated blood vessel

Stopping an attack
Ergotamine and 5HT$_1$ agonists taken during a migraine attack return the dilated blood vessels in the scalp to their normal size.

COMMON DRUGS

Drugs to prevent migraine
Amitriptyline ✳
Cyproheptadine
Fremanezumab
Pizotifen ✳
Propranolol ✳
Sodium valproate ✳
Verapamil ✳

5HT$_1$ agonists
Almotriptan
Eletriptan
Frovatriptan

Naratriptan
Rizatriptan
Sumatriptan ✳
Zolmitriptan

Other drugs to relieve migraine
Codeine ✳
Ergotamine ✳
NSAIDs (see p.74)
Paracetamol ✳
Tolfenamic acid

✳ See Part 3

ANTI-EMETICS

Drugs used to treat or prevent vomiting or the feeling of sickness (nausea) are known as anti-emetics. Vomiting is a reflex action for getting rid of harmful substances, but it may also be a symptom of disease. Vomiting and nausea are often caused by a digestive tract infection, travel sickness, pregnancy, or vertigo (a balance disorder involving the inner ear). They can also occur as a side effect of some drugs, especially those used for cancer, radiation therapy, or general anaesthesia.

Commonly used anti-emetics include metoclopramide, domperidone, cyclizine, haloperidol, ondansetron, granisetron, prochlorperazine, promethazine, and cinnarizine. The phenothiazine and butyrophenone drug groups are also used as antihistamines (see p.82) and to treat some types of mental illness (see Antipsychotic drugs, p.41).

Why they are used

Doctors usually diagnose the cause of vomiting before prescribing an anti-emetic because vomiting may be due to an infection of the digestive tract or some other condition of the abdomen that might require treatment such as surgery. Treating only the vomiting and nausea might delay diagnosis, correct treatment, and recovery. Anti-emetics may be taken to prevent travel sickness (using one of the antihistamines), to relieve vomiting resulting from anticancer (see p.112) and other drug treatments (metoclopramide, haloperidol, domperidone, ondansetron, and prochlorperazine), to help the nausea in vertigo (see right), and occasionally to relieve cases of severe vomiting during pregnancy. You should not take an anti-emetic during pregnancy except on medical advice.

No anti-emetic drug should be taken for longer than a couple of days without consulting your doctor.

How they work

Nausea and vomiting occur when the vomiting centre in the brain is stimulated by signals from three places in the body: the digestive tract, the part of the inner ear controlling balance, and the brain itself via thoughts and emotions and via its

chemoreceptor trigger zone, which responds to harmful substances in the blood. Anti-emetic drugs may act at one or more of these places (see Action of anti-emetics, left). Some help the stomach to empty its contents into the intestine. A combination may be used that works at different sites and has an additive effect.

How they affect you

As well as treating vomiting and nausea, many anti-emetic drugs may make you feel drowsy. However, for preventing travel sickness on long journeys, a sedating antihistamine may be an advantage.

Some anti-emetics (in particular, the phenothiazines and antihistamines) can block the parasympathetic nervous system (see p.35), causing dry mouth, blurred vision, or difficulty in passing urine. The phenothiazines may also lower blood pressure, leading to dizziness or fainting.

Risks and special precautions

Because some antihistamines can make you drowsy, it may be advisable not to drive while taking them. Phenothiazines, butyrophenones, and metoclopramide can produce uncontrolled movements of the face and tongue, so they are used with caution in people with parkinsonism.

ACTION OF ANTI-EMETICS

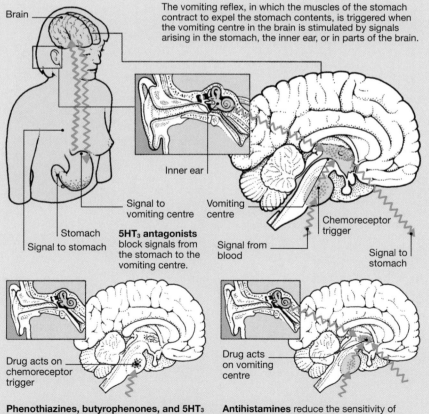

Brain

The vomiting reflex, in which the muscles of the stomach contract to expel the stomach contents, is triggered when the vomiting centre in the brain is stimulated by signals arising in the stomach, the inner ear, or in parts of the brain.

Inner ear

Signal to vomiting centre

Stomach
Signal to stomach

5HT₃ antagonists block signals from the stomach to the vomiting centre.

Vomiting centre

Signal from blood

Chemoreceptor trigger

Signal to stomach

Drug acts on chemoreceptor trigger

Drug acts on vomiting centre

Phenothiazines, butyrophenones, and 5HT₃ antagonists prevent the chemoreceptor trigger from stimulating vomiting.

Antihistamines reduce the sensitivity of the vomiting centre.

COMMON DRUGS

Antihistamines
Cinnarizine *
Cyclizine
Meclozine
Promethazine *

Phenothiazines
Chlorpromazine *
Levomepromazine
Perphenazine
Prochlorperazine *
Trifluoperazine

5HT₃ antagonists
Granisetron
Ondansetron *
Palonosetron

Butyrophenones
Haloperidol *

Other drugs
Aprepitant
Betahistine *
Dexamethasone *
Domperidone *
Hyoscine
hydrobromide *
Metoclopramide *
Nabilone

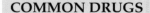
* See Part 3

RESPIRATORY SYSTEM

The respiratory system consists of the lungs and the passageways, such as the trachea and bronchi, by which air reaches them. Through the process of inhaling and exhaling air – breathing – the body is able to obtain the oxygen necessary for survival, and to expel carbon dioxide, which is the waste product of the basic human biological process.

What can go wrong

Difficulty in breathing may be due to narrowing of the air passages, from spasm, as in asthma and bronchitis, or from swelling of the linings of the air passages, as in bronchiolitis and bronchitis. Breathing difficulties may also be due to an infection of the lung tissue, as in pneumonia, or to damage to the small air sacs (alveoli) from emphysema or scarring (fibrosis), or from inhaled dusts or moulds, which cause pneumoconiosis and farmer's lung. Smoking and air pollution can affect the respiratory system in many ways, leading to diseases such as lung cancer and bronchitis.

Sometimes difficulty in breathing may be due to congestion of the lungs from heart disease, to an inhaled object such as a peanut, or to infection or inflammation of the throat. Symptoms of breathing difficulties often include a cough and a tight feeling in the chest.

Why drugs are used

Drugs with a variety of actions are used to clear the air passages, soothe inflammation, and reduce the production of mucus. Some can be bought without a prescription as single-ingredient or combined-ingredient preparations, often with an analgesic.

Decongestants (p.51) reduce the swelling inside the nose, thereby making it possible to breathe more freely. If the cause of the congestion is an allergic response, an antihistamine (p.82) is often recommended to relieve symptoms or to prevent attacks. Bacterial infections of the respiratory tract are usually treated with antibiotics (p.86), although most respiratory tract infections are viral.

Bronchodilators are drugs that widen the bronchi (p.48). They are used to prevent and relieve asthma attacks. Corticosteroids (p.99) reduce inflammation in the swollen inner layers of the airways. They are used to prevent asthma attacks. Other drugs, such as sodium cromoglicate, may be used for treating allergies and preventing asthma attacks but they are not effective once an asthma attack has begun.

A variety of drugs are used to relieve a cough, depending on the type of cough involved. Some drugs make it easier to eliminate phlegm; others suppress the cough by inhibiting the cough reflex.

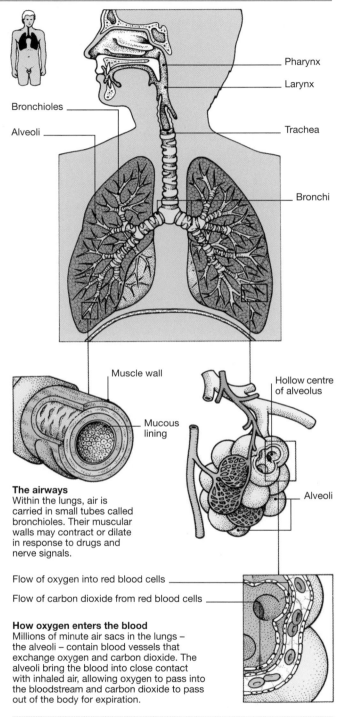

Pharynx

Larynx

Bronchioles

Alveoli

Trachea

Bronchi

Muscle wall

Mucous lining

Hollow centre of alveolus

Alveoli

The airways
Within the lungs, air is carried in small tubes called bronchioles. Their muscular walls may contract or dilate in response to drugs and nerve signals.

Flow of oxygen into red blood cells

Flow of carbon dioxide from red blood cells

How oxygen enters the blood
Millions of minute air sacs in the lungs – the alveoli – contain blood vessels that exchange oxygen and carbon dioxide. The alveoli bring the blood into close contact with inhaled air, allowing oxygen to pass into the bloodstream and carbon dioxide to pass out of the body for expiration.

MAJOR DRUG GROUPS

Bronchodilators
Drugs for asthma
Decongestants
Drugs to treat coughs

See also sections on Allergy (p.81) and Infections (p.84)

BRONCHODILATORS

Air entering the lungs passes through narrow tubes called bronchioles. In asthma and bronchitis the bronchioles become narrower, either as a result of contraction of the muscles in their walls, or as a result of mucus congestion. This narrowing of the bronchioles obstructs the flow of air into and out of the lungs and causes breathlessness.

Bronchodilators are prescribed to widen the bronchioles and improve breathing. There are three main groups of bronchodilators: sympathomimetics, anticholinergics, and xanthine drugs (which are related to caffeine). They are all used for relief of symptoms, and do not affect the underlying disease process. Anticholinergics are thought to be more effective in, and are used particularly for, bronchitis. In chronic asthma, they are less effective, and are usually prescribed as additional therapy when control with other drugs is inadequate. Sympathomimetics are the first-choice drugs in the management of asthma, and are frequently used in bronchitis. Xanthines have been used for many years, both for asthma and for bronchitis. They usually need precise adjustment of dosage to be effective while avoiding side effects. This makes them more difficult to use,

and they are reserved for people whose condition cannot be controlled by other bronchodilators alone.

Why they are used

Bronchodilators help to dilate the bronchioles of people suffering from asthma and bronchitis. However, they are of little benefit to those suffering from severe chronic bronchitis.

Bronchodilators are usually taken when they are needed in order to relieve an attack of breathlessness that is in progress. Some people find it helpful to take an extra dose of their bronchodilator immediately before undertaking any activity that is likely to provoke an attack of breathlessness. A patient who requires treatment with a sympathomimetic inhaler more than twice a week or at night should see their doctor about preventative treatment with an inhaled corticosteroid.

Sympathomimetic drugs are mainly used for the rapid relief of breathlessness; anticholinergic and xanthine drugs are used both for acute attacks and long-term.

How they work

Bronchodilator drugs act by relaxing the muscles surrounding the bronchioles. Sympathomimetic and anticholinergic

drugs achieve this by interfering with nerve signals passed to the muscles through the autonomic nervous system (see p.35). Xanthine drugs are thought to relax the muscle in the bronchioles by a direct effect on the muscle fibres, but their precise action is not known.

Bronchodilator drugs usually improve breathing within a few minutes of administration. Corticosteroids act more slowly and it may be several days before the capacity for exercise increases substantially. Eventually the corticosteroids should reduce the need for bronchodilators.

Because sympathomimetic drugs stimulate a branch of the autonomic nervous system that controls heart rate, they may sometimes cause palpitations and trembling. Typical side effects of anticholinergic drugs include dry mouth, blurred vision, and difficulty in passing urine. Xanthine drugs may cause headaches and nausea.

Risks and special precautions

Since most bronchodilators are not taken by mouth but inhaled, they do not commonly cause serious side effects. However, because of their possible effect on heart rate, xanthine and sympathomimetic drugs need to be prescribed with caution to people with heart problems, high blood pressure, or an overactive thyroid gland. Smoking tobacco and drinking alcohol increase excretion of xanthines from the body, reducing their effects. Stopping smoking after being stabilized on a xanthine may result in a rise in blood concentration, and an increased risk of side effects. It is advisable to stop smoking before starting treatment. The anticholinergic drugs may not be suitable for people with urinary retention or those who have a tendency to glaucoma.

ACTION OF BRONCHODILATORS

When the bronchioles are narrowed following contraction of the muscle layer and swelling of the mucous lining, the passage of air is impeded. Bronchodilators act on the nerve signals that govern muscle activity. Sympathomimetics enhance the action of neurotransmitters that encourage muscle relaxation. Anticholinergics block the neurotransmitters that trigger muscle contraction and reduce production of mucus. Xanthines promote muscle relaxation by a direct effect on the muscles.

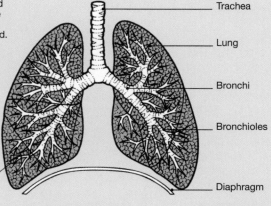

- Trachea
- Lung
- Bronchi
- Bronchioles
- Diaphragm

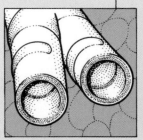

Normal bronchioles
The muscle surrounding the bronchioles is relaxed, thus leaving the airway open.

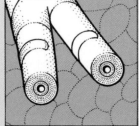

Asthma attack
The bronchiole muscle contracts and the lining swells, narrowing the airway.

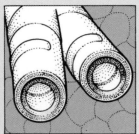

After drug treatment
The muscles relax, thereby opening the airway, but the lining remains swollen.

COMMON DRUGS

Sympathomimetics	Anticholinergics
Bambuterol	Aclidinium
Ephedrine ✳	Glycopyrronium
Epinephrine ✳	Ipratropium
Fenoterol	bromide ✳
Formoterol	Tiotropium ✳
Indacaterol	Umeclidinium
Salbutamol ✳	
Salmeterol ✳	**Xanthines**
Terbutaline ✳	Theophylline/
Vilanterol	aminophylline ✳

✳ See Part 3

DRUGS FOR ASTHMA

Asthma is a chronic lung disease characterized by episodes in which the bronchioles constrict due to oversensitivity. The attacks are usually, but not always, reversible; asthma is also known as reversible airways obstruction. It often starts in childhood, although it may also first develop in adulthood, and can affect people of any age. Sometimes the inflammation causing the constriction is due to an identifiable allergen in the atmosphere, such as house dust mite, but often there is no obvious trigger. Breathlessness is the main symptom, and wheezing, coughing, and chest tightness are common. People with asthma often have attacks during the night and wake up with breathing difficulty. The illness varies in severity, and it can be life threatening.

There are a number of drugs that are used in the control of asthma. Where drugs are needed only to control an occasional attack, a sympathomimetic bronchodilator will probably be used in inhaler form. When a person needs continuous preventative treatment there are a number of choices: often an inhaled corticosteroid may be used (with a sympathomimetic inhaler if attacks persist). More severe cases may require higher-dose corticosteroids or the addition of a long-acting sympathomimetic bronchodilator. If this is not adequate, the addition of an anticholinergic drug, or theophylline, or these in combination with others already tried may be needed. There are also leukotriene antagonists, which may be used alone or with

corticosteroids; they are less effective in severe cases when patients are taking high doses of other drugs. Some people who suffer from very severe asthma may need such large doses of corticosteroids that tablets have to be taken. Antihistamines have been prescribed for asthma in the past but this has not proved to be a successful treatment.

Why they are used

In asthma, the airways (bronchioles) constrict, making it difficult to get air in or out of the lungs. Bronchodilators (sympathomimetics, anticholinergics, and theophylline) relax the constricted muscles around the bronchioles (p.48). Short-acting sympathomimetics act within a few minutes when inhaled and are used to provide relief of symptoms during an attack, and in more severe cases the long-acting sympathomimetics may be used to help with continuous protective cover. They are particularly useful for preventing symptoms overnight. Theophylline/aminophylline must be given by mouth or injection; the tablets are used for regular continuous dosing, and the injection is used in hospital to gain control of severe asthma. Drugs that are not bronchodilators, such as corticosteroids and leukotriene receptor antagonists (see p.50), are effective for long-term protection. Corticosteroids are also given orally for severe acute attacks. Although they have a delayed onset of action (12–24 hours), they help to prevent a

recurrence of symptoms in the days after the acute attack.

In some cases, an intravenous injection of magnesium sulfate may be given to treat a severe asthma attack.

How they work

Inhaling a drug directly into the lungs is the best way of getting benefit without excessive side effects. A selection of devices for delivering the drug into the airways is illustrated below.

Inhalers or puffers release a small dose when they are pressed, but require some skill to use effectively. If you have a pressurized metered-dose inhaler, a large hollow plastic "spacer" can help you to inhale your drug more easily. Some devices are triggered by an inward breath and may be easier to use than a puffer.

In severe attacks, nebulizers pump compressed air through a solution of drug to produce a fine mist that is inhaled through a face mask. They deliver large doses of the drug to the lungs, rapidly relieving breathing difficulty.

Bronchodilators act by relaxing the muscles surrounding the bronchioles (see p.48). Corticosteroids are used for their anti-inflammatory properties. By suppressing airway inflammation they reduce swelling (oedema) inside the bronchioles, complementing relaxation of the walls by the bronchodilators in opening up the tubes. Reducing the inflammation also has the effect of reducing the amount of mucus produced, and this again helps to clear the airways. Corticosteroids

DIFFERENT TYPES OF INHALER

Inhalers are used to deliver drugs to relieve or prevent the symptoms of asthma. A wide range of different types of inhaler is available and the most commonly prescribed ones are shown here. Many people are prescribed a reliever and a preventer drug, and these are often given in combination in a single inhaler. Although every inhaler works on the same broad principle to deliver the drug directly to the bronchioles through a mouthpiece, there are individual differences in the actions required. Therefore, it is important to read the instructions carefully and practise using the

inhaler before you need it in an emergency. Some inhalers are activated by taking in a breath, and these may be easier for some people to use. However, some, such as the turbohaler, require forceful inhalation, which may be challenging for some people. If you have trouble operating an inhaler, you can ask your doctor for a spacer (see p.50); this requires less coordination between releasing the drug and breathing in, and is particularly suitable for children, older people, or those with coordination difficulties.

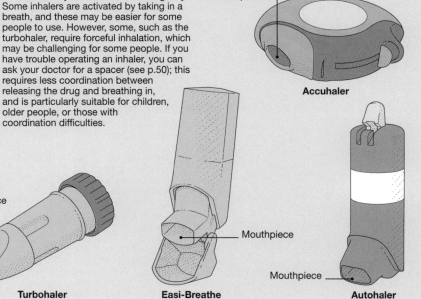

Mouthpiece

Accuhaler

Easi-Breathe
Mouthpiece

Mouthpiece
Autohaler

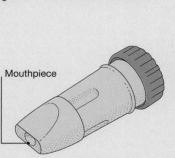

Mouthpiece
Turbohaler

Mouthpiece
Metered-dose

DRUGS FOR ASTHMA continued

HOW TO USE A SPACER

A spacer is a large, hollow plastic device that has a mouthpiece at one end and a slot for a metered-dose inhaler at the other; it can be split in two for easy cleaning and transporting. A spacer is ideal for groups such as children and older people as it avoids special breathing techniques and allows the patient to breathe in the drug at a normal rate. For small children and very sick people, the mouthpiece can be fitted with a mask that covers the mouth and nose. The spacer should be cleaned once a week to remove deposits and reduce the build-up of static electricity because this can reduce the amount of drug that reaches the airways.

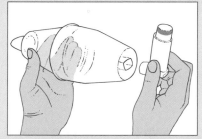

1 Click the two halves of the spacer together securely. Remove the cap from the inhaler's mouthpiece and shake the inhaler.

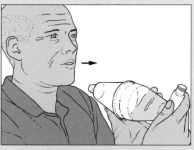

2 Push the mouthpiece of the inhaler into the slot at the blunt end of the spacer. Breathe out as deeply as possible; prepare to place the spacer in your mouth.

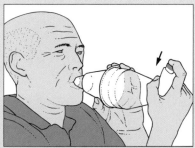

3 Press the canister to release a dose of the drug. Breathe in, hold breath for 10 seconds, breathe out into the spacer, and repeat. Another dose can be taken.

HOW TO USE A METERED-DOSE INHALER

The metered-dose inhaler is one of the most commonly prescribed devices for treating asthma, and is used to deliver a range of drugs. It is easy to use, and it takes only a matter of seconds for the drug to reach the airways and relieve breathing. Practise the technique before you need to use the inhaler in an emergency.

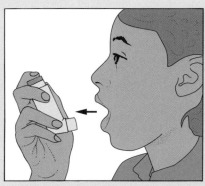

1 Remove the cap from the mouthpiece and shake the inhaler. Breathe out gently. Get ready to place the mouthpiece in the mouth.

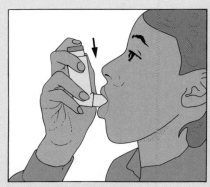

2 Tilt back the head, breathe in slowly and deeply, and at the same time press the canister. Hold breath for 10 seconds.

usually start to increase the user's capacity for exercise within a few days, and most people find that the frequency of their attacks of breathlessness is greatly reduced.

Leukotrienes occur naturally in the body; they used to be called "slow reacting substances". They are chemically related to the prostaglandins, but much more potent in producing an inflammatory reaction; they are also much more potent than histamine at causing bronchoconstriction. Leukotrienes seem to play an important part in asthma. Drugs have been developed that block their receptors (leukotriene receptor antagonists) and therefore reduce the inflammation and bronchoconstriction of asthma. Cromoglicate and nedocromil act by stabilizing mast cells in the lungs, preventing them from releasing histamine, leukotrienes, and other inflammation-causing chemicals.

Risks and special precautions

The drugs taken by inhalation act locally and are used in much lower doses than would be needed as tablets. They do not commonly cause serious side effects, but the dry powder inhalations can cause a reflex bronchospasm as the powder hits the lining of the airways; this can be avoided by first using a short-acting sympathomimetic. Inhaled corticosteroids may encourage fungal growth in the mouth and throat (thrush). This can be minimized by using a spacer and by rinsing your mouth out and gargling after each inhalation. High doses of inhaled corticosteroids may suppress adrenal gland function, reduce bone density, cause bruising, increase the risk of glaucoma, and retard growth in children. Sympathomimetics and theophylline by mouth may affect heart rate, and should be prescribed with caution to people with heart problems, high blood pressure, or an overactive thyroid gland. The effects of theophylline may last longer if you have a viral infection, heart failure, or liver cirrhosis. The drugs also interact with many other drugs. Anticholinergics must be used with caution in patients who have prostate problems or urinary retention. Leukotriene receptor antagonists may rarely produce a syndrome with several potentially serious effects including worsening lung function and heart complications.

COMMON DRUGS

Sympathomimetics
Bambuterol
Ephedrine *
Epinephrine *
Fenoterol
Formoterol
Salbutamol *
Salmeterol *
Terbutaline *

Anticholinergics
Ipratropium
bromide *
Tiotropium *

Leukotriene antagonists
Montelukast *
Zafirlukast

Corticosteroids
Beclometasone *
Budesonide *
Ciclesonide
Fluticasone *
Mometasone *
Prednisolone *

Xanthines
Theophylline/
aminophylline *

Other drugs
Nedocromil
Sodium
cromoglicate *

* See Part 3

DECONGESTANTS

The usual cause of a blocked nose is swelling of the delicate mucous membrane that lines the nasal passages and excessive production of mucus as a result of inflammation. This may be caused by an infection (for example, a common cold) or it may be caused by an allergy – for example, to pollen – a condition known as allergic rhinitis or hay fever. Congestion can also occur in the sinuses (the air spaces in the skull), resulting in sinusitis. Decongestants are drugs that reduce swelling of the mucous membrane and suppress the production of mucus, helping to clear blocked nasal passages and sinuses. Antihistamines counter the allergic response in allergy-related conditions (see p.82). If the symptoms are persistent, either topical corticosteroids (see p.99) or sodium cromoglicate (p.397) may be preferred.

Why they are used

Most common colds and blocked noses do not need to be treated with decongestants. Simple home remedies, such as steam inhalation, possibly with the addition of an aromatic oil – such as menthol or eucalyptus – are often effective. Decongestants are used when such measures are ineffective or when there is a particular risk from untreated congestion – for example, in people who experience recurrent middle-ear or sinus infections.

Decongestants are available in the form of drops or sprays applied directly into the nose (topical decongestants), or they can be taken by mouth. Small quantities of decongestant drugs are added to many over-the-counter cold remedies (see p.52).

How they work

When the mucous membrane lining the nose is irritated by infection or allergy, the blood vessels supplying the membrane become enlarged. This leads to fluid accumulation in the surrounding tissue and encourages the production of larger-than-normal amounts of mucus.

Most decongestants belong to the sympathomimetic group of drugs, which stimulate the sympathetic branch of the autonomic nervous system (see p.35).

ACTION OF DECONGESTANTS

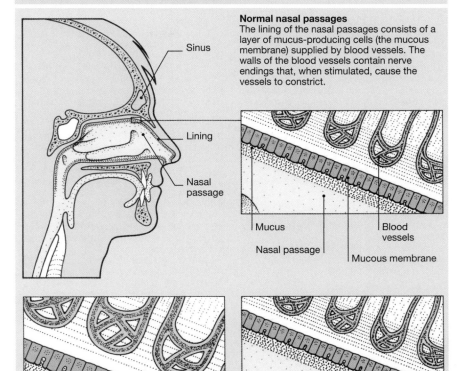

Normal nasal passages
The lining of the nasal passages consists of a layer of mucus-producing cells (the mucous membrane) supplied by blood vessels. The walls of the blood vessels contain nerve endings that, when stimulated, cause the vessels to constrict.

Sinus
Lining
Nasal passage
Mucus
Nasal passage
Blood vessels
Mucous membrane

Congested nasal lining
When the blood vessels enlarge in response to infection or irritation, increased amounts of fluid pass into the mucous membrane, which swells and produces more mucus.

Effect of decongestants
Decongestants enhance the action of chemicals that stimulate constriction of the blood vessels. Narrowing of the blood vessels reduces swelling and mucus production.

One effect of this action is to constrict the blood vessels, so reducing swelling of the lining of the nose and sinuses.

How they affect you

When applied topically in the form of drops or sprays, these drugs start to relieve congestion within a few minutes. Decongestants by mouth take a little longer to act, but their effect may also last longer.

Used in moderation, topical decongestants have few adverse effects, because they are not absorbed by the body in large amounts.

Used for too long or in excess, topical decongestants can, after giving initial relief, do more harm than good, causing a "rebound congestion" (see left). This effect can be prevented by taking the minimum effective dose and by using decongestant preparations only when absolutely necessary. Decongestants taken by mouth do not cause rebound congestion but are more likely to cause other side effects.

REBOUND CONGESTION

This can happen when decongestant nose drops and sprays are withdrawn or overused. The result is a sudden increase in congestion due to widening of the blood vessels in the nasal lining because blood vessels are no longer constricted by the decongestant.

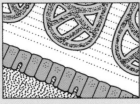

Congestion before drug treatment

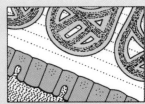

Congestion after stopping drug treatment

COMMON DRUGS

Used topically
Ephedrine *
Ipratropium *
Oxymetazoline
Phenylephrine
Xylometazoline

Taken by mouth
Ephedrine *
Phenylephrine
Pseudoephedrine

* See Part 3

DRUGS TO TREAT COUGHS

Coughing is a natural response to irritation of the lungs and air passages, designed to expel harmful substances from the respiratory tract. Common causes of coughing include infection of the respiratory tract (for example, bronchitis or pneumonia), inflammation of the airways caused by asthma, reflux of stomach acid, or exposure to irritant substances such as smoke or chemical fumes. Depending on their cause, coughs may be productive – that is, phlegm-producing – or they may be dry.

In most cases coughing is a helpful reaction that assists the body in ridding itself of excess phlegm and substances that irritate the respiratory system; suppressing the cough may actually delay recovery. However, repeated bouts of coughing can be distressing, and may increase irritation of the air passages. In such cases, medication to ease the cough may be recommended.

There are two main groups of cough remedies, according to whether the cough is productive or dry.

Productive coughs

Mucolytics and expectorants are sometimes recommended for productive coughs when simple home remedies such as steam inhalation have failed to "loosen" the cough and make it easier to cough up phlegm. Mucolytics alter the consistency of the phlegm, making it less sticky and easier to cough up. These are often given by inhalation. However, there

is little evidence that they are effective. Dornase alfa may be given to people who suffer from cystic fibrosis; the drug, given by inhalation via a nebulizer, is an enzyme that improves lung function by thinning the mucus. Expectorant drugs are taken by mouth to loosen a cough. There is some evidence that guaifenesin is effective but, overall, evidence of benefit is poor. Expectorants are included in many over-the-counter cough remedies.

Dry coughs

In dry coughs, no advantage is gained from promoting the expulsion of phlegm. Drugs used for dry coughs are given to suppress the coughing mechanism by calming the part of the brain that governs the coughing reflex. Antihistamines are often given for mild coughs, particularly in children. A demulcent, such as a simple linctus, can be used to soothe a dry, irritating cough. For persistent coughs, mild opioid drugs such as codeine may be prescribed (see also Analgesics, p.36). All cough suppressants have a generally sedating effect on the brain and nervous system and commonly cause drowsiness and other side effects.

Selecting a cough medication

There is a bewildering variety of over-the-counter medications available for the treatment of coughs. Most consist of a syrupy base to which active ingredients and flavourings are added. Many contain a number of different active ingredients,

COLD CURES

Many preparations are available over the counter to treat different symptoms of the common cold. The main ingredient in most preparations is a mild analgesic such as aspirin or paracetamol, accompanied by a decongestant (p.51), an antihistamine (p.82), and sometimes caffeine. Often the dose of each added ingredient is too low to provide any benefit. There is no evidence that vitamin C (see p.443) speeds recovery, but zinc supplements (see p.445) may be effective in shortening the cold's duration.

While some people find these drugs help to relieve symptoms, over-the-counter "cold cures" do not alter the course of the illness. Most doctors recommend using a product with a single analgesic, as the best way of alleviating symptoms. Other decongestants or antihistamines may be taken if needed, although antihistamines may cause sedation. These medicines are not harmless: take care to avoid overdose if using different brands.

sometimes with contradictory effects: it is not uncommon to find an expectorant (for a productive cough) and a decongestant included in the same preparation.

It is important to select the correct type of medication for your cough to avoid the risk of making your condition worse. For example, using a cough suppressant for a productive cough may prevent you getting rid of excess infected phlegm and may delay your recovery. It is best to choose a preparation with a single active ingredient that is appropriate for your type of cough. People with diabetes may need to select a sugar-free product. If you are in any doubt about which product to choose, ask your doctor or pharmacist for advice. Since there is a danger that use of over-the-counter cough remedies to alleviate symptoms may delay the diagnosis of a more serious underlying disorder, it is important to seek medical advice for any cough that persists for longer than a few days or if a cough is accompanied by additional symptoms such as fever or blood in the phlegm.

ACTION OF COUGH REMEDIES

Cough remedies are divided into two main groups: those that alter the consistency or production of phlegm (mucolytics and expectorants); and those that suppress the coughing reflex (opioid and non-opioid cough suppressants). Mucolytics are usually given by inhalation and act directly on the lungs and airways. Expectorants are taken by mouth, and are supposed to help bring up phlegm. Cough suppressants are taken by mouth and they act on the coughing centre in the brain.

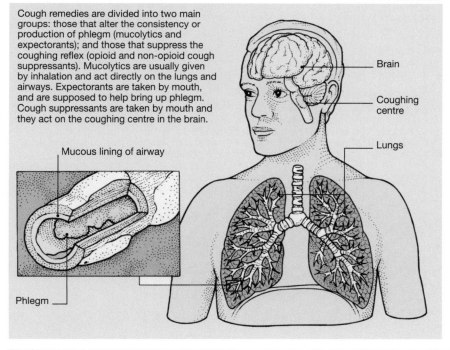

Brain

Coughing centre

Lungs

Mucous lining of airway

Phlegm

COMMON DRUGS

Expectorants
Ammonium chloride
Guaifenesin

Mucolytics
Carbocisteine
Dornase alfa
Mecysteine

Steam inhalation
Eucalyptus
Menthol

Opioid cough suppressants
Codeine *
Dextromethorphan
Methadone *
Pholcodine

Non-opioid cough suppressants
Antihistamines
(see p.82)

* See Part 3

HEART AND CIRCULATION

The blood transports oxygen, nutrients, and heat, contains chemical messages in the form of drugs and hormones, and carries away waste products for excretion by the kidneys. It is pumped by the heart to and from the lungs, and then in a separate circuit to the rest of the body, including the brain, digestive organs, muscles, kidneys, and skin.

What can go wrong

The efficiency of the circulation may be impaired by weakening of the heart's pumping action (heart failure) or irregularity of heart rate (arrhythmia). In addition, the blood vessels may be narrowed and clogged by fatty deposits (atherosclerosis). This may reduce blood supply to the brain, the extremities (peripheral vascular disease), or the heart muscle (coronary heart disease), causing angina. These last disorders can be complicated by the formation of clots that may block a blood vessel. A clot in the arteries supplying the heart muscle is known as coronary thrombosis; a clot in an artery inside the brain is the most frequent cause of stroke.

One common circulatory disorder is abnormally high blood pressure (hypertension), in which the pressure of circulating blood on the vessel walls is increased for reasons not yet fully understood. One factor may be loss of elasticity of the vessel walls (arteriosclerosis). Several other conditions, such as migraine and Raynaud's disease, are caused by temporary alterations to blood vessel size.

Why drugs are used

Because people with heart disease often have more than one problem, several drugs may be prescribed at once. Many act directly on the heart to alter the rate and rhythm of the heart beat. These are known as anti-arrhythmics and include beta blockers, calcium channel blockers, and digoxin.

Other drugs affect the diameter of the blood vessels, either dilating them (vasodilators) to improve blood flow and reduce blood pressure, or constricting them (vasoconstrictors).

Drugs may also reduce blood volume and fat levels, and alter clotting ability. Diuretics (used in the treatment of hypertension and heart failure) increase the body's excretion of salt and water. Lipid-lowering drugs reduce blood cholesterol levels, thereby minimizing the risk of atherosclerosis. Drugs to reduce blood clotting are administered if there is a risk of abnormal blood clots forming in the heart, veins, or arteries. Drugs that increase clotting are given when the body's natural clotting mechanism is defective.

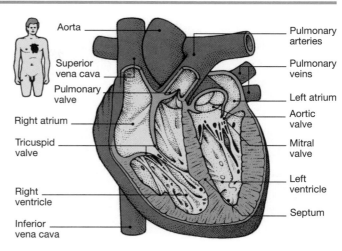

The heart
The heart is a pump with four chambers. The atrium and ventricle on the left side pump oxygenated blood to the body, while the chambers on the right pump deoxygenated blood to the lungs. Backflow of blood is stopped by valves at the chamber exits.

How blood circulates
Deoxygenated blood is carried to the heart from all parts of the body. It is then pumped to the lungs, where it becomes oxygenated. The oxygenated blood returns to the heart and from there is pumped throughout the body.

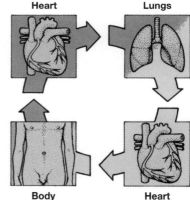

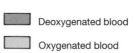
Deoxygenated blood

Oxygenated blood

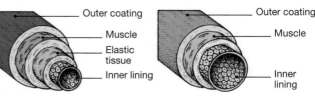

Arteries
Arteries carry blood away from the heart. Muscle walls contract and dilate in response to nerve signals.

Veins
Veins carry blood back to the heart. The walls are less elastic than artery walls.

MAJOR DRUG GROUPS

Digitalis drugs
Beta blockers
Vasodilators
Diuretics
Anti-arrhythmics
Anti-angina drugs

Antihypertensive drugs
Lipid-lowering drugs
Drugs that affect blood
   clotting

DIGITALIS DRUGS

Digitalis is the collective term for the naturally occurring substances (also called cardiac glycosides) that are found in the leaves of plants of the foxglove family and used to treat certain heart disorders. The principal drugs in this group are digoxin and digitoxin. Digoxin is more commonly used because it is shorter acting and dosage is easier to adjust (see also Risks and special precautions, below).

Why they are used

Digitalis drugs do not cure heart disease but improve the heart's pumping action and so relieve many of the symptoms that result from poor heart function. They are useful for treating conditions in which the heart beats irregularly or too rapidly (notably in atrial fibrillation; see Anti-arrhythmic drugs, p.58), when it pumps too weakly (in congestive heart failure), or when the heart muscle is damaged and weakened following a heart attack.

Digitalis drugs can be used for a short period when the heart is working poorly, but in many cases they have to be taken indefinitely. Their effect does not diminish with time. In heart failure, digitalis drugs are often given together with a vasodilator or diuretic drug (see pp.56–57).

How they work

The normal heart beat results from electrical impulses generated in nerve tissue within the heart. These cause the heart muscle to contract and pump blood. By reducing the flow of electrical impulses in the heart, digitalis makes the heart beat more slowly.

The force with which the heart muscle contracts depends on chemical changes in the heart muscle. By promoting these chemical changes, digitalis increases the force of muscle contraction each time the heart is stimulated. This compensates for the loss of power that occurs when some of the muscle is damaged following a heart attack. The stronger heart beat increases blood flow to the kidneys. This increases urine production and helps to remove the excess fluid that often accumulates as a result of heart failure.

How they affect you

Digitalis relieves the symptoms of heart failure – fatigue, breathlessness, and swelling of the legs – and increases your capacity for exercise. The frequency with which you need to pass urine may also be increased initially.

Risks and special precautions

Digitalis drugs can be toxic and, if blood levels rise too high, they may produce symptoms of digitalis poisoning. These include excessive tiredness, confusion, loss of appetite, nausea, vomiting, visual disturbances, and diarrhoea. If such symptoms occur, it is important to report them to your doctor promptly.

Digoxin is normally removed from the body by the kidneys; if kidney function is impaired, the drug is more likely to accumulate in the body and cause toxic effects. Digitoxin, which is broken down in the liver, is sometimes preferred in such cases. Digitoxin can accumulate after repeated dosage if liver function is severely impaired.

Both digoxin and digitoxin are more toxic when blood potassium levels are low. Potassium deficiency is commonly caused by diuretic drugs, so that people taking these along with digitalis drugs need to have the effects of both drugs and blood potassium levels carefully monitored. Potassium supplements may be required.

ACTION OF DIGITALIS DRUGS

The heart beat is triggered by electrical impulses that are generated by the pacemaker, a small mass of nerve tissue in the right atrium. Electrical signals are passed from the pacemaker to the atrioventricular node. From here a wave of impulses spreads throughout the heart muscle, causing it to contract and pump blood to the body. The pumping action of the heart can become weak if the heart muscle is damaged or if the heart beat is too fast, as in atrial fibrillation. In this condition (shown right), rapid signals from the pacemaker trigger fast and inefficient contractions of both the atria and the ventricles.

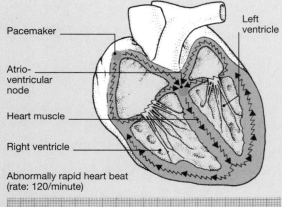

Pacemaker

Left ventricle

Atrio-ventricular node

Heart muscle

Right ventricle

Abnormally rapid heart beat (rate: 120/minute)

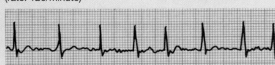

The effect of digitalis
Digitalis drugs reduce the flow of electrical impulses through the atrioventricular node so that the ventricles contract less often. In addition, by promoting the chemical changes in muscle cells necessary for muscular contraction, these drugs increase the force with which the heart muscle contracts and thereby improve the efficiency of each heart beat.

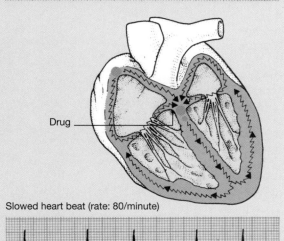

Drug

Slowed heart beat (rate: 80/minute)

COMMON DRUGS

Digitoxin
Digoxin *

⁕ See Part 3

BETA BLOCKERS

Beta blockers are drugs that interrupt the transmission of stimuli through the beta receptors of the body. Since the actions they block originate in the adrenal glands (and elsewhere) they are also sometimes called beta adrenergic blocking agents. Used mainly in heart disorders, these drugs are occasionally prescribed for other conditions.

Why they are used

Beta blockers are used for treating angina (see p.59) and irregular heart rhythms (see p.58). They may also be used for treating hypertension (see p.60) but are not usually used to initiate treatment. They are often given after a heart attack to reduce the likelihood of abnormal heart rhythms or further damage to the heart muscle. They are also prescribed to improve heart function in heart muscle disorders, known as cardiomyopathies.

Beta blockers may also be given to prevent migraine headaches (see p.45), or to reduce the physical symptoms of anxiety (see p.39). These drugs may be given to control symptoms of an overactive thyroid gland. A beta blocker is sometimes given in the form of eye drops in glaucoma to lower the fluid pressure inside the eye (see p.128).

How they work

By occupying the beta receptors, beta blockers nullify the stimulating action of norepinephrine (noradrenaline), the main

THE USES AND EFFECTS OF BETA BLOCKERS

Blocking the transmission of signals through beta receptors in different parts of the body produces a wide variety of benefits and side effects depending on the disease being treated. The illustration (right) shows the main areas and body systems affected by the action of beta blockers.

Brain
Dilation of the blood vessels surrounding the brain is inhibited, so preventing migraine.

Eye
Beta blocker eye drops reduce fluid production and so lower pressure inside the eye.

Heart
Slowing of the heart rate and reduction of the force of the heart beat reduces the workload of the heart, helping to prevent angina and abnormal heart rhythms.

Lungs
Constriction of the airways may provoke breathlessness in people with asthma or chronic bronchitis.

Blood vessels
Constriction of the blood vessels may cause coldness of the hands and feet.

Blood pressure
This is lowered because the rate and force at which the heart pumps blood into the circulatory system is reduced.

Muscles
Muscle tremor due to anxiety or to overactivity of the thyroid gland is reduced.

BETA RECEPTORS

Signals from the sympathetic nervous system are carried by norepinephrine (noradrenaline), a neurotransmitter produced in the adrenal glands and at the ends of the sympathetic nerve fibres. Beta blockers stop the signals from the neurotransmitter.

Neurotransmitter

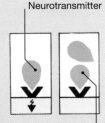

Beta blocker

Types of beta receptor
There are two types of beta receptor: beta 1 and beta 2. Beta 1 receptors are located mainly in the heart muscle; beta 2 receptors are found in the airways and blood vessels. Cardioselective drugs act mainly on beta 1 receptors; non-cardioselective drugs act on both types of receptor.

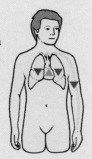

▲ Beta 1 receptors
▼ Beta 2 receptors

"fight or flight" hormone. As a result, they reduce the force and speed of the heart beat and prevent the dilation of the blood vessels surrounding the brain and leading to the extremities. The effect of this "beta blockade" in a variety of disorders is shown in the box above.

How they affect you

Beta blockers are taken to treat angina. They reduce the frequency and severity of attacks. As part of the treatment for hypertension, beta blockers help to lower blood pressure and thus reduce the risks that are associated with this condition. Beta blockers help to prevent severe attacks of arrhythmia, in which the heart beat is wild and uncontrolled.

Because beta blockers affect many parts of the body, they often produce minor side effects. By reducing heart rate and air flow to the lungs, they may reduce capacity for strenuous exercise, although this is unlikely to be noticed by somebody whose physical activity was previously limited by heart problems. Many people experience cold hands and feet while taking these drugs as a result of the reduction in the blood supply to the limbs. Reduced circulation can also lead to temporary erectile dysfunction during treatment.

Risks and special precautions

The main risk of beta blockers is that of provoking breathing difficulties as a result of their blocking effect on beta receptors in the lungs. Cardioselective beta blockers, which act principally on the heart, are thought less likely than non-cardioselective ones to cause such problems. But all beta blockers are prescribed with caution for people who have asthma, bronchitis, or other forms of respiratory disease.

Beta blockers are not commonly prescribed to people who have poor circulation in the limbs because they reduce blood flow and may aggravate such conditions. They are of definite benefit in heart failure, but treatment is usually initiated by specialists. People with diabetes who need to take beta blockers should be aware that they may notice a change in the warning signs of low blood sugar; in particular, they may find that symptoms such as palpitations and tremor are suppressed.

Beta blockers should not be stopped suddenly after prolonged use; this may provoke a sudden and severe recurrence of symptoms of the original disorder, even a heart attack. The blood pressure may also rise markedly. When treatment with beta blockers needs to be stopped, it should be withdrawn gradually under medical supervision.

COMMON DRUGS

Cardioselective	Non-cardioselective
Acebutolol	Carvedilol
Atenolol ✳	Labetalol
Betaxolol	Nadolol
Bisoprolol ✳	Oxprenolol
Celiprolol	Pindolol
Esmolol	Propranolol ✳
Metoprolol ✳	Sotalol ✳
Nebivolol	Timolol ✳

✳ See Part 3

VASODILATORS

Vasodilators are drugs that widen blood vessels. Their most obvious use is to reverse narrowing of blood vessels when this leads to reduced blood flow and a lower oxygen supply to parts of the body. This problem occurs in angina, when narrowing of the coronary arteries reduces blood supply to the heart muscle. Vasodilators are often used to treat high blood pressure (hypertension).

Why they are used

Vasodilators improve the blood flow and thus the oxygen supply to areas of the body where they are most needed. In angina, dilation of the blood vessels throughout the body reduces the force with which the heart needs to pump and so eases its workload (see also Anti-angina drugs, p.59). This may also be helpful in treating congestive heart failure when other treatments are not effective.

Because blood pressure is dependent partly on the diameter of blood vessels, vasodilators are often helpful in treating hypertension (see p.60).

In peripheral vascular disease, narrowed blood vessels in the legs cannot supply sufficient blood to the extremities, often leading to pain in the legs during exercise. As the narrowing is due to atherosclerosis, vasodilators have little effect.

How they work

Vasodilators widen the blood vessels by relaxing the muscles surrounding them, either by affecting the action of the muscles directly (nitrates, hydralazine, and calcium channel blockers), or by interfering with the nerve signals that govern contraction of the blood vessels (alpha blockers). ACE (angiotensin-converting enzyme) inhibitors block the activity of an enzyme in the blood that is responsible for producing angiotensin II, a powerful vasoconstrictor. Angiotensin II blockers prevent angiotensin II from constricting

the blood vessels by blocking its receptors within the vessels. Sacubitril blocks another enzyme that degrades natriuretic peptides, thus prolonging the vasodilating effects of these peptides. Sacubitril is often given combined with the angiotensin II blocker valsartan.

How they affect you

Vasodilators can have many minor side effects related to their action on the circulation. Flushing and headaches are common at the start of treatment. Dizziness and fainting may also occur as a result of lowered blood pressure, which is often worse on standing. Dilation

of the blood vessels can also cause fluid build-up, leading to swelling, particularly of the ankles.

Risks and special precautions

The major risk is of blood pressure falling too low; vasodilators are used with caution in people with unstable blood pressure. It is also advisable to sit or lie down after taking the first dose of a vasodilator.

ACTION OF VASODILATORS

The diameter of blood vessels is governed by the contraction of the surrounding muscle. The muscle contracts in response to signals from the sympathetic nervous system (p.35). Vasodilators encourage the muscles to relax, thus increasing the size of blood vessels.

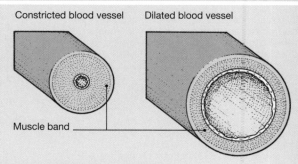

Constricted blood vessel   Dilated blood vessel

Muscle band

Where they act
Each type of vasodilator acts on a different part of the mechanism controlling blood vessel size in order to prevent contraction of the surrounding layer of muscles.

Nerves – Alpha blockers interfere with nerve signals to the muscles.

Muscle layer – Nitrates and calcium channel blockers act directly on the muscle to inhibit contraction.

Blood – ACE inhibitors block enzyme activity in the blood; angiotensin II blockers block receptors in the vessels (see box below).

COMMON DRUGS

ACE inhibitors
Captopril *
Cilazapril
Enalapril *
Fosinopril
Lisinopril *
Perindopril *
Quinapril
Ramipril *
Trandolapril

Angiotensin II blockers
Candesartan *
Irbesartan *
Losartan *
Telmisartan

Alpha blockers
Doxazosin *
Indoramin
Prazosin
Terazosin

Potassium channel activators
Nicorandil *

Nitrates
Glyceryl trinitrate *
Isosorbide dinitrate/ mononitrate *

Calcium channel blockers
Amlodipine *
Diltiazem *
Felodipine *
Lacidipine
Lercanidipine
Nicardipine
Nifedipine *
Verapamil *

Other drugs
Hydralazine
Minoxidil *
Sacubitril/ valsartan *

Peripheral vasodilators
Cilostazol
Naftidrofuryl *
Pentoxifylline

* See Part 3

ACE INHIBITORS AND ANGIOTENSIN II BLOCKERS

ACE inhibitors block the action of ACE (an enzyme in the blood that is responsible for converting the chemical angiotensin I into angiotensin II). Angiotensin II encourages the blood vessels to constrict; its absence permits them to dilate. Angiotensin II blockers do not prevent angiotensin II from being produced, but they block its receptors, preventing it from acting on the blood vessels to constrict them.

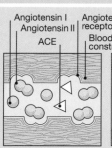

Before drugs
Angiotensin I is converted by the enzyme into angiotensin II. The blood vessel constricts.

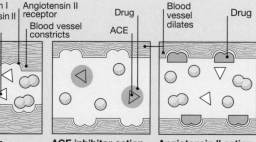

ACE inhibitor action
ACE inhibitors block enzyme activity, thereby preventing the formation of angiotensin II. The blood vessel dilates.

Angiotensin II action
Angiotensin II blockers block the receptors, preventing angiotensin II from acting on the blood vessel. The blood vessel dilates.

DIURETICS

Diuretic drugs help to turn excess body water into urine. As the urine is expelled, two disorders are relieved: excess water in tissues (oedema) is lessened, and the heart action improves because it has to pump a smaller volume of blood. There are several classes of diuretics, each of which has different uses, modes of action, and effects (see Types of diuretic, below). But all diuretics act on the kidneys, the organs that govern the water content of the body.

Why they are used

Diuretics are most commonly used in the treatment of high blood pressure (hypertension). By removing a larger amount of water than usual from the bloodstream, the kidneys reduce the total volume of blood circulating. This drop in volume causes a reduction of the pressure within the blood vessels (see Antihypertensive drugs, p.60).

Diuretics are also widely used to treat heart failure in which the heart's pumping mechanism has become weak. In the treatment of this disorder, they remove fluid that has accumulated in the tissues and lungs. The resulting drop in blood volume reduces the work of the heart.

Other conditions for which diuretics are often prescribed include nephrotic syndrome (a kidney disorder that causes oedema), cirrhosis of the liver (in which fluid may accumulate in the abdominal cavity), and premenstrual syndrome (when hormonal activity can lead to fluid retention and bloating).

Less commonly, diuretics are used to treat glaucoma (see p.128) and Ménière's disease (see p.46).

How they work

The kidneys' normal filtration process takes water, salts (mainly potassium and sodium), and waste products out of the bloodstream. Most of the salts and water are returned to the bloodstream, but some are expelled from the body together with the waste products in the urine. Diuretics interfere with this filtration process by reducing the amounts of sodium and water taken back into the

ACTION OF DIURETICS

As blood passes through the kidney, water, sodium and potassium salts, and waste products are filtered out of the bloodstream. Most of the water and filtered salts are then reabsorbed by the bloodstream from the tubule; the remainder is excreted as urine.

By blocking the movement of sodium back into the bloodstream, diuretics prevent the reabsorption of water, so that more is expelled from the body as urine. Different diuretic drugs act on different parts of the tubule (see right).

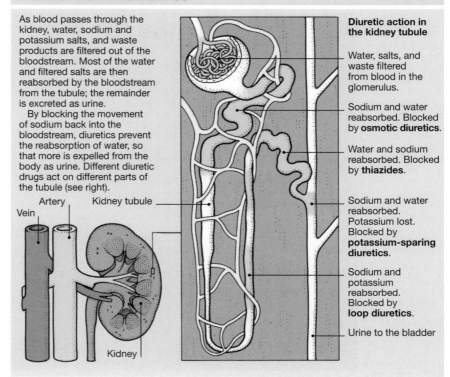

Artery Kidney tubule
Vein
Kidney

Diuretic action in the kidney tubule

Water, salts, and waste filtered from blood in the glomerulus.

Sodium and water reabsorbed. Blocked by **osmotic diuretics**.

Water and sodium reabsorbed. Blocked by **thiazides**.

Sodium and water reabsorbed. Potassium lost. Blocked by **potassium-sparing diuretics**.

Sodium and potassium reabsorbed. Blocked by **loop diuretics**.

Urine to the bladder

bloodstream, thus increasing the volume of urine produced. Modifying the filtration process in this way means that the water content of the blood is reduced; less water in the blood causes excess water present in the tissues to be drawn out and eliminated in urine.

How they affect you

All diuretics increase the frequency with which you need to pass urine. This is most noticeable at the start of treatment. People who have suffered from oedema may notice that swelling – particularly of the ankles – is reduced, and those with heart failure may find that breathlessness is relieved.

Risks and special precautions

Diuretics can cause blood chemical imbalances, of which a fall in potassium levels (hypokalaemia) is the most common. Hypokalaemia can cause confusion and weakness, and trigger abnormal heart rhythms (especially in people taking digitalis drugs). Potassium supplements or a potassium-sparing diuretic usually corrects the imbalance. A diet that is rich in potassium (containing plenty of fresh fruits and vegetables) may be helpful.

Some diuretics may raise blood levels of uric acid, increasing the risk of gout. They may also raise blood sugar levels, causing problems for people with diabetes.

TYPES OF DIURETIC

Thiazides The diuretics most commonly prescribed, thiazides may lead to potassium deficiency and they are, therefore, sometimes given together with a potassium supplement or in conjunction with a potassium-sparing diuretic (see right).

Loop diuretics These fast-acting, powerful drugs increase the output of urine for a few hours, and are therefore sometimes used in emergencies. They may cause excessive loss of potassium, which may need to be countered as for thiazides. Large doses given into a vein may disturb hearing.

Potassium-sparing diuretics These mild diuretics are usually used in conjunction with a thiazide or a loop diuretic to prevent excessive potassium loss.

Osmotic diuretics Prescribed only rarely, these drugs are used to maintain the flow of urine through the kidneys after surgery or injury, and to reduce pressure rapidly within fluid-filled cavities.

Acetazolamide This mild diuretic drug is used principally in the treatment of acute glaucoma (see p.128).

COMMON DRUGS

Loop diuretics
Bumetanide *
Furosemide/
  frusemide *
Torasemide

Potassium-sparing diuretics
Amiloride *
Eplerenone
Spironolactone *
Triamterene *

Thiazides
Bendroflumethiazide *
Chlortalidone
Cyclopenthiazide
Hydrochlorothiazide *
Hydroflumethiazide
Indapamide *
Metolazone
Xipamide

* See Part 3

ANTI-ARRHYTHMICS

The heart contains two upper and two lower chambers, which are known as the atria and ventricles (see p.53). The pumping actions of these two sets of chambers are normally coordinated by electrical impulses that originate in the pacemaker and then travel along conducting pathways so that the heart beats with a regular rhythm. If this coordination breaks down, the heart will beat abnormally, either irregularly or faster or slower than usual. The general term for abnormal heart rhythm is arrhythmia.

Arrhythmias may occur as a result of a birth defect, coronary heart disease, or other less common heart disorders. A variety of more general conditions, including overactivity of the thyroid gland, and certain drugs – such as caffeine and anticholinergic drugs – can also disturb heart rhythm.

SITES OF DRUG ACTION

Anti-arrhythmic drugs either slow the flow of electrical impulses to the heart muscle or inhibit the muscle's ability to contract. Beta blockers reduce the ability of the pacemaker to pass electrical signals to the atria. Digitalis drugs reduce the passage of signals from the atrioventricular node. Calcium channel blockers interfere with the ability of the heart muscle to contract by impeding the flow of calcium into muscle cells. Other drugs such as quinidine and disopyramide reduce the sensitivity of muscle cells to electrical impulses.

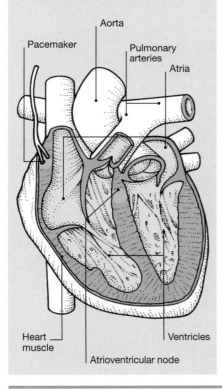

Aorta

Pacemaker

Pulmonary arteries

Atria

Heart muscle

Ventricles

Atrioventricular node

A broad selection of drugs is used to regulate heart rhythm, including beta blockers, digitalis drugs, and calcium channel blockers. Other drugs used are disopyramide, lidocaine, and procainamide.

Why they are used

Minor disturbances of heart rhythm are common and do not usually require drug treatment. However, if the pumping action of the heart is seriously affected, the circulation of blood throughout the body may become inefficient, and drug treatment may be necessary.

Drugs may be taken to treat individual attacks of arrhythmia, or they may be taken on a regular basis to prevent or control abnormal heart rhythms. The particular drug prescribed depends on the type of arrhythmia to be treated, but because people differ in their response, it may be necessary to try several in order to find the most effective one. When the arrhythmia is sudden and severe, it may be necessary to inject a drug immediately to restore normal heart function.

How they work

The heart's pumping action is governed by electrical impulses under the control of the sympathetic nervous system (see Autonomic nervous system, p.35). These signals pass through the heart muscle, causing the two pairs of chambers – the atria and ventricles – to contract in turn (see Sites of drug action, left).

All anti-arrhythmic drugs alter the conduction of electrical signals in the heart. However, each drug or drug group has a different effect on the sequence of events controlling the pumping action. Some block the transmission of signals to the heart (beta blockers); some affect the way in which signals are conducted within the heart (digitalis drugs); others affect the response of the heart muscle to the signals received (calcium channel blockers, disopyramide, and procainamide).

How they affect you

These drugs usually prevent symptoms of arrhythmia and may restore a regular heart rhythm. Although they do not prevent all arrhythmias, they usually reduce the frequency and severity of any symptoms.

Unfortunately, as well as suppressing arrhythmias, many of these drugs tend to depress normal heart function, and may produce dizziness on standing up, or increased breathlessness on exertion. Mild nausea and visual disturbances are also fairly frequent. Verapamil can cause constipation, especially when it is prescribed in high doses. Disopyramide may interfere with the parasympathetic nervous system (see p.35), resulting in a number of anticholinergic effects.

TYPES OF ARRHYTHMIA

Atrial fibrillation In this common type of arrhythmia, the atria contract irregularly at such a high rate that the ventricles cannot keep pace. It is treated with digoxin, verapamil, amiodarone, or a beta blocker.

Ventricular tachycardia This condition arises from abnormal electrical activity in the ventricles that causes the ventricles to contract rapidly. Treatment with disopyramide, procainamide, or amiodarone may be effective, although implanted defibrillators are replacing drug treatment for this condition.

Supraventricular tachycardia This condition occurs when extra electrical impulses arise in the pacemaker or atria. These extra impulses stimulate the ventricles to contract rapidly. Attacks may disappear on their own without treatment, but drugs such as adenosine, digoxin, verapamil, or a beta blocker may be given.

Heart block When impulses are not conducted from the atria to the ventricles, the ventricles start to beat at a slower rate. Some cases of heart block do not require treatment. For more severe heart block accompanied by dizziness and fainting, it is usually necessary to fit the patient with an artificial pacemaker.

Risks and special precautions

These drugs may further disrupt heart rhythm under certain circumstances and therefore they are used only when the likely benefit outweighs the risks.

Amiodarone may accumulate in the tissues over time, and may lead to light-sensitive rashes, changes in thyroid function, and lung problems.

COMMON DRUGS

Beta blockers
(see also p.55)
Sotalol *

Calcium channel blockers
Felodipine *
Verapamil *

Digitalis drugs
(see also p.54)
Digitoxin
Digoxin *

Other drugs
Adenosine
Amiodarone *
Disopyramide
Flecainide
Lidocaine
Mexiletine
Moracizine
Procainamide
Propafenone

* See Part 3

ANTI-ANGINA DRUGS

Angina is chest pain produced when insufficient oxygen reaches the heart muscle. This is usually caused by a narrowing of the blood vessels (coronary arteries) that carry blood and oxygen to the heart muscle. In the most common type of angina (classic angina), pain usually occurs during physical exertion or emotional stress. In variant angina, pain may also occur at rest. In classic angina, the narrowing of the coronary arteries results from deposits of fat – called atheroma – on the walls of the arteries. In the variant type, however, angina is caused by contraction (spasm) of the muscle fibres in the artery walls.

Atheroma deposits build up more rapidly in the arteries of smokers and people who eat a high-fat diet. This is why, as a basic component of angina treatment, doctors recommend that smoking should be given up and the diet changed. Overweight people are also advised to lose weight in order to reduce the demands placed on the heart. While such changes in lifestyle often produce an improvement in symptoms, drug treatment to relieve angina is also frequently necessary.

The drugs used to treat angina include beta blockers, nitrates, calcium channel blockers, and potassium channel openers.

Why they are used

Frequent episodes of angina can be disabling and, if left untreated, can lead to an increased risk of a heart attack. Drugs can be used both to relieve angina attacks and to reduce their frequency. People who experience only occasional episodes are usually prescribed a rapid-acting drug to take at the first signs of an attack, or before an activity that is known to bring on an attack. A rapid-acting nitrate – glyceryl trinitrate – is usually prescribed for this purpose.

If attacks become more frequent or more severe, regular preventative treatment may be advised. Beta blockers, long-acting nitrates, and calcium channel blockers are used as regular medication to prevent attacks. The introduction of adhesive patches to administer nitrates through the patient's skin has extended the duration of action of glyceryl trinitrate, making treatment easier.

Drugs can often control angina for many years, but they cannot cure the disorder. When severe angina cannot be controlled by drugs, then surgery to increase the blood flow to the heart may be recommended.

How they work

Nitrates and calcium channel blockers dilate blood vessels by relaxing the muscle layer in the blood vessel walls (see also Vasodilators, p.56). Blood is more easily pumped through the dilated vessels, reducing the strain on the heart.

Beta blockers reduce heart muscle stimulation during exercise or stress by interrupting signal transmission in the heart. Decreased heart muscle stimulation means less oxygen is required, reducing the risk of angina attacks. For further information on beta blockers, see p.55.

How they affect you

Treatment with one or more of these medicines usually effectively controls angina. Drugs to prevent attacks allow people with angina to undertake more strenuous activities without provoking pain, and if an attack does occur, nitrates usually provide effective relief.

ACTION OF ANTI-ANGINA DRUGS

Angina pain occurs when the heart muscle runs short of oxygen as it pumps blood round the circulatory system. Nitrates, calcium channel blockers, and potassium channel openers reduce the heart's work by dilating blood vessels. Beta blockers impede the stimulation of heart muscle, reducing its oxygen requirement, thus relieving angina.

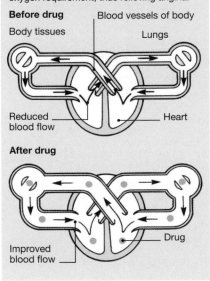

Before drug
Body tissues
Blood vessels of body
Lungs
Reduced blood flow
Heart

After drug
Improved blood flow
Drug

These drugs do not usually cause serious adverse effects, but they can produce a variety of minor symptoms. By dilating blood vessels throughout the body, the nitrates and calcium channel blockers can cause dizziness (especially when standing) and may cause fainting. Other possible side effects are headaches at the start of treatment, flushing of the skin (especially of the face), and ankle swelling. Beta blockers often cause cold hands and feet, and sometimes they may produce tiredness and a feeling of heaviness in the legs.

COMMON DRUGS

Beta blockers (see p.55)	Calcium channel blockers
Nitrates	Amlodipine ✳
Glyceryl trinitrate ✳	Diltiazem ✳
Isosorbide dinitrate/	Felodipine ✳
mononitrate ✳	Nicardipine
	Nifedipine ✳
Potassium channel opener	Verapamil ✳
Nicorandil ✳	**Heparin/low molecular weight heparins** ✳
Other drugs	Dalteparin
Aspirin ✳	Enoxaparin
Ezetimibe ✳	
Ivabradine	
Ranolazine	✳ See Part 3
Simvastatin ✳	

CALCIUM CHANNEL BLOCKERS

The passage of calcium through special channels into muscle cells is a vital part of the mechanism of muscle contraction (see right). Calcium channel blockers prevent movement of calcium in the muscles of the blood vessels and so encourage them to dilate (see far right). The action helps to reduce blood pressure and relieves the strain on the heart muscle in angina by making it easier for the heart to pump blood throughout the body (see Action of anti-angina drugs, above right). Verapamil also slows the passage of nerve signals through the heart muscle. This can be helpful for correcting certain arrhythmias.

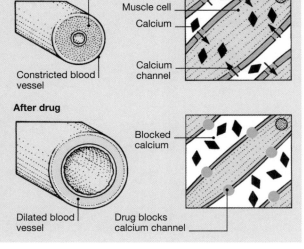

Before drug
Muscle
Muscle cell
Calcium
Constricted blood vessel
Calcium channel

After drug
Blocked calcium
Dilated blood vessel
Drug blocks calcium channel

ANTIHYPERTENSIVE DRUGS

Blood pressure is the force exerted by the blood against the walls of the arteries. Two measurements are taken: one indicates force while the heart's ventricles are contracting (systolic pressure); this reading is a higher figure than the other one, which measures the blood pressure during ventricle relaxation (diastolic pressure). Blood pressure varies among individuals and normally increases with age. If a person's blood pressure is higher than normal on at least three separate occasions, a doctor may diagnose the condition as hypertension.

Blood pressure may be elevated as a result of an underlying disorder, which the doctor will try to identify. Usually, however, it is not possible to determine a cause. This condition is referred to as essential hypertension.

Although hypertension does not usually cause any symptoms, severely raised blood pressure may produce headaches, palpitations, and general feelings of ill-health. It is important to reduce high blood pressure because it can have serious consequences, including stroke, heart attack, heart failure, and kidney damage. Certain groups are particularly at risk from high blood pressure. These risk groups include people with diabetes, smokers, people with pre-existing heart damage, and those whose blood contains a high level of fat. High blood pressure is more common among people of Black African or Caribbean descent, and in countries where the diet is high in salt.

A small reduction in blood pressure may be brought about by lifestyle changes, including regular exercise, reducing weight, and lowering salt intake. But for more severely raised blood pressure, one or more antihypertensive drugs may be prescribed. Several classes of drugs have antihypertensive properties, including the centrally acting antihypertensives, diuretics (p.57), beta blockers (p.55), calcium channel blockers (p.59), ACE (angiotensin-converting enzyme) inhibitors (p.56), angiotensin II blockers, and alpha blockers. See also Vasodilators, p.56.

Why they are used

Antihypertensive drugs are prescribed when lifestyle changes have not brought about an adequate reduction in blood pressure, and your doctor sees a risk of serious consequences if left untreated. These drugs do not cure hypertension and have to be taken indefinitely.

How they work

Blood pressure depends not only on the force with which the heart pumps blood, but also on the diameter of blood vessels and volume of blood in circulation: blood pressure is increased either if the vessels are narrow or if the volume of blood is high. Antihypertensives lower blood pressure either by dilating the blood vessels or by reducing blood volume. Antihypertensive drugs work in different ways and some have more than one action (see Action of antihypertensive drugs, left).

Choice of drug

Drug treatment depends on the severity of the hypertension. At the beginning of treatment for mild or moderately high blood pressure, a single drug is used. A thiazide diuretic is often chosen for initial treatment, but it is increasingly common to use a calcium channel blocker or an ACE inhibitor. For those over 50 or of Black African or Caribbean descent, a calcium channel blocker is usually the first-line treatment. If a single drug does not reduce the blood pressure sufficiently, a combination of these drugs may be used. Some people with more severe hypertension require an additional drug, in which case an alpha blocker, beta blocker, or aldosterone blocking drug may be added.

Severe hypertension is usually controlled with a combination of drugs, which may need to be given in high doses. Your doctor may need to try a number of drugs before finding a combination that controls blood pressure without unacceptable side effects.

How they affect you

Treatment with antihypertensive drugs relieves symptoms such as headache and palpitations. However, since most people with hypertension have few, if any, symptoms, side effects may be more noticeable than any immediate beneficial effect. Some antihypertensive drugs may cause dizziness and fainting at the start of treatment because they can sometimes cause an excessive fall in blood pressure. It may take a while for your doctor to determine a dosage that avoids such effects. For detailed information on the adverse effects of drugs used to treat hypertension, consult the individual drug profiles in Part 3.

Risks and special precautions

Because your doctor needs to know exactly how treatment with a particular drug affects your hypertension – the benefits as well as the side effects – it is important for you to keep using the antihypertensive medication as prescribed, even though you may feel the problem is under control. Sudden withdrawal of some of these drugs may cause a potentially dangerous rebound increase in blood pressure. To stop treatment, the dose needs to be reduced gradually under medical supervision.

ACTION OF ANTI-HYPERTENSIVE DRUGS

Each type of antihypertensive drug acts on a different part of the body to lower blood pressure.

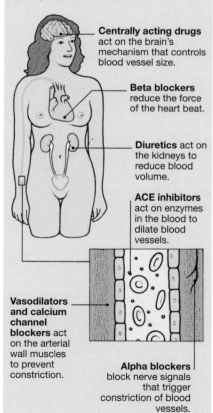

Centrally acting drugs act on the brain's mechanism that controls blood vessel size.

Beta blockers reduce the force of the heart beat.

Diuretics act on the kidneys to reduce blood volume.

ACE inhibitors act on enzymes in the blood to dilate blood vessels.

Vasodilators and calcium channel blockers act on the arterial wall muscles to prevent constriction.

Alpha blockers block nerve signals that trigger constriction of blood vessels.

COMMON DRUGS

ACE inhibitors (see p.56)

Angiotensin II blockers
Candesartan *
Irbesartan *
Losartan *
Olmesartan

Beta blockers (see p.55)

Calcium channel blockers (see p.59)
Amlodipine *
Diltiazem *
Felodipine *
Isradipine
Lacidipine
Lercanidipine
Nicardipine

Nifedipine *
Verapamil *

Centrally acting antihypertensives
Clonidine
Methyldopa
Moxonidine *

Diuretics (see p.57)

Alpha blockers
Doxazosin *
Indoramin
Prazosin
Terazosin

Vasodilators (see p.56)

Aldosterone blockers
Eplerenone
Spironolactone *

* See Part 3

LIPID-LOWERING DRUGS

The blood contains several types of fats, or lipids. They are necessary for normal body function but can be damaging in excess, particularly saturated fats such as cholesterol. The main risk is atherosclerosis, in which fatty deposits (atheroma) build up in the arteries, restricting and disrupting blood flow. This can increase the likelihood of abnormal blood clots forming, leading to potentially fatal disorders such as stroke and heart attack.

For most people, cutting down the amount of fat in the diet is sufficient to reduce the risk of atherosclerosis; but for those with an inherited tendency to high blood levels of fat (hyperlipidaemia), lipid-lowering drugs may also be recommended.

Why they are used

Lipid-lowering drugs are generally used only when dietary measures have failed to control hyperlipidaemia. They may be prescribed at an earlier stage to people at increased risk of atherosclerosis – such as people with diabetes and those who already have circulatory disorders. The drugs may help the body to remove existing atheroma in the blood vessels and prevent accumulation of new deposits. Low-dose simvastatin is available over the counter to help lower cholesterol levels in certain people.

For maximum benefit, lipid-lowering drugs are used in conjunction with a low-fat diet and a reduction in other risk factors such as obesity and smoking. The choice of drug depends on the type of lipid causing problems, so a full medical history, examination, and laboratory analysis of blood samples are needed before drug treatment is prescribed.

How they work

Cholesterol and triglycerides are two of the major fats in the blood. One or both may be raised, influencing the choice of drug. Bile salts contain a large amount of cholesterol and are normally released into the bowel to aid digestion before being reabsorbed into the blood. Drugs that bind to bile salts reduce cholesterol levels by blocking their reabsorption, allowing them to be lost from the body.

Other drugs act on the liver. Fibrates can reduce the level of both cholesterol and triglycerides in the blood. Statins block cholesterol synthesis in the liver. This causes increased uptake of LDL cholesterol from the blood, thereby lowering blood cholesterol levels. The uptake of LDL cholesterol is also stimulated by the newer anti-PCSK9 drugs, such as evolocumab and alirocumab.

Lipid-lowering drugs do not correct the underlying cause of raised levels of fat in the blood, so it is usually necessary to continue with diet and drug treatment indefinitely. Stopping treatment usually leads to a return of high blood lipid levels.

ACTION OF LIPID-LOWERING DRUGS

Lipid-lowering drugs reduce the levels of fats in the blood by interfering with the absorption of bile salts in the bowel, or by altering the way in which the liver converts fatty acids in the blood into different types of lipids.

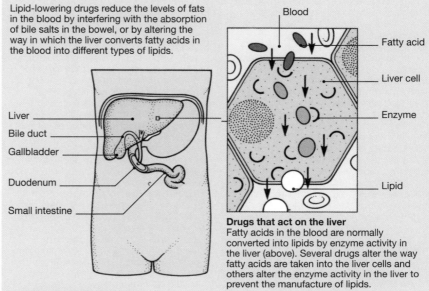

Liver
Bile duct
Gallbladder
Duodenum
Small intestine

Blood
Fatty acid
Liver cell
Enzyme
Lipid

Drugs that act on the liver
Fatty acids in the blood are normally converted into lipids by enzyme activity in the liver (above). Several drugs alter the way fatty acids are taken into the liver cells and others alter the enzyme activity in the liver to prevent the manufacture of lipids.

Drugs that bind to bile salts
Bile is produced by the liver and released into the small intestine via the bile duct to aid digestion. Salts in the bile carry large amounts of cholesterol and are normally reabsorbed from the intestine into the bloodstream during digestion (right). Some drugs bind to bile salts in the intestine and prevent their reabsorption (far right). This action reduces the levels of bile salts in the blood, and triggers the liver to convert more cholesterol into bile salts, thus reducing blood cholesterol levels.

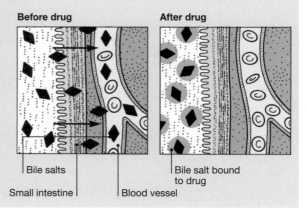

Before drug

After drug

Bile salts
Small intestine

Bile salt bound to drug
Blood vessel

How they affect you

Because hyperlipidaemia and athero-sclerosis are usually without symptoms, you are unlikely to notice any short-term benefits from these drugs. Rather, the aim of treatment is to reduce long-term complications. There may be minor side effects from some of these drugs.

The statin drugs appear to be well tolerated and are widely used to lower cholesterol levels when diet alone is not effective.

Risks and special precautions

Drugs that bind to bile salts can limit absorption of some fat-soluble vitamins, so vitamin supplements may be needed. The fibrates can increase susceptibility to gallstones and occasionally upset the balance of fats in the blood. Statins are used with caution in people with reduced kidney or liver function, and monitoring

of blood samples is often advised. You should consult your doctor or pharmacist before taking simvastatin.

COMMON DRUGS

Statins
Atorvastatin ✳
Pravastatin ✳
Rosuvastatin ✳
Simvastatin ✳

Drugs that bind to or reduce bile salts
Colestipol
Colestyramine ✳
Ezetimibe ✳
Ispaghula

Fibrates
Bezafibrate ✳
Fenofibrate
Gemfibrozil

Other drugs acting on the liver
Alirocumab
Evolocumab ✳
Omega-3 acid ethyl esters

✳ See Part 3

DRUGS THAT AFFECT BLOOD CLOTTING

When bleeding occurs from injury or surgery, the body normally acts swiftly to stem the flow by sealing the breaks in the blood vessels. This occurs in two stages – first when cells called platelets accumulate as a plug at the opening in the blood vessel wall, and then when these platelets produce chemicals that activate clotting factors in the blood to form a protein called fibrin. Vitamin K plays an important role in this process (see The clotting mechanism, below). An enzyme in the blood called plasmin ensures that clots are broken down when the injury has been repaired.

Some disorders interfere with this process, either preventing clot formation or creating clots uncontrollably. If the blood does not clot, there is a danger of excessive blood loss. Inappropriate development of clots may block the supply of blood to a vital organ.

Drugs used to promote blood clotting

Fibrin formation depends on the presence in the blood of several clotting-factor proteins. When Factor VIII is absent or at low levels, the condition is known as haemophilia A. Factor IX deficiency causes another bleeding condition, haemophilia B (previously known as Christmas disease). Both conditions are inherited and almost always affect only males. Lack of these clotting factors can lead to uncontrolled bleeding or excessive bruising following even minor injuries.

Regular drug treatment for haemophilia is not normally required. However, if severe bleeding or bruising occurs, a concentrated form of the missing factor, extracted from normal blood, may be injected in order to promote clotting and thereby halt bleeding. Injections may need to be repeated for several days after injury.

It is sometimes useful to promote blood clotting in people who do not have haemophilia when bleeding is difficult to stop (for example, after surgery). In such cases, blood clots are sometimes stabilized by reducing the action of plasmin with an antifibrinolytic (or haemostatic) drug like tranexamic acid; this is also occasionally given to people with haemophilia before minor surgery such as tooth extraction.

A tendency to bleed may also occur as a consequence of vitamin K deficiency (see the box below).

Drugs used to prevent abnormal blood clotting

Blood clots normally form only as a response to injury. In some people, however, there is a tendency for clots to form in the blood vessels without apparent cause. Disturbed blood flow occurring as a result of the presence of fatty deposits – atheroma – inside the blood vessels increases the risk of the formation of this type of abnormal clot (or thrombus). In addition, a portion of a blood clot (known as an embolus) formed in response to injury or surgery may sometimes break off and be removed in the bloodstream. The likelihood of this happening is increased by long periods of little or no activity. When an abnormal clot forms, there is a risk that it may become lodged in a blood vessel, thereby blocking the blood supply to a vital organ such as the brain or heart.

THE CLOTTING MECHANISM

When a blood vessel wall is damaged, platelets accumulate at the site of damage and form a plug (1). Platelets clumped together release chemicals that activate blood clotting factors (2). These factors together with vitamin K act on a substance called fibrinogen and convert it to fibrin (3). Strands of fibrin become enmeshed in the platelet plug to form a blood clot (4).

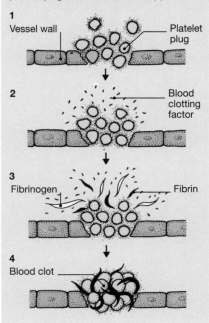

1
Vessel wall — Platelet plug

2
Blood clotting factor

3
Fibrinogen — Fibrin

4
Blood clot

VITAMIN K

Vitamin K is required for the production of several blood clotting factors. It is absorbed from the intestine in fats, but some diseases of the small intestine or pancreas cause fat to be poorly absorbed. As a result, the level of vitamin K in the circulation is low, causing impaired blood clotting. A similar problem sometimes occurs in newborn babies due to an absence of the vitamin. Injections of phytomenadione, a vitamin K preparation, are used to restore normal levels.

ACTION OF ANTIPLATELET DRUGS

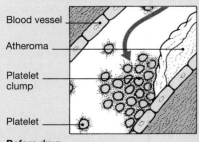

Blood vessel
Atheroma
Platelet clump
Platelet

Before drug
Where the blood flow is disrupted by a patch of atheroma in the blood vessels, platelets tend to clump together.

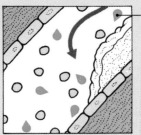

Antiplatelet drug

After drug
Antiplatelet drugs reduce the ability of platelets to stick together and so prevent clot formation.

Three main types of drug are used to prevent and disperse clots: antiplatelet drugs, anticoagulants, and thrombolytics.

Antiplatelet drugs

Taken regularly by people with a tendency to form clots in the fast-flowing blood of the heart and arteries, these drugs are also given to prevent clots from forming after heart surgery. They reduce the tendency of platelets to stick together when blood flow is disrupted (see Action of antiplatelet drugs, above).

The most widely used antiplatelet drug is aspirin (see also Analgesics, p.36). This drug has an antiplatelet action even when given in much lower doses than would be necessary to reduce pain. In these low doses adverse effects that may occur when aspirin is given in pain-relieving doses are unlikely. Other antiplatelet drugs are clopidogrel and dipyridamole.

Anticoagulants

Anticoagulants help to maintain normal blood flow in people at risk from clot formation. They can either prevent the formation of blood clots in the veins or stabilize an existing clot so that it does not break away and become a circulation-stopping embolism. All anticoagulants reduce the activity of certain blood clotting factors, but each drug's mode of action differs (see Action of anticoagulant drugs, right). These medicines do not dissolve clots that have already formed, however: these are treated with thrombolytic drugs (below).

Anticoagulants fall into two groups: those that are given by intravenous injection and act immediately, and those that are given by mouth and take effect after a few days.

Injected anticoagulants
Heparin is the most widely used drug of this type and it is used mainly in hospital during or after surgery. In addition, it is also given during kidney dialysis to prevent clots from forming in the dialysis equipment. Because heparin cannot be taken by mouth, it is less suitable for long-term treatment in the home.

A number of synthetic injected anticoagulants have recently been developed. Some act for a longer time than heparin, and others are alternatives for people who react adversely to heparin.

Oral anticoagulants
Warfarin is the most widely used of the oral anticoagulants. These drugs are mainly prescribed to prevent the formation of clots in veins and in the chambers of the heart (they are less likely to prevent clot formation in arteries). Oral anticoagulants may be given following injury or surgery (in particular, heart valve replacement) when there is a high risk of embolism. They are also given long-term as preventative treatment to people at risk of strokes. A common problem with these drugs is that overdosage may lead to bleeding from the nose or gums, or in the urinary tract. For this reason, the dosage needs to be

ACTION OF ANTICOAGULANT DRUGS

Anticoagulant drugs block the action of certain blood clotting factors that convert fibrinogen into fibrin, the protein that binds platelets into blood clots.

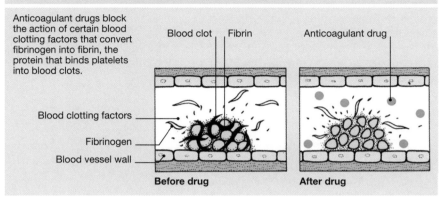

Before drug — After drug

carefully calculated; regular blood tests are performed to ensure that the clotting mechanism is correctly adjusted, although this is not necessary with newer oral anticoagulants such as dabigatran and rivaroxaban.

The action of oral anticoagulants may be affected by many other drugs and it may therefore be necessary to alter the dosage of anticoagulant when other drugs also need to be given. In particular, no anticoagulant should be taken together with aspirin except on the direction of a doctor.

Thrombolytics
Also known as fibrinolytics, these drugs are used to dissolve clots that have already formed. They are usually given in hospital intravenously to clear a blocked blood vessel – for example, in coronary thrombosis. The sooner they are given after the start of symptoms, the more likely they are to reduce the size and severity of a

heart attack. Thrombolytic drugs may be given either intravenously or directly into the blocked blood vessel. The main thrombolytics are streptokinase and alteplase, which act by increasing the blood level of plasmin, the enzyme that breaks down fibrin (see Action of thrombolytic drugs, below). When given promptly, alteplase appears to be tolerated better than streptokinase.

The most common problems with these drugs are increased susceptibility to bleeding and bruising, and allergic reactions to streptokinase, such as rashes or breathing difficulty. Once streptokinase has been given, patients are given a card indicating this, because further treatment with the same drug may be less effective, and an alternative (such as alteplase) used instead.

COMMON DRUGS

Blood clotting factors	Fondaparinux
Factor VIIa	Heparin ✳
Factor VIII	Lepirudin
Factor IX	
Fresh frozen plasma	**Heparin/low molecular weight heparins** ✳
Antifibrinolytic drugs	Dalteparin
Tranexamic acid	Enoxaparin
	Tinzaparin
Vitamin K	**Oral anti-coagulants**
Phytomenadione	Acenocoumarol/
	nicoumalone
Antiplatelet drugs	Apixaban
Abciximab	Dabigatran ✳
Aspirin ✳	Rivaroxaban ✳
Clopidogrel ✳	Warfarin ✳
Dipyridamole ✳	
Eptifibatide	**Thrombolytic drugs**
Prasugrel	Alteplase ✳
Tirofiban	Reteplase
	Streptokinase
Injected anticoagulants	Tenecteplase
Danaparoid	
Epoprostenol	✳ See Part 3

ACTION OF THROMBOLYTIC DRUGS

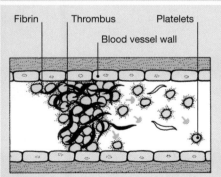

Fibrin   Thrombus   Platelets
Blood vessel wall

Before drug
When platelets accumulate in a blood vessel and are reinforced by strands of fibrin, the resultant blood clot, which is known as a thrombus, cannot be dissolved either by antiplatelet drugs or by anticoagulant drugs.

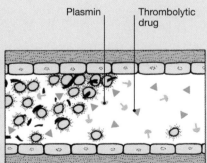

Plasmin   Thrombolytic drug

After drug
Thrombolytic drugs boost the action of plasmin, an enzyme in the blood that breaks up the strands of fibrin that bind the clot together. This allows the accumulated platelets to disperse and restores normal blood flow.

GASTROINTESTINAL TRACT

The gastrointestinal tract, also known as the digestive or alimentary tract, is the pathway through which food passes as it is processed to enable the nutrients it contains to be absorbed for use by the body. It consists of the mouth, oesophagus, stomach, duodenum, small intestine, large intestine (including the colon and rectum), and anus. In addition, a number of other organs are involved in the digestion of food: the salivary glands in the mouth, the liver, pancreas, and gallbladder. These organs, together with the gastrointestinal tract, form the digestive system.

The digestive system breaks down the large, complex chemicals – proteins, carbohydrates, and fats – present in the food we eat into simpler molecules that can be used by the body (see also Nutrition, p.106). Undigested or indigestible material, together with some of the body's waste products, pass to the large intestine, and, when a sufficient mass of such matter has accumulated, it is expelled from the body as faeces.

What can go wrong

Inflammation of the lining of the stomach or intestine (gastroenteritis) is usually the result of an infection or parasitic infestation. Damage may also be done by the inappropriate production of digestive juices, leading to minor complaints like acidity and major disorders like peptic ulcers. The lining of the intestine can be damaged by abnormal functioning of the immune system (inflammatory bowel disease). The rectum and anus can become painful and irritated by damage to the lining, tears in the skin at the opening of the anus (anal fissure), or enlarged veins (haemorrhoids).

The most frequently experienced gastrointestinal complaints – constipation, diarrhoea, and irritable bowel syndrome – usually occur when something disrupts the normal muscle contractions that propel food residue through the bowel.

Why drugs are used

Many drugs for gastrointestinal disorders are taken by mouth and act directly on the digestive tract without first entering the bloodstream. Such drugs include certain antibiotics and other drugs used to treat infestations. Some antacids for peptic ulcers and excess stomach acidity, and the bulk-forming agents for constipation and diarrhoea, also pass through the system unabsorbed.

However, for many disorders, drugs with a systemic effect are required, including anti-ulcer drugs, opioid antidiarrhoeal drugs, and some of the drugs for inflammatory bowel disease.

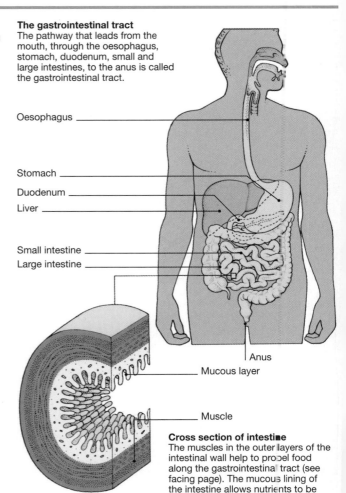

The gastrointestinal tract
The pathway that leads from the mouth, through the oesophagus, stomach, duodenum, small and large intestines, to the anus is called the gastrointestinal tract.

Oesophagus

Stomach

Duodenum

Liver

Small intestine

Large intestine

Anus

Mucous layer

Muscle

Cross section of intestine
The muscles in the outer layers of the intestinal wall help to propel food along the gastrointestinal tract (see facing page). The mucous lining of the intestine allows nutrients to be absorbed into the bloodstream.

Pancreas
The pancreas produces enzymes that digest fats, carbohydrates, and proteins into simpler substances. Pancreatic juices neutralize acidity of the stomach contents.

Gallbladder
Bile produced by the liver is stored in the gallbladder and released into the small intestine. Bile assists the digestion of fats by reducing them to smaller units that are more easily acted upon by digestive enzymes.

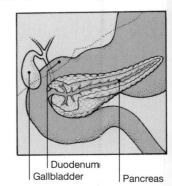

Duodenum

Gallbladder

Pancreas

MAJOR DRUG GROUPS

Antacids
Anti-ulcer drugs
Antidiarrhoeal drugs
Laxatives
Drugs for inflammatory bowel disease

Drugs for rectal and anal disorders
Drug treatment for gallstones

The lining of the gastrointestinal tract

The lining of the different sections of the gastrointestinal tract varies according to the function of that part, depending, for example, on whether its principal role is to secrete digestive juices or to absorb nutrients.

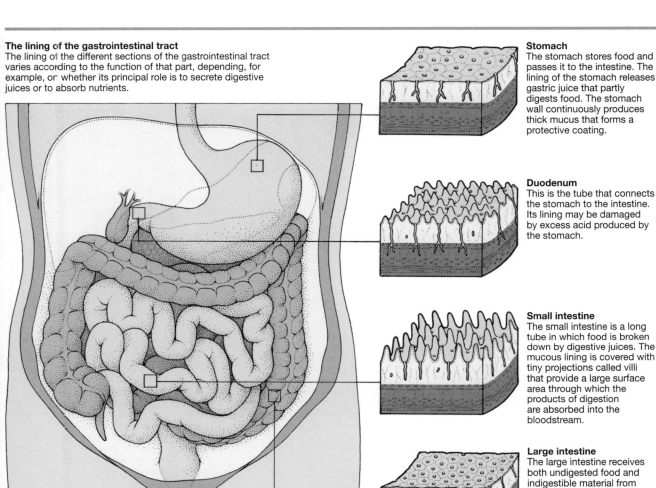

Stomach
The stomach stores food and passes it to the intestine. The lining of the stomach releases gastric juice that partly digests food. The stomach wall continuously produces thick mucus that forms a protective coating.

Duodenum
This is the tube that connects the stomach to the intestine. Its lining may be damaged by excess acid produced by the stomach.

Small intestine
The small intestine is a long tube in which food is broken down by digestive juices. The mucous lining is covered with tiny projections called villi that provide a large surface area through which the products of digestion are absorbed into the bloodstream.

Large intestine
The large intestine receives both undigested food and indigestible material from the small intestine. Water and mineral salts pass through the lining into the bloodstream.

MOVEMENT OF FOOD THROUGH THE GASTROINTESTINAL TRACT

Food is propelled through the gastrointestinal tract by rhythmic waves of muscular contraction called peristalsis. The illustration shows how peristaltic contractions of the bowel wall push food through the intestine.

Muscle contraction in the tract is controlled by the autonomic nervous system (see p.35) and is therefore easily disrupted by drugs that either stimulate or inhibit the activity of the autonomic nervous system. Excessive peristaltic action may cause diarrhoea; slowed peristalsis may cause constipation.

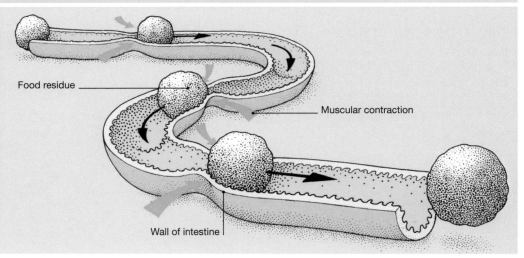

Food residue

Muscular contraction

Wall of intestine

ANTACIDS

Digestive juices in the stomach contain acid and enzymes that break down food before it passes into the intestine. The wall of the stomach is normally protected from the action of digestive acid by a layer of mucus that is constantly secreted by the stomach lining. Problems arise when the stomach lining is damaged or too much acid is produced and eats away at the mucous layer.

Excess acid that leads to discomfort, commonly referred to as indigestion, may result from anxiety, overeating or eating certain foods, coffee, alcohol, or smoking. Some drugs, notably aspirin and non-steroidal anti-inflammatory drugs, can irritate the stomach lining and even cause ulcers to develop.

Antacids are used to neutralize acid and thus relieve pain. They are simple chemical compounds that are mildly alkaline and some also act as chemical buffers. Their chalky taste is often disguised with flavourings.

Why they are used

Antacids may be needed when simple remedies (such as a change in diet or a glass of milk) fail to relieve indigestion. They are especially useful following a meal to neutralize the acid surge that sometimes occurs after a meal.

Doctors prescribe these drugs in order to relieve dyspepsia (pain in the chest or upper abdomen caused by or aggravated by acid) in disorders such as inflammation or ulceration of the oesophagus, stomach lining, and duodenum. Antacids usually relieve pain resulting from ulcers in the oesophagus, stomach, or duodenum within a few minutes. Regular treatment with antacids reduces the acidity of the stomach, thereby encouraging the healing of any ulcers that may have formed.

ACTION OF ANTACIDS

Excess acid in the stomach may eat away at the layer of mucus that protects the stomach. When this occurs, or when the mucous lining is damaged, for example by an ulcer, stomach acid comes into contact with the underlying tissues, causing pain and inflammation (right). Antacids combine with stomach acid to reduce the acidity of the digestive juices. This helps to prevent pain and inflammation, and allows the mucous layer to repair itself (far right).

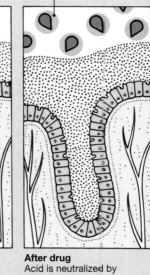

Acid   Drug

Mucus _____

Mucous lining _____

Stomach wall _____

Before drug
Acid damages mucous layer of stomach lining.

After drug
Acid is neutralized by antacid action.

How they work

By neutralizing stomach acid, antacids prevent inflammation, relieve pain, and allow the mucous layer and lining to mend. When used in the treatment of ulcers, they prevent acid from attacking damaged stomach lining and so allow the ulcer to heal.

How they affect you

If antacids are taken according to the instructions, they are usually effective in relieving abdominal discomfort caused by acid. The speed of action, dependent on the ability to neutralize acid, varies.

Their duration of action also varies; the short-acting drugs may have to be taken quite frequently.

Although most antacids have few serious side effects when used only occasionally, some may cause diarrhoea, and others may cause constipation (see Types of antacid, below).

Risks and special precautions

Antacids should not be taken to prevent abdominal pain on a regular basis except under medical supervision, as they may suppress the symptoms of stomach cancer. Your doctor is likely to want to arrange tests such as endoscopy or barium X-rays before prescribing long-term treatment.

Antacids can interfere with the absorption of other drugs. If you are taking a prescription medicine, you should check with your doctor or pharmacist before taking an antacid.

TYPES OF ANTACID

Aluminium compounds These drugs have a prolonged action and are widely used, especially for indigestion and dyspepsia. They may cause constipation, but this is often countered by combining this type of antacid with one that contains magnesium. Aluminium compounds can interfere with the absorption of phosphate from the diet, causing weakness and bone damage if taken in high doses over a long period. A high blood level of aluminium may build up in people with kidney failure, causing a dementia-like illness.

Magnesium compounds Like the aluminium compounds, these have a prolonged action. In large doses they can cause diarrhoea, and in people who have impaired kidney function a high blood magnesium level may build up, causing weakness, lethargy, and drowsiness.

Sodium bicarbonate This antacid acts quickly, but its effect soon passes. It reacts

with stomach acids to produce gas, which may cause bloating and belching. Sodium bicarbonate is not advised for people with heart or kidney disease, as it can lead to the accumulation of water (oedema) in the legs and lungs, or serious changes in the acid-base balance of the blood.

Combined preparations Antacids may be combined with other substances called alginates and antifoaming agents. Alginates are intended to float on the contents of the stomach and produce a neutralizing layer to subdue acid that can otherwise rise into the oesophagus, causing heartburn. Antifoaming agents are intended to relieve flatulence. In some preparations a local anaesthetic is combined with the antacid to relieve discomfort in oesophagitis. The value of these additives is dubious.

COMMON DRUGS

Antacids	Antifoaming agents
Aluminium hydroxide ✱	Dimeticone
Calcium carbonate	Simeticone
Hydrotalcite	
Magnesium carbonate	**Other drugs**
Magnesium hydroxide ✱	Alginates ✱
Magnesium trisilicate	
Sodium bicarbonate	

✱ See Part 3

ANTI-ULCER DRUGS

Normally, the linings of the oesophagus, stomach, and duodenum are protected from the irritant action of stomach acids or bile by a thin covering layer of mucus. If this is damaged, or if large amounts of stomach acid are formed, the underlying tissue may become eroded, causing a peptic ulcer. An ulcer often leads to abdominal pain, vomiting, and changes in appetite. The most common type of ulcer occurs just beyond the stomach, in the duodenum. The exact cause of peptic ulcers is not understood, but a

number of risk factors have been identified, including heavy smoking, the regular use of aspirin or similar drugs, and family history. An organism found in almost all patients who have peptic ulcers, *Helicobacter pylori*, is believed to be the main causative agent.

The symptoms caused by ulcers may be relieved by an antacid (see facing page), but healing is slow. The usual treatment is with an anti-ulcer drug, such as a proton pump inhibitor, bismuth, or sucralfate, although an H₂ blocker may

be used. The anti-ulcer drug is usually combined with antibiotics to eradicate *Helicobacter pylori* infection.

Why they are used
Anti-ulcer drugs are used to relieve symptoms and heal the ulcer. Untreated ulcers may erode blood vessel walls or perforate the stomach or duodenum.

Eradication of *Helicobacter pylori* by an antisecretory drug (such as a proton pump inhibitor) combined with two antibiotics (triple therapy) may provide a cure in one to two weeks. Surgery is reserved for complications such as obstruction, perforation, haemorrhage, and when there is a possibility of cancer.

How they work
Drugs protect ulcers from the action of stomach acid, allowing the tissue to heal. H₂ blockers, misoprostol, and proton pump inhibitors reduce the amount of acid released; bismuth and sucralfate form a protective coating over the ulcer. Bismuth also has an antibacterial effect.

How they affect you
These drugs begin to reduce pain in a few hours and usually allow the ulcer to heal in four to eight weeks. They produce few side effects, although H₂ blockers such as cimetidine can cause confusion in older people. Bismuth may cause blackened faeces; sucralfate may cause constipation; misoprostol may lead to diarrhoea; and proton pump inhibitors may cause either constipation or diarrhoea. Triple therapy is given for one or two weeks. If *Helicobacter pylori* is eradicated, maintenance therapy should not be necessary. Sucralfate is usually prescribed for up to 12 weeks, and bismuth and misoprostol for four to eight weeks. Because they may mask symptoms of stomach cancer, H₂ blockers and proton pump inhibitors are normally prescribed only when tests have ruled out this disorder.

ACTION OF ANTI-ULCER DRUGS

Proton pump inhibitors
Acid secretion by the cells lining the stomach depends on an enzyme system (also known as the proton pump) that transports hydrogen ions across the cell walls. Omeprazole, lansoprazole, and

similar drugs work by blocking the proton pump. They can stop stomach acid production until a new supply of the enzyme can be made by the body and, therefore, have a long duration of action.

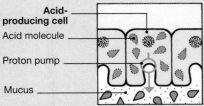

The proton pump
This enzyme system transports hydrogen ions across the cell wall into the stomach, thereby stimulating acid secretion.

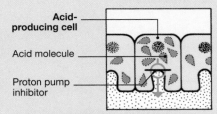

The action of proton pump inhibitors
Proton pump inhibitors block the enzyme system, stopping the transport of hydrogen ions and, thus, the secretion of acid.

H₂ blockers
Histamine is a chemical released by mast cells (see Allergies, p.81) that can produce a number of effects in different parts of the body. In the stomach, histamine stimulates H₂ receptors, causing acid production. To control stomach acid production, a class of

antihistamine drugs was developed that acts by blocking the H₂ receptors. These drugs are known as H₂ blockers to distinguish them from antihistamines used for allergic disorders (see p.82), which are sometimes called H₁ blockers because they block H₁ receptors.

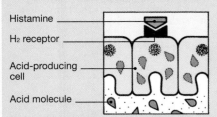

The action of histamine on the stomach
Histamine binds to specialized H₂ receptors and stimulates acid-producing cells in the stomach wall to release acid.

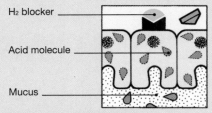

The action of H₂ blockers
H₂ blockers occupy H₂ receptors, preventing histamine from triggering the production of acid. This allows the mucous lining to heal.

Sucralfate and bismuth
Sucralfate forms a coating over the ulcer, protecting it from the action of stomach acid and allowing it to heal. Bismuth may stimulate production of prostaglandins or bicarbonate, and also kills the bacteria that are thought to cause most peptic ulcers.

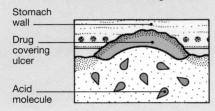

COMMON DRUGS

Proton pump inhibitors
Esomeprazole
Lansoprazole ✱
Omeprazole ✱
Pantoprazole
Rabeprazole ✱

H₂ blockers
Cimetidine ✱
Famotidine
Nizatidine
Ranitidine ✱

Other drugs
Antacids (see p.66)
Antibiotics (see p.86)
Carbenoxolone
Misoprostol ✱
Sucralfate ✱
Tripotassium dicitrato-bismuthate (bismuth chelate)

✱ See Part 3

ANTIDIARRHOEAL DRUGS

Diarrhoea is an increase in the fluidity and frequency of bowel movements. In some cases diarrhoea protects the body from harmful substances in the intestine by hastening their removal. The most common causes are viral infection, food poisoning, and parasites. But it also occurs as a symptom of other illnesses. It can be a side effect of some drugs and may follow radiation therapy for cancer. Diarrhoea may also be caused by anxiety.

An attack of diarrhoea usually clears up quickly without medical attention. The best treatment is to abstain from food and to drink plenty of clear fluids. Rehydration solutions containing sugar as well as potassium and sodium salts are widely recommended for preventing dehydration and chemical imbalances, particularly in children. You should consult your doctor if: the condition does not improve within 48 hours; the diarrhoea contains blood; severe abdominal pain and vomiting are present; you have just returned from a foreign country; or if the diarrhoea occurs in a small child or an older adult.

Severe diarrhoea can impair absorption of drugs, and anyone taking a prescribed drug should seek advice from a doctor or pharmacist. A woman taking oral contraceptives may need additional contraceptive measures (see p.121).

The main types of drug used to relieve non-specific diarrhoea are opioids, and bulk-forming and adsorbent agents. Antispasmodic drugs may also be used to relieve accompanying pain (see Drugs for irritable bowel syndrome, below).

Why they are used

An antidiarrhoeal drug may be prescribed to provide relief when simple remedies are not effective, and once it is certain the diarrhoea is neither infectious nor toxic.

Opioid drugs are the most effective antidiarrhoeals. They are used when the diarrhoea is severe and debilitating. The bulking and adsorbent agents have

ACTION OF ANTIDIARRHOEAL DRUGS

Opioid antidiarrhoeals
These drugs reduce the transmission of nerve signals to the intestinal muscles, thus reducing muscle contraction. This allows more time for water to be absorbed from the food residue and therefore reduces the fluidity as well as the frequency of bowel movements.

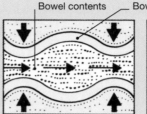
Bowel contents — Bowel wall

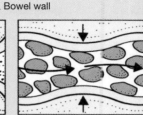

Before drug
Rapid bowel contraction prevents water from being absorbed.

After drug
Slowed bowel action allows more water to be absorbed.

Bulk-forming agents
These preparations contain particles that swell up as they absorb water from the large intestine. This makes the faeces firmer and less fluid. It is thought that bulk-forming agents may absorb irritants and harmful chemicals along with excess water.

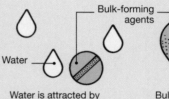
Water

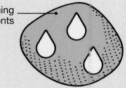
Bulk-forming agents

Water is attracted by bulk-forming agent.

Bulk-forming agent swells as water is absorbed.

a milder effect and are often used when it is necessary to regulate bowel action over a prolonged period – for example, in people with colostomies or ileostomies.

How they work

Opioids decrease the muscles' propulsive activity so that faecal matter passes more slowly through the bowel.

Bulk-forming agents and adsorbents absorb water and irritants present in the bowel, thereby producing larger and firmer stools at less frequent intervals.

How they affect you

Drugs that are used to treat diarrhoea reduce the urge to move the bowels. Opioids and antispasmodics may relieve

abdominal pain. All antidiarrhoeals may cause constipation if used in excess.

Risks and special precautions

Used in relatively low doses for a limited period of time, opioid drugs are unlikely to produce adverse effects. However, these drugs are not recommended for acute diarrhoea in children and should be used with caution when diarrhoea is caused by an infection, since they may slow the elimination of microorganisms from the intestine. All antidiarrhoeals should be taken with plenty of water. It is important not to take a bulk-forming agent together with an opioid or antispasmodic drug, because a bulky mass could form and obstruct the bowel.

DRUGS FOR IRRITABLE BOWEL SYNDROME

Irritable bowel syndrome is a common stress-related condition in which the normal coordinated waves of muscular contraction responsible for moving the bowel contents smoothly through the intestines become strong and irregular, often causing pain, and associated with diarrhoea or constipation.

Symptoms are often relieved by adjusting the amount of fibre in the diet, although medication may also be required. Bulk-forming agents may be given to regulate the consistency of the bowel contents. If pain is severe, an antispasmodic drug may be prescribed. These anticholinergic drugs reduce the transmission of nerve signals to the bowel wall, thus preventing spasm. Tricyclic antidepressants are sometimes used because their anticholinergic action has a calming effect on the bowel.

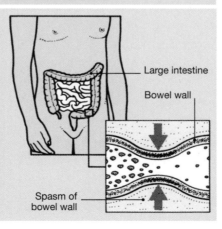
Large intestine

Bowel wall

Spasm of bowel wall

COMMON DRUGS

Antispasmodics
Alverine
Atropine *
Dicycloverine
(dicyclomine) *
Hyoscine
butylbromide *
Mebeverine *
Peppermint oil
Propantheline

Opioids
Codeine *
Co-phenotrope *
Loperamide *
Morphine/
diamorphine *

Antibacterials
Ciprofloxacin *

Bulk-forming agents and adsorbents
Ispaghula
Kaolin
Methylcellulose *
Sterculia

Other drugs
Aluminium
hydroxide *
Colestyramine *

* See Part 3

LAXATIVES

When your bowels do not move as frequently as usual and the faeces are hard and difficult to pass, you are suffering from constipation. The most common cause is lack of sufficient fibre in your diet; fibre supplies the bulk that makes the faeces soft and easy to pass. The simplest remedy is more fluid and a diet that contains plenty of foods that are high in fibre, but laxative drugs may also be used.

Ignoring the urge to defecate can also cause constipation, because the faeces become dry, hard to pass, and too small to stimulate the muscles that propel them through the intestine.

Certain drugs may be constipating: for example, opioid analgesics, tricyclic antidepressants, and antacids containing aluminium. Some diseases, such as hypothyroidism (underactive thyroid gland) and scleroderma (a rare disorder of connective tissue characterized by the hardening of the skin), can also lead to constipation.

The onset of constipation in a middle-aged or older person may be an early symptom of bowel cancer. Consult your doctor about any persistent change in bowel habit.

Why they are used

Since prolonged use is harmful, laxatives should be used for very short periods only. They may prevent pain and straining in people suffering from either hernias or haemorrhoids (p.71). Doctors may prescribe laxatives for the same reason after childbirth or abdominal surgery. Laxatives are also used to clear the bowel before investigative procedures such as colonoscopy. They may be prescribed for patients who are older or confined to bed because lack of exercise can often lead to constipation.

How they work

Laxatives act on the large intestine by increasing the speed with which faecal matter passes through the bowel, or increasing its bulk and/or water content.

ACTION OF LAXATIVES

Bulk-forming agents
Taken after a meal, these agents are not absorbed as they pass through the digestive tract. They contain particles that absorb many times their own volume of water. By doing so, they increase the bulk of the bowel movements and thus encourage bowel action.

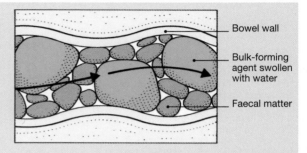

Bowel wall

Bulk-forming agent swollen with water

Faecal matter

Stimulant laxatives
These laxatives are thought to encourage bowel movements by acting on nerve endings in the wall of the intestines that trigger contraction of the intestinal muscles. This speeds the passage of faecal matter through the large intestine, allowing less time for water to be absorbed. Thus faeces become more liquid and are passed more frequently.

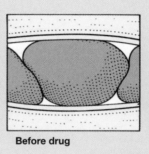

Increased contractions speed passage of faecal matter

Before drug

After drug

Stimulants encourage the bowel muscles to contract, increasing the speed at which faecal matter goes through the intestine. Bulk-forming laxatives absorb water in the bowel, thereby increasing the volume of faeces, making them softer and easier to pass. Lactulose also causes fluid to accumulate in the intestine. Osmotic laxatives act by keeping water in the bowel, thereby making the bowel movements softer. This also increases the bulk of the faeces and enables them to be passed more easily. Lubricant liquid paraffin preparations make bowel movements softer and easier to pass

without increasing their bulk. Prolonged use can interfere with absorption of some essential vitamins.

Risks and special precautions

Laxatives can cause diarrhoea if taken in overdose, and constipation if overused. The most serious risk of prolonged use is developing dependence on the laxative for normal bowel action. Use of any laxative should therefore be discontinued as soon as normal bowel movements have been re-established. Children should not be given laxatives except in special circumstances on the advice of a doctor.

TYPES OF LAXATIVE

Bulk-forming agents These are relatively slow acting but are less likely than other laxatives to interfere with normal bowel action. For constipation accompanied by abdominal pain they should be taken only after consultation with your doctor, because of the risk of intestinal obstruction.

Stimulant (contact) laxatives These are for occasional use when other treatments have failed or when rapid onset of action is needed. Stimulant laxatives should not normally be used for longer than a week as they can cause abdominal cramps and diarrhoea.

Softening agents These are often used when hard bowel movements cause pain on defecation – for example, when haemorrhoids

are present, or after surgery when straining must be avoided. Liquid paraffin was once used for the relief of faecal impaction (blockage of the bowel by faecal material), but it can cause side effects and has generally been replaced by docusate sodium.

Osmotic laxatives Preparations containing magnesium carbonate or citrate may be used to evacuate the bowel before investigative procedures or surgery. They are not normally used for long-term relief because they can cause chemical imbalances in the blood.

Lactulose is an alternative to bulk-forming laxatives for the long-term treatment of chronic constipation. It may cause stomach cramps and flatulence but is usually well tolerated.

COMMON DRUGS

Stimulant laxatives
Bisacodyl
Dantron
Docusate
Glycerol
Senna
Sodium picosulfate

Bulk-forming agents
Bran
Ispaghula
Methylcellulose *
Sterculia

Softening agents
Arachis oil
Liquid paraffin

Osmotic laxatives
Lactulose *
Macrogols
Magnesium citrate
Magnesium hydroxide *
Magnesium sulfate
Sodium acid phosphate

* See Part 3

DRUGS FOR INFLAMMATORY BOWEL DISEASE

Inflammatory bowel disease is the term used for disorders in which inflammation of the intestinal wall causes recurrent attacks of abdominal pain, general feelings of ill-health, and frequently diarrhoea, with blood and mucus in the faeces. Loss of appetite and poor absorption of food may often result in weight loss.

There are two main types of inflammatory bowel disease: Crohn's disease and ulcerative colitis. In Crohn's disease (also called regional enteritis), any part of the digestive tract may become inflamed, although the small intestine is the most commonly affected site. In ulcerative colitis, it is the large intestine (colon) that becomes inflamed and ulcerated, often producing bloodstained diarrhoea (see right).

The exact cause of these disorders is unknown, although stress-related, dietary, infectious, and genetic factors may all be important.

Establishing a proper diet and a less stressful lifestyle may help to alleviate these conditions. Bed rest during attacks is also advisable. However, these simple measures alone do not usually relieve or prevent attacks, and drug treatment is often necessary.

Three types of drug are used to treat inflammatory bowel disease: corticosteroids (p.99), immunosuppressants (p.115), and aminosalicylate anti-inflammatory drugs such as sulfasalazine. Nutritional supplements (used especially for Crohn's disease) and antidiarrhoeal drugs (p.68) may also be used. Surgery to remove damaged areas of the intestine may be needed in severe cases.

SITES OF BOWEL INFLAMMATION

The two main types of bowel inflammation are ulcerative colitis and Crohn's disease. The former occurs in the large intestine. Crohn's disease can occur anywhere along the gastrointestinal tract, but it most often affects the small intestine.

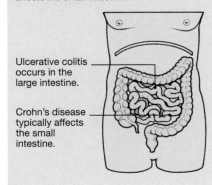

Ulcerative colitis occurs in the large intestine.

Crohn's disease typically affects the small intestine.

Why they are used

Drugs cannot cure inflammatory bowel disease, but treatment is needed, not only to control symptoms, but also to prevent complications, especially severe anaemia and perforation of the intestinal wall. Aminosalicylates are used to treat acute attacks of ulcerative colitis and Crohn's disease, and they may be continued as maintenance therapy. People who have severe bowel inflammation are usually prescribed a course of corticosteroids, particularly during a sudden flare-up.

Once the disease is under control, an immunosuppressant may be prescribed to prevent a relapse. Therapeutic antibodies that block a molecule called tumour necrosis factor (TNF) are used increasingly for this purpose.

How they work

Corticosteroids and sulfasalazine damp down the inflammatory process, allowing the damaged tissue to recover. They act in different ways to prevent migration of white blood cells into the bowel wall, which may be responsible in part for the inflammation of the bowel.

How they affect you

Taken to treat attacks, these drugs relieve symptoms within a few days, and general health improves gradually over a period of a few weeks. Aminosalicylates usually provide long-term relief from symptoms.

Immunosuppressants may take several months to produce an improvement, and regular blood tests to monitor possible drug side effects are often required.

Risks and special precautions

Immunosuppressant and corticosteroid drugs can cause serious adverse effects and are only prescribed when potential benefits outweigh the risks involved.

The side effects of corticosteroids can be reduced by the use of budesonide in a topical preparation (enema) that releases the drug at the site of inflammation.

It is important to continue taking these drugs as instructed because stopping them abruptly may cause a sudden flare-up of the disorder. Doctors usually supervise a gradual reduction in dosage when such drugs are stopped, even when they are given as a short course for an attack. Antidiarrhoeal drugs should not be taken on a routine basis because they may mask signs of deterioration or cause sudden bowel dilation or rupture.

How they are administered

Antidiarrhoeal drugs are usually taken in the form of tablets, although mild ulcerative colitis in the last part of the large intestine may be treated with suppositories or an enema containing a corticosteroid or aminosalicylate.

ACTION OF DRUGS IN ULCERATIVE COLITIS

The most common form of inflammatory bowel disease is ulcerative colitis. It affects the large intestine, causing ulceration of the lining and producing pain and violent blood-stained diarrhoea. It is often treated with corticosteroids and aminosalicylates.

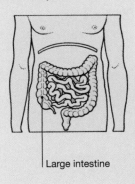

Large intestine

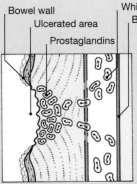

Bowel wall
Ulcerated area
Prostaglandins

White blood cell
Blood vessel

Corticosteroid drug
Aminosalicylate drug

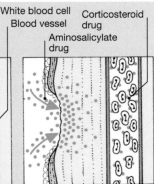

Before drug
Damage to the bowel lining provokes the formation of prostaglandins, chemicals that trigger the migration of white blood cells into the ulcerated area. The build-up of white blood cells in the intestinal wall causes inflammation.

Drug action
Aminosalicylate drugs pass into the ulcerated area from inside the bowel. They prevent prostaglandins from forming in the damaged tissue. Corticosteroids in the bloodstream reduce the ability of white blood cells to pass into the bowel wall.

COMMON DRUGS

Corticosteroids
Budesonide *
Hydrocortisone *
Prednisolone *

Immunosuppressants
Azathioprine *
Mercaptopurine *
Methotrexate *

See Part 3

Aminosalicylates
Balsalazide
Mesalazine *
Olsalazine
Sulfasalazine *

Other drugs
Adalimumab
Colestyramine *
Etanercept *
Infliximab *
Metronidazole *

DRUGS FOR RECTAL AND ANAL DISORDERS

The most common disorder affecting the rectum (the last part of the large intestine) and anus (the opening from the rectum) is haemorrhoids, commonly known as piles. They occur when haemorrhoidal veins become swollen or irritated, often due to prolonged pressure on the area – for example, from pregnancy or long hours of sitting. Haemorrhoids may cause irritation and pain, especially on defecation, and they are aggravated by constipation and straining during defecation. In some cases haemorrhoids may bleed, and occasionally clots form in the swollen veins, leading to severe pain, a condition called thrombosed haemorrhoids.

Other common disorders include anal fissure (painful cracks in the anus) and pruritus ani (itching around the anus). Anal disorders of all kinds occur less frequently in people who have soft, bulky stools.

A number of both over-the-counter and prescription-only preparations are available for the relief of such disorders.

Why they are used

Preparations for relief of haemorrhoids and anal discomfort fall into three main groups: creams or suppositories that act locally to relieve inflammation and irritation; glyceryl trinitrate ointment, which reduces pain by relieving anal pressure and increasing blood flow; and measures designed to relieve constipation, which contributes to the formation of, and discomfort from, haemorrhoids and anal fissure.

Preparations from the first group often contain a soothing agent with antiseptic, astringent, or vasoconstrictor properties. Ingredients of this type include zinc oxide, bismuth, hamamelis (witch hazel), and Peru balsam. Some of these products

DISORDERS OF THE RECTUM AND ANUS

The rectum and anus form the last part of the digestive tract. Common conditions affecting the area include swelling of the veins around the anus (haemorrhoids), cracks in the anus (anal fissure), and inflammation or irritation of the anus and surrounding area (pruritus ani).

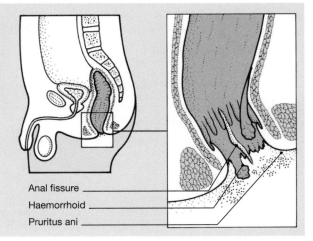

Anal fissure

Haemorrhoid

Pruritus ani

also include a mild local anaesthetic (see p.36) such as lidocaine. In some cases a doctor may prescribe an ointment containing a corticosteroid to relieve inflammation around the anus (see Topical corticosteroids, p.134).

People who have haemorrhoids or anal fissure are generally advised to include in their diets plenty of fluids and fibre-rich foods, such as fresh fruits, vegetables, and whole grain products, both to prevent constipation and to ease defecation. A mild bulk-forming or softening laxative may also be prescribed (see p.69).

Neither of these treatments can shrink large haemorrhoids, although they may provide relief while anal fissures heal naturally. Severe, persistently painful haemorrhoids that continue to be

troublesome in spite of these measures may need to be removed surgically or, more commonly, by banding with specially applied small rubber bands (see below left).

How they affect you

The treatments described above usually relieve discomfort, especially during defecation. Most people experience no adverse effects, although preparations containing local anaesthetics may cause irritation or even a rash in the anal area. It is rare for ingredients in locally acting preparations to be absorbed into the body in sufficient quantities to cause generalized side effects.

The main risk is that self-treatment of haemorrhoids may delay diagnosis of bowel cancer. It is therefore always wise to consult your doctor if symptoms of haemorrhoids are present, especially if you have noticed bleeding from the rectum or a change in bowel habits.

SITES OF TREATMENT

The illustration below shows how and where drugs for the treatment of rectal disorders act to relieve symptoms.

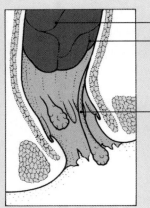

Faecal matter

Laxatives
These act in the large intestine to soften and ease the passage of faeces.

Creams, ointments, and suppositories
Astringents reduce the swelling and restrict blood supply, helping to relieve haemorrhoids. Local anaesthetics numb pain signals from the anus. Topical corticosteroids relieve inflammation.

Banding treatment
A small rubber band is applied tightly to a haemorrhoid, thereby blocking off its blood supply. The haemorrhoid will eventually wither away.

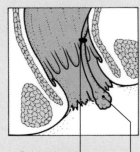

Rubber band

Haemorrhoid

COMMON DRUGS

Soothing and astringent agents
Aluminium acetate
Bismuth
Peru balsam
Zinc oxide

Topical corticosteroids
Hydrocortisone *

Local anaesthetics
(see p.36)

Laxatives
(see p.69)

Other drugs
Glyceryl trinitrate *

* See Part 3

DRUG TREATMENT FOR GALLSTONES

The formation of gallstones is the most common disorder of the gallbladder, which is the storage and concentrating unit for bile, a digestive juice produced by the liver. During digestion, bile passes from the gallbladder via the bile duct into the small intestine, where it assists in the digestion of fats. Bile is composed of several ingredients, including bile acids, bile salts, and bile pigments. It also has a significant amount of cholesterol, which is dissolved in bile acid. If the amount of cholesterol in the bile increases, or if the amount of bile acid is reduced, a proportion of the cholesterol cannot remain dissolved, and under certain circumstances this excess accumulates in the gallbladder as gallstones.

Gallstones may be present in the gallbladder for years without causing symptoms. However, if they become lodged in the bile duct they cause pain and block the flow of bile. If the bile accumulates in the blood, it may cause an attack of jaundice, or the gallbladder may become infected and inflamed.

Drug treatment with ursodeoxycholic acid is only effective against stones made principally of cholesterol (some contain other substances), and even these take many months to dissolve. Therefore, surgery and ultrasound have become widely used, especially the use of laparoscopic ("keyhole") surgery. Surgery and ultrasound treatments are always used to remove stones blocking the bile duct.

Why they are used

Even if you have not experienced any symptoms, once gallstones have been diagnosed your doctor may advise treatment because of the risk of blockage of the bile duct. Drug treatment is usually preferred to surgery for small cholesterol stones or when there is a possibility that surgery may be risky.

How they work

Ursodeoxycholic acid is a substance that is naturally present in bile. It acts on chemical processes in the liver to regulate the amount of cholesterol in the blood by controlling the amount that passes into the bile. Once the cholesterol level in the bile is reduced, the bile acids

DIGESTION OF FATS

The digestion of fats (or lipids) in the small intestine is assisted by the action of bile, a digestive juice produced by the liver and stored in the gallbladder. A complex sequence of chemical processes enables fats to be absorbed through the intestinal wall, broken down in the liver, and converted for use in the body. Cholesterol, a lipid present in bile, plays an important part in this chain.

2 Bile salts act on fats to enable them to pass from the small intestine into the bloodstream, either directly or via the lymphatic system.

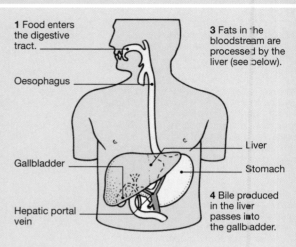

1 Food enters the digestive tract.

Oesophagus

3 Fats in the bloodstream are processed by the liver (see below).

Liver

Gallbladder

Stomach

4 Bile produced in the liver passes into the gallbladder.

Hepatic portal vein

How fats are processed in the liver

Fat molecules are broken down in the liver into fatty acids and glycerol. Glycerol, as well as some of the fatty acids, pass back into the bloodstream. Other fatty acids are used to form cholesterol, some of which in turn is used to make bile salts. Unchanged cholesterol is dissolved in the bile, which then passes into the gallbladder.

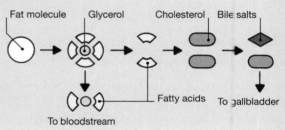

Fat molecule   Glycerol   Cholesterol   Bile salts

Fatty acids   To gallbladder

To bloodstream

---

are able to start dissolving the stones in the gallbladder. To achieve maximum effect, ursodeoxycholic acid treatment usually needs to be accompanied by adherence to a low-cholesterol, high-fibre diet.

How they affect you

Drug treatment may often take years to dissolve gallstones completely. You will not, therefore, feel any immediate benefit from the drug, but you may have some minor side effects, the most usual of which is diarrhoea. If this occurs, your doctor may adjust the dosage. The effect of drug treatment on the gallstones is usually monitored at regular intervals by means of ultrasound or X-ray examinations.

Even after successful treatment with drugs, gallstones often recur when the drug is stopped. In some cases drug treatment and dietary restrictions may be continued even after the gallstones have dissolved, to prevent a recurrence.

Although the drug reduces cholesterol in the gallbladder, it increases the level in the blood because it reduces the excretion of cholesterol in the bile. Doctors therefore prescribe it with caution to people who have atherosclerosis (fatty deposits in the blood vessels) The drug is not usually given to people who have liver disorders because it can interfere with normal liver function. Surgical or ultrasound treatment is used for people with liver problems.

AGENTS USED IN DISORDERS OF THE PANCREAS

The pancreas releases certain enzymes into the small intestine that are necessary for digestion of a range of foods. If the release of pancreatic enzymes is impaired (caused by, for example, chronic pancreatitis or cystic fibrosis), enzyme replacement therapy may be necessary. Replacement of enzymes does not cure the underlying disorder, but it restores normal digestion. Pancreatic enzymes should be taken just before or with

meals, and usually take effect immediately. Your doctor will probably advise you to eat a diet that is high in protein and carbohydrates and low in fat.

Pancreatin, the generic name for those preparations containing pancreatic enzymes, is extracted from pig pancreas. Treatment must be continued indefinitely as long as the pancreatic disorder persists.

COMMON DRUGS

Pancreatic enzymes
Amylase
Lipase
Pancreatin
Protease

Drugs for gallstones
Ursodeoxycholic acid

Other drugs
Colestyramine *

* See Part 3

MUSCLES, BONES, AND JOINTS

The basic architecture of the human body relies on 206 bones, over 600 muscles, and a complex assortment of other tissues – ligaments, tendons, and cartilage – that enable the body to move with remarkable efficiency.

What can go wrong

Although tough, these structures often suffer damage. Muscles, tendons, and ligaments can be strained or torn by violent movement, which may cause inflammation, making the affected tissue swollen and painful. Joints, especially those that bear the body's weight – hips, knees, ankles, and vertebrae – are prone to wear and tear. The cartilage covering the bone ends may tear, causing pain and inflammation. Joint damage also occurs in rheumatoid arthritis, which is thought to be a form of autoimmune disorder. Gout, in which uric acid crystals form in some joints, may also cause inflammation, a condition known as gouty arthritis.

Another problem affecting the muscles and joints includes nerve injury or degeneration, which alters nerve control over muscle contraction. Myasthenia gravis, in which transmission of signals between nerves and muscles is reduced, affects muscle control as a result. Bones may also be weakened by vitamin, mineral, or hormone deficiencies.

Why drugs are used

A simple analgesic drug or one that has an anti-inflammatory effect will provide pain relief in most of the above conditions. For severe inflammation, a doctor may inject a drug with a more powerful anti-inflammatory effect, such as a corticosteroid, into the affected site. In cases of severe progressive rheumatoid arthritis, antirheumatic drugs may halt the disease's progression and relieve symptoms.

Drugs that reduce the production of uric acid or speed its elimination are often prescribed to treat gout. Muscle relaxants that inhibit transmission of nerve signals to the muscles are used to treat muscle spasm. Drugs that increase nervous stimulation of the muscle are prescribed for myasthenia gravis. Bone disorders in which the mineral content of bone is reduced are treated with supplements of minerals, vitamins, and hormones.

MAJOR DRUG GROUPS

Non-steroidal anti-inflammatory drugs
Antirheumatic drugs
Locally acting corticosteroids
Drugs for gout

Muscle relaxants
Drugs used for myasthenia gravis
Drugs for bone disorders

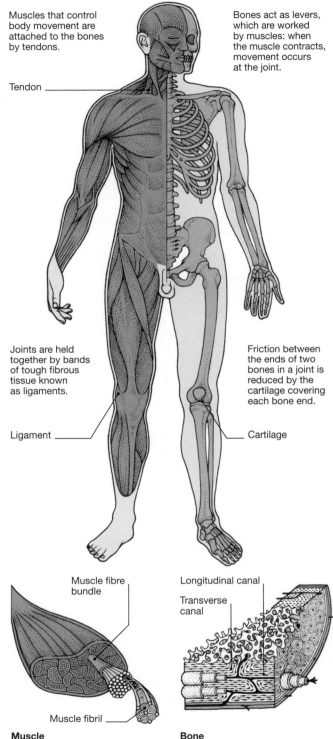

Muscles that control body movement are attached to the bones by tendons.

Tendon

Bones act as levers, which are worked by muscles: when the muscle contracts, movement occurs at the joint.

Joints are held together by bands of tough fibrous tissue known as ligaments.

Ligament

Friction between the ends of two bones in a joint is reduced by the cartilage covering each bone end.

Cartilage

Muscle fibre bundle

Longitudinal canal

Transverse canal

Muscle fibril

Muscle
Each muscle is made of thick bundles of fibres; each bundle in turn is made of fibrils. Tiny nerves and blood vessels enable the muscle to function.

Bone
Long bones, such as the femur, contain a network of longitudinal and transverse canals to carry blood, nerves, and lymph vessels through the bone.

NON-STEROIDAL ANTI-INFLAMMATORY DRUGS

These drugs (also called NSAIDs) are used to relieve the pain, stiffness, and inflammation of conditions affecting the muscles, bones, and joints. NSAIDs are called "non-steroidal" to distinguish them from corticosteroid drugs (see p.99), which also damp down inflammation.

Why they are used

NSAIDs are widely prescribed for the treatment of osteoarthritis, rheumatoid arthritis, and other rheumatic conditions. They reduce pain and inflammation in the joints, but they do not alter the progress of these diseases.

The response to the various drugs in this group varies between individuals. It is sometimes necessary to try several different NSAIDs before finding the one that best suits a particular individual.

Because NSAIDs do not change the progress of a disease, additional treatment is often necessary, particularly for rheumatoid arthritis (see facing page).

NSAIDs are also commonly prescribed to relieve back pain, headaches, gout (p.77), menstrual pain (p.120), mild pain following surgery, and pain from soft tissue injuries, such as sprains and strains (see also Analgesics, p.36).

How they work

Prostaglandins are chemicals released by the body at the site of injury. They are responsible for producing inflammation and pain following tissue damage. NSAIDs block an enzyme, cyclo-oxygenase (COX), which is involved in the production of prostaglandins, and thus reduce pain and inflammation (see p.37).

How they affect you

NSAIDs are rapidly absorbed from the digestive system and most start to relieve pain within an hour. When used regularly they reduce pain, inflammation, and stiffness and may restore or improve the function of a damaged or painful joint.

Most NSAIDs are short acting and need to be taken a few times a day for optimal pain relief. Some need to be taken only twice daily. Others, such as piroxicam, are very slowly eliminated from the body and are effective when taken once a day.

Risks and special precautions

Most NSAIDs carry a low risk of serious adverse effects although nausea, indigestion, and altered bowel action are common. The main risk from NSAIDs is that, occasionally, they can cause bleeding in the stomach or duodenum; to avoid this, the lowest effective dose is given for the shortest duration. NSAIDs should be avoided altogether by people who have had peptic ulcers.

Most NSAIDs are not recommended during pregnancy or for breast-feeding mothers. Caution is also advised for people with kidney or liver abnormalities

ACTION OF NSAIDs IN OSTEOARTHRITIS

Non-steroidal anti-inflammatory drugs (NSAIDs) are often prescribed to diminish the pain and stiffness associated with osteoarthritis, a disorder in which, typically, a weight-bearing joint such as the hip is damaged by wear and tear or other factors.

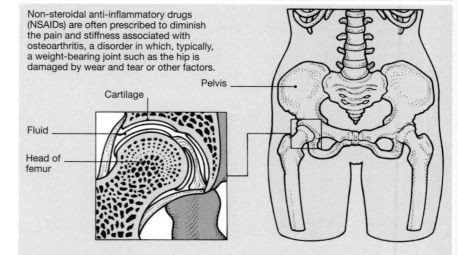

Pelvis

Cartilage

Fluid

Head of femur

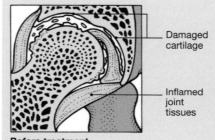

Damaged cartilage

Inflamed joint tissues

Before treatment
The protective layers of cartilage surrounding the joint are worn away and the joint becomes inflamed and painful.

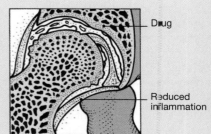

Drug

Reduced inflammation

Effect of NSAIDs
NSAIDs reduce inflammation and may thus relieve pain, but damage to the joint remains and symptoms are likely to worsen or recur if the drug is stopped.

or heart disease, or those people with a history of hypersensitivity to other drugs.

NSAIDs may impair blood clotting and are, therefore, prescribed with caution for people with bleeding disorders or who are taking drugs that reduce blood clotting.

Misoprostol

An NSAID may cause bleeding when its antiprostaglandin action occurs in the digestive tract. To protect against this side effect, a drug called misoprostol is sometimes combined with the NSAID. Misoprostol is also used to help heal peptic ulcers (see p.67).

COX-2 inhibitors

NSAIDs block two types of COX, COX-1 and COX-2, at different sites in the body; blocking COX-1 leads to the upper gastrointestinal tract irritation of NSAIDs, while blocking COX-2 leads to the anti-inflammatory effect. COX-2 inhibitors block COX-2 but not COX-1. COX-2 inhibitors are not prescribed to anyone who has had a heart attack or stroke,

however, because they significantly increase the risk of recurrence, nor are they prescribed to people with peripheral artery disease (poor circulation). They are prescribed with caution to anyone at risk of any of these conditions.

COMMON DRUGS

Aceclofenac	Meloxicam
Acemetacin	Nabumetone
Aspirin *	Naproxen *
Diclofenac *	Piroxicam *
Felbinac	Sulindac
Fenbufen	Tenoxicam
Fenoprofen	Tiaprofenic acid
Flurbiprofen	
Ibuprofen *	**COX-2 inhibitors**
Indometacin	Celecoxib *
(indomethacin)	Etodolac
Ketoprofen *	Etoricoxib
Mefenamic acid *	

* See Part 3

ANTIRHEUMATIC DRUGS

These drugs are used in the treatment of various rheumatic disorders, the most crippling and deforming being rheumatoid arthritis, an autoimmune disease in which the body's mechanism for fighting infection contributes to the damage of its own joint tissue. There is pain, stiffness, and swelling of the joints that, over many months, can lead to deformity. Flare-ups of rheumatoid arthritis also cause a general feeling of being unwell, fatigue, and loss of appetite.

Treatments for rheumatoid arthritis include drugs, rest, physiotherapy, changes in diet, and immobilization of joints. The disorder cannot yet be cured, but in many cases it does not progress to permanent disability. It also sometimes subsides spontaneously for prolonged periods.

Why they are used

The aim of drug treatment is to relieve the symptoms of pain and stiffness, maintain mobility, and prevent deformity. Drugs for rheumatoid arthritis fall into two main categories: those that alleviate symptoms, and those that modify, halt, or slow the underlying disease process. Drugs in the first category include aspirin (p.162) and other non-steroidal anti-inflammatory drugs (NSAIDs, facing page). These drugs are usually prescribed as a first treatment.

Drugs in the second category are known collectively as disease-modifying antirheumatic drugs (DMARDs). They may be given if rheumatoid arthritis is severe or if initial drug treatment has proved to be ineffective. DMARDs may prevent further joint damage and disability, but they are not prescribed routinely because the disease may stop spontaneously and because they have potentially severe adverse effects (see Some types of Disease-Modifying Antirheumatic Drug, below, for information on individual drugs).

Corticosteroids (p.99) are sometimes used in treating rheumatoid arthritis, but are used only for limited periods because they depress the immune system, increasing susceptibility to infection.

THE EFFECTS OF ANTIRHEUMATIC DRUGS

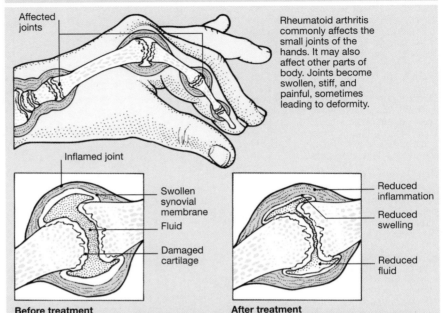

Rheumatoid arthritis commonly affects the small joints of the hands. It may also affect other parts of body. Joints become swollen, stiff, and painful, sometimes leading to deformity.

Affected joints

Inflamed joint

Swollen synovial membrane
Fluid
Damaged cartilage

Reduced inflammation
Reduced swelling
Reduced fluid

Before treatment
The synovial membrane surrounding the joint is inflamed and thickened, producing increased fluid within the joint. The surrounding tissue is inflamed and joint cartilage damaged.

After treatment
Treatment with antirheumatic drugs relieves pain, swelling, and inflammation. Damage to cartilage and bone may be halted so that further deformity is minimized.

How they work

It is not known precisely how most DMARDs stop or slow the disease process. Some may reduce the body's immune response, which is thought to be partly responsible for the disease (see also Immunosuppressant drugs, p.115). Monoclonal antibodies such as infliximab combine with a body protein known as tumour necrosis factor alpha (TNF), which is overactive in rheumatoid arthritis. By reducing the level of TNF activity, they can improve the arthritis. When effective, DMARDs prevent damage to the cartilage and bone, thereby reducing progressive deformity and disability. The effectiveness of each drug varies depending on individual response.

How they affect you

DMARDs are generally slow acting; it may be four to six months before any benefit is noticed. So, treatment with aspirin or other NSAIDs is usually continued until remission occurs. Prolonged treatment with DMARDs can markedly improve symptoms. Arthritic pain is relieved, joint mobility increased, and general symptoms of ill health fade. Side effects (which vary between individual drugs) may be noticed before beneficial effects, so patience is required. Regular monitoring of the kidneys, liver and bone marrow are needed. Severe adverse effects may require treatment to be abandoned.

SOME TYPES OF DISEASE-MODIFYING ANTIRHEUMATIC DRUG

Chloroquine was originally developed to treat malaria (see p.95). It and related drugs are less effective than penicillamine or gold. Since prolonged use may cause eye damage, regular eye checks are needed.

Immunosuppressants such as methotrexate (p.320) are given if other drugs do not provide relief and if rheumatoid arthritis is severe and disabling. Regular observation and blood tests must be carried out because these drugs can cause severe complications.

Sulfasalazine is used mainly for ulcerative colitis (p.70), but was originally introduced to treat mild to moderate rheumatoid arthritis. It slows the disease's progress in some cases and has a low risk of serious adverse effects.

Gold-based drugs are now seldom used but may be given orally or by injection. Side effects can include a rash and digestive disturbances. Gold may sometimes damage the kidneys, which recover on stopping treatment; regular urine tests are usually carried out. It can also suppress blood cell production in bone marrow, so periodic blood tests are also carried out.

Monoclonal antibodies such as infliximab (p.283) and adalimumab target a particular body protein responsible for rheumatoid arthritis. These drugs often cause allergy-type reactions, especially at the start of treatment. Infections, especially of the upper respiratory and urinary tracts, are common.

COMMON DRUGS

Immunosuppressants	DMARDs
Azathioprine ✳	Adalimumab
Ciclosporin ✳	Chloroquine ✳
Cyclophosphamide ✳	Etanercept ✳
Leflunomide	Hydroxychloroquine
Methotrexate ✳	Infliximab ✳
	Penicillamine
NSAIDs	Sodium
(see facing page)	aurothiomalate
	Sulfasalazine ✳
✳ See Part 3	

LOCALLY ACTING CORTICOSTEROIDS

The adrenal glands, which lie on the top of the kidneys, produce a number of important hormones. Among these are the corticosteroids, so named because they are made in the outer part (cortex) of the glands. The corticosteroids play an important role, influencing the immune system and regulating the carbohydrate and mineral metabolism of the body. A number of drugs that mimic the natural corticosteroids have been developed.

These drugs have many uses and are discussed in detail under Corticosteroids (p.99). This section concentrates on those corticosteroids injected into an affected site to treat joint disorders.

Why they are used

Corticosteroids given by injection are particularly useful for treating joint disorders – notably rheumatoid arthritis and osteoarthritis – when one or only a few joints are involved, and when pain and inflammation have not been relieved by other drugs. In such cases, it is possible to relieve symptoms by injecting each of the affected joints individually. Corticosteroids may also be injected to relieve pain and inflammation caused by strained or contracted muscles, ligaments, and/or tendons – for example, in frozen shoulder or tennis elbow. They may also be given for bursitis, tendinitis, or swelling that is compressing a nerve. Corticosteroid injections are sometimes used in order to relieve pain and stiffness sufficiently to permit physiotherapy.

How they work

Corticosteroid drugs have two important actions believed to account for their effectiveness. They block the production of prostaglandins – chemicals responsible for triggering inflammation and pain – and depress the accumulation and activity of the white blood cells that cause the inflammation (below). Injection of these drugs concentrates their effects at the site of the problem, thus giving the maximum benefit where it is most needed.

How they affect you

Corticosteroids usually produce dramatic relief from symptoms when the drug is injected into a joint. Often a single injection is sufficient to relieve pain and swelling, and to improve mobility. When used to treat muscle or tendon pain, they may not always be effective because it is difficult to position the needle so that the drug reaches the right spot. In some cases, repeated injections are necessary.

Because these drugs are concentrated in the affected area, rather than being dispersed in significant amounts in the body, the generalized adverse effects that sometimes occur when corticosteroids are taken by mouth are unlikely. Minor side effects, such as loss of skin pigment at the injection site, are uncommon. Occasionally, a temporary increase in pain (steroid flare) may occur. In such cases, rest, local application of ice, and analgesic medication may relieve the condition. Sterile injection technique is critically important.

COMMON INJECTION SITES

Corticosteroids are often injected into joints affected by osteo- and rheumatoid arthritis. Joints commonly treated in this way are knee, shoulder, and finger joints.

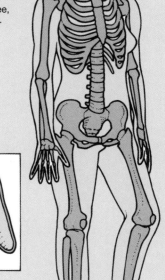

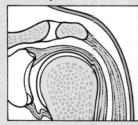
Shoulder joint

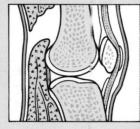
Knee joint

Finger joints

ACTION OF CORTICOSTEROIDS ON INFLAMED JOINTS

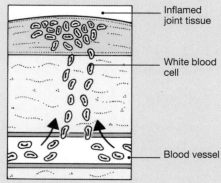

Inflamed joint tissue

White blood cell

Blood vessel

Inflamed tissue
Inflammation occurs when disease or injury causes large numbers of white blood cells to accumulate in the affected area. In joints this leads to swelling and stiffness.

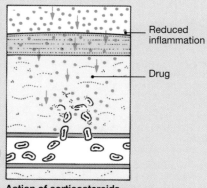

Reduced inflammation

Drug

Action of corticosteroids
Corticosteroids injected into the joint permeate the lining (synovial membrane), blocking prostaglandin production and preventing white blood cells accumulating.

COMMON DRUGS

Dexamethasone ✳   Prednisolone ✳
Hydrocortisone ✳   Triamcinolone
Methylprednisolone

✳ See Part 3

DRUGS FOR GOUT

Gout is a disorder that arises when the blood contains increased levels of uric acid, which is a by-product of normal body metabolism. When its concentration in the blood is excessive, uric acid crystals may form in various parts of the body, especially in the joints of the foot (most often the big toe), the knee, and the hand, causing intense pain and inflammation known as gout. Crystals may form as white masses, known as tophi, in soft tissue, and in the kidneys as stones. Attacks of gout can recur, and may lead to damaged joints and deformity, known as gouty arthritis. Kidney stones can cause kidney damage.

An excess of uric acid can be caused either by increased production or by decreased elimination by the kidneys, which normally remove it from the body. The disorder tends to run in families and is far more common in men than women. The risk of attack is increased by high alcohol intake, the consumption of certain foods (red meat, sardines, anchovies, yeast extract, and offal such as liver, brains, and sweetbreads), and obesity. An attack may be triggered by drugs such as thiazide diuretics (see p.57) or anticancer drugs (see p.112), or excessive intake of alcohol, especially beer. Changes in diet and a reduction in alcohol consumption may be important parts of treatment.

Drugs to treat acute attacks of gout include non-steroidal anti-inflammatory drugs (NSAIDs, see p.74), and colchicine. Other drugs, which lower the blood level of uric acid, are used for the long-term prevention of gout. These include uricosuric drugs (such as sulfinpyrazone) and allopurinol, the drug of choice. Aspirin is not prescribed for pain relief because it slows excretion of uric acid.

Why they are used

Drugs may be prescribed either to treat an attack of gout or to prevent recurrent attacks that could lead to deformity of affected joints and kidney damage. NSAIDs and colchicine are both used to treat an attack of gout and should be taken as soon as an attack begins. Because colchicine is relatively specific in relieving the pain and inflammation arising from gout, doctors sometimes administer it in order to confirm their diagnosis of the condition before prescribing an NSAID.

If symptoms recur, your doctor may advise long-term treatment with either allopurinol or a uricosuric drug. One of these drugs must usually be taken indefinitely. Since they can trigger attacks of gout at the beginning of treatment, colchicine is sometimes given with these drugs for a few months.

How they work

Allopurinol and febuxostat reduce the level of uric acid in the blood by interfering with the activity of xanthine oxidase, an enzyme involved in the production of uric acid in the body. Sulfinpyrazone increases the rate at which uric acid is excreted by the kidneys. The process by which colchicine reduces inflammation and relieves pain is poorly understood. The actions of NSAIDs are described on p.74.

How they affect you

Drugs used in the long-term treatment of gout are usually successful in preventing attacks and joint deformity. However, response may be slow.

Colchicine can disturb the digestive system, causing diarrhoea, in which case treatment is stopped.

Risks and special precautions

Since they increase the output of uric acid through the kidneys, uricosuric drugs can cause crystals of uric acid salts (urates) to form in the kidneys. They are not, therefore, usually prescribed for those people who already have impaired kidney function or urate stones. In such cases, allopurinol may be preferred. It is important to drink plenty of fluids while taking drugs for gout in order to prevent kidney crystals from forming. Regular blood tests to monitor levels of uric acid in the blood may be required.

ACTION OF URICOSURIC DRUGS

Uric acid is removed from the blood by the kidneys and excreted in the urine. Excess uric acid, caused by increased production or impaired kidney function, requires treatment with uricosuric drugs, which increase the rate at which uric acid is expelled.

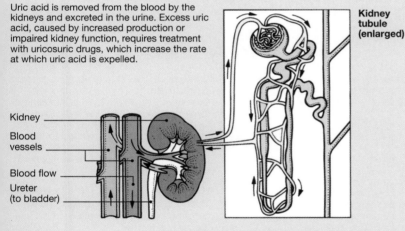

Kidney tubule (enlarged)

Kidney

Blood vessels

Blood flow

Ureter (to bladder)

Uric acid and gout
Gout occurs when uric acid crystals form in a joint, often a toe, knee, or hand, causing inflammation and pain. This is the result of excessively high levels of uric acid in the blood. In some cases this is caused by overproduction of uric acid, while in others it is the result of reduced excretion of uric acid by the kidneys.

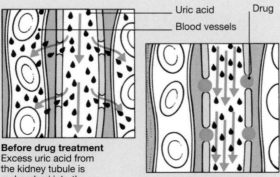

Uric acid

Blood vessels

Drug

Before drug treatment
Excess uric acid from the kidney tubule is reabsorbed into the surrounding blood vessels. This leads to the formation of uric acid crystals, which can cause gout.

After drug treatment
By blocking the reabsorption of uric acid into the blood vessels, the amount of uric acid excreted in the urine is increased.

COMMON DRUGS

Drugs to treat attacks
Colchicine *
NSAIDs (see p.74) (but not aspirin)

Drugs to treat high uric acid caused by cytotoxic drugs
Rasburicase

Drugs to prevent attacks
Allopurinol *
Febuxostat
Sulfinpyrazone

* See Part 3

MUSCLE RELAXANTS

Several drugs are available to treat muscle spasm – the involuntary, painful contraction of a muscle or a group of muscles that can stiffen an arm or leg, or make it nearly impossible to straighten your back. There are various causes. It can follow an injury, or come on without warning. It may also be brought on by a disorder like osteoarthritis, the pain in the affected joint triggering abnormal tension in a nearby muscle.

Spasticity is another form of muscle tightness seen in some neurological disorders, such as multiple sclerosis, stroke, or cerebral palsy. Spasticity can sometimes be helped by physiotherapy, but in severe cases drugs may be used to relieve symptoms.

Why they are used

Muscle spasm resulting from direct injury is usually treated with a non-steroidal anti-inflammatory drug (see p.74) or an analgesic (see p.36). However, if the spasm is severe, a muscle relaxant may also be tried for a short period.

In spasticity, the legs may become so stiff and uncontrollable that walking unaided is impossible. In such cases, a drug may be used to relax the muscles. Relaxation of the muscles often permits physiotherapy to be given for longer-term relief from spasms.

The muscle relaxant botulinum toxin may be injected locally to relieve muscle spasm in small groups of accessible muscles, such as those around the eye or in the neck.

How they work

Muscle-relaxant drugs work in one of several ways. The centrally acting drugs damp down the passage of the nerve signals from the brain and spinal cord that cause muscles to contract, thus reducing excessive stimulation of muscles as well as unwanted muscular contraction. Dantrolene reduces the sensitivity of the muscles to nerve signals. When

injected locally, botulinum toxin prevents transmission of impulses between nerves and muscles.

How they affect you

Drugs taken regularly for a spastic disorder of the central nervous system usually reduce stiffness and improve mobility. They may restore the use of the arms and legs when this has been impaired by muscle spasm.

Unfortunately, most centrally acting drugs can have a generally depressant effect on nervous activity and produce

drowsiness, particularly at the beginning of treatment. Too high a dosage can excessively reduce the muscles' ability to contract and can therefore cause weakness. For this reason, the dosage needs to be carefully adjusted to find a level that controls symptoms but which, at the same time, maintains sufficient muscle strength.

Risks and special precautions

The main long-term risk associated with centrally acting muscle relaxants is that the body becomes dependent. If the drugs are withdrawn suddenly, the stiffness may become worse than before drug treatment.

Rarely, dantrolene can cause serious liver damage. Anyone who is taking this drug should have their blood tested regularly to assess liver function.

Unless used very cautiously, botulinum toxin can paralyse unaffected muscles, and might interfere with functions such as speech and swallowing.

SITES OF ACTION OF MUSCLE RELAXANTS

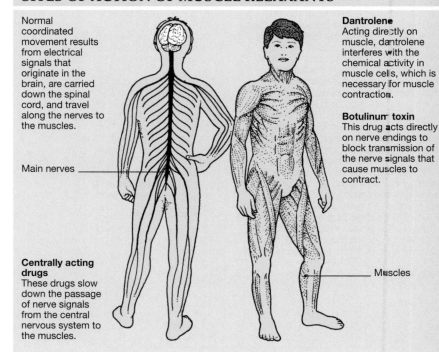

Normal coordinated movement results from electrical signals that originate in the brain, are carried down the spinal cord, and travel along the nerves to the muscles.

Main nerves

Centrally acting drugs
These drugs slow down the passage of nerve signals from the central nervous system to the muscles.

Dantrolene
Acting directly on muscle, dantrolene interferes with the chemical activity in muscle cells, which is necessary for muscle contraction.

Botulinum toxin
This drug acts directly on nerve endings to block transmission of the nerve signals that cause muscles to contract.

Muscles

ACTION OF CENTRALLY ACTING DRUGS

Centrally acting muscle relaxants restrict passage of nerve signals to the muscles by occupying a proportion of the receptors in the central nervous system that are normally used by neurotransmitters to transmit such impulses. Reduced nervous stimulation allows the muscles to relax; however, if the dose of the drug is too high, this action may give rise to excessive muscle weakness.

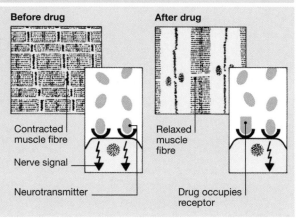

Before drug

Contracted muscle fibre

Nerve signal

Neurotransmitter

After drug

Relaxed muscle fibre

Drug occupies receptor

COMMON DRUGS

Centrally acting drugs	Other drugs
Baclofen *	Botulinum toxin *
Diazepam *	Dantrolene
Orphenadrine *	
Tizanidine	

* See Part 3

DRUGS USED FOR MYASTHENIA GRAVIS

Myasthenia gravis is a disorder that occurs when the immune system (see p.110) becomes defective and produces antibodies that disrupt the signals being transmitted between the nervous system and muscles that are under voluntary control. As a result, the body's muscular response is progressively weakened. The first muscles to be affected are those controlling the eyes, eyelids, face, pharynx, and larynx, with muscles in the arms and legs becoming involved as the disease progresses. The disease is often linked to a disorder of the thymus gland, which is the source of the destructive antibodies concerned.

Various methods can be used in the treatment of myasthenia gravis, including removal of the thymus gland (called a thymectomy) or temporarily clearing the blood of antibodies (a procedure known as plasmapheresis, or plasma exchange). Drugs that improve muscle function, principally neostigmine and pyridostigmine, may be prescribed. They may be used alone or together with other drugs that depress the immune system – usually azathioprine (see Immunosuppressant drugs, p.115) or corticosteroids (see p.99). Intravenous immunoglobulins may also be used in severe cases where there are breathing and swallowing problems.

Why they are used

Drugs that improve the muscle response to nerve impulses have several uses. One such drug, edrophonium, acts very quickly and, once administered intravenously, brings about a dramatic improvement in symptoms. This effect is used to confirm the diagnosis of myasthenia gravis. However, because of its short duration of action, edrophonium is not used for long-term treatment. Pyridostigmine and neostigmine are preferred for long-term treatment, especially when removal of the thymus gland is not feasible or does not provide adequate relief. These drugs may

be given to non-myasthenic patients after surgery to reverse the effects of a muscle-relaxant drug given as part of the general anaesthetic.

How they work

Normal muscle action occurs when a nerve impulse triggers a nerve ending to release a neurotransmitter, which combines with a specialized receptor on the muscle cells and causes the muscles to contract. In myasthenia gravis, the body's immune system destroys many of these receptors, so that the muscle is less responsive to nervous stimulation. Drugs used to treat the disorder increase the amount of neurotransmitter at the nerve ending by blocking the action of an

enzyme that normally breaks it down. Increased levels of the neurotransmitter permit the remaining receptors to function more efficiently (see Action of drugs used for myasthenia gravis, below).

How they affect you

These drugs usually restore the muscle function to a normal or near-normal level, particularly when the disease takes a mild form. Unfortunately, the drugs can produce unwanted muscular activity by enhancing the transmission of nerve impulses elsewhere in the body.

Common side effects include vomiting, nausea, diarrhoea, and muscle cramps in the arms, legs, and abdomen.

Risks and special precautions

Muscle weakness can suddenly worsen even when being treated with drugs. Should this occur, it is important not to take larger doses of the drug to try to relieve the symptoms, since excessive levels can interfere with transmission of nerve impulses to muscles, causing further weakness. Administration of other drugs, including some antibiotics, can also markedly increase the symptoms of myasthenia gravis. If your symptoms suddenly worsen, consult your doctor.

THE EFFECTS OF MYASTHENIA GRAVIS

Myasthenia gravis initially causes weakness of the muscles in the face and throat, affecting the muscles around the eyes and the mouth. In the later stages, arms and legs may be affected.

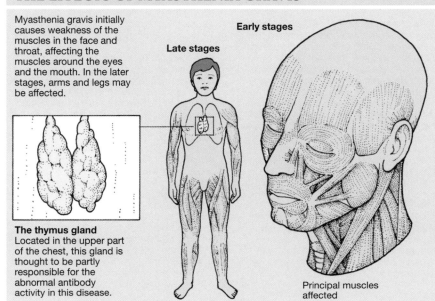

Late stages

Early stages

The thymus gland
Located in the upper part of the chest, this gland is thought to be partly responsible for the abnormal antibody activity in this disease.

Principal muscles affected

ACTION OF DRUGS USED FOR MYASTHENIA GRAVIS

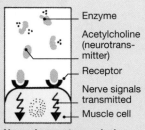

- Enzyme
- Acetylcholine (neurotransmitter)
- Receptor
- Nerve signals transmitted
- Muscle cell

Normal nerve transmission
Muscles contract when a neurotransmitter (acetylcholine) binds to receptors on muscle cells. An enzyme breaks down acetylcholine.

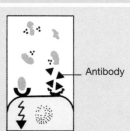

- Antibody

In myasthenia gravis
Abnormal antibody activity destroys many receptors, reducing stimulation of the muscle cells and weakening the muscle action.

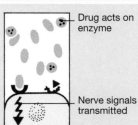

- Drug acts on enzyme
- Nerve signals transmitted

Drug action
Anticholinesterase drugs block enzyme action, increasing acetylcholine and prolonging the muscle cell response to nervous stimulation.

COMMON DRUGS

Azathioprine ✱	Neostigmine
Corticosteroids	Pyridostigmine ✱
(see p.99)	
Distigmine	✱ See Part 3
Edrophonium	

DRUGS FOR BONE DISORDERS

Bone is a living structure. Its hard, mineral quality is created by the action of the bone cells. These cells continuously deposit and remove phosphorus and calcium, stored in a honeycombed protein framework called the matrix. Because the rates of deposit and removal (the bone metabolism) are about equal in adults, the bone mass remains fairly constant.

Removal and renewal is regulated by hormones and influenced by a number of factors, notably the level of calcium in the blood, which depends on the intake of calcium and vitamin D from the diet, the actions of various hormones, plus everyday movement and weight-bearing stress. When normal bone metabolism is altered, various bone disorders result.

Osteoporosis

In osteoporosis, the strength and density of bone are reduced. Such wasting occurs when the rate of removal of mineralized bone exceeds the rate of deposit. In most people, bone density decreases very gradually from the age of 30. But bone loss can dramatically increase when a person is immobilized for a period, and this is an important cause of osteoporosis in older people. Hormone deficiency is another important cause, commonly occurring in women with lowered oestrogen levels after the menopause or removal of the ovaries. Osteoporosis also occurs in disorders in which there is excess production of adrenal or thyroid hormones. In addition, osteoporosis can result from long-term treatment with corticosteroid drugs.

People with osteoporosis often have no symptoms but, if the vertebrae become so weakened that they are unable to bear the body's weight, they may collapse spontaneously or after a minor accident. Subsequently, the affected person develops back pain, reduced height, and a round-shouldered appearance. Osteoporosis also makes a fracture of an arm, leg, or hip more likely.

Most doctors emphasize the need to prevent the disorder by an adequate intake of protein and calcium and by regular exercise throughout adult life. Oestrogen supplements are no longer usually recommended to prevent osteoporosis.

The condition of bones damaged by osteoporosis cannot usually be improved, although drug treatment can help prevent further deterioration and help fractures to heal. For people whose diet is deficient in calcium or vitamin D, supplements may be prescribed. However, these are of limited value and are often less useful than drugs that inhibit removal of calcium from the bones. In the past, the hormone calcitonin was used, but it has now been largely superseded by drugs such as alendronate. These drugs, known as bisphosphonates, bind very tightly to the bone matrix, preventing its removal by bone cells.

Osteomalacia and rickets

In osteomalacia (called rickets when it affects children) lack of vitamin D leads to loss of calcium, resulting in softening of the bones. There is pain and tenderness and a risk of fracture and bone deformity. In children, growth is retarded.

Osteomalacia is most commonly caused by a lack of vitamin D. This can result from an inadequate diet, inability to absorb the vitamin, or insufficient exposure of the skin to sunlight (the action of the sun on the skin produces vitamin D inside the body). Individuals at special risk include those whose absorption of vitamin D is impaired by an intestinal disorder, like Crohn's disease or coeliac disease. People with dark skins living in northern Europe or North America are also susceptible. Chronic kidney disease is an important cause of rickets in children and osteomalacia in adults, since healthy kidneys play an essential role in the body's metabolism of vitamin D.

Long-term relief depends on treating the underlying disorder where possible. In rare cases, treatment may be lifelong.

Vitamin D

A number of substances that are related to vitamin D may be used in the treatment of bone disorders. These drugs include alfacalcidol, calcitriol, and ergocalciferol. The one prescribed depends on the underlying problem (see also p.444).

BONE WASTING

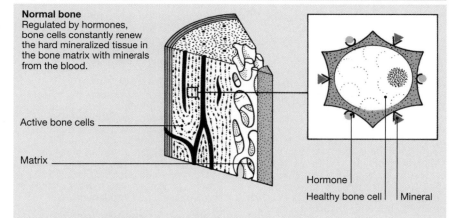

Normal bone
Regulated by hormones, bone cells constantly renew the hard mineralized tissue in the bone matrix with minerals from the blood.

Active bone cells

Matrix

Hormone

Healthy bone cell   Mineral

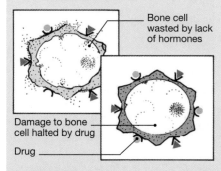

Bone cell wasted by lack of hormones

Damage to bone cell halted by drug

Drug

In osteoporosis
Hormonal disturbance leads to wasting of active bone cells. The bones become less dense and more fragile. Treatment with drugs such as bisphosphonates or, rarely, HRT usually only prevents further bone loss.

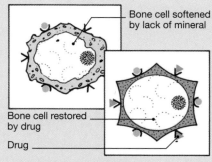

Bone cell softened by lack of mineral

Bone cell restored by drug

Drug

In osteomalacia
Deficiency of calcium or vitamin D causes softening of the bone tissue. The bones become weaker and sometimes deformed. Drug treatment with vitamin D and minerals usually restores bone stregth.

COMMON DRUGS

Alendronic acid ✱	Ergocalciferol
Alfacalcidol	Fluorice
Calcitonin	Pamidronate
Calcitriol	Risedronate ✱
Calcium carbonate	Salcatonin (salmon
Conjugated	calcitonin)
oestrogens ✱	Strontium ranelate ✱
	Teriparatide
	Vitamin D ✱

✱ See Part 3

ALLERGY

Allergy, which is a hypersensitivity to certain substances, is a extreme reaction of the body's immune system. Through a variety of mechanisms (see Malignant and immune disease, p.110), the immune system protects the body by eliminating foreign substances that it does not recognize, such as microorganisms (bacteria or viruses).

One way in which the immune system acts is through the production of antibodies. When the body encounters a particular foreign substance (or allergen) for the first time, one type of white blood cell, the lymphocyte, produces antibodies that attach themselves to another type of white blood cell, the mast cell. If the same substance is encountered again, the allergen binds to the antibodies on the mast cells, causing the release of chemicals known as mediators.

The most important mediator is histamine. This can produce a rash, swelling, narrowing of the airways, and a drop in blood pressure. Although these effects are important in protecting the body against infection, they may also be triggered inappropriately in an allergic reaction.

What can go wrong

One of the most common allergic disorders, hay fever, is caused by an allergic reaction to inhaled pollen leading to allergic rhinitis – swelling and irritation of the nasal passages and watering of the nose and eyes. Other substances, such as house-dust mites, animal fur, and feathers, may cause a similar reaction in susceptible people.

Asthma, another allergic disorder, may result from the action of leukotrienes rather than histamine. Other allergic conditions include urticaria (hives) or other rashes (sometimes in response to a drug), some forms of eczema and dermatitis, and allergic alveolitis (farmer's lung). Anaphylaxis is a serious systemic allergic reaction (p.520) that occurs when an allergen reaches the bloodstream.

Why drugs are used

Antihistamines and drugs that inhibit mast cell activity are used to prevent and treat allergic reactions. Other drugs minimize allergic symptoms, such as decongestants (p.51) to clear the nose in allergic rhinitis, bronchodilators (p.48) to widen the airways of those with asthma, and corticosteroids applied to skin affected by eczema (p.139).

MAJOR DRUG GROUPS

Antihistamines	Corticosteroids (see p.99)
Leukotriene antagonists	Drugs for asthma (see p.49)

Allergic response
Lymphocytes produce antibodies to allergens and these attach to mast cells. If the allergen enters the body again, it binds to the antibodies, and the mast cells release histamine.

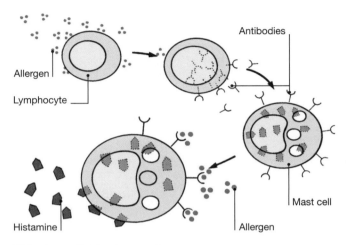

Allergen
Lymphocyte
Antibodies
Mast cell
Histamine
Allergen

Histamine and histamine receptors
Histamine, released in response to injury or the presence of allergens, acts on H_1 receptors in the skin, blood vessels, nasal passages, and airways, and on H_2 receptors in the stomach lining, salivary glands, and lacrimal (tear) glands. It provokes dilation of blood vessels, inflammation and swelling of tissues, and narrowing of the airways.

In some cases a reaction called anaphylactic shock may occur, caused by a dramatic fall in blood pressure, which may lead to collapse. Antihistamine drugs block the H_1 receptors, and H_2 blockers block the H_2 receptors (see also Antihistamines, p.82, and Anti-ulcer drugs, p.67).

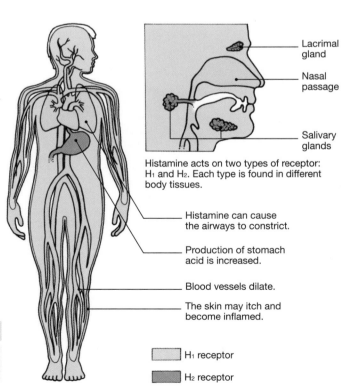

Lacrimal gland
Nasal passage
Salivary glands

Histamine acts on two types of receptor: H_1 and H_2. Each type is found in different body tissues.

Histamine can cause the airways to constrict.

Production of stomach acid is increased.

Blood vessels dilate.

The skin may itch and become inflamed.

H_1 receptor

H_2 receptor

ANTIHISTAMINES

Antihistamines are the most widely used drugs in the treatment of allergic reactions of all kinds. They can be subdivided according to their chemical structure, each subgroup having slightly different actions and characteristics (see table on facing page). Their main action is to counter the effects of histamine, one of the chemicals released in the body when there is an allergic reaction. (For a full explanation of the allergy mechanism, see p.81.)

Histamine is also involved in other body functions, including blood vessel dilation and constriction, contraction of muscles in the respiratory and gastrointestinal tracts, and the release of digestive juices in the stomach. The antihistamine drugs described here are also known as H₁ blockers because they only block the action of histamine on certain receptors, known as H₁ receptors. Another group of antihistamines, known as H₂ blockers, is used in the treatment of peptic ulcers (see Anti-ulcer drugs, p.67).

Some antihistamines have a significant anticholinergic action. This is used to advantage in a variety of conditions, but it also accounts for certain undesired side effects.

Why they are used

Antihistamines relieve allergy-related symptoms when it is not possible or practical to prevent exposure to the substance that has provoked the reaction. They are most commonly used in the prevention of allergic rhinitis (hay fever), the inflammation of the nose and upper airways that results from an allergic reaction to a substance such as pollen, house dust, or animal fur. Antihistamines are more effective when taken before the start of an attack. If they are taken only after an attack has begun, beneficial effects may be delayed.

Antihistamines are not usually effective in asthma caused by similar allergens because the symptoms of this allergic disorder are not solely caused by the action of histamine, but are likely to be the result of more complex mechanisms. Antihistamines are usually the first drugs to be tried in the treatment of allergic disorders, but there are alternatives that can be prescribed (see below).

Antihistamines are also prescribed to relieve the itching, swelling, and redness that are characteristic of allergic reactions involving the skin – for example, urticaria (hives), infantile eczema, and other forms of dermatitis. Irritation from chickenpox may be reduced by these drugs. Allergic reactions to insect stings may also be reduced by antihistamines. In such cases the drug may be taken by mouth or applied topically. Applied as drops, antihistamines can reduce inflammation and irritation of the eyes and eyelids in allergic conjunctivitis.

An antihistamine is often included as an ingredient in cough and cold preparations (see p.52), when the anticholinergic effect of drying mucus secretions and their sedative effect on the coughing mechanism may be helpful.

Because most antihistamines have a depressant effect on the brain, they are sometimes used to promote sleep, especially when discomfort from itching is disturbing sleep (see also Sleeping drugs, p.38). The depressant effect of antihistamines on the brain also extends to the centres that control nausea and vomiting. Antihistamines are therefore often effective for preventing and controlling these symptoms (see Anti-emetics, p.46).

Occasionally, antihistamines are used to treat fever, rash, and breathing difficulties that may occur in adverse reactions to blood transfusions and allergic reactions to drugs. Promethazine and alimemazine may also be used as premedication to provide sedation and to dry secretions during surgery, particularly in children.

How they work

Antihistamines block the action of histamine on H₁ receptors. These are found in various body tissues,

SITES OF ACTION

Antihistamines act on a variety of sites and systems throughout the body. Their main action is on the muscles surrounding the small blood vessels that supply the skin and mucous membranes. They also act on the airways in the lungs and on the brain.

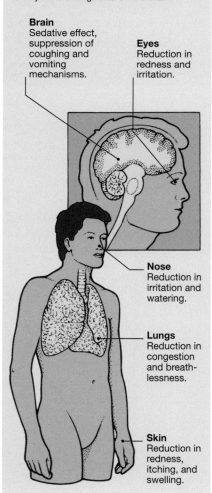

Brain
Sedative effect, suppression of coughing and vomiting mechanisms.

Eyes
Reduction in redness and irritation.

Nose
Reduction in irritation and watering.

Lungs
Reduction in congestion and breathlessness.

Skin
Reduction in redness, itching, and swelling.

OTHER ALLERGY TREATMENTS

Sodium cromoglicate
This drug (p.397) prevents the release of histamine from mast cells (see p.81) in response to exposure to an allergen, thus preventing the physical symptoms of allergies. It is commonly given by inhaler for the prevention of allergy-induced rhinitis (hay fever) or asthma attacks and by drops for the treatment of allergic eye disorders.

Leukotriene antagonists
Like histamines, leukotrienes are substances that occur naturally in the body and seem to play an important part in asthma. Drugs such as montelukast (p.333) and zafirlukast, known as leukotriene antagonists, have been developed to prevent asthma attacks. They are not bronchodilators and will not relieve an existing attack (see Drugs for asthma, p.50).

Corticosteroids
These drugs (p.99) are used to treat allergic rhinitis and asthma. They are given by inhaler, which supplies much lower doses than tablets.

Desensitization
This may be tried in conditions such as allergic rhinitis due to pollen sensitivity and insect venom hypersensitivity, when avoidance, antihistamines, and other treatments have not been effective and tests have shown one or two specific allergens to be responsible. Desensitization often provides incomplete relief and can be time consuming.

Treatment involves giving a series of injections containing gradually increasing doses of an extract of the allergen. The way in which this prevents allergic reactions is poorly understood. Perhaps controlled exposure triggers the immune system into producing increasing levels of antibodies so that the body no longer responds dramatically when the allergen is encountered naturally.

Desensitization must be carried out under medical supervision because it can provoke a severe allergic response. It is important to remain near emergency medical facilities for at least one hour after each injection.

COMPARISON OF ANTIHISTAMINES

Although antihistamines have broadly similar effects and uses, differences in their strength of anticholinergic action and the amount of drowsiness they produce, as well as in their duration of action, affect the uses for which each drug is commonly selected. The table indicates the main uses of some of the common antihistamines and gives an indication of the relative strengths of their anticholinergic and sedative effects and of their duration of action.

- ● Drug used
- ■ Strong
- ◣ Medium
- □ Minimal
- ▲ Long (over 12 hours)
- ◭ Medium (6–12 hours)
- △ Short (4–6 hours)

Drugs	Common uses / Allergic rhinitis	Skin allergy	Sedation	Premedication	Nausea/vomiting	Cough/cold remedies	Actions and effects / Drowsiness	Anticholinergic action	Duration of action
Alimemazine		●	●	●			■	□	◭
Acrivastine	●	●					□	◣	△
Cetirizine	●	●					□	□	▲
Chlorphenamine	●	●	●			●	◣	◣	△
Cyclizine					●		◣	◣	◭
Diphenhydramine			●		●	●	◣	◣	△
Hydroxyzine		●	●				■	◣	▲
Loratadine	●	●					□	□	▲
Promethazine	●	●	●	●	●		■	◣	◭

particularly the small blood vessels in the skin, nose, and eyes. This helps prevent the dilation of the vessels, thus reducing the redness, watering, and swelling. In addition, the anticholinergic action of these drugs contributes to this effect by reducing the secretions from tear glands and nasal passages.

Antihistamine drugs pass from the blood into the brain. In the brain, the blocking action of the antihistamines on histamine activity may produce general sedation and depression of various brain functions, including the vomiting and coughing mechanisms.

How they affect you

Antihistamines frequently cause a degree of drowsiness and may adversely affect coordination, leading to clumsiness. Some of the newer drugs have little or no sedative effect (see table above).

Anticholinergic side effects, including dry mouth, blurred vision, and difficulty passing urine, are common. Most side effects diminish with continued use and can often be helped by an adjustment in dosage or a change to a different drug.

Risks and special precautions

It may be advisable to avoid driving or operating machinery while taking antihistamines, particularly those that are more likely to cause drowsiness (see table above). The sedative effects of alcohol, sleeping drugs, opioid analgesics, and anti-anxiety drugs can also be increased by antihistamines.

In high doses, or in children, some antihistamines can cause excitement, agitation, and even, in extreme cases, hallucinations and seizures. Abnormal heart rhythms have occurred after high doses with some antihistamines (mostly now discontinued) or when drugs that interact with them, such as antifungals and antibiotics, have been taken at the same time. Heart rhythm problems may also affect people with liver disease, electrolyte disturbances, or abnormal heart activity. A person who has these conditions, or who has glaucoma or prostate trouble, should seek medical advice before taking antihistamines because their various drug actions may make such conditions worse.

ANTIHISTAMINES AND ALLERGIC RHINITIS

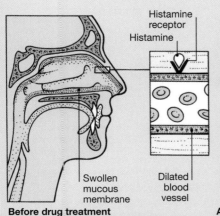

Histamine receptor
Histamine

Swollen mucous membrane | Dilated blood vessel

Before drug treatment
In allergic rhinitis, histamine released in response to an allergen acts on histamine receptors and produces dilation of the blood vessels supplying the lining of the nose, leading to swelling and increased mucus production. There is also irritation that causes sneezing, and often redness and watering of the eyes.

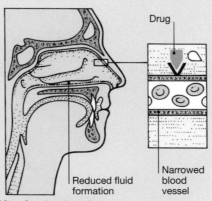

Drug

Reduced fluid formation | Narrowed blood vessel

After drug treatment
Antihistamine drugs prevent histamine from attaching to histamine receptors, thereby preventing the body from responding to allergens. Over a period of time, the swelling, irritation, sneezing, and watery discharge are reduced, and further contact with the allergen responsible usually produces only minor allergic symptoms.

COMMON DRUGS

Non-sedating
Acrivastine
Cetirizine ✱
Fexofenadine
Levocetirizine
Loratadine/
   Desloratadine ✱
Mizolastine

Sedating
Alimemazine
Chlorphenamine ✱
Cinnarizine ✱
Clemastine
Diphenhydramine
Hydroxyzine
Promethazine ✱

✱ See Part 3

INFECTIONS AND INFESTATIONS

The human body provides a suitable environment for the growth of many types of microorganism, including bacteria, viruses, fungi, yeasts, and protozoa. It may also become the host for animal parasites such as insects, worms, and flukes.

Microorganisms (microbes) exist all around us and can be transmitted from person to person in many ways: direct contact, inhalation of infected air, and consumption of contaminated food or water (see Transmission of infection, facing page). Not all microorganisms cause disease; many types of bacteria exist on the skin surface or in the bowel without causing ill effects, while others cannot live either in or on the body.

Normally the immune system protects the body from infection. Invading microbes are killed before they can multiply in sufficient numbers to cause serious disease. (See also Malignant and immune disease, p.110.)

What can go wrong

Infectious diseases occur when the body is invaded by microbes. This may be caused by the body having little or no natural immunity to the invading organism, or the number of invading microbes being too great for the body's immune system to overcome. Serious infections can occur when the immune system does not function properly or when a disease weakens or destroys the immune system, as occurs in AIDS (acquired immune deficiency syndrome).

Infections (such as childhood infectious diseases or those with flu-like symptoms) can cause generalized illness, or they may affect a specific part of the body (as in wound infections). Some parts are more susceptible to infection than others – respiratory tract infections are relatively common, whereas bone and muscle infections are rare.

Some symptoms are the result of damage to body tissues by the infection, or by toxins released by the microbes. In other cases, the symptoms result from the body's defence mechanisms.

Most bacterial and viral infections cause fever. Bacterial infections may also cause inflammation and pus formation in the affected area.

Why drugs are used

Treatment of an infection is necessary only when the type or severity of symptoms shows that the immune system has not overcome the infection.

Bacterial infection can be treated with antibiotic or antibacterial drugs. Some of these drugs actually kill the infecting bacteria, whereas others merely prevent them from multiplying.

Types of infecting organism

Bacteria

A typical bacterium (right) consists of a single cell that has a protective wall. Some bacteria are aerobic – that is, they require oxygen – and therefore are more likely to infect surface areas such as the skin or respiratory tract. Others are anaerobic and multiply in oxygen-free surroundings such as the bowel or deep puncture wounds.

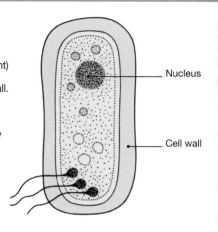

Nucleus

Cell wall

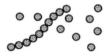

Cocci (spherical)
Streptococcus (above) can cause sore throats and pneumonia.

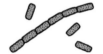

Bacilli (rod-shaped)
Mycobacterium tuberculosis (above) causes tuberculosis.

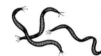

Spirochaete (spiral-shaped)
This group includes bacteria that cause syphilis and gum infections.

Viruses

These infectious agents are smaller than bacteria and consist simply of a core of genetic material surrounded by a protein coat. A virus can multiply only in a living cell, by using the host tissue's replicating material.

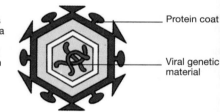

Protein coat

Viral genetic material

Protozoa

These single-celled parasites are slightly bigger than bacteria. Many protozoa live in the human intestine and are harmless. However, some types cause malaria, sleeping sickness, and dysentery.

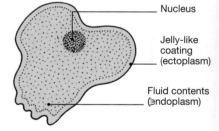

Nucleus

Jelly-like coating (ectoplasm)

Fluid contents (endoplasm)

Unnecessary use of antibiotics may result in the development of resistant bacteria (see p.86).

Some antibiotics can be used to treat a broad range of infections, while others are effective against a particular type of bacterium or in a certain part of the body. Antibiotics are most commonly given by mouth, or by injection in severe infections, but they may be applied topically for a local action.

Antiviral drugs are used for severe viral infections that threaten body organs or survival. Antivirals may

How bacteria affect the body

Bacteria can cause symptoms of disease in two principal ways: first, by releasing toxins that harm body cells; second, by provoking an inflammatory response in the infected tissues.

Effects of toxins

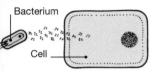

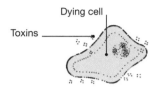

The invading bacterium gives off poisons (toxins) that attack the body cell.

The toxins emanating from the bacterium break through the cell structure and destroy the cell.

Inflammatory response

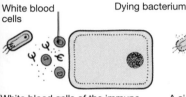

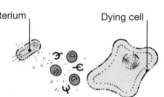

White blood cells of the immune system attack the bacterium directly by releasing inflammatory substances and, later, antibodies.

A side effect of this attack of the immune system on the bacterium is damage to, and inflammation of, the body's own cells.

Transmission of infection

Infecting organisms can enter the human body through a variety of routes, including direct contact between an infected person and someone else and eating or inhaling infected material.

Droplet infection
Coughing and sneezing spread infected secretions.

Insects
Insect bites may transmit infection.

Physical contact
Everyday contact may spread infection.

Sexual contact
Certain infections and infestations may be spread by genital contact.

Food
Many infecting organisms can be ingested in food.

Water
Infections can be spread in polluted water.

be used in topical preparations, given by mouth, or administered by injection, usually in hospital.

Other drugs used in the fight against infection include antiprotozoal drugs for protozoal infections such as malaria; antifungal drugs for infection by fungi and yeasts, including *Candida* (thrush); and anthelmintics to eradicate worm and fluke infestations. Cases of infestation by skin parasites are usually treated with the topical application of insecticides (see p.136).

INFESTATIONS

Invasion by parasites that live on the body (such as lice) or in the body (such as tapeworms) is known as infestation. Since the body lacks strong natural defences against infestation, antiparasitic treatment is necessary. Infestations are often associated with tropical climates and poor standards of hygiene.

Tapeworms and roundworms live in the intestines and may cause diarrhoea and anaemia. Roundworm eggs may be passed in faeces. Hookworm larvae in infected soil usually enter the body through the skin. Tapeworms may grow to 9m (30 feet) and infection occurs through undercooked meat containing larvae.

Flukes are of various types. The liver fluke (acquired from infected vegetation) lives near the bile duct in the liver and can cause jaundice. A more serious type (which lives in small blood vessels supplying the bladder or intestines) causes schistosomiasis and is acquired from contact with infected water.

Lice and scabies spread by direct contact. Head, clothing, and pubic lice need human blood to survive and die away from the body. Dried faeces of clothing lice spread typhus by infecting wounds or being inhaled. Scabies (caused by a tiny mite that does not carry disease) makes small, itchy tunnels in the skin.

Life cycle of a roundworm

Many roundworms have a complex life cycle. The life cycle of the roundworm that causes the group of diseases known as filariasis is illustrated below.

A mosquito ingests the filarial larvae and bites a human, thereby transmitting the larvae.

The mature larvae enter the lymph glands and vessels and reproduce there, often causing no ill effects.

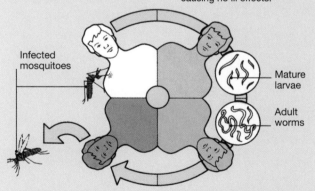

Infected mosquitoes

Mature larvae

Adult worms

The infestation is spread by mosquitoes biting infected people and restarting the cycle.

The larvae grow into adult worms, which release larvae into the bloodstream.

MAJOR DRUG GROUPS

Antibiotics
Antibacterial drugs
Antituberculous drugs
Antiviral drugs
Vaccines and immunization

Antiprotozoal drugs
Antimalarial drugs
Antifungal drugs
Anthelmintic drugs

ANTIBIOTICS

One out of every six prescriptions that British doctors write every year is for antibiotics. These drugs are usually safe and effective in the treatment of bacterial disorders ranging from minor infections, like conjunctivitis, to life-threatening diseases like pneumonia, meningitis, and septicaemia. They are similar in function to the antibacterial drugs (see p.89), but the early antibiotics all had a natural origin in moulds and fungi, although most are now synthesized.

Since the 1940s, when penicillin was introduced, many different classes of antibiotic have been developed. Each one has a different chemical composition and is effective against a particular range of bacteria. None is effective against viral infections (see Antiviral drugs, p.91).

Some of the antibiotics have a broad spectrum of activity against a wide variety of bacteria. Others are used in the treatment of infection by only a few specific organisms. For a description of each common class of antibiotic, see Classes of antibiotics, p.88.

Why they are used

We are surrounded by bacteria – in the air we breathe, on the mucous membranes of our mouth and nose, on our skin, and in our intestines – but we are protected, most of the time, by our immunological defences. When these break down, or when bacteria already present migrate to a vulnerable new site, or when harmful

ANTIBIOTIC RESISTANCE

The increasing use of antibiotics in the treatment of infection has led to resistance in certain types of bacteria to the effects of particular antibiotics. This resistance to the drug usually occurs when bacteria develop mechanisms of growth and reproduction that are not disrupted by the effects of the antibiotics. In other cases, bacteria produce enzymes that neutralize the antibiotics.

Antibiotic resistance may develop in a person during prolonged treatment when a drug has failed to eliminate the infection quickly. The resistant strain of bacteria is able to multiply, thereby prolonging the illness.

It may also infect other people, and result in the spread of resistant infection. One particularly important example is methicillin-resistant *Staphylococcus aureus*, which resists most antibiotics but can be treated with other drugs such as teicoplanin and vancomycin.

Doctors try to prevent the development of antibiotic resistance by selecting the drug most likely to eliminate the bacteria present in each individual case as quickly and as thoroughly as possible. Failure to complete a course of antibiotics that has been prescribed by your doctor increases the likelihood that the infection will recur in a resistant form.

bacteria not usually present invade the body, infectious disease sets in.

The bacteria multiply uncontrollably, destroying tissue, releasing toxins, and, in some cases, threatening to spread via the bloodstream to such vital organs as the heart, brain, lungs, and kidneys. The symptoms of infectious disease vary widely, depending on the site of the infection and the type of bacteria.

Confronted with a sick person and suspecting a bacterial infection, the doctor will need to identify the organism causing the disease before prescribing any drug. However, tests to analyse blood, sputum, urine, stool, or pus usually take 24 hours or more. In the meantime, especially if the person is in discomfort

or pain, the doctor usually makes a preliminary drug choice, something of an educated guess as to the causative organism. In starting this empirical treatment, as it is called, the doctor is guided by the site of the infection, the nature and severity of the symptoms, the likely source of infection, and the prevalence of any similar illnesses in the community at that time.

In such circumstances, pending laboratory identification of the trouble-making bacteria, the doctor may initially prescribe a broad-spectrum antibiotic, which is effective against a wide variety of bacteria. As soon as tests provide more exact information, the doctor may switch the person to the recommended antibiotic treatment for the identified bacteria. In some cases, more than one antibiotic is prescribed, to be sure of eliminating all strains of bacteria.

In most cases, antibiotics can be given by mouth. However, in serious infections when high blood levels of the drug are needed rapidly, or when a type of antibiotic is needed that cannot be given by mouth, the drug may be given by injection. Antibiotics are also included in topical preparations for localized skin, eye, and ear infections (see also Anti-infective skin preparations, p.135, and Drugs for ear disorders, p.131).

How they work

Depending on the type of drug and the dosage, antibiotics are either bactericidal, killing organisms directly, or bacteriostatic, halting the multiplication of bacteria and enabling the body's natural defences to overcome the remaining infection.

Penicillins and cephalosporins are bactericidal, destroying bacteria by preventing them from making normal cell walls; most other antibiotics act inside the bacteria by interfering with the chemical activities essential to their life cycle.

How they affect you

Antibiotics stop most common types of infection within days. Because they do not relieve symptoms directly, your doctor

ACTION OF ANTIBIOTICS

Penicillins and cephalosporins
Drugs from these groups are bactericidal – that is, they kill growing or dividing bacteria. They interfere with the chemicals needed by bacteria to form normal cell walls (right). The cell's outer lining disintegrates and the bacterium dies (far right).

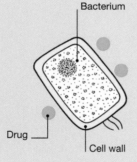

Bacterium

Drug

Cell wall

Disintegrating cell wall

Other antibiotics
These drugs alter chemical activity inside the bacteria, thereby preventing the production of proteins that the bacteria need to multiply and survive (right). This may have a bactericidal effect in itself, or it may have bacteriostatic action, preventing reproduction (far right).

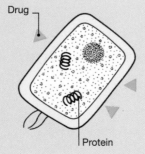

Drug

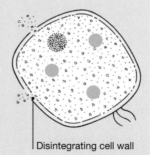

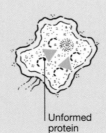

Protein

Unformed protein

USES OF ANTIBIOTICS

The table below shows which common drugs in each class of antibiotic are used for the treatment of infections in different parts of the body. For the purposes of comparison, this table also includes (in the Other drugs category) some antibacterial drugs that are discussed on page 89. This table is not intended to be used as a guide to prescribing but indicates the possible applications of each drug. Some drugs have a wide range of possible uses; this table concentrates on the most common ones.

Antibiotic / Site of infection	Ear, nose, throat, and mouth	Respiratory tract	Skin and soft tissue	Gastrointestinal tract	Eye	Kidney and urinary tract	Brain and nervous system	Heart and blood	Bones and joints	Genital tract
Penicillins										
Amoxicillin	●	●	●			●		●	●	
Ampicillin	●	●	●			●	●		●	
Benzylpenicillin	●	●	●				●	●		●
Co-amoxiclav	●	●	●			●				
Flucloxacillin	●	●						●	●	
Phenoxymethylpenicillin	●	●	●							
Cephalosporins										
Cefaclor	●	●				●				
Cefalexin		●	●			●				
Cefotaxime		●		●			●	●		
Macrolides										
Azithromycin	●	●	●							●
Clarithromycin	●	●	●	●						
Erythromycin	●	●	●	●	●				●	●
Tetracyclines										
Doxycycline	●	●	●			●				●
Oxytetracycline	●	●	●							
Tetracycline	●	●	●		●	●				●
Aminoglycosides										
Amikacin		●	●	●		●	●		●	
Gentamicin		●	●	●	●	●	●	●	●	
Neomycin			●	●						
Streptomycin		●						●		
Tobramycin		●	●	●		●	●		●	
Sulfonamide										
Co-trimoxazole		●				●				
Other drugs										
Chloramphenicol	●				●		●			
Ciprofloxacin		●		●	●	●				●
Clindamycin		●	●	●					●	
Colistin		●								
Dapsone		●								
Fusidic acid		●			●			●	●	
Levofloxacin	●	●	●			●				
Linezolid		●	●							
Metronidazole	●		●	●				●	●	●
Nalidixic acid						●				
Nitrofurantoin						●				
Teicoplanin			●					●	●	
Trimethoprim						●				
Vancomycin			●					●	●	

ANTIBIOTICS continued

may advise additional medication, such as analgesics (see p.36), to relieve pain and fever until the antibiotics take effect.

It is important to complete the course of medication as it has been prescribed, even if all your symptoms have disappeared. Failure to do this can lead to a resurgence of the infection in an antibiotic-resistant form (see Antibiotic resistance, p.86).

Most antibiotics used in the home do not cause any adverse effects if taken in the recommended dosage. In people who do experience adverse effects, nausea and diarrhoea are among the more common ones. Some people may be hypersensitive to certain types of antibiotic, which can result in a variety of serious adverse effects.

DRUG TREATMENT FOR MENINGITIS

Meningitis is inflammation of the meninges (the membranes surrounding the brain and spinal cord) and is caused by both bacteria and viruses. Bacterial meningitis can kill previously well individuals within hours.

If bacterial meningitis is suspected, intravenous antibiotics are needed immediately and admission to hospital is arranged. In cases of bacterial meningitis caused by *Haemophilus influenzae* or *Neisseria meningitidis*, close contacts of these patients are advised to have a preventative course of antibiotics, usually rifampicin or ciprofloxacin.

Risks and special precautions

Most antibiotics used for short periods outside a hospital setting are safe for most people. The most common risk, particularly with cephalosporins and penicillins, is an allergic reaction that causes a rash. Very rarely, the reaction may be severe, causing swelling of the throat and face, breathing difficulty, and circulatory collapse – a potentially fatal condition called anaphylactic shock. If you have an allergic reaction, the drug should be stopped and immediate medical advice sought. If you have had a previous allergic reaction to an antibiotic, all other drugs in that class and related classes should be avoided. It is therefore important to inform your doctor if you have previously had an adverse reaction to an antibiotic (with the exception of minor bowel disturbances).

Another risk of antibiotic treatment, especially if it is prolonged, is that the balance among microorganisms normally inhabiting the body may be disturbed. In particular, antibiotics may destroy the bacteria that normally limit the growth of *Candida*, a yeast that is often present in the body in small amounts. This can lead to overgrowth of *Candida* (thrush) in the mouth, vagina, or bowel, and an antifungal drug (p.96) may be needed.

A rarer, but more serious, result of disruption of normal bacterial activity in the body is a disorder known as pseudomembranous colitis, in which bacteria (called *Clostridium difficile*)

resistant to the antibiotic multiply in the bowel, causing violent, bloody diarrhoea. This potentially fatal disorder can occur with any antibiotic, but is most common with cephalosporins and clindamycin.

COMMON DRUGS

Aminoglycosides
Amikacin
Gentamicin *
Neomycin
Streptomycin
Tobramycin

Cephalosporins
Cefaclor
Cefadroxil
Cefalexin *
Cefixime
Cefpodoxime
Ceftazidime

Tetracyclines
Doxycycline *
Minocycline *
Oxytetracycline
Tetracycline/
lymecycline *

Macrolides
Azithromycin
Clarithromycin *
Erythromycin *

Penicillins
Amoxicillin/
co-amoxiclav *
Benzylpenicillin
Co-fluampicil
Flucloxacillin *
Phenoxymethyl-
penicillin *
Piperacillin/
tazobactam

Lincosamides
Clindamycin *

Other drugs
Aztreonam
Chloramphenicol *
Ciprofloxacin *
Colistin
Fusidic acid
Imipenem
Levofloxacin *
Linezolic
Metronidazole *
Rifampicin *
Teicoplanin
Trimethoprim *
Vancomycin

* See Part 3

CLASSES OF ANTIBIOTIC

Penicillins First introduced in the 1940s, penicillins are still widely used to treat many common infections. Some penicillins are not effective when they are taken by mouth and therefore have to be given by injection, usually in hospital. Unfortunately, certain strains of bacteria are resistant to penicillin treatment, and other drugs may have to be substituted.

Cephalosporins These are broad-spectrum antibiotics that are similar to the penicillins. Cephalosporins are often used when penicillin treatment has proved ineffective. Some cephalosporins can be given by mouth, but others are only given by injection. About 10 per cent of people who are allergic to penicillins may be allergic to cephalosporins. Some cephalosporins can occasionally damage the kidneys, particularly if used with aminoglycosides.

Macrolides Erythromycin is the most common drug in this group. It is a broad-spectrum antibiotic that is often prescribed as an alternative to penicillins or cephalosporins. Erythromycin is also effective against certain diseases, such as Legionnaires' disease (a rare type of pneumonia), that cannot be treated with other antibiotics. The main risk with erythromycin is that it can occasionally impair liver function.

Tetracyclines These have a broader spectrum of activity than other classes of antibiotic. However, increasing bacterial resistance (see Antibiotic resistance, p.86) has limited their use, although they are still widely prescribed. As well as being used for the treatment of infections, tetracyclines are also used in the long-term treatment of acne, although this application is probably not entirely due to their antibacterial action. A major drawback to the use of tetracycline antibiotics in young children and in pregnant women is that they are deposited in developing bones and teeth.

With the exception of doxycycline, drugs from this group are poorly absorbed through the intestines, and when given by mouth they have to be administered in high doses in order to reach effective levels in the blood. Such high doses increase the likelihood of diarrhoea as a side effect. The absorption of tetracyclines can be further reduced by interaction with calcium and other minerals. Drugs from this group should not therefore be taken with iron tablets or milk products.

Aminoglycosides These potent drugs are effective against a broad range of bacteria. However, they are not as widely used as some other antibiotics since they have to be given by injection and they have potentially

serious side effects, especially or the kidneys and middle ear. Their use is therefore limited to hospital treatment of serious infections. They are often given with other antibiotics.

Lincosamides The lincosamide clindamycin is not commonly used as it is more likely to cause serious disruption of bacterial activity in the bowel than other antibiotics. It is mainly reserved for the treatment of bone, joint, abdominal, and pelvic infections that do not respond well to other antibiotics. Clindamycin is also used topically for acne and vaginal infections.

Quinolones (see p.89) This group of drugs consists of nalidixic acid and substances chemically related to it, including the fluoroquinolones. Fluoroquinolones have a broad spectrum of activity. They are used to treat urinary infections and acute diarrhoeal diseases, including that caused by *Salmonella*, as well as in the treatment of enteric fever.

Their absorption is reduced by antacids containing magnesium and aluminium. Fluoroquinolones are generally well tolerated but may cause seizures in some people. These drugs are less frequently used in children because there is a theoretical risk of damage to the developing joints.

ANTIBACTERIAL DRUGS

This broad classification of drugs comprises agents that are similar to the antibiotics (p.86) in function but dissimilar in origin. The original antibiotics were derived from living organisms – for example, moulds and fungi. Antibacterials were developed from chemicals. The sulfonamides were the first drugs to be given for the treatment of bacterial infections and provided the mainstay of the treatment of infection before penicillin (the first antibiotic) became generally available. Increasing bacterial resistance and the development of antibiotics that are more effective and less toxic have reduced the use of sulfonamides.

Why they are used

Sulfonamides are less commonly used these days, and co-trimoxazole is reserved for rare cases of pneumonia in immunocompromised patients.

Trimethoprim is used for chest and urinary tract infections. The drug used to be combined with sulfamethoxazole as co-trimoxazole, but because of the side effects of sulfamethoxazole, trimethoprim on its own is usually preferred now.

Antibacterials used for tuberculosis are discussed on p.90. Other types of antibacterial sometimes classified as antimicrobials include metronidazole, which is prescribed for a variety of genital infections and for some serious infections of the abdomen, pelvic region, heart, and central nervous system. Other antibacterials are used to treat urinary infections. These include nitrofurantoin and drugs in the quinolone group (see Classes of antibiotic, facing page) such as nalidixic acid, which can be used to cure or prevent recurrent infections.

DRUG TREATMENT FOR LEPROSY

Leprosy, also known as Hansen's disease, is a bacterial infection caused by *Mycobacterium leprae*. It is rare in the United Kingdom, but relatively common in parts of Africa, Asia, and Latin America.

The disease progresses slowly, first affecting the peripheral nerves and causing loss of sensation in the hands and feet. This leads to frequent unnoticed injuries or burns and consequent scarring. Later, the nerves of the face may also be affected.

Treatment uses three drugs together to prevent the development of resistance. Usually, dapsone, rifampicin, and clofazimine will be given for at least 2 years. If one of these cannot be used, then a second-line drug (ofloxacin, minocycline, or clarithromycin) might be substituted. Complications during treatment sometimes require the use of prednisolone, aspirin, chloroquine, or even thalidomide.

ACTION OF SULFONAMIDES AND TRIMETHOPRIM

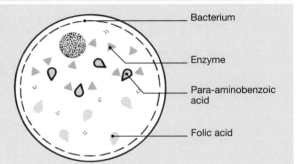

Before drug treatment
Folic acid, a chemical that is necessary for the growth of bacteria, is produced within bacterial cells by enzymes that act on a chemical called para-aminobenzoic acid.

Bacterium

Enzyme

Para-aminobenzoic acid

Folic acid

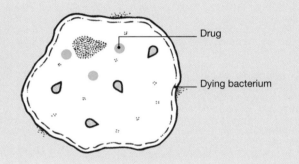

After drug treatment
Sulfonamides and trimethoprim interfere with the action of the enzymes, and with the production of folic acid. The bacterium is therefore unable to function properly and dies.

Drug

Dying bacterium

The quinolones are effective against a broad spectrum of bacteria. More potent relatives of nalidixic acid include norfloxacin, which is used to treat urinary tract infections, and ciprofloxacin, levofloxacin, and ofloxacin. These are all also used to treat many serious bacterial infections.

How they work

Most antibacterials act by preventing the growth and multiplication of bacteria (see Action of antibiotics, p.86, and Action of sulfonamides and trimethoprim, above).

How they affect you

Antibacterial drugs usually take several days to eliminate bacteria. During this time your doctor may recommend additional medication to alleviate pain and fever.

Risks and special precautions

Like antibiotics, most antibacterials can cause allergic reactions in susceptible people. Possible symptoms that should always be brought to your doctor's attention include rashes and fever. If such symptoms occur, a change to another drug is likely to be necessary.

Possible side effects of sulfonamides include loss of appetite, nausea, a rash, and drowsiness. Treatment with sulfonamides also carries a number of serious, but uncommon risks. Some drugs in this group can cause crystals

to form in the kidneys, a risk that can be reduced by drinking adequate amounts of fluid during prolonged treatment. Because sulfonamides may also occasionally damage the liver, they are not usually prescribed for people with impaired liver function. These drugs are also less frequently used in children because there is a theoretical risk of damage to the developing joints.

COMMON DRUGS

Quinolones
Ciprofloxacin ✳
Levofloxacin ✳
Moxifloxacin
Nalidixic acid
Norfloxacin
Ofloxacin

Sulfonamides
Co-trimoxazole ✳
Sulfadiazine

Other drugs
Clofazimine
Dapsone
Daptomycin
Linezolid
Metronidazole ✳
Nitrofurantoin
Thalidomide ✳
Tinidazole
Trimethoprim ✳

✳ See Part 3

ANTITUBERCULOUS DRUGS

Tuberculosis is an infectious bacterial disease acquired, often in childhood, by inhaling the tuberculosis bacilli present in the spray caused by a sneeze or cough from someone who is actively infected. It may also, rarely, be acquired from infected unpasteurized cow's milk. The disease usually starts in a lung and takes one of two forms: either primary infection or reactivated infection.

In 90 to 95 per cent of those with a primary infection, the body's immune system suppresses the infection but does not kill the bacilli. The infection is said to be latent and the dormant bacilli can be reactivated. After they are reactivated, the tuberculosis bacilli may spread via the lymphatic system and bloodstream throughout the body (see Sites of infection, below).

The first symptoms of the primary infection may include a cough, fever, tiredness, night sweats, and weight loss. Tuberculosis is confirmed through clinical investigations, which may include a chest X-ray, isolation of the bacilli from the person's sputum, and a positive reaction (localized inflammation) to a skin test in which tuberculin (a protein extracted from tuberculosis bacilli) is injected into the skin.

In adults, the gradual emergence of the destructive and progressive form of tuberculosis is caused by the reactivated infection. It occurs in 5 to 10 per cent of those who have had a previous primary infection. Another form, reinfection tuberculosis, occurs when someone with the dormant primary form is reinfected. Reinfection tuberculosis is clinically identical to the reactivated form.

Reactivation tuberculosis is more likely in people whose immune system is suppressed, such as older adults, those taking corticosteroids or other immuno-suppressants, patients receiving anti-tumour necrosis factor (anti-TNF) drugs such as infliximab, and those with AIDS. Reactivation may start in any part of the body seeded with the bacilli. It is most often first seen in the upper lobes of the lung, and is frequently diagnosed after a chest X-ray. The early symptoms may be identical to those of primary infection: a cough, tiredness, night sweats, fever, and weight loss.

If it is left untreated, tuberculosis continues to destroy tissue, spreading throughout the body and eventually causing death. It was one of the most common causes of death in the United Kingdom until the 1940s, but the disease is now on the increase again worldwide. Vulnerable groups are people with suppressed immune systems and people who are homeless.

Why they are used

A person who has been diagnosed with tuberculosis is likely to be treated with three or four antituberculous drugs. This helps to overcome the risk of drug-resistant strains of the bacilli emerging (see Antibiotic resistance, p.86).

The standard drug combination for the treatment of tuberculosis consists of rifampicin, isoniazid, pyrazinamide, and ethambutol. However, other drugs may be substituted if initial treatment fails or drug sensitivity tests indicate that the bacilli are resistant to these drugs.

The standard duration of treatment for a newly diagnosed tuberculosis infection is a six-month regimen as follows: isoniazid, rifampicin, pyrazinamide, and ethambutol daily for two months, followed by isoniazid and rifampicin for four months. The duration of treatment can be extended from nine months to up to two years in people at particular risk, such as those with a suppressed immune system or those in whom tuberculosis has infected the central nervous system.

Corticosteroids may be added to the treatment, if the patient does not have a suppressed immune system, to reduce the amount of tissue damage.

Both the number of drugs required and the long duration of treatment may make treatment difficult, particularly for those who are homeless. To help with this problem, supervised administration of treatment is available when required, both in the community and in hospital.

Tuberculosis in patients with HIV infection or AIDS is treated with the standard antituberculous drug regimen; but lifelong preventative treatment with isoniazid may be necessary.

How they work

Antituberculous drugs act in the same way as other antibiotics, by either killing bacilli or preventing them from multiplying (see Action of antibiotics, p.86).

How they affect you

Although the drugs start to combat the disease within days, benefits of drug treatment are not usually noticeable for a few weeks. As the infection is eradicated, the body repairs the damage caused by the disease. Symptoms such as fever and coughing gradually subside, and appetite and general health improve.

Risks and special precautions

Antituberculous drugs may cause adverse effects (nausea, vomiting, and abdominal pain), and they occasionally lead to serious allergic reactions. When this happens, another drug is substituted.

Rifampicin and isoniazid may affect liver function; isoniazid may adversely affect the nerves as well. Ethambutol can cause changes in colour vision. Dosage is carefully monitored, especially in children, older adults, and people with reduced kidney function.

SITES OF INFECTION

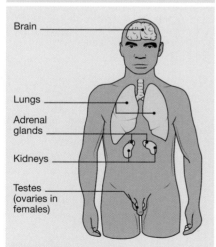

Brain

Lungs

Adrenal glands

Kidneys

Testes (ovaries in females)

Tuberculosis usually affects only part of one lung at first. However, later outbreaks usually spread to both lungs and may also affect the kidneys, leading to pyelonephritis; the adrenal glands, causing Addison's disease; and the membranes surrounding the brain, which may lead to meningitis. The testes (in men) and the ovaries (in women) may also be affected.

TUBERCULOSIS PREVENTION

A vaccine prepared from an artificially weakened strain of cattle tuberculosis bacteria can provide immunity from tuberculosis by provoking the development of natural resistance to the disease (see Vaccines and immunization, p.92). The BCG (Bacille Calmette-Guérin) vaccine is a form of tuberculosis bacillus that provokes the body's immune response but does not cause the illness because it is not infectious. The vaccine is no longer given as part of the routine immunization schedule but is offered to certain high-risk groups, for example newborn babies in areas where there is a high rate of tuberculosis.

How it is done
The vaccine is usually injected into the upper arm. A small pustule usually appears 6–12 weeks later, by which time the person can be considered immune.

COMMON DRUGS

Amikacin	Cycloserine
Capreomycin	Ethambutol *
Ciprofloxacin *	Isoniazid *
Clarithromycin *	Pyrazinamide
	Rifabutin
	Rifampicin *
* See Part 3	Streptomycin

ANTIVIRAL DRUGS

Viruses are simpler and smaller organisms than bacteria and are less able to sustain themselves. These organisms can survive and multiply only by penetrating body cells (see Action of antiviral drugs, right). Because viruses perform few functions independently, medicines that disrupt or halt their life cycle without harming human cells have been difficult to develop.

There are many different types of virus, and viral infections cause illnesses with various symptoms and degrees of severity. Common viral illnesses include the cold, influenza, and flu-like illnesses, cold sores, and childhood diseases such as chickenpox, mumps, and measles. Throat infections, pneumonia, acute bronchitis, gastroenteritis, and meningitis are often, but not always, caused by a virus.

Fortunately, the natural defences of the body are usually strong enough to overcome infections such as these, with drugs given to ease pain and lower fever. However, the more serious viral diseases, such as pneumonia and meningitis, need close medical supervision.

Another difficulty with viral infections is the speed with which the virus multiplies. By the time symptoms appear, the viruses are so numerous that antiviral drugs have little effect. Antiviral agents must be given early in the course of a viral infection, or they may be used prophylactically (as a preventative). Some viral infections can be prevented by vaccination (see p.92).

Why they are used

Antiviral drugs are helpful in the treatment of various conditions caused by the herpes virus: cold sores, encephalitis, genital herpes, chickenpox, and shingles.

Aciclovir and penciclovir are applied topically to treat outbreaks of cold sores, herpes eye infections, and genital herpes. They can reduce the severity and duration of an outbreak but do not eliminate the infection permanently. Aciclovir, famciclovir, and valaciclovir are given by mouth, or in exceptional circumstances by injection, to prevent chickenpox or severe, recurrent attacks of the herpes virus infections in those people who are already weakened by other conditions.

Influenza may sometimes be prevented or treated using oseltamivir or zanamivir. Oseltamivir may also be used to treat the symptoms of influenza in at-risk people, such as those over 65 or with respiratory diseases such as chronic obstructive pulmonary disease (COPD) or asthma, cardiovascular disease, kidney disease, immunosuppression, or diabetes mellitus.

The interferons are proteins produced by the body and involved in the immune response. Interferon is effective in reducing the activity of hepatitis B and hepatitis C. Hepatitis B replication can be controlled with tenofovir, and hepatitis C can be cured in most cases by antivirals such as ledipasvir and sofosbuvir.

ACTION OF ANTIVIRAL DRUGS

In order to reproduce, a virus requires a living host cell. The invaded cell eventually dies and the new viruses are released, spreading and infecting other cells. Most antiviral drugs act to prevent the virus from using the host cell's genetic material, DNA, to multiply. Unable to divide, the virus dies and the spread of infection is halted.

Before drug

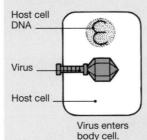
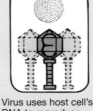
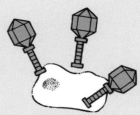

Host cell DNA

Virus

Host cell

Virus enters body cell.

Virus uses host cell's DNA to reproduce.

Host cell dies and new viruses are released.

After drug

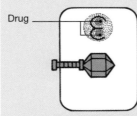
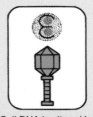
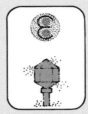

Drug

Virus enters cell that has absorbed an antiviral drug.

Cell DNA is altered by drug action and virus cannot use it.

Virus dies and spread of infection is thereby halted.

Ganciclovir is sometimes used for cytomegalovirus (CMV). Respiratory syncytial virus (RSV) has been treated with ribavirin, and prevented by palivizumab. Drug treatment for AIDS is discussed on p.116.

How they work

Some antivirals act by altering the building blocks for the cells' genetic material (DNA), so that the virus cannot multiply. Others stop viruses multiplying by blocking enzyme activity within the host cell. Halting multiplication prevents the virus from spreading to uninfected cells and improves symptoms rapidly. However, in herpes infections, it does not eradicate the virus from the body, so infection may flare up again in future.

How they affect you

Topical antiviral drugs usually start to act immediately. Providing that the treatment is applied early enough, an outbreak of herpes can be cut short. Symptoms usually clear up within two to four days.

Antiviral ointments may cause irritation and redness. Antiviral drugs given by mouth or injection can occasionally cause nausea and dizziness.

Risks and special precautions

Because some of these drugs may affect the kidneys adversely, they are prescribed with caution for people with reduced kidney function. Some antiviral drugs can adversely affect the activity of normal body cells, particularly those in the bone marrow. Idoxuridine is, for this reason, available only for topical application.

COMMON DRUGS

Aciclovir ✳	Peginterferon alfa
Amantadine	Penciclovir
Cidofovir	Ribavirin
Daclatasvir	Sofosbuvir
Famciclovir	Tenofovir ✳
Foscarnet	Valaciclovir
Ganciclovir	Valganciclovir
Inosine pranobex	Zanamivir
Ledipasvir	Zidovudine/
Oseltamivir ✳	Lamivudine ✳
Palivizumab	

✳ See Part 3

See also Drugs for HIV, p.116

VACCINES AND IMMUNIZATION

Many infectious diseases, including most common viral infections, occur only once during a person's lifetime. This is because the antibodies produced in response to the disease remain in the body afterwards to combat any future invasion by the infectious organisms. The duration of such immunity varies, but can last a lifetime.

Protection against many infections can be provided artificially by using vaccines derived from altered forms of the infecting organism. These vaccines stimulate the immune system in the same way as a genuine infection, and provide lasting, active immunity. Because each type of microbe stimulates the production of a specific antibody, a different vaccine must be given for each disease.

Another type of immunization, called passive immunization, relies on giving antibodies (see Immunoglobulins, below).

Why they are used

Some infectious diseases cannot be treated effectively or are so serious that prevention is the best course. Routine immunization not only protects the individual but may gradually eradicate the disease completely, as with smallpox.

Newborn babies receive antibodies for many diseases from their mothers, but this protection lasts only for about three months. Most children are vaccinated against common childhood infectious diseases. Additionally, travellers are advised to be vaccinated against diseases common in the areas they are visiting.

Effective lifelong immunization can sometimes be achieved by a single dose of the vaccine. However, in many cases reinforcing doses (boosters) are needed later to maintain reliable immunity.

Vaccines do not provide immediate protection and it may be up to four weeks before full immunity develops. When immediate protection is needed, it may be necessary to establish passive immunity with immunoglobulins (see below).

How they work

Vaccines provoke the immune system into creating antibodies that help the body to resist specific infectious diseases. Some vaccines (live vaccines) are made from artificially weakened forms of the

ACTIVE AND PASSIVE IMMUNIZATION

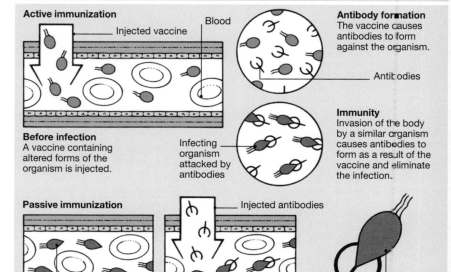

Active immunization

Injected vaccine — Blood

Before infection
A vaccine containing altered forms of the organism is injected.

Antibody formation
The vaccine causes antibodies to form against the organism.

— Antibodies

Infecting organism attacked by antibodies

Immunity
Invasion of the body by a similar organism causes antibodies to form as a result of the vaccine and eliminate the infection.

Passive immunization

Injected antibodies

— Infecting organisms

Infecting organism attacked by antibodies

After infection
Passive immunization may be needed when the infection has entered the blood.

Immunoglobulin injection
A serum containing antibodies (immunoglobulin) extracted from donated blood is injected. This helps the body to fight the infection.

disease-causing organism. Others rely on inactive (or killed) disease-causing organisms, or inactive derivatives of those organisms. Whatever their type, all vaccines stimulate antibody production and establish active immunity.

How they affect you

The degree of protection varies among different vaccines. Some provide reliable lifelong immunity; others may not give full protection against a disease, or the effects may last for as little as six months. Influenza vaccines usually protect only against the strains of virus causing the latest outbreaks of flu.

Any vaccine may cause side effects but they are usually mild and soon disappear. The most common reactions are a red,

slightly raised, tender area at the site of injection, and a slight fever or a flu-like illness lasting for one or two days.

Risks and special precautions

Serious reactions are rare, and for most people the risk is far outweighed by the protection given. A family or personal history of seizures is not necessarily a contraindication to immunization, but immunization may be delayed if the condition is unstable. Children who have any infection more severe than a common cold will not be given any routine vaccination until they have recovered.

Live vaccines should not be given during pregnancy because they may affect the developing baby, nor should they be given to people whose immune systems are weakened. It is also advisable for those taking high doses of corticosteroids to delay vaccinations until the end of drug treatment.

The risk of fever following the DTaP/IPV/Hib/HepB (diphtheria, tetanus, acellular pertussis, inactivated polio, Haemophilus influenzae type b, and hepatitis B) vaccine can be reduced by giving paracetamol at the time of the vaccination. The pertussis vaccine may rarely cause a mild seizure, which is brief, usually associated with fever, and stops without treatment. Children who have experienced such seizures recover completely.

IMMUNOGLOBULINS

Antibodies, which can result from exposure to snake and insect venom as well as infectious disease, are carried around the body in the serum of the blood (the fluid part remaining after the red cells and clotting agents are removed). The concentrated serum of people who have survived diseases or poisonous bites is called immunoglobulin, and when it is given by injection it creates passive immunity. Immunoglobulins may be obtained from human donors or extracted from horse blood following repeated doses of the toxin.

Because immunoglobulins do not stimulate the body to produce its own antibodies, continued protection requires repeated injections of immunoglobulins.

Adverse effects from immunoglobulins are uncommon. Some people are sensitive to horse globulins, and about a week after the injection they may experience a reaction known as serum sickness, with fever, a rash, joint swelling, and pain. This usually ends in a few days but should be reported to your doctor before any further immunization.

COMMON VACCINATIONS

Infection	How given	When/to whom given	General information
Diphtheria/tetanus/pertussis/polio/ *Haemophilus influenzae* type b (Hib)/ hepatitis E (DTaP/IPV/Hib/HepB) Rotavirus infection Meningitis B (MenB)	1 injection 1 oral dose 1 injection	8 weeks	Rotavirus can cause diarrhoea, sickness, and severe dehydration in infants. MenB protects against types of meningitis and septicaemia caused by meningococcal B bacteria
Diphtheria/tetanus/pertussis/polio/Hib/ hepatitis B (DTaP/IPV/Hib/HepB) Pneumococcal infection (PCV – pneumococcal conjugate vaccine) Rotavirus infection	1 injection 1 injection 1 oral dose	12 weeks	PCV protects against pneumonia, septicaemia, and meningitis caused by pneumococcal infection. A different pneumococcal vaccine (PPV) is used in adults over 65 and those at risk due to long-term health problems
Diphtheria/tetanus/pertussis/polio/Hib/ hepatitis B (DTaP/IPV/Hib/HepB) Meningitis B (MenB)	1 injection 1 injection	16 weeks	Hib vaccine protects against meningitis, epiglottitis, and septicaemia caused by *Haemophilus influenzae* type b
Hib/meningitis C (Hib/MenC) Measles/mumps/rubella (MMR) Pneumococcal infection (PCV) Meningitis B (Men B)	1 injection 1 injection 1 injection 1 injection	1 year	Rubella is important because it can damage the fetus if it affects a woman in early pregnancy. MenC protects against types of meningitis and septicaemia caused by meningococcal C bacteria
Childhood influenza	1 dose of nasal spray	2–10 years (annually). Also offered annually to those aged 2–17 years who are at risk due to long-term health conditions	Children unable to have the nasal spray may be offered injectable influenza vaccine instead (see below)
Diphtheria/tetanus/pertussis/polio (DTaP/IPV or dTaP/IPV) Measles/mumps/rubella (MMR)	1 injection 1 injection	3 years 4 months or soon after	Diphtheria is most serious in very young children or older adults
Human papillomavirus (HPV)	2 injections, 6–24 months apart	11–14 years (girls and boys)	HPV is linked to a number of cancers including those of the cervix, vagina, vulva, penis, and anus
Meningitis A, C, W, and Y (MenACWY) Diphtheria/tetanus/polio (Td/IPV)	1 injection 1 injection	14 years	MenACWY is recommended for all teenagers and university students up to the age of 25
Influenza	1 injection	Offered routinely from the age of 65. Also offered to pregnant women, at-risk babies aged 6 months to 2 years, and at-risk adults over 18	Long-term immunity against all strains of influenza is impossible. Annual vaccinations protect against the strains of influenza prevalent that year
Pneumococcal infection (PPV – pneumococcal polysaccharide vaccine)	1 injection	Single dose offered to those aged 65 or over. Also offered to those at risk due to health problems, including children who cannot have the PCV vaccine	People at risk include those who are immunodeficient, have had their spleen removed, or have certain long-term health conditions, such as diabetes or chronic liver or lung disease
Shingles	1 injection	Single dose offered to those aged 70 and over	Shingles is a painful rash caused by reactivation of the chickenpox virus in those previously infected with the virus
Tuberculosis (TB)	1 injection	Infants and children at high risk of contracting TB or recently arrived from an area with a high level of TB; unimmunized people under 35 in certain high-risk groups (e.g. some healthcare workers)	No further immunizations should be given in the same arm for at least 3 months due to the risk of a reaction in the lymph nodes
Chickenpox	2 injections, 4–8 weeks apart	Recommended for non-immune people in close contact with those at risk of serious illness (see right)	Chickenpox can be serious in certain groups of people, especially those with a weakened immune system
Pertussis (whooping cough)	1 injection	Advised for pregnant women at 16–32 weeks' gestation, to protect baby in first 8 weeks of life	Cases in the UK have risen since 2011. Pertussis can cause pneumonia, brain damage, or even death in infants

ANTIPROTOZOAL DRUGS

Protozoa are single-celled organisms that are present in soil and water. They may be transmitted to or between humans through contaminated food or water, sexual contact, or insect bites. There are many types of protozoal infection, each of which causes a different disease depending on the organism involved. Trichomoniasis, toxoplasmosis, cryptosporidium, giardiasis, and pneumocystis pneumonia are probably the most common protozoal infections seen in the United Kingdom. The rarer infections are usually contracted as a result of exposure to infection in another part of the world.

Many types of protozoa infect the bowel, causing diarrhoea and generalized symptoms of ill-health. Others may infect the genital tract or skin. Some protozoa may penetrate vital organs such as the lungs, brain, and liver. Prompt diagnosis and treatment are important in order to limit the spread of the infection within the body and, in some cases, prevent it from spreading to other people. Increased attention to hygiene is an important factor in controlling the spread of the disease.

A variety of medicines is used in the treatment of these diseases. Some, such as metronidazole and tetracycline, are also commonly used for their antibacterial action (see p.89). Others, such as pentamidine, are rarely used except in treating specific protozoal infections.

How they affect you

Protozoa are often difficult to eradicate from the body. Drug treatment may therefore need to be continued for several months in order to eliminate the infecting organisms completely and thus prevent recurrence of the disease. In addition, unpleasant side effects such as nausea, diarrhoea, and abdominal cramps are often unavoidable because of the limited choice of drugs and the need to maintain dosage levels that will effectively cure the disease. For detailed information on the risks and adverse effects of individual antiprotozoals, consult the appropriate drug profile in Part 3 of the book.

The table below describes the principal protozoal infections and some of the drugs used in their treatment. Malaria, probably the most common protozoal disease in the world today, is discussed on the facing page.

SUMMARY OF PROTOZOAL DISEASES

Disease	Protozoan	Description	Drugs
Amoebiasis (amoebic dysentery)	*Entamoeba histolytica*	Infection of the bowel and sometimes of the liver and other organs. Usually transmitted in contaminated food or water. Major symptom is violent, sometimes bloody, diarrhoea.	Diloxanide Metronidazole Tinidazole
Balantidiasis	*Balantidium coli*	Infection of the bowel, specifically the colon. Usually transmitted through contact with infected pigs. Possible symptoms include diarrhoea and abdominal pain.	Tetracycline/metronidazole/ di-iodohydroxyquinoline
Cryptosporidiosis	*Cryptosporidium*	Infection of the bowel, also occasionally of the respiratory tract and bile ducts. Symptoms include diarrhoea and abdominal pain.	No specific drugs but paromomycin, azithromycin, eflornithine may be effective
Giardiasis (lambliasis)	*Giardia lamblia*	Infection of the bowel. Usually transmitted in contaminated food or water but may also be spread by some types of sexual contact. Major symptoms are general ill health, diarrhoea, flatulence, and abdominal pain.	Metronidazole Tinidazole
Leishmaniasis	*Leishmania*	A mainly tropical and subtropical disease caused by organisms spread through sandfly bites. It affects the mucous membranes of the mouth, nose, and throat, and may in its severe form invade organs such as the liver.	Paromomycin Sodium stibogluconate Pentamidine Amphotericin
Pneumocystis pneumonia	*Pneumocystis jiroveci* (formerly called *Pneumocystis carinii*)	Potentially fatal lung infection that usually affects only those with reduced resistance to infection, such as those who are HIV-positive. The symptoms include cough, breathlessness, fever, and chest pain.	Atovaquone/Co-trimoxazole Pentamidine/Dapsone with trimethoprim
Toxoplasmosis	*Toxoplasma gondii*	Infection is usually spread via cat faeces or by eating undercooked meat. Although usually symptomless, infection may cause generalized ill-health, mild fever, and eye inflammation. Treatment is necessary only if the eyes are involved or if the patient is immunosuppressed (such as in HIV). It may also pass from mother to baby during pregnancy, leading to severe disease in the fetus.	Pyrimethamine with sulfadiazine or with azithromycin, clarithromycin, or clindamycin/spiramycin (during pregnancy)
Trichomoniasis	*Trichomonas vaginalis*	Infection most often affects the vagina, causing irritation and an offensive discharge. In men, infection may occur in the urethra. The disease is usually sexually transmitted.	Metronidazole Tinidazole
Trypanosomiasis	*Trypanosoma*	African trypanosomiasis (sleeping sickness) is spread by the tsetse fly and causes fever, swollen glands, and drowsiness. South American trypanosomiasis (Chagas' disease) is spread by assassin bugs and causes inflammation, enlargement of internal organs, and infection of the brain.	Pentamidine (sleeping sickness), Suramin eflornithine melarsoprol (sleeping sickness), Primaquine (Chagas' disease), Nifurtimox (Chagas' disease)

ANTIMALARIAL DRUGS

Malaria is one of the main killing diseases in the tropics (see map below). It is most likely to affect people who live in or travel to such places.

The disease is caused by protozoa (see also facing page) whose life cycle is far from simple. The malaria parasite, which is called *Plasmodium*, lives in and depends on the female *Anopheles* mosquito during one part of its life cycle. It lives in and depends on human beings during other parts of its life cycle.

Transferred to humans in the saliva of the female mosquito as she penetrates ("bites") the skin, the malaria parasite enters the bloodstream and settles in the liver, where it multiplies asexually.

Following its stay in the liver, the parasite (or plasmodium) enters another phase of its life cycle, circulating in the bloodstream, penetrating and destroying red blood cells, and reproducing again. If the plasmodia then transfer back to a female *Anopheles* mosquito via another "bite", they breed sexually, and are again ready to start a human infection.

Following the emergence of plasmodia from the liver, the symptoms of malaria occur: episodes of high fever and profuse sweating alternate with equally agonizing episodes of shivering and chills. One of the four strains of malaria (*Plasmodium falciparum*) can produce a single severe attack that can be fatal unless treated.

The others cause recurrent attacks, sometimes extending over many years.

A number of drugs are available for preventing malaria (see box, below), depending on the region in which the disease can be contracted and the resistance to the commonly used drugs. In most areas, *Plasmodium falciparum* is resistant to chloroquine. In all regions, four drugs are commonly used for treating malaria: quinine, mefloquine, proguanil with atovaquone (Malarone), and artemether with lumefantrine (Riamet).

Why they are used

The medical response to malaria takes three forms: prevention, treatment of attacks, and the complete eradication of the plasmodia (radical cure).

For someone planning a trip to an area where malaria is prevalent, drugs are given that destroy the parasites as they enter the liver. This preventative treatment needs to start up to 3 weeks before departure and continue for 1–4 weeks after returning (the exact timings depend on the drugs taken).

Antimalarials such as mefloquine and Riamet can produce a radical cure, but chloroquine does not. After chloroquine treatment of non-falciparum malaria, a 14- to 21-day course of primaquine is administered. Although highly effective in destroying plasmodia in the liver, the drug is weak against the plasmodia in the blood. Primaquine is recommended only after a person leaves the malarial area because of the high risk of reinfection.

How they work

Taken to prevent the disease, the drugs kill the plasmodia in the liver, preventing them from multiplying. Once plasmodia have multiplied, the same drugs may be used in higher doses to kill plasmodia that re-enter the bloodstream. If these drugs are not effective, primaquine may be used to destroy any plasmodia that are still present in the liver.

How they affect you

The low doses of antimalarial drugs taken for prevention rarely produce noticeable effects. Drugs taken for an attack usually begin to relieve symptoms within a few hours. Most of them can cause nausea, vomiting, and diarrhoea. Quinine can cause disturbances in vision and hearing. Mefloquine can cause sleep disturbance, dizziness, and difficulties in coordination.

Risks and special precautions

When drugs are given, the full course of treatment must be taken. No drugs give long-term protection; a new course of treatment is needed for each journey.

Most of these drugs do not produce severe adverse effects, but primaquine can cause the blood disorder haemolytic anaemia, particularly in people with glucose-6-phosphate dehydrogenase (G6PD) deficiency. Blood tests are taken before treatment to identify susceptible individuals. Mefloquine is not prescribed for those who have had psychological disorders or seizures.

Other protective measures

Because *Plasmodium* strains continually develop resistance to the available drugs, prevention using drugs is not absolutely reliable. Protection from mosquito bites is of the highest priority. Such protection includes the use of insect repellents and mosquito nets impregnated with permethrin insecticide, as well as covering any exposed skin after dark.

PREVENTION OF MALARIA

Malaria is found in more than 100 countries across the world, mainly in tropical and subtropical regions. The vast majority of cases (over 90%) occur in Africa, but the disease also occurs in Southeast Asia and the eastern Mediterranean countries, as well as in India, China, Central America, and northern South America. Babies, children under 5 years, pregnant women, and immunocompromised people (particularly those with HIV/AIDS) are most at risk of infection with malaria and of developing severe symptoms.

The incidence of the disease is declining, but malaria is still a serious problem; in 2019 the World Health Organization estimated that there had been 229 million cases worldwide. In addition, drug resistance in the malarial organisms, and insecticide resistance in malaria-carrying mosquitoes, have become problems. For example, resistance to chloroquine (see p.193) and proguanil (see p.368) has developed in some parts of the world. However, such resistance may be countered by giving combinations of drugs, such as proguanil with atovaquone.

There are generally two preventative regimens in use, which differ according to the area to be visited; these are outlined in the table below. The main drugs used are proguanil with atovaquone, doxycycline (see p.238), and mefloquine (see p.315). However, recommendations for malaria prevention change frequently, and you should seek specific medical advice before travelling. The websites below the table contain information about preventing or minimizing the risk of malaria infection.

Regimen	Recommendation for malaria prevention
Low risk	Preventative drugs not usually advised but mosquito bites should be avoided
High risk	Proguanil with atovaquone (Malarone), or doxycycline, or mefloquine
Useful websites:	https://www.fitfortravel.nhs.uk/advice/malaria.aspx
	https://bnf.nice.org.uk/treatment-summary/malaria-prophylaxis.html
	https://www.cdc.gov/malaria/travelers/country_table/a.html
	https://www.who.int/malaria/travellers/en/

COMMON DRUGS

Drugs for prevention	Drugs for treatment
Chloroquine ✳	Artemether with lumefantrine (Riamet)
Doxycycline ✳	
Mefloquine ✳	Chloroquine ✳
Proguanil	Mefloquine ✳
Proguanil with atovaquone (Malarone) ✳	Primaquine
	Proguanil with atovaquone (Malarone) ✳
	Pyrimethamine with sulfadoxine ✳
✳ See Part 3	Quinine ✳

ANTIFUNGAL DRUGS

We are continually exposed to fungi – in the air we breathe, the food we eat, and the water we drink. Fortunately, most of them cannot live in the body, and few are harmful. But some can grow in the mouth, skin, hair, or nails, causing irritating or unsightly changes, and a few can cause serious and possibly fatal disease. The most common fungal infections are caused by the tinea group. These include tinea pedis (athlete's foot), tinea cruris (jock itch), tinea corporis (ringworm), and tinea capitis (scalp ringworm). Caused by a variety of organisms, they are spread by direct or indirect contact with infected humans or animals. Infection is encouraged by warm, moist conditions.

Problems may also result from the proliferation of a fungus normally present in the body; the most common example is excessive growth of *Candida*, a yeast that causes thrush infection of the mouth, vagina, and bowel. It can also infect other organs if it spreads through the body via the bloodstream. Overgrowth of *Candida* may occur in people taking antibiotics (p.86) or oral contraceptives (p.121), in pregnant women, or in those with diabetes or immune system disorders such as HIV.

Superficial fungal infections (those that attack only the outer layer of the skin and mucous membranes) are relatively common and, although irritating, do not usually present a threat to general health. Internal fungal infections (for example, of the lungs, heart, or other organs) are very rare, but may be serious and prolonged.

As antibiotics and other antibacterial drugs have no effect on fungi and yeasts, a different type of drug is needed. Drugs for fungal infections are either applied topically to treat minor infections of the skin, nails, and mucous membranes, or they are given by mouth or injection to eliminate serious fungal infections of the internal organs and nails.

Why they are used

Drug treatment is necessary for most fungal infections since they rarely improve alone. Measures such as careful washing and drying of affected areas may help but are not a substitute for antifungal drugs. The use of over-the-counter preparations to increase the acidity of the vagina is not usually effective except when it is accompanied by drug treatment.

Fungal infections of the skin and scalp are usually treated with a cream or shampoo. Drugs for vaginal thrush are most often applied in the form of vaginal pessaries or cream applied with a special applicator. For very severe or persistent vaginal infections, fluconazole or itraconazole may be given as a short course by mouth. Mouth infections are usually eliminated by lozenges dissolved in the mouth or an antifungal solution or gel applied to the affected areas. For severe or persistent nail infections, griseofulvin or terbinafine are given by mouth until the infected nails have grown out.

In the rare cases of fungal infections of internal organs, such as the blood, the heart, or the brain, potent drugs such as fluconazole and itraconazole are given by mouth, or amphotericin and flucytosine are given by injection. These drugs pass into the bloodstream to fight the fungi.

How they work

Most antifungals alter the permeability of the fungal cell's walls. Chemicals needed for cell life leak out and the fungal cell dies.

ACTIONS OF ANTIFUNGAL DRUGS

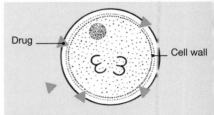

Drug — Cell wall

Stage one
The drug acts on the wall of the fungal cell.

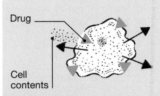

Drug —
Cell contents

Stage two
The drug damages the cell wall and the cell contents leak out. The cell dies.

How they affect you

The speed with which antifungal drugs provide benefit varies with the type of infection. Most fungal or yeast infections of the skin, mouth, and vagina improve within a week. The condition of nails affected by fungal infections improves only when new nail growth occurs, which takes months. Systemic infections of the internal organs can take weeks to cure.

Antifungal drugs applied topically rarely cause side effects, although they may irritate the skin. However, treatment by mouth or injection for systemic and nail infections may produce more serious side effects. Amphotericin, injected in cases of life-threatening systemic infections, can cause potentially dangerous effects, including kidney damage.

COMMON DRUGS

Amorolfine
Amphotericin B *
Caspofungin
Clotrimazole *
Econazole
Fluconazole *

Flucytosine
Griseofulvin
Itraconazole
Ketoconazole *
Miconazole *
Nystatin *
Terbinafine *
Tioconazole
Voriconazole

* See Part 3

CHOICE OF ANTIFUNGAL DRUG

The table below shows the range of uses for some antifungal drugs. The particular drug chosen in each case depends on the precise nature and site of the infection. The usual route of administration for each drug is also indicated.

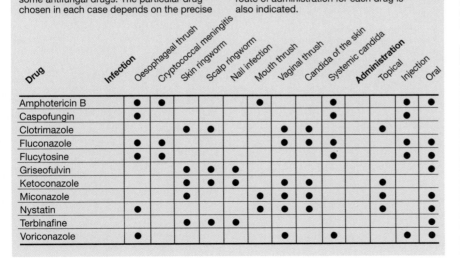

Drug	Oesophageal thrush	Cryptococcal meningitis	Skin ringworm	Scalp ringworm	Nail infection	Mouth thrush	Vaginal thrush	Candida of the skin	Systemic candida	Topical	Injection	Oral
Amphotericin B	•	•				•			•		•	•
Caspofungin	•								•		•	
Clotrimazole			•	•		•	•			•		
Fluconazole	•	•				•	•	•			•	•
Flucytosine	•	•							•			•
Griseofulvin			•	•	•							•
Ketoconazole			•	•		•	•			•		•
Miconazole			•			•	•	•		•		•
Nystatin	•					•	•	•		•		•
Terbinafine			•	•	•							•
Voriconazole	•								•	•		•

ANTHELMINTIC DRUGS

Anthelmintics are drugs that are used to eliminate the many types of worm (helminths) that can enter the body and live there as parasites, producing a general weakness in some cases and serious harm in others. The body may be host to many different worms (see Choice of drug, below). Most species spend part of their life cycle in another animal, and the infestation is often passed on to humans in food contaminated with the eggs or larvae. In some cases, such as hookworm, larvae enter the body through the skin. Larvae or adults may attach themselves to the intestinal wall and feed on the bowel contents; others feed off the intestinal blood supply, causing anaemia. Worms can also infest the bloodstream or lodge in the muscles or internal organs.

Many people have worms at some time during their life, especially during childhood; most can be effectively eliminated with anthelmintic drugs.

Why they are used

Most worms common in the United Kingdom cause only mild symptoms and usually do not pose a serious threat to general health. Anthelmintic drugs are usually necessary, however, because the body's natural defences against infection are not effective against most worm infestations. Certain types of infestation must always be treated since they can cause serious complications. In some cases, such as threadworm infestation, doctors may recommend anthelmintic treatment for the whole family to prevent reinfection. If worms have invaded tissues and formed cysts, they may have to be removed surgically. Laxatives are given with some anthelmintics to hasten expulsion of worms from the bowel. Other drugs may be prescribed to ease symptoms or to compensate for any blood loss or nutritional deficiency.

How they work

The anthelmintic drugs act in several ways. Many of them kill or paralyse the worms, which pass out of the body in the faeces. Others, which act systemically, are used to treat infection in the tissues.

Many anthelmintics are specific for particular worms, and the doctor must identify the nature of the infection before selecting the most appropriate treatment (see Choice of drug, below). Most of the common intestinal infestations are easily treated, often with only one or two doses of the drug. However, tissue infections may require more prolonged treatment.

How they affect you

Once the drug has eliminated the worms, symptoms caused by infestation rapidly disappear. Taken as a single dose or a short course, anthelmintics do not usually produce side effects. However, treatment can disturb the digestive system, causing abdominal pain, nausea, and vomiting.

COMMON DRUGS

Albendazole	Mebendazole ✳
Diethylcarbamazine	Niclosamide
Ivermectin	Praziquantel
Levamisole	Tiabendazole

✳ See Part 3

CHOICE OF DRUG

Threadworm (enterobiasis)
The most common worm infection in the United Kingdom, particularly among young children. The worm lives in the intestine, but it travels to the anus at night to lay eggs. This causes itching; scratching leaves eggs on the fingers, usually under the fingernails. These eggs are transferred to the mouth, often by sucking the fingers or eating food with unwashed hands. Keeping nails short and good hygiene, including washing the hands after using the toilet and before each meal, and an early morning bath to remove the eggs, are all important elements in the eradication of infection.
Drugs Mebendazole. All members of the family should be treated simultaneously.

Common roundworm (ascariasis)
The most common worm infection worldwide. Transmitted to humans in contaminated raw food or in soil. Infects the intestine. The worms are large and dense clusters of them can block the intestine.
Drugs Levamisole, mebendazole

Tropical threadworm (strongyloidiasis)
Occurs in the tropics and southern Europe. Larvae from contaminated soil penetrate skin, pass into the lungs, and are swallowed into the gut.
Drugs Albendazole, tiabendazole, ivermectin

Whipworm (trichuriasis)
Mainly occurs in tropical areas as a result of eating contaminated raw vegetables. Worms infest the intestines.
Drugs Mebendazole

Hookworm (uncinariasis)
Mainly found in tropical areas. Worm larvae penetrate skin and pass via the lymphatic system and bloodstream to the lungs. They then travel up the airways, are swallowed, and attach themselves to the intestinal wall, where they feed off the intestinal blood supply.
Drugs Mebendazole

Pork roundworm (trichinosis)
Transmitted in infected undercooked pork. Initially worms lodge in the intestines, but larvae may invade muscle to form cysts that are often resistant to drug treatment and may require surgery.
Drugs Mebendazole, tiabendazole

Toxocariasis (visceral larva migrans)
Usually results from eating soil or eating with fingers contaminated with dog or cat faeces. Eggs hatch in the intestine and may travel to the lungs, liver, kidney, brain, and eyes. Treatment is not always effective.
Drugs Mebendazole, tiabendazole, diethylcarbamazine

Creeping eruption (cutaneous larva migrans)
Mainly occurs in tropical areas and coastal areas of southeastern United States as a result of skin contact with larvae from cat and dog faeces. Infestation is usually confined to the skin.
Drugs Tiabendazole, ivermectin, albendazole

Filariasis (including onchocerciasis and loiasis)
Tropical areas only. Infection by this group of worms is spread by bites of insects that are carriers of worm larvae or eggs. May affect the lymphatic system, blood, eyes, and skin.
Drugs Diethylcarbamazine, ivermectin

Flukes
Sheep liver fluke (fascioliasis) is indigenous to the United Kingdom. Infestation usually results from eating watercress grown in contaminated water. Mainly affects the liver and biliary tract. Other flukes only found abroad may infect the lungs, intestines, or blood.
Drugs Praziquantel

Tapeworms (including beef, pork, fish, and dwarf tapeworms)
Depending on the type, may be carried by cattle, pigs, or fish and transmitted to humans in undercooked meat. Most types affect the intestines. Larvae of the pork tapeworm may form cysts in muscle and other tissues.
Drugs Niclosamide, praziquantel

Hydatid disease (echinococciasis)
Eggs are transmitted in dog faeces. Larvae may form cysts over many years, commonly in the liver. Surgery is the usual treatment for cysts.
Drugs Albendazole

Bilharzia (schistosomiasis)
Occurs in polluted water in tropical areas. Larvae may be swallowed or penetrate the skin, and pass to the liver; adult worms live in the bladder.
Drugs Praziquantel

HORMONES AND ENDOCRINE SYSTEM

The endocrine system is a collection of glands located throughout the body that produce hormones and release them into the bloodstream. Each endocrine gland produces one or more hormones, each of which governs a particular body function, including growth and repair of tissues, sexual development and reproductive function, and the body's response to stress.

Most hormones are released continuously from birth, but the amount produced fluctuates with the body's needs. Others are produced mainly at certain times – for example, growth hormone is released mainly during childhood and adolescence. Sex hormones are produced by the testes and ovaries from puberty onwards (see p.118).

Many endocrine glands release their hormones in response to triggering hormones produced by the pituitary gland. The pituitary releases a variety of pituitary hormones, each of which, in turn, stimulates the appropriate endocrine gland to produce its hormone.

A feedback system usually regulates blood hormone levels: if the blood level rises too high, the pituitary responds by reducing the amount of stimulating hormone produced, thereby allowing the blood hormone level to return to normal.

What can go wrong

Endocrine disorders, usually resulting in too much or too little of a particular hormone, have a variety of causes. Some are congenital in origin; others may be caused by autoimmune disease (including some forms of diabetes mellitus), malignant or benign tumours, injury, or certain drugs.

Why drugs are used

Natural hormone preparations or their synthetic versions are often prescribed to treat deficiency. Sometimes drugs are given to stimulate increased hormone production in the endocrine gland, such as oral antidiabetic drugs, which act on the insulin-producing cells of the pancreas. When too much hormone is produced, drug treatment may reduce the activity of the gland.

Hormones or related drugs are also used to treat certain other conditions. Corticosteroids related to adrenal hormones are prescribed to relieve inflammation and to suppress immune system activity (see p.115). Several types of cancer are treated with sex hormones (see p.112). Female sex hormones are used as contraceptives (see p.121) and to treat menstrual disorders (see p.120).

The pituitary gland produces hormones that regulate growth, sexual, and reproductive development, and also stimulate other endocrine glands (see p.103).

The thyroid gland regulates metabolism. Hyperthyroidism or hypothyroidism may occur if the thyroid does not function well (see p.102).

The adrenal glands produce hormones that regulate the body's mineral and water content and reduce inflammation (see p.99). They also produce stress hormones and male sex hormones.

The pancreas produces insulin, to regulate blood sugar levels, and glucagon, which helps the liver and muscles to store glucose (see p.100).

The kidneys produce a hormone, erythropoietin, needed for red blood cell production. Patients with kidney failure become anaemic because they lack this hormone (see p.246).

The ovaries (in women) secrete oestrogen and progesterone, responsible for female sexual and physical development (see p.105).

The testes (in men) produce testosterone, which controls the development of male sexual and physical characteristics (see p.104).

MAJOR DRUG GROUPS

Corticosteroids	Drugs for pituitary disorders
Drugs used in diabetes	Female sex hormones
Drugs for thyroid disorders	Male sex hormones

CORTICOSTEROIDS

Corticosteroid drugs – often referred to simply as steroids – are derived from, or are synthetic variants of, the natural corticosteroid hormones formed in the outer part (cortex) of the adrenal glands, situated on top of each kidney.

Corticosteroids produced by the body may have either mainly mineralocorticoid or mainly glucocorticoid effects. The main mineralocorticoid effects are the regulation of the balance of mineral salts and of the water content in the body. Glucocorticoid effects include the maintenance of normal levels of sugar in the blood and the promotion of recovery from injury and stress. The release of glucocorticoid hormones is governed by the pituitary gland (see p.103). When present in large amounts, glucocorticoids act to reduce inflammation and suppress allergic reactions and immune system activity. They are distinct from another group of steroid hormones, the anabolic steroids (see p.104).

Although corticosteroids have broadly similar actions to each other, they vary in

their relative strength and duration of action. The mineralocorticoid effects of these drugs also vary in strength.

Why they are used

Glucocorticoid-type corticosteroids are used primarily for their effect in controlling inflammation, whatever its cause. Topical preparations containing corticosteroids are often used to treat many inflammatory skin disorders (see p.134). These drugs may also be injected directly into a joint or around a tendon to relieve inflammation caused by injury or disease (see p.76). However, if these local treatments are either not possible or not effective, corticosteroids may be given systemically by mouth or by intravenous injection.

Corticosteroids are commonly used in many disorders in which inflammation is thought to be caused by excessive or inappropriate immune system activity. These disorders include inflammatory bowel disease (p.70), rheumatoid arthritis (p.75), glomerulonephritis (a kidney disease), and some rare connective tissue disorders, such as systemic lupus erythematosus. In these conditions corticosteroids relieve symptoms and may also temporarily halt the disease.

Corticosteroids may be given regularly by mouth or inhaler to treat asthma, although their effect on relieving acute asthma attacks is delayed by a few hours (see Bronchodilators, p.48 and Drugs for asthma, p.49).

An important use of oral corticosteroids is to correct the deficiency of natural hormones resulting from reduced adrenal gland function, as in Addison's disease. In these cases, the drugs most closely resembling the actions of the natural hormones are selected and a combination of these may be used.

Some cancers of the lymphatic system (lymphomas) and the blood (leukaemias) may also respond to corticosteroid treatment. These drugs are also widely used to prevent or treat rejection of organ transplants, usually in conjunction with other drugs, such as azathioprine (see Immunosuppressants, p.115).

How they work

Given in high doses, corticosteroid drugs reduce inflammation by blocking the action of chemicals such as prostaglandins that trigger the inflammatory response. These drugs also temporarily depress the immune system by reducing the activity of certain types of white blood cell. In addition, they may be used to treat severe allergic reactions or anaphylaxis.

How they affect you

Corticosteroid drugs often produce a dramatic improvement in symptoms. Given systemically, they may also act on the brain to produce a heightened sense of well-being and, in some people, a sense

of euphoria. Troublesome day-to-day side effects are rare. Long-term corticosteroid treatment, however, carries a number of serious risks for the patient.

Risks and special precautions

In the treatment of Addison's disease, corticosteroids can be considered as "hormone replacement therapy", with drugs replacing the natural hormone hydrocortisone. This physiological replacement means that adverse effects are rarely seen.

Drugs with strong mineralocorticoid effects, such as fludrocortisone, may cause water retention, swelling (especially of the ankles), and an increase in blood pressure. Because corticosteroids reduce the effect of insulin (among their other effects), they may create problems in people with diabetes and may even give rise to diabetes in susceptible people. They can also cause peptic ulcers.

Because corticosteroids suppress the immune system's activity, they increase susceptibility to infection. They also suppress symptoms of infectious disease. People taking them should avoid exposure to chickenpox or shingles; if they catch either disease, drugs such as aciclovir tablets may be prescribed. With long-term use, corticosteroids may cause various adverse effects (see left). Doctors try to avoid long-term use of corticosteroids for children because it may retard growth.

Long-term use of corticosteroids suppresses production of the body's own corticosteroid hormones. For this reason, treatment that lasts for more than a few weeks should be withdrawn gradually to give the body time to adjust. If stopped abruptly, the lack of corticosteroid hormones may lead to fatigue, nausea, vomiting, or even sudden collapse.

People taking corticosteroids by mouth for longer than one month are advised to carry a warning card. If someone who is taking steroids long-term has a serious accident or surgery, their defences against shock may need to be supported with extra hydrocortisone, administered intravenously.

ADVERSE EFFECTS OF CORTICOSTEROIDS

Corticosteroids with glucocorticoid properties are effective and useful, often providing benefit in cases where other drugs are ineffective. However, long-term use of high doses can lead to various unwanted effects on the body, as shown below.

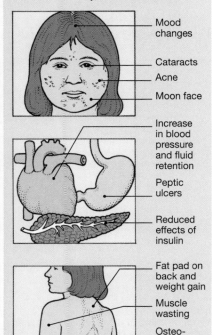

Mood changes

Cataracts

Acne

Moon face

Increase in blood pressure and fluid retention

Peptic ulcers

Reduced effects of insulin

Fat pad on back and weight gain

Muscle wasting

Osteo-porosis

Easy bruising

COMMON DRUGS

Alclometastone	Flunisolide
Beclometasone ✱	Fluocinolone
Betamethasone ✱	Fluocinonide
Budesonide ✱	Fluocortolone
Clobetasol ✱	Fluticasone ✱
Clobetasone	Hydrocortisone ✱
Deflazacort	Methylprednisolone
Dexamethasone ✱	Mometasone
Diflucortolone	Prednisolone ✱
Fludrocortisone	Triamcinolone
Fludroxycortide	
Flumetasone	

✱ See Part 3

DRUGS USED IN DIABETES

The body obtains most of its energy from glucose, a simple form of sugar formed in the gut from the breakdown of starch and other sugars or by metabolic processes in the liver, fat, and muscle. Insulin, one of the hormones produced in the pancreas, enables body tissues to take up glucose from the blood, either to use it for energy or to store it. In diabetes mellitus, there is either a complete lack of insulin or too little is produced. This results in reduced uptake of glucose by the tissues and thus an abnormal rise in the blood glucose level. A high blood glucose level is medically known as hyperglycaemia.

There are two main types of diabetes mellitus. Type 1 (insulin-dependent) diabetes usually appears in young people, 50 per cent of cases occurring around the time of puberty. The insulin-secreting cells in the pancreas are gradually destroyed. An autoimmune condition (where the body mis-identifies its pancreas as "foreign" and tries to eliminate it) or a childhood viral infection is the most likely cause. Although the decline in insulin production is slow, the condition often appears suddenly, brought on by periods of stress (for example, infection or puberty) when the body's insulin requirements are high. Symptoms of Type 1 diabetes include extreme thirst, increased urination, lethargy, and weight loss. This type of diabetes is fatal if it is left untreated.

In Type 1 diabetes, insulin treatment is the only treatment option. It has to be continued for the rest of the patient's life. Several types of insulin are available, which are broadly classified by their duration of action (short-, medium-, and long-acting).

Type 2 diabetes, formerly known as non-insulin-dependent diabetes mellitus (NIDDM) or maturity-onset diabetes, tends to appear at an older age (usually in people over 40, although it has become increasingly common in younger age groups) and to come on much more gradually – there may be a delay in its diagnosis for several years because of the gradual onset of symptoms. In this type of diabetes, the levels of insulin in the

ADMINISTRATION OF INSULIN

A healthy person's body produces a background level of insulin, with additional insulin being produced as required during meals. The insulin delivery systems currently available for people with diabetes cannot mimic this precisely. In people with Type 1 diabetes, short-acting insulin is usually given before meals, and medium-acting insulin is given either before the evening meal or at bedtime. Insulin pen injectors are particularly useful for administration during the day because they are discreet and easy to use. In people with Type 2 diabetes who need insulin, a mixture of short- and medium-acting insulin may be given twice a day. Pumps that deliver continuous subcutaneous insulin are now used in some people with Type 1 diabetes and some who find it difficult to control their insulin levels with injections. Some new types of insulin called insulin analogues (e.g. Insulin lispro) may be better at mimicking the insulin-producing behaviour of a healthy pancreas.

Duration of action of types of insulin

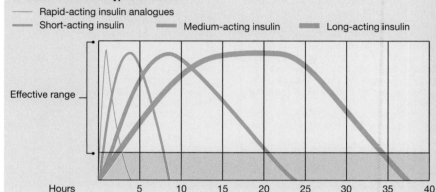

— Rapid-acting insulin analogues
— Short-acting insulin
— Medium-acting insulin
— Long-acting insulin

Effective range

Hours   5   10   15   20   25   30   35   40

blood are usually high. However, the cells of the body are resistant to the effects of insulin and have a reduced glucose uptake despite the high insulin levels. This results in hyperglycaemia. Obesity is the most common cause of Type 2 diabetes.

In both types of diabetes, an alteration in diet is vital. A healthy diet that is low in fats and simple sugars (cakes, sweets) and high in fibre and foods with complex sugars and a low glycaemic index (brown rice, wholewheat pasta), is advised.

In Type 2 diabetes, a reduction in weight alone may be sufficient to lower the body's energy requirements and restore blood glucose to normal levels. If an alteration in diet fails, oral antidiabetic drugs, such as metformin, acarbose, or sulfonylureas, are prescribed. Insulin may

need to be given to people with Type 2 diabetes if the above treatments fail, or in pregnancy, during severe illness, and before the patient undergoes any surgery requiring a general anaesthetic.

Importance of treating diabetes

If diabetes is left untreated, the continual high blood glucose levels damage various parts of the body. The major problems are caused by atherosclerosis, in which a build-up of fatty deposits in the arteries narrows them, reducing the flow of blood. This can result in heart attacks, blindness, stroke, kidney failure, reduced circulation in the legs, and even gangrene. The risk of these conditions is greatly reduced with treatment. Careful control of diabetes in young people, during puberty and afterwards, is essential in reducing the risk of possible long-term complications. Good diabetic control before conception reduces the chance of miscarriage or abnormalities in the baby.

How antidiabetic drugs work

Insulin treatment directly replaces the natural hormone that is deficient in diabetes mellitus. Synthetic human insulins are now the preferred forms. Insulin cannot be taken by mouth because it is broken down in the digestive tract before it reaches the bloodstream. Regular injections are therefore necessary (see Administration of insulin, above).

Sulfonylurea oral antidiabetic drugs encourage the pancreas to produce

ACTION OF SULFONYLUREA DRUGS

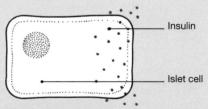

Before drug treatment
In Type 2 diabetes, the islet cells of the pancreas secrete insufficient insulin to meet the body's needs.

Insulin

Islet cell

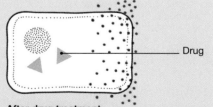

After drug treatment
The drug stimulates the islet cells to release increased amounts of insulin.

Drug

insulin. They are therefore effective only when some insulin-secreting cells remain active; this is why they are ineffective in the treatment of Type 1 diabetes. Metformin alters the way in which the body metabolizes sugar. Acarbose slows digestion of starch and sugar. Both slow the increase in blood sugar that occurs after a meal. Nateglinide and repaglinide stimulate insulin release. Pioglitazone reduces the body's resistance to insulin. Exenatide and sitagliptin stimulate insulin release and block the release of glucagon (a substance that raises blood glucose), thereby helping to prevent the rise in blood sugar after a meal. The new gliflozin drugs (such as dapagliflozin) block reabsorption of sugar by the kidney, so it is lost in the urine.

Insulin treatment and you

The insulin requirements in diabetes vary greatly between individuals and also depend on physical activity and calorie intake. Hence, insulin regimens are tailored to particular needs, and the person is encouraged to take an active role in their own management.

A regular record of home blood glucose monitoring should be kept. This is the basis on which insulin doses are adjusted, preferably by the person with diabetes.

A person with diabetes should learn to recognize warning signs of a "hypo", or attack of hypoglycaemia (low blood sugar): hunger, anxiety, slurred speech, tremor, cold sweats, blurred vision, and headache. The symptoms disappear when glucose is administered, so anyone with diabetes should always carry glucose tablets or sweets. Recurrent "hypos" at specific times may require a reduction of insulin dose. Rarely, undetected low glucose levels may lead to coma. The injection of glucagon rapidly reverses this, so a carer or relative should be shown how to give the injection.

Repeated injection at the same site may disturb the fat layer beneath the skin, producing either swelling or dimpling. This alters the rate of insulin absorption. However, it can be avoided by regularly rotating injection sites.

Insulin requirements are increased during illness and pregnancy. During an illness, the urine or blood should be checked for ketones, substances that are produced in the body when there is insufficient insulin to permit the normal uptake of glucose by the tissues. If high ketone levels occur in the urine during an illness, urgent medical advice should be sought. The combination of high blood sugars, high urinary ketones, and vomiting is a diabetic emergency, and the affected person should be taken to an Accident and Emergency department without delay.

Exercise increases the body's need for glucose, and therefore extra calories may be needed before and during exertion. The effects of vigorous exercise on blood sugar levels may last up to 18–24 hours, and the subsequent (post-exercise) doses of insulin may need to be reduced by 10–25 per cent to avoid hypoglycaemia.

It is advisable for those with diabetes to carry a card or bracelet detailing their condition and treatment. This will be useful in a medical emergency.

SITES OF INJECTION

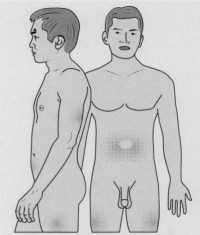

The shaded areas indicate suitable sites for the injection of insulin.

Antidiabetic drugs and you

The sulfonylureas may lower the blood glucose too much. This can be avoided by starting treatment with low doses and ensuring a regular food intake. Rarely, these drugs cause a decrease in the blood cell count, a rash, or intestinal or liver disturbances. Interactions may occur with other drugs, so your doctor should be informed of your treatment before prescribing any medicines for you.

Unlike the sulfonylureas, metformin does not cause hypoglycaemia. Its most common side effects are nausea, weight loss, abdominal distension, and diarrhoea. It should not be used in people with liver, kidney, or heart problems. Acarbose does not cause hypoglycaemia if used on its own. The tablets must either be chewed with the first mouthful of food at meal times or swallowed whole with a little liquid immediately before food. Sitagliptin is taken orally once a day, either with or without food. Exenatide, used mainly in obese patients, is given by injection twice a day before meals.

MONITORING BLOOD GLUCOSE

People with diabetes need to check either their blood or their urine glucose level at home. Blood tests give the most accurate results. There are many types of meter for measuring blood glucose, but they all work in basically the same way.

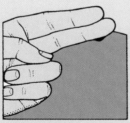

1 Prick your finger to give a large drop of blood.

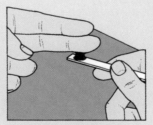

2 Touch the blood on to the test pads of the special testing strip.

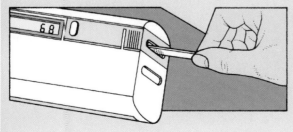

3 Insert the test strip into the meter. Your blood glucose reading will appear as a digital readout.

COMMON DRUGS

Sulfonylurea drugs
Glibenclamide *
Gliclazide *
Glimepiride
Glipizide
Tolbutamide *

Other drugs
Acarbose
Dapagliflozin *
Dulaglutide *
Exenatide *
Glucagon *

Insulin *
Insulin aspart
Insulin glargine
Insulin glulisine
Insulin lispro
Liraglutide
Metformin *
Nateglinide
Pioglitazone *
Repaglinide *
Sitagliptin *

| * See Part 3 |

DRUGS FOR THYROID DISORDERS

The thyroid gland produces the hormone thyroxine, which regulates the body's metabolism. During childhood, thyroxine is essential for normal physical and mental development. Calcitonin, also produced by the thyroid, regulates calcium metabolism and is used as a drug for certain bone disorders (p.80).

Hyperthyroidism

In this condition (also called thyrotoxicosis), the thyroid is overactive and produces too much thyroxine. Women are more commonly affected than men. Symptoms include anxiety, palpitations, weight loss, increased appetite, heat intolerance, diarrhoea, and menstrual disturbances. Graves' disease is the most common form of hyperthyroidism. This is an autoimmune disease in which the body produces antibodies that stimulate the thyroid to make excess thyroxine. Affected people may develop abnormally protuberant eyes (exophthalmos) or a swelling involving the skin over the shins (pretibial myxoedema). Hyperthyroidism can be caused by a benign tumour of the thyroid (an adenoma) or a pre-existing multinodular goitre (see right). Rarely, an overactive thyroid may follow a viral infection, a condition called thyroiditis, or use of certain medications (such as amiodarone or alemtuzumab). Inflammation of the gland leads to the release of stored thyroxine.

Management of hyperthyroidism

There are three possible treatments: antithyroid drugs, radioactive iodine (radio-iodine), and surgery. The most commonly used antithyroid drug is carbimazole, which inhibits the formation of thyroid hormones and reduces their levels to normal over about 4–8 weeks. In the early stage of treatment, a beta blocker (see p.55) may be prescribed to control symptoms. This should be stopped once thyroid function returns to normal. Long-term carbimazole is usually given for 12–18 months to prevent relapse. A "block and replace" regimen may also be used. In this treatment, the thyroid gland is blocked by high doses of carbimazole, and thyroxine is added when the blood level of thyroid hormone falls below normal.

Carbimazole may produce minor side effects such as nausea, vomiting, skin rashes, or headaches. Rarely, the drug may reduce the white blood cell count. Propylthiouracil may be used as an alternative antithyroid drug.

Radio-iodine is often used as a first-line therapy, especially in older people, or as a second choice if hyperthyroidism recurs following use of carbimazole. It acts by destroying thyroid tissue. Hypothyroidism occurs in up to 80 per cent of people within 20 years after treatment. Long-term studies show radio-iodine to be safe, but it should be avoided during pregnancy and breast-feeding, and in patients with thyroid eye disease.

Surgery is a third-line therapy. It may be favoured for patients with a large goitre (see above right), particularly one that causes difficulty in swallowing or breathing. Thyroid eye disease may require corticosteroids (p.99) or other immunomodulatory drugs.

Hypothyroidism

This is a condition resulting from too little thyroxine. Sometimes it may be caused

ACTION OF DRUGS FOR THYROID DISORDERS

Thyroid hormone production
Iodine combines with certain other chemicals (precursors) in the thyroid gland to make thyroid hormones.

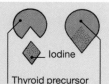

Iodine

Thyroid precursor

Thyroid hormone

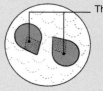

Thyroid hormone

Normal output of thyroid hormones
Thyroid output is normally regulated according to the body's needs.

After drug

Before drug

Drug

Action of antithyroid drugs
In hyperthyroidism, antithyroid drugs partly reduce the production of thyroid hormones by preventing iodine from combining with thyroid precursors in the thyroid gland.

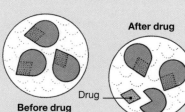

Before drug **After drug**

Synthetic thyroid hormone

Action of thyroid hormones
In hypothyroidism, when the thyroid gland is underactive, supplements of synthetic or (rarely) natural thyroid hormones restore hormone levels to normal.

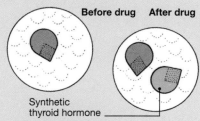

TREATMENT FOR GOITRE

A goitre is a swelling of the thyroid gland. It may occur only temporarily, during puberty or pregnancy, or it may be due to an abnormal growth of thyroid tissue that requires surgical removal. It may rarely be brought about by iodine deficiency. This last cause is treated with iodine supplements (see also p.437).

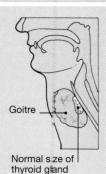

Goitre

Normal size of thyroid gland

by an autoimmune disorder, in which the immune system attacks the thyroid gland. Other cases may follow treatment for hyperthyroidism. In newborn babies, hypothyroidism may be the result of an inborn enzyme disorder. In the past, it also arose from a lack of iodine in the diet.

The symptoms of adult hypothyroidism develop slowly and include weight gain, mental slowness, dry skin, hair loss, increased sensitivity to cold, and heavy menstrual periods. In babies, low levels of thyroxine cause permanent mental and physical retardation and, for this reason, babies are tested for hypothyroidism within a week of birth.

Management of hypothyroidism

Lifelong oral treatment with synthetic thyroid hormones (thyroxine (levothyroxine), or rarely liothyronine) is the only option. Blood tests are done regularly to monitor the treatment and permit the dose to be adjusted. In older people and those with heart disease, thyroxine is introduced gradually to prevent heart strain.

In severely ill patients, thyroid hormone may be given by injection. Hormone injections may also be used for newborn infants with low levels of thyroxine.

Symptoms of thyrotoxicosis may appear if excess thyroxine replacement is given. Otherwise, no adverse events occur since treatment is adjusted to replace the natural hormone that the body should normally produce itself.

COMMON DRUGS

Drugs for hypothyroidism	Drugs for hyperthyroidism
Levothyroxine (thyroxine) *	Carbimazole *
Liothyronine	Iodine *
	Nadolol
	Propranolol *
	Propylthiouracil *
	Radioactive iodine (radio-iodine)

* See Part 3

DRUGS FOR PITUITARY DISORDERS

The pituitary gland, which lies at the base of the brain, produces a number of hormones that regulate physical growth, metabolism, sexual development, and reproductive function. Many of these hormones act indirectly by stimulating other glands, such as the thyroid, adrenal glands, ovaries, and testes, to release their own hormones. A summary of the actions and effects of each pituitary hormone is given below.

An excess or a lack of one of the pituitary hormones may produce serious effects, the nature of which depends on the hormone involved. Abnormal levels of a particular hormone may be caused by a pituitary tumour, which may be treated surgically, with radiotherapy, or with drugs. In other cases, drugs may be used to correct the hormonal imbalance.

The more common pituitary disorders that can be treated with drugs are those involving growth hormone, antidiuretic hormone, prolactin, adrenal hormones, and the gonadotrophins. The first three are discussed below. For information on the use of drugs to treat infertility arising from inadequate levels of gonadotrophins, see p.124. Lack of corticotrophin, leading to inadequate production of adrenal hormones, is usually treated with corticosteroids (see p.99).

Drugs for growth hormone disorders

Growth hormone (somatotropin) is the principal hormone required for normal growth in childhood and adolescence.

Lack of growth hormone impairs normal physical growth. Doctors administer hormone treatment only after tests have proven that a lack of this hormone is the cause of the disorder. If treatment is started at an early age, regular injections of somatropin, a synthetic form of natural growth hormone, administered until the end of adolescence usually allow normal growth and development to take place.

Growth hormone deficiency in adults is rare but may cause loss of strength and stamina, reduced bone mass, weight gain, and psychological symptoms such as poor memory and depression. In some cases it may be treated with somatotropin.

Less often, the pituitary produces an excess of growth hormone. In children this can result in pituitary gigantism; in adults, it can produce a disorder known as acromegaly. This disorder, which is usually the result of a pituitary tumour, is characterized by thickening of the skull, face, hands, and feet, and enlargement of some internal organs.

The pituitary tumour may either be surgically removed or destroyed by radiotherapy. In frail or older people, drugs are used to reduce growth hormone levels. Drugs may also be used as an adjunctive treatment before surgery and in those with increased growth hormone levels occurring after surgery. People who have undergone surgery and/or radiotherapy may require long-term replacement with other hormones (such as sex hormones, thyroid hormone, or corticosteroids).

Drugs for diabetes insipidus

Antidiuretic hormone (also called ADH or vasopressin) acts on the kidneys to control the amount of water retained in the body and returned to the blood. Defective ADH function can be caused by pituitary damage reducing production, or by defects in the kidneys' response to ADH. Both cause the rare condition of diabetes insipidus, in which the kidneys cannot retain water and large quantities pass into the urine. The chief symptoms of diabetes insipidus are constant thirst and production of large volumes of urine.

Diabetes insipidus due to pituitary damage is treated with ADH or a related synthetic drug, desmopressin. These replace naturally produced ADH. If it is due to the kidneys not responding to ADH (nephrogenic diabetes insipidus), other drugs such as thiazide diuretics (p.57) or non-steroidal anti-inflammatory drugs (p.74) may be used. These drugs usually increase urine production, but in diabetes insipidus they have the opposite effect.

Drugs to reduce prolactin levels

Prolactin, also called lactogenic hormone, is produced in both men and women. In women, it controls the secretion of breast milk following childbirth. Its function in men is not understood, although it seems to be necessary for sperm production.

The disorders associated with prolactin are all to do with overproduction. High levels in women can cause lactation that is not associated with pregnancy and birth (galactorrhoea), lack of menstruation (amenorrhoea), and infertility. Excess levels in men may cause galactorrhoea, gynaecomastia (growth of breast tissue), erectile dysfunction, or infertility.

Some drugs, notably methyldopa, oestrogen, metoclopramide, domperidone, and antipsychotics, can raise the prolactin level in the blood. More often, however, increased prolactin results from a pituitary tumour and is usually treated with a dopamine mimetic such as cabergoline to inhibit prolactin production.

THE EFFECTS OF PITUITARY HORMONES

The pituitary gland produces a large number of hormones, many of which control the activities of other glands. The illustration shows the principal sites of action of the major pituitary hormones.

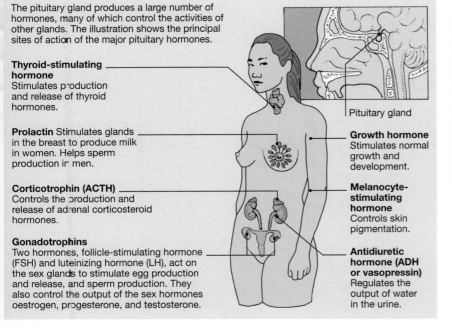

Thyroid-stimulating hormone
Stimulates production and release of thyroid hormones.

Prolactin Stimulates glands in the breast to produce milk in women. Helps sperm production in men.

Corticotrophin (ACTH)
Controls the production and release of adrenal corticosteroid hormones.

Gonadotrophins
Two hormones, follicle-stimulating hormone (FSH) and luteinizing hormone (LH), act on the sex glands to stimulate egg production and release, and sperm production. They also control the output of the sex hormones oestrogen, progesterone, and testosterone.

Pituitary gland

Growth hormone
Stimulates normal growth and development.

Melanocyte-stimulating hormone
Controls skin pigmentation.

Antidiuretic hormone (ADH or vasopressin)
Regulates the output of water in the urine.

COMMON DRUGS

Drugs for growth hormone disorders
Bromocriptine ✱
Lanreotide
Octreotide
Pegvisomant
Somatropin

Drugs for diabetes insipidus
Carbamazepine ✱
Chlortalidone
Desmopressin ✱
Vasopressin (ADH)

Drugs to reduce prolactin levels
Bromocriptine ✱
Cabergoline
Quinagolide

✱ See Part 3

MALE SEX HORMONES

Male sex hormones (androgens) are responsible for the development of male sexual characteristics. The principal androgens are testosterone, produced by the testes, and its more active conversion product dihydrotestosterone, produced in other tissues. Women produce small amounts of testosterone in their adrenal glands and ovaries. In both sexes, androgens stimulate libido (sex drive).

Testosterone has two major effects: an androgenic effect and an anabolic effect. Its androgenic effect is to stimulate the development of the secondary sexual characteristics at puberty, such as growth of body hair, deepening of the voice, and an increase in genital size. Its anabolic effects are to increase muscle mass, bone density, and growth rate in adolescents.

There are several synthetic derivatives of testosterone that produce varying degrees of the androgenic and anabolic effects mentioned above. Derivatives with a mainly anabolic effect are called anabolic steroids (see box below).

Testosterone and its derivatives have been used medically in both men and women to treat a number of conditions.

Why they are used

Male sex hormones are mainly given to men to promote the development of, or maintain, male sexual characteristics when hormone production is deficient. Deficiency may result from abnormality or absence of the testes or inadequate production of the pituitary hormones that stimulate the testes to release testosterone. Androgens are sometimes given to adolescent boys if the onset of puberty is delayed by pituitary problems. The treatment may also help to stimulate development of secondary male sexual characteristics and to increase libido in men with inadequate testosterone levels. This has been found to reduce sperm production, however. (For information on the drug treatment of male infertility, see p.124.) An anti-androgen (a substance that inhibits the effects of androgens) may be used in the treatment of prostate cancer or of benign prostatic hyperplasia, or BPH (an enlarged prostate gland).

EFFECTS OF MALE SEX HORMONES

Anabolic effects
These are the tissue-building effects of male sex hormones.

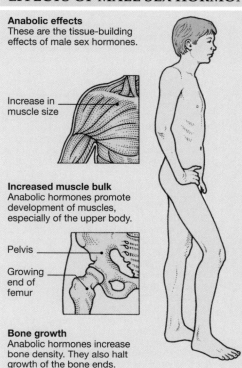

Increase in muscle size

Increased muscle bulk
Anabolic hormones promote development of muscles, especially of the upper body.

Pelvis

Growing end of femur

Bone growth
Anabolic hormones increase bone density. They also halt growth of the bone ends.

Androgenic effects
These are the effects of male sex hormones on the development of secondary male sexual characteristics.

Voice changes
Androgenic hormones cause enlargement of the larynx and thus deepen the voice.

Facial hair

Larynx

Facial and body hair
Androgenic hormones stimulate hair growth on face and body areas.

Penis

Testis

Genital development
Androgenic hormones stimulate enlargement of the testes and penis.

Androgens may also be prescribed for women to treat certain types of cancer of the breast and uterus (see Anticancer drugs, p.112). Testosterone can be given by injection, as a gel to rub into the skin, or as a nasal spray.

How they work

Taken in low doses as part of replacement therapy when natural production is low, male sex hormones act in the same way as the natural hormones. In adolescents suffering from delayed puberty, hormone treatment produces both androgenic and anabolic effects (above), initiating the development of secondary sexual characteristics over a few months; full

sexual development usually takes place over three to four years. When sex hormones are given to adult men, the effects on physical appearance and libido may begin to be felt within a few weeks.

Risks and special precautions

The main risks with these drugs occur when they are given to boys with delayed puberty and to women with breast cancer. Given to initiate the onset of puberty, they may stunt growth by prematurely sealing the growing ends of the long bones. Doctors normally try to avoid prescribing hormones in these circumstances until growth is complete. High doses given to women have various masculinizing effects, including increased facial and body hair, and a deeper voice. The drugs may also produce enlargement of the clitoris, changes in libido, and acne.

ANABOLIC STEROIDS

Anabolic steroids are synthetically produced variants that mimic the anabolic effects of the natural hormones. They increase muscle bulk and body growth.

Doctors very occasionally prescribe anabolic steroids and a high-protein diet to promote recovery after serious illness or major surgery. The steroids may also help to increase the production of blood cells in some forms of anaemia and to reduce itching in chronic obstructive jaundice.

Anabolic steroids have been misused in sports such as athletics, weight-lifting, and

body-building, because these drugs are perceived by some users to enhance athletic performance, especially with regard to muscle power and overall endurance. The use of anabolic steroids by sportspeople to improve their performance is condemned by doctors and banned by many athletic organizations because of the risks to health, particularly for women. The side effects range from acne and baldness to fluid retention, reduced fertility in men and women, hardening of the arteries, a long-term risk of liver disease, and certain forms of cancer.

COMMON DRUGS

Primarily androgenic
Mesterolone
Testosterone ✳

Primarily anabolic
Nandrolone

Anti-androgens
Cyproterone ✳
Dutasteride
Finasteride ✳

✳ See Part 3

FEMALE SEX HORMONES

There are two types of female sex hormone: oestrogen and progesterone. In women, these hormones are secreted by the ovaries from puberty until the menopause and by the placenta during pregnancy. Production of oestrogen and progesterone is regulated by the two gonadotrophin hormones (FSH and LH), produced by the pituitary gland (see p.103). Each month (in non-pregnant women) the levels of oestrogen and progesterone fluctuate, producing the menstrual cycle (see p.119).

In girls, oestrogen is responsible for the development of secondary sexual characteristics at puberty, including breast development and widening of the pelvis. During the menstrual cycle, progesterone prepares the lining of the uterus for implantation of a fertilized egg. Progesterone is also important for the maintenance of pregnancy.

Synthetic forms of these hormones, known as oestrogens and progestogens, are used medically to treat a number of conditions. They can be given as tablets, patches, gels, implants, and intravaginal creams, pessaries, and rings.

Why they are used

The best-known use of oestrogens and progestogens is in oral contraceptives (see p.121). Other uses include the treatment of menstrual disorders (p.120) and certain hormone-sensitive cancers (p.112), and the management of gender reassignment. This page discusses the drug treatments that are used for natural hormone deficiency.

Hormone deficiency

Deficiency of female sex hormones may result from deficiency of gonadotrophins, which in turn may be due to a pituitary disorder or to abnormal development of the ovaries or to abnormal development of the ovaries (ovarian failure). This may lead to the absence of menstruation and lack of sexual development. If tests show a deficiency of gonadotrophins, preparations of these hormones may be prescribed (see p.124). These trigger the release of oestrogen and progesterone from the ovaries. If pituitary function is normal and ovarian failure is diagnosed as the cause of hormone deficiency, oestrogens and progestogens may be given as supplements. In this situation, these supplements ensure development of normal female sexual characteristics but cannot stimulate ovulation.

Menopause

A decline in the levels of oestrogen and progesterone occurs naturally following the menopause, when the ovaries stop functioning and the menstrual cycle ceases. The sudden reduction in levels of oestrogen can cause various symptoms, often including hot flushes, sweating, and palpitations. Many doctors suggest that hormone supplements be used around the time of the menopause (see below). Such hormone replacement therapy (HRT) may also be prescribed for women who have undergone early or premature menopause – for example, as a result of surgical removal of the ovaries or radiotherapy for ovarian cancer.

HRT helps to reduce menopausal symptoms, including hot flushes and vaginal dryness. It is not normally recommended for long-term use or for the treatment of osteoporosis (p.80), however, because of the increased risk of disorders such as breast cancer, stroke, and thromboembolism occurring. In HRT, oestrogen is used together with a progestogen unless the woman has had a hysterectomy, in which case oestrogen alone is used. If dryness of the vagina is a particular problem, a cream containing an oestrogen drug may be prescribed for short-term use.

How they affect you

Hormones that are given to treat ovarian failure or delayed puberty take three to six months to produce a noticeable effect on sexual development. Taken for menopausal symptoms, they can dramatically reduce the number of hot flushes within a week.

Both oestrogens and progestogens can cause fluid retention, and oestrogens may cause nausea, vomiting, breast tenderness, headache, dizziness, and depression. Progestogens may cause breakthrough bleeding between menstrual periods. In the comparatively low doses used to treat these disorders, however, side effects are unlikely.

Risks and special precautions

Because oestrogens increase the risk of hypertension (raised blood pressure), thrombosis (abnormal blood clotting), and breast cancer, there are risks associated with long-term HRT. Treatment is used with caution in women who have heart or circulatory disorders, and in those who are overweight or who smoke. HRT given via patches or gels does not carry an increased risk of blood clots. Tibolone has both oestrogenic and progestogenic properties and may be used on its own.

The use of oestrogens and progestogens as replacement therapy in ovarian failure carries few risks for otherwise healthy young women.

EFFECTS OF HORMONE REPLACEMENT THERAPY (HRT)

HRT is primarily used to relieve symptoms related to menopause, such as hot flushes, mood swings, night sweats, and vaginal dryness. It may also be used to prevent or treat osteoporosis (p.80). However, the benefits must be weighed against increased health risks associated with its use, such as breast cancer, thromboembolism, and stroke.

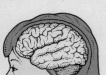

Brain
HRT increases the risk of stroke.

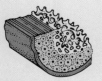

Bones
HRT reduces the thinning of bone that occurs in osteoporosis and thus protects against fractures.

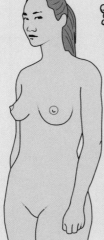

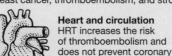

Heart and circulation
HRT increases the risk of thromboembolism and does not prevent coronary artery disease.

Breasts
There is a slightly increased risk of breast cancer with HRT (apart from vaginal oestrogen).

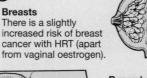

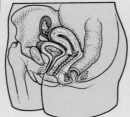

Reproductive organs
HRT can prevent thinning and dryness of the vaginal tissues leading to painful intercourse.

COMMON DRUGS

Oestrogens
Conjugated oestrogens ✳
Estradiol ✳
Estriol
Estrone
Ethinylestradiol ✳

Progestogens
Desogestrel ✳
Dydrogesterone ✳
Levonorgestrel ✳
Medroxyprogesterone ✳
Norethisterone ✳
Norgestrel
Progesterone

Other drugs
Raloxifene ✳

✳ See Part 3

NUTRITION

Food provides energy (as calories) and materials called nutrients needed for growth and renewal of tissues. Protein, carbohydrate, and fat are the three major nutrient components of food. Vitamins and minerals are found only in small amounts in food, but are very important for normal function of the body. Fibre, found only in foods from plants, is needed for the digestive system to work well.

During digestion, large molecules of food are broken down into smaller molecules, releasing nutrients that are absorbed into the bloodstream. Carbohydrate and fat are then metabolized by body cells to produce energy. They may also be incorporated with protein into the cell structure. Each metabolic process is promoted by a specific enzyme and often requires the presence of a particular vitamin or mineral.

Why drugs are used

Dietary deficiency of essential nutrients can lead to illness. In poorer countries where there is a shortage of food, marasmus (resulting from lack of food energy) and kwashiorkor (from lack of protein) are common. In rich countries, however, excessive food intake leading to obesity is more common. Nutritional deficiencies in developed countries result from poor food choices and usually stem from a lack of a specific vitamin or mineral, such as in iron-deficiency anaemia.

Some nutritional deficiencies may be caused by an inability of the body to absorb nutrients from food (malabsorption) or to utilize them once they have been absorbed. Malabsorption may be caused by lack of an enzyme or an abnormality of the digestive tract. Errors of metabolism are often inborn and are not yet fully understood. They may be caused by failure of the body to produce the chemicals required to process nutrients for use.

Why supplements are used

Deficiencies such as kwashiorkor or marasmus are usually treated by dietary improvement and, in some cases, food supplements, rather than drugs. Vitamin and mineral deficiencies are usually treated with appropriate supplements. Malabsorption disorders may require changes in diet or long-term use of supplements. Metabolic errors are not easily treated with supplements or drugs, and a special diet may be the main treatment.

The preferred treatment of obesity is reduction of food intake, altered eating patterns, and increased exercise. When these methods are not effective, and the body mass index (BMI) is 30 or more, an anti-obesity drug may be used.

Major food components

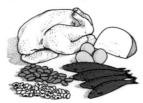

Proteins
Vital for tissue growth and repair. In meat and dairy products, cereals, and pulses. Moderate amounts required.

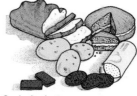

Carbohydrates
A major energy source, stored as fat when taken in excess. In cereals, sugar, and vegetables. Starchy foods preferable to sugar.

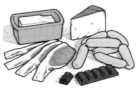

Fats
A concentrated energy form that is needed only in small quantities. In animal products such as butter and in plant oils.

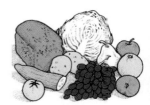

Fibre (non-starch polysaccharides)
The indigestible part of any plant product that, although it contains no nutrients, adds bulk to faeces.

Absorption of nutrients
Food passes through the mouth, oesophagus, and stomach to the small intestine. The lining of the small intestine secretes many enzymes and is covered by tiny projections (villi) that enable nutrients to pass into the blood.

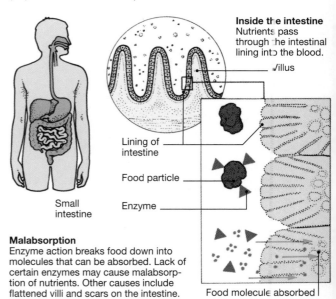

Inside the intestine
Nutrients pass through the intestinal lining into the blood.
— Villus

Lining of intestine

Food particle

Enzyme

Small intestine

Malabsorption
Enzyme action breaks food down into molecules that can be absorbed. Lack of certain enzymes may cause malabsorption of nutrients. Other causes include flattened villi and scars on the intestine.

Food molecule absorbed

MAJOR DRUG GROUPS

Vitamins

VITAMINS

Vitamins are complex chemicals that are essential for a variety of body functions. With the exception of vitamin D, the body cannot manufacture these substances itself and therefore we need to include them in our diet. There are 13 major vitamins: A, C, D, E, K; the B complex vitamins – thiamine (B1), riboflavin (B2), niacin (B3), pantothenic acid (B5), pyridoxine (B6), and cobalamin (B12); folic acid; and biotin. Most vitamins are required in very small amounts, and each vitamin is present in one or more foods (see Main food sources of vitamins, p.108). Vitamin D is also produced in the body when the skin is exposed to sunlight. Vitamins fall into two groups, depending on whether they dissolve in fat or water (see Fat-soluble and water-soluble vitamins, p.109).

A number of vitamins (such as vitamins A, C, and E) have now been recognized as having strong antioxidant properties. Antioxidants neutralize the effect of free radicals, substances produced during the body's normal processes that may be potentially harmful if they are not neutralized. Free radicals are believed to play a role in cardiovascular disease, ageing, and cancer.

A balanced diet that includes a variety of different types of food is likely to contain adequate amounts of all the vitamins. Inadequate intake of any vitamin over an extended period can lead to symptoms of deficiency. The nature of these symptoms depends on the vitamin concerned.

A doctor may recommend taking supplements of one or more vitamins in a variety of circumstances: to prevent vitamin deficiency occurring in people who are considered at special risk, to treat symptoms of deficiency, and in the treatment of certain medical conditions.

Why they are used
Preventing deficiency
Most people in the United Kingdom obtain sufficient quantities of vitamins in their diet, and it is therefore not usually necessary to take additional vitamins in the form of supplements. People who are unsure if their present diet is adequate are advised to look at the table on p.108 to check that foods that are rich in vitamins are eaten regularly. Vitamin intake can often be boosted simply by increasing the quantities of fresh foods and raw fruit and vegetables in the diet. Certain groups in the population are, however, at increased

risk of vitamin deficiency. These include people who have an increased need for certain vitamins that may not be met from dietary sources – in particular, women who are pregnant or breast-feeding, and infants and young children. Older people who may not be eating a varied diet may also be at risk. Strict vegetarians, vegans, and others on restricted diets may not receive adequate amounts of all vitamins.

In addition, people who suffer from disorders in which absorption of nutrients from the bowel is impaired, or who need to take drugs that reduce the absorption of vitamins (for example, some types of lipid-lowering drugs), are usually given additional vitamins.

In these cases, the doctor is likely to advise supplements of one or more vitamins. Although most preparations are available without a prescription, it is important to seek specialist advice before starting a course of vitamin supplements, so that a proper assessment is made of your individual requirements.

Vitamin supplements should not be used as a general tonic to improve well-being – they are not effective for this purpose – nor should they ever be used as a substitute for a balanced diet.

PRIMARY FUNCTIONS OF VITAMINS

The role of vitamins in the body is not yet fully understood; much of our knowledge is based on the evidence that is provided by symptoms resulting from deficiency of a particular vitamin. Most vitamins have been found to have a number of important actions on one or more body systems or functions. Many are involved in the activity of enzymes (substances that promote or enable biochemical reactions in the body). This illustration (right) indicates the organs and body systems on which each vitamin has its principal effect.

Brain and nervous system
Folic acid, pyridoxine, pantothenic acid, thiamine, vitamin B12, vitamin C

Eyes
Riboflavin, vitamin A

Blood vessels
Vitamin E

Lungs
Vitamin A, vitamin E

Heart
Thiamine, vitamin E

Adrenal hormones
Pantothenic acid, riboflavin, vitamin C

Fertility
Folic acid, vitamin A

Skin
Niacin, pyridoxine, riboflavin, vitamin A, vitamin E

Muscles
Pyridoxine, thiamine, vitamin E

Connective tissue
Vitamin C

Teeth and gums
Vitamin A, vitamin C, vitamin D

Digestion
Pantothenic acid, pyridoxine

Bones
Vitamin A, vitamin C, vitamin D

Metabolism
Biotin, folic acid, riboflavin, niacin, pantothenic acid, pyridoxine, thiamine, vitamin B12, vitamin E

Growth
Folic acid, vitamin A, vitamin B12

Immune system
Vitamin C, vitamin D

Blood
Folic acid, pantothenic acid, pyridoxine, vitamin B12, vitamin E, vitamin K

VITAMINS continued

MAIN FOOD SOURCES OF VITAMINS AND MINERALS

The table below indicates which foods are especially good sources of particular vitamins and minerals. Ensuring that you regularly select foods from a variety of categories helps to maintain adequate intake for most people, without a need for supplements. It is important to remember that processed and overcooked foods are likely to contain fewer vitamins than fresh, raw, or lightly cooked foods.

Vitamins	Red meat	Poultry	Liver	Milk	Cheese	Butter/margarine	Eggs	Fish	Cereals and bread	Green vegetables	Root vegetables	Pulses/legumes	Nuts	Fruit	Other	
Biotin			●				●					●	●			Especially peanuts. Cauliflower and mushrooms are good sources.
Folic acid			●				●			●					●	Wheat germ and mushrooms are rich sources.
Niacin as nicotinic acid	●	●	●					●	●			●	●			Protein-rich foods such as milk and eggs contain tryptophan, which can be converted to niacin in the body.
Pantothenic acid			●					●	●							Each food group contributes some pantothenic acid.
Pyridoxine	●	●	●					●	●	●						Especially white meat (poultry), fish, and wholemeal cereals.
Riboflavin			●	●	●		●		●	●	●				●	Found in most foods.
Thiamine	●		●						●	●	●					Brewer's yeast, wheat germ, and bran are also good sources.
Vitamin A			●	●	●	●	●			●	●				●	Fish liver oil, dark green leafy vegetables such as spinach, and orange or yellow-orange vegetables and fruits such as carrots, apricots, and peaches are especially good sources of vitamin A.
Vitamin B$_{12}$	●		●	●	●		●	●								Obtained only from animal products, especially liver and red meat.
Vitamin C										●	●				●	Especially citrus fruits, tomatoes, potatoes, broccoli, strawberries, and melon.
Vitamin D				●		●	●	●								Fish liver oils, margarine, and milk are the best sources, but the vitamin is also produced when the skin is exposed to sunlight.
Vitamin E						●	●		●	●		●	●			Vegetable oils, wholemeal cereals, and wheat germ are the best sources.
Vitamin K										●	●					Green leafy vegetables are the best source. Also found in small amounts in fruits, seeds, root vegetables, dairy products, and meat.
Minerals																
Calcium				●	●				●			●	●			Dark green leafy vegetables, soya bean products, and nuts are good non-dairy alternatives. Also present in hard, or alkaline, water supplies.
Chromium	●				●				●	●						Especially unrefined wholemeal cereals.
Copper	●	●	●					●	●	●		●	●			Especially shellfish, wholemeal cereals, and mushrooms.
Fluoride								●								Primarily obtained from fluoridated water supplies. Also in seafood and tea.
Iodine				●	●			●	●							Provided by iodized table salt, but adequate amounts can be obtained without using table salt from dairy products, saltwater fish, and bread.
Iron	●	●	●				●	●	●	●						Especially liver, red meat, and enriched or whole grains.
Magnesium				●				●	●	●		●	●			Dark green leafy vegetables such as spinach are rich sources. Also present in alkaline water supplies.
Phosphorus	●	●	●	●	●		●	●	●	●	●	●	●		●	Common food additive. Large amounts found in some carbonated beverages.
Potassium									●	●		●			●	Best sources are fruits and vegetables, especially oranges, bananas, and potatoes.
Selenium	●		●	●				●	●							Seafood is the richest source. Amounts in most foods are variable depending on soil where plants were grown and animals grazed.
Sodium	●	●	●	●	●	●	●	●	●	●	●	●	●		●	Sodium is present in all foods, especially table salt, processed foods, potato crisps, crackers, pickled, cured, or smoked meats, seafood, and vegetables. Also present in softened water.
Zinc	●				●			●	●			●				Highest amounts in wholemeal breads and cereals.

Vitamin deficiency

It is rare for a diet to be totally lacking in a particular vitamin, but if intake of a vitamin is regularly lower than the body's requirements, over a period of time the body's stores of that vitamin may become depleted and symptoms of deficiency may appear. In the UK, vitamin deficiency disorders are most common among homeless people, those who misuse alcohol, and those on low incomes who fail to eat an adequate diet. Deficiencies of water-soluble vitamins are more likely since most of these are not stored in large quantities in the body. For descriptions of individual deficiency disorders, see the vitamin profiles in Part 3.

Dosages of vitamins prescribed to treat vitamin deficiency are likely to be larger than those used to prevent deficiency. Medical supervision is required when correcting vitamin deficiency.

Other medical uses of vitamins

Various claims have been made for the value of vitamins in the treatment of medical disorders other than vitamin deficiency. High doses of vitamin C have been said to be effective in the prevention and treatment of the common cold, but such claims are not yet proved; zinc, however, may be helpful for this purpose. Vitamin and mineral supplements do not improve IQ in well-nourished children, but quite small dietary deficiencies can cause poor academic performance.

Certain vitamins have recognized medical uses apart from their nutritional role. Vitamin D has long been used to treat bone-wasting disorders (see p.80). Niacin is sometimes used (in the form of nicotinic acid) as a lipid-lowering drug (see p.61). Derivatives of vitamin A (retinoids) are an established part of the

MINERALS

Minerals are chemical elements (the simplest form of substances), many of which are vital in trace amounts for normal metabolic processes. A balanced diet usually contains all of the minerals that the body requires; mineral deficiency diseases, except iron-deficiency anaemia, are uncommon.

Dietary supplements are necessary only when a doctor has diagnosed a specific deficiency or in preventing or treating a medical disorder. Doctors often prescribe minerals for people with intestinal diseases that reduce the absorption of minerals from the diet. Iron supplements are often advised for pregnant or breast-feeding women, and iron-rich foods are recommended for infants over six months.

Much of the general advice given for vitamins also applies to minerals: taking supplements unless under medical direction is not advisable, exceeding the body's daily requirements is not beneficial, and large doses may be harmful.

CALCULATING DAILY VITAMIN REQUIREMENTS

Everyone needs a minimum amount of each vitamin to maintain their health. This may vary with age, sex, and, in women, pregnancy or breast-feeding. For example, women planning a pregnancy need to have sufficient folic acid (see p.436) before conceiving and during pregnancy to prevent a neural tube defect in the baby. Guidelines for assessing nutritional values in diets are called Reference Nutrient Intakes or Reference Intakes (RNIs or RIs). These are based on how much of a nutrient is enough to meet the needs of about 97 per cent of people. Those consuming much less than the RNI on a daily basis may be at risk of getting less than their minimum needs.

For further information, see the individual vitamin profiles in Part 3, or see the British Nutrition Foundation at www.nutrition.org.uk.

Reference Nutrient Intakes of vitamins for adults (aged 19–50)

Vitamin (unit)	Reference Nutrient Intake	
	Men	Women
Biotin (mcg)	10–200*	10–200*
Folic acid as folate (mcg)	200	200
Niacin as nicotinic acid (mg)	17	13
Pantothenic acid (mg)	3–7*	3–7*
Pyridoxine (mg)	1.4	1.2
Riboflavin (mg)	1.3	1.1
Thiamine (mg)	1.0	0.8
Vitamin A (mcg)	700	600
Vitamin B_{12} (mcg)	1.5	1.5
Vitamin C (mg)	40	40
Vitamin D (mcg)	10 Ø	10 Ø
Vitamin E (mg)	10†	8†

✳ Estimated requirement;　Ø See also Vitamin D, p.444;　† US figure

treatment for severe acne (see p.137). Many women who have pre-menstrual syndrome take pyridoxine (vitamin B_6) supplements to relieve their symptoms; see Drugs for menstrual disorders, p.120.

Risks and special precautions

Vitamins are essential for health, and supplements can be taken without risk by most people. It is important, however, not to exceed the recommended dosage, particularly in the case of fat-soluble vitamins, which may accumulate in the body. Dosage needs to be carefully calculated, taking into account the degree of deficiency, the dietary intake, and the duration of treatment. Overdosage has at best no therapeutic value, and at worst it may carry the risk of serious harmful effects. Multivitamin preparations containing a large number of different vitamins are widely available. Fortunately, the amounts of each vitamin contained in each tablet are not usually large and are not likely to be harmful unless the dose is greatly exceeded. However, single vitamin supplements can be harmful because an excess of one vitamin may increase requirements for others; hence, they should be used only on medical advice. For specific information on each vitamin, see Part 3, pp.433–445.

FAT-SOLUBLE AND WATER-SOLUBLE VITAMINS

Fat-soluble vitamins
Vitamins A, D, E, and K are absorbed from the intestine into the bloodstream together with fat (see also How drugs pass through the body, p.17). Deficiency of these vitamins may occur as a result of any disorder that affects the absorption of fat (for example, coeliac disease). These vitamins are stored in the liver, and reserves of some of them may last for several years. Taking an excess of a fat-soluble vitamin for a long period may cause it to build up to a harmful level in the body. Ensuring that foods rich in these vitamins are regularly included in the diet usually provides a sufficient supply without the risk of overdosage.

Water-soluble vitamins
Vitamin C and the B vitamins dissolve in water. Most are stored in the body for only a short period and are rapidly excreted by the kidneys if taken in higher amounts than the body requires. Vitamin B_{12} is the exception; it is stored in the liver, which may hold up to six years' supply. For these reasons, foods containing water-soluble vitamins need to be eaten daily. They are easily lost in cooking, so uncooked foods containing these vitamins should be eaten regularly. An overdose of water-soluble vitamins does not usually cause toxic effects, but adverse reactions to large dosages of vitamin C and pyridoxine (vitamin B_6) have been reported.

MALIGNANT AND IMMUNE DISEASE

The body constantly needs to produce new cells to replace those that wear out and die naturally and to repair injured tissue. Normally, the rate at which cells are created is carefully regulated. However, sometimes abnormal cells are formed that multiply uncontrollably. These cells may form lumps of abnormal tissue, or tumours.

Usually, tumours are confined to one place and cause few problems; these are benign growths, such as warts. In other types of tumour, cells may invade or destroy the structures around the tumour, and abnormal cells may spread to other parts of the body, forming satellite or metastatic tumours. These are malignant growths, also called cancers.

Opposing the development of tumours is the body's immune system. This can recognize as foreign not only invading bacteria and viruses but also transplanted tissue and cells that have become cancerous. The immune system relies on different types of white blood cell produced in the lymph glands and the bone marrow. The white blood cells respond to foreign cells in a variety of ways, which are described on the facing page.

What can go wrong

No single cause for cancer has been identified, and an individual's risk of developing cancer may depend both upon genetic predisposition (some families seem prone to cancers of one or more types) and upon exposure to external risk factors, known as carcinogens. These include tobacco smoke, which increases the risk of lung cancer, and ultraviolet light, which makes skin cancer more likely in those who spend long periods in the sun. Long-term suppression of the immune system by disease (as in AIDS) or by drugs – for example, those given to prevent rejection of transplanted organs – increases the risk of developing infections and also certain cancers. This demonstrates the importance of the immune system in removing abnormal cells with the potential to cause a tumour.

Overactivity of the immune system may also cause problems. It may respond excessively to an innocuous stimulus, as in hay fever (see Allergy, p.81), or may mount a reaction against normal tissues (autoimmunity), leading to disorders known as autoimmune diseases. These include rheumatoid arthritis, systemic lupus erythematosus, pernicious anaemia, and some forms of hypothyroidism. Immune system activity can also be troublesome following a transplant, when it may lead to rejection of the foreign tissue. Medication is then needed to damp down the immune system and enable the body to accept the foreign tissue.

Types of cancer
Inappropriate multiplication of cells leads to the formation of tumours that may be benign or malignant. Benign tumours do not spread to other tissues; however, malignant (cancerous) tumours do. Some of the main types of cancer are defined below.

Type of cancer	Tissues affected
Carcinoma	Skin and glandular tissue lining cells of internal organs
Sarcoma	Muscles, bones, and fibrous tissues and lining cells of blood vessels
Leukaemia	White blood cells
Lymphoma	Lymph glands

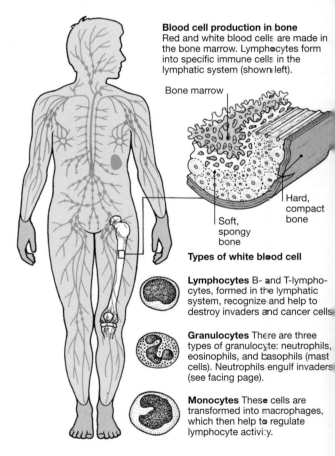

Blood cell production in bone
Red and white blood cells are made in the bone marrow. Lymphocytes form into specific immune cells in the lymphatic system (shown left).

Bone marrow

Hard, compact bone

Soft, spongy bone

Types of white blood cell

Lymphocytes B- and T-lymphocytes, formed in the lymphatic system, recognize and help to destroy invaders and cancer cells

Granulocytes There are three types of granulocyte: neutrophils, eosinophils, and basophils (mast cells). Neutrophils engulf invaders (see facing page).

Monocytes These cells are transformed into macrophages, which then help to regulate lymphocyte activity.

Why drugs are used

In cancer treatment, conventional chemotherapy involves using cytotoxic (cell-killing) drugs to eliminate abnormally dividing cells. These slow the growth rate of tumours and sometimes lead to their complete disappearance. However, because these drugs act against all rapidly dividing cells, they also reduce the number of normal cells, including blood cells, being produced from bone marrow. This can

Types of immune response

A specific response occurs when the immune system recognizes an invader. Two types of specific response, humoral and cellular, are described below. Phagocytosis, a non-specific response that does not depend on recognition of the invader, is also described below.

Humoral response

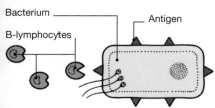

B-lymphocytes are activated by unfamiliar proteins (antigens) on the surface of the invading bacterium.

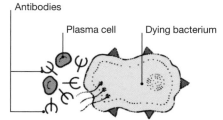

The activated B-lymphocytes form plasma cells, which release antibodies that bind to the invader and kill it.

Cellular response

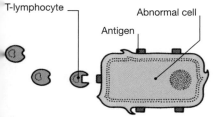

T-lymphocytes recognize the antigens on abnormal or invading cells.

The T-lymphocytes bind to the abnormal cell and destroy it by altering chemical activity within the cell.

Engulfing invaders (phagocytosis)

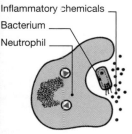

Certain cells, such as neutrophils, are attracted by inflammatory chemicals to an area of bacterial infection.

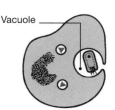

The neutrophil flows around the bacterium, enclosing it within a fluid-filled space called a vacuole.

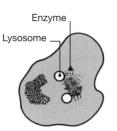

When the vacuole is formed, enzymes from areas called lysosomes in the neutrophil destroy the bacterium.

INTERFERONS

Interferons are natural proteins that limit viral infection by inhibiting viral replication within body cells. These substances may also assist in the destruction of cancer cells.

Effect on viral infection

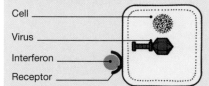

Interferon binds to receptors on a virus-infected cell.

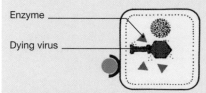

The presence of interferon triggers the release of enzymes that block viral replication. The virus is thus destroyed.

Effect on cancer cells

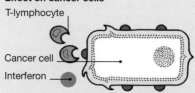

Interferon produced in response to a cancer cell activates T-lymphocytes.

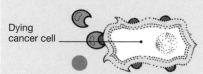

T-lymphocytes attack and destroy the cancer cell.

---

produce serious adverse effects such as anaemia and neutropenia in cancer patients, but it can be useful in limiting white cell activity in autoimmune disorders. Newer anticancer drugs are more selective in the cells they target. For example, trastuzumab (Herceptin) targets a specific protein produced by certain types of breast cancer cell.

Other drugs that have immunosuppressant effects include corticosteroids, azathioprine, and ciclosporin, which are used after transplant surgery. No drugs are yet available that directly stimulate the entire immune system. However, growth factors may be used to increase the number and activity of some white blood cells, and antibody infusions may help those with deficient production or be used against specific targets in organ transplantation and cancer.

MAJOR DRUG GROUPS

Anticancer drugs
Immunosuppressant drugs
Drugs for HIV and AIDS

ANTICANCER DRUGS

Cancer is a general term that covers a wide range of disorders, ranging from the leukaemias (blood cancers) to solid tumours of the lung, breast, and other organs. In all cancers, a group of cells escape from the normal controls on cell growth and multiplication. As a result, the cancerous (malignant) cells begin to crowd out the normal cells and a tumour develops. Cancerous cells are frequently unable to perform their usual functions, and this may lead to progressively impaired function of the organ or area concerned. Cancers may develop from cells of the blood, skin, muscle, or any other tissue.

Malignant tumours spread into nearby structures, blocking blood vessels and compressing nerves and other structures. Fragments of the tumour may become detached and carried in the bloodstream to other parts of the body, where they form secondary growths (metastases).

Many different factors, or a combination of them, can provoke cancerous changes in cells. These include an individual's genetic background, immune system failure, and exposure to cancer-causing agents (carcinogens). Known carcinogens include ultraviolet light, tobacco smoke, radiation, certain chemicals, viruses, and dietary factors.

Treating cancer is a complicated process that depends on the type of cancer, its stage of development, and the patient's condition and wishes. Any of the following treatments may be used alone or in combination with the others: surgery, radiotherapy, and drug therapy.

Until recently, drug treatment of cancer relied heavily on hormonal drugs and cytotoxic agents (usually referred to as chemotherapy). Hormone treatments are suitable for only a few types of cancer, and cytotoxic drugs, although valuable, can have severe side effects because of the damage that they do to normal tissues. However, as understanding of cancer biology has increased, new drugs have been developed. These targeted agents predominantly take the forms of small molecule inhibitors, which target growth and survival signals arising within cancer cells, and monoclonal antibodies, which affect growth and survival signals arising outside the cancer cells. In addition, immunomodulatory drugs (immunotherapies), pioneered by agents such as interleukin-2, are now entering the mainstream.

Why they are used

Cytotoxic drugs can cure rapidly growing cancers and are the treatment of choice for leukaemias, lymphomas, and certain cancers of the testis. They are less effective against slow-growing solid tumours, such as those of the breast and bowel, but they can relieve symptoms and prolong life when given as palliative chemotherapy (treatment that relieves symptoms but does not cure the disease). Adjuvant chemotherapy is increasingly being used following surgery, especially for breast and bowel tumours, to prevent regrowth of the cancer from cells left behind after the surgery. Neoadjuvant or primary chemotherapy is sometimes used before surgery to reduce the size of the tumour.

Hormone treatment is offered in cases of hormone-sensitive cancer, such as breast, uterine, and prostatic cancers, where they can be used to relieve disease

SUCCESSFUL CHEMOTHERAPY

Not all cancers respond to treatment with anticancer drugs. Some cancers can be cured by drug treatment. In others, drug treatment can slow or temporarily halt the progress of the disease. The list on the right summarizes the main cancers that fall into each of these two groups. In certain individual cases, drug treatment has no beneficial effect, but in some of these, other treatments, such as surgery, often produce significant benefits.

Successful drug treatment of cancer usually requires repeated courses of anticancer drugs because the treatment needs to be halted periodically to allow the blood-producing cells in the bone marrow to recover. The diagram below shows the number of cancer cells and normal blood cells before and after each course of treatment with cytotoxic anticancer drugs during successful chemotherapy. Both cancer cells and blood cells are reduced, but the blood cells recover quickly between courses of drug treatment. When treatment is effective, the number of cancer cells is reduced, so they no longer cause symptoms.

Response to chemotherapy

Cancers that can be cured by drugs
Some cancers of the lymphatic system
    (including Hodgkin's disease)
Acute leukaemias (forms of blood cancer)
Choriocarcinoma (cancer of the placenta)
Germ cell tumours (cancers affecting sperm
    and egg cells)
Wilms' tumour (a rare form of kidney cancer
    that affects children)
Cancer of the testis

**Cancers in which drugs produce
worthwhile benefits**
Breast cancer
Ovarian cancer
Some leukaemias
Multiple myeloma (a bone marrow cancer)
Many types of lung cancer
Head and neck cancers
Cancer of the stomach
Cancer of the prostate
Some cancers of the lymphatic system
Bladder cancer
Endometrial cancer (cancer affecting
    the lining of the uterus)
Cancer of the large intestine
Cancer of the oesophagus
Cancer of the pancreas
Cancer of the cervix

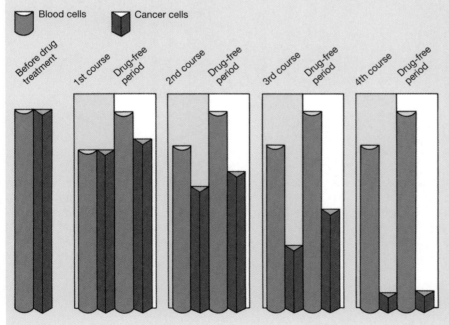

Blood cells   Cancer cells

Before drug treatment | 1st course | Drug-free period | 2nd course | Drug-free period | 3rd course | Drug-free period | 4th course | Drug-free period

ACTION OF CYTOTOXIC ANTICANCER DRUGS

Each type of cytotoxic drug affects a separate stage of the cancer cell's development, and each type of drug kills the cell by a different mechanism of action. The action of some of the principal classes of cytotoxic drugs is described below.

Alkylating agents and cytotoxic antibiotics
These act within the cell's nucleus to damage the cell's genetic material, DNA. This prevents the cell from growing and dividing.

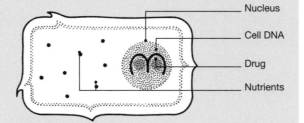

Nucleus
Cell DNA
Drug
Nutrients

Antimetabolites
These drugs mainly interfere with the production of RNA and DNA; they prevent the cell from metabolizing (processing) nutrients and other substances that are necessary for normal activity in the cell.

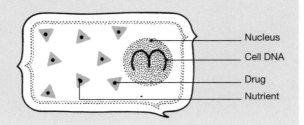

Nucleus
Cell DNA
Drug
Nutrient

symptoms or provide palliative treatment in advanced disease.

Targeted agents such as small molecule inhibitors and monoclonal antibodies are increasingly useful when used alone or in combination with other therapies to induce disease responses or maintain remission. There is gathering data that immunotherapies may give prolonged responses akin to cure even in cases of metastatic cancer.

Most anticancer drugs, especially cytotoxic drugs, have side effects, which are sometimes severe, and so treatment decisions have to balance possible benefits against the side effects. Often a combination of several drugs is used. Special regimes of different drugs used together and in succession have been devised to maximize their activity and minimize side effects.

How they work
Anticancer drugs work in many different ways. The main groups of drugs and how they work are described below.

Cytotoxic drugs
There are several classes of cytotoxic drugs, including the alkylating agents, antimetabolites, taxanes, and cytotoxic antibiotics. Each class has a different mechanism of action, but all act by interfering with basic processes of cell replication and division. They are particularly potent against rapidly dividing cells. These include cancer cells but also certain normal cells, especially those in the hair follicles, gut lining, and bone

marrow. This action explains their side effects and why treatment needs careful scheduling (see box on facing page).

Hormone therapies
Hormone treatments counteract the effects of the hormone that is promoting growth of the cancer. For example, some breast cancers are stimulated by the female sex hormone oestrogen; the action of oestrogen is opposed by the drug tamoxifen. Other cancers, by contrast, are damaged by very high doses of a particular sex hormone. An example is medroxyprogesterone, a progesterone that is often used to halt the spread of endometrial cancer.

Monoclonal antibodies
Antibodies are a fundamental building block of the immune system. They recognize and bind very specifically to foreign proteins on the surface of bacteria, viruses, and parasites, marking them out for destruction by other parts of the immune system. Monoclonal antibodies are produced in tissue culture using cells genetically engineered to make antibodies against a particular target protein. If the target is carefully selected, the antibodies can be used to identify cancer cells for destruction. If the target is found only on cancer cells, or on the cancer cells and the normal tissue from which it arose, the damage to healthy tissues during treatment is limited.

Monoclonal antibodies are being used increasingly in cancer treatment. Examples include trastuzumab (Herceptin), which

binds to a protein produced by certain types of breast cancer cell, and alemtuzumab and rituximab, which recognize different types of proteins on white blood cells and are used to treat leukaemias and lymphomas. These antibodies are very specific for certain types of cancer, and they cause little of the toxicity of conventional chemotherapy. They can, however, cause allergy-type reactions, especially at the beginning of treatment.

Growth factor inhibitors
The growth of cells is controlled by a complex network of growth factors that bind very specifically to receptor sites on the cell surface. This triggers a complex series of chemical reactions that transmit the "grow" message to the nucleus, triggering cell growth and replication. In many cancers, this system is faulty and there are either too many receptors on the cell surface or other abnormalities that result in inappropriate "grow" messages. The extra or abnormal cell surface receptors can be used as targets for monoclonal antibodies (see above).

Other defects in this system are being used as the basis for further new drugs. For example, imatinib very selectively interferes with an abnormal version of an enzyme that is found in certain leukaemic cells. This abnormal enzyme results in the cell nucleus receiving a "grow" signal continuously, resulting in the uncontrolled growth of cancer. By stopping the enzyme working, it is possible to selectively "turn off" the growth of the abnormal cells. Imatinib is proving very successful in treating certain types of leukaemia, with few serious side effects.

Another new area of cancer treatment is the use of drugs that inhibit the growth of new blood vessels to tumours (anti-angiogenesis agents), thereby depriving the tumours of the nutrients and oxygen they need to grow. One example is bevacizumab, a monoclonal antibody that blocks vascular endothelial growth factor (VEGF), a protein produced by certain tumours that promotes blood vessel growth. Bevacizumab is used to treat advanced cancer of the bowel, breast, lung, or kidney. Other new drugs are being developed that work in similar ways.

How they affect you
Cytotoxic drugs are generally associated with more side effects than other types of anticancer drug. At the start of treatment, adverse effects of the drugs may be more noticeable than benefits. The most common side effect is nausea and vomiting, for which an anti-emetic drug (see p.46) will usually be prescribed. Effects on the blood are also common. Many cytotoxic drugs cause hair loss because of the effect of their activity on

ANTICANCER DRUGS continued

ACTION OF MONOCLONAL ANTIBODIES

Antibodies are a vital part of the body's immune system. They identify rogue cells, which are then destroyed in different ways by the action of the immune system; killer leukocytes are one type of immune response. Monoclonal antibodies are manufactured antibodies in the form of drugs that are designed to bind to proteins on the surface of specific cancer cells. The antibodies can be designed to trigger the immune system and target the tagged cancer cells for destruction while minimizing harm to nearby normal cells.

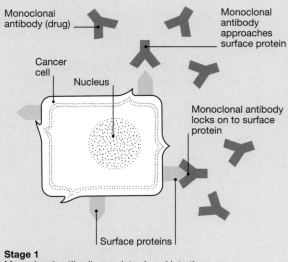

Monoclonal antibody (drug)

Cancer cell

Nucleus

Monoclonal antibody approaches surface protein

Monoclonal antibody locks on to surface protein

Surface proteins

Killer leukocyte is attracted to attached monoclonal antibody

Antibody-recognition sites

Nucleus

Cancer cell begins to disintegrate

Killer leukocyte is attached to cancer cell via monoclonal antibody

Stage 1
Monoclonal antibodies are introduced into the body. They are attracted to the surface proteins on a cancer cell and lock on to them. When sufficient antibodies have attached, the cell is recognized as rogue.

Stage 2
The tagged cancer cell becomes a target for destruction by killer leukocytes. Their antibody-recognition sites lock on to the monoclonal antibodies. This initiates destruction of the cell.

the hair follicle cells, but the hair usually starts to grow back after chemotherapy has been completed. Individual drugs may produce other side effects. Cytotoxic drugs are, in most cases, administered in the highest doses that can be tolerated in order to kill as many cancer cells as quickly as possible.

The unpleasant side effects of intensive chemotherapy, combined with a delay of several weeks before any benefits are seen, and the seriousness of the disease often lead to depression in those receiving anticancer drugs. Specialist counselling, support from family and friends, and, in some cases, treatment with antidepressant drugs may be helpful.

Risks and special precautions

All cytotoxic anticancer drugs interfere with the activity of non-cancerous cells, and for this reason they often produce serious adverse effects during long-term treatment. In particular, these drugs often adversely affect rapidly dividing cells such as the blood-producing cells in the bone marrow. The numbers of red and white blood cells and of platelets (particles in the blood responsible for clotting) may all be reduced. In some cases, symptoms of anaemia (weakness and fatigue) and an increased risk of abnormal or excessive bleeding may arise as a result of treatment

with anticancer drugs. A reduction in the number of white blood cells may result in increased susceptibility to infection. Even a simple infection such as a sore throat may be a sign of depressed white cell production in a patient taking anticancer drugs, and it must be reported to the doctor without delay. In addition, wounds may take longer to heal, and susceptible people can develop gout as a result of increased uric acid production due to cells being broken down.

Several short courses of drug treatment are usually given, to give the bone marrow time to recover in the period between courses (see Successful chemotherapy, p.112). Blood tests are done regularly. When necessary, blood transfusions, antibiotics, or other forms of treatment are used to overcome the adverse effects. When relevant, contraceptive advice is given early in treatment because most anticancer drugs can damage a developing baby. Eggs or sperm may be harvested before chemotherapy for later in vitro fertilization (IVF) after the chemotherapy is completed.

In addition to these general effects, individual drugs may have adverse effects on particular organs. These are described under individual drug profiles in Part 3.

By contrast, other anticancer drugs, such as hormonal drugs, antibodies, and

small molecule inhibitors, are more selective in their actions and tend to have less serious side effects.

COMMON DRUGS

Alkylating agents
Chlorambucil
Cyclophosphamide *
Melphalan

Antimetabolites
Azathioprine *
Capecitabine
Cytarabine
Fluorouracil *
Mercaptopurine *
Methotrexate *

Cytotoxic antibiotics
Doxorubicin *
Epirubicin

Hormone treatments
Anastrozole *
Bicalutamide
Cyproterone *
Flutamide *
Goserelin *
Letrozole
Leuprorelin
Medroxy-
    progesterone *

Megestrol
Tamoxifen *

Immunotherapies
Interferon alfa *
Interleukin 2

Taxanes
Docetaxel
Paclitaxel

Monoclonal antibodies
Alemtuzumab
Bevacizumab *
Rituximab *
Trastuzumab *

Growth factor inhibitors
Erlotinib
Imatinib *

Other drugs
Carboplatin
Cisplatin *
Etoposide
Irinotecan

| * See Part 3 |

IMMUNOSUPPRESSANT DRUGS

The body is protected against attack from bacteria, fungi, and viruses by specialized cells and proteins in the blood and tissues that make up the immune system (see p.110). White blood cells known as lymphocytes kill invading organisms directly or produce proteins (antibodies) to destroy them. These mechanisms are also responsible for eliminating abnormal or unhealthy cells that could otherwise multiply and develop into a cancer.

In certain conditions it is medically necessary to damp down the activity of the immune system. These include a number of autoimmune disorders, in which the immune system attacks normal body tissue. Autoimmune disorders may affect a single organ – for example, the kidneys in Goodpasture's syndrome or the thyroid gland in Hashimoto's disease – or they may result in widespread damage: for example, in rheumatoid arthritis or systemic lupus erythematosus.

Immune system activity may also need to be reduced following an organ transplant, when the body's defences would otherwise attack and reject the transplanted tissue.

Several types of drug are used as immunosuppressants: anticancer drugs (see p.112), corticosteroids (see p.99), ciclosporin (see p.196), and monoclonal antibodies (see p.113).

Why they are used

Immunosuppressant drugs are given to treat autoimmune disorders, such as rheumatoid arthritis, when symptoms are severe and other treatments have not provided adequate relief. Corticosteroids are usually prescribed initially. Their pronounced anti-inflammatory effect, as well as their immunosuppressant action, helps to promote healing of tissue damaged by abnormal immune system activity. Anticancer drugs such as methotrexate (see p.320) may be used in addition to corticosteroids if these do not produce sufficient improvement or if their effect wanes (see also Antirheumatic drugs, p.75).

Immunosuppressant drugs are given before and after organ and other tissue transplants. Treatment may have to be continued indefinitely to prevent rejection. A number of drugs and drug combinations are used, depending on which organ is being transplanted and the underlying condition of the patient. However, ciclosporin (see p.196), along with the related drug tacrolimus (see p.405), is now the most widely used drug for preventing organ rejection. It is also increasingly used to treat autoimmune disorders. It is often used in combination with a corticosteroid or the more specific drug mycophenolate mofetil.

Monoclonal antibodies, which destroy specific cells of the immune system, are also used to aid transplantation and are increasingly being used to treat autoimmune disorders. For example, infliximab (see p.283) is used to treat certain types of arthritis, while rituximab (see p.385) is also used for systemic lupus erythematosus and vasculitis.

How they work

Immunosuppressant drugs reduce the effectiveness of the immune system, either by depressing the production of lymphocytes or by altering their activity.

How they affect you

When immunosuppressants are given to treat an autoimmune disorder, they reduce the severity of the symptoms and may temporarily halt the progress of the disease. However, they cannot restore major tissue damage.

Immunosuppressant drugs can produce a variety of unwanted side effects. The side effects of corticosteroids are described in more detail on p.99. Anticancer drugs, when prescribed as immunosuppressants, are given in low doses that produce only mild side effects. They may cause nausea and vomiting, for which an anti-emetic drug (p.46) may be prescribed. Hair loss is rare and regrowth usually occurs when the drug treatment is discontinued. Ciclosporin may cause increased growth of facial hair, swelling of the gums, and tingling in the hands.

Risks and special precautions

All of these drugs may produce potentially serious adverse effects. By reducing the activity of the patient's immune system, immunosuppressant drugs can affect the body's ability to fight invading microorganisms, thereby increasing the risk of serious infections. Because lymphocyte activity is also important for preventing the multiplication of abnormal cells, there is an increased risk of certain types of cancer. A major drawback of anticancer drugs is that, in addition to their effect on lymphocyte production, they interfere with the growth and division of other blood cells in the bone marrow. Reduced production of red blood cells can cause anaemia; when the production of blood platelets is suppressed, blood clotting may be less efficient.

Although ciclosporin is more specific in its action than either corticosteroids or anticancer drugs, it can cause kidney damage and, in too high a dose, may affect the brain, causing hallucinations or seizures. Ciclosporin also tends to raise blood pressure, and another drug may be required to counteract this effect (see Antihypertensive drugs, p.60).

ACTION OF IMMUNOSUPPRESSANTS

Before treatment
Many types of blood cell, each with a distinct role, form in the bone marrow. Lymphocytes respond to infection and foreign tissue. B-lymphocytes produce antibodies to attack invading organisms, whereas T-lymphocytes directly attack invading cells. Other blood cells help the action of the B- and T-cells.

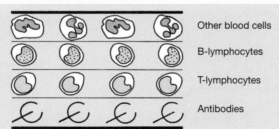

Other blood cells

B-lymphocytes

T-lymphocytes

Antibodies

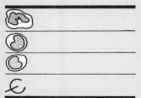

Anticancer drugs
These drugs slow the production of all cells in the bone marrow.

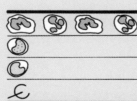

Corticosteroids
These drugs reduce the activity of both B- and T-lymphocytes.

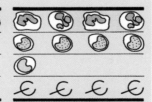

Ciclosporin
This inhibits the activity of T-lymphocytes only, and not the activity of B-lymphocytes.

COMMON DRUGS

Anticancer drugs
Azathioprine *
Chlorambucil
Cyclophosphamide *
Methotrexate *

Corticosteroids
(see p.99)

Antibodies
Adalimumab
Anti-lymphocyte globulin
Basiliximab
Infliximab *
Rituximab *

Other drugs
Ciclosporin *
Mycophenolate mofetil
Tacrolimus *

* See Part 3

DRUGS FOR HIV AND AIDS

AIDS (acquired immune deficiency syndrome) is caused by infection with the human immunodeficiency virus (HIV). This virus invades certain cells of the immune system, particularly the white blood cells called T-helper lymphocytes (or CD_4 cells), which normally activate other immune cells to fight infection. HIV kills T-helper lymphocytes, so that the body cannot fight the virus or subsequent infections, resulting in immune deficiency. In recent years the number of drugs to treat HIV has increased considerably, as well as knowledge about how best to use them in combination.

Why they are used

Drugs can be divided into treatments for the initial HIV infection and treatment of complications associated with AIDS.

Drugs that act directly against HIV are called antiretrovirals. The two most common groups work by interfering with enzymes vital for virus replication. The first group inhibit an enzyme called reverse transcriptase. They are divided into nucleoside inhibitors (also called nucleoside analogues), nucleotide inhibitors (nucleotide analogues), and non-nucleoside inhibitors. The second group interfere with an enzyme called protease. Integrase inhibitors prevent the virus from injecting its DNA into the cell nucleus and are joining first-line therapy combinations. Entry inhibitors inhibit the entry of the virus into the cell. Further groups are being developed to target the receptor sites for entry into cells.

Antiretrovirals are much more effective in combination. Treatment usually starts with two nucleoside transcriptase inhibitors plus a non-nucleoside drug, integrase inhibitor, or protease inhibitor. If combination antiretroviral therapy (ART) is started before the immune system is too damaged, it can dramatically reduce the level of HIV in the body and improve the outlook for HIV-infected people, although it is not a cure and such people remain infectious. The mainstay of treatment for AIDS-related diseases are antimicrobial drugs for the bacterial, viral, fungal, and protozoal infections to which people with AIDS are particularly susceptible. These drugs include antituberculous drugs (p.90), co-trimoxazole for pneumocystis pneumonia, and ganciclovir to treat cytomegalovirus (CMV) infection.

HIV INFECTION AND POSSIBLE TREATMENTS

The illustrations below show how the human immunodeficiency virus (HIV) enters T-helper white blood cells containing the CD_4 protein and a co-receptor protein and replicates itself. The actions of existing drugs, and possible actions of future drugs, are also described.

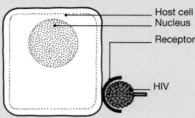

Stage 1
The virus binds to a specialized set of receptors on a T-helper cell with CD_4 protein.

Host cell
Nucleus
Receptor
HIV

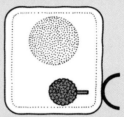

Stage 2
The virus enters the cell.

Possible drug intervention
Drugs such as enfuvirtide and dolutegravir block the entry of HIV into T-helper cells. Drugs that block the receptor site include maraviroc, which blocks the co-receptor.

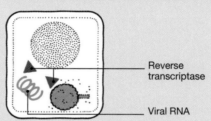

Reverse transcriptase
Viral RNA

Stage 3
The virus loses its protective coat and releases RNA, its genetic material, and an enzyme known as reverse transcriptase.

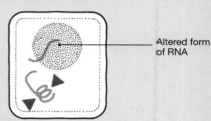

Altered form of RNA

Stage 4
The enzyme reverse transcriptase converts viral RNA into a form that can enter the host cell's nucleus and become integrated with the cell's genetic material.

Drug intervention
The reverse transcriptase inhibitors, such as zidovudine, efavirenz, and tenofovir, act at this point.

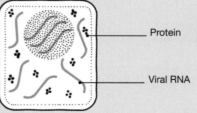

Protein
Viral RNA

Stage 5
The host cell starts to produce new viral RNA and protein from the viral material that has been integrated into its nucleus.

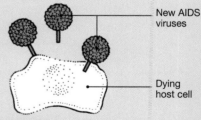

New AIDS viruses
Dying host cell

Stage 6
The new viral RNA and proteins assemble to produce new viruses. These leave the host cell (which then dies) and are free to attack other cells in the body.

Drug intervention
The protease inhibitors prevent formation of viral proteins and viral assembly.

COMMON DRUGS

Nucleoside reverse transcriptase inhibitors (nucleoside analogues)
Abacavir
Emtricitabine ✷
Lamivudine
Stavudine
Zidovudine (AZT)/
  lamivudine ✷

Nucleotide reverse transcriptase inhibitor (nucleotide analogue)
Tenofovir ✷

✷ See Part 3

Non-nucleoside reverse transcriptase inhibitors
Efavirenz ✷
Nevirapine

Integrase inhibitors
Dolutegravir
Raltegravir

Protease inhibitors
Atazanavir
Darunavir
Lopinavir/ritonavir ✷
Saquinavir

Entry/fusion inhibitors
Enfuvirtide
Maraviroc

ANTIRETROVIRAL DRUGS

Drug name	Class of drug	Formulation	Standard adult dose	Additional information
Abacavir Ziagen	Nucleoside analogue (NA)	Tablets (300mg). Oral solution (20mg/ml)	300mg twice daily	Abacavir can cause a severe allergic-type reaction (see additional product information)
Abacavir, lamivudine Kivexa	Nucleoside analogues (NAs)	Kivexa contains abacavir (600mg) and lamivudine (300mg)	1 tablet once daily	Abacavir can cause a severe allergic-type reaction (see additional product information)
Abacavir, lamivudine, zidovudine (AZT) Trizivir	Nucleoside analogues (NAs)	Trizivir contains abacavir (300mg), lamivudine (150mg), and zidovudine (300mg)	1 tablet twice daily	The abacavir contained in Trizivir can cause a severe allergic-type reaction (see additional product information)
Emtricitabine Emtriva	Nucleoside analogue (NA)	Capsules (200mg). Oral solution (10mg/ml)	200mg capsule once daily or 240mg oral solution once daily	
Lamivudine (3TC) Epivir	Nucleoside analogue (NA)	Tablets (300mg, 150mg). Oral solution (50mg/5ml)	300mg in 1 or 2 divided doses	Lamivudine can also be used to treat hepatitis B
Stavudine (d4T) Zerit	Nucleoside analogue (NA)	Capsules (40mg, 30mg, 20mg). Oral solution (1mg/ml)	Adults over 60kg: 40mg twice daily. Adults under 60kg: 30mg twice daily	
Zidovudine (AZT) Retrovir	Nucleoside analogue (NA)	Capsules (250mg, 100mg). Syrup (50mg/5ml). Injection (10mg/ml)	500–600mg in 2–3 divided doses	
Zidovudine (AZT), lamivudine Combivir	Nucleoside analogues (NAs)	Combivir contains zidovudine (300mg) and lamivudine (150mg)	1 tablet twice daily	
Tenofovir disoproxil Viread	Nucleotide analogue (NA)	Tablets (245mg as disoproxil fumarate = 300mg tenofovir)	1 tablet once daily	Tenofovir should be taken with food
Tenofovir disoproxil, emtricitabine Truvada	Nucleotide analogue and nucleoside analogue (NA)	Truvada contains tenofovir (245mg) and emtricitabine (200mg)	1 tablet once daily	
Efavirenz Sustiva	Non-nucleoside reverse transcriptase inhibitor (NNRTI)	Capsules (200mg, 50mg). Tablets (600mg)	600mg once daily	Efavirenz can cause a severe allergic-type rash (see additional product information)
Nevirapine Viramune	Non-nucleoside reverse transcriptase inhibitor (NNRTI)	Tablets (200mg). Suspension (50mg/5ml)	200mg once daily for 2 weeks then 200mg twice daily	Nevirapine can cause a severe allergic-type reaction (see additional product information)
Atazanavir Reyataz	Protease inhibitor (PI)	Capsules (200mg, 150mg, 100mg)	300mg once daily	
Darunavir Prezista	Protease inhibitor (PI)	Tablets (400mg, 600mg, 800mg). Oral solution (100mg/ml)	600mg twice daily	Co-administered with a pharmacokinetic enhancer such as low-dose ritonavir
Indinavir Crixivan	Protease inhibitor (PI)	Capsules (400mg, 200mg)	800mg every 8 hours	Indinavir should be taken with a low-fat meal or 1 hour before or 2 hours after any other meal
Lopinavir with ritonavir Kaletra	Protease inhibitors (PIs)	Tablets (200mg lopinavir, 50mg ritonavir). Capsules (133mg, 33mg). Oral solution (400mg, 100mg/5ml)	2 tablets or 3 capsules twice daily or 5ml twice daily	
Ritonavir Norvir	Protease inhibitor (PI)	Capsules (100mg). Oral solution (400mg/5ml)	600mg twice daily	Doses should be taken with food
Saquinavir Invirase	Protease inhibitor (PI)	Capsules (200mg). Tablets (500mg)	1g every 12 hours	Doses should be taken within 2 hours of a full meal
Dolutegravir Tivicay	Integrase inhibitor (INI)	Tablets (10mg, 25mg, 50mg)	50mg once daily	
Raltegravir Isentress	Integrase inhibitor (INI)	Tablets (400mg, 600mg)	400mg twice daily	
Enfuvirtide Fuzeon	Fusion inhibitor	Subcutaneous injection (90mg) powder for reconstitution	Subcutaneous injection (90mg) twice daily	Caution in liver impairment, including hepatitis B or C
Maraviroc Celsentri	Entry inhibitor	Tablets (25mg, 75mg, 150mg, 300mg)	300mg twice daily	

REPRODUCTIVE & URINARY TRACTS

The reproductive systems of men and women consist of those organs that produce and release sperm (male), or store and release eggs and then nurture a fertilized egg until it develops into a baby (female).

The urinary system filters wastes and water from the blood, producing urine, which is then expelled from the body. The reproductive and urinary systems of men are partially linked, but those of women form two physically close but functionally separate systems.

The female reproductive organs comprise the ovaries, fallopian tubes, and uterus (womb). The uterus opens via the cervix (neck of the uterus) into the vagina. The principal male reproductive organs are the two sperm-producing glands, the testes (testicles), which lie within the scrotum, and the penis. Other parts of the system in males include the prostate gland and several tubular structures – the tightly coiled epididymides (singular: epididymis), the vas deferens, the seminal vesicles, and the urethra (see right).

The urinary organs in both sexes comprise the kidneys, which filter the blood and excrete urine (see also p.57); the ureters, down which urine passes; and the bladder, where urine is stored until it is released from the body via the urethra.

What can go wrong

The reproductive and urinary tracts are both subject to infection. Such infections (apart from those transmitted by sexual activity) are relatively uncommon in men because the long male urethra prevents bacteria and other organisms passing easily to the bladder and upper urinary tract, and to the male sex organs. The shorter female urethra does allow urinary tract infections, especially of the bladder (cystitis) and of the urethra (urethritis), to occur commonly. The female reproductive tract is also vulnerable to infection, which in some cases is sexually transmitted.

Reproductive function may also be disrupted by hormonal disturbances that lead to reduced fertility. Women may also develop symptoms arising from normal activity of the reproductive organs, including menstrual disorders as well as problems associated with childbirth.

The most common urinary problems apart from infection are those related to bladder function. Urine may be released involuntarily (incontinence), or it may be retained in the bladder. Such urinary disorders are usually the result of abnormal nerve signals to the bladder or sphincter muscle. The filtering action of the kidneys may be affected by

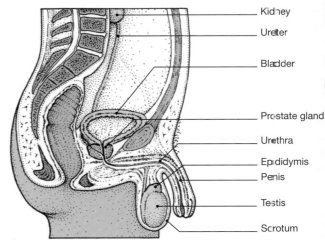

Male reproductive system
Sperm produced in each testis pass into the epididymis, a tightly coiled tube in which the sperm mature before passing along the vas deferens to the seminal vesicle. Sperm are stored in the seminal vesicle until they are ejaculated from the penis via the urethra, together with seminal fluid and secretions from the prostate gland.

Kidney
Ureter
Bladder
Prostate gland
Urethra
Epididymis
Penis
Testis
Scrotum

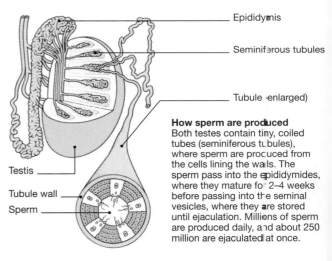

Epididymis
Seminiferous tubules
Tubule (enlarged)
Testis
Tubule wall
Sperm

How sperm are produced
Both testes contain tiny, coiled tubes (seminiferous tubules), where sperm are produced from the cells lining the walls. The sperm pass into the epididymides, where they mature for 2–4 weeks before passing into the seminal vesicles, where they are stored until ejaculation. Millions of sperm are produced daily, and about 250 million are ejaculated at once.

alteration in the composition of the blood or the hormones that regulate urine production, or by damage to the filtering units themselves from infection or inflammation.

Why drugs are used

Antibiotic drugs (p.86) are used to eliminate both urinary and reproductive tract infections (including sexually transmitted infections). In addition, certain infections of the vagina are caused by fungi or yeasts and require antifungal drugs (p.96).

Hormone drugs are used both to reduce fertility deliberately (oral contraceptives) and to increase fertility in certain conditions in which it has not been

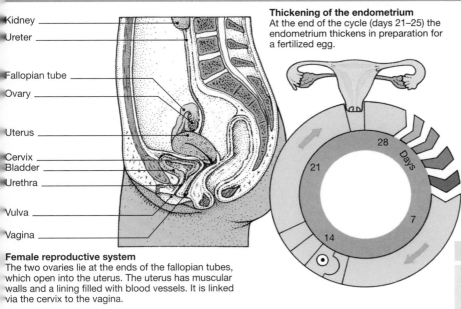

Kidney
Ureter
Fallopian tube
Ovary
Uterus
Cervix
Bladder
Urethra
Vulva
Vagina

Thickening of the endometrium
At the end of the cycle (days 21–25) the endometrium thickens in preparation for a fertilized egg.

28
Days
21
7
14

Menstrual cycle
A monthly cycle of hormone interactions allows an egg to be released and creates the correct environment for the egg, if fertilized, to implant in the uterus. Major body changes occur, the most obvious being menstruation. The cycle usually starts between the ages of 11 and 14 years and continues until the menopause, which occurs at around 50. After the menopause, childbearing is no longer possible. The cycle is usually 28 days, but this varies with individuals.

Menstruation
If no egg is fertilized, the endometrium is shed (days 1–5).

Fertile period
Conception may take place in the two days after ovulation (days 14–16).

Female reproductive system
The two ovaries lie at the ends of the fallopian tubes, which open into the uterus. The uterus has muscular walls and a lining filled with blood vessels. It is linked via the cervix to the vagina.

URINARY SYSTEM

The kidneys extract waste and excess water from the blood. The waste liquid (urine) passes into the bladder, from which it is expelled via the urethra.

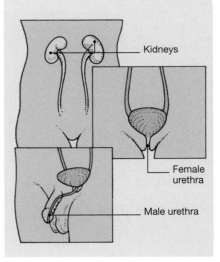

Kidneys
Female urethra
Male urethra

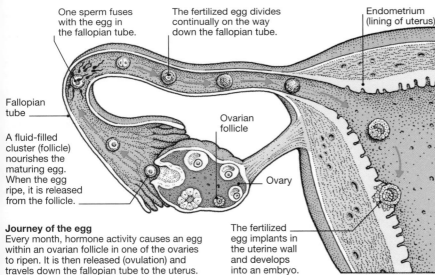

One sperm fuses with the egg in the fallopian tube.

The fertilized egg divides continually on the way down the fallopian tube.

Endometrium (lining of uterus)

Fallopian tube

A fluid-filled cluster (follicle) nourishes the maturing egg. When the egg ripe, it is released from the follicle.

Ovarian follicle

Ovary

The fertilized egg implants in the uterine wall and develops into an embryo.

Journey of the egg
Every month, hormone activity causes an egg within an ovarian follicle in one of the ovaries to ripen. It is then released (ovulation) and travels down the fallopian tube to the uterus.

possible for a couple to conceive. Hormones may also be used to regulate menstruation when it is irregular or excessively painful or heavy. Analgesic drugs (see p.36) are used to treat menstrual period pain and are also widely used for pain relief in labour. Other drugs used in labour include those that increase contraction of the muscles of the uterus and those that limit blood loss after the birth. Drugs may also be employed to halt premature labour.

Drugs that alter the transmission of nerve signals to the bladder muscles have an important role in the treatment of urinary incontinence and retention. Drugs that increase the kidneys' filtering action are commonly used to reduce blood pressure and fluid retention (see Diuretics, p.57). Other drugs may alter the composition of the urine – for example, the uricosuric drugs that are used in the treatment of gout (see p.77) increase the amount of uric acid.

MAJOR DRUG GROUPS

Drugs used to treat menstrual disorders
Oral contraceptives
Drugs for infertility
Drugs used in labour
Drugs used for urinary disorders

DRUGS USED TO TREAT MENSTRUAL DISORDERS

The menstrual cycle results from the actions of female sex hormones that cause ovulation (the release of an egg) and thickening of the endometrium (the lining of the uterus) each month in preparation for pregnancy. Unless the egg is fertilized, the endometrium will be shed about two weeks later during menstruation (see also p.119).

The main problems associated with menstruation that may require medical treatment are excessive blood loss (menorrhagia), pain during menstruation (dysmenorrhoea), and distressing physical and psychological symptoms occurring prior to menstruation (premenstrual syndrome). The absence of periods (amenorrhoea) is discussed under female sex hormones (p.105).

The drugs most commonly used to treat the menstrual disorders described above include oestrogens, progestogens, and analgesics.

Why they are used

Drug treatment for menstrual disorders is undertaken only when the doctor has ruled out the possibility of an underlying gynaecological disorder, such as a pelvic infection or fibroids. In some cases, especially in women over the age of 35, a D and C (dilatation and curettage) may be recommended. When no underlying reason for the problem is found, drug treatment aimed primarily at the relief of symptoms is usually prescribed.

Dysmenorrhoea

Painful menstrual periods are usually treated initially with a simple analgesic drug (see p.36). Non-steroidal anti-inflammatory drugs (NSAIDs; see p.74) are often most effective because they counter the effects of prostaglandins, chemicals that are partly responsible for transmission of pain to the brain. The NSAID mefenamic acid has the additional ability to reduce the excessive blood loss of menorrhagia (see below).

When these drugs are not sufficient to provide adequate pain relief, hormonal drug treatment may be recommended. If contraception is also required, treatment may involve an oral contraceptive pill containing both an oestrogen and a progestogen, or a progestogen alone. However, non-contraceptive progestogen preparations may also be prescribed. These are usually taken for only a few days during each month. The treatment of dysmenorrhoea that occurs as a result of endometriosis is described in the box above right.

Menorrhagia

Excessive blood loss during menstruation can sometimes be reduced by some NSAIDs. Tranexamic acid, an antifibrinolytic drug (see p.63), is an effective treatment for menorrhagia. Alternatively, danazol, a

drug that reduces production of the female sex hormone oestrogen, may be prescribed to reduce blood loss.

Premenstrual syndrome

This is a collection of psychological and physical symptoms that affect many women to some degree in the days before menstruation. Psychological symptoms include mood changes such as increased irritability, depression, and anxiety. Principal physical symptoms are bloating, headache, and breast tenderness. Combined oral contraceptives may be prescribed and, for severe premenstrual syndrome, SSRI antidepressants (see p.40) are sometimes given. Other drugs sometimes used include pyridoxine (vitamin B$_6$), diuretics (see p.57) if bloating due to fluid retention is a problem, and bromocriptine when breast tenderness is the major symptom.

How they work

Drugs used to treat menstrual disorders act in a variety of ways. Hormonal treatments are aimed at suppressing the pattern of hormonal changes that is causing troublesome symptoms. Contraceptive preparations override the woman's normal menstrual cycle. Ovulation does not occur, and the endometrium does not thicken normally. Bleeding that occurs at the end of a cycle is less likely to be abnormally heavy, to be accompanied by severe discomfort, or to be preceded by distressing symptoms. For further information on oral contraceptives, see facing page.

ENDOMETRIOSIS

Endometriosis is a condition in which fragments of endometrial tissue (uterine lining) occur outside the uterus in the pelvic cavity. This disorder can cause severe pain during menstruation or intercourse, as well as cyclical gastrointestinal or urinary symptoms, and may sometimes lead to infertility.

Drugs used for this disorder are similar to those prescribed for heavy periods (menorrhagia). However, in this case the intention is to suppress endometrial development for an extended period so that the abnormal tissue eventually withers away. Progesterone supplements that suppress endometrial thickening may be prescribed throughout the menstrual cycle. Alternatively, danazol, which suppresses endometrial development by reducing oestrogen production, may be prescribed. Any drug treatment usually needs to be continued for a minimum of six months.

When drug treatment is unsuccessful, surgical removal of the abnormal tissue is usually necessary.

Sites of endometriosis

Ovary — Wall of uterus — Fallopian tube — Bladder wall — Bowel wall

☐ Endometrial tissue

Non-contraceptive progestogen preparations taken in the days before menstruation do not suppress ovulation. Increased progesterone during this time reduces premenstrual symptoms and prevents excessive thickening of the endometrium.

Danazol, a potent drug, prevents the thickening of the endometrium, thereby correcting excessively heavy periods. Blood loss is reduced, and in some cases menstruation ceases altogether during treatment.

COMMON DRUGS

Oestrogens and progestogens
(see p.105)

NSAID analgesics
Aspirin *
Dexibuprofen
Dexketoprofen
Diclofenac *
Flurbiprofen
Ibuprofen *
Indometacin
Ketoprofen *
Mefenamic acid *
Naproxen *

Diuretics
(see p.57)

Other drugs
Bromocriptine *
Buserelin
Danazol
Gestrinone
Goserelin *
Leuprorelin
Nafarelin
Pyridoxine *
Tranexamic acid
Triptorelin

★ See Part 3

ORAL CONTRACEPTIVES

There are many different methods of ensuring that conception and pregnancy do not follow sexual intercourse, but for many women oral contraception is the preferred method because it is highly effective (see table, right), convenient, and unobtrusive during sexual intercourse. About 30 per cent of the women who seek contraceptive protection in Britain choose a form of oral contraceptive.

There are three main types of oral contraceptive: the combined pill, the progestogen-only pill (POP), and the phased pill. All three types contain a progestogen (a synthetic form of the female sex hormone progesterone). Both the combined and phased pills also contain a natural or synthetic oestrogen (see also Female sex hormones, p.105).

Why they are used

The combined pill
The combined pill is the most widely prescribed form of oral contraceptive and has the lowest failure rate in terms of unwanted pregnancies. It is referred to as the "pill" and is the type thought most suitable for young women who want to use a hormonal form of contraception. The combined pill is particularly suitable for those women who regularly experience exceptionally painful, heavy, or prolonged periods (see Drugs used to treat menstrual disorders, facing page).

There are many different products available containing a fixed dose of an oestrogen and a progestogen drug. They are divided generally into three groups according to their oestrogen content (see table, below). Low-dose products are chosen when possible to minimize the risk of adverse effects.

COMPARISON OF RELIABILITY OF DIFFERENT METHODS OF CONTRACEPTION

The table indicates the number of pregnancies that occur with each method of contraception among 100 women using that method in a year. The figures in the first column are for correct usage; if a contraceptive is used incorrectly, the failure rate will be higher as shown in the second column. The wide variation in figures for the morning after pill reflects differences in effectiveness depending on how soon it is taken after unprotected sex.

Method	Perfect use ✳	Typical use ✳
Combined and phased pills	Less than 1	9
Progestogen-only pill	About 1	9
IUD (intrauterine device)	Less than 1	Less than 1
Male condom	About 2	18
Female condom	About 5	21
Diaphragm with spermicide	4–8	12–29
Cap with spermicide	4–8	12–29
IUS (intrauterine system)	Less than 1	Less than 1
Contraceptive implant	Less than 1	Less than 1
Contraceptive injection	Less than 1	6
Morning after pill	About 2–42	N/A

✳ Pregnancies per 100 users per year

Progestogen-only pill
The progestogen-only pill (POP) is often recommended for women who react adversely to the oestrogen in the combined pill or for whom the combined pill is not considered suitable because of their age or medical history (see Risks and special precautions, p.123). It is also prescribed for breast-feeding women, since it does not reduce milk production. For maximum contraceptive effectiveness, the progestogen-only pill must be taken at precisely the same time each day. It works by changing the quality of the endometrium (the lining of the uterus), making implantation of a fertilized egg less likely. However, Cerazette (a brand of the progestogen desogestrel) also inhibits ovulation, making it more reliable than other POPs.

Phased pills
The third form of oral contraceptive is a pack of pills divided into two or three groups or phases. Each phase contains a different proportion of an oestrogen and a progestogen. The aim is to provide a hormonal balance that closely resembles the fluctuations of a normal menstrual cycle. Phased pills provide effective protection for many women who suffer side effects from other available forms of oral contraceptive.

How they work
In a normal menstrual cycle, the ripening and release of an egg and preparation of the uterus for implantation of a fertilized egg result from a complex interplay between the natural female sex hormones, oestrogen and progesterone, and the pituitary hormones, follicle-stimulating hormone (FSH) and luteinizing hormone (LH) (see also p.105). The oestrogen and progestogens in oral contraceptives disrupt the normal menstrual cycle in such a way that conception is less likely.

With combined and phased pills, the increased levels of oestrogen and progesterone produce similar effects to the hormonal changes of pregnancy. The actions of the hormones inhibit the production of FSH and LH, thereby preventing the egg from ripening in the ovary and from being released.

The progestogen-only pill has a slightly different effect. It does not always prevent release of an egg; its main contraceptive action may be to thicken the mucus that lines the cervix, preventing sperm from crossing it. This effect occurs to some extent with combined and phased pills. Cerazette, additionally, inhibits ovulation.

How they affect you
Each course of combined and phased pills lasts for 21 days, followed by a pill-free seven days, during which time

HORMONE CONTENT OF COMMON ORAL CONTRACEPTIVES

The oestrogen-containing forms are classified according to oestrogen content as follows: low: 20 micrograms; standard: 30–35 micrograms; high: 50 micrograms; phased pills: 30–40 micrograms. Morning after: 1.5 milligrams (levonorgestrel), 30 milligrams (ulipristal).

Type of pill (oestrogen content)	Brand names
Combined (20mcg)	Loestrin 20, Femodette, Gedarel 20/150, Mercilon, Millinette 20/75, Sunya 20/75
(30–35mcg)	Brevinor, Cilest, Femodene, Femodene ED, Gedarel 30/150, Katya 30/75, Levest, Loestrin 30, Marvelon, Microgynon 30, Microgynon 30 ED, Millinette 30/75, Norimin, Ovranette, Rigevidon, Yasmin
(50mcg)	Norinyl-1 (as Mestranol)
Phased (30–40mcg)	Logynon, Logynon ED, Synphase, TriRegol
Progestogen-only (no oestrogen)	Cerazette, Cerelle, Feanolla, Micronor, Norgeston, Noriday
Postcoital (morning after) (no oestrogen)	EllaOne, Levonelle 1500, Levonelle One Step

ORAL CONTRACEPTIVES continued

BALANCING THE RISKS AND BENEFITS OF ORAL CONTRACEPTIVES

Oral contraceptives are safe for the vast majority of young women. However, every woman who is considering oral contraception should discuss with her doctor the risks and possible adverse effects of the drugs before deciding whether a hormonal method is the most suitable in her case. A variety of factors must be taken into account, including the woman's age, her own medical history and that of her close relatives, and factors such as whether she is a smoker. The importance of such factors varies depending on the type of contraceptive. The table below gives the main advantages and disadvantages of oestrogen-containing and progestogen-only pills.

Type of oral contraceptive	Oestrogen-containing combined and phased	Progestogen-only
Advantages	<ul><li>Very reliable</li><li>Convenient/unobtrusive</li><li>Regularizes menstruation</li><li>Reduces menstrual pain and blood loss</li><li>Reduces risk of: benign breast disease endometriosis ectopic pregnancy ovarian cysts pelvic infection ovarian and endometrial cancer</li></ul>	<ul><li>Very reliable</li><li>Convenient/unobtrusive, but timing of doses is more critical than with combined and phased pills (see What to do if you miss a pill, opposite page)</li><li>Suitable during breast-feeding</li><li>Avoids oestrogen-related side effects and risks</li><li>Allows rapid return to fertility</li><li>Suitable for women in whom use of oestrogen-containing contraception is not possible</li></ul>
Side effects	<ul><li>Weight gain</li><li>Depression</li><li>Breast swelling</li><li>Reduced sex drive</li><li>Headaches</li><li>Increased vaginal discharge</li><li>Nausea</li></ul>	<ul><li>Irregular menstruation</li><li>Nausea</li><li>Headaches</li><li>Breast discomfort</li><li>Depression</li><li>Changes in libido</li><li>Weight changes</li></ul>
Risks	<ul><li>Thromboembolism</li><li>Heart disease</li><li>High blood pressure</li><li>Liver impairment/cancer of the liver (rare)</li><li>Gallstones</li><li>Breast and/or cervical cancer (risk is low)</li></ul>	<ul><li>Ectopic pregnancy</li><li>Ovarian cysts</li><li>Breast cancer (risk is low)</li></ul>
Factors that may prohibit use	<ul><li>Previous thrombosis *</li><li>Heart disease</li><li>High levels of lipid in blood</li><li>Liver disease</li><li>Blood disorders</li><li>High blood pressure</li><li>Unexplained vaginal bleeding</li><li>Migraine</li><li>Otosclerosis</li><li>Presence of several risk factors (below)</li></ul>	<ul><li>Previous ectopic pregnancy</li><li>Heart or circulatory disease</li><li>Unexplained vaginal bleeding</li><li>History of breast cancer</li></ul>
Factors that increase risks	<ul><li>Smoking *</li><li>Obesity *</li><li>Increasing age</li><li>Diabetes mellitus</li><li>Family history of heart or circulatory disease *</li><li>Current treatment with other drugs</li></ul>	<ul><li>As for oestrogen-containing pills, but to a lesser degree</li></ul>

* Products containing desogestrel or gestodene have a higher excess risk with these factors than other progestogens.

How to minimize your health risks while taking the pill
- Do not smoke.
- Maintain a healthy weight and diet.
- Have regular blood pressure and blood lipid checks.
- Have regular cervical screening tests.
- Remind your doctor that you are taking oral contraceptives before taking other prescription drugs.
- Stop taking oestrogen-containing oral contraceptives four weeks before planned major surgery (use alternative contraception).

menstruation occurs. Some brands contain additional inactive pills. With these, the new course directly follows the last so that the habit of taking the pill daily is not broken. Progestogen-only pills are taken for 28 days each month. Menstruation usually occurs during the last few days of the menstrual cycle.

Women taking oral contraceptives, especially drugs that contain oestrogen, usually find that their menstrual periods are lighter and relatively pain-free. Some women cease to menstruate altogether. This is not a cause for concern in itself, provided no pills have been missed, but it may make it difficult to determine if pregnancy has occurred. An apparently missed period probably indicates a light one, rather than pregnancy. However, if you have missed two consecutive periods and you feel that you may be pregnant, it is advisable to have a pregnancy test.

All forms of oral contraceptive may cause spotting of blood in mid-cycle (breakthrough bleeding), especially at first, but this can be a particular problem with the progestogen-only pill.

Oral contraceptives that contain oestrogen may produce any of a large number of mild side effects depending on the dose. Symptoms similar to those experienced early in pregnancy may occur, particularly in the first few months of pill use: some women complain of nausea and vomiting, weight gain, depression, altered libido, increased appetite, and cramps in the legs and abdomen. The pill may also affect the circulation, producing minor headaches and dizziness. All these effects usually disappear within a few months, but if they persist, it may be advisable to change to a brand containing a lower dose of oestrogen or to some other contraceptive method.

Risks and special precautions

All oral contraceptives need to be taken regularly for maximum protection against pregnancy. Contraceptive protection can be reduced by missing a pill (see What to do if you miss a pill, below). It may also be reduced by vomiting or diarrhoea. If you vomit within two hours of taking a pill, take another one. If vomiting and diarrhoea persist, follow the instructions on the packet or consult your doctor or pharmacist. Many drugs may also affect the action of oral contraceptives, and it is essential to tell your doctor that you are taking oral contraceptives before taking additional prescribed medications.

Oral contraceptives, particularly those containing an oestrogen, have been found to carry a number of risks. These are summarized in the box on the facing page. One of the most serious potential adverse effects of oestrogen-containing pills is development of a thrombus (blood clot) in a vein or artery. The thrombus may travel to the lungs or cause a stroke or heart attack. The risk of thrombus formation increases with age and other factors, notably obesity, high blood pressure, and smoking. Doctors assess these risk factors for each person when prescribing oral contraceptives. A woman who is over 35 may be advised against

POSTCOITAL CONTRACEPTION

Pregnancy following sexual intercourse without contraception may be avoided by taking a postcoital (morning after) pill. The drugs contained in this pill (levonorgestrel and ulipristal) are synthetic progestogens that work by inhibiting ovulation and also by changing the endometrium (uterine lining) to reduce the likelihood of a fertilized egg implanting. The drugs should be taken as soon as possible after unprotected sex; levonorgestrel is only effective if taken within 72 hours, ulipristal if taken within 120 hours. The high progestogen dose required makes this method unsuitable for regular use. It also has a higher failure rate than the usual oral contraceptives. Having a coil (IUD) inserted within 120 hours of unprotected intercourse can also prevent pregnancy.

taking a combined pill, especially if she smokes or has an underlying medical condition such as diabetes mellitus. Some studies have found that women who take a combined oral contraceptive containing desogestrel or gestodene are at greater risk of developing a venous thromboembolism. The risk is still very small, however, and is lower than the risk of developing a venous thromboembolism during pregnancy. The combined oral contraceptives that contain desogestrel include Marvelon and Mercilon; those containing gestodene include Femodene, Femodette, Katya 30/75, Millinette 20/75 and 30/75, and Sunya 20/75.

High blood pressure is a possible complication of oral contraceptives for some women. Measurement of blood pressure before the pill is prescribed and every six months after the woman starts taking oral contraceptives is advised for all women taking oral contraceptives.

Some very rare liver cancers have occurred in pill-users, and breast cancer and cervical cancer may be slightly more common, but cancers of the ovaries and uterus are less common.

Although there is no evidence that oral contraceptives reduce a woman's fertility or damage babies conceived after they are discontinued, doctors recommend waiting for at least one normal menstrual period before you attempt to conceive.

WHAT TO DO IF YOU MISS A PILL

Contraceptive protection may be reduced if blood levels of the hormones in the body fall as a result of missing a pill. It is particularly important to ensure that the progestogen-only pills are taken punctually. The table below is a guide to what you should do if you miss a pill. The action you take depends on the degree of lateness and the type of pill being used. You should consult your doctor or pharmacist if you are unsure.

Combined and phased pills *		Progestogen-only pills	
Less than 24 hours late	Take the missed pill now, and take the next one on time.	Less than 3 hours late (12 hours for Cerazette)	Take the missed pill now, and take the next one on time.
More than 24 hours late	The pill may not work. Take the missed pill now, and take the next one on time. If more than one pill has been missed, just take one, then take the next on time (even if on the same day). Take extra precautions for the next 7 days. If the 7 days extends into the pill-free (or inactive pill) period, start the next packet without a break (or without taking inactive pills).	More than 3 hours late (12 hours for Cerazette)	Take the missed pill now and take the next pill one on time. If more than one pill has been missed, just take one, then take the next pill on time (even if on the same day). In either case you are not protected and will need to take extra precautions for the next 7 days.

* Except Qlaira, Zoely, Eloine, and Daylette; refer to patient information leaflet.

COMMON DRUGS

Progestogens	Norgestimate
Desogestrel *	Ulipristal *
Dienogest	
Drospirenone	**Oestrogens**
Gestodene	Estradiol *
Levonorgestrel *	Ethinylestradiol *
Nomegestrol	Mestranol
Norethisterone *	

* See Part 3

DRUGS FOR INFERTILITY

Conception and the establishment of pregnancy require a healthy reproductive system in both partners. The man must be able to produce sufficient numbers of healthy sperm; the woman must be able to produce a healthy egg that is able to pass freely down the fallopian tube to the uterus. The lining of the uterus must be in a condition that allows the implantation of the fertilized egg.

The cause of infertility may sometimes remain undiscovered, but in the majority of cases it is due to one of the following factors: intercourse taking place at the wrong time during the menstrual cycle; the man producing too few or unhealthy sperm; the woman either failing to ovulate (release an egg) or having blocked fallopian tubes perhaps as a result of previous pelvic infection. Alternatively, production of gonadotrophin hormones – follicle-stimulating hormone (FSH) and luteinizing hormone (LH) – needed for ovulation and implantation of the egg may be affected by illness or psychological stress.

If no simple explanation can be found, the man's semen will be analysed. If these tests show that abnormally low numbers of sperm are being produced, or if a large proportion of the sperm produced are unhealthy, drug treatment may be tried.

If no abnormality of sperm production is discovered, the woman will be given a thorough medical examination. Ovulation is monitored and blood tests may be performed to assess hormone levels. If ovulation does not occur, the woman may be offered drug treatment.

Why they are used

In men, the evidence is poor for the treatment of low sperm production with gonadotrophins – FSH or human chorionic gonadotrophin (hCG) – or a pituitary-stimulating drug (for example, clomifene) and corticosteroids.

In women, drugs are useful in helping to achieve pregnancy only when a hormone defect inhibiting ovulation has been diagnosed. Treatment may continue for months and does not always produce

ACTION OF FERTILITY DRUGS

Ovulation (release of an egg) and implantation are governed by hormones that are produced by the pituitary gland. FSH stimulates ripening of the egg follicle. LH triggers ovulation and ensures that progesterone is produced to prepare the uterus for the implantation of the egg. Drugs for female infertility boost the actions of these hormones.

FSH and hCG FSH adds to the action of the natural FSH early in the menstrual cycle. hCG mimics the action of natural LH at mid-cycle.

Clomifene Normally, oestrogen suppresses the pituitary gland's output of FSH and LH. Clomifene opposes the action of oestrogen so that FSH and LH continue to be produced.

Comparison of normal hormone fluctuation and timing of drug treatment

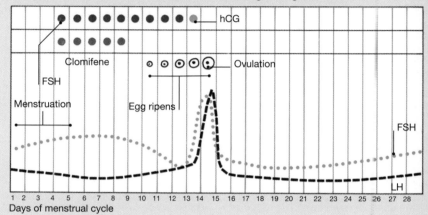

Days of menstrual cycle

a pregnancy. Women in whom the pituitary gland produces some FSH and LH may be given courses of clomifene for several days during each month. Usually, up to three courses may be tried. An effective dose produces ovulation five to ten days after the last tablet is taken.

Clomifene may thicken the cervical mucus, impeding the passage of sperm, but the advantage of achieving ovulation outweighs the risk of this side effect. If treatment with clomifene fails to produce ovulation, or if a disorder of the pituitary gland prevents the production of FSH and LH, treatment with FSH and LH together, FSH alone, or hCG may be given. In menstruating women, FSH is started within the first 7 days of the menstrual cycle.

How they work

Fertility drugs raise the chance of ovulation by boosting levels of LH and FSH. Clomifene stimulates the pituitary gland to increase its output of these hormones. Artificial FSH and hCG mimic the action of naturally produced FSH and LH, respectively. Both treatments, when successful, stimulate ovulation and implantation of the fertilized egg.

How they affect you

Clomifene may produce hot flushes, nausea, headaches, and, rarely, ovarian cysts and visual disturbance, while hCG can cause tiredness, headaches, and mood changes. FSH can cause the ovaries to enlarge, producing abdominal discomfort. These drugs increase the likelihood of multiple births, usually twins.

DRUGS FOR ERECTILE DYSFUNCTION

Erectile dysfunction (also known as impotence) is defined as the inability to achieve or maintain an erection. The penis contains three cylinders of erectile tissue, the two corpora cavernosa and the corpus spongiosum. Normally, when a man is sexually aroused, the arteries in the penis relax and widen, allowing more blood than usual to flow into the organ, filling the corpora cavernosa and the corpus spongiosum. As these tissues expand and harden, the veins that carry blood out of the penis become compressed, reducing outflow and resulting in an erection. In some forms

of erectile dysfunction, this does not happen. Drugs can then be used that will increase the blood flow into the penis to produce an erection.

Sildenafil and tadalafil not only increase the blood flow into the penis but also prevent the muscle wall from relaxing, so the blood does not drain out of the blood vessels and the penis remains erect.

Alprostadil is a prostaglandin drug that helps men achieve an erection by widening the blood vessels, but it must be injected directly into the penis, or applied into the urethra using a special syringe.

COMMON DRUGS

Bromocriptine ✱
Buserelin
Cetrorelix
Chorionic
   gonadotrophin
   (hCG)
Clomifene ✱
Follitropin (FSH)
Ganirelix
Goserelin ✱
Lutropin (LH)

Menopausal
   gonadotrophins
   (Menotrophin)
Nafarelin
Tamoxifen ✱

Drugs for erectile dysfunction
Alprostadil
Sildenafil/tadalafil ✱
Vardenafil

✱ See Part 3

DRUGS USED IN LABOUR

Normal labour has three stages. In the first stage, the uterus begins to contract, initially irregularly and then gradually more regularly and powerfully, while the cervix dilates until it is fully stretched. During the second stage, powerful contractions of the uterus push the baby down the mother's birth canal and out of her body. The third stage involves delivery of the placenta.

Drugs may be required during one or more stages of labour for any of the following reasons: to induce or augment labour; to delay premature labour (see Uterine muscle relaxants, below right); and to relieve pain. The administration of some drugs may be viewed as part of normal obstetric care; for example, the uterine stimulants ergometrine and oxytocin may be injected routinely before the third stage of labour to prevent excessive bleeding. Other drugs are administered only when the condition of the mother or baby requires intervention. The possible adverse effects of the drug on both mother and baby are always carefully balanced against the benefits.

Drugs to induce or augment labour

Induction of labour may be advised when a doctor considers it risky for the mother or baby for the pregnancy to continue – for example, if natural labour does not occur within two weeks of the due date or when a woman has pre-eclampsia. Other common reasons for inducing labour include premature rupture of the membrane surrounding the baby (breaking of the waters), slow growth of the baby due to poor nourishment by the placenta, or death of the fetus in the uterus.

When labour needs to be induced, oxytocin may be given intravenously. Alternatively, a prostaglandin pessary may be administered to soften and dilate the cervix. If these methods are ineffective or cannot be used because of potential adverse effects (see Risks and special

DRUGS USED TO TERMINATE PREGNANCY

Drugs may be used to terminate a pregnancy or to empty the uterus after the death of the baby. The principal drugs used are mifepristone and a prostaglandin (usually gemeprost or misoprostol). The effect of these drugs is to stimulate a miscarriage. Mifepristone blocks the action of progesterone, which is necessary for continuation of pregnancy, and ripens the cervix. The prostaglandin causes the uterine lining to break down and be shed from the body, causing bleeding. Surgical methods of termination, such as suction termination or surgical dilation and evacuation, can be used either instead of drugs or when a drug-induced termination is unsuccessful; these may be carried out under local or general anaesthesia.

precautions, below), a caesarean delivery may have to be performed.

Oxytocin may also be used to strengthen the force of contractions in labour that has started spontaneously but has not continued normally.

A combination of oxytocin and another uterine stimulant, ergometrine, is given to most women as the baby is being born or immediately following birth to prevent excessive bleeding after the delivery of the placenta. This combination encourages the uterus to contract after delivery, which restricts the flow of blood.

Risks and special precautions

When oxytocin is used to induce labour, the dosage is carefully monitored throughout to prevent the possibility of excessively violent contractions. It is administered to women who have had surgery of the uterus only with careful monitoring. The drug is not known to affect the baby adversely. Ergometrine is not given to women who have had high blood pressure during pregnancy or those who have cardiovascular disease.

Drugs used for pain relief
Opioid analgesics

Pethidine, morphine, or other opioids may be given once active labour has been established (see Analgesics, p.36). Possible side effects in the mother include drowsiness, nausea, and vomiting. Opioid drugs may cause breathing difficulties for the new baby, but these problems may be reversed by the antidote naloxone.

Epidural anaesthesia

This provides pain relief during labour and birth by numbing the nerves leading to the uterus and pelvic area. It is often used during a planned caesarean delivery, thus enabling the mother to be fully conscious for the birth.

An epidural involves injection of a local anaesthetic (see p.36) into the epidural space, between the spinal cord and the vertebrae. An epidural may block the mother's urge to push during the second stage, and a forceps delivery may be necessary. Headaches may occasionally occur following epidural anaesthesia.

Oxygen and nitrous oxide

These gases are combined to produce a mixture that reduces the pain caused by contractions. During the first and second stages of labour, gas is self-administered by inhalation through a mouthpiece or mask. If it is used over too long a period, it may produce nausea, confusion, and dehydration in the mother.

Local anaesthetics

These drugs are injected inside the vagina or near the vaginal opening and are used to numb sensation during forceps delivery, before an episiotomy

WHEN DRUGS ARE USED IN LABOUR

The drugs used in each stage of labour are described below.

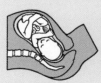

Before labour
Oxytocin
Prostaglandins

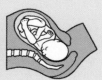

First stage
Epidural anaesthetics
Morphine
Oxytocin
Pethidine

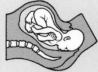

Second stage
Local anaesthetics
Nitrous oxide
Oxytocin

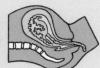

Third stage
Ergometrine
Oxytocin

(an incision made to enlarge the vaginal opening), and when stitches are necessary. Side effects are rare.

Uterine muscle relaxants

When contractions of the uterus start before the 34th week of pregnancy, doctors usually advise bed rest and may also administer a drug that relaxes the muscles of the uterus, halting labour. Initially, the drug is given in hospital by injection, but it may be continued orally at home. These drugs work by stimulating the sympathetic nervous system (see Autonomic nervous system, p.35) and may cause palpitations and anxiety in the mother. They have not been shown to have adverse effects on the baby.

COMMON DRUGS

Prostaglandins
Carboprost
Dinoprostone
Gemeprost
Misoprostol ✳

Pain relief
Entonox® (oxygen
  and nitrous oxide)
Fentanyl
Morphine ✳
Pethidine

Antiprogestogen
Mifepristone

Uterine muscle relaxants
Atosiban
Salbutamol ✳
Terbutaline ✳

Uterine stimulants
Ergometrine
Oxytocin

Local anaesthetics
Bupivacaine
Lidocaine
  (lignocaine)

✳ See Part 3

125

DRUGS USED FOR URINARY DISORDERS

Urine is produced by the kidneys and stored in the bladder. As the urine accumulates, the bladder walls stretch and pressure within the bladder increases. Eventually, the stretching stimulates nerve endings that produce the urge to urinate. The ring of muscle (sphincter) around the bladder neck normally keeps the bladder closed until it is consciously relaxed, allowing urine to pass via the urethra out of the body.

A number of disorders can affect the urinary tract. The most common of these disorders are infection in the bladder (cystitis) or the urethra (urethritis), and loss of reliable control over urination (urinary incontinence). A less common problem is inability to expel urine (urinary retention). Drugs used to treat these problems include antibiotics (see p.86) and antibacterial drugs (p.89), analgesics (p.36), drugs to increase the acidity of the urine, and drugs that act on nerve control over the bladder and sphincter muscles.

Drugs for urinary infection

Nearly all infections of the bladder are caused by bacteria. Symptoms include a continual urge to urinate, although often nothing is passed; pain on urinating; and lower abdominal pain. Many antibiotics and antibacterials are used to treat urinary tract infections. Among the most widely used, owing to their effectiveness, are cephalosporins, amoxicillin, and trimethoprim (see Antibiotics, p.86, and Antibacterial drugs, p.89).

Measures are also sometimes taken to increase the acidity of the urine, thereby making it hostile to bacteria. Ascorbic acid (vitamin C) and acid fruit juices have this effect, although making the urine less acidic with potassium or sodium citrate during an attack of cystitis helps to relieve the discomfort. Symptoms are commonly relieved within a few hours of the start of treatment.

For maximum effect, all drug treatments prescribed for urinary tract infections need to be accompanied by increased fluid intake.

Drugs for urinary incontinence

Urinary incontinence can occur for a several reasons. A weak sphincter muscle allows the involuntary passage of urine when abdominal pressure is raised by coughing or physical exertion. This is known as stress incontinence and commonly affects women who have had children. Urgency – the sudden need to urinate – stems from oversensitivity of the bladder muscle; small quantities of urine stimulate the urge to urinate frequently.

Incontinence can also occur due to loss of nerve control in neurological disorders such as multiple sclerosis. In children, inability to control urination at night (nocturnal enuresis) is also a form of urinary incontinence.

Drug treatment is not necessary or appropriate for all forms of incontinence. In stress incontinence, exercises to strengthen the pelvic floor muscles or surgery to tighten stretched ligaments may be effective. In urgency, regular emptying of the bladder can often avoid the need for medical intervention. Incontinence caused by loss of nerve control is unlikely to be helped by drug treatment. Frequency of urination in urgency may be reduced by anticholinergic and antispasmodic drugs. These reduce nerve signals from the muscles in the bladder, allowing greater volumes of urine to accumulate without stimulating the urge to pass urine. Tricyclic antidepressants, such as imipramine (see p.281), have a strong anticholinergic action, and have been prescribed for nocturnal enuresis in children, but many doctors believe the risk of overdosage is unacceptable. Desmopressin, a synthetic derivative of antidiuretic hormone (see p.103), is also used for nocturnal enuresis.

Drugs for urinary retention

Urinary retention is the inability to empty the bladder. This usually results from the failure of the bladder muscle to contract sufficiently to expel accumulated urine. Possible causes include an enlarged prostate gland or tumour, or a long-standing neurological disorder. Some drugs can cause urinary retention.

Most cases of urinary retention need to be relieved by inserting a tube (catheter) into the urethra. Surgery may be needed to prevent a recurrence of the problem. Drugs that relax the sphincter or stimulate bladder contraction are now rarely used in the treatment of urinary retention, but two types of drug are used in the long-term management of prostatic enlargement. Finasteride prevents production of male hormones that stimulate prostatic growth, and alpha blockers, such as prazosin, tamsulosin, and terazosin, relax prostatic and urethral smooth muscle, thereby improving urine outflow. Long-term drug treatment can relieve symptoms and delay the need for surgery.

ACTION OF DRUGS ON URINATION

Normal bladder action
Urination occurs when the sphincter keeping the exit from the bladder into the urethra closed is consciously relaxed in response to signals from the bladder indicating that it is full. As the sphincter opens, the bladder wall contracts and urine is expelled.

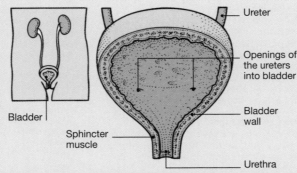

Ureter

Openings of the ureters into bladder

Bladder wall

Bladder

Sphincter muscle

Urethra

How drugs act to improve bladder control

Anticholinergic drugs relax the bladder muscle by interfering with the passage of nerve impulses to the muscle.

Sympathomimetics act directly on the sphincter muscle, causing it to contract.

How drugs act to relieve urinary retention

Parasympathomimetics (cholinergics) stimulate contraction of the bladder wall.

Alpha blockers relax the muscle of the sphincter.

COMMON DRUGS

Antibiotics and antibacterials
(see pp.86–89)

Anticholinergics
Flavoxate
Imipramine *
Oxybutynin *
Propantheline
Propiverine
Solifenacin
Tolterodine *
Trospium

Parasympatho-mimetic
Bethanechol
Distigmine

Alpha blockers
Alfuzosin
Doxazosin *
Indoramin
Prazosin
Tamsulosin *
Terazosin

Other drugs
Desmopressin *
Dimethyl sulfoxide
Duloxetine
Finasteride *
Potassium citrate
Sodium bicarbonate/ citrate
Vitamin C *

* See Part 3

EYES AND EARS

The eye and ear are the two sense organs that provide us with the most information about the world around us. The eye is the organ of vision that converts light into nerve signals, which are transmitted to the brain for interpretation into images. The ear not only provides the means by which sound is detected and communicated to the brain, but it also contains the organ of balance that tells the brain about the position and movement of the body. It is divided into three parts – outer, middle, and inner ear.

What can go wrong

The most common eye and ear disorders are infection and inflammation (sometimes caused by allergy). Many parts of the eye may be affected, notably the conjunctiva (the membrane that covers the front of the eye and lines the eyelids) and the iris. The middle and outer ear are more commonly affected by infection than the inner ear.

The eye may also be damaged by glaucoma, a disorder in which the optic nerve, which connects the eye to the brain, becomes damaged. Glaucoma is usually caused by fluid building up in the front part of the eye and may eventually threaten the vision. Eye problems such as retinopathy (disease of the retina) or cataracts (clouding of the lens) may occur as a result of diabetes or for other reasons, but both of these eye problems are now treatable.

Other disorders affecting the ear include build-up of wax (cerumen) in the outer ear canal and disturbances to the balance mechanism (see Vertigo and Ménière's disease, p.46).

Why drugs are used

Doctors usually prescribe antibiotics (see p.86) to clear ear and eye infections. These drugs may be given by mouth or topically. Topical eye and ear preparations may contain a corticosteroid (p.99) to reduce inflammation. When inflammation has been caused by allergy, antihistamines (p.82) may also be taken. Decongestant drugs (p.51) are often prescribed to help clear the eustachian tube (see right) in middle ear infections.

Various drugs are used to reduce fluid pressure in glaucoma. These include diuretics (p.57), beta blockers (p.55), and miotics (drugs to narrow the pupil). In other cases, the pupil may need to be widened by mydriatic drugs.

MAJOR DRUG GROUPS

Drugs for glaucoma   Drugs for ear disorders
Drugs affecting the pupil

How the eye works
Light enters the eye through the cornea. The muscles of the iris control pupil size and thus the amount of light passing into the eye. In the eye, light hits the retina, which converts it to nerve signals that are carried by the optic nerve to the brain.

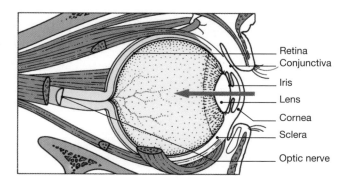

Retina
Conjunctiva
Iris
Lens
Cornea
Sclera
Optic nerve

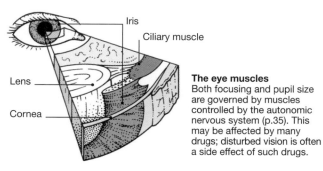

Iris
Ciliary muscle
Lens
Cornea

The eye muscles
Both focusing and pupil size are governed by muscles controlled by the autonomic nervous system (p.35). This may be affected by many drugs; disturbed vision is often a side effect of such drugs.

The ear
The outer ear canal is separated from the middle ear by the eardrum. Three bones in the middle ear connect it to the inner ear. This contains the cochlea (organ of hearing) and the labyrinth (organ of balance).

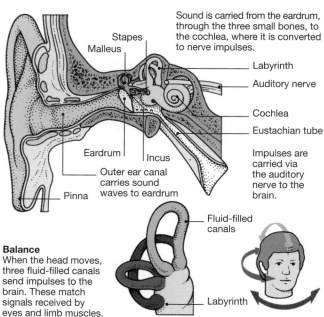

Sound is carried from the eardrum, through the three small bones, to the cochlea, where it is converted to nerve impulses.

Stapes
Malleus
Labyrinth
Auditory nerve
Cochlea
Eustachian tube

Impulses are carried via the auditory nerve to the brain.

Eardrum
Incus
Outer ear canal carries sound waves to eardrum
Pinna

Fluid-filled canals

Balance
When the head moves, three fluid-filled canals send impulses to the brain. These match signals received by eyes and limb muscles.

Labyrinth

DRUGS FOR GLAUCOMA

Glaucoma is the name given to a group of conditions that damage the optic nerve, which transmits vision signals from the eye to the brain. One of the main modifiable risk factors for glaucoma is abnormally high fluid pressure inside the eye, which in turn compresses the blood vessels that supply the optic nerve. This problem may result in irreversible nerve damage and permanent loss of vision.

In the most common form, chronic (or open-angle) glaucoma, reduced drainage of fluid from the eye causes pressure in the eye to build up slowly. Progressive reduction in the peripheral field of vision may take months or years to be noticed.

Acute (or closed-angle) glaucoma occurs when the drainage angle between the iris and cornea (see below) is suddenly blocked by the iris. Fluid pressure usually builds up quite suddenly, blurring vision in the affected eye (see below). The eye becomes red and painful, and there may be a headache and sometimes vomiting.

The main attack is often preceded by milder warning attacks, such as seeing haloes around lights, in the previous weeks or months. Older, long-sighted people are particularly at risk of developing acute glaucoma. The angle may also narrow suddenly following injury or after taking certain drugs, such as anticholinergics. Closed-angle glaucoma may develop more slowly (chronic closed-angle glaucoma).

Drugs are used in the treatment of both types of glaucoma. These include miotics (see Drugs affecting the pupil, p.130) and beta blockers (p.55), as well as certain diuretics (carbonic anhydrase inhibitors and osmotics, p.57).

Why they are used

Chronic (open-angle) glaucoma

In this condition, drugs are used to reduce pressure inside the eye. They will prevent further deterioration of vision, but cannot repair damage that has already occurred and may therefore be required for life. In most patients, treatment is begun with eye drops containing a beta blocker to reduce fluid production in the eye. Miotic drops to constrict the pupil and improve fluid drainage may be given. Prostaglandin analogues, such as latanoprost (p.296), are also used to increase fluid outflow. If these drugs are not effective, dipivefrine, apraclonidine, or brimonidine (p.177) may be tried to reduce secretion and help outflow. Sometimes a carbonic anhydrase inhibitor such as acetazolamide or dorzolamide may be given to reduce fluid production. Laser treatment and surgery may also be used to improve drainage.

Acute (closed-angle) glaucoma

Acute glaucoma needs immediate medical treatment to prevent total loss of vision. Drugs are used initially to bring down the pressure within the eye. Laser treatment or surgery is then carried out to prevent any recurrence so that long-term drug treatment is seldom required.

WHAT HAPPENS IN GLAUCOMA

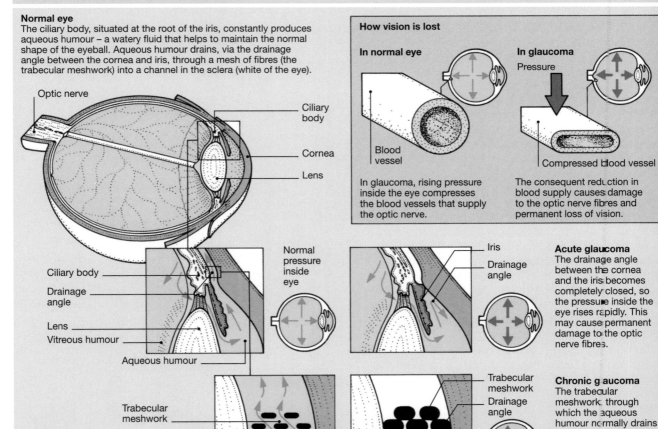

Normal eye
The ciliary body, situated at the root of the iris, constantly produces aqueous humour – a watery fluid that helps to maintain the normal shape of the eyeball. Aqueous humour drains, via the drainage angle between the cornea and iris, through a mesh of fibres (the trabecular meshwork) into a channel in the sclera (white of the eye).

Optic nerve

Ciliary body

Cornea

Lens

Ciliary body

Drainage angle

Lens

Vitreous humour

Aqueous humour

Trabecular meshwork

Drainage angle

How vision is lost

In normal eye

In glaucoma

Pressure

Blood vessel

Compressed blood vessel

In glaucoma, rising pressure inside the eye compresses the blood vessels that supply the optic nerve.

The consequent reduction in blood supply causes damage to the optic nerve fibres and permanent loss of vision.

Normal pressure inside eye

Iris

Drainage angle

Trabecular meshwork

Drainage angle

Acute glaucoma
The drainage angle between the cornea and the iris becomes completely closed, so the pressure inside the eye rises rapidly. This may cause permanent damage to the optic nerve fibres.

Chronic glaucoma
The trabecular meshwork through which the aqueous humour normally drains from the eye, slowly closes off, so that fluid pressure builds up gradually and damages the optic nerve.

Acetazolamide is often the first drug administered when the condition is diagnosed. It may be injected into a vein for rapid effect and thereafter administered by mouth. Frequent applications of eye drops containing pilocarpine or carbachol are given. An osmotic diuretic such as mannitol may be administered. This draws fluid out of all body tissues, including the eye, and reduces pressure within the eye.

How they work

Drugs for glaucoma act in various ways to reduce fluid pressure inside the eye. Miotics improve the drainage of the fluid out of the eye. In chronic glaucoma, this is achieved by increasing the outflow of aqueous humour through the drainage channel called the trabecular meshwork (see facing page). In acute glaucoma, the pupil-constricting effect of miotics pulls the iris away from the drainage channel, allowing the aqueous humour to flow out. Prostaglandin analogues act by increasing fluid flow from the eye. Beta blockers and carbonic anhydrase inhibitors act on the fluid-producing cells inside the eye to reduce the production of aqueous humour. Sympathomimetic drugs such as brimonidine and apraclonidine are also thought to act partly in this way and partly by improving fluid drainage.

How they affect you

Drugs for acute glaucoma relieve pain and other symptoms within a few hours of being used. The benefits of drug treatment in chronic glaucoma, however, may not be immediately apparent since treatment is only able to halt a further deterioration of vision.

People receiving miotic eye drops are likely to notice darkening of vision and difficulty seeing in the dark. Increased shortsightedness may be noticeable. Some miotics also cause irritation and redness of the eyes.

Beta blocker eye drops have few day-to-day side effects but carry risks for a few people (see right). Oral acetazolamide usually causes an increase in frequency of urination and thirst. Nausea and a pins-and-needles sensation are also common.

ACTION OF DRUGS FOR GLAUCOMA

Miotics
These act on the circular muscle in the iris to reduce the size of the pupil. In acute glaucoma, this relieves any obstruction to the flow of aqueous humour by pulling the iris away from the cornea (right). In chronic glaucoma, miotic drugs act directly to increase the outflow of aqueous humour.

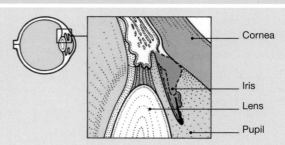

Cornea

Iris

Lens

Pupil

Beta blockers
The fluid-producing cells in the ciliary body are stimulated by signals passed through beta receptors (see p.35). Beta blocking drugs prevent the transmission of signals through these receptors, thereby reducing the stimulus to produce fluid.

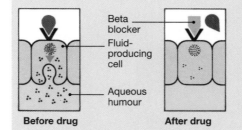

Beta blocker

Fluid-producing cell

Aqueous humour

Before drug

After drug

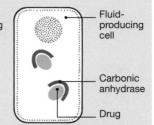

Fluid-producing cell

Carbonic anhydrase

Drug

Carbonic anhydrase inhibitors
These block the enzyme carbonic anhydrase, involved in the production of aqueous humour in the ciliary body.

Risks and special precautions

Miotics can cause alteration in vision. Beta blockers are absorbed into the body and can affect the lungs, heart, and circulation. As a result, cardioselective beta blockers, such as betaxolol, are prescribed with caution to people with asthma or certain circulatory disorders and, in some cases, may be withheld altogether. The amount of the drug absorbed into the body can be reduced by applying the drops carefully (see left). Acetazolamide may cause troublesome adverse effects, including tingling of the hands and feet, the formation of kidney stones, and, rarely, kidney damage. People with existing kidney problems are not usually given this drug.

APPLYING EYE DROPS IN GLAUCOMA

To reduce the amount of drug absorbed into the blood via the lacrimal (tear) duct, apply eye drops as shown here. This also improves the effectiveness of the drug.

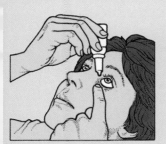

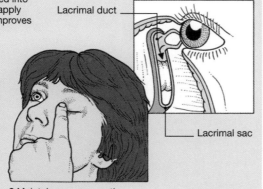

Lacrimal duct

Lacrimal sac

1 Press firmly on the lacrimal sac in the corner of the eye and apply the number of drops prescribed by your doctor.

2 Maintain pressure on the lacrimal sac for a few moments after applying the drops.

COMMON DRUGS

Miotics
Carbachol
Pilocarpine *

Carbonic anhydrase inhibitors
Acetazolamide
Brinzolamide *
Dorzolamide *

Prostaglandin analogues
Bimatoprost
Latanoprost *
Travoprost

Beta blockers
Betaxolol
Carteolol
Levobunolol
Metipranolol
Timolol *

Sympathomimetics
Apraclonidine
Brimonidine *
Dipivefrine

| * See Part 3 |

DRUGS AFFECTING THE PUPIL

The pupil of the eye is the circular opening in the centre of the iris (the coloured part of the eye) through which light enters. It continually changes in size to adjust to variations in the intensity of light; in bright light it becomes quite small (constricts), but in dim light the pupil enlarges (dilates).

Eye drops containing drugs that act on the pupil are widely used by specialists. They are grouped into two categories: mydriatics, which dilate the pupil, and miotics, which constrict it.

Why they are used

Mydriatics are most often used to allow the doctor to view the inside of the eye – particularly the retina, the optic nerve head, and the blood vessels that supply the retina. Many of these drugs cause a temporary paralysis of the eye's focusing mechanism, a state called cycloplegia. This state is sometimes induced to help identify any focusing errors, especially in babies and young children. By producing cycloplegia, it is possible to determine the precise optical prescription required for a child, especially in the case of a squint.

Dilation of the pupil is part of the treatment for uveitis, an inflammatory disease of the iris and focusing muscle. In uveitis, the inflamed iris may stick to the lens, causing severe damage to the eye. This complication can be prevented by early dilation of the pupil so that the iris is no longer in contact with the lens.

Constriction of the pupil with miotic drugs is often required in the treatment of glaucoma (see p.129). Miotics can also be used to restore the pupil to a normal size after dilation is induced by mydriatics.

How they work

The size of the pupil is controlled by two separate sets of muscles in the iris – the circular muscle and the radial muscle. The two sets of muscles are governed by separate branches of the autonomic nervous system (see p.35): the radial muscle is controlled by the sympathetic nervous system, and the circular muscle

is controlled by the parasympathetic nervous system.

Individual mydriatic and miotic drugs affect different branches of the autonomic nervous system, and cause the pupil to dilate or to contract, depending on the type of drug used (see above).

How they affect you

Mydriatic drugs – especially the long-acting types – impair the ability to focus the eye(s) for several hours or even days

after use. This interferes particularly with close activities such as reading. Bright light may cause discomfort. Miotics often interfere with night vision and may cause temporary short sight.

Normally, these eye drops produce few serious adverse effects. Sympathomimetic mydriatics may raise blood pressure and are used with caution in people with hypertension or heart disease. Miotics may irritate the eyes, but rarely cause generalized effects.

ACTION OF DRUGS AFFECTING THE PUPIL

The muscles of the iris
Pupil size is controlled by the coordinated action of the circular and radial muscles in the iris. The circular muscle forms a ring around the pupil; when this muscle contracts, the pupil becomes smaller. The radial muscle is composed of fibres that run from the pupil to the base of the iris like the spokes of a wheel. Contraction of these fibres causes the pupil to become larger.

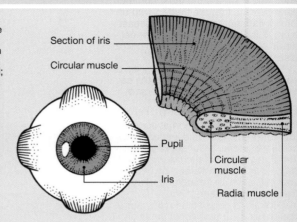

Section of iris
Circular muscle
Pupil
Circular muscle
Radial muscle
Iris

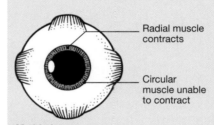

Radial muscle contracts
Circular muscle unable to contract

Mydriatics
Mydriatics enlarge the pupil in one of two ways. The sympathomimetics stimulate the radial muscle to contract. The anticholinergics prevent the circular muscle from contracting.

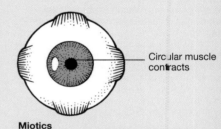

Circular muscle contracts

Miotics
Most miotics reduce the size of the pupil by stimulating the activity of the parasympathetic nervous system, which causes the circular muscle to contract.

ARTIFICIAL TEAR PREPARATIONS

Tears are continually produced to keep the front of the eye covered with a thin, moist film. This is essential for clear vision and for keeping the front of the eye free from dirt and other irritants. In some conditions, known collectively as dry eye syndromes (for example, Sjögren's syndrome), inadequate tear production may make the eyes feel dry and sore. Sore eyes can also occur in disorders where the eyelids do not close properly, causing the eye to become dry.

Why they are used
Since prolonged deficiency of natural tears can damage the cornea, regular application of

artificial tears in the form of eye drops is recommended for all of the conditions described above. Artificial tears may also be used to provide temporary relief from any feeling of discomfort and dryness in the eye caused by irritants, exposure to wind or sun, or following the initial wearing of contact lenses.

Although artificial tears are non-irritating, they often contain a preservative (for example, thiomersal or benzalkonium chloride) that may cause irritation. This risk of irritation is increased for wearers of soft contact lenses, who should ask their optician for advice before using any type of eye drops.

COMMON DRUGS

Sympathomimetic mydriatics
Phenylephrine

Miotics
Carbachol
Pilocarpine *

Anticholinergic mydriatics
Atropine *
Cyclopentolate
Homatropine
Tropicamide

* See Part 3

DRUGS FOR EAR DISORDERS

Inflammation and infection of the outer and middle ear are the most common ear disorders that are treated with drugs. Drug treatment for Ménière's disease, a condition that affects the inner ear, is described under Vertigo and Ménière's disease, p.46.

The type of drug treatment given for ear inflammation depends on the cause of the trouble and the site affected.

Inflammation of the outer ear

Inflammation of the external ear canal (otitis externa) can be caused by eczema or by a bacterial or fungal infection. The risk of inflammation is increased by swimming in dirty water, accumulation of wax in the ear, or scratching or poking too frequently at the ear.

Symptoms vary, but in many cases there is itching, pain (which may be severe if there is a boil in the ear canal), tenderness, and possibly some loss of hearing. If the ear is infected there will probably be a discharge.

Drug treatment

A corticosteroid drug (see p.99) in the form of ear drops may be used to treat inflammation of the outer ear when there is no infection. Aluminium acetate solution, as drops or applied on a piece of gauze, may also be used. Relief is usually obtained within a day or two. Prolonged use of corticosteroids is not advisable because they may reduce the ear's resistance to infection.

If there is both inflammation and infection, your doctor may prescribe ear drops containing an antibiotic (see p.86) combined with a corticosteroid to relieve the inflammation. Usually, a combination of antibiotics is prescribed to make the treatment effective against a wide range of bacteria. Commonly used antibiotics include framycetin, neomycin, and polymyxin B. These antibiotics are not used if the eardrum is perforated. They

EAR WAX REMOVAL

Ear wax (cerumen) is a natural secretion from the outer ear canal that keeps it free from dust and skin debris. Occasionally, wax may build up in the outer ear canal and become hard, leading to irritation and/or hearing loss.

Various over-the-counter remedies are available to soften ear wax and hasten its expulsion. These products may contain irritating substances that can cause inflammation. Doctors advise application of olive or almond oil instead. A cotton wool plug should be inserted to retain the oil in the outer ear. If ear wax is not dislodged by such home treatment, a doctor may syringe the ear with warm water. Do not use a stick or cotton wool bud.

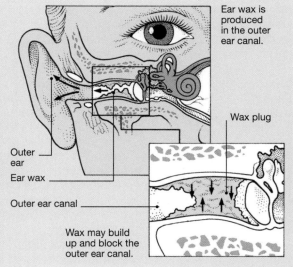

Ear wax is produced in the outer ear canal.

Outer ear

Ear wax

Outer ear canal

Wax plug

Wax may build up and block the outer ear canal.

are not usually applied for long periods because prolonged application can irritate the skin that lines the ear canal.

Sometimes an antibiotic given in the form of drops is not effective, and another type of antibiotic may also have to be taken by mouth.

Infection of the middle ear

Infection of the middle ear (otitis media) often causes severe pain and hearing loss. It is particularly common in young children in whom infecting organisms are able to spread easily into the middle ear from the nose or throat via the eustachian tube (see p.127).

Viral infections of the middle ear usually cure themselves and are less serious than those caused by bacteria. Bacterial ear infections are treated with antibiotics

given by mouth or injection. Bacterial infections often cause the eustachian tube to swell and become blocked. When a blockage occurs, pus builds up in the middle ear and puts pressure on the eardrum, which may perforate as a result.

Drug treatment

Doctors usually prescribe a decongestant (see p.51) or antihistamine (see p.82) to reduce swelling in the eustachian tube, thus allowing the pus to drain out of the middle ear. Usually, an antibiotic is also given by mouth to clear the infection.

Although antibiotics are not effective against viral infections, it is often difficult to distinguish between a viral and a bacterial infection of the middle ear, so your doctor may prescribe an antibiotic as a precautionary measure. Paracetamol, an analgesic (see p.36), may be given to relieve pain.

HOW TO USE EAR DROPS

Ear drops for outer ear disorders are more easily and efficiently administered if you have someone to help you. Lie on your side while the other person drops the medication into the ear cavity, ensuring that the dropper does not touch the ear. If possible, it is advisable to remain lying in that position for a few minutes in order to allow the drops to bathe the ear canal. Ear drops should be discarded when the course of treatment has been completed.

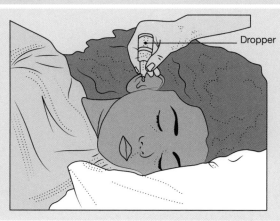

Dropper

COMMON DRUGS

Antibiotic and antibacterial ear drops
Chloramphenicol *
Clioquinol
Clotrimazole *
Framycetin
Gentamicin *
Neomycin

Decongestants
Ephedrine *
Oxymetazoline
Xylometazoline

Corticosteroids
Betamethasone *
Dexamethasone *
Flumetasone
Hydrocortisone *
Prednisolone *
Triamcinolone

Other drugs
Aluminium acetate
Antihistamines
(see p.82)
Choline salicylate

| * See Part 3 |

SKIN

The skin waterproofs, cushions, and protects the rest of the body and is, in fact, its largest organ. It provides a barrier against innumerable infections and infestations, it helps the body to retain its vital fluids, it plays a major role in temperature control, and it houses the sensory nerves of touch.

The skin consists of two main layers: a thin, tough top layer, the epidermis, and below it a thicker layer, the dermis. The epidermis also has two layers: the skin surface, or stratum corneum (horny layer) consisting of dead cells, and below, a layer of active cells. The cells in the active layer divide and eventually die, maintaining the horny layer. Living cells produce keratin, which toughens the epidermis and is the basic substance of hair and nails. Some living cells in the epidermis produce melanin, a pigment released in increased amounts following exposure to sunlight.

The dermis contains different types of nerve ending for sensing pain, pressure, and temperature; sweat glands to cool the body; sebaceous glands, which release an oil (sebum) that lubricates and waterproofs the skin; and white blood cells, which help to keep the skin clear of infection.

What can go wrong
Most skin complaints are not serious, but they may be distressing if visible. They include infection, inflammation and irritation, infestation by skin parasites, and changes in skin structure and texture (for example, psoriasis, eczema, and acne).

Why drugs are used
Skin problems often resolve themselves without drug treatment. Over-the-counter preparations containing active ingredients are available, but doctors generally advise against their use without medical supervision because they could aggravate some skin conditions if used inappropriately. The drugs prescribed by doctors, however, are often highly effective, including antibiotics (p.86) for bacterial infections, antifungal drugs (p.96) for fungal infections, anti-infestation agents for skin parasites (p.136), and topical corticosteroids (p.134) for inflammatory conditions. Specialized drugs are available for conditions such as psoriasis and acne.

Although many drugs are topical medications, they must be used carefully because, like drugs taken orally, they can cause adverse effects.

Structure of the skin
The epidermis contains keratin and melanin, while the dermis contains sweat glands, sebaceous glands, and nerve endings that sense pain, temperature, and pressure.

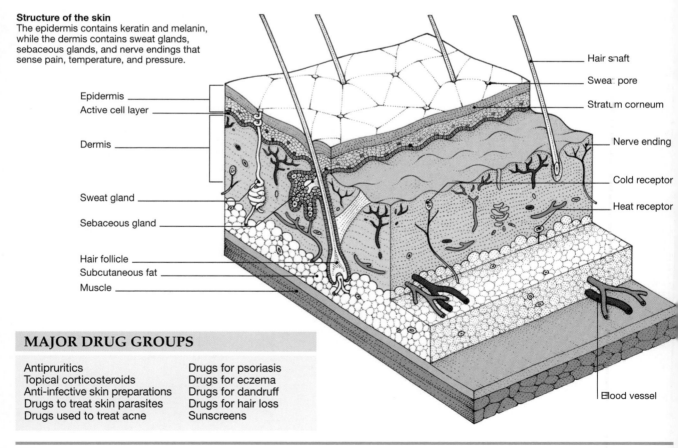

Epidermis
Active cell layer
Dermis
Sweat gland
Sebaceous gland
Hair follicle
Subcutaneous fat
Muscle

Hair shaft
Sweat pore
Stratum corneum
Nerve ending
Cold receptor
Heat receptor
Blood vessel

MAJOR DRUG GROUPS

Antipruritics	Drugs for psoriasis
Topical corticosteroids	Drugs for eczema
Anti-infective skin preparations	Drugs for dandruff
Drugs to treat skin parasites	Drugs for hair loss
Drugs used to treat acne	Sunscreens

ANTIPRURITICS

Itching (irritation of the skin that creates the urge to scratch), also known as pruritus, most often occurs as a result of minor physical irritation or chemical changes in the skin caused by disease, inflammation, allergy, or exposure to irritant substances. People differ in their tolerance to itch, and a person's threshold can be altered by stress and other psychological factors.

Itching is a common symptom of many skin disorders, including eczema and psoriasis, and allergic conditions such as urticaria (hives). It is sometimes caused by a localized fungal infection or parasitic infestation. Diseases such as chickenpox may also cause itching. Less commonly, itching may occur as a symptom of diabetes mellitus, jaundice, kidney failure, or drug reactions.

In many cases, generalized itching is caused by dry skin. Itching in particular parts of the body is often caused by a specific problem. For example, itching around the anus (pruritus ani) may result from haemorrhoids or worm infestation, while genital itching in women (pruritus vulvae) may be caused either by vaginal infection or, in postmenopausal women, may be due to a hormone deficiency.

Although scratching frequently provides temporary relief, it can often increase skin inflammation and make the condition worse. Continued scratching of an area of irritated skin may occasionally lead to a vicious "itch-scratch" cycle that continues long after the original cause of the trouble has been removed.

There are several different types of medicine used to relieve skin irritation. These products include soothing topical preparations applied to the affected skin and drugs that are taken by mouth. The main drugs used in antipruritic products include corticosteroids (see Topical corticosteroids, p.134), antihistamines (p.82), and local anaesthetics (p.36). Simple emollient or cooling creams or ointments, which do not contain active ingredients, are often recommended, especially if there is associated dry skin.

Why they are used

For mild itching arising from sunburn, urticaria, or insect bites, a cooling lotion such as calamine, perhaps containing menthol, phenol, or camphor, may be the most appropriate treatment. Local anaesthetic creams are sometimes helpful for small areas of irritation, such as insect bites, but are unsuitable for widespread itching. The itching caused by dry skin is often soothed by a simple emollient. Avoiding excessive bathing and using moisturizing bath oils may also help.

Severe itching from eczema or other inflammatory skin conditions may be treated with a topical corticosteroid preparation. When the irritation prevents sleep, a doctor may prescribe a sedating antihistamine drug, such as hydroxyzine, to promote sleep as well as to relieve itching (see also Sleeping drugs, p.38). Antihistamines are also sometimes included in topical preparations to relieve skin irritation, but their effectiveness when administered in this way is doubtful. For the treatment of pruritus ani, see Drugs for rectal and anal disorders (p.71). Postmenopausal pruritus vulvae may be helped by vaginal creams containing oestrogen; for further information, see Female sex hormones (p.105). Itching due to an underlying systemic illness cannot be helped by skin creams and requires treatment for the principal disorder.

Risks and special precautions

The main risk from any antipruritic, with the exception of simple emollients and soothing preparations, is skin irritation, and therefore aggravated itching, that is caused by prolonged or heavy use. Antihistamine and local anaesthetic creams are especially likely to cause a reaction, and must be stopped if they do so. Antihistamines taken by mouth to relieve itching may cause drowsiness. The special risks of topical corticosteroids are discussed on p.134.

Because itching can be a symptom of many underlying conditions, self-treatment should be continued for no longer than a week before seeking medical advice.

ACTION OF ANTIPRURITICS

Irritation of the skin causes the release of substances, such as histamine, that cause blood vessels to dilate and fluid to accumulate under the skin, which results in itching and inflammation. Antipruritic drugs act either by reducing inflammation, and therefore irritation, or by numbing the nerve impulses that transmit sensation to the brain.

Corticosteroids applied to the skin surface reduce itching caused by allergy within a few days, although the soothing effect of the cream may produce an immediate improvement. They pass into the underlying tissues and blood vessels and reduce the release of histamine, the chemical that causes itching and inflammation.

Antihistamines act within a few hours to reduce allergy-related skin inflammation. Applied to the skin, they pass into the underlying tissue and block the effects of histamine on the blood vessels beneath the skin. Taken by mouth, they also act on the brain to reduce the perception of irritation.

Local anaesthetics absorbed through the skin numb the transmission of signals from the nerves in the skin to the brain.

Soothing and emollient creams Calamine lotion and similar preparations applied to the skin reduce inflammation and itching by cooling the skin. Emollient creams lubricate the skin surface and prevent dryness.

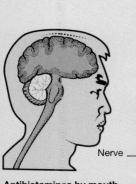

Antihistamines by mouth
The action of these drugs on histamine in the brain reduces the response to signals from irritated skin.

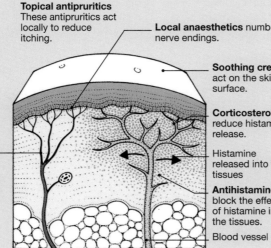

Topical antipruritics
These antipruritics act locally to reduce itching.

Local anaesthetics numb nerve endings.

Soothing creams act on the skin surface.

Corticosteroids reduce histamine release.

Histamine released into the tissues

Antihistamines block the effects of histamine in the tissues.

Blood vessel

Nerve

COMMON DRUGS

Antihistamines
(see also p.82)
Cetirizine *
Chlorphenamine *
Diphenhydramine
Fexofenadine
Hydroxyzine

Corticosteroids
(see also p.99)
Betamethasone *
Hydrocortisone *

Local anaesthetics
Benzocaine
Lidocaine
Tetracaine

Emollient and cooling preparations
Aqueous cream
Calamine lotion
Cold cream
Emulsifying ointment

Other drugs
Colestyramine *
Crotamiton
Doxepin

| * See Part 3 |

TOPICAL CORTICOSTEROIDS

Corticosteroid drugs (often simply called steroids) are related to the hormones produced by the adrenal glands. For a full description of these drugs, see p.99. Topical preparations containing a corticosteroid drug are often used to treat skin conditions in which inflammation is a prominent feature.

Why they are used

Corticosteroid creams and ointments are most commonly given to relieve itching and inflammation associated with skin diseases such as eczema and dermatitis. Corticosteroid preparations may also be prescribed for some other skin conditions, including psoriasis (see p.138).

Corticosteroids do not affect the underlying cause of skin irritation, and the condition is therefore likely to recur unless the substance (an allergen or irritant) that has provoked the irritation is removed, or the underlying condition is treated.

In most cases, treatment is started with a preparation containing a low concentration of a mild corticosteroid drug. A stronger preparation may be prescribed subsequently if the first product is ineffective.

How they affect you

Corticosteroids prevent the release of substances that trigger inflammation (see Action of corticosteroids on the skin, above right). Conditions treated with these drugs typically improve within a few days of starting the drug. Applied topically, corticosteroids rarely cause side effects, although the stronger drugs used in high concentrations have certain risks.

Risks and special precautions

Prolonged use of potent corticosteroids in high concentrations can lead to permanent changes in the skin. Applying them sparingly and only to the affected area minimizes this risk.

ACTION OF CORTICOSTEROIDS ON THE SKIN

Skin inflammation
Irritation of the skin, caused by allergens or irritant factors, provokes white blood cells to release substances that dilate the blood vessels. This makes the skin hot, red, and swollen.

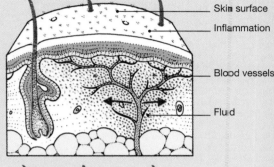

Drug action
Applied to the skin surface, corticosteroids are absorbed into the underlying tissue. There they inhibit the action of the substances that cause inflammation, allowing the blood vessels to return to normal and reducing the swelling.

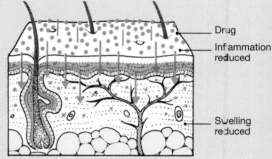

The most common side effect is thinning of the skin, sometimes resulting in permanent stretch marks. Fine blood vessels under the skin surface may become prominent (this condition is known as telangiectasia). Because the skin on the face is especially vulnerable to such damage, only milder corticosteroids should be prescribed for use on the face. Dark-skinned people may sometimes experience a temporary reduction in pigmentation at the site of application. When corticosteroids have been used on the skin for a prolonged period, abrupt discontinuation may cause a reddening of the skin called rebound erythema. This effect may be avoided by a gradual reduction in dosage.

Corticosteroids suppress the body's immune system (see p.115), thereby increasing the risk of infection. For this reason, they are never used alone to treat skin inflammation that is caused by bacterial or fungal infection. However, corticosteroids are sometimes included in topical preparations that also contain an antibiotic or antifungal agent (see Anti-infective skin preparations, facing page).

LONG-TERM EFFECTS OF TOPICAL CORTICOSTEROIDS

Prolonged use of topical corticosteroids causes thinning of the epidermis, so that tiny blood vessels close to the skin surface become visible. In addition, long-term use of these drugs weakens the underlying connective tissue of the dermis, causing the skin to become increasingly susceptible to developing stretch marks.

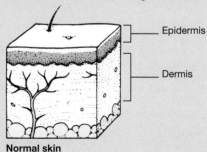

Normal skin

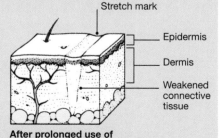

After prolonged use of topical corticosteroids

COMMON DRUGS

Very potent
Clobetasol ✳

Potent
Beclometasone ✳
Betamethasone ✳
Fluocinolone
Fluocinonide
Fluticasone ✳
Mometasone ✳
Triamcinolone

Moderate
Alclometasone
Clobetasone
Fludroxycortide
Fluocortolone

Mild
Hydrocortisone ✳

✳ See Part 3

ANTI-INFECTIVE SKIN PREPARATIONS

The skin is the body's first line of defence against infection. Yet the skin can also become infected itself, especially if the outer layer (epidermis) is damaged by a burn, cut, scrape, insect bite, or an inflammatory skin condition – for example, eczema or dermatitis.

Several different types of organism may infect the skin, including bacteria, viruses, fungi, and yeasts. This page concentrates on drugs applied topically to treat bacterial skin infections. These drugs include antiseptics, antibiotics, and other antibacterial agents. Infection by other organisms is covered elsewhere (see Antiviral drugs, p.91, Antifungal drugs, p.96, and Drugs used to treat skin parasites, p.136).

Why they are used

Bacterial infection of a skin wound can usually be prevented by thorough cleansing of the damaged area and the application of antiseptic creams or lotions as described in the box (right). If infection does occur, the wound usually becomes inflamed and swollen, and pus may form. If you develop these signs, you should see your doctor. The usual treatment for a wound infection is an antibiotic taken orally, although often an antibiotic cream is also prescribed.

An antibiotic or antibacterial skin cream may also be used to prevent infection when your doctor considers this to be a particular risk – for example, in the case of severe burns.

Other skin disorders in which topical antibiotic treatment may be prescribed include impetigo and infected eczema, bedsores, and nappy rash.

Often, a preparation containing two or more antibiotics is used in order to ensure

ANTISEPTICS

Antiseptics (sometimes called germicides or skin disinfectants) are chemicals that kill or prevent the growth of microorganisms. They are weaker than household disinfectants, which are irritating to the skin.

Antiseptic lotions, creams, gels, and solutions may be effective for preventing infection following wounds to the surface of the skin. Solutions can be added to water to clean wounds (if they are used undiluted, they may cause inflammation and increase the risk of infection). Creams may be applied to wounds after cleansing.

Antiseptics are included in some soaps and shampoos for the prevention of acne and dandruff, but their benefit in these disorders is doubtful. They are also included in some throat lozenges, but their effectiveness in curing throat infections is unproven.

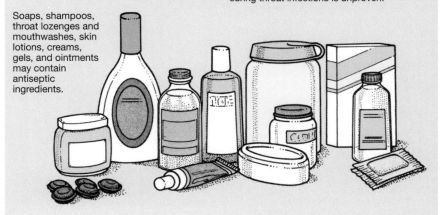

Soaps, shampoos, throat lozenges and mouthwashes, skin lotions, creams, gels, and ointments may contain antiseptic ingredients.

that all bacteria are eradicated. The antibiotics selected for inclusion in topical preparations are usually drugs that are poorly absorbed through the skin (such as aminoglycosides). Thus the drug remains concentrated on the surface and in the skin's upper layers, where it is intended to have its effect. However, if the infection is deep under the skin, or is causing fever and malaise, antibiotics may need to be given by mouth or injection.

Risks and special precautions

Any topical antibiotic product can irritate the skin or cause an allergic reaction. Irritation is sometimes provoked by another ingredient of the preparation rather than the active drug: for example, a preservative contained in the product. An allergic reaction causing swelling and reddening of the skin is more likely to be caused by the antibiotic drug itself. Any adverse reaction of this kind should be reported to your doctor, who may substitute another drug, or prescribe a different preparation.

Always follow your doctor's instructions on how long the treatment with antibiotics should be continued. Stopping too soon may cause the infection to flare up again.

Never use a skin preparation that has been prescribed for someone else, since it may aggravate your condition. Always throw away any unused medication.

BASES FOR SKIN PREPARATIONS

Drugs that are applied to the skin are usually in a preparation known as a base (or vehicle), such as a cream, lotion, ointment, gel, or paste. Many bases are beneficial on their own.

Creams These have an emollient effect. They usually consist of an oil-in-water emulsion and are used in the treatment of dry skin disorders, such as psoriasis and eczema. They may also contain other ingredients, such as camphor or menthol.

Ointments These are usually greasy and are suitable for treating eczema and very dry chronic lesions.

Gels These are jelly-like in consistency and are often water-based. They are used increasingly for a wide variety of topical skin treatments because they are easy to apply, usually non-greasy, and more rapidly absorbed than ointments.

Collodions These are preparations that, when they are applied to damaged areas of the skin such as ulcers and minor wounds, dry to form

a protective film. Collodions are sometimes used to keep a dissolved drug in contact with the skin.

Barrier preparations These may be creams or ointments. They protect the skin against water and irritating substances. They may be used in the treatment of nappy rash or to protect the skin around an open sore. They may contain powders and water-repellent substances, such as silicones.

Lotions These thin, semi-liquid preparations are often used to cool and soothe inflamed skin. They are most suitable for use on large, hairy areas. Preparations known as shake lotions contain fine powder that remains on the surface of the skin when the liquid has evaporated. They encourage scabs to form.

Pastes These are ointments containing large amounts of finely powdered solids such as starch or zinc oxide. Pastes protect the skin and absorb unwanted moisture. They are used for skin conditions that affect clearly defined areas, such as psoriasis.

COMMON DRUGS

Antibiotics	Oxytetracycline
Bacitracin	Polymyxin B
Colistin	**Antiseptics and**
Framycetin	**other antibacterials**
Fusidic acid	Cetrimide
Gramicidin	Chlorhexidine
Metronidazole ✳	Povidone iodine
Mupirocin	Silver sulfadiazine
Neomycin	Triclosan

| ✳ See Part 3 |

DRUGS TO TREAT SKIN PARASITES

Mites and lice are the most common parasites that live on the skin. One common mite causes the skin disease scabies. The mite burrows into the skin and lays eggs, causing intense itching. Scratching the affected area results in bleeding and scab formation, as well as increasing the risk of infection.

There are three types of lice, each of which infests a different part of the human body: the head louse, the body (or clothes) louse, and the crab louse, which often infests the pubic areas but is also sometimes found on other hairy areas such as the eyebrows. All of these lice cause itching and lay eggs (nits) that look like white grains attached to hairs.

Both mites and lice are passed on by direct contact with an infected person (during sexual intercourse in the case of pubic lice) or, particularly in the case of body lice, by contact with infected bedding or clothing.

The drugs most often used to eliminate skin parasites are insecticides that kill both the adult insects and their eggs. The most effective drugs for scabies are malathion and permethrin; benzyl benzoate is occasionally used. Very severe scabies may require oral ivermectin as well. For lice infestations, malathion, permethrin, and phenothrin are used.

Why they are used

Skin parasites do not represent a serious threat to health, but they require prompt treatment since they can cause severe irritation and spread rapidly if untreated. Drugs are used to eradicate the parasites from the body, but bedding, clothing, and other items may need to be disinfected to avoid the possibility of reinfestation.

How they are used

Lotions for treating scabies are applied to the whole body, apart from the head and neck, after a bath or shower. Many people

SITES AFFECTED BY SKIN PARASITES

Scabies
The female scabies mite burrows into the skin and lays its eggs under the skin surface. After hatching, larvae travel to the skin surface, where they mature for 10–17 days before starting the cycle again.

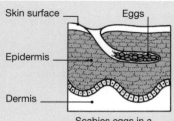

Scabies eggs in a burrow under the skin

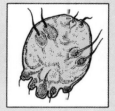

Scabies mite

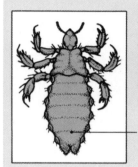

Head lice
These tiny brown insects are transmitted from person to person (commonly among children). Their bites often cause itching.

Head louse

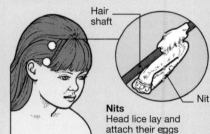

Hair shaft

Nit

Nits
Head lice lay and attach their eggs near the base of the hair shaft, especially around the ears.

find the lotions messy to use, but they should not be washed off for 8–12 hours (permethrin), 24 hours (malathion), or 48 hours (benzyl benzoate), otherwise they will not be effective. It is probably most convenient to apply permethrin or malathion before going to bed. The lotion may then be washed off the next morning.

Two treatments one week apart are normally sufficient to remove the scabies mites. However, the itch associated with scabies may persist after the mite has been removed, so it may be necessary to use a soothing cream or medication containing an antipruritic drug (see p.133) to ease this. People who have direct

skin-to-skin contact with someone who has scabies, such as family members and sexual partners, should also be treated with antiparasitic preparations at the same time. Head and pubic lice infestations are usually treated by applying a preparation of one of the products and washing it off with water when and as instructed by the leaflet given with the preparation. If the skin has become infected as a result of scratching, a topical antibiotic (see Anti-infective skin preparations, p.135) may also be prescribed.

Risks and special precautions

Lotions prescribed to control parasites can cause irritation and stinging that may be intense if the medication is allowed to come into contact with the eyes, mouth, or other moist membranes. Therefore, lotions and shampoos should be applied carefully, following the instructions of your doctor or the manufacturer.

Because they are applied topically, antiparasitic drugs do not usually have generalized effects. Nevertheless, it is important not to apply these preparations more often than directed.

ELIMINATING PARASITES FROM BEDDING AND CLOTHING

Most skin parasites may also infest bedding and clothing that has been next to an infected person's skin. Therefore, to avoid reinfestation following removal of the parasites from the body, any insects and eggs lodged in the bedding or clothing must be eradicated.
Washing
Since all skin parasites are killed by heat, washing affected items of clothing and bedding in hot water and drying them in a hot dryer is an effective and convenient method of dealing with the problem.
Non-washable items
Items that cannot be washed should be isolated in plastic bags. The insects and their eggs cannot survive long without their human hosts and die within days. The length of time

they can survive, and therefore the period of isolation, varies depending on the type of parasite (see the table below).

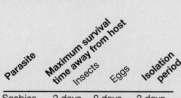

Parasite	Maximum survival time away from host — Insects	Maximum survival time away from host — Eggs	Isolation period
Scabies	2 days	0 days	2 days
Head lice	2 days	10 days	10 days
Crab lice	1 day	10 days	10 days
Body lice	10 days	30 days	30 days

COMMON DRUGS

Benzyl benzoate
Crotamiton
Dimeticone
Ivermectin

Malathion ✱
Permethrin ✱
Phenothrin

✱ See Part 3

DRUGS USED TO TREAT ACNE

Acne, known medically as acne vulgaris, is a common condition caused by excess production of the skin's natural oil (sebum), leading to blockage of hair follicles (see What happens in acne, right). It chiefly affects adolescents but it may occur at any age, due to taking certain drugs, exposure to industrial chemicals, oily cosmetics, or hot, humid conditions.

Acne primarily affects the face, neck, back, and chest. The primary skin signs are blackheads, papules (inflamed spots), and pustules (raised pus-filled spots with a white centre). Mild acne may produce only blackheads and an occasional papule or pustule. Moderate cases are characterized by larger numbers of pustules and papules. In severe cases of acne, painful, inflamed cysts also develop. These can cause permanent pitting and scarring.

Medication for acne can be divided into two groups: topical preparations applied directly to the skin and systemic treatments taken by mouth.

Why they are used

Mild acne usually does not need medical treatment; instead, it can be controlled simply by regular washing. Over-the-counter antibacterial soaps and lotions are limited in use and may cause irritation.

When a doctor or dermatologist thinks acne is severe enough to need medical treatment, he or she usually recommends a topical preparation containing benzoyl

CLEARING BLOCKED HAIR FOLLICLES

The most common treatment for acne is the application of keratolytic skin ointments. These encourage the layer of dead and hardened skin cells that form the skin surface to peel off. At the same time, this clears blackheads that block hair follicles and give rise to the formation of acne spots.

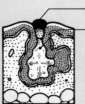

Blackhead

Trapped sebum

Blocked hair follicle
A hair follicle blocked by a plug of skin debris and sebum is ideal for acne spot formation.

Freed sebum

Cleared hair follicle
Once the follicle is unblocked, sebum can escape and air can enter, thereby limiting bacterial activity.

WHAT HAPPENS IN ACNE

In normal, healthy skin, sebum produced by a sebaceous gland attached to a hair follicle is able to flow out of the follicle along the hair. An acne spot forms when the flow of the sebum from the sebaceous gland is blocked by a plug of skin debris and hardened sebum, leading to an accumulation of sebum.

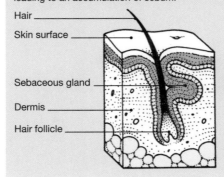

Hair

Skin surface

Sebaceous gland

Dermis

Hair follicle

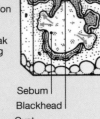

Acne papules and pustules
Bacterial activity leads to the formation of pustules and papules. Irritant substances may leak into the surrounding skin, causing inflammation.

Sebum

Blackhead

Cyst

Cystic acne
When acne is severe, cysts may form in the inflamed dermis. These are pockets of pus enclosed within scar tissue.

peroxide or salicylic acid. If this does not produce an improvement, preparations containing tretinoin, a drug related to vitamin A (see p.442); azelaic acid; or the antibiotics clindamycin, erythromycin, or tetracycline may be prescribed.

If the acne is severe or does not respond to topical treatments, a doctor may prescribe a course of antibiotics by mouth (usually a tetracycline). If these measures are unsuccessful, the more powerful vitamin A-like drug isotretinoin, taken by mouth, may be prescribed.

Oestrogen-containing drugs may have a beneficial effect on acne. A woman with acne who also needs contraception may be given an oestrogen-containing oral contraceptive (p.121). In severe cases, a preparation containing an oestrogen and cyproterone (a drug that opposes male sex hormones) may be prescribed.

How they work

Drugs used to treat acne act in different ways. Some have a keratolytic effect – that is, they loosen the dead cells on the skin surface (see Clearing blocked hair follicles, left). Other drugs work by countering bacterial activity in the skin or reducing sebum production.

Topical preparations, such as benzoyl peroxide, salicylic acid, and tretinoin, have a keratolytic effect. Benzoyl peroxide also has an antibacterial effect. Topical or systemic tetracyclines reduce bacteria but may also have a direct anti-inflammatory effect on the skin. Isotretinoin reduces sebum production, soothes inflammation, and helps to unblock hair follicles.

How they affect you

Keratolytic preparations often cause soreness of the skin, especially at the

start of treatment. If this persists, a change to a milder preparation may be recommended. Day-to-day side effects are rare with antibiotics.

Treatment with isotretinoin often causes dry and scaly skin, particularly on the lips. The skin may become itchy and some hair loss may occur.

Risks and special precautions

Antibiotics in skin ointments may, in rare cases, provoke an allergic reaction requiring discontinuation of treatment. The tetracyclines, which are some of the most commonly used antibiotics for acne, have the advantage of being effective both topically and systemically. However, they are not suitable for use by mouth in pregnancy since they can affect the bones and teeth of the developing baby.

Isotretinoin sometimes increases levels of lipids in the blood. More seriously, the drug is known to damage the developing baby if taken during pregnancy. Women taking this drug need to make sure that they avoid conception during treatment.

COMMON DRUGS

Topical treatments	Oral and topical antibiotics
Adapalene	Clindamycin ✳
Azelaic acid	Doxycycline ✳
Benzoyl peroxide ✳	Erythromycin ✳
Isotretinoin ✳	Tetracycline ✳
Nicotinamide	Trimethoprim ✳
(Niacin) ✳	**Other oral drugs**
Salicylic acid	Co-cyprindiol
Tretinoin	(women only)
	Isotretinoin ✳

✳ See Part 3

DRUGS FOR PSORIASIS

The skin is constantly being renewed; as fast as dead cells in the outermost layer (epidermis) are shed, they are replaced by cells from the base of the epidermis. Psoriasis occurs when the production of new cells increases while the shedding of old cells remains normal. As a result of increased cell production, the live skin cells accumulate and produce patches of inflamed, thickened skin covered by silvery scales. In some cases, the area of skin affected is extensive and causes severe embarrassment and physical discomfort. Psoriasis may occasionally be accompanied by arthritis, in which the joints become swollen and painful.

The underlying cause of psoriasis is not well understood. The disorder first occurs between the ages of 15 and 30, with a second peak between 50 and 60 years, and may recur through life. Flares of the disorder may be triggered by emotional stress, skin damage, drugs, and physical illness. Psoriasis can also recur as a result of the withdrawal of corticosteroid drugs.

There is no complete cure. Simple measures, such as avoiding trigger factors and regular use of an emollient cream (see Antipruritics, p.133) may relieve symptoms and improve the condition. However, often drug therapy is needed.

Why they are used

Drugs are used to decrease the size of affected skin areas and to reduce scaling and inflammation. Mild and moderate psoriasis are usually treated with a topical preparation. Coal tar preparations, which are available in the form of creams, pastes, or bath additives, are often helpful. Dithranol is also occasionally used. Once it has been applied to the affected areas, the preparation is left for a few minutes or overnight (depending on the product), before being washed off. Both dithranol and coal tar can stain clothing and bed linen.

If these agents alone do not produce adequate benefit, ultraviolet light therapy in the form of regulated exposure to natural sunlight or specialist phototherapy treatment with UVB light or PUVA (see box, above right) may be advised. Salicylic acid may be applied to help remove thick scale and crusts, especially from the scalp.

Topical corticosteroids (see p.134) may be used as a treatment for psoriasis. This is often in combination with other agents, such as vitamin D analogues like calcitriol or calcipotriol (see p.181).

If the psoriasis is severe and other treatments have not been effective, specialist treatment may involve the use of more potent drugs. These may include vitamin A derivatives (e.g. acitretin), methotrexate (see p.320), ciclosporin (see p.193), apremilast (a drug that modulates the inflammatory process in cells), or monoclonal antibodies (see p.114).

PUVA

PUVA is the combined use of a psoralen drug (e.g. methoxsalen) and ultraviolet A light (UVA). The drug is applied topically or taken by mouth some hours before exposure to UVA, which enhances the effect of the drug on skin cells.

This therapy is given two to three times a week and produces an improvement in skin condition within about four to six weeks.

Possible adverse effects include nausea, itching, and painful reddening of the normal areas of skin. More seriously, there is a risk of the skin ageing prematurely and a long-term risk of skin cancer, particularly in fair-skinned people. For these reasons, PUVA therapy is generally recommended only for severe psoriasis, when other treatments have failed.

In psoriasis
Skin cells form at the base of the epidermis faster than they can be shed from the skin surface. This causes the formation of patches of thickened, inflamed skin covered by a layer of flaking dead skin.

Normal skin   **Skin in psoriasis**

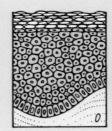
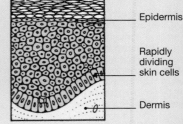

- Epidermis
- Rapidly dividing skin cells
- Dermis

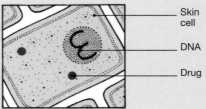
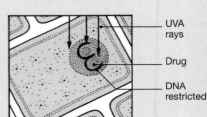

- Skin cell
- DNA
- Drug

- UVA rays
- Drug
- DNA restricted

Psoralen drugs
In PUVA, psoralen drugs administered by mouth or as ointment penetrate the skin cells.

Ultraviolet light
The drug is activated by exposure of the skin to ultraviolet light. It acts on the cell's genetic material (DNA) to regulate its rate of division.

How they work

Dithranol and methotrexate slow down the rapid rate of cell division that causes skin thickening. Acitretin and calcipotriol also reduce production of keratin, the hard protein that forms in the outer layer of skin. Salicylic acid and coal tar remove the layers of dead skin cells. Corticosteroids, ciclosporin, apremilast, and monoclonal antibodies reduce inflammation of underlying skin.

How they affect you

Appropriate treatment of psoriasis usually improves the appearance of the skin. However, since drugs cannot cure the underlying cause of the disorder, psoriasis tends to recur, even following successful treatment of a recurrence.

Individual drugs may cause side effects. Topical preparations can cause stinging and inflammation, especially if applied to normal skin. Coal tar increases the skin's sensitivity to sunlight; excessive sunbathing or overexposure to artificial ultraviolet light may damage skin and worsen the condition.

Acitretin, ciclosporin, and methotrexate can have several serious side effects, including gastrointestinal upsets, liver damage (acitretin and methotrexate), kidney damage (ciclosporin), and bone marrow damage (methotrexate). Acitretin, apremilast, and methotrexate are contraindicated in pregnancy, and women are advised not to become pregnant for three years after completing treatment with acitretin. Topical corticosteroids may cause rebound worsening of psoriasis when these drugs are stopped.

COMMON DRUGS

Acitretin
Adalimumab
Calcipotriol *
Calcitriol
Ciclosporin *
Coal tar
Dithranol *
Etanercept *

Hydroxycarbamide
Infliximab *
Methotrexate *
Methoxsalen
Salicylic acid
Secukinumab
Topical cortico- steroids (see p.134)
Ustekinumab

| * See Part 3 |

DRUGS AND OTHER TREATMENTS FOR ECZEMA

Eczema is a skin condition causing a dry, itchy rash that may be inflamed and blistered. There are several types, some of which are called dermatitis. Eczema can be triggered by allergy but often occurs for no known reason. In the long term, it can thicken (or lichenify) the skin as a result of persistent scratching.

The most common type, atopic eczema, may appear in infancy, but many children grow out of it. There is often a family history of eczema, asthma, or allergic rhinitis. Atopic eczema commonly appears on the hands, due to their exposure to detergents, and the feet, due to the warm, moist conditions of enclosed footwear.

Irritant contact dermatitis, another common form of eczema, is caused by chemicals, detergents, or soap. It may only appear after repeated exposure to the substance, but strong acids or alkalis can cause a reaction within minutes. It can also result from irritation of the skin by traces of detergent on clothes and bedding.

Allergic contact dermatitis can appear days or even years after initial contact with triggers such as nickel, hair dyes, rubber, elastic, or drugs (e.g. antibiotics, antihistamines, antiseptics, or local anaesthetics). Sunlight can also trigger the dermatitis following use of perfumes or some components of sunscreens.

Nummular (or discoid) eczema causes round, dry, scaly, itchy patches to appear anywhere on the body, with bacteria often found in the areas. The cause is unknown.

Seborrhoeic dermatitis mainly affects the scalp and face (see Dandruff and hair loss p.140). A yeast called *Malassezia* is thought to play a role in its development.

Why they are used

Emollients are used to soften and moisten the skin. Oral antihistamines (p.82) may be prescribed for a particularly itchy rash (topical antihistamines make the skin

PATCH TESTING

Low concentrations of the suspected substances are applied as spots to the skin of the back and held in place with nonabsorbent adhesive tape. This method allows a number of potential allergens (substances that can cause an allergic reaction) to be tested at the same time.

After 48 hours, the adhesive tape is removed and the skin inspected for any redness, swelling, or blistering that has developed. The skin is then assessed again after a further 48 hours. Reactions present at the second assessment usually indicate a true contact allergy.

Patches being applied

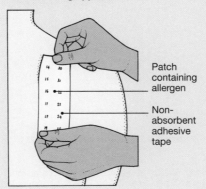

Patch containing allergen

Non-absorbent adhesive tape

Results of patch test

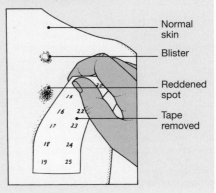

Normal skin

Blister

Reddened spot

Tape removed

more sensitive and should not be used). Coal tar or ichthammol may be used for chronic atopic eczema, but topical corticosteroids (p.134) may be needed to help control a flare. Rarely, severe treatment-resistant cases may need the immunosuppressant ciclosporin (p.196). A short course of oral corticosteroids may be used to treat severe contact dermatitis. Nummular eczema requires treatment with topical corticosteroids and a thick moisturizing ointment.

How they work

Emollients make the skin less dry and itchy. They are available as ointments, creams, lotions, soap substitutes, or bath oils. The effect is not long-lasting, so they need to be applied frequently. Emollients do not usually contain an active drug.

Antihistamines block the action of histamine (see p.81). Histamine dilates the blood vessels in the skin, causing redness and swelling of the surrounding tissue due to fluid leaking from the circulation. The drugs also prevent histamine from irritating the nerve fibres to cause itching.

Topical corticosteroids are absorbed into the tissues to relieve itching and inflammation. The least potent one that is effective is given. Hydrocortisone 1 per cent is often used in 1–2-week courses.

Oral or topical antibiotics destroy the bacteria sometimes present in broken, oozing, or blistered skin.

Ciclosporin blocks the action of white blood cells, which are involved in the immune response. The drug is given in short courses to gain control of severe eczema. Other oral medications for

chronic eczema include methotrexate and azathioprine. An injectable drug called dupilumab has been approved for severe treatment-resistant eczema.

Risks and special precautions

All types of eczema can become infected, and antibiotics may be needed. Herpes virus may infect atopic eczema, so direct contact with infected people, such as those with a cold sore, should be avoided. Ciclosporin and other oral drugs may produce some adverse effects.

Preventing eczema

Triggers identified by patch testing (see above) should be avoided. PVC gloves should be worn to protect the hands from detergents. Cotton clothing should be worn next to the skin. Moisturizers that contain perfumes and other sensitizers should be avoided.

COMMON SUBSTANCES THAT CAN CAUSE ECZEMA

Some substances produce an allergic reaction and some irritate the skin, causing eczema. The most common are listed below.

Allergens	Irritants
● Nickel, chromium	● Detergents
● Perfumes	● Soaps
● Plants	● Disinfectants
● Drugs	● Household cleaning products
● Rubber, elastic	● Paints
● Sticking plasters (especially zinc oxide ones)	● Glues and resins
● Cats and dogs	● Vegetable and fruit juices
● Tanning agents and dyes in leather and clothing	● Extremes of weather

COMMON DRUGS

Emollient and cooling preparations	Corticosteroids (see also p.134)
Aqueous cream	Betamethasone ✳
Cold cream	Hydrocortisone ✳
Emulsifying ointment	
Calamine lotion	**Other drugs**
	Azathioprine ✳
Antihistamines	Ciclosporin ✳
(see also p.82)	Coal tar
Cetirizine ✳	Ichthammol
Chlorphenamine ✳	Mycophenolate mofetil
Clemastine	Pimecrolimus
Fexofenadine	Tacrolimus ✳
	✳ See Part 3

DRUGS FOR DANDRUFF

Dandruff is an irritating, but harmless, condition that involves an acceleration in the normal shedding of skin cells from the scalp (see right).

Extensive dandruff is considered to be a mild form of a type of dermatitis known as seborrhoeic dermatitis, which is caused by an overgrowth of a yeast organism that lives in the scalp. In severe cases, a rash and reddish-yellow, scaly pimples appear along the hairline and on the face.

Why they are used

Frequent washing with a detergent shampoo usually keeps the scalp free of dandruff, but more persistent dandruff can be treated with a shampoo containing the antifungal drug ketoconazole (see p.291), medicated shampoos containing zinc pyrithione or selenium sulfide (see p.441), or shampoos containing coal tar or salicylic acid. Ointments containing coal tar and salicylic acid are also available. Corticosteroid lotions and gels may be needed to treat an itchy rash, especially in cases of severe seborrhoeic dermatitis.

How they work

Coal tar and salicylic acid preparations reduce the overproduction of new

WHAT HAPPENS IN DANDRUFF

All skin cells are replaced regularly as new cells grow from the epidermis. They gradually flatten as they die, and are shed on reaching the surface. Increased rate of production and

sticking together of the cells produces dandruff. In children, dandruff may produce thick scaly flakes that can be 1–2 cm across. In adults, smaller flakes are produced.

Normal shedding

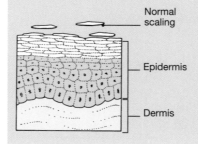

Dandruff

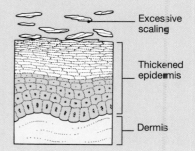

skin cells and break down flakes and scales, which can then be washed off while shampooing. Antifungal drugs (see p.96) reduce the overgrowth of yeast on the scalp by altering the permeability of the fungal cell walls. Corticosteroids (see p.99) help to relieve an itchy rash by reducing inflammation of the underlying skin.

COMMON DRUGS

Antifungals	Other drugs
Ketoconazole ✳	Arachis oil
Pyrithione zinc	Coal tar
	Corticosteroids
✳ See Part 3	Salicylic acid
	Selenium sulfide ✳

DRUGS FOR HAIR LOSS

Hair loss (alopecia) is the result of greater than normal shedding of hairs, or reduced hair production. Hair loss can be caused by a number of skin conditions, including autoimmune disorders such as lupus erythematosus and alopecia areata.

Other forms of hair loss are due to a disorder of the follicles themselves and may be a response to illness, malnutrition,

or a reaction to some drugs, such as anticancer drugs or anticoagulants. The hair loss may be diffuse or in a pattern, as in male-pattern baldness, which is caused by oversensitivity to testosterone.

Why they are used

If the hair loss is due to a skin disorder such as scalp ringworm, an antifungal

drug will be used as treatment. If male-pattern baldness is a response to the male hormone testosterone, finasteride may be used to reduce the hormone's effect. The antihypertensive drug minoxidil (see p.328) can also be applied to the scalp to promote hair growth.

How they work

Some forms of hair loss are reversible, but this depends on the underlying cause. Finasteride by mouth inhibits conversion of testosterone to its more active form and reduces sensitivity to androgens. The role of minoxidil in hair growth is not fully understood, but it is thought to stimulate the hair follicles (see left).

Risks and special precautions

Finasteride can lead to loss of libido or erectile dysfunction. For minoxidil, anyone with a history of heart disease or high blood pressure should consult their doctor before using the drug.

HAIR REGROWTH IN MALE-PATTERN BALDNESS

Follicles on the scalp have periods of activity and rest. During the rest phase, the bottom of the hair detaches from the follicle and the hair

falls out. Regular applications of minoxidil, the antihypertensive drug, stimulate follicles to produce new hair growth.

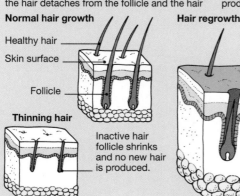

Normal hair growth

Healthy hair

Skin surface

Follicle

Thinning hair

Inactive hair follicle shrinks and no new hair is produced.

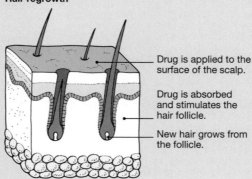

Hair regrowth

Drug is applied to the surface of the scalp.

Drug is absorbed and stimulates the hair follicle.

New hair grows from the follicle.

COMMON DRUGS

Antifungals	Other drugs
Griseofulvin	Finasteride ✳
Ketoconazole ✳	Minoxidil ✳
Terbinafine ✳	
	✳ See Part 3

SUNSCREENS

Sunscreens and sunblocks are chemicals, usually formulated as creams or oils, that protect the skin from the damaging effects of ultraviolet radiation from the sun.

People vary in their sensitivity to sunlight. Fair-skinned people generally have the least tolerance and tend to burn easily when exposed to the sun, while those with darker skin can withstand exposure to the sun for longer periods.

In a few cases, the skin's sensitivity to sunlight is increased by a disease such as pellagra (see p.438) or herpes simplex infection. Some drugs, such as thiazide diuretics, phenothiazine antipsychotics, psoralens, sulfonamide antibacterials, tetracycline antibiotics, and nalidixic acid, can also increase the skin's sensitivity.

Apart from sunburn and premature ageing of the skin, the most serious health risk from sunlight is skin cancer. Reducing the skin's exposure to sunlight (and avoiding the use of sunbeds) can help to prevent skin cancers.

How they work

Sunlight consists of different wavelengths of radiation. Of these, ultraviolet (UV) radiation is particularly harmful to the skin, causing ageing and burning. Excessive exposure also increases the risk of developing skin cancer. UV radiation is mainly composed of UVA and UVB rays, both of which age the skin. In addition, UVA rays cause tanning and UVB rays cause burning. People with fair skins and those taking immunosuppressant drugs are especially vulnerable to skin damage.

ACTION OF SUNSCREENS

Fair skin that is unprotected by a sunscreen becomes damaged as ultraviolet rays pass through to the layers beneath, causing pain and inflammation. Sunscreens act by blocking out some of these ultraviolet rays, while allowing a proportion of them to pass through the skin surface to the epidermis to stimulate the production of melanin – the pigment that gives the skin a tan and helps to protect it during further exposure to the sun.

Skin unprotected

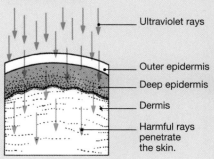

- Ultraviolet rays
- Outer epidermis
- Deep epidermis
- Dermis
- Harmful rays penetrate the skin.

Skin protected by sunscreen

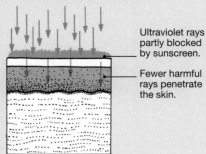

- Ultraviolet rays partly blocked by sunscreen.
- Fewer harmful rays penetrate the skin.

Sunscreens absorb some of the UVB radiation, ensuring that less of it reaches the skin. Sunscreens are graded using the Sun Protection Factor (SPF) (see below). Some preparations contain chemicals such as zinc oxide and titanium dioxide, which reflect both UVB and UVA rays; these preparations are often referred to as sunblocks.

A sunscreen is particularly advisable for visitors to tropical, subtropical, and mountainous areas, and for those who wish to sunbathe, because sunscreens can prevent burning while allowing the skin to tan. Sunscreens must be applied before exposure to the sun and reapplied every 2 hours. People with fair skin should use a sunscreen with a higher SPF than people with darker skin.

Risks and special precautions

Sunscreens only form a physical barrier to the passage of UV radiation. They do not alter the skin to make it more resistant to sunlight. Sunscreen lotions must therefore be applied thickly and frequently during exposure to the sun to maintain protection. People who have very fair skin or those who are known to be very sensitive to sunlight should never expose their skin to direct sunlight, even if they are using a sunscreen, since not even sunscreens with high SPF values give complete protection.

Sunscreens can irritate the skin, and some preparations may cause an allergic rash. People who are sensitive to some drugs, such as procaine and benzocaine, and to some hair dyes, might develop a rash after applying sunscreen containing aminobenzoic acid or a benzophenone derivative such as oxybenzone.

SUN PROTECTION FACTORS

Sun protection factor (SPF) is the degree of protection that a sunscreen gives against sunburn. It is a measure of the amount of UVB radiation that a sunscreen absorbs. The higher the number, the greater the protection. The table below shows the major skin types and the minimum SPF recommended for each.

This number only defines protection against UVB radiation. Some sunscreens protect against UVA radiation as well; these are often called sunblocks. The term "broad spectrum" is used to describe sunscreens that offer both UVA and UVB protection.

Some sunscreens use a "star" classification. The stars indicate a ratio of UVA to UVB protection. A rating of 4 stars means that the product gives balanced protection against both UVA and UVB. Sunscreens with a rating of 1, 2, or 3 stars give more protection against UVB than UVA.

Skin type	Type 1	Type 2	Type 3	Type 4	Type 5/6
Skin/hair tone	Pale skin, fair or red hair, freckles	Fair skin, fair or dark hair	Medium fair skin, brown hair	Olive skin, dark hair and eyes	Brown/ black skin, dark hair and eyes
Sun sensitivity	Always burns easily, never tans	Burns easily, tans eventually	Tans slowly, burns sometimes	Tans easily, burns occasionally	Very rarely burns
Minimum SPF	SPF 50	SPF 25 + SPF 50 for vulnerable areas	SPF 25	SPF 15 + SPF 25 for vulnerable areas	May not need; SPF 15 if at risk of burning

COMMON DRUGS

Ingredients in sunscreens and sunblocks	
Aminobenzoic acid	Methylbenzylidene camphor
Benzones	Octocrilene
Dibenzoylmethanes	Oxybenzone
Drometizole trisiloxane	Padimate-O
Ethylhexyl methoxy-cinnamate	Titanium dioxide
	Zinc oxide

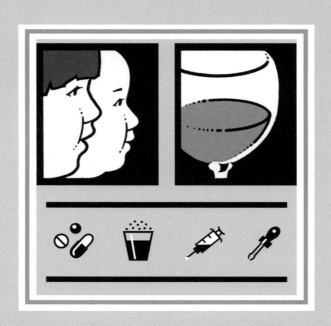

A–Z OF MEDICAL DRUGS

The drug profiles in this section give information and practical advice on 285 individual drugs. They are designed to provide reference and guidance for non-medical readers taking drug treatment. However, it is impossible for this kind of book to take into account every variation in individual circumstances; readers should always follow their doctor's or pharmacist's instructions in instances where these differ from the advice in this section.

The entries have been selected to provide representative coverage of the principal classes of drugs in medical use today. In the case of disorders for which a number of drugs are available, the most commonly used drugs have been selected. The emphasis is on drugs likely to be prescribed by a GP or bought over the counter, although in some cases drugs administered only in hospital have been included if the drug has been judged to be of sufficient general interest. At the end of this section there are supplementary profiles on vitamins and minerals (pp.433–445) and on selected drugs of abuse (pp.446–456), as well as information on complementary and alternative medicine (p.457), and medicines and travel (pp.458–459).

Each drug profile is organized in the same way, using standard headings (see sample page, below). To help you make the most of the information provided, the terms used and the instructions given under each heading are discussed and explained on the following pages.

HOW TO UNDERSTAND THE PROFILES

For ease of reference, the information on each drug is arranged in a consistent format under standard headings.

Drug name
Tells you the drug's generic name, brand names under which the drug is marketed, and any combined preparations that contain the drug.

General information
Gives you a brief summary of the drug's important characteristics.

Information for users
Practical information on how and when to take the drug, the usual recommended dosage, how soon it takes effect, how long it is active, and advice on diet, storage, missed doses, and stopping the drug.

Possible adverse effects
Indicates adverse effects that you may experience with the drug.

Interactions
Tells you how the drug may interact with other drugs or substances taken at the same time.

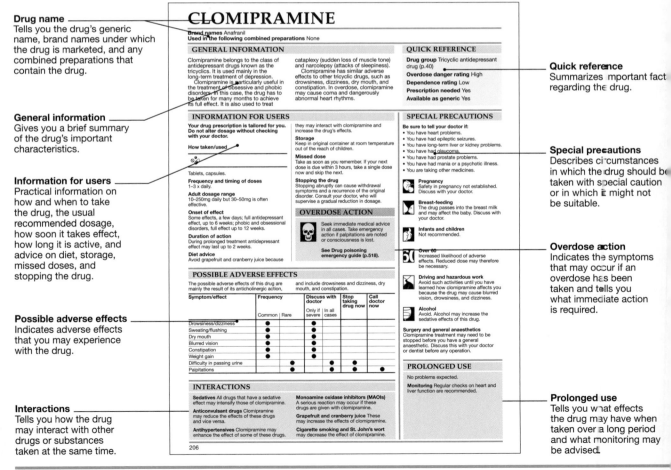

Quick reference
Summarizes important facts regarding the drug.

Special precautions
Describes circumstances in which the drug should be taken with special caution or in which it might not be suitable.

Overdose action
Indicates the symptoms that may occur if an overdose has been taken and tells you what immediate action is required.

Prolonged use
Tells you what effects the drug may have when taken over a long period and what monitoring may be advised.

DRUG NAME

Generic name

The main heading on the page is the drug's shortest generic name, unless the short name causes confusion with another drug, in which case the full generic name is given. For example, amiodarone hydrochloride (a drug for abnormal heart rhythms) is listed as amiodarone because there is no other generic drug of this name. However, magnesium hydroxide, an antacid, is listed under its full name to avoid confusing it with the mineral magnesium or other compounds, such as magnesium sulfate. If the drug has an alternative name, this appears in brackets.

Brand names

Under the generic name are the brand names of products in which the drug is the major single active ingredient. If there are many different brand names for the drug, only the most commonly used ones are given owing to limitations of space. The names of the principal preparations, if any, in which the drug is combined with other drugs, are also listed. For more information about brand names and generic names, see p.13.

ACICLOVIR

Brand names Action Cold Sore Cream, Boots
Used in the following combined preparation

GENERAL INFORMATION

GENERAL INFORMATION

The information here gives an overall picture of the drug. It may include notes on the drug's history (for example, when it was first introduced) and the principal disorders for which it is prescribed. This section also discusses the drug's major advantages and disadvantages.

Used in the following combined prepa

GENERAL INFORMATION

Dexamethasone is a long-acting, potent corticosteroid drug used to suppress inflammatory and allergic disorders, shock, and brain swelling (as a result of injury or tumour), and to relieve the lung

QUICK REFERENCE

The text in this box summarizes the important facts regarding your drug, and is organized under five headings, which are explained in detail below.

Drug group

This tells you which of the major groups the drug belongs to, and the page on which you can find out more about the drugs in that group and the various disorders or conditions they are used to treat. Where a drug belongs to more than one group, each group mentioned in the book is listed. For example, interferon is listed as an antiviral drug (p.91) and an anticancer drug (p.112).

Overdose danger rating

The information in this box gives an indication of the seriousness of the drug's effects if the dosage prescribed by your doctor, or that recommended on the label of an over-the-counter drug, is exceeded.

QUICK REFERENCE

Drug group Male sex hormone (p.104)

Overdose danger rating Low

Dependence rating Low

Prescription needed Yes

The ratings – low, medium, and high – are explained more fully on p.146.
- **Low** Symptoms unlikely. Death unknown.
- **Medium** Medical advice needed. Death rare.
- **High** Medical attention needed urgently. Potentially fatal.

If you do exceed the dose, advice is given in an "Overdose action" panel, as well as in "Exceeding the dose" (p.30).

Dependence rating

Drugs are rated low, medium, or high on the basis of the risk of dependence (p.23).
- **Low** Dependence unknown.
- **Medium** Rare risk of dependence.
- **High** Dependence likely with long-term use.

Prescription needed

This tells you whether or not you need a prescription to obtain the drug. Some drugs are available over the counter in lower-strength preparations or restricted amounts but require a prescription for higher doses or larger amounts. Certain other prescription drugs are subject to government regulations (see How drugs are classified, p.13).

Available as generic

Tells you if the drug is available as a generic product.

INFORMATION FOR USERS (for common forms of each medication)

This section contains information on the following: administration, i.e. the forms in which the drug is available; dosage frequency and amount; effects and actions; and advice on diet, storage, missed doses, stopping drug treatment, and overdose. All the information is generalized and should not be taken as a recommendation for an individual dosing schedule. Always follow your doctor's instructions carefully when taking prescription drugs, and instructions from the manufacturer or pharmacist when you buy over-the-counter medications.

How used/taken

The symbols in the box show how drugs can be administered. They are a visual back-up to the written information below the box.

Tablets/capsules; slow-release (SR)/ modified release (MR) tablets/capsules

Oral liquid (as syrup, drops, suspension, or solution)

Depot, implant, or pen injection; infusion

Inhaler (powder/ capsules/spray); nebulizer (nebules/liquid)

Eye, ear, or nose drops

Transdermal patch

Lozenges; pastilles; chewing gum; chewable tablets; orosoluble tablets (wafers, melts, or buccal/ sublingual tablets)

Soluble/ dispersible tablets; granules; powder

Suppository; pessary; foam; enema; bladder irrigation

Cream; ointment; topical liquid, lotion, gel, solution, or powder; shampoo; scalp application

A–Z OF MEDICAL DRUGS continued

INFORMATION FOR USERS continued

Frequency and timing of doses

This refers to the standard number of times each day that the drug should be taken and, where relevant, whether it should be taken with liquid, with meals, or on an empty stomach.

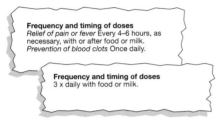

Frequency and timing of doses
Relief of pain or fever Every 4–6 hours, as necessary, with or after food or milk.
Prevention of blood clots Once daily.

Frequency and timing of doses
3 x daily with food or milk.

Dosage range

This is generally given as the normal dosage range for an adult. In cases where the dosages for specific age groups vary significantly from the normal adult dosage, these will also be given. Where dosage varies according to use, the dosage for each is included.

The vast majority of drug dosages are expressed in metric units, usually milligrams (mg) or micrograms (mcg). In a few, dosage is given in units (u) or international units (IU). See also Weights and measures, facing page.

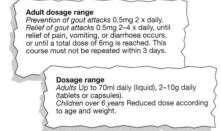

Adult dosage range
Prevention of gout attacks 0.5mg 2 x daily.
Relief of gout attacks 0.5mg 2–4 x daily, until relief of pain, vomiting, or diarrhoea occurs, or until a total dose of 6mg is reached. This course must not be repeated within 3 days.

Dosage range
Adults Up to 70ml daily (liquid), 2–10g daily (tablets or capsules).
Children over 6 years Reduced dose according to age and weight.

Onset of effect

The onset of effect is the time it takes for the drug to become active in the body. This sometimes coincides with the onset of beneficial effects, but there may sometimes be an interval between the time when a drug is pharmacologically active and when you start to notice improvement in your symptoms or your underlying condition.

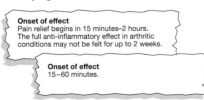

Onset of effect
Pain relief begins in 15 minutes–2 hours. The full anti-inflammatory effect in arthritic conditions may not be felt for up to 2 weeks.

Onset of effect
15–60 minutes.

Duration of action

The information given here refers to the length of time that one dose of the drug remains active in the body.

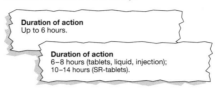

Duration of action
Up to 6 hours.

Duration of action
6–8 hours (tablets, liquid, injection); 10–14 hours (SR-tablets).

Diet advice

With some drugs, it is important to avoid certain foods, either because they reduce the effect of the drug or because they interact adversely with that drug. This section of the profile tells you what, if any, dietary changes are necessary.

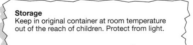

Diet advice
Avoid foods that are high in potassium – for example, dried fruit, bananas, tomatoes, and "low salt" salt substitutes.

Storage

Drugs will deteriorate and may become inactive if they are not stored under suitable conditions. The advice usually given is to store in a cool, dry place out of the reach of children. Some drugs must also be protected from light. Others, especially liquid medications, need to be kept in a refrigerator, but should not be frozen. For further advice on storing drugs, see p.29.

Storage
Keep in original container at room temperature out of the reach of children. Protect from light.

Missed dose

This section gives advice on what to do if you forget a dose of your drug, so that the effectiveness and safety of your treatment is maintained as far as possible. If you forget to take several doses in succession, consult your doctor. You can read more about missed doses on p.28.

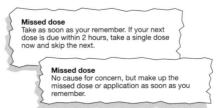

Missed dose
Take as soon as your remember. If your next dose is due within 2 hours, take a single dose now and skip the next.

Missed dose
No cause for concern, but make up the missed dose or application as soon as you remember.

Stopping the drug

If you are taking a drug regularly, you need to know how and when you can safely stop taking it. Some drugs can be safely stopped as soon as you feel better, or as soon as your symptoms have disappeared. Others must not be stopped until the full course of treatment has been completed, or they must be gradually withdrawn under the supervision of a doctor. Failure to comply with instructions for stopping a drug may lead to adverse effects. It may also cause your condition to worsen or your symptoms to reappear. See also Ending drug treatment, p.28.

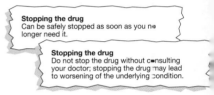

Stopping the drug
Can be safely stopped as soon as you no longer need it.

Stopping the drug
Do not stop the drug without consulting your doctor; stopping the drug may lead to worsening of the underlying condition.

Exceeding the dose

The information in this section expands on that in the quick reference box on the drug's overdose danger rating. It explains possible consequences of exceeding the dose and what to do if an overdose is taken. Examples of wording used for low, medium, and high overdose ratings are:

Low
An occasional extra dose is unlikely to be a cause for concern. But if you notice any unusual symptoms, or if a large overdose has been taken, notify your doctor.

Medium
An occasional extra dose is unlikely to cause problems. Large overdoses may cause [symptoms listed]. Notify your doctor.

High
Seek immediate medical advice in all cases. Take emergency action if [relevant symptoms listed] occur.

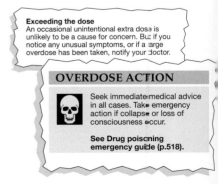

Exceeding the dose
An occasional unintentional extra dose is unlikely to be a cause for concern. But if you notice any unusual symptoms, or if a large overdose has been taken, notify your doctor.

OVERDOSE ACTION
Seek immediate medical advice in all cases. Take emergency action if collapse or loss of consciousness occur.

See Drug poisoning emergency guide (p.518).

SPECIAL PRECAUTIONS

Many drugs need to be used with care by people who have a history of particular conditions The profile lists conditions that you should tell your doctor about when you are prescribed a drug, or about which you should consult your doctor or pharmacist before taking an over-the-counter drug. Certain groups (pregnant women, breast-feeding mothers, children, and people over age 60) may also be at special risk from drug treatment. Advice for each of these groups is given in every profile. Information is also included about driving, undertaking hazardous work, and drinking alcohol.

SPECIAL PRECAUTIONS

Be sure to tell your doctor if:
- You have long-term liver or kidney problems.
- You have a history of gallbladder disease.
- You are taking other medicines.

 Pregnancy
Safety in pregnancy not established. Discuss with your doctor.

 Breast-feeding
The drug may pass into the breast milk and affect the baby. Discuss with your doctor.

 Infants and children
Not recommended.

 Over 60
No special problems.

 Driving and hazardous work
Avoid such activities until you have learned how the drug affects you because rarely it may cause drowsiness.

 Alcohol
Avoid. Alcohol may further reduce blood pressure, causing dizziness or other symptoms.

POSSIBLE ADVERSE EFFECTS

The adverse effects discussed in the drug profile are symptoms or reactions that may arise when you take the drug. The emphasis is on symptoms that you, the patient, are likely to notice, rather than on the findings of laboratory tests that your doctor may order. The bulk of the section is in the form of a table that lists the adverse effects and indicates how commonly they occur, when to tell your doctor about them, and when to stop the drug. The headings in the table are explained below.

Frequency

This column shows you whether the adverse effect is common or rare. Common effects are listed first.

Discuss with doctor

The marker in this section indicates any circumstances in which you need to inform your doctor about an adverse effect you are experiencing.

Only if severe A marker in this column means that the symptom is unlikely to be serious, but that you should seek your doctor's advice if it troubles you.
In all cases Adverse effects that have a marker in this column require prompt, but not necessarily emergency, medical attention. (See also Call doctor now, below.)

Stop taking drug now

In cases where certain unpleasant or dangerous adverse effects of a drug may override its beneficial effects, you are advised to stop taking the drug immediately, if necessary before seeing your doctor.

Call doctor now

Effects marked in this column require immediate medical help. They indicate a potentially dangerous response to the drug treatment, for which you should seek emergency medical attention.

Symptom/effect	Frequency		Discuss with doctor		Stop taking drug now	Call doctor now
	Common	Rare	Only if severe	In all cases		
Nausea	●			●		
Diarrhoea/abdominal pain	●			●		
Hearing disorders/dizziness		●		●		
Hair loss/depigmentation		●		●		
Blurred vision/rash		●		●	●	●

INTERACTIONS

The interactions that are discussed here are those that may occur between the drug under discussion and other drugs. Information includes the name of the interacting drug or group of drugs and the effect of the interaction.

INTERACTIONS

Antidiabetic drugs Dexamethasone reduces the action of these drugs. Dosage may need to be adjusted accordingly to prevent abnormally high blood sugar

PROLONGED USE

The information given here concerns the adverse, and sometimes beneficial, effects of the drug that may occur during long-term use. These may differ from those listed under Possible adverse effects. This section of the profile also includes information on monitoring the effects of the drug during long-term treatment, explaining the tests that you may be given if your doctor thinks they are necessary.

PROLONGED USE

Apart from an increased risk of gout in the first weeks or months, no problems are expected.

Monitoring Periodic checks on uric acid levels in the blood are usually performed, and the dose of allopurinol adjusted if necessary.

WEIGHTS AND MEASURES

Equivalents of metric measurements used in this book:

1,000mcg (microgram) = 1mg (milligram)
1,000mg = 1g (gram)
1,000ml (millilitre) = 1l (litre)

Units or international units
Units (u) and international units (IU) are also used to express drug dosages. They represent the biological activity of a drug (its effect on the body). This ability cannot be measured in terms of weight or volume, but must be calculated in a laboratory.

ACICLOVIR

Brand names Action Cold Sore Cream, Boots Avert, Cymex Ultra, Lypsyl Aciclovir 5%, Virasorb, Zovirax
Used in the following combined preparations None

GENERAL INFORMATION

Aciclovir is an antiviral drug used in the treatment of herpes infections, which can cause cold sores and genital herpes. It is available as tablets, a liquid, a cream, eye ointment, and injection. The cream is commonly used to treat cold sores, and can speed up the healing of these lesions, provided it is started as soon as symptoms occur and as the lesions appear. The tablets and injection are used to treat severe herpes infections, shingles, chickenpox, and genital herpes. The tablets can also be used to prevent the development of herpes infection in people who have reduced immunity. Herpes infection affecting the eye can be treated with an eye ointment.

QUICK REFERENCE

Drug group Antiviral drug (p.91)
Overdose danger rating Low
Dependence rating Low
Prescription needed No (cold sore cream); Yes (other preparations)
Available as generic Yes

INFORMATION FOR USERS

Follow instructions on the label. Call your doctor if symptoms worsen.

How taken/used

Tablets, liquid, injection, cream, eye ointment.

Frequency and timing of doses
2–5 x daily. Start as soon as possible.

Adult dosage range
Tablets, liquid 1–4g daily (treatment); 800mg–1.6g daily (prevention).
Injection 5–10mg per kg body weight 3 x daily.
Cream, eye ointment 5 x daily.

Onset of effect
Within 24 hours.

Duration of action
Up to 8 hours.

Diet advice
It is necessary to drink plenty of water when taking high doses by mouth or injection.

Storage
Keep in original container at room temperature out of the reach of children. Protect from light.

Missed dose
Tablets/liquid Take as soon as you remember.
Cream, eye ointment Do not apply the missed dose. Apply your next dose as usual.

Stopping the drug
Complete the full course as directed.

Exceeding the dose
An occasional unintentional extra dose is unlikely to be a cause for concern. But if you notice any unusual symptoms, or if a large overdose has been taken, notify your doctor.

SPECIAL PRECAUTIONS

Be sure to consult your doctor or pharmacist before taking this drug if:
- You have a long-term kidney problem.
- You have reduced immunity.
- You are taking other medicines.

 Pregnancy
Topical preparations carry negligible risk. Oral and injectable forms may be prescribed if the benefits outweigh the risks. Discuss with your doctor.

 Breast-feeding
No evidence of risk with topical forms but avoid using on the breast area. The drug passes into the breast milk following injection or oral administration. Discuss with your doctor.

 Infants and children
Reduced dose necessary in young children.

 Over 60
Reduced dose may be necessary.

 Driving and hazardous work
No known problems with topical forms. High doses of oral and injectable forms may cause drowsiness; if so, avoid driving and hazardous activities.

 Alcohol
No known problems.

POSSIBLE ADVERSE EFFECTS

Serious adverse effects are rare. The cream commonly causes discomfort at the site of application. Confusion and hallucinations occur rarely with injections.

Symptom/effect	Frequency		Discuss with doctor		Stop taking drug now	Call doctor now
	Common	Rare	Only if severe	In all cases		
Topical applications						
Burning/stinging/itching	●		●			
Rash		●		●	●	
By mouth						
Nausea/vomiting		●	●			
Dizziness		●		●		
Rash		●		●	●	
Confusion/hallucinations		●		●	●	●
Injection						
Inflammation at injection site		●		●	●	●
Confusion/hallucinations		●		●	●	●

PROLONGED USE

Aciclovir is usually given as single courses of treatment and is not given long term, except for people with reduced immunity.

INTERACTIONS (by mouth or injection only)

General note Any drug that affects the kidneys increases the risk of side effects with aciclovir.

Probenecid and cimetidine These drugs may increase the level of aciclovir in the blood.

Mycophenolate mofetil Aciclovir may increase the levels of this drug in the blood and vice versa.

Ciclosporin Aciclovir may increase the levels of this drug in the blood and increase the risk of kidney problems.

ALENDRONIC ACID

Brand names Binosto, Fosamax, Fosamax Once Weekly
Used in the following combined preparation Fosavance

GENERAL INFORMATION

Alendronic acid is prescribed to treat osteoporosis. It is also used to treat or prevent corticosteroid-induced osteoporosis and to prevent post-menopausal osteoporosis in women at risk of developing the disease. A calcium supplement and vitamin D may also be prescribed if dietary intake is inadequate, but calcium should not be taken at the same time as alendronic acid because calcium reduces its absorption. Combined use of alendronic acid with HRT in post-menopausal women is more effective than either treatment alone. Alendronic acid tablets should be taken first thing in the morning, swallowed whole with a full glass of tap water (not even mineral water is acceptable because of the minerals' possible effect on absorption). After taking the tablet(s), remain upright for at least 30 minutes to prevent the drug from sticking in the oesophagus, where it could cause ulcers or irritation. Those with poor dental health should have a dental check-up before starting alendronic acid.

QUICK REFERENCE

Drug group Drug for bone disorders (p.80)

Overdose danger rating Medium

Dependence rating Low

Prescription needed Yes

Available as generic Yes

INFORMATION FOR USERS

Your drug prescription is tailored for you. Do not alter dosage without checking with your doctor.

How taken/used

Tablets.

Frequency and timing of doses
Once daily, first thing in the morning. Once weekly, first thing in the morning (post-menopausal women). Take with water.

Adult dosage range
Treatment: 10mg daily (for all indications) or 70mg taken once weekly.

Onset of effect
It may take some months before you notice any improvement.

Duration of action
Some effects may persist for months or years.

Diet advice
Do not eat or take other medicines for at least 30 minutes after doses.

Storage
Keep in original container at room temperature out of the reach of children.

Missed dose
Take the next dose at the usual time next morning.

Stopping the drug
Do not stop the drug without consulting your doctor. Stopping the drug may lead to worsening of the underlying condition.

Exceeding the dose
An occasional unintentional extra dose is unlikely to cause problems. However, large overdoses may cause stomach problems including heartburn, irritation, and ulcers. If you have taken a large overdose, notify your doctor at once, and try to remain upright.

SPECIAL PRECAUTIONS

Be sure to tell your doctor if:
- You have pain or difficulty in swallowing, or problems with your oesophagus.
- You have significant dental health problems.
- You have a history of peptic ulcers or stomach problems.
- You have long-term kidney problems.
- You have low calcium levels in your blood.
- You may be, or plan to become, pregnant.
- You are unable to sit or stand upright for at least 30 minutes.
- You are taking other medicines.

 Pregnancy
Not recommended.

 Breast-feeding
Not recommended.

 Infants and children
Not recommended.

 Over 60
No special problems.

 Driving and hazardous work
No special problems.

 Alcohol
Avoid. May cause further stomach irritation.

POSSIBLE ADVERSE EFFECTS

The most frequent adverse effect caused by alendronic acid is abdominal pain or indigestion as a result of irritation to the oesophagus, stomach, or small intestine.

Symptom/effect	Frequency		Discuss with doctor		Stop taking drug now	Call doctor now
	Common	Rare	Only if severe	In all cases		
Abdominal pain/distension	●		●			
Diarrhoea/constipation	●		●			
Muscle/bone/joint pain	●		●			
Headache	●		●			
Nausea/vomiting		●	●			
Rash/photosensitivity		●		●		
Eye inflammation		●		●		
Jaw pain/ear pain		●		●		
Pain on/difficulty in swallowing	●			●	●	
New or worsening heartburn	●			●	●	

INTERACTIONS

Antacids and products containing calcium or iron These reduce the absorption of alendronic acid and should be taken at a different time of day.

PROLONGED USE

Alendronic acid is usually prescribed long-term, but the need for continued treatment should be reassessed periodically (especially after five years) to ensure that the benefits continue to outweigh the risks in each individual case. Inappropriate prolonged use may lead to complications such as atypical bone fractures.

Monitoring Blood and urine tests may be carried out at intervals.

ALGINATES

Brand names [dressings] Algisite M, Kaltostat, Kendall, Melgisorb, Sorbalgon, Sorbsan; [oral] Gaviscon Infant
Used in the following combined preparations Acidex, Gastrocote, Gaviscon, Peptac liquid aniseed, Rennie heartburn relief

GENERAL INFORMATION

"Alginates" is a group term that refers to a mixture of compounds extracted from brown algae (seaweeds). When the powder extract is mixed with water, alginates become a thick, viscous fluid or gel depending on the chemicals used. Alginates combined with antacids form a "raft" that floats on the surface of the stomach contents, which reduces reflux and protects the lining of the oesophagus from attack by acid

regurgitated from the stomach. Many of these combined antacid preparations of alginates are used to treat mild gastro-oesophageal reflux disease. A number of indigestion remedies on sale to the public also contain alginates.

The properties of alginates are also used in wound dressings where, in the form of a woven pad, they absorb fluids from the surface of the wound, keeping it moist and allowing it to heal.

INFORMATION FOR USERS

Follow instructions on the label. Inform your doctor if you have no relief after 7 days of intake or if symptoms worsen.

How taken/used

Chewable tablets, liquid, powder.

Frequency and timing of doses
4 x daily after meals and at bedtime (as oral solution).

Adult dosage range
800–2,000mg daily.

Onset of effect
10–20 minutes.

Duration of action
3–4 hours.

Diet advice
None.

Storage
Keep in original container at room temperature out of the reach of children.

Missed dose
Take as soon as you remember, if you need it.

Stopping the drug
Alginates can be safely stopped as soon as you no longer need them.

Exceeding the dose
Overdose of alginates is likely to produce abdominal distension, without any other symptoms. Notify your doctor if symptoms are severe.

SPECIAL PRECAUTIONS

Be sure to tell your doctor if:
• You are on a salt-restricted diet.
• You are taking other medicines.
• You have renal failure.

Pregnancy
No evidence of risk to baby. Some products can be used in pregnancy.

Breast-feeding
No evidence of risk.

Infants and children
Reduced dose necessary.

Over 60
No special problems.

Driving and hazardous work
No known problems.

Alcohol
No known problems.

POSSIBLE ADVERSE EFFECTS

The antacid salts used in combined oral preparations of alginates may cause abdominal discomfort and distension.

Symptom/effect	Frequency		Discuss with doctor		Stop taking drug now	Call doctor now
	Common	Rare	Only if severe	In all cases		
Stomach distension	●		●			
Nausea		●	●			

INTERACTIONS

Other medications A time interval of 2 hours should be considered between taking alginate antacid medication and taking any other medicinal products, especially tetracyclines, digoxin, fluoroquinolone, iron salt, ketoconazole, antipsychotic drugs, thyroid hormones, penicillamine, beta-blockers (atenolol, metoprolol, propanolol), glucocorticoid, chloroquine, and bisphosphonates.

Sodium bicarbonate Due to effects at the renal level, sodium bicarbonate may reduce plasma lithium levels and increase plasma quinidine levels.

PROLONGED USE

This medicine should not be taken as an antacid for more than 2 weeks. If symptoms persist after this time, discuss them with your doctor, to rule out more serious possible problems such as cancer of the oesophagus or stomach.

ALLOPURINOL

Brand names Caplenal, Cosuric, Rimapurinol, Zyloric
Used in the following combined preparations None

GENERAL INFORMATION

Allopurinol is used to prevent gout, which is caused by deposits of uric acid crystals in joints. Allopurinol blocks an enzyme called xanthine oxidase that is involved in forming uric acid. It is also used to lower high uric acid levels (hyperuricaemia) caused by other drugs and sometimes for preventing uric acid kidney stones. Allopurinol should never be started until several weeks after an acute attack has subsided because it may cause a further episode. Treatment should continue indefinitely to prevent further attacks. At the start of treatment, an acute attack may occur and colchicine or an anti-inflammatory drug may also be given until uric acid levels fall. If an acute attack occurs while on allopurinol, treatment should continue along with an anti-inflammatory drug.

QUICK REFERENCE

Drug group Drug for gout (p.77)
Overdose danger rating Medium
Dependence rating Low
Prescription needed Yes
Available as generic Yes

INFORMATION FOR USERS

Your drug prescription is tailored for you. Do not alter dosage without checking with your doctor.

How taken/used

Tablets.

Frequency and timing of doses
1–3 x daily after food.

Adult dosage range
100–900mg daily.

Onset of effect
Within 24–48 hours. Full effect may not be felt for several weeks.

Duration of action
Up to 30 hours. Some effect may last for 1–2 weeks after the drug has been stopped.

Diet advice
A high fluid intake (2 litres of fluid daily) is recommended.

Storage
Keep in original container at room temperature out of the reach of children.

Missed dose
If your next dose is not due for another 12 hours or more, take a dose as soon as you remember and take the next one as usual. Otherwise skip the missed dose and take your next dose on schedule.

Stopping the drug
Do not stop the drug without consulting your doctor; symptoms may recur.

Exceeding the dose
An occasional unintentional extra dose is unlikely to cause problems. Large overdoses may cause nausea, vomiting, abdominal pain, diarrhoea, and dizziness. Notify your doctor.

POSSIBLE ADVERSE EFFECTS

Adverse effects of allopurinol are not very common. The most serious is an allergic rash that may require the drug to be stopped and an alternative treatment substituted. Nausea can be avoided by taking allopurinol after food.

Symptom/effect	Frequency		Discuss with doctor		Stop taking drug now	Call doctor now
	Common	Rare	Only if severe	In all cases		
Nausea	●		●			
Rash/itching	●			●	●	
Drowsiness/dizziness		●	●			
Headache		●	●			
Taste/visual disturbances		●		●		
Sore throat		●		●	●	
Fever and chills		●		●	●	

INTERACTIONS

ACE inhibitors Allopurinol may increase the risk of toxicity from these drugs.

Anticoagulant drugs Allopurinol may increase the effects of these drugs.

Ciclosporin Allopurinol may increase the effects of this drug.

Didanosine Allopurinol increases levels of this drug.

Mercaptopurine and azathioprine Allopurinol blocks the breakdown of these drugs, requiring a reduction in their dosage.

Theophylline Allopurinol may increase levels of this drug.

SPECIAL PRECAUTIONS

Be sure to tell your doctor if:
- You have long-term liver or kidney problems.
- You have had a previous sensitivity reaction to allopurinol.
- You have a current attack of gout.
- You are taking other medicines.

 Pregnancy
Safety in pregnancy not established. Discuss with your doctor.

 Breast-feeding
The drug passes into the breast milk but is not known to be harmful to the baby. Discuss with your doctor.

 Infants and children
Reduced dose necessary.

 Over 60
Reduced dose may be necessary.

 Driving and hazardous work
Avoid such activities until you have learned how allopurinol affects you because the drug can cause drowsiness.

 Alcohol
Avoid. Alcohol may worsen gout.

PROLONGED USE

Apart from an increased risk of gout in the first weeks or months, no problems are expected.

Monitoring Periodic checks on uric acid levels in the blood are usually performed, and the dose of allopurinol adjusted if necessary.

ALTEPLASE

Brand name Actilyse
Used in the following combined preparations None

GENERAL INFORMATION

Alteplase belongs to a group of drugs called thrombolytics, which act by dissolving blood clots that have formed in blood vessels. Synthesized by genetically modified bacteria, alteplase works by dissolving the fibrin (see p.62) in blood clots. It is used to treat a number of conditions caused by clots in blood vessels, including heart attacks due to clots in the arteries of the heart, pulmonary embolism due to clots in the lungs' blood vessels, and acute stroke from a clot in an artery of the brain.

Alteplase is administered via a catheter inserted into an artery or vein and works rapidly. It is given within a few hours of a heart attack or stroke to reduce damage to the heart or brain. As with other thrombolytics, alteplase is associated with a risk of bleeding, which may occasionally be life-threatening, so treatment is closely supervised.

INFORMATION FOR USERS

This drug is given only under medical supervision and is not for self-administration.

How taken/used

Injection, infusion.

Frequency and timing of doses
Usually given as a single intravenous injection followed by a continuous intravenous infusion over several hours.

Adult dosage range
Dosage is determined individually based on the condition being treated and the patient's body weight.

Onset of effect
30 minutes.

Duration of action
60 minutes.

Diet advice
None.

Storage
Not applicable. The drug is not normally kept at home.

Missed dose
Not applicable. The drug is given only in hospital under close supervision.

Stopping the drug
The drug is usually given over several hours and then stopped.

Exceeding the dose
Overdose is unlikely as treatment is closely monitored by medical staff.

SPECIAL PRECAUTIONS

Alteplase is only prescribed under close medical supervision, usually in life-threatening circumstances. Your doctor will usually go through a checklist of questions before administering the drug to assess your risk of bleeding.

Pregnancy
Safety not established. Alteplase carries a risk of bleeding for the mother and baby and may damage the placenta. Discuss with your doctor.

Breast-feeding
Safety not established. Breast milk should not be used for 24 hours after treatment with alteplase. Discuss with your doctor.

Infants and children
Not recommended.

Over 60
Increased risk of bleeding. Close observation required.

Driving and hazardous work
Not applicable.

Alcohol
Not applicable.

PROLONGED USE

Alteplase is never used long term.

POSSIBLE ADVERSE EFFECTS

Alteplase is given under strict supervision, and adverse effects are closely monitored. The main adverse effect is bleeding, which is common where the catheter is inserted but may occur anywhere in the body.

Symptom/effect	Frequency		Discuss with doctor		Stop taking drug now	Call doctor now
	Common	Rare	Only if severe	In all cases		
Bleeding/bruising	●			●		
Nausea/vomiting	●			●		
Collapse		●		●	●	●
Rash		●		●	●	●
Wheezing		●		●	●	●
Swelling of lips/face		●		●	●	●

INTERACTIONS

Anticoagulant drugs (e.g. warfarin, heparin) There is an increased risk of bleeding when these are taken before, during, or soon after alteplase is used.

Antiplatelet drugs (e.g. aspirin, clopidogrel) There is an increased risk of bleeding when these are taken before, during, or soon after alteplase is used.

ALUMINIUM HYDROXIDE

Brand name Alu-Cap, Alu-Tab, Amphojel, Dialume
Used in the following combined preparations Algicon, Aludrox, Asilone, Co-magaldrox, Maalox, Mucogel, Topal, and others

GENERAL INFORMATION

Aluminium hydroxide is a common ingredient of many over-the-counter remedies for indigestion and heartburn. Because the drug is constipating (it is sometimes used to treat diarrhoea), it is usually combined with a magnesium-containing antacid with a balancing laxative effect. The combination is sometimes referred to by the generic name of co-magaldrox.

The prolonged action of the drug makes it useful in preventing the pain of stomach and duodenal ulcers or heartburn. Aluminium hydroxide can also promote the healing of ulcers.

The drug may be more effective as an antacid in liquid form rather than as tablets. Some antacid preparations include large amounts of sodium, and these should be used with caution by those on low-sodium diets.

In the intestine, aluminium hydroxide binds with, and thereby reduces the absorption of, phosphate. This makes it helpful in treating high blood phosphate (hyperphosphataemia), which occurs in some people with impaired kidney function. However, prolonged heavy use can lead to phosphate deficiency and a consequent weakening of the bones.

QUICK REFERENCE

Drug group Antacid (p.66)
Overdose danger rating Low
Dependence rating Low
Prescription needed No
Available as generic Yes

INFORMATION FOR USERS

Follow instructions on the label. Call your doctor if symptoms worsen.

How taken/used

Capsules, chewable tablets, liquid (suspension). The tablets should be well chewed.

Frequency and timing of doses
As antacid 4 x daily as needed, or 1 hour before and after meals.
Peptic ulcer 4 x daily.
Hyperphosphataemia 3–4 x daily with meals.

Dosage range
Adults Up to 70ml daily (liquid), 2–10g daily (tablets or capsules).
Children over 6 years Reduced dose according to age and weight.

Onset of effect
Within 15 minutes.

Duration of action
2–4 hours.

Diet advice
For hyperphosphataemia, a low-phosphate diet may be advised in addition to aluminium hydroxide treatment.

Storage
Keep in original container at room temperature out of the reach of children.

Missed dose
Do not take the missed dose. Take your next dose as usual.

Stopping the drug
Can be safely stopped as soon as you no longer need it (indigestion). When taken as ulcer treatment or for hyperphosphataemia resulting from kidney failure, do not stop without consulting your doctor.

Exceeding the dose
An occasional unintentional extra dose is unlikely to be a cause for concern. But if you notice any unusual symptoms, or if a large overdose has been taken, notify your doctor.

POSSIBLE ADVERSE EFFECTS

Constipation is common with aluminium hydroxide; nausea and vomiting may occur due to the granular, powdery nature of the drug. Bone pain occurs only when large doses have been taken regularly for a period of months or years.

Symptom/effect	Frequency		Discuss with doctor		Stop taking drug now	Call doctor now
	Common	Rare	Only if severe	In all cases		
Constipation	●		●			
Nausea		●	●			
Vomiting		●		●		

INTERACTIONS

General note Aluminium hydroxide may interfere with the absorption or excretion of many drugs, including oral anticoagulants, digoxin, many antibiotics, penicillamine, corticosteroids, antipsychotics, and phenytoin. It should only be taken at least 2 hours before or after other drugs.

Enteric-coated tablets Aluminium hydroxide may lead to the break-up of the enteric coating of tablets (e.g. bisacodyl, or enteric-coated prednisolone) before they leave the stomach, leading to stomach irritation.

SPECIAL PRECAUTIONS

Be sure to consult your doctor or pharmacist before taking this drug if:
- You have a long-term kidney problem.
- You have heart problems.
- You have high blood pressure.
- You have constipation.
- You have a bone disease.
- You have porphyria.
- You are taking other medicines.

Pregnancy
Safety in pregnancy not established. Discuss with your doctor.

Breast-feeding
No evidence of risk.

Infants and children
Not recommended under 6 years except on the advice of a doctor.

Over 60
No special problems.

Driving and hazardous work
No known problems.

Alcohol
No known problems.

PROLONGED USE

Aluminium hydroxide should not be used for longer than 4 weeks without consulting your doctor. Prolonged use of high doses in people with normal kidney function may deplete blood phosphate and calcium levels, leading to weakening of the bones and fractures. In people with kidney disease, long-term treatment may lead to accumulation of aluminium in the brain, causing dementia.

AMILORIDE

Brand name None
Used in the following combined preparations Co-amilofruse, Co-amilozide, Frumil, Moduretic, Navispare, and others

GENERAL INFORMATION

Amiloride is a diuretic. It acts on the kidneys to increase the amount of urine that is passed, although the diuretic effect of amiloride is very mild. The drug is used in the treatment of oedema (fluid retention), which can result from heart failure or liver disease, and for hypertension (high blood pressure).

The effect that amiloride has on urine flow may last for several hours, so the drug should be taken in the morning.

Amiloride causes the kidneys to conserve potassium (it is a potassium-sparing diuretic) and it should not be used when there is a high blood level of potassium. The drug is prescribed with caution in people taking potassium supplements or those with kidney disease. Amiloride is often combined with other diuretics such as furosemide (co-amilofruse) and hydrochlorothiazide (co-amilozide).

INFORMATION FOR USERS

Your drug prescription is tailored for you. Do not alter dosage without checking with your doctor.

How taken/used

Tablets, liquid.

Frequency and timing of doses
Once or twice daily, usually in the morning.

Adult dosage range
5–20mg daily.

Onset of effect
Within 2–4 hours.

Duration of action
12 hours.

Diet advice
Avoid foods that are high in potassium – for example, dried fruit, bananas, tomatoes, and "low salt" salt substitutes.

Storage
Keep in original container at room temperature out of the reach of children.

Missed dose
Take as soon as you remember. However, if it is late in the day, do not take the missed dose, or you may need to get up at night to pass urine. Take the next scheduled dose as usual.

Stopping the drug
Do not stop the drug without consulting your doctor; symptoms may recur.

Exceeding the dose
An occasional unintentional extra dose is unlikely to be a cause for concern. But if you notice any unusual symptoms, or if a large overdose has been taken, notify your doctor.

SPECIAL PRECAUTIONS

Be sure to tell your doctor if:
- You have long-term liver or kidney problems.
- You are taking other medicines.

 Pregnancy
Not usually prescribed. May cause a reduction in the blood supply to the developing baby. Discuss with your doctor.

 Breast-feeding
Not usually prescribed during breast-feeding. Discuss with your doctor.

 Infants and children
Not recommended.

 Over 60
Increased likelihood of adverse effects. Reduced dose may be necessary.

 Driving and hazardous work
No known problems.

 Alcohol
No special problems.

PROLONGED USE

Monitoring Blood tests may be carried out to monitor levels of body salts.

POSSIBLE ADVERSE EFFECTS

Amiloride has few adverse effects; the main problem is the possibility that potassium may be retained by the body or excessive sodium lost in the urine, causing muscle weakness or heart rhythm problems.

Symptom/effect	Frequency		Discuss with doctor		Stop taking drug now	Call doctor now
	Common	Rare	Only if severe	In all cases		
Digestive disturbance		●	●			
Confusion		●		●		
Muscle weakness/cramps		●		●		
Dry mouth/thirst		●		●		
Dizziness		●		●		
Rash		●		●	●	

INTERACTIONS

Lithium Amiloride may increase the blood levels of lithium, leading to an increased risk of lithium toxicity.

ACE inhibitors, angiotensin II blockers, renin inhibitors (e.g. aliskiren), ciclosporin, drosperinone, tacrolimus, and NSAIDs These drugs may increase the risk of potassium retention if taken with amiloride.

AMIODARONE

Brand name Cordarone X
Used in the following combined preparations None

GENERAL INFORMATION

Amiodarone is used for a variety of abnormal heart rhythms (arrhythmias). It works by slowing nerve impulses in the heart muscle. The drug is given to prevent recurrent atrial and ventricular fibrillation (irregular heart beat) and to treat ventricular and supraventricular tachycardias (overly fast heart beat) and Wolff-Parkinson-White syndrome (persistent tachycardia due to an abnormal extra electrical connection in the heart). Often the last choice when other treatments have failed, especially for long-term use, it has serious adverse effects including liver damage, thyroid problems, and eye and lung damage. Treatment should be started only under specialist supervision or in hospital.

QUICK REFERENCE

Drug group Anti-arrhythmic drug (p.58)

Overdose danger rating High

Dependence rating Low

Prescription needed Yes

Available as generic Yes (tablets)

INFORMATION FOR USERS

Your drug prescription is tailored for you. Do not alter dosage without checking with your doctor.

How taken/used

Tablets, injection.

Frequency and timing of doses
3 x daily or by injection initially, then reduced to twice daily, then once daily or every other day (maintenance dose).

Adult dosage range
600mg daily, reduced to 400mg, then 100–200mg daily.

Onset of effect
By mouth, some effects may occur in 72 hours; full benefits may take some weeks to show. By injection, effects may occur within 30 minutes.

Duration of action
3–12 months.

Diet advice
Grapefruit juice should be avoided.

Storage
Keep in original container at room temperature out of the reach of children. Protect from light.

Missed dose
Take as soon as you remember. If your next dose is due within 12 hours, do not take the missed dose. Take your next scheduled dose as usual.

Stopping the drug
Do not stop the drug without consulting your doctor; symptoms may recur.

OVERDOSE ACTION

Seek immediate medical advice in all cases. Take emergency action if collapse or loss of consciousness occur.

See Drug poisoning emergency guide (p.518).

POSSIBLE ADVERSE EFFECTS

Amiodarone has a number of unusual side effects, including a metallic taste in the mouth, a greyish skin colour, and increased sensitivity of the skin to sunlight (photosensitivity).

Symptom/effect	Frequency		Discuss with doctor		Stop taking drug now	Call doctor now
	Common	Rare	Only if severe	In all cases		
Nausea/vomiting	●		●			
Liver damage	●			●		
Photosensitivity	●			●		
Visual disturbances	●			●		
Thyroid problems		●		●		
Heart rate disturbances		●		●		
Numb, tingling extremities		●		●		
Shortness of breath/cough		●		●		
Headache/weakness/fatigue		●		●		
Grey skin colour		●		●		

INTERACTIONS

General note Consult your doctor or pharmacist before taking other medications.

Diuretics Some cause potassium loss and increase the toxic effects of amiodarone.

Other anti-arrhythmics Amiodarone may increase the effects of these drugs.

Warfarin Amiodarone may increase the anticoagulant effect of warfarin.

Anti-hepatitis C drugs Use with amiodarone raises the risk of bradycardia or heart block.

SPECIAL PRECAUTIONS

Be sure to tell your doctor if:
- You have long-term liver problems.
- You have heart problems.
- You have eye disease.
- You have a lung disorder such as asthma or bronchitis.
- You have a thyroid disorder.
- You are sensitive to iodine.
- You are taking other medicines.

 Pregnancy
Not recommended. Discuss with your doctor.

 Breast-feeding
The drug passes into the breast milk and may affect the baby. Safety not established. Discuss with your doctor.

 Infants and children
Not recommended.

 Over 60
Increased likelihood of adverse effects. Reduced dose may therefore be necessary.

 Driving and hazardous work
Avoid these activities until you have learned how amiodarone affects you because the drug can cause the eyes to be dazzled by bright light.

 Alcohol
No known problems.

PROLONGED USE

Prolonged use of this drug may cause a number of adverse effects on the eyes, heart, skin, nervous system, lungs, thyroid gland, and liver.

Monitoring A chest X-ray may be taken before treatment starts. Blood tests are done before treatment starts and then every 6 months to check thyroid and liver function. Regular eye examinations are required.

AMISULPRIDE/SULPIRIDE

Brand names [amisulpride] Solian; [sulpiride] Dolmatil
Used in the following combined preparations None

GENERAL INFORMATION

Amisulpride and sulpiride are antipsychotic drugs used to treat acute and chronic schizophrenia, in which a person experiences "positive" symptoms such as delusions, hallucinations, and thought disorders, and/or "negative" symptoms such as emotional and social withdrawal. Patients who have mainly positive symptoms are treated with higher doses; patients with mainly negative symptoms are given lower doses. Sulpiride has also been used in the treatment of Tourette's syndrome.

An advantage of amisulpride, a so-called atypical antipsychotic, is that it is less likely than older antipsychotic drugs to cause the movement disorders parkinsonism or tardive dyskinesia.

QUICK REFERENCE

Drug group Antipsychotic drug (p.41)

Overdose danger rating Medium

Dependence rating Low

Prescription needed Yes

Available as generic Yes

INFORMATION FOR USERS

Your drug prescription is tailored for you. Do not alter dosage without checking with your doctor.

How taken/used

Tablets, liquid.

Frequency and timing of doses
1–2 x daily (doses of up to 300mg of amisulpride may be 1 x daily).

Dosage range
Amisulpride 50–300mg daily (mainly negative symptoms); 400–1,200mg daily (mainly positive symptoms).
Sulpiride 400–800mg daily (mainly negative symptoms); 400–2,400mg daily (mainly positive symptoms).

Onset of effect
1 hour.

Duration of action
12–24 hours.

Diet advice
None.

Storage
Keep in original container at room temperature out of the reach of children.

Missed dose
Take as soon as you remember. If your next dose is due within 2 hours, take a single dose now and skip the next dose.

Stopping the drug
Do not stop taking the drug without consulting your doctor; symptoms may recur.

Exceeding the dose
An occasional unintentional extra dose is unlikely to cause problems. Large overdoses may cause drowsiness and low blood pressure. Notify your doctor immediately.

SPECIAL PRECAUTIONS

Be sure to tell your doctor if:
- You have liver or kidney problems.
- You have heart problems or hypertension.
- You have epilepsy.
- You have Parkinson's disease.
- You have a pituitary tumour or breast cancer.
- You have phaeochromocytoma.
- You have had blood problems.
- You are taking other medicines.

Pregnancy
Short-term nervous system problems may occur in babies when the drug is taken in the third trimester. Discuss with your doctor.

Breast-feeding
Safety not established. Discuss with your doctor.

Infants and children
Not recommended.

Over 60
Reduced dose may be necessary.

Driving and hazardous work
Avoid such activities until you have learned how amisulpride and sulpiride affect you; the drugs can slow reaction times and may occasionally cause drowsiness or loss of concentration.

Alcohol
Avoid. Alcohol increases the sedative effects of these drugs.

PROLONGED USE

An adverse effect called tardive dyskinesia, in which there are involuntary movements of the tongue and face, may rarely occur during long-term use.

POSSIBLE ADVERSE EFFECTS

Most of the side effects of antipsychotic drugs such as amisulpride and sulpiride are mild; insomnia is the most common problem.

Symptom/effect	Frequency		Discuss with doctor		Stop taking drug now	Call doctor now
	Common	Rare	Only if severe	In all cases		
Sleep disturbances	●		●			
Drowsiness	●		●			
Anxiety/agitation	●		●			
Weight gain		●	●			
Nausea/vomiting		●	●			
Breast swelling		●		●		
Parkinsonism		●		●		
Loss of libido		●		●		
Menstrual irregularities		●		●		

INTERACTIONS

Amiodarone, disopyramide, diuretics, droperidol, erythromycin, methadone, and sotalol These drugs increase the risk of abnormal heart rhythms when taken with amisulpride or sulpiride.

Antihypertensive drugs Amisulpride and sulpiride may reduce the blood-pressure-lowering effect of certain of these drugs.

Central nervous system depressants These drugs may all increase the sedative effects of amisulpride and sulpiride.

AMITRIPTYLINE

Brand names None
Used in the following combined preparation Triptafen

GENERAL INFORMATION

Amitriptyline belongs to the tricyclic group of antidepressants. These drugs are effective for long-term depression but are poorly tolerated and dangerous in overdose, so they are second-line choices after SSRI antidepressants (see p.40). The sedative effect of amitriptyline is useful if depression is accompanied by anxiety or insomnia. Taken at night, the drug encourages sleep and reduces the need for additional sleeping drugs. Amitriptyline is sometimes used to treat nocturnal enuresis (bedwetting) in children. It may also be used to treat neuropathic pain such as postherpetic neuralgia after shingles and to prevent tension headache and migraine. In overdose, amitriptyline may cause abnormal heart rhythms, seizures, and coma.

INFORMATION FOR USERS

Your drug prescription is tailored for you. Do not alter dosage without checking with your doctor.

How taken/used

Tablets, liquid.

Frequency and timing of doses
1–3 x daily, usually as a single dose at night.

Adult dosage range
10–150mg daily.

Onset of effect
Sedation can appear within hours, although full antidepressant effect may not be felt for 2–4 weeks.

Duration of action
Antidepressant effect may last for 6 weeks; common adverse effects gone within 1 week.

Diet advice
None.

Storage
Keep in original container at room temperature out of the reach of children. Protect from light.

Missed dose
Take as soon as you remember. If your next dose is due within 3 hours, take a single dose now and skip the next.

Stopping the drug
An abrupt stop can cause withdrawal symptoms and recurrence of the original trouble. Consult your doctor, who may supervise a gradual reduction in dosage over at least 4 weeks.

OVERDOSE ACTION

 Seek immediate medical advice in all cases. Take emergency action if palpitations are noted or consciousness is lost.

See Drug poisoning emergency guide (p.518).

POSSIBLE ADVERSE EFFECTS

The possible adverse effects of this drug are mainly the result of its anticholinergic action and its blocking action on the transmission of signals through the heart.

Symptom/effect	Frequency		Discuss with doctor		Stop taking drug now	Call doctor now
	Common	Rare	Only if severe	In all cases		
Drowsiness	●		●			
Sweating	●		●			
Dry mouth/constipation	●		●			
Blurred vision	●			●		
Dizziness/fainting	●			●	●	
Difficulty in passing urine		●		●		
Confusion		●		●	●	
Palpitations		●		●	●	●

INTERACTIONS

Monoamine oxidase inhibitors (MAOIs)
In the rare cases where these drugs are given with amitriptyline, there is a possibility of serious interactions.

Anticonvulsants The effects of these drugs are reduced by amitriptyline as it lowers the threshold for seizures.

Sedatives All drugs that have sedative effects intensify those of amitriptyline.

Anti-arrhythmic drugs There is an increased risk of abnormal heart rhythms when these drugs are taken with amitriptyline.

SPECIAL PRECAUTIONS

Be sure to tell your doctor if:
- You have heart problems.
- You have had epileptic seizures.
- You have long-term liver or kidney problems.
- You have glaucoma.
- You have prostate trouble.
- You have thyroid disease.
- You have had mania or a psychotic illness.
- You are taking other medicines.

 Pregnancy
Avoid if possible. Discuss with your doctor.

 Breast-feeding
The drug passes into the breast milk, but at normal doses adverse effects are unlikely. Discuss with your doctor.

 Infants and children
Not recommended under 16 years for depression, or under 6 years for enuresis.

 Over 60
Reduced dose may be necessary because older patients are more sensitive to adverse reactions.

 Driving and hazardous work
Avoid such activities until you have learned how amitriptyline affects you because the drug may cause blurred vision and reduced alertness.

 Alcohol
Avoid. Alcohol may increase the sedative effects of this drug.

Surgery and general anaesthetics
Amitriptyline treatment may need to be stopped before you have a general anaesthetic. Discuss this with your doctor or dentist before any operation.

PROLONGED USE

No problems expected.

AMLODIPINE

Brand name Istin
Used in the following combined preparations Exforge, Sevikar

GENERAL INFORMATION

Amlodipine belongs to a group of drugs known as calcium channel blockers, which interfere with the conduction of signals in the muscles of the heart and blood vessels.

Amlodipine is used in the treatment of angina to help prevent attacks of chest pain. Unlike some other anti-angina drugs (such as beta blockers), it can be used safely by people with asthma and those with diabetes who require insulin. Amlodipine is also used to reduce raised blood pressure (hypertension). Like other drugs of its class, amlodipine may cause blood pressure to fall too low at the start of treatment. In rare cases, angina may become worse at the start of amlodipine treatment.

QUICK REFERENCE

Drug group Anti-angina drug (p.59) and antihypertensive drug (p.60)

Overdose danger rating Medium

Dependence rating Low

Prescription needed Yes

Available as generic Yes

INFORMATION FOR USERS

Your drug prescription is tailored for you. Do not alter dosage without checking with your doctor.

How taken/used

Tablets, liquid (oral solution).

Frequency and timing of doses
Once daily.

Adult dosage range
5–10mg daily.

Onset of effect
6–12 hours.

Duration of action
24 hours.

Diet advice
Avoid grapefruit juice because it may interact with amlodipine and increase the drug's effects.

Storage
Keep in original container at room temperature out of the reach of children.

Missed dose
If you miss a dose and you remember it within 12 hours, take it as soon as you remember. However, if you do not remember until later, do not take the missed dose and do not double up the next one. Instead, go back to your regular schedule.

Stopping the drug
Do not stop taking the drug without consulting your doctor; stopping the drug may lead to worsening of the underlying condition.

Exceeding the dose
An occasional unintentional extra dose is unlikely to cause problems. Large overdoses may cause a marked lowering of blood pressure. Notify your doctor immediately.

SPECIAL PRECAUTIONS

Be sure to tell your doctor if:
- You have long-term liver problems.
- You have heart failure or aortic stenosis.
- You have diabetes.
- You are taking other medicines.

Pregnancy
Safety in pregnancy not established. Discuss with your doctor.

Breast-feeding
It is not known if the drug passes into the breast milk. Discuss with your doctor.

Infants and children
Not recommended.

Over 60
No special problems.

Driving and hazardous work
Avoid such activities until you have learned how amlodipine affects you because the drug can cause dizziness owing to lowered blood pressure.

Alcohol
Avoid. Alcohol may further reduce blood pressure, causing dizziness or other symptoms.

Surgery and general anaesthetics
Amlodipine may interact with some general anaesthetics, causing a fall in blood pressure. Discuss this with your doctor or dentist before any surgery.

PROLONGED USE

No problems expected.

POSSIBLE ADVERSE EFFECTS

Amlodipine can cause a variety of minor adverse effects, but the most serious effect is the rare possibility of angina becoming worse after starting amlodipine treatment. This should be reported to your doctor.

Symptom/effect	Frequency		Discuss with doctor		Stop taking drug now	Call doctor now
	Common	Rare	Only if severe	In all cases		
Leg and ankle swelling	●		●			
Headache	●		●			
Dizziness/fatigue	●		●			
Flushing	●		●			
Nausea/abdominal pain	●			●		
Palpitations	●			●		
Skin rash		●		●	●	
Breathing difficulties		●		●		
Worsening of angina		●		●	●	●

INTERACTIONS

Ketoconazole, itraconazole, and ritonavir These drugs may increase blood levels and adverse effects of amlodipine.

St John's wort This reduces the blood level of amlodipine.

Grapefruit juice This may increase the effects of amlodipine.

Alpha blockers, beta blockers, ACE inhibitors, and diuretics Amlodipine may increase the effects of these drugs and vice versa.

Antimalarials Taken with amlodipine, some antimalarials may cause abnormally slow heart beat.

AMOXICILLIN/CO-AMOXICLAV

Brand name Amoxil
Used in the following combined preparations Augmentin, Co-amoxiclav

GENERAL INFORMATION

Amoxicillin is a penicillin antibiotic. It is given to treat a variety of infections, but is particularly useful for treating ear, nose, and throat infections, respiratory tract infections, cystitis, uncomplicated gonorrhoea, and certain skin and soft tissue infections. The drug is sometimes combined with clavulanic acid (as co-amoxiclav) to prevent bacteria from breaking down the amoxicillin; this makes it effective against a wider range of bacteria than amoxicillin alone. Doses of co-amoxiclav are given as two numbers (e.g. 500/125 is 500mg amoxicillin plus 125mg clavulanic acid).

Amoxicillin/co-amoxiclav can cause minor stomach upsets and a rash. It can also provoke a severe allergic reaction with fever, swelling of the mouth and tongue, itching, and breathing difficulties.

QUICK REFERENCE

Drug group Penicillin antibiotic (p.86)
Overdose danger rating Low
Dependence rating Low
Prescription needed Yes
Available as generic Yes

INFORMATION FOR USERS

Your drug prescription is tailored for you. Do not alter dosage without checking with your doctor.

How taken/used

Tablets, capsules, liquid, powder (dissolved in water), injection.

Frequency and timing of doses
Normally 3 x daily.

Dosage range
Adults 750mg–1.5g (of amoxicillin) daily. In some cases a short course of up to 6g (of amoxicillin) daily is given. A single dose of 3g (of amoxicillin) may be given as a preventative. However, dosage range depends on preparation and condition being treated
Children Reduced dose according to age and weight.

Onset of effect
1–2 hours.

Duration of action
Up to 8 hours.

Diet advice
Make sure you keep well hydrated.

Storage
Keep in original container at room temperature out of the reach of children.

Missed dose
Take as soon as you remember. Take your next dose at the scheduled time.

Stopping the drug
Take the full course. Even if you feel better, the original infection may still be present if treatment is stopped too soon.

Exceeding the dose
An occasional unintentional extra dose is unlikely to be a cause for concern. But if you notice any unusual symptoms, or if a large overdose has been taken, notify your doctor.

SPECIAL PRECAUTIONS

Be sure to tell your doctor if:
- You are allergic to penicillin antibiotics or cephalosporin antibiotics.
- You have glandular fever (infectious mononucleosis).
- You have a history of allergy.
- You have liver problems, or have had previous liver problems with amoxicillin/co-amoxiclav.
- You have a kidney problem.
- You are taking other medicines.

 Pregnancy
No evidence of risk.

 Breast-feeding
No evidence of risk.

 Infants and children
Reduced dose necessary.

 Over 60
No known problems.

 Driving and hazardous work
No known problems.

 Alcohol
No known problems.

PROLONGED USE

Amoxicillin and co-amoxiclav are usually given only for short courses of treatment.

POSSIBLE ADVERSE EFFECTS

The most common adverse effects are gastrointestinal. If you develop a rash, itching, wheezing or breathing difficulties, swollen joints (signs of an allergic reaction), or jaundice (which may occur weeks or even months after finishing treatment), call your doctor.

Symptom/effect	Frequency		Discuss with doctor		Stop taking drug now	Call doctor now
	Common	Rare	Only if severe	In all cases		
Diarrhoea/nausea	●		●			
Rash	●			●		
Abdominal pain		●		●		
Bruising		●		●		
Sore throat/fever		●		●		
Itching		●		●	●	●
Breathing difficulties/wheezing		●		●	●	●
Jaundice		●		●	●	●

INTERACTIONS

Anticoagulant drugs Amoxicillin and co-amoxiclav may alter the anticoagulant effect of these drugs.

Allopurinol Amoxicillin may increase the likelihood of allergic skin reactions.

Oral typhoid vaccine Amoxicillin and co-amoxiclav inactivate this vaccine. Avoid taking these drugs for 3 days before and after having the vaccine.

AMPHOTERICIN (B)

Brand names Abelcet, AmBisome, Fungizone
Used in the following combined preparations None

GENERAL INFORMATION

Amphotericin is a highly effective and powerful antifungal drug. Although it was previously given by mouth to treat candida (thrush) infections of the mouth or intestines, it is now only given by intravenous infusion to treat serious systemic fungal infections. All of the oral formulations have been discontinued in the UK. Administration of amphotericin is carefully supervised, usually in hospital, because of potentially serious adverse effects. A test dose for allergy may be given before treatment is started. The newer formulations of amphotericin appear to be less toxic than the original ones.

INFORMATION FOR USERS

Your drug prescription is tailored for you. Do not alter dosage without checking with your doctor.

How taken/used

Intravenous infusion.

Frequency and timing of doses
Once daily.

Dosage range
The dosage is determined individually.

Onset of effect
Improvement may be noticed after 2–4 days.

Duration of action
Up to several days.

Diet advice
The drug may reduce the levels of potassium and magnesium in the blood. To correct this, mineral supplements may be recommended by your doctor.

Storage
Not applicable. The drug is not normally kept in the home.

Missed dose
If you miss your scheduled dose, contact your doctor as soon as possible.

Stopping the drug
Discuss with your doctor. Stopping the drug prematurely may lead to worsening of the underlying condition.

Exceeding the dose
Overdosage is unlikely since treatment is carefully monitored and supervised.

POSSIBLE ADVERSE EFFECTS

Amphotericin is given only by infusion under close medical supervision. Any adverse effects that develop are thus monitored closely and treated promptly.

Symptom/effect	Frequency		Discuss with doctor		Stop taking drug now	Call doctor now
	Common	Rare	Only if severe	In all cases		
Nausea/vomiting	●			●		
Headache/fever	●			●		
Rash	●			●		
Unusual bleeding		●		●		
Muscle and joint pain		●		●		
Palpitations		●		●	●	●
Difficulty in breathing		●		●	●	●

INTERACTIONS

Digitalis drugs Amphotericin may increase the toxicity of digoxin.

Diuretics Amphotericin increases the risk of low potassium levels with diuretics.

Aminoglycoside antibiotics Taken with amphotericin, these drugs increase the likelihood of kidney damage.

Corticosteroids may increase loss of potassium from the body caused by amphotericin.

Ciclosporin and tacrolimus increase the likelihood of kidney damage.

SPECIAL PRECAUTIONS

Be sure to tell your doctor if:
- You have a long-term liver or kidney problem.
- You have previously had an allergic reaction to amphotericin.
- You are taking other medicines.

Pregnancy
The drug is given only when the infection is very serious.

Breast-feeding
It is not known whether the drug passes into the breast milk. Discuss with your doctor.

Infants and children
Reduced dose may be necessary.

Over 60
No special problems.

Driving and hazardous work
No known problems.

Alcohol
No known problems.

PROLONGED USE

The drug may cause a reduction in blood levels of potassium and magnesium. It may also damage the kidneys and cause blood disorders.

Monitoring Regular blood tests to monitor liver and kidney function, blood cell counts, and potassium and magnesium levels are advised during treatment.

ANASTROZOLE

Brand name Arimidex
Used in the following combined preparations None

GENERAL INFORMATION

Anastrozole is a potent non-steroidal inhibitor of the enzyme that makes oestradiol (natural oestrogen) in the body. The drug can reduce oestradiol production by more than 80 per cent. It works by blocking production in peripheral body tissues such as fat, rather than in the ovary, so is generally not suitable for use in premenopausal women where the ovaries are still producing oestrogen. The drug is used in postmenopausal women for types of breast cancer in which the tumour cells have oestrogen receptors (oestrogen-receptor-positive breast cancer).

Anastrozole is generally well tolerated; any adverse effects are principally gastrointestinal or gynaecological and similar to menopausal symptoms. If there is any doubt about whether a woman to be treated is postmenopausal, a blood test may be performed.

QUICK REFERENCE

Drug group Anticancer drug (p.112)
Overdose danger rating Low
Dependence rating Low
Prescription needed Yes
Available as generic Yes

INFORMATION FOR USERS

Your drug prescription is tailored for you. Do not alter dosage without checking with your doctor.

How taken/used

Tablets.

Frequency and timing of doses
Once daily.

Adult dosage range
1mg.

Onset of effect
A few hours.

Duration of action
More than 24 hours.

Diet advice
None.

Storage
Keep in original container at room temperature out of the reach of children.

Missed dose
Take as soon as you remember. If your next dose is due within 2 hours, take a single dose now and skip the next.

Stopping the drug
Do not stop the drug without consulting your doctor. Stopping the drug may lead to worsening of the underlying condition.

Exceeding the dose
An occasional unintentional extra dose is unlikely to be a cause for concern. But if you notice any unusual symptoms, or if a large overdose has been taken, notify your doctor.

SPECIAL PRECAUTIONS

Be sure to tell your doctor if:
• You are premenopausal.
• You have osteoporosis.
• You have kidney or liver problems.
• You are allergic to anastrozole.
• You are taking other medicines.

Pregnancy
Not prescribed in pregnancy.

Breast-feeding
Not prescribed when breast-feeding.

Infants and children
Not recommended.

Over 60
No special problems.

Driving and hazardous work
Do not drive until you know how the drug affects you. It can cause drowsiness.

Alcohol
No known problems.

PROLONGED USE

No known problems.

Monitoring Women with osteoporosis or at risk of osteoporosis will have their bone mineral density assessed at the start of treatment and at regular intervals. Cholesterol levels may also be monitored.

POSSIBLE ADVERSE EFFECTS

Anastrozole is usually well tolerated and any side effects tend to be relatively minor, except for the increased risk of osteoporosis and bone fracture.

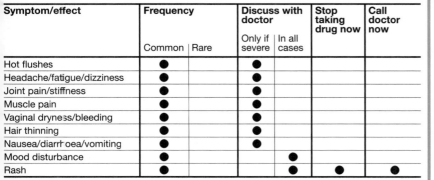

Symptom/effect	Frequency		Discuss with doctor		Stop taking drug now	Call doctor now
	Common	Rare	Only if severe	In all cases		
Hot flushes	●			●		
Headache/fatigue/dizziness	●			●		
Joint pain/stiffness	●			●		
Muscle pain	●			●		
Vaginal dryness/bleeding	●			●		
Hair thinning	●			●		
Nausea/diarrhoea/vomiting	●			●		
Mood disturbance	●		●			
Rash	●		●		●	●

INTERACTIONS

Tamoxifen and oestrogens oppose the effects of anastrozole and should be avoided.

ASPIRIN

Brand names Aspro, Danamep, Disprin, Nu-Seals Aspirin, and others
Used in the following combined preparations Anadin, Beechams Powders, Codis, Migramax, and others

GENERAL INFORMATION

In use for over a century, aspirin relieves pain, reduces fever, and alleviates the symptoms of arthritis. In low doses, it helps to prevent blood clots, particularly in atherosclerosis or angina due to coronary artery disease, and it reduces the risk of heart attacks and strokes.

It is present in many medicines for colds, flu, headaches, menstrual period pains, and joint or muscular aches.

Aspirin may irritate the stomach and even cause peptic ulcers or bleeding. Another drawback of aspirin is that it can provoke asthma attacks.

In children, aspirin can cause Reye's syndrome, a rare but serious brain and liver disorder. For this reason, aspirin should not be given to children under the age of 16 years, except on the advice of a doctor.

INFORMATION FOR USERS

Follow instructions on the label. Call your doctor if symptoms worsen.

How taken/used

Tablets, SR capsules, suppositories.

Frequency and timing of doses
Relief of pain or fever Every 4–6 hours, as necessary, with or after food or milk.
Prevention of blood clots Once daily.

Adult dosage range
Relief of pain or fever 300–900mg per dose.
Prevention of blood clots 75–300mg daily.

Onset of effect
30–60 minutes (regular aspirin); 1½–8 hours (coated tablets or SR capsules).

Duration of action
Up to 12 hours. Effect persists for 7–10 days when used to prevent blood clotting.

Diet advice
Take with or immediately after food.

Storage
Keep in original container at room temperature out of the reach of children.

Missed dose
Take as soon as you remember. If your next dose is due within 2 hours, take a single dose now and skip the next.

Stopping the drug
If you have been prescribed aspirin by your doctor for a long-term condition, you should seek medical advice before stopping the drug. Otherwise it can be safely stopped.

OVERDOSE ACTION

Seek immediate advice in all cases. Take emergency action if there is restlessness, sweating, ringing noises in the ears, blurred vision, or vomiting.

See Drug poisoning emergency guide (p.518).

SPECIAL PRECAUTIONS

Be sure to consult your doctor or pharmacist before taking this drug if:
- You have long-term liver or kidney problems.
- You have asthma.
- You are allergic to aspirin or any non-steroidal anti-inflammatory drug (NSAID).
- You have a blood clotting disorder.
- You have a history of peptic ulcer.
- You have glucose-6-phosphate dehydrogenase (G6PD) deficiency.
- You are taking other medicines.

Pregnancy
Not usually recommended but may be prescribed to prevent pre-eclampsia if high risk. Discuss with your doctor.

Breast-feeding
Avoid. It passes into breast milk and can cause Reye's syndrome in babies.

Infants and children
Do not give to children under 16 years, except on a doctor's advice.

Over 60
Adverse effects more likely.

Driving and hazardous work
No special problems.

Alcohol
Avoid. Alcohol increases the likelihood of stomach irritation with this drug.

Surgery and general anaesthetics
Regular aspirin treatment may need to be stopped about a week before surgery. Talk to your doctor or dentist before any operation.

POSSIBLE ADVERSE EFFECTS

Adverse effects are more likely to occur with high doses of aspirin, but may be reduced by taking the drug with food or in buffered or enteric coated forms.

Symptom/effect	Frequency		Discuss with doctor		Stop taking drug now	Call doctor now
	Common	Rare	Only if severe	In all cases		
Indigestion	●		●			
Nausea/vomiting		●		●		
Rash		●		●	●	
Breathlessness/wheezing		●		●		
Blood in vomit/black faeces		●		●		●
Ringing in the ears/dizziness		●	●		●	●

INTERACTIONS

Anticoagulants Aspirin may add to the anticoagulant effect of such drugs, leading to an increased risk of abnormal bleeding.

Drugs for gout Aspirin may reduce the effect of these drugs.

NSAIDs may increase the likelihood of stomach irritation with aspirin.

Methotrexate Aspirin may increase the toxicity of this drug.

Sulfonylurea antidiabetic drugs Aspirin may increase the effect of these drugs.

Corticosteroids and some SSRI antidepressants These may increase the risk of gastrointestinal bleeding with aspirin.

PROLONGED USE

Aspirin should not be taken in high doses for prolonged periods. When taken long term, all doses of aspirin increase the risk of peptic ulcers and gastrointestinal bleeding, so regular use should be avoided. Exceptions include long-term use of low dose aspirin to prevent blood clots in people who are at high risk of cardiovascular disease, where this benefit outweighs the risk of bleeding.

ATENOLOL

Brand name Tenormin
Used in the following combined preparations Beta-Adalat, Co-tenidone, Kalten, Tenif, Tenoret, Tenoretic

GENERAL INFORMATION

Atenolol is a cardioselective beta blocker (see p.55). It prevents the heart from beating too quickly and is used mainly to treat irregular heart rhythms (arrhythmias) and chest pain (angina). It may be given following a heart attack to protect the heart from further damage. Atenolol is also used to treat high blood pressure but is not usually used to initiate treatment. It is less likely than non-cardioselective beta blockers to provoke breathing difficulties, but, nevertheless, it is not usually given to patients with asthma. It may slow the body's response to low blood sugar in people with diabetes who are on insulin.

INFORMATION FOR USERS

Your drug prescription is tailored for you. Do not alter dosage without checking with your doctor.

How taken/used

Tablets, liquid, injection.

Frequency and timing of doses
1–2 x daily.

Adult dosage range
25–100mg daily.

Onset of effect
2–4 hours.

Duration of action
20–30 hours.

Diet advice
None.

Storage
Keep in original container in a cool, dry place out of the reach of children. Protect from light.

Missed dose
Take as soon as you remember. If your next dose is due within 6 hours, omit the missed dose but take the next scheduled dose.

Stopping the drug
Do not stop taking the drug without consulting your doctor; sudden withdrawal may lead to dangerous worsening of the underlying condition. It should be withdrawn gradually.

OVERDOSE ACTION

Seek immediate medical advice. Take emergency action if breathing difficulties, collapse, or loss of consciousness occur.

See Drug poisoning emergency guide (p.518).

SPECIAL PRECAUTIONS

Be sure to tell your doctor if:
- You have heart problems.
- You have a long-term kidney problem.
- You have diabetes.
- You have a lung disorder such as asthma or bronchitis.
- You have psoriasis.
- You are taking other medicines.

 Pregnancy
Safety in pregnancy not established. Discuss with your doctor.

 Breast-feeding
The drug passes into the breast milk. Discuss with your doctor.

 Infants and children
Not recommended.

 Over 60
No special problems. Reduced dose may be necessary if there is impaired kidney function.

 Driving and hazardous work
Avoid such activities until you have learned how atenolol affects you because the drug can cause dizziness.

 Alcohol
Avoid excessive intake. Alcohol may increase the blood-pressure-lowering effects of atenolol.

Surgery and general anaesthetics
Occasionally, atenolol may need to be stopped before you have a general anaesthetic, but only do this after discussion with your doctor or dentist.

POSSIBLE ADVERSE EFFECTS

Atenolol's adverse effects are common to most beta blockers, and tend to diminish with long-term use. Fainting may be a sign that the drug has slowed the heart beat excessively.

Symptom/effect	Frequency		Discuss with doctor		Stop taking drug now	Call doctor now
	Common	Rare	Only if severe	In all cases		
Lethargy/fatigue	●			●		
Cold hands and feet	●			●		
Nausea/vomiting		●		●		
Nightmares/vivid dreams		●		●		
Rash/dry eyes		●		●	●	
Visual disturbances		●		●	●	
Fainting/palpitations		●		●	●	●
Breathlessness/wheeze		●		●	●	●

PROLONGED USE

No special problems expected.

INTERACTIONS

Antihypertensive drugs Atenolol may enhance the blood-pressure-lowering effect.

Calcium channel blockers may cause low blood pressure, a slow heartbeat, and heart failure if used with atenolol.

Non-steroidal anti-inflammatory drugs (NSAIDs) may reduce the antihypertensive effect of atenolol.

Cardiac glycosides (e.g. digoxin) may increase the heart-slowing effect of atenolol.

Antidiabetic drugs used with atenolol may increase the risk of low blood sugar or mask its symptoms.

Decongestants used with atenolol may increase blood pressure and heart rate.

ATORVASTATIN

Brand name Lipitor
Used in the following combined preparations None

GENERAL INFORMATION

Atorvastatin is a member of the statin group of lipid-lowering drugs. It is used to treat hypercholesterolaemia (high blood cholesterol levels) in patients who have not responded to other treatments, such as a special diet or lifestyle changes, and who have, or are at risk of developing, heart disease. Atorvastatin is also used in patients with diabetes who are at high risk of heart attack or stroke. It blocks the action in the liver of an enzyme that is needed for the manufacture of cholesterol. As a result, blood levels of cholesterol are lowered, which can help to prevent coronary heart disease.

Rarely, atorvastatin can cause muscle pain, inflammation, and muscle damage.

INFORMATION FOR USERS

Your drug prescription is tailored for you. Do not alter dosage without checking with your doctor.

How taken/used

Tablets, chewable tablets.

Frequency and timing of doses
Once daily.

Adult dosage range
10–80mg.

Onset of effect
Within 2 weeks. Full beneficial effects are usually seen within 4 weeks.

Duration of action
20–30 hours.

Diet advice
A low-fat diet is usually recommended. Do not drink more than 2 small glasses of grapefruit juice per day.

Storage
Keep in original container at room temperature out of the reach of children.

Missed dose
Take as soon as you remember. If your next dose is due within 8 hours, do not take the missed dose, but take the next one on schedule.

Stopping the drug
Do not stop taking the drug without consulting your doctor. Stopping the drug may lead to a recurrence of the original condition.

Exceeding the dose
An occasional unintentional extra dose is unlikely to cause problems. Large overdoses may cause liver problems. Notify your doctor.

SPECIAL PRECAUTIONS

Be sure to tell your doctor if:
- You have had liver problems.
- You have kidney problems.
- You are a heavy drinker.
- You have an underactive thyroid.
- You or a family member have a muscle disorder.
- You have had muscle problems or other reactions with other lipid-lowering drugs.
- You are taking other medicines.

Pregnancy
Not recommended. May affect fetal development. Discuss with your doctor if you are pregnant or intend to become pregnant.

Breast-feeding
Safety not established. Discuss with your doctor.

Infants and children
Not recommended.

Over 60
No special problems.

Driving and hazardous work
No special problems.

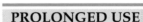

Alcohol
Avoid excessive amounts. Alcohol may increase the risk of developing liver problems with atorvastatin.

POSSIBLE ADVERSE EFFECTS

Adverse effects of atorvastatin are usually mild and transient. Muscle damage is a rare side effect, and muscle aching or weakness should be reported to your doctor promptly.

Symptom/effect	Frequency		Discuss with doctor		Stop taking drug now	Call doctor now
	Common	Rare	Only if severe	In all cases		
Nausea/constipation/diarrhoea	●		●			
Headache/dizziness/tiredness	●		●			
Insomnia	●		●			
Back/joint pain	●		●			
Jaundice		●		●		
Skin rash		●		●	●	
Muscle pain/weakness		●		●	●	●

INTERACTIONS

Warfarin Atorvastatin may reduce the anticoagulant effect of warfarin. The dose of warfarin may need adjustment.

Macrolide antibiotics (e.g. erythromycin, clarithromycin), fusidic acid, and antifungals Taken with atorvastatin, these drugs may increase the risk of muscle damage.

Other lipid-lowering drugs Taken with atorvastatin, these drugs may increase the risk of muscle damage.

Ciclosporin and other immuno-suppressant drugs Atorvastatin is not usually prescribed with these drugs because of the increased risk of muscle damage.

Oral contraceptives Atorvastatin increases blood levels of ethinylestradiol and norethisterone. The dose of these drugs may need adjustment.

Digoxin Atorvastatin increases blood levels of digoxin.

PROLONGED USE

Long-term use of atorvastatin may affect liver function.

Monitoring Regular blood tests to check liver function are needed. Tests of muscle function may be carried out if problems are suspected.

ATROPINE

Brand name Minims Atropine
Used in the following combined preparations Co-phenotrope, Lomotil, Minims Atropine

GENERAL INFORMATION

Atropine is an anticholinergic drug. Because of its antispasmodic action, which relaxes the muscle wall of the gut, the drug may be used to ease abdominal cramps in irritable bowel syndrome. It may be prescribed in combination with diphenoxylate, an antidiarrhoeal drug; however, the benefit may be outweighed by atropine-related side effects. This combination can also be dangerous in overdose, particularly in young children.

Atropine eye drops are used to enlarge the pupil during eye examinations and to treat inflammatory eye disorders such as uveitis. Atropine may also be used as part of premedication before a general anaesthetic, injected to treat heart block (p.58), or given with pralidoxime to treat poisoning with organophosphates.

Atropine must be used with caution in children and older adults due to their sensitivity to the drug's effects.

INFORMATION FOR USERS

Your drug prescription is tailored for you. Do not alter dosage without checking with your doctor.

How taken/used

Tablets, injection, eye ointment, eye drops.

Frequency and timing of doses
Once only, or up to 4 times daily according to condition (eye drops); as directed (other forms).

Adult dosage range
1–2 drops as directed (eye drops); as directed (other forms).

Onset of effect
Varies according to method of administration. 30 minutes (eye drops).

Duration of action
7 days or longer (eye drops); several hours (other forms).

Diet advice
None.

Storage
Keep in original container at room temperature out of the reach of children. Protect from light.

Missed dose
Take as soon as you remember. If your next dose is due within 2 hours, take a single dose now and skip the next.

Stopping the drug
Do not stop the drug without consulting your doctor.

OVERDOSE ACTION

Seek immediate medical advice in all cases. Take emergency action if palpitations, tremor, delirium, seizures, or loss of consciousness occur.

See Drug poisoning emergency guide (p.518).

SPECIAL PRECAUTIONS

Be sure to tell your doctor if:
- You have long-term liver or kidney problems.
- You have prostate problems.
- You have gastro-oesophageal reflux.
- You have glaucoma.
- You have urinary difficulties.
- You have ulcerative colitis.
- You wear contact lenses (eye drops).
- You have heart problems.
- You are taking other medicines.

 Pregnancy
Safety in pregnancy not established. Discuss with your doctor.

 Breast-feeding
The drug may pass into the breast milk and affect the baby. Discuss with your doctor.

 Infants and children
Combination with diphenoxylate not recommended under 4 years; reduced dose necessary in older children.

 Over 60
Increased likelihood of adverse effects.

 Driving and hazardous work
Avoid such activities until you have learned how atropine affects you because the drug can cause blurred vision and may impair concentration.

Alcohol
Avoid. Alcohol increases the likelihood of confusion and affects your concentration when taken with atropine.

PROLONGED USE

No problems expected.

POSSIBLE ADVERSE EFFECTS

The use of this drug is limited by the frequency of anticholinergic effects. In addition to these effects, atropine eye drops may cause stinging.

Symptom/effect	Frequency		Discuss with doctor		Stop taking drug now	Call doctor now
	Common	Rare	Only if severe	In all cases		
Blurred vision/dry mouth/thirst	●		●			
Constipation	●		●			
Flushing/dry skin	●		●			
Difficulty in passing urine		●		●		
Nausea/vomiting		●	●			
Dizziness		●	●			
Rash		●		●	●	
Eye pain and irritation		●		●	●	●
Palpitations/confusion		●		●	●	●

INTERACTIONS

General note Atropine delays stomach emptying and may therefore alter the absorption of other drugs.

Ketoconazole Atropine reduces the absorption of this drug from the digestive tract. Increased dose may be necessary.

Anticholinergic drugs Atropine increases the risk of side effects from drugs that also have anticholinergic effects.

AZATHIOPRINE

Brand name Azapress, Imuran
Used in the following combined preparations None

GENERAL INFORMATION

Azathioprine is an immunosuppressant drug used to prevent immune-system rejection of transplanted organs. It is also used to modify, halt, or slow the underlying disease process in severe rheumatoid arthritis (see Antirheumatic drugs, p.75) that has failed to respond to conventional drug therapy.

Autoimmune and collagen diseases (including polymyositis, systemic lupus erythematosus, myasthenia gravis, and dermatomyositis) may be treated with azathioprine, usually in combination with corticosteroids. Azathioprine is also occasionally used for other skin disorders, such as severe atopic eczema.

Azathioprine is administered only under close supervision because of the risk of serious adverse effects, including reduced production of blood cells. For this reason, blood counts may be carried out before and during treatment.

QUICK REFERENCE

Drug group Disease-modifying antirheumatic drug (p.75) and immunosuppressant drug (p.115)
Overdose danger rating Medium
Dependence rating Low
Prescription needed Yes
Available as generic Yes

INFORMATION FOR USERS

Your drug prescription is tailored for you. Do not alter dosage without checking with your doctor.

How taken/used

Tablets, injection.

Frequency and timing of doses
Usually once daily. Tablets taken 1 hour before or 3 hours after food.

Dosage range
Initially according to body weight and disorder, then adjusted according to response.

Onset of effect
2–4 weeks. Antirheumatic effect may not be felt for 8 weeks or more.

Duration of action
Immunosuppressant effects may last for several weeks after the drug is stopped.

Diet advice
None.

Storage
Keep in original container at room temperature out of the reach of children. Protect from light.

Missed dose
Take as soon as you remember, then return to your normal schedule. If more than 2 doses are missed, consult your doctor.

Stopping the drug
Do not stop taking the drug without first consulting your doctor. If taken to prevent graft transplant rejection, stopping treatment could provoke the rejection of the transplant.

Exceeding the dose
An occasional unintentional extra dose is unlikely to cause problems. Large overdoses may cause nausea, vomiting, abdominal pains, and diarrhoea. Notify your doctor.

SPECIAL PRECAUTIONS

Be sure to tell your doctor if:
- You have long-term liver or kidney problems.
- You have had a previous allergic reaction to azathioprine or 6-mercaptopurine.
- You have hepatitis B infection or have recently had shingles or chickenpox.
- You have an infection.
- You have a blood disorder.
- You are taking other medicines.

 Pregnancy
Azathioprine has been taken in pregnancy without problems but safety is not certain. Discuss with your doctor.

 Breast-feeding
Not recommended.

 Infants and children
No special problems.

 Over 60
Increased likelihood of adverse effects. Reduced dose necessary.

 Driving and hazardous work
Avoid such activities until you have learned how azathioprine affects you because the drug can cause dizziness.

 Alcohol
No known problems.

POSSIBLE ADVERSE EFFECTS

Digestive disturbances and adverse effects on the blood that could lead to sore throat, fever, and weakness are common with azathioprine. Unusual bleeding or bruising while taking this drug may be a sign of reduced levels of platelets in the blood.

Symptom/effect	Frequency		Discuss with doctor		Stop taking drug now	Call doctor now
	Common	Rare	Only if severe	In all cases		
Nausea/vomiting	●		●			
Hair loss	●		●			
Loss of appetite	●			●		
Weakness/fatigue		●		●		
Unusual bleeding/bruising		●		●		●
Jaundice		●		●	●	●
Rash		●		●	●	●
Fever/chills		●		●	●	●

INTERACTIONS

Allopurinol This drug increases the effects and toxicity of azathioprine.

Warfarin Azathioprine may reduce the effect.

Live vaccines increase risk of generalized infection when given with azathioprine.

Co-trimoxazole, mesalazine, olsalazine, trimethoprim, ribavirin, and sulfasalazine These drugs may increase the risk of blood problems if taken with azathioprine.

Corticosteroids may increase the risk of infections and bowel problems.

PROLONGED USE

Prolonged use of azathioprine may reduce bone marrow activity, leading to a reduction of all types of blood cells. Some people have a genetic susceptibility to this effect. There is also a small increase in the risk of cancers affecting the immune system. Avoiding excessive exposure to sunlight may help to prevent adverse skin effects.

Monitoring Regular checks on blood chemistry and blood cell counts are carried out.

BACLOFEN

Brand names Lioresal, Lyflex
Used in the following combined preparations None

GENERAL INFORMATION

Baclofen is a muscle relaxant that acts on the central nervous system, including the spinal cord. The drug relieves the spasms, cramping, and muscle rigidity (spasticity) caused by various disorders, including multiple sclerosis, spinal cord injury, brain injury, cerebral palsy, or stroke. Although it does not cure any of these disorders, baclofen increases mobility, allowing other treatment, such as physiotherapy, to be carried out. It may also be used to treat hiccups due to distension of the stomach.

Baclofen is less likely to cause muscle weakness than similar drugs, and its side effects, such as dizziness or drowsiness, are usually temporary. Older people are more susceptible to side effects, especially during early stages of treatment.

INFORMATION FOR USERS

Your drug prescription is tailored for you. Do not alter dosage without checking with your doctor.

How taken/used

Tablets, liquid, injection (specialist use).

Frequency and timing of doses
3 x daily with food or milk.

Adult dosage range
15mg daily (starting dose). Daily dose may be increased by 15mg every 3 days as necessary. Maximum daily dose: 100mg.

Onset of effect
Some benefits may appear after 1–3 hours but full benefits may not be felt for several weeks. A dose 1 hour before a task will improve mobility.

Duration of action
Up to 8 hours.

Diet advice
None.

Storage
Keep in original container at room temperature out of the reach of children. Protect liquid preparations from light.

Missed dose
Take as soon as you remember. If your next dose is due within 2 hours, take a single dose now and skip the next.

Stopping the drug
Do not stop taking the drug without consulting your doctor, who will supervise a gradual reduction in dosage. Abrupt cessation may cause hallucinations, confusion, anxiety, seizures, and worsening spasticity.

Exceeding the dose
An occasional unintentional extra dose is unlikely to cause problems. Large overdoses may cause weakness, vomiting, and severe drowsiness. Notify your doctor.

SPECIAL PRECAUTIONS

Be sure to tell your doctor if:
- You have long-term liver or kidney problems.
- You have difficulty in passing urine.
- You have had a peptic ulcer.
- You have had epileptic seizures or a stroke.
- You have diabetes.
- You are being treated for hypertension.
- You have porphyria.
- You have Parkinson's disease.
- You have a history of psychiatric illness.
- You have breathing problems.
- You are taking other medicines.

 Pregnancy
Safety in pregnancy not established. Discuss with your doctor.

 Breast-feeding
The drug passes into the breast milk, but at normal doses adverse effects are unlikely. Discuss with your doctor.

 Infants and children
Reduced dose necessary.

 Over 60
Increased likelihood of adverse effects at start of treatment. Reduced initial dose may therefore be necessary.

 Driving and hazardous work
Avoid until you have learned how baclofen affects you; the drug can cause drowsiness, decreased alertness, and blurred vision.

 Alcohol
Avoid. Alcohol may increase the sedative effects of this drug.

Surgery and general anaesthetics
Be sure to inform your doctor or dentist that you are taking baclofen before you have a general anaesthetic.

POSSIBLE ADVERSE EFFECTS

The common adverse effects are related to the sedative effects of the drug. Such effects are minimized by starting with a low dose that is gradually increased.

Symptom/effect	Frequency		Discuss with doctor		Stop taking drug now	Call doctor now
	Common	Rare	Only if severe	In all cases		
Dizziness	●		●			
Drowsiness	●		●			
Nausea	●		●			
Muscle fatigue/weakness	●		●			
Confusion	●			●		
Depression or euphoria	●			●		
Difficulty in passing urine		●	●			
Constipation/diarrhoea		●	●			
Headache		●	●			
Blurred vision		●		●		

INTERACTIONS

Antihypertensive and diuretic drugs Baclofen may increase the blood-pressure-lowering effect of such drugs.

Drugs for parkinsonism Some drugs used for parkinsonism may cause confusion and hallucinations if taken with baclofen.

Sedatives All drugs with a sedative effect on the central nervous system may increase the sedative properties of baclofen.

Tricyclic antidepressants may increase the effects of baclofen, leading to muscle weakness.

PROLONGED USE

No problems expected.

BECLOMETASONE

Brand names Asmabec, Beclazone, Becodisks, Beconase, Clenil Modulite, Clipper, Pulvinal, Qvar, and others
Used in the following combined preparation Fostair

GENERAL INFORMATION

Beclometasone is a corticosteroid drug that is prescribed to relieve the symptoms of allergic rhinitis (as a nasal spray) and to control asthma (as an inhalant). It controls nasal symptoms by reducing inflammation and mucus production in the nose. It also helps to reduce chest symptoms, such as wheezing and coughing. People with asthma may take it regularly to reduce the severity and frequency of attacks. However, once an attack has started, the drug does not relieve symptoms. Beclometasone is given primarily to people whose asthma has not responded to treatment with bronchodilators alone (see p.48).

Beclometasone is also used orally to help treat acute ulcerative colitis if there is an inadequate response to aminosalicylates such as mesalazine.

There are few serious adverse effects associated with beclometasone when it is given topically by nasal spray or inhaler. Fungal infections of the mouth and throat (thrush) are a possible side effect of inhaling beclometasone. These can be mitigated by using a spacer device and by rinsing the mouth and gargling with water after use.

INFORMATION FOR USERS

Your drug prescription is tailored for you. Do not alter dosage without checking with your doctor.

How taken/used

Inhaler, nasal spray, tablets.

Frequency and timing of doses
2–4 x daily.

Dosage range
Adults 1–2 puffs 2–4 x daily according to preparation used (asthma); 1–2 sprays in each nostril 2–4 x daily (allergic rhinitis); 5mg daily orally for a maximum of 4 weeks.
Children Reduced dose according to age and weight. Tablets not recommended.

Onset of effect
Within 1 week (asthma); 1–3 days (allergic rhinitis). Full benefit may not be felt for up to 4 weeks (all conditions being treated).

Duration of action
Several days after stopping the drug.

Diet advice
None.

Storage
Keep in original container at room temperature out of the reach of children. Protect from light.

Missed dose
Take as soon as you remember. If your next dose is due within 2 hours, take a single dose now and skip the next.

Stopping the drug
Do not stop the drug without consulting your doctor; symptoms may recur. Sometimes a gradual reduction in dosage is recommended.

Exceeding the dose
An occasional unintentional extra dose is unlikely to cause problems. But if you notice any unusual symptoms, or if a large overdose has been taken, notify your doctor. Adverse effects may occur if the recommended dose is regularly exceeded over a prolonged period.

SPECIAL PRECAUTIONS

Be sure to tell your doctor if:
- You have had tuberculosis or another nasal or respiratory infection.
- You have a skin infection (cream/ointment).
- You have had recent nasal ulcers or nasal surgery.

 Pregnancy
No evidence of risk.

 Breast-feeding
No evidence of risk.

 Infants and children
Reduced dose necessary.

 Over 60
No known problems.

 Driving and hazardous work
No known problems.

 Alcohol
No known problems.

POSSIBLE ADVERSE EFFECTS

The occurrence and severity of side effects depend on the dose and duration of use. The main side effect of the inhaler is thrush of the throat and mouth, and irritation of the nose and throat for the nasal spray.

Symptom/effect	Frequency		Discuss with doctor		Stop taking drug now	Call doctor now
	Common	Rare	Only if severe	In all cases		
Inhaler/nasal spray						
Nasal discomfort/irritation	●		●			
Cough	●		●			
Bruising	●		●			
Sore throat/hoarseness	●			●		
Nosebleed	●			●		

INTERACTIONS

None.

PROLONGED USE

Long-term use can lead to peptic ulcers, glaucoma, muscle weakness, osteoporosis, growth retardation in children, and, rarely, adrenal gland suppression. However, courses of oral beclometasone lasting more than 4 weeks are not generally recommended, which minimizes the risk of these side effects. Patients on long-term treatment should carry a steroid card or wear a MedicAlert bracelet.

Monitoring Periodic checks on adrenal gland function may be required if large doses are being taken. Children should have their height monitored.

BENDROFLUMETHIAZIDE (BENDROFLUAZIDE)

Brand name Aprinox
Used in the following combined preparation Prestim

GENERAL INFORMATION

Bendroflumethiazide belongs to the thiazide diuretic group of drugs, which increase the amount of salt and water the kidneys remove from the body. It is used predominantly for treating high blood pressure (see Antihypertensive drugs, p.60). The drug may also be used for reducing oedema (water retention) caused by heart, kidney, or liver conditions, and for treating premenstrual oedema. As with all thiazides, this drug increases the loss of potassium in the urine, which can cause various symptoms (see p.57), and increases the likelihood of irregular heart rhythms, particularly if taken with digoxin for heart failure. Although this effect is rare with low doses, potassium supplements may be given with bendroflumethiazide as a precaution.

INFORMATION FOR USERS

Your drug prescription is tailored for you. Do not alter dosage without checking with your doctor.

How taken/used

Tablets.

Frequency and timing of doses
Once daily, early in the day. (Sometimes 1–3 x per week.)

Adult dosage range
2.5–10g daily.

Onset of effect
Within 2 hours but takes weeks to produce maximum effect on blood pressure.

Duration of action
6–18 hours.

Diet advice
Use of this drug may reduce potassium in the body, so you should eat plenty of fresh fruit and vegetables. Discuss with your doctor the advisability of reducing salt intake as a further precaution for hypertension.

Storage
Keep in original container at room temperature out of the reach of children.

Missed dose
No cause for concern, but take as soon as you remember. However, if it is late in the day do not take the missed dose, or you may need to get up during the night to pass urine. Take the next scheduled dose as usual.

Stopping the drug
Do not stop taking the drug without consulting your doctor; symptoms may recur.

Exceeding the dose
An occasional unintentional extra dose is unlikely to be a cause for concern. But if you notice any unusual symptoms, or if a large overdose has been taken, notify your doctor.

SPECIAL PRECAUTIONS

Be sure to tell your doctor if:
- You have long-term liver or kidney problems.
- You have or have had gout.
- You have diabetes.
- You have Addison's disease.
- You have hyperparathyroidism.
- You have lactose intolerance.
- You have systemic lupus erythematosus.
- You are taking other medicines.

 Pregnancy
Not usually prescribed. Safety in pregnancy not established. Discuss with your doctor.

 Breast-feeding
The drug passes into breast milk but the level is usually too low to harm the baby. Discuss with your doctor.

 Infants and children
Not usually prescribed. Reduced dose necessary.

 Over 60
Reduced dose may be necessary.

 Driving and hazardous work
No special problems.

 Alcohol
No problems expected if consumption is kept low.

POSSIBLE ADVERSE EFFECTS

Adverse effects resulting from potassium loss can be corrected with potassium supplements. Bendroflumethiazide may precipitate gout in susceptible people, and diabetes may become more difficult to control. Blood cholesterol level may rise slightly.

Symptom/effect	Frequency		Discuss with doctor		Stop taking drug now	Call doctor now
	Common	Rare	Only if severe	In all cases		
Dizziness		●	●			
Nausea/diarrhoea/constipation		●	●			
Lethargy/fatigue		●	●			
Leg cramps		●	●			
Erectile dysfunction		●	●			
Rash	●			●	●	

INTERACTIONS

Non-steroidal anti-inflammatory drugs (NSAIDs) may reduce diuretic and anti-hypertensive effect of bendroflumethiazide, and bendroflumethiazide may increase kidney toxicity of NSAIDs.

Digoxin The effects of digoxin may be increased if excessive potassium is lost.

Anti-arrhythmic drugs Low potassium levels may increase these drugs' toxicity.

Lithium Bendroflumethiazide may increase lithium levels in the blood.

Corticosteroids These drugs further increase potassium loss when they are taken with bendroflumethiazide. Potassium supplements may be necessary to correct the deficiency. Corticosteroids may also reduce the diuretic effect of bendroflumethiazide.

PROLONGED USE

Prolonged use of this drug can lead to excessive loss of potassium and imbalances of other salts.

Monitoring Blood tests may be performed periodically to check kidney function and levels of potassium and other salts.

BENZOYL PEROXIDE

Brand names Acnecide, Brevoxyl, Oxy 10, Oxy On-the-Spot, PanOxyl
Used in the following combined preparations Duac Once Daily, Epiduo, Quinoderm

GENERAL INFORMATION

Benzoyl peroxide is used in a variety of topical preparations for the treatment of acne. Available over the counter, it comes in concentrations of varying strengths for mild to moderate acne.

Benzoyl peroxide works by softening and shedding the top layer of skin and unblocking the sebaceous glands. It can also reduce inflammation of blocked hair follicles by killing the bacteria that infect them.

Benzoyl peroxide may cause irritation due to its drying effect on the skin, but this generally diminishes with time. The drug should be applied to the affected areas as directed on the label. Washing the area prior to application greatly enhances the drug's beneficial effects.

Side effects are less likely if treatment is started with a preparation containing a low concentration of benzoyl peroxide, and changed to a stronger preparation gradually and only if necessary. Marked dryness and peeling of the skin may occur, but can usually be controlled by reducing the frequency of application. Care should be taken to avoid contact of the drug with the eyes, mouth, and mucous membranes. It is also advisable to avoid excessive exposure to sunlight. Preparations of benzoyl peroxide can bleach clothing and hair.

QUICK REFERENCE

Drug group Drug for acne (p.137)
Overdose danger rating Low
Dependence rating Low
Prescription needed No (most preparations)
Available as generic Yes

INFORMATION FOR USERS

Follow instructions on the label. Call your doctor if symptoms worsen.

How taken/used

Cream, body wash, gel, lotion.

Frequency and timing of doses
1–2 x daily (after washing with soap and water).

Dosage range
Start with the lowest strength preparation (2.5 per cent) and, if necessary, increase gradually to highest strength (10 per cent).

Onset of effect
Reduces oiliness of skin immediately. Acne usually improves within 4–6 weeks.

Duration of action
24–48 hours.

Diet advice
None.

Storage
Keep in original container at room temperature out of the reach of children.

Missed dose
Apply as soon as you remember.

Stopping the drug
Can be safely stopped as soon as you no longer need it.

Exceeding the dose
A single extra application is unlikely to cause problems. Regular overuse may result in extensive irritation, peeling, redness, and swelling of the skin.

SPECIAL PRECAUTIONS

Be sure to tell your doctor or pharmacist before using this drug if:
- You have eczema.
- You have sunburn.
- You have had a previous allergic reaction to benzoyl peroxide.
- You are taking other medicines.

Pregnancy
No evidence of risk.

Breast-feeding
No evidence of risk.

Infants and children
Not usually recommended under 12 years except under medical supervision.

Over 60
Not usually required.

Driving and hazardous work
No known problems.

Alcohol
No known problems.

POSSIBLE ADVERSE EFFECTS

Application of benzoyl peroxide may cause temporary burning or stinging of the skin. Redness, peeling, and swelling may result from excessive drying of the skin and usually clears up if the treatment is stopped or used less frequently. If severe burning, blistering, or crusting occur, stop using benzoyl peroxide and consult your doctor.

Symptom/effect	Frequency		Discuss with doctor		Stop taking drug now	Call doctor now
	Common	Rare	Only if severe	In all cases		
Skin irritation	●		●			
Dryness/peeling	●		●			
Stinging/redness	●		●			
Blistering/crusting/swelling		●		●	●	

PROLONGED USE

Benzoyl peroxide usually takes 4–6 weeks to produce an effect. If the acne has not improved after 6 weeks, consult your doctor.

INTERACTIONS

Skin-drying preparations Medicated cosmetics, soaps, toiletries, and other anti-acne preparations increase the likelihood of dryness and irritation of the skin with benzoyl peroxide.

BETAHISTINE

Brand name Serc
Used in the following combined preparations None

GENERAL INFORMATION

Betahistine, a drug that resembles the naturally occurring substance histamine in some of its effects, was introduced in the 1970s as a treatment for Ménière's disease, which is caused by the pressure of excess fluid in the inner ear.

Taken regularly, betahistine reduces both the frequency and the severity of the nausea and vertigo attacks that characterize this condition. It may also be used to treat tinnitus (ringing in the ears) and hearing loss due to Ménière's disease. Betahistine is thought to work by reducing pressure in the inner ear, possibly by improving blood flow in the small blood vessels in the area. Drug treatment is not successful in all cases, however, and surgery may be needed.

QUICK REFERENCE

Drug group Drug for Ménière's disease (p.46)
Overdose danger rating High
Dependence rating Low
Prescription needed Yes
Available as generic Yes

INFORMATION FOR USERS

Your drug prescription is tailored for you. Do not alter dosage without checking with your doctor.

How taken/used

Tablets.

Frequency and timing of doses
3 x daily with or after food.

Adult dosage range
24–48mg daily.

Onset of effect
Usually within 1 hour, but full effect may not be reached for some time.

Duration of action
6–12 hours.

Diet advice
None.

Storage
Keep in original container at room temperature out of the reach of children.

Missed dose
Take as soon as you remember. If your next dose is due within 2 hours, take a single dose now and skip the next.

Stopping the drug
Do not stop the drug without consulting your doctor; symptoms may recur.

OVERDOSE ACTION

Seek immediate medical advice in all cases. Large overdoses may cause collapse and seizures requiring emergency action.

See Drug poisoning emergency guide (p.518).

POSSIBLE ADVERSE EFFECTS

Adverse effects from betahistine are minor and rarely cause problems.

Symptom/effect	Frequency		Discuss with doctor		Stop taking drug now	Call doctor now
	Common	Rare	Only if severe	In all cases		
Nausea	●		●			
Indigestion	●		●			
Headache		●	●			
Itching		●	●			
Rash		●		●		

INTERACTIONS

Antihistamines Although unproven, there is a possibility that betahistine may reduce the effects of these drugs, and antihistamines may reduce the effects of betahistine.

SPECIAL PRECAUTIONS

Be sure to tell your doctor if:
- You have asthma.
- You have a history of peptic ulcers.
- You have lactose intolerance.
- You have phaeochromocytoma.
- You are taking other medicines.

Pregnancy
Safety in pregnancy not established. Discuss with your doctor.

Breast-feeding
The drug may pass into the breast milk, and effects on the baby are unknown, but at normal doses adverse effects are unlikely. Discuss with your doctor.

Infants and children
Not recommended.

Over 60
No special problems.

Driving and hazardous work
Avoid such activities until you have learned how the drug affects you because rarely it may cause drowsiness.

Alcohol
No special problems.

PROLONGED USE

No special problems.

BETAMETHASONE

Brand names Betacap, Betesil, Betnelan, Betnesol, Betnovate, Bettamousse, Diprosone, Vistamethasone
Used in the following combined preparations Betnesol-N, Betnovate-C, Diprosalic, Dovobet, Enstilar, Fucibet, Lotriderm

GENERAL INFORMATION

Betamethasone is a corticosteroid drug used to treat a variety of conditions. When injected directly into the joints it relieves joint inflammation and the pain and stiffness of rheumatoid arthritis. It is given by mouth or injection to treat certain endocrine conditions affecting the pituitary and adrenal glands, and some blood disorders. It is also used topically (p.134) to treat skin disorders such as eczema and psoriasis.

When taken for short periods, low or moderate doses of betamethasone rarely cause serious side effects. High dosages or prolonged use can lead to many adverse effects (see table below).

INFORMATION FOR USERS

Your drug prescription is tailored for you. Do not alter dosage without checking with your doctor.

How taken/used

Tablets, injection, cream, ointment, rectal ointment, lotion, scalp solution, eye ointment, eye/ear/nose drops.

Frequency and timing of doses
Usually once daily in the morning (systemic). Otherwise varies according to disorder being treated.

Dosage range
Varies; follow your doctor's instructions.

Onset of effect
Within 30 minutes (injection); within 48 hours (other forms).

Duration of action
Up to 24 hours.

Diet advice
A low-sodium and high-potassium diet may be recommended when the oral form of the drug is prescribed for extended periods. Follow the advice of your doctor.

Storage
Keep in original container at room temperature out of the reach of children. Protect from light.

Missed dose
Take as soon as you remember. If your next dose is due within 2 hours, take a single dose now and skip the next.

Stopping the drug
Do not stop tablets without consulting your doctor, who may supervise a gradual reduction in dosage. Abrupt cessation after long-term treatment may cause problems with the pituitary and adrenal gland system.

Exceeding the dose
An occasional unintentional extra dose is unlikely to cause problems. But if you notice any unusual symptoms, or if a large overdose has been taken, notify your doctor.

SPECIAL PRECAUTIONS

Be sure to tell your doctor if:
- You have a psychiatric disorder.
- You have a heart condition.
- You have glaucoma.
- You have high blood pressure.
- You have a history of epilepsy.
- You have had a peptic ulcer.
- You have had tuberculosis.
- You have any infection.
- You have diabetes.
- You have liver or kidney problems.
- You are taking other medicines.

Pregnancy
No evidence of risk with topical preparations. Taken as tablets in low doses, harm to the baby is unlikely. Discuss with your doctor.

Breast-feeding
No risk with topical preparations. Normal doses of tablets are unlikely to have adverse effects on the baby. Discuss with your doctor

Infants and children
Reduced dose necessary.

Over 60
Reduced dose may be necessary.

Driving and hazardous work
No known problems.

Alcohol
Keep consumption low. Betamethasone tablets increase the risk of peptic ulcers.

Infection
Avoid exposure to chickenpox, measles, or shingles if you are on betamethasone tablets.

POSSIBLE ADVERSE EFFECTS

Serious adverse effects occur only when high doses are taken by mouth for long periods. Topical preparations are unlikely to cause adverse effects unless overused.

Symptom/effect	Frequency		Discuss with doctor		Stop taking drug now	Call doctor now
	Common	Rare	Only if severe	In all cases		
Indigestion	●			●		
Weight gain		●		●		
Acne		●		●		
Muscle weakness		●		●		
Mood changes		●		●		
Blood in faeces/tarry faeces		●		●	●	●

INTERACTIONS

Insulin, antidiabetic drugs, and oral anticoagulant drugs Betamethasone may alter insulin requirements and the effects of these drugs.

Antifungal drugs (e.g. itraconazole) may increase the effects of betamethasone.

Antihypertensive drugs and drugs used in myasthenia gravis Betamethasone may reduce the effects of these drugs.

Anticonvulsants and barbiturates These drugs may reduce the effects of betamethasone.

Vaccines Betamethasone can interact with some vaccines. Discuss with your doctor before having any vaccinations.

PROLONGED USE

Prolonged use by mouth can lead to peptic ulcers, glaucoma, osteoporosis, muscle weakness, and growth retardation in children. Prolonged use of topical treatment may also lead to skin thinning. People taking betamethasone tablets regularly should carry a steroid treatment card or wear a MedicAlert bracelet.

BEVACIZUMAB

Brand name Avastin, Zirabev
Used in the following combined preparations None

GENERAL INFORMATION

Bevacizumab is a monoclonal antibody (see p.113) used with other anticancer drugs for treating advanced cancer of the bowel, breast, lung, ovary, or kidney. It blocks vascular endothelial growth factor (VEGF), a protein produced by cancer metastases that promotes the growth of new blood vessels (angiogenesis). Blocking VEGF inhibits blood vessel growth and deprives metastases of nutrients and oxygen.

But bevacizumab does not destroy tumours and the cancer will eventually progress. On average, the drug improves survival for a few months.

A portion of the bevacizumab molecule is marketed separately under the generic name ranibizumab. This has the same anti-angiogenesis properties as bevacizumab and, given by injection into the eye, is used to treat wet age-related macular degeneration.

(see p.113)

QUICK REFERENCE

Drug group Anticancer drug (p.112)
Overdose danger rating Medium
Dependence rating Low
Prescription needed Yes
Available as generic Not currently (will be available from 2022)

(p.112)

INFORMATION FOR USERS

This drug is given only under medical supervision and is not for self-administration.

How taken/used

Intravenous infusion.

Frequency and timing of doses
Once every 2–3 weeks.

Adult dosage range
Dosage is determined individually according to the type of cancer and the patient's body weight.

Onset of effect
4–6 hours.

Duration of action
18–20 days.

Diet advice
Bevacizumab can cause nausea and vomiting so it is advisable not to eat or drink for a few hours before treatment.

Storage
Not applicable. This drug is not normally kept in the home.

Missed dose
If you miss your scheduled dose, contact your doctor as soon as possible.

Stopping the drug
Discuss with your doctor. Stopping the drug prematurely may lead to a worsening of the underlying condition.

Exceeding the dose
Overdosage is unlikely since treatment is carefully monitored and supervised.

POSSIBLE ADVERSE EFFECTS

Bevacizumab frequently causes fatigue and gastrointestinal symptoms; increased blood pressure is also common. More serious and rarer side effects include internal bleeding from the cancer, stroke, and heart attack. Normal wound healing is also impaired and there is a risk of jaw bone problems, causing pain and swelling in the jaw.

Symptom/effect	Frequency		Discuss with doctor		Stop taking drug now	Call doctor now
	Common	Rare	Only if severe	In all cases		
Diarrhoea/nausea/vomiting	●		●			
Chest pain/breathlessness		●		●		●
Jaw pain/swelling		●		●		
Seizures/loss of vision		●		●	●	●
Blood in faeces/coughing up blood		●		●	●	●
Severe abdominal pain		●		●	●	●

INTERACTIONS

Bisphosphonates Those who have previously been treated with intravenous bisphosphonates or who are currently being treated with bisphosphonates are at increased risk of jaw bone problems if also being treated with bevacizumab.

Live vaccines (e.g. influenza; measles, mumps, rubella (MMR)) These are predicted to increase the risk of generalized infection if given with bevacizumab.

Anticoagulation drugs (e.g. rivaroxaban, apixaban) are predicted to increase the risk of bleeding when given with bevacizumab.

SPECIAL PRECAUTIONS

Be sure to tell your doctor if:
- You have a history of colitis or have previously had a bowel perforation or fistula.
- You have recently had major surgery.
- You have high blood pressure, heart failure, or a history of thromboembolism, stroke, or heart attacks.
- You have liver or kidney problems.
- You have a blood clotting disorder.
- You are pregnant, planning a pregnancy, or breast-feeding.
- You are taking other medicines, especially anticoagulants.

Pregnancy
Must not be used during pregnancy. Women of childbearing age must use contraception during treatment and for up to 6 months afterwards.

Breast-feeding
Women must not breast-feed during treatment and for at least six months afterwards.

Infants and children
Unlikely to be necessary as the conditions for which the drug is used occur almost exclusively in adults.

Over 60
Increased risk of adverse effects.

Driving and hazardous work
No known problems.

Alcohol
No known problems.

PROLONGED USE

Prolonged treatment increases the risks of severe hypertension (high blood pressure), bleeding or clotting problems, and bowel perforation. The risks increase with the dose and duration of treatment.

Monitoring You will have blood tests to check your blood cell count and clotting, and regular checks of your blood pressure. Your urine will be tested for protein. You may need to have a dental check-up before beginning treatment.

BEZAFIBRATE

Brand names Bezalip, Bezalip-Mono, Caberzol XL, Fibrazate (bezatard) XL
Used in the following combined preparations None

GENERAL INFORMATION

Bezafibrate belongs to a group of drugs, usually called fibrates, that lower lipid (fat) levels in the blood. Fibrates are particularly effective in decreasing levels of triglycerides in the blood. They also reduce blood levels of cholesterol. Raised levels of lipids in the blood are associated with atherosclerosis (deposition of fat in blood vessel walls). This can lead to coronary heart disease (for example, angina and heart attacks) and cerebrovascular disease (for example, stroke). When bezafibrate is taken with a diet low in saturated fats, there is modest evidence that the risk of coronary heart disease is reduced. Bezafibrate should not be used with statins (another group of lipid-lowering drugs) due to the increased risk of muscle damage.

QUICK REFERENCE

Drug group Lipid-lowering drug (p.61)

Overdose danger rating Low

Dependence rating Low

Prescription needed Yes

Available as generic Yes

INFORMATION FOR USERS

Your drug prescription is tailored for you. Do not alter dosage without checking with your doctor.

How taken/used

Tablets.

Frequency and timing of doses
1–3 x daily with a little liquid after a meal.

Adult dosage range
400–600mg daily.

Onset of effect
It may take weeks for blood fat levels to be reduced, and it takes months or years for fat deposits in the arteries to be reduced. Treatment should be withdrawn if no adequate response is obtained within 3–4 months.

Duration of action
About 6–24 hours. This may vary according to the individual.

Diet advice
A low-fat and low-carbohydrate diet will have been recommended. Follow the advice of your doctor.

Storage
Keep in original container at room temperature out of the reach of children.

Missed dose
Take as soon as you remember. If your next dose is due within 4 hours (and you take it once daily), take a single dose now and skip the next. If you take 2–3 times daily, take the next dose as normal.

Stopping the drug
Do not stop the drug without consulting your doctor.

Exceeding the dose
An occasional unintentional extra dose is unlikely to be a cause for concern. But if you notice unusual symptoms, notify your doctor.

SPECIAL PRECAUTIONS

Be sure to tell your doctor if:
- You have long-term liver or kidney problems.
- You have a history of gallbladder disease.
- You are taking other medicines.

Pregnancy
Safety in pregnancy not established. Discuss with your doctor.

Breast-feeding
The drug may pass into the breast milk and may affect the baby. Discuss with your doctor.

Infants and children
Not usually prescribed.

Over 60
No special problems expected.

Driving and hazardous work
Avoid such activities until you have learned how bezafibrate affects you because the drug can cause dizziness.

Alcohol
No special problems.

POSSIBLE ADVERSE EFFECTS

The most common adverse effects are those involving the gastrointestinal tract, such as loss of appetite and nausea. These effects normally diminish as treatment continues.

Symptom/effect	Frequency		Discuss with doctor		Stop taking drug now	Call doctor now
	Common	Rare	Only if severe	In all cases		
Nausea/loss of appetite	●		●			
Diarrhoea		●	●			
Dizziness/fatigue		●	●			
Skin rash		●		●		
Headache		●		●		
Muscle pain/cramp/weakness		●		●		
Abdominal pain		●		●		

INTERACTIONS

Anticoagulants Bezafibrate may increase the effect of anticoagulants such as warfarin. Your anticoagulant dose will be reduced when starting bezafibrate.

Monoamine oxidase inhibitors (MAOIs) There is a risk of liver damage when bezafibrate is taken with an MAOI.

Antidiabetic drugs These may interact with bezafibrate to lower blood sugar.

Simvastatin and other lipid-lowering drugs whose name ends in "statin" There is an increased risk of muscle damage if bezafibrate is taken with these drugs.

Ciclosporin This may interact with bezafibrate to impair kidney function. Bezafibrate may also raise blood levels of ciclosporin.

PROLONGED USE

No problems expected, but patients with kidney disease will need special care as there is a high risk of muscle problems developing.

Monitoring Blood tests will be performed occasionally to monitor the effect of the drug on lipids in the blood.

BISOPROLOL

Brand names Cardicor
Used in the following combined preparations None

GENERAL INFORMATION

Bisoprolol is a cardioselective beta blocker (see p.55). It is used in the treatment of angina and, usually in combination with an ACE inhibitor (see p.56) and a diuretic (see p.57), for treating heart failure. It is also used to treat high blood pressure, but is not usually used to initiate treatment.

Bisoprolol is less likely than non-cardioselective beta blockers to provoke breathing difficulties, but, nevertheless, it is not usually given to patients with asthma. It may also slow the body's response to low blood sugar if you have diabetes and you are taking insulin.

QUICK REFERENCE

Drug group Beta blocker (p.55)
Overdose danger rating High
Dependence rating Low
Prescription needed Yes
Available as generic Yes

INFORMATION FOR USERS

Your drug prescription is tailored for you. Do not alter dosage without checking with your doctor.

How taken/used

Tablets.

Frequency and timing of doses
Once daily.

Adult dosage range
Heart failure 1.25mg per day (initial dose), increasing to 10mg.
Hypertension and angina 5–20mg.

Onset of effect
2 hours. Full antihypertensive effect seen after 2 weeks.

Duration of action
24 hours.

Diet advice
None.

Storage
Keep in original container in a cool dry place, out of the reach of children.

Missed dose
If your next dose is due within 12 hours, take a single dose now. If more than 12 hours have passed, skip the missed dose and take the next dose at the scheduled time.

Stopping the drug
Do not stop taking the drug without consulting your doctor; abrupt cessation may lead to worsening of the underlying condition. The drug should be withdrawn gradually.

OVERDOSE ACTION

Seek immediate medical advice. Take emergency action if breathing difficulties, collapse, or loss of consciousness occur.

See Drug poisoning emergency guide (p.518).

POSSIBLE ADVERSE EFFECTS

Bisoprolol has adverse effects that are common to most beta blockers. Symptoms are usually temporary and tend to diminish with long-term use.

Symptom/effect	Frequency		Discuss with doctor		Stop taking drug now	Call doctor now
	Common	Rare	Only if severe	In all cases		
Dizziness	●		●			
Lethargy/fatigue	●			●		
Cold hands and feet	●			●		
Nausea/vomiting	●			●		
Nightmares/vivid dreams		●		●	●	
Rash/dry eyes		●		●		
Fainting/palpitations		●		●	●	●
Breathlessness/wheeze		●		●	●	●

SPECIAL PRECAUTIONS

Be sure to tell your doctor if:
- You have, or have had, asthma.
- You have heart problems.
- You have liver or kidney problems.
- You have diabetes.
- You have psoriasis.
- You have phaeochromocytoma.
- You are taking other medicines.

Pregnancy
Not normally prescribed. May affect the developing baby. Discuss with your doctor.

Breast-feeding
The drug passes into breast milk but the small amount present is unlikely to affect your baby. Discuss with your doctor.

Infants and children
Not recommended.

Over 60
No special problems.

Driving and hazardous work
Avoid such activities until you have learned how bisoprolol affects you because the drug can cause fatigue and dizziness.

Alcohol
Avoid excessive intake. Alcohol may increase the blood-pressure-lowering effect of bisoprolol.

Surgery and general anaesthetics
Occasionally, bisoprolol may need to be stopped before you have a general anaesthetic, but only do this after discussion with your doctor or dentist.

INTERACTIONS

Other antihypertensives may enhance bisoprolol's blood-pressure-lowering effect and some may worsen heart failure.

Non-steroidal anti-inflammatory drugs (NSAIDs) may reduce the blood-pressure-lowering effect of bisoprolol.

Insulin and oral antidiabetics Bisoprolol may increase the blood-sugar-lowering effect of these drugs and may also mask symptoms of low blood sugar.

Cardiac glycosides (e.g. digoxin) These may increase the heart-slowing effect of bisoprolol.

Calcium channel blockers These may cause low blood pressure, a slow heartbeat, and heart failure if taken with bisoprolol.

PROLONGED USE

No special problems.

BOTULINUM TOXIN

Brand names Azzalure, Bocouture, Botox, Dysport, NeuroBloc, Xeomin
Used in the following combined preparations None

GENERAL INFORMATION

Botulinum toxin is a neurotoxin (nerve poison) produced naturally by the bacterium *Clostridium botulinum*. The toxin causes botulism, a rare but serious form of food poisoning.

Research has found that there are several slightly different components in the toxin. Two are used medically: botulinum A toxin and botulinum B toxin. They are used therapeutically to treat conditions in which there are painful muscle spasms – for example, spastic foot deformity, blepharospasm (spasm of the eyelids, causing them almost to close), hemifacial spasm, and spasmodic torticollis (spasms of the neck muscles, causing the head to jerk). Toxin A is also used to treat very resistant and distressing cases of hyperhidrosis (excessive sweating). The effects produced by the toxins may last for 2–3 months, until new nerve endings have formed.

Botulinum toxin is used cosmetically to remove facial wrinkles by paralysing the muscles under the skin.

INFORMATION FOR USERS

This drug is given only under medical supervision and is not for self-administration.

How taken/used

Injection.

Frequency and timing of doses
Every 2–3 months, depending on response.

Adult dosage range
Dose depends on the particular condition being treated. Individual injections may range from 1.25 units to 100 units. The number of injection sites depends on the size and number of the muscles to be paralysed. Specialist judgement is necessary.

Onset of effect
Within 3 days to 2 weeks.

Duration of action
2–3 months.

Diet advice
None.

Storage
Not applicable as the drug is not normally kept in the home.

Missed dose
Attend for treatment at the next possible time.

Stopping the drug
If having botulinum toxin for medical reasons, discuss with your doctor whether you should stop receiving the drug. Cosmetic use of the drug can be stopped safely at any time.

Exceeding the dose
When used for medical reasons, overdose is unlikely since treatment is carefully monitored. If the drug was injected into your face for cosmetic reasons, the effects of an overdose will develop gradually over several days; you should be especially alert for any weakness in your neck or swallowing difficulty and, if they occur, you should contact your doctor immediately.

SPECIAL PRECAUTIONS

Be sure to tell your doctor if:
- You have any difficulty in swallowing.
- You are taking an anticoagulant drug or have a bleeding disorder.
- You are allergic to botulinum toxin.
- You are taking other medicines.

 Pregnancy
Not prescribed.

 Breast-feeding
Not prescribed.

 Infants and children
Reduced dose necessary

 Over 60
No special problems.

 Driving and hazardous work
Do not drive until you know how botulinum toxin affects you; the drug may impair ability.

 Alcohol
No known problems.

PROLONGED USE

To maintain the desired effects, the drug may have to be administered at regular intervals.

POSSIBLE ADVERSE EFFECTS

Some of the adverse effects depend on the site of injection. Misplaced injections may paralyse unintended muscle groups. All paralyses are likely to be long lasting.

Symptom/effect	Frequency		Discuss with doctor		Stop taking drug now	Call doctor now
	Common	Rare	Only if severe	In all cases		
Reduced blinking/dry eye	●			●		
Painful swallowing	●			●		
Pain at site/local weakness	●			●		
Glaucoma/painful eye		●		●		
Headache	●		●			
Neck weakness/head tremor		●		●		
Hypersensitivity reactions		●		●		
Difficulty in swallowing		●		●	●	●

INTERACTIONS

Aminoglycoside antibiotics and other drugs affecting neuromuscular transmission (e.g. curare-like muscle relaxant drugs) can intensify the effect of botulinum toxin.

BRIMONIDINE

Brand names Alphagan, Mirvaso
Used in the following combined preparations Combigan (with timolol), Simbrinza (with brinzolamide)

GENERAL INFORMATION

Brimonidine is a sympathomimetic drug (alpha-adrenoceptor agonist; see p.35) that is available for use in the form of eye drops or gel.

As eye drops, brimonidine is used to reduce intra-ocular (inside the eye) pressure in the treatment of glaucoma, when patients cannot tolerate topical beta blockers (such as timolol). It may also be used in conjunction with other topical agents, when lower intra-ocular pressure is not achieved by a single agent. It works by reducing the production and increasing the outflow of the fluid inside the eye.

As a gel, it is used for symptomatic treatment of facial redness caused by rosacea in adult patients. Side effects of brimonidine are usually limited to the local area where the drug is applied; however, systemic side effects such as slowing of the heart rate, low blood pressure, and dizziness may occur. Care should be taken to minimize application just to irritated or damaged skin when applying gel preparations.

QUICK REFERENCE

Drug group Drug for glaucoma (p.128)

Overdose danger rating Medium

Dependence rating Low

Prescription needed Yes

Available as generic Yes

INFORMATION FOR USERS

Your drug prescription is tailored for you. Do not alter dosage without checking with your doctor.

How taken/used

Eye drops, gel.

Frequency and timing of doses
Twice daily (eye drops); once daily (gel to skin). If more than one type of eye drops is to be used, the different drugs should be instilled at least 5 minutes apart. Similarly, the gel should be applied only to the face; any other products can be applied after the gel has dried. Wash hands thoroughly after application.

Adult dosage range
1 drop per eye, twice daily (eye drops). Once daily, max 1 g (pea-size drop) per application (gel). Treatment should be initiated with a smaller amount of gel for at least 1 week; it can then be gradually increased.

Onset of effect
0.5–2 hours.

Duration of action
12 hours.

Diet advice
None.

Storage
Keep the eye drops in the outer cardboard package to protect from light. Store at room temperature, out of reach of children. Discard any unused solution 4 weeks after opening.

Missed dose
Apply the next dose as normal.

Stopping the drug
Do not stop taking the drug without consulting your doctor; symptoms may recur.

Exceeding the dose
An occasional unintentional extra application is unlikely to cause problems. Excessive use may irritate the eye and produce adverse effects in other parts of your body, notably low blood pressure, lethargy, and slow heart rate.

POSSIBLE ADVERSE EFFECTS

The most common side effects are redness, burning, or stinging of the eye, and mouth dryness. These are usually transient and not severe enough to require stopping treatment.

Symptom/effect	Frequency		Discuss with doctor		Stop taking drug now	Call doctor now
	Common	Rare	Only if severe	In all cases		
Eye irritation	●		●			
Blurred vision	●		●			
Eye pain/eye discharge	●		●			
Eye/mouth dryness	●		●			
Headache/drowsiness	●		●			
Lack of energy/fatigue	●		●			
Rash/itching	●			●		
Eye/facial swelling		●		●	●	●

INTERACTIONS

Monoamine oxidase inhibitors (MAOIs)
When used with brimonidine, may result in an increased systemic side effect such as hypotension (low blood pressure).

Tricyclic antidepressants (e.g. amitriptyline, imipramine) and mianserin
When used with brimonidine, may result in an increased systemic side effect such as hypotension (low blood pressure).

SPECIAL PRECAUTIONS

Be sure to tell your doctor if:
- You wear contact lenses or have dry eyes.
- You are allergic to brimonidine or any of the ingredients in the formulation.
- You have heart or blood vessel problems (such as Raynaud's phenomenon).
- You are taking any other medicines, notably monoamine oxidase inhibitor (MAOI) therapy or antidepressants.

 Pregnancy
Safety in pregnancy not established. Discuss with your doctor.

 Breast-feeding
Safety in breast-feeding not established. Discuss with your doctor.

 Infants and children
Not recommended for children under the age of 12 (eye drops) or 18 (gel).

 Over 60
No dose adjustment required.

 Driving and hazardous work
Eye drops may cause fatigue, drowsiness, and blurred vision. Wait until the symptoms have cleared before such activities.

 Alcohol
Avoid. Alcohol may increase the sedative effect of the drug.

PROLONGED USE

There is no evidence that prolonged use of brimonidine causes any specific problems.

Monitoring Your doctor will continue to monitor the control of the glaucoma.

BRINZOLAMIDE

Brand name Azopt
Used in the following combined preparations Azarga (with timolol), Simbrinza (with brimonidine)

GENERAL INFORMATION

Brinzolamide is a carbonic anhydrase inhibitor (a type of diuretic; see p.57) used in the form of eye drops to treat glaucoma and/or ocular hypertension (high pressure inside the eye). The drug inhibits the action of the enzyme carbonic anhydrase inside the eye; this decreases the amount of fluid produced inside the eye, so lowering the intra-ocular pressure.

Brinzolamide is used on its own in cases where beta blockers (see p.55) such as timolol are contraindicated, or as combined therapy with beta blockers or prostaglandin analogues when a beta blocker alone does not lower the pressure sufficiently. Most side effects are local to the eye, but systemic effects may occur occasionally if enough of the drug is absorbed into the bloodstream.

QUICK REFERENCE

Drug group Drug for glaucoma (p.128)

Overdose danger rating Low

Dependence rating Low

Prescription needed Yes

Available as generic Yes

INFORMATION FOR USERS

Your drug prescription is tailored for you. Do not alter dosage without checking with your doctor.

How taken/used

Eye drops.

Frequency and timing of doses
2–3 x daily.

Adult dosage range
One drop in the affected eye(s) or as directed. If using additional eye drops, allow 5 minutes between using brinzolamide and applying the different drops into each eye.

Onset of effect
0.5–2 hours.

Duration of action
6–9 hours.

Diet advice
None.

Storage
Keep in original container at room temperature out of reach of children. Protect from light. Discard eye drops 4 weeks after opening.

Missed dose
Use the next dose as normal. Do not exceed one drop in the eye(s) three times daily.

Stopping the drug
Do not stop the drug without consulting with your doctor; symptoms may recur.

Exceeding the dose
An occasional unintentional extra dose is not likely to cause problems. Excessive use may irritate the eye and cause adverse effects in other body systems; discuss with your doctor.

SPECIAL PRECAUTIONS

Be sure to tell your doctor if:
- You wear contact lenses or have dry eyes.
- You are allergic to brinzolamide, sulfonamides (such as in co-trimoxazole), or any of the ingredients in the formulation including benzalkonium chloride.
- You have severe kidney problems.
- You are taking any other medicines.

 Pregnancy
Safety in pregnancy not established. Discuss with your doctor.

 Breast-feeding
Safety in breast-feeding not established. Discuss with your doctor.

 Infants and children
Safety has not been established, so not recommended for children and adolescents under the age of 17.

 Over 60
No special problems.

 Driving and hazardous work
Avoid such activities until you have learned how brinzolamide affects you because the drug can cause temporary blurred vision.

 Alcohol
No special problems.

POSSIBLE ADVERSE EFFECTS

The most common side effects are temporary blurred vision and a bitter or unusual taste. The taste is likely to be due to drops dripping into the nose and throat via the nasolacrimal canal. Pressing the inner corner of the eye (see p.129) or gently closing the eyelid after instillation may help to prevent it. Systemic side effects may also occur but are rare.

Symptom/effect	Frequency		Discuss with doctor		Stop taking drug now	Call doctor now
	Common	Rare	Only if severe	In all cases		
Burning/stinging eyes	●		●			
Blurred vision/runny eyes	●		●			
Red, painful eyes	●		●			
Bitter taste in the mouth	●		●			
Hair loss		●		●		
Fainting/palpitations		●		●	●	●
Rash/breathing difficulties		●		●	●	●
Swollen lips/tongue		●		●	●	●

INTERACTIONS

Other carbonic anhydrase inhibitors taken orally Metabolic acid-base disturbance has been reported as there is a potential for additive effect (i.e. the drugs may enhance the effect of brinzolamide).

Antifungals (ketoconazole, itraconazole, clotrimazole) and ritonavir may increase the level of brinzolamide.

PROLONGED USE

No particular problems associated with prolonged use.

Monitoring Your doctor will continue to monitor the control of the glaucoma.

BROMOCRIPTINE

Brand name Parlodel
Used in the following combined preparations None

GENERAL INFORMATION

Bromocriptine stimulates dopamine receptors in the brain, causing a reduction in the secretion of the hormone prolactin from the pituitary gland. Hence it is used in the treatment of conditions associated with excessive prolactin production, such as some types of female infertility and, occasionally, male infertility. It is also used to reduce the size of prolactin-secreting tumours in the brain, and may be used to suppress lactation in women who do not wish to breast-feed.

Bromocriptine may also be used to treat Parkinson's disease, especially when the disease is not controlled by levodopa. In addition, bromocriptine reduces the release of growth hormone and can therefore be used to treat acromegaly (see p.103).

QUICK REFERENCE

Drug group Drug for parkinsonism (p.43) and pituitary agent (p.103)

Overdose danger rating Low

Dependence rating Low

Prescription needed Yes

Available as generic Yes

INFORMATION FOR USERS

Your drug prescription is tailored for you. Do not alter dosage without checking with your doctor.

How taken/used

Tablets, capsules.

Frequency and timing of doses
1–4 x daily with food.

Adult dosage range
The dose given depends on the condition being treated and your response. In most cases treatment starts with a daily dose of 1–1.25mg. This is gradually increased until a satisfactory response is achieved.

Onset of effect
Variable depending on the condition.

Duration of action
8–12 hours.

Diet advice
None.

Storage
Keep in original container at room temperature out of the reach of children. Protect from light.

Missed dose
Take as soon as you remember. If your next dose is due within 2 hours, take a single dose now and skip the next.

Stopping the drug
Do not stop the drug without consulting your doctor; symptoms may recur.

Exceeding the dose
An occasional unintentional extra dose is unlikely to be a cause for concern. If you notice any unusual symptoms, or if a large overdose has been taken, notify your doctor.

SPECIAL PRECAUTIONS

Be sure to tell your doctor if:
- You have a history of peptic ulcers.
- You have a history of psychiatric disorders.
- You have high blood pressure.
- You have porphyria.
- You have heart disease.
- You have liver disease.
- You are taking other medicines.

 Pregnancy
Safety in pregnancy not established. Discuss with your doctor.

 Breast-feeding
The drug suppresses milk production, and prevents it completely if given within 12 hours of delivery. If you wish to breast-feed, consult your doctor.

 Infants and children
Not usually prescribed under 15 years.

 Over 60
Reduced dose may be necessary.

 Driving and hazardous work
Avoid such activities until you have learned how bromocriptine affects you because the drug may cause dizziness and drowsiness.

 Alcohol
Avoid. Alcohol increases the likelihood of confusion and reduces tolerance to bromocriptine.

POSSIBLE ADVERSE EFFECTS

Adverse effects are usually related to the dose. When it is used to treat Parkinson's disease, bromocriptine may cause abnormal movements. Rarely, the drug may cause hypersexuality and behavioural problems, such as compulsive gambling. When used for long periods, there is a small risk of fibrosis (see below right).

Symptom/effect	Frequency		Discuss with doctor		Stop taking drug now	Call doctor now
	Common	Rare	Only if severe	In all cases		
Nausea/vomiting	●		●			
Constipation	●		●			
Confusion/dizziness/headache	●			●		
Abnormal movements		●		●		
Sudden drowsiness		●		●		
Compulsive behaviour		●		●		
Palpitations/breathlessness		●		●		
Back pain/swollen legs or feet		●		●		

INTERACTIONS

Antipsychotic drugs oppose the action of bromocriptine and increase the risk of parkinsonism.

Phenylpropanolamine, ephedrine, and pseudoephedrine These drugs are found in some over-the-counter cough and cold remedies. Use of these with bromocriptine may lead to severe adverse effects.

Erythromycin and other macrolide antibiotics These drugs may lead to increased levels of bromocriptine and the risk of adverse effects.

Domperidone and metoclopramide These drugs may reduce some of the effects of bromocriptine.

PROLONGED USE

Rarely, long-term use is associated with fibrosis (thickening of connective tissue) of the heart valves, lungs, and lining of the chest and abdominal cavities.

Monitoring Periodic blood tests may be performed to check hormone levels. To check for fibrosis, echocardiography may be carried out when starting treatment and at intervals during the treatment. Other tests, such as lung function tests, kidney function tests, or kidney scans, may also be carried out.

BUDESONIDE

Brand names Benacort, Budelin Novolizer, Budenofalk, Cortiment, Entocort, Jorveza, Pulmicort, Rhinocort Aqua
Used in the following combined preparation DuoResp Spiromax, Fobumix, Symbicort

GENERAL INFORMATION

Budesonide is a corticosteroid drug used in the form of slow-release capsules to relieve the symptoms of Crohn's disease, as an enema to treat ulcerative colitis, and via an inhaler as a maintenance treatment for asthma. The inhaled corticosteroid is administered either on its own or in combination with a bronchodilator. Budesonide is also given in a nasal spray to relieve the symptoms of allergic rhinitis and to treat nasal polyps.

Side effects are fewer and less serious with the inhaler or nasal spray because less of the drug is absorbed than with oral forms. Mouth and throat irritation can occur with the inhaler, but these effects can be minimized by thoroughly rinsing the mouth and gargling with water after each inhalation.

INFORMATION FOR USERS

Your drug prescription is tailored for you. Do not alter dosage without checking with your doctor.

How taken/used

SR capsules, enema, inhaler, powder for inhalation, nasal spray.

Frequency and timing of doses
1–3 x daily (capsules); once daily at bedtime (enema); twice daily (inhaler); once or twice daily (nasal spray).

Dosage range
3–9mg (capsules); 2mg (enema); 200–1,600mcg (inhaler); 100–200mcg (nasal spray).

Onset of effect
Asthma Within 1 week.
Other conditions 1–3 days.

Duration of action
12–24 hours.

Diet advice
None.

Storage
Keep in original container at room temperature out of the reach of children.

Missed dose
Take as soon as you remember. If your next dose is due within 2 hours, take a single dose now and skip the next.

Stopping the drug
Do not stop taking the drug without consulting your doctor; symptoms may recur. The SR capsules used in Crohn's disease should be withdrawn gradually.

Exceeding the dose
An occasional extra dose is unlikely to be a cause for concern. But if you notice any unusual symptoms, or if a large overdose has been taken, notify your doctor.

POSSIBLE ADVERSE EFFECTS

As with other corticosteroids, the principal side effects of inhalers and nasal spray are confined to the nasal passages and the mouth. Capsules and enemas can cause gastrointestinal disturbances and rashes. High doses of budesonide by any route can cause weight gain and other long-term side effects associated with corticosteroids.

Symptom/effect	Frequency		Discuss with doctor		Stop taking drug now	Call doctor now
	Common	Rare	Only if severe	In all cases		
Inhalers and nasal spray						
Cough	●		●			
Nasal irritation	●		●			
Bruising	●		●			
Sore throat/hoarseness	●			●		
Nosebleed		●		●		
Capsules and enema						
Diarrhoea/constipation	●		●			
Rash/itching		●		●		
All preparations						
Weight gain		●		●		

INTERACTIONS

Itraconazole, ritonavir, and telaprevir may increase the blood level of budesonide and the risk of adrenal gland suppression.

SPECIAL PRECAUTIONS

Be sure to tell your doctor if:
- You have had tuberculosis or another respiratory infection.
- You are taking other medicines.

Pregnancy
Discuss with your doctor, especially if used for Crohn's disease.

Breast-feeding
Discuss with your doctor, especially if used for Crohn's disease.

Infants and children
Reduced dose necessary.

Over 60
No special problems.

Driving and hazardous work
No special problems.

Alcohol
No special problems.

Infection
Avoid exposure to chickenpox.

PROLONGED USE

Asthma prevention is the condition for which prolonged use may be required. High doses inhaled for a prolonged period can lead to peptic ulcers, osteoporosis, glaucoma, muscle weakness, and growth retardation in children. Patients taking the drug long term are advised to carry a steroid card or wear a MedicAlert bracelet.

Monitoring If budesonide is being taken in large doses, periodic checks may be needed to make sure that the adrenal glands are working properly. Children using inhalers should have their growth (height) monitored regularly.

BUMETANIDE

Brand name Burinex
Used in the following combined preparations None

GENERAL INFORMATION

Bumetanide is a powerful, short-acting loop diuretic used to treat oedema (accumulation of fluid in tissue spaces) resulting from heart failure, nephrotic syndrome, and cirrhosis of the liver. Bumetanide is particularly useful in treating people with impaired kidney function who do not respond well to thiazide diuretics. Bumetanide increases potassium loss in the urine, which can result in a wide variety of symptoms (see p.57). For this reason, potassium supplements or a potassium-sparing diuretic may be given with the drug.

INFORMATION FOR USERS

Your drug prescription is tailored for you. Do not alter dosage without checking with your doctor.

How taken/used

Tablets, liquid.

Frequency and timing of doses
Usually once daily in the morning. In some cases, twice daily.

Dosage range
1–5mg daily. Dose may be increased if kidney function is impaired.

Onset of effect
Within 30 minutes.

Duration of action
2–4 hours.

Diet advice
Use of this drug may reduce potassium in the body. Eat plenty of fresh fruit and vegetables, such as bananas and tomatoes.

Storage
Keep in original container at room temperature out of the reach of children. Protect from light.

Missed dose
No cause for concern, but take as soon as you remember. However, if it is late in the day do not take the missed dose, or you may need to get up during the night to pass urine. Take the next scheduled dose as usual.

Stopping the drug
Do not stop the drug without consulting your doctor; symptoms may recur.

Exceeding the dose
An occasional unintentional extra dose is unlikely to be a cause for concern. But if you notice any unusual symptoms, or if a large overdose has been taken, notify your doctor.

POSSIBLE ADVERSE EFFECTS

Adverse effects are caused mainly by the rapid fluid loss produced by bumetanide. These diminish as the body adjusts to the drug.

Bumetanide may precipitate gout in susceptible individuals and can affect the control of diabetes.

Symptom/effect	Frequency		Discuss with doctor		Stop taking drug now	Call doctor now
	Common	Rare	Only if severe	In all cases		
Dizziness/fainting	●		●			
Lethargy/fatigue		●	●			
Muscle cramps		●	●			
Rash/photosensitivity		●		●		
Nausea/vomiting		●		●		

INTERACTIONS

Anti-arrhythmic drugs Low potassium levels may increase these drugs' toxicity.

Antibacterials Very high doses of bumetanide can increase the ear damage that is caused by some antibiotics.

Digoxin Excessive potassium loss may increase the adverse effects of digoxin.

Non-steroidal anti-inflammatory drugs (NSAIDs) These drugs may reduce the diuretic effect of bumetanide.

Lithium Bumetanide may increase the blood levels of lithium, leading to an increased risk of lithium toxicity.

Amisulpride, sertindole, and pimozide Low potassium levels increase the risk of abnormal heart rhythms with these antipsychotic drugs.

Thiazides Extremely large amounts of urine may be produced when these drugs are taken with bumetanide.

SPECIAL PRECAUTIONS

Be sure to tell your doctor if:
- You have a long-term liver or kidney problem.
- You have prostate problems.
- You have gout.
- You have diabetes.
- You have low blood pressure.
- You are taking other medicines.

 Pregnancy
Not usually prescribed. May reduce blood supply to the developing baby. Discuss with your doctor.

 Breast-feeding
This drug may reduce your milk supply. Discuss with your doctor.

 Infants and children
Not usually prescribed. Reduced dose necessary.

 Over 60
Dosage is often reduced.

 Driving and hazardous work
Avoid until you know how bumetanide affects you because the drug may cause dizziness and faintness.

 Alcohol
Increases the likelihood of dehydration and hangovers. Keep intake low.

PROLONGED USE

Serious problems are unlikely, but the levels of certain salts in the body may occasionally become abnormal during prolonged use.

Monitoring Regular blood tests may be performed to check on kidney function and levels of body salts.

BUPROPION

Brand name Zyban
Used in the following combined preparations None

GENERAL INFORMATION

Bupropion (also called amfebutamone) is an antidepressant, although it is chemically unrelated to other classes of antidepressant. It has been used to treat depression but is generally used as an aid to giving up tobacco smoking. The person being treated must commit in advance to a date for stopping smoking. Treatment is started while the patient is still smoking, and the "target stop date" is decided on within the first 2 weeks of treatment. Bupropion will be stopped after 7 weeks if the smoker has not given up smoking completely by then.

The drug should not be prescribed for people with a history of seizures or eating disorders, or those who are withdrawing from benzodiazepines or alcohol. In addition it should not be used by people with bipolar disorder or psychosis because there is a risk of mania developing.

QUICK REFERENCE

Drug group Smoking cessation aid
Overdose danger rating High
Dependence rating Low
Prescription needed Yes
Available as generic No

INFORMATION FOR USERS

Your drug prescription is tailored for you. Do not alter dosage without checking with your doctor.

How taken/used

SR tablets.

Frequency and timing of doses
1–2 x daily. Swallow the tablets whole.

Adult dosage range
150–300mg.

Onset of effect
Up to 4 weeks for full effect.

Duration of action
12 hours.

Diet advice
None.

Storage
Keep in original container at room temperature out of the reach of children.

Missed dose
Take as soon as you remember. If your next dose is due within 2 hours, take a single dose now and skip the next.

Stopping the drug
Do not stop the drug without consulting your doctor. The doctor may want to reduce the dose gradually.

OVERDOSE ACTION

Seek immediate medical advice in all cases. Take emergency action if consciousness is lost.

See Drug poisoning emergency guide (p.518).

SPECIAL PRECAUTIONS

Be sure to tell your doctor if:
- You have had a head injury or have a history of seizures or epilepsy.
- You have an eating disorder.
- You have cancer of the nervous system.
- You have diabetes.
- You have high blood pressure.
- You have bipolar disorder (manic depressive disorder) or a psychosis.
- You have kidney or liver problems.
- You are withdrawing from alcohol or benzodiazepine dependence.
- You are taking other medicines.

Pregnancy
Safety not established. Try to give up smoking without using drugs.

Breast-feeding
Safety not established. The drug passes into the breast milk and may affect the baby. Discuss with your doctor.

Infants and children
Not recommended.

Over 60
Increased sensitivity to the drug's effects. Reduced dose may therefore be necessary.

Driving and hazardous work
Avoid until you have learned how bupropion affects you. The drug may cause impaired concentration and dizziness.

Alcohol
Avoid. Alcohol will increase any sedative effects.

POSSIBLE ADVERSE EFFECTS

Some effects, such as agitation, tremor, sweating, and insomnia, may be due to the withdrawal of nicotine rather than to the effects of bupropion itself.

Symptom/effect	Frequency		Discuss with doctor		Stop taking drug now	Call doctor now
	Common	Rare	Only if severe	In all cases		
Insomnia/poor concentration	●		●			
Headache/dizziness/tremor	●		●			
Nausea/vomiting/constipation	●		●			
Rash/itch/fever	●			●		
Depression	●			●		
Confusion/anxiety		●		●		
Jaundice		●		●		●
Palpitations/fainting/chest pain		●		●	●	
Seizures		●		●	●	

INTERACTIONS

General note A wide range of drugs increases the likelihood of seizures when taken with bupropion. Check with your doctor if you are on other medications.

Ritonavir, amantadine, levodopa, and monoamine oxidase inhibitors increase the risk of adverse effects with bupropion.

Anticonvulsants Phenytoin and carbamazepine may reduce the blood levels and effects of bupropion. Valproate may increase its blood levels and effects.

Tamoxifen Bupropion may reduce blood levels and effects of tamoxifen.

PROLONGED USE

Bupropion is used for up to 9 weeks for cessation of smoking.

Monitoring Progress will be reviewed after about 3–4 weeks, and the drug continued only if it is having some effect. The drug may increase blood pressure, so this should be monitored.

CALCIPOTRIOL

Brand name Dovonex
Used in the following combined preparations Dovobet, Enstilar, Xamiol

GENERAL INFORMATION

Calcipotriol is a synthetic derivative of vitamin D used in the treatment of plaque psoriasis affecting the skin and scalp. Although similar to vitamin D, outside the skin calcipotriol is weak compared to vitamin D. In the skin, it is thought to work by reducing production of the skin cells that cause skin thickening and scaling, which are the most common symptoms of psoriasis. Because this drug is related to vitamin D, excessive use can lead to a rise of calcium levels in the body, although this is very uncommon;

otherwise calcipotriol is unlikely to cause any serious adverse effects.

Calcipotriol is applied to the affected areas in the form of cream, ointment, foam, or scalp solution. It should not be used on the face, and it is important to wash the hands following application to the affected area to avoid accidental transfer of the drug to unaffected areas. Local irritation may occur during the early stages of treatment. Excessive exposure to sunlight should be avoided while using calcipotriol.

QUICK REFERENCE

Drug group Drug for psoriasis (p.138)

Overdose danger rating Low

Dependence rating Low

Prescription needed Yes

Available as generic Yes

INFORMATION FOR USERS

Your drug prescription is tailored for you. Do not alter dosage without checking with your doctor.

How taken/used

Cream, ointment, scalp solution, foam.

Frequency and timing of doses
1–2 x daily.

Adult dosage range
Maximum 100g each week (cream, ointment); maximum 60ml each week (scalp solution); maximum 15g each day (foam); less if more than one preparation is used together.

Onset of effect
Improvement is seen within 2 weeks.

Duration of action
One application of cream, ointment, or scalp solution lasts up to 12 hours; one application of foam lasts up to 24 hours. Beneficial effects are longer lasting.

Diet advice
None.

Storage
Store in original container at room temperature out of the reach of children.

Missed dose
Apply the next dose at the scheduled time.

Stopping the drug
Do not stop the drug without consulting your doctor; symptoms may recur.

Exceeding the dose
Excessive prolonged use may lead to an increase in blood calcium levels, which can cause nausea, constipation, thirst, abdominal pain, weakness, tiredness, and frequent urination. Notify your doctor.

SPECIAL PRECAUTIONS

Be sure to tell your doctor if:
- You have a metabolic disorder.
- You have previously had a hypersensitivity reaction to the drug.
- You have long-term liver or kidney problems.
- You are taking other medicines.

 Pregnancy
Safety in pregnancy not established. Discuss with your doctor.

 Breast-feeding
Not known if excreted into breast milk. Discuss with your doctor.

 Infants and children
Not recommended.

 Over 60
No problems expected.

 Driving and hazardous work
No problems expected.

 Alcohol
No problems expected.

POSSIBLE ADVERSE EFFECTS

Temporary local irritation may occur when treatment is started. The other effects are uncommon and usually due to heavy or prolonged use, leading to high blood calcium levels.

Symptom/effect	Frequency		Discuss with doctor		Stop taking drug now	Call doctor now
	Common	Rare	Only if severe	In all cases		
Local irritation/itching	●		●			
Dry skin	●		●			
Rash on face/mouth		●		●		
Thirst/frequent urination		●		●		
Nausea/constipation		●		●		
Light-sensitive rash		●		●		
Abdominal pain		●		●	●	
Weakness/tiredness		●		●	●	
Confusion		●	●		●	
Worsening psoriasis		●		●	●	

PROLONGED USE

No problems expected from use of calcipotriol in low doses. If the effects of the skin preparation decline after several weeks, they may be regained by suspending use for a few weeks and then recommencing treatment.

Monitoring Regular checks on calcium levels in the blood or urine are required only during prolonged or heavy use.

INTERACTIONS

None known.

CANDESARTAN

Brand name Amias, Atacand
Used in the following combined preparations None

GENERAL INFORMATION

Candesartan belongs to the group of vasodilator drugs known as angiotensin II blockers and is used to treat hypertension (high blood pressure) and heart failure (inability of the heart muscle to cope with its workload). It works by blocking the action of angiotensin II (a hormone that constricts blood vessels). This relaxes the blood vessels, thereby lowering blood pressure and easing the heart's workload.

Unlike ACE inhibitors, candesartan does not cause a persistent dry cough or angioedema (tissue swelling) of the larynx or throat, and may be a useful alternative for people who have to discontinue treatment with an ACE inhibitor for those reasons.

QUICK REFERENCE

Drug group Vasodilator (p.56) and antihypertensive drug (p.60)

Overdose danger rating Low

Dependence rating Low

Prescription needed Yes

Available as generic No

INFORMATION FOR USERS

Your drug prescription is tailored for you. Do not alter dosage without checking with your doctor.

How taken/used

Tablets.

Frequency and timing of doses
Once daily.

Adult dosage range
4mg initially, increased to maximum of 32mg.

Onset of effect
2 hours.

Duration of action
24 hours.

Diet advice
None.

Storage
Keep in original container at room temperature out of the reach of children.

Missed dose
Take as soon as you remember. If your next dose is due within 8 hours, take a single dose now and skip the next.

Stopping the drug
Do not stop taking the drug without consulting your doctor. Stopping the drug may lead to worsening of the underlying condition.

Exceeding the dose
An occasional unintentional extra dose is unlikely to cause problems. Large overdoses may cause dizziness and fainting. Notify your doctor.

SPECIAL PRECAUTIONS

Be sure to tell your doctor if:
- You have heart problems, including heart failure.
- You have kidney problems or stenosis of the kidney's arteries.
- You have liver problems.
- You have lactose/galactose intolerance or glucose/galactose malabsorption.
- You are taking other medicines.

 Pregnancy
Not prescribed. If you become pregnant during treatment consult your doctor without delay.

 Breast-feeding
Safety not established. Discuss with your doctor.

 Infants and children
Not prescribed.

 Over 60
Increased risk of adverse effects. Reduced dose may therefore be necessary.

 Driving and hazardous work
Do not undertake such activities until you have learned how candesartan affects you because the drug can cause dizziness and fatigue.

 Alcohol
Regular intake of excessive alcohol may raise blood pressure and reduce the effectiveness of candesartan.

POSSIBLE ADVERSE EFFECTS

Adverse effects are usually mild and transient; common effects include dizziness, headache, flushing, and nausea.

Symptom/effect	Frequency		Discuss with doctor		Stop taking drug now	Call doctor now
	Common	Rare	Only if severe	In all cases		
Dizziness/headache	●		●			
Flushing	●		●			
Nausea	●		●			
Muscle or joint pain		●	●			
Swollen face or lips		●		●	●	●
Jaundice		●		●	●	●

INTERACTIONS

ACE inhibitors (e.g. enalapril, captopril, lisinopril, or ramipril) may increase potassium levels when taken with candesartan. However, the combination of ACE inhibitor with candesartan is not generally recommended.

Diuretics There is a risk of a sudden fall in blood pressure if these drugs are taken when candesartan treatment is started. They may also affect sodium and potassium levels in the blood.

NSAIDs (e.g. diclofenac or ibuprofen) may reduce candesartan's effectiveness.

Lithium Levels of this drug may be increased when it is combined with candesartan, leading to toxicity.

Ciclosporin may increase potassium levels when combined with candesartan.

Potassium salts may increase risk of high potassium levels with candesartan.

PROLONGED USE

No special problems.

Monitoring Periodic checks on blood potassium levels and kidney function may be performed.

CANNABIDIOL

Brand name Epidyolex, Sativex
Used in the following combined preparations None

GENERAL INFORMATION

Cannabinoids are chemicals produced by the cannabis plant (*Cannabis sativa*) that affect signalling processes in the brain and nervous system.

In the UK two products are licensed: Epidyolex and Sativex. Epidyolex is an oral solution containing cannabidiol but lacking tetrahydrocannabinol (THC), the psychoactive chemical from the cannabis plant. It is used to treat rare forms of epilepsy, usually in combination with another anticonvulsant (clobazam). In contrast, Sativex contains both THC and cannabidiol. It is used to treat moderate to severe muscle spasms and stiffness in people with multiple sclerosis who have not derived benefit from other antispasmodic drugs.

QUICK REFERENCE

Drug group Anticonvulsants (p.42)
Overdose danger rating Medium
Dependence rating Low
Prescription needed Yes
Available as generic No

INFORMATION FOR USERS

Your drug prescription is tailored for you. Do not alter dosage without checking with your doctor.

How taken/used

Oral solution (Epidyolex); oral spray (Sativex).

Frequency and timing of doses
Epidyolex: twice daily via measuring syringe. Sativex: 1–12 sprays a day inside cheeks or under tongue; dose is titrated for maximum relief with least side effects. Separate each spray by at least 15 minutes.

Adult dosage range
Epidyolex: 2.5mg/kg to 10mg/kg twice daily. Sativex: two or more doses in a day.

Onset of effect
Sativex: within 30 minutes, but may take weeks to stabilize.

Duration of action
Both Epidyolex and Sativex have a duration of up to a week once the effect is stabilized.

Diet advice
Epidyolex: take consistently with/without food.

Storage
Epidyolex: no special conditions. Sativex: if unopened, store upright in a refrigerator. If opened, discard after 42 days. For both, ask pharmacist to dispose of unused drug.

Missed dose
Epidyolex: take the next dose at the correct time. Sativex: use as soon as you remember or if you need it.

Stopping the drug
Epidyolex should be discontinued gradually.

Exceeding the dose
Epidyolex may cause diarrhoea and sleepiness; Sativex may cause dizziness, hallucinations, paranoia, altered heart rate, low blood pressure. Seek medical attention in all cases.

SPECIAL PRECAUTIONS

Be sure to tell your doctor if:
- You have a history of psychiatric disorders.
- You are allergic to cannabis, or (with Epidyolex) to alcohol or sesame oil.
- You have heart disease including fainting or an abnormal ECG.
- You have epilepsy.
- You have kidney or liver problems.
- You are taking any other medicines.
- You have previously abused any drug or other substance.
- You cannot take alcohol (Sativex).

Pregnancy
Avoid. Use reliable barrier contraception with Sativex.

Breast-feeding
Avoid. The drug may pass into breast milk and harm the baby.

Infants and children
Sativex not recommended. Epidyolex can be used in children over 2 years.

Over 60
Increased risk of adverse effects involving the central nervous system.

Driving and hazardous work
Cannabidiol may affect your ability to drive or work. Do not drive until you are on a stable dose and know how the medicine affects you.

Alcohol
Avoid. The drug can impair reactions, concentration, and coordination.

Legal and safety information
Taking cannabinoids is illegal in many countries.

Both men and women should take reliable contraception until 3 months after stopping therapy. Patients who are on Sativex and taking hormonal contraceptives should add a barrier method.

POSSIBLE ADVERSE EFFECTS

Both products affect mood and thinking, but many of the side effects settle over time.

Epidyolex can lead to liver injury and may also cause fever, rash, and respiratory symptoms.

Symptom/effect	Frequency		Discuss with doctor		Stop taking drug now	Call doctor now
	Common	Rare	Only if severe	In all cases		
Impaired concentration/memory	●		●			
Tiredness/impaired sleep	●			●		
Suicidal thoughts/hallucinations/paranoia		●		●	●	●
Altered appetite or taste	●		●			
Dry/painful/blistered mouth	●		●			
Change in mouth/teeth colour		●		●		
Nausea/constipation/diarrhoea	●			●		
Fainting		●		●		●
Feeling dizzy/agitated/drunk	●		●			
Heart rate/blood pressure rise	●		●			
More frequent seizures		●		●		
Fever, cough, sore throat	●			●		
Jaundice, itching, dark urine		●		●	●	●

INTERACTIONS

Many drugs, including antibiotics, sedatives, hormonal contraceptives, anticonvulsants, and antidepressants, may increase or reduce the effects of cannibidiol. Discuss with your doctor or pharmacist before taking other medications.

PROLONGED USE

The value of continued treatment should be re-evaluated periodically.

Monitoring Liver function tests are monitored periodically for those on Epidyolex.

CAPTOPRIL

Brand names Noyada
Used in the following combined preparations None

GENERAL INFORMATION

Captopril belongs to the class of drugs called ACE inhibitors, used to treat high blood pressure and heart failure. The drug works by relaxing the muscles around blood vessels, allowing them to dilate and thereby easing blood flow.

Captopril lowers blood pressure rapidly but may require several weeks to achieve full effect. People with heart failure may be given captopril in addition to diuretics. It can achieve dramatic results, relaxing muscle in blood vessel walls and reducing the heart's workload.

The first dose is usually very small and taken while lying down as there is a risk of a sudden fall in blood pressure. Various minor side effects may occur. Some people experience loss of taste, while others get a persistent dry cough. The cough may be severe enough to necessitate switching to an angiotensin-blocking drug, such as losartan.

INFORMATION FOR USERS

Your drug prescription is tailored for you. Do not alter dosage without checking with your doctor.

How taken/used

Tablets, oral solution.

Frequency and timing of doses
2–3 x daily.

Adult dosage range
6.25–25mg daily initially, gradually increased to 37.5–150mg daily.

Onset of effect
30–60 minutes; full beneficial effect may take several weeks.

Duration of action
6–8 hours.

Diet advice
Your doctor may advise you to reduce your salt intake to help control your blood pressure.

Storage
Keep in original container at room temperature out of the reach of children.

Missed dose
Take as soon as you remember. If your next dose is due within 2 hours, take a single dose now and skip the next.

Stopping the drug
Do not stop the drug without consulting your doctor; the underlying condition may worsen.

Exceeding the dose
An occasional unintentional extra dose is not likely to cause problems. Large overdoses may cause dizziness or fainting. Notify your doctor.

SPECIAL PRECAUTIONS

Be sure to tell your doctor if:
- You have long-term kidney or liver problems.
- You have heart problems.
- You have had angioedema or a previous allergic reaction to ACE inhibitors.
- You are pregnant or intend to become pregnant.
- You are taking other medicines.

Pregnancy
Not prescribed. Evidence of harm to fetus in second and third trimesters.

Breast-feeding
Safety not established. Discuss with your doctor.

Infants and children
Not recommended.

Over 60
Reduced dose may be necessary.

Driving and hazardous work
Avoid such activities until you have learned how captopril affects you because the drug can cause dizziness and fainting.

Alcohol
Avoid. Alcohol may increase the blood-pressure lowering and adverse effects of the drug.

Surgery and general anaesthetics
Captopril may need to be stopped before you have a general anaesthetic. Discuss with your doctor or dentist before any operation.

POSSIBLE ADVERSE EFFECTS

Captopril causes a variety of minor adverse effects, primarily rashes and gastrointestinal symptoms. These usually disappear soon after treatment has started.

Symptom/effect	Frequency		Discuss with doctor		Stop taking drug now	Call doctor now
	Common	Rare	Only if severe	In all cases		
Loss of taste	●		●			
Rash	●			●		
Persistent dry cough	●			●		
Mouth ulcers/sore mouth		●		●		
Dizziness		●		●		
Sore throat/fever		●		●		
Swelling of mouth/lips		●		●	●	●
Breathing difficulty		●		●	●	●

INTERACTIONS

Non-steroidal anti-inflammatory drugs (NSAIDs) may reduce the effectiveness of captopril. There is also a risk of kidney damage when they are taken with captopril.

Vasodilators, diuretics, and other antihypertensives These drugs may increase the blood-pressure-lowering effect of captopril.

Potassium supplements and potassium-sparing diuretics increase the risk of high potassium levels when taken with captopril.

Ciclosporin This drug increases the risk of high potassium levels in the blood when taken with captopril.

Lithium Blood levels of lithium may be raised by captopril.

PROLONGED USE

No problems expected.

Monitoring Periodic checks on potassium levels, white blood cell count, kidney function, and urine are usually performed.

CARBAMAZEPINE

Brand names Carbagen SR, Curatil, Epimaz, Tegretol, Tegretol Retard
Used in the following combined preparations None

GENERAL INFORMATION

Carbamazepine is used to treat several forms of epilepsy as it reduces the likelihood of seizures caused by abnormal nerve signals in the brain.

The drug is also prescribed to relieve the intermittent severe pain caused by irritation of the cranial nerves in trigeminal neuralgia. It is prescribed to stabilize mood in bipolar disorder (manic depression), to reduce urine output in diabetes insipidus, and to relieve pain in diabetic neuropathy. Rarely, it may be used in the management of acute alcohol withdrawal.

In order to avoid side effects, carbamazepine therapy is usually commenced at a low dose and is gradually increased. It is recommended that patients stick to the same brand of carbamazepine prescribed.

QUICK REFERENCE

Drug group Anticonvulsant drug (p.42)

Overdose danger rating Medium

Dependence rating Low

Prescription needed Yes

Available as generic Yes

INFORMATION FOR USERS

Your drug prescription is tailored for you. Do not alter dosage without checking with your doctor.

How taken/used

Tablets, chewable tablets, liquid, suppositories.

Frequency and timing of doses
1–2 x daily.

Adult dosage range
Epilepsy 100–2,000mg daily (low starting dose that is slowly increased every 2 weeks).
Pain relief 100–1,600mg daily.
Psychiatric disorders 400–1,600mg daily.

Onset of effect
Within 4 hours.

Duration of action
12–24 hours.

Diet advice
None.

Storage
Keep in original container at room temperature out of the reach of children.

Missed dose
Take as soon as you remember. If your next dose is due within 2 hours, take a single dose now and skip the next.

Stopping the drug
Do not stop the drug without consulting your doctor; symptoms may recur.

Exceeding the dose
An occasional unintentional extra dose is unlikely to cause problems. Large overdoses may cause tremor, seizures, and coma. Notify your doctor.

POSSIBLE ADVERSE EFFECTS

Most people experience very few adverse effects with this drug, but when blood levels get too high, adverse effects are common and the dose may need to be reduced.

Symptom/effect	Frequency		Discuss with doctor		Stop taking drug now	Call doctor now
	Common	Rare	Only if severe	In all cases		
Dizziness/unsteadiness	●		●			
Drowsiness	●		●			
Nausea/loss of appetite	●		●			
Blurred vision	●			●		
Jaundice		●		●		
Ankle swelling		●		●		
Sore throat/hoarseness		●		●	●	
Rash/fever/bruising		●		●	●	●

INTERACTIONS

General note Many drugs may increase or reduce the effects of carbamazepine. In addition, carbamazepine itself may reduce the blood levels and effectiveness of other drugs. Discuss with your doctor or pharmacist before taking other medications.

Other anticonvulsant drugs Complex and variable interactions can occur between these drugs and carbamazepine.

Contraceptive pill Carbamazepine may reduce the effectiveness of the contraceptive pill. Discuss this with your doctor.

SPECIAL PRECAUTIONS

Be sure to tell your doctor if:
• You have a long-term liver or kidney problem.
• You have heart problems.
• You have had blood problems with other drugs.
• You are taking other medicines.

Pregnancy
Avoid if possible. Associated with abnormalities in the unborn baby. Folic acid supplements should be taken before and during pregnancy. Discuss with your doctor.

Breast-feeding
The drug passes into the breast milk and can affect the baby. Discuss with your doctor.

Infants and children
Reduced dose necessary.

Over 60
May cause confused or agitated behaviour in older people. Reduced dose may be necessary.

Driving and hazardous work
Discuss with your doctor. Your underlying condition, as well as the possibility of reduced alertness while taking carbamazepine, may make such activities inadvisable.

Alcohol
Avoid. Alcohol may increase the sedative effects of this drug.

PROLONGED USE

There is a slight risk of changes in liver function or of skin or blood abnormalities occurring during prolonged use.

Monitoring Periodic blood tests are usually performed to monitor levels of the drug, blood cell counts, and liver and kidney function.

CARBIMAZOLE

Brand names None
Used in the following combined preparations None

GENERAL INFORMATION

Carbimazole is an antithyroid drug that suppresses the formation of thyroid hormones and is used to manage overactivity of the thyroid gland (hyperthyroidism). In Graves' disease, which is the most common cause of hyperthyroidism, a course of carbimazole alone or combined with thyroxine (so-called "block and replace" therapy) – usually given for 6–18 months – may cure the disorder. In other conditions, carbimazole is given until other treatments, such as surgery or radioiodine, take effect. If other treatments are not possible or are declined by the patient, carbimazole can be given long term. The full effect of the drug may take several weeks, and beta blockers may be given during this period to control symptoms.

The most important adverse effect is a reduction in white blood cells (agranulocytosis), increasing the risk of infection. Although this is rare, if you develop a sore throat, mouth ulcers, or a fever, you should see your doctor immediately to have your white blood cell count checked.

QUICK REFERENCE

Drug group Antithyroid drug (p.102)
Overdose danger rating Medium
Dependence rating Low
Prescription needed Yes
Available as generic Yes

INFORMATION FOR USERS

Your drug prescription is tailored for you. Do not alter dosage without checking with your doctor.

How taken/used

Tablets.

Frequency and timing of doses
1–3 x daily.

Adult dosage range
15–40mg daily (occasionally a larger dose may be needed). Once control is achieved, dosage is reduced gradually to a maintenance dose of 5–15mg for about 18 months.

Onset of effect
Some improvement is usually felt within 1–3 weeks. Full beneficial effects usually take 4–8 weeks.

Duration of action
12–24 hours.

Diet advice
Your doctor may advise you to avoid foods that are high in iodine, such as cod and mackerel.

Storage
Keep in original container at room temperature out of the reach of children.

Missed dose
Take as soon as you remember. If your next dose is due, take both doses together.

Stopping the drug
Do not stop the drug without consulting your doctor; symptoms may recur.

Exceeding the dose
An occasional unintentional extra dose is unlikely to cause problems. Large overdoses may cause nausea, vomiting, and headache. Notify your doctor.

SPECIAL PRECAUTIONS

Be sure to tell your doctor if:
• You have a long-term liver problem.
• You are pregnant.
• You are taking other medicines.

 Pregnancy
May be associated with defects in the baby. Discuss with your doctor.

 Breast-feeding
The drug passes into the breast milk, but mothers may breast-feed as long as the lowest effective dose is used and the baby is carefully monitored. Discuss with your doctor.

 Infants and children
Reduced dose necessary.

 Over 60
No special problems.

 Driving and hazardous work
Avoid such activities until you have learned how carbimazole affects you because the drug may cause dizziness.

 Alcohol
No known problems.

POSSIBLE ADVERSE EFFECTS

The most important side effect is a rare life-threatening reduction in white blood cells (agranulocytosis). This may be indicated by a sore throat or fever and should be reported to your doctor immediately.

Symptom/effect	Frequency		Discuss with doctor		Stop taking drug now	Call doctor now
	Common	Rare	Only if severe	In all cases		
Headache/dizziness/nausea	●		●			
Joint pain	●		●			
Rash/itching	●			●		
Hair loss	●			●		
Loss of sense of taste		●	●			
Bleeding/bruising		●		●		●
Jaundice		●		●		●
Sore throat/fever/mouth ulcers		●		●	●	●

PROLONGED USE

Carbimazole may rarely cause a reduction in the number of white blood cells.

Monitoring Periodic tests of thyroid function are usually required. If you have a sore throat, fever, or mouth ulcers, your white blood cell count must be checked.

INTERACTIONS

Theophylline Blood levels of this drug may increase when taken with carbimazole.

Erythromycin and prednisolone Blood levels of these drugs may decrease when taken with carbimazole.

CEFALEXIN

Brand names Keflex
Used in the following combined preparations None

GENERAL INFORMATION

Cefalexin is a cephalosporin antibiotic that is prescribed for a variety of mild to moderate infections. It does not have such a wide range of uses as some other antibiotics, but it is helpful in treating respiratory tract infections, cystitis, ear infections, and certain skin and soft tissue infections. In some cases it is prescribed as follow-up treatment for severe infections after a more powerful cephalosporin has been given by injection.

Diarrhoea is the most common adverse effect of cefalexin. Although this tends to be less severe than with other cephalosporins, the risk of the more dangerous *Clostridium difficile* diarrhoea is much higher for older adult patients who are taking cefalexin (or any other cephalosporin) than other classes of antibiotic. Some people may also find they are allergic to cefalexin, especially if they are sensitive to penicillin.

INFORMATION FOR USERS

Your drug prescription is tailored for you. Do not alter dosage without checking with your doctor.

How taken/used

Tablets, capsules, granules, liquid.

Frequency and timing of doses
2–4 x daily.

Dosage range
Adults 1–4g daily.
Children Reduced dose according to age and weight.

Onset of effect
Within 1 hour

Duration of action
6–12 hours.

Diet advice
None.

Storage
Keep tablets, capsules, and granules in original container at room temperature; refrigerate liquid, but do not freeze, and keep for no longer than 10 days. Keep out of the reach of children and protect from light.

Missed dose
Take as soon as you remember. If your next dose is due at this time, take both doses now.

Stopping the drug
Take the full course. Even if you feel better, the original infection may still be present and may recur if treatment is stopped too soon.

Exceeding the dose
An occasional unintentional extra dose is unlikely to be a cause for concern. But if you notice any unusual symptoms, or if a large overdose has been taken, notify your doctor.

POSSIBLE ADVERSE EFFECTS

Most people do not suffer serious adverse effects while taking cefalexin. Diarrhoea is common but it tends not to be severe. The rarer adverse effects are usually due to an allergic reaction and may necessitate stopping the drug.

Symptom/effect	Frequency		Discuss with doctor		Stop taking drug now	Call doctor now
	Common	Rare	Only if severe	In all cases		
Diarrhoea	●		●			
Nausea/vomiting		●	●			
Abdominal pain		●		●		
Rash		●		●	●	●
Itching/swelling/wheezing		●		●	●	●

INTERACTIONS

Probenecid This drug increases the level of cefalexin in the blood. The dosage of cefalexin may need to be adjusted accordingly.

Oral contraceptives Cefalexin may reduce the contraceptive effect of these drugs. Discuss with your doctor.

SPECIAL PRECAUTIONS

Be sure to tell your doctor if:
- You have a long-term kidney problem.
- You have had a previous allergic reaction to a penicillin or cephalosporin antibiotic.
- You have a history of blood disorders.
- You are taking other medicines.

Pregnancy
No evidence of risk to the developing baby.

Breast-feeding
The drug passes into the breast milk but at normal doses adverse effects on the baby are unlikely. Discuss with your doctor.

Infants and children
Reduced dose necessary.

Over 60
Avoid. Increased risk of *Clostridium difficile* diarrhoea.

Driving and hazardous work
No known problems.

Alcohol
No known problems.

PROLONGED USE

Cefalexin is usually given only for short courses of treatment.

CELECOXIB

Brand name Celebrex
Used in the following combined preparations None

GENERAL INFORMATION

Celecoxib is a type of non-steroidal anti-inflammatory drug (NSAID) called a cyclo-oxygenase-2 (COX-2) inhibitor; these drugs were originally thought to have a lower risk of irritating the upper gastrointestinal tract than other NSAIDs, but this is now disputed.

Celecoxib reduces pain, stiffness, and inflammation caused by rheumatoid arthritis, osteoarthritis, or ankylosing spondylitis. Older people may be more sensitive to its effects, so they are usually given a low dose to begin with.

Celecoxib is not prescribed to anyone who has had a heart attack or stroke, because it slightly increases the risk of recurrence, nor is it given to people with peripheral artery disease (poor circulation). It is prescribed with caution to anyone at risk of these conditions.

QUICK REFERENCE

Drug group Analgesic (p.36) and non-steroidal anti-inflammatory drug (p.74)

Overdose danger rating Medium

Dependence rating Low

Prescription needed Yes

Available as generic Yes

INFORMATION FOR USERS

Your drug prescription is tailored for you. Do not alter dosage without checking with your doctor.

How taken/used

Capsules.

Frequency and timing of doses
1–2 x daily.

Adult dosage range
200–400mg daily.

Onset of effect
1 hour.

Duration of action
8 hours.

Diet advice
None.

Storage
Keep in original container at room temperature out of the reach of children.

Missed dose
Take as soon as you remember. If your next dose is due within 4 hours, take a single dose now and skip the next.

Stopping the drug
If being used short term, the drug can safely be stopped as soon as you no longer need it. If prescribed for long-term use, you should not stop taking the drug without consulting your doctor.

Exceeding the dose
An occasional unintentional extra dose is unlikely to cause problems. Large overdoses may cause stomach and intestinal pain and damage. Notify your doctor.

SPECIAL PRECAUTIONS

Be sure to tell your doctor if:
- You have liver or kidney problems.
- You have epilepsy.
- You have asthma.
- You are allergic to aspirin or other NSAIDs.
- You are allergic to sulfonamides.
- You have a history of peptic ulcers.
- You have high blood pressure.
- You have ankle swelling.
- You have heart problems.
- You have had a heart attack or stroke.
- You have inflammatory bowel disease.
- You are taking other medicines.

 Pregnancy
Not prescribed.

 Breast-feeding
Not prescribed.

 Infants and children
Not recommended.

 Over 60
Older people may be more sensitive to the drug's effects. Lower doses may be necessary.

 Driving and hazardous work
Avoid until you know how the drug affects you. It can cause dizziness, vertigo, and sleepiness.

 Alcohol
Avoid. Alcohol may increase drowsiness and the risk of stomach irritation.

POSSIBLE ADVERSE EFFECTS

Gastrointestinal, nervous, and respiratory symptoms are the most likely adverse effects.

Symptom/effect	Frequency		Discuss with doctor		Stop taking drug now	Call doctor now
	Common	Rare	Only if severe	In all cases		
Indigestion/abdominal pain	●		●			
Diarrhoea/flatulence/nausea	●		●			
Dizziness/insomnia	●		●			
Rash	●			●		
Swollen ankles		●		●		
Palpitations		●		●		●
Wheezing/breathlessness		●		●	●	●
Pain in chest/groin/leg		●		●	●	●
Black/bloody vomit/faeces		●		●	●	●
Loss of consciousness		●		●	●	●

INTERACTIONS

General note Celecoxib interacts with a wide range of drugs, including ACE inhibitors, SSRI antidepressants, antihypertensives, diuretics, and drugs that increase the risk of bleeding and/or peptic ulcers (e.g. aspirin and other NSAIDs).

Lithium Levels and effects of this drug are increased when taken with celecoxib.

Carbamazepine, fluconazole, rifampicin, and barbiturates reduce the effects of celecoxib.

PROLONGED USE

Long-term use increases the risk of a stroke or heart attack, so the lowest effective dose is given for the shortest duration.

Monitoring Periodic tests of kidney function may be performed.

CETIRIZINE/LEVOCETIRIZINE

Brand names [cetirizine] Benadryl, Boots Hayfever and Allergy Relief, Piriteze, Pollenshield Hayfever, Zirtek; [levocetirizine] Xyzal
Used in the following combined preparations None

GENERAL INFORMATION

Cetirizine and levocetirizine are long-acting antihistamines. Their main use is in the treatment of allergic rhinitis, particularly hay fever. Both drugs are also used to treat a number of allergic skin conditions, such as urticaria (hives).

The principal difference between these medicines and traditional antihistamines such as chlorphenamine (chlorpheniramine) is that they have less sedative effect on the central nervous system and may therefore be suitable for people when they need to avoid sleepiness (for example, when driving or at work). However, because these drugs can cause drowsiness in some people, you should learn how cetirizine and levocetirizine affect you before you undertake any activities that require concentration.

INFORMATION FOR USERS

Your drug prescription is tailored for you. Do not alter dosage without checking with your doctor.

How taken/used

Tablets, liquid.

Frequency and timing of doses
1–2 x daily.

Dosage range
Cetirizine 10mg daily (adults and children over 12 years); 5mg twice daily (children 6–12 years); 2.5mg twice daily (children 2–6 years)
Levocetirizine 5mg daily.

Onset of effect
1–3 hours. Some effects may not be felt for 1–2 days.

Duration of action
Up to 24 hours.

Diet advice
None.

Storage
Keep in original container at room temperature out of the reach of children.

Missed dose
No cause for concern, but take as soon as you remember. If your next dose is due within 8 hours, take a single dose now and skip the next.

Stopping the drug
Can be safely stopped as soon as you no longer need it.

Exceeding the dose
An occasional unintentional extra dose is unlikely to cause problems. Large overdoses may cause nausea or drowsiness and have adverse effects on the heart. Notify your doctor.

SPECIAL PRECAUTIONS

Be sure to tell your doctor if:
• You have long-term liver or kidney problems.
• You have glaucoma.
• You are taking other medicines.

Pregnancy
Safety in pregnancy not established. Discuss with your doctor.

Breast-feeding
The drug passes into the breast milk. Discuss with your doctor.

Infants and children
Not recommended under 2 years (cetirizine): not recommended under 6 years (levocetirizine).

Over 60
No problems expected.

Driving and hazardous work
Avoid such activities until you have learned how cetirizine and levocetirizine affect you because the drug can cause drowsiness in some people.

Alcohol
Keep consumption low.

POSSIBLE ADVERSE EFFECTS

The most common adverse effects are drowsiness, dry mouth, and fatigue. Side effects may be reduced if the dose of cetirizine is taken as 5mg twice a day.

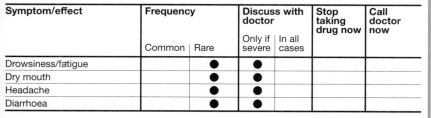

Symptom/effect	Frequency		Discuss with doctor		Stop taking drug now	Call doctor now
	Common	Rare	Only if severe	In all cases		
Drowsiness/fatigue	●			●		
Dry mouth	●			●		
Headache	●			●		
Diarrhoea	●			●		

PROLONGED USE

No problems expected.

INTERACTIONS

Anticholinergic drugs The anticholinergic effects of cetirizine and levocetirizine may be increased by all drugs that have anticholinergic effects (see p.35), including antipsychotics, tricyclic antidepressants, and some drugs for parkinsonism.

Sedatives Cetirizine and levocetirizine may increase the sedative effects of anti-anxiety drugs, sleeping drugs, antidepressants, and antipsychotic drugs.

Allergy tests Antihistamines should be discontinued about 3 days before allergy skin testing. Discuss details in advance with your allergy clinic; timings of discontinuation vary from clinic to clinic.

CHLORAMPHENICOL

Brand names Boots Antibiotic Eye Drops, Brochlor, Chloromycetin, Kemicetine, Minims Chloramphenicol, Optrex Infected Eyes
Used in the following combined preparation Actinac

GENERAL INFORMATION

Chloramphenicol is an antibiotic used topically to treat eye and ear infections. Eye drops are available over the counter. Given by mouth or injection, the drug is used in treating meningitis and brain abscesses. It is also effective in acute infections such as typhoid, pneumonia, epiglottitis, or meningitis caused by bacteria resistant to other antibiotics. Although most people experience few adverse effects, chloramphenicol occasionally causes serious or even fatal blood disorders. For this reason, chloramphenicol by mouth or injection is normally only given (usually in hospital) to treat life-threatening infections that do not respond to safer drugs.

QUICK REFERENCE

Drug group Antibiotic (p.86)

Overdose danger rating Low

Dependence rating Low

Prescription needed Yes (except some eye drops)

Available as generic Yes

INFORMATION FOR USERS

Your drug prescription is tailored for you. Do not alter dosage without checking with your doctor.

How taken/used

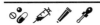

Capsules, injection, lotion, eye ointment, eye and ear drops.

Frequency and timing of doses
Every 6 hours (by mouth or injection); every 2–6 hours (eye preparations); 2–3 x daily (ear drops).

Adult dosage range
Varies according to preparation and condition. Follow your doctor's instructions.

Onset of effect
1–3 days, depending on the condition and preparation.

Duration of action
6–8 hours.

Diet advice
None.

Storage
Keep in original container at room temperature out of the reach of children.

Missed dose
For skin, eye, and ear preparations, apply as soon as you remember. Other preparations are usually given in hospital.

Stopping the drug
Take the full course. Even if you feel better the infection may still be present and may recur if treatment is stopped too soon.

Exceeding the dose
An occasional unintentional extra dose is unlikely to be a cause for concern. But if you notice any unusual symptoms, or if a large overdose has been taken, notify your doctor.

POSSIBLE ADVERSE EFFECTS

Transient irritation may occur with eye or ear drops. Sore throat, fever, and unusual tiredness with any form of chloramphenicol may be signs of blood abnormalities and should be reported to your doctor without delay, even if treatment has been stopped.

Symptom/effect	Frequency		Discuss with doctor		Stop taking drug now	Call doctor now
	Common	Rare	Only if severe	In all cases		
Burning/stinging (drops)		●	●			
Nausea/vomiting/diarrhoea		●	●			
Numb/tingling hands/feet		●		●		
Rash/itching		●		●		
Impaired vision		●		●	●	●
Sore throat		●		●	●	●
Fever/weakness		●		●	●	●
Painful mouth/tongue		●		●	●	●
Easy bruising		●		●	●	●

INTERACTIONS (oral and injection only)

General note Chloramphenicol may increase the effect of certain drugs, such as phenytoin, oral anticoagulants, and oral antidiabetics; phenobarbital or rifampicin may reduce the effect of chloramphenicol.

Antidiabetic drugs Chloramphenicol may increase the effect of sulfonylurea drugs.

Ciclosporin, tacrolimus, and sirolimus Chloramphenicol capsules, injection, or liquid may raise blood levels of these drugs.

Clozapine and other bone marrow suppressive drugs may increase the risk of bone marrow suppression (neutropenia) if used with chloramphenicol.

SPECIAL PRECAUTIONS

Be sure to tell your doctor if:
- You have long-term liver or kidney problems.
- You have a blood disorder.
- You have porphyria.
- You are taking other medicines.

Pregnancy
No evidence of risk with eye or ear preparations. Safety in pregnancy of other methods of administration not established. Discuss with your doctor.

Breast-feeding
No evidence of risk with eye or ear preparations. Taken by mouth, the drug passes into the breast milk and may increase the risk of blood disorders in the baby. Discuss with your doctor. Avoid unless essential.

Infants and children
Over-the-counter preparations should not be used in infants under 2 years. Other preparations are rarely used in infants and children, and then only under medical supervision.

Over 60
No problems expected.

Driving and hazardous work
Avoid such activities until you have learned how chloramphenicol eye drops affect your vision; the drug can cause transient stinging or blurred vision after application.

Alcohol
No known problems.

PROLONGED USE

Rarely, prolonged or repeated use may increase the risk of serious blood disorders. Prolonged or repeated use of eye drops may make the drug less effective at treating eye infections.

Monitoring Patients given the drug by mouth or injection may have periodic blood cell counts and eye tests. In the rare cases when chloramphenicol is given to infants by mouth or injection, blood levels of the drug are usually monitored.

CHLOROQUINE

Brand names Avloclor, Malarivon
Used in the following combined preparation chloroquine with proguanil, Paludrine/Avloclor

GENERAL INFORMATION

Chloroquine is used for the prevention and treatment of malaria. It usually clears an attack in three days. Injections may be given for a severe attack. To prevent malaria, a low dose is given once weekly, starting one week before visiting a high-risk area and continuing for four weeks after leaving. Chloroquine is not suitable for use in all parts of the world as resistance to the drug has developed in some areas. The other main use is in treating autoimmune diseases, such as rheumatoid arthritis and lupus erythematosus.

Common side effects include nausea, headache, diarrhoea, and abdominal cramps. Occasionally a rash develops. Chloroquine can damage the retina during prolonged treatment, causing blurred vision that may progress to blindness. Regular eye examinations are performed to detect early changes.

INFORMATION FOR USERS

Follow instructions on the label. Call your doctor if symptoms worsen.

How taken/used

Tablets, liquid, injection.

Frequency and timing of doses
By mouth 1 x weekly (prevention of malaria); 1–2 x daily (treatment of malaria); 1 x daily (arthritis); 1–2 x daily (lupus erythematosus).

Adult dosage range
Prevention of malaria 310mg (2 tablets) as a single dose on the same day each week. Start 1 week before entering endemic area, and continue for 4 weeks after leaving. *Treatment of malaria* Initial dose 620mg (4 tablets) and following doses 310mg. *Rheumatoid arthritis* 150mg (1 tablet) per day.

Onset of effect
2–3 days. In rheumatoid arthritis, full effect may not be felt for up to 6 months.

Duration of action
Up to 1 week

Diet advice
None.

Storage
Keep in original container at room temperature out of the reach of children.

Missed dose
Take as soon as you remember but if your next dose is due within 24 hours (1 x weekly schedule), or 6 hours (1–2 x daily schedule), take a single dose now and skip the next.

Stopping the drug
Do not stop the drug without consulting your doctor.

OVERDOSE ACTION

Seek immediate medical advice in all cases. Take emergency action if breathing difficulties, seizures, or loss of consciousness occur.

See Drug poisoning emergency guide (p.518).

SPECIAL PRECAUTIONS

Be sure to tell your doctor or pharmacist before taking this drug if:
- You have liver or kidney problems.
- You have heart problems.
- You have glucose-6-phosphate dehydrogenase (G6PD) deficiency.
- You have eye or vision problems.
- You have psoriasis.
- You have a history of epilepsy.
- You suffer from porphyria.
- You are taking other medicines.

 Pregnancy
No evidence of risk with low doses. High doses may affect the baby. Discuss the benefits versus the risks of malaria prevention with your doctor.

 Breast-feeding
The drug may pass into breast milk in small amounts. At normal doses, effects on the baby are unlikely. At high doses in the long term, discuss with your doctor.

 Infants and children
Reduced dose necessary.

 Over 60
No special problems, except that it may be difficult to tell between changes in eyesight due to ageing and those that are drug induced.

 Driving and hazardous work
Avoid such activities until you have learned how chloroquine affects you because the drug may cause dizziness and changes in vision.

 Alcohol
Keep consumption low.

POSSIBLE ADVERSE EFFECTS

Side effects such as nausea, diarrhoea, and abdominal pain might be avoided by taking the drug with food. Changes in vision should be reported promptly.

Symptom/effect	Frequency		Discuss with doctor		Stop taking drug now	Call doctor now
	Common	Rare	Only if severe	In all cases		
Nausea	●		●			
Diarrhoea/abdominal pain	●		●			
Hearing disorders/dizziness		●		●		
Hair loss/depigmentation		●		●		
Blurred vision/rash		●		●	●	●

INTERACTIONS

Ciclosporin and digoxin Chloroquine increases blood levels of these drugs.

Anticonvulsant drugs Chloroquine may reduce the effect of these drugs.

Mefloquine may increase the risk of seizures if taken with chloroquine.

Thyroxine For chloroquine with proguanil, thyroxine dose may need to be increased.

Amiodarone, bosutinib, droperidol, and moxifloxacin Chloroquine may increase the risk of abnormal heart rhythms if taken with these drugs.

PROLONGED USE

Prolonged use may cause eye damage and blood disorders.

Monitoring Periodic eye tests and blood counts must be done. People taking chloroquine with proguanil and thyroxine need their thyroid function monitored.

CHLORPHENAMINE (CHLORPHENIRAMINE)

Brand names Allercalm, Allerief, Boots Allergy Relief, Hayleve, Numark, Piriton, Pollenase
Used in the following combined preparations Galpseud Plus, Haymine

GENERAL INFORMATION

Chlorphenamine has been used for over 30 years to treat allergies such as hay fever, allergic conjunctivitis, urticaria (hives), insect bites and stings, and angioedema (allergic swellings). It is included in several over-the-counter cold remedies (see, p.52).

Like other antihistamines, it relieves allergic skin symptoms such as itching, swelling, and redness. It also reduces sneezing and the runny nose and itching eyes of hay fever. Chlorphenamine also has a mild anticholinergic action, which suppresses mucus secretion.

Chlorphenamine may also be used to prevent or treat allergic reactions to blood transfusions or X-ray contrast material, and can be given with epinephrine (adrenaline) injections for acute allergic shock (anaphylaxis).

QUICK REFERENCE

Drug group Antihistamine (p.82)
Overdose danger rating Medium
Dependence rating Low
Prescription needed No (tablets and liquid); Yes (injection)
Available as generic Yes

INFORMATION FOR USERS

Follow instructions on the label. Call your doctor if symptoms worsen.

How taken/used

Tablets, liquid, injection.

Frequency and timing of doses
4–6 x daily (tablets, liquid); single dose as needed (injection).

Dosage range
Adults 12–24mg daily (by mouth); up to 40mg daily (injection).
Children Reduced dose according to age and weight.

Onset of effect
Within 60 minutes (by mouth); within 20 minutes (injection).

Duration of action
4–6 hours (tablets, liquid, injection).

Diet advice
None.

Storage
Keep in original container at room temperature out of the reach of children.

Missed dose
Take as soon as you remember. If your next dose is due within 2 hours, take a single dose now and skip the next.

Stopping the drug
Can be safely stopped as soon as you no longer need it.

Exceeding the dose
An occasional unintentional extra dose is unlikely to cause problems. Large overdoses may cause drowsiness or agitation, seizures, or heart problems. Notify your doctor.

SPECIAL PRECAUTIONS

Be sure to tell your doctor or pharmacist before taking this drug if:
- You have a long-term liver problem.
- You have had epileptic seizures
- You have glaucoma.
- You have urinary difficulties.
- You are taking other medicines.

 Pregnancy
Safety in pregnancy not established. Discuss with your doctor.

 Breast-feeding
The drug passes into the breast milk and may cause drowsiness and poor feeding in the baby. Discuss with your doctor.

 Infants and children
Reduced dose necessary.

 Over 60
Reduced dose may be necessary. Increased likelihood of adverse effects.

 Driving and hazardous work
Avoid such activities until you have learned how chlorphenamine affects you because the drug can cause drowsiness, dizziness, and blurred vision.

 Alcohol
Avoid. Alcohol may increase the sedative effects of this drug.

POSSIBLE ADVERSE EFFECTS

Drowsiness is the most common adverse effect of chlorphenamine; other side effects are rare. Some of these, such as dryness of the mouth, blurred vision, and difficulty passing urine, are due to its anticholinergic effects. Gastrointestinal irritation may be reduced by taking the tablets or liquid with food or drink.

Symptom/effect	Frequency		Discuss with doctor		Stop taking drug now	Call doctor now
	Common	Rare	Only if severe	In all cases		
Drowsiness/dizziness	●			●		
Blurred vision	●			●		
Digestive disturbances		●	●			
Difficulty in passing urine		●	●			
Dry mouth	●			●		
Headache	●			●		
Excitation (children)		●		●	●	
Rash		●		●	●	

PROLONGED USE

No problems expected.

INTERACTIONS

Anticholinergic drugs All drugs, including some drugs for parkinsonism, that have an anticholinergic effect (see p.35) are likely to increase the anticholinergic effect of chlorphenamine.

Phenytoin The effects of phenytoin may be enhanced by chlorphenamine.

Monoamine oxidase inhibitors (MAOIs) and tricyclic antidepressants These drugs may increase the side effects of chlorphenamine.

Sedatives All drugs with a sedative effect are likely to increase the sedative properties of chlorphenamine.

CHLORPROMAZINE

Brand name Largactil
Used in the following combined preparations None

GENERAL INFORMATION

Chlorpromazine was the first anti-psychotic drug to be marketed and it is still used today. It has a calming and sedative effect that is useful in the short-term treatment of anxiety, agitation, and aggressive behaviour.

Chlorpromazine is prescribed for the treatment of schizophrenia, psychosis, and mania. Other uses of this drug include the treatment of nausea and vomiting, especially when caused by drug or radiation treatment; and treating severe, prolonged hiccups.

Chlorpromazine can produce a number of adverse effects, some of which may be serious. After continuous use of the drug over several years, eye changes and skin discoloration may occur.

INFORMATION FOR USERS

Your drug prescription is tailored for you. Do not alter dosage without checking with your doctor.

How taken/used

Tablets, liquid, injection, suppositories (specialist manufacturers only).

Frequency and timing of doses
1–6 x daily.

Adult dosage range
Mental illness 75–300mg daily; dose is started low and gradually increased. Some patients may need up to 1g daily.
Nausea and vomiting 40–150mg daily.

Onset of effect
30–60 minutes (by mouth); 15–20 minutes (injection); up to 30 minutes (suppository).

Duration of action
8–12 hours (by mouth or injection); 3–4 hours (suppository). Some effects may persist for up to 3 weeks when stopping the drug after regular use.

Diet advice
None.

Storage
Keep in original container at room temperature out of the reach of children. Protect from light. Healthcare professionals should avoid direct contact with the drug because of the risk of contact sensitization; tablets should not be crushed and liquids should be handled carefully.

Missed dose
Take as soon as you remember. If your next dose is due within 2 hours, do not take the missed dose. Take your next scheduled dose as usual.

Stopping the drug
Do not stop taking the drug without consulting your doctor; symptoms may recur.

Exceeding the dose
An occasional unintentional extra dose is unlikely to cause problems. Larger overdoses may cause unusual drowsiness, fainting, abnormal heart rhythms, muscle rigidity, and agitation. Notify your doctor.

SPECIAL PRECAUTIONS

Be sure to tell your doctor if:
- You have long-term liver or kidney problems.
- You have had heart problems or blood clots.
- You have Parkinson's disease or have had epileptic seizures or a stroke.
- You have any blood disorders.
- You have glaucoma.
- You have an underactive thyroid gland.
- You have prostate or urethra problems.
- You are taking other medicines.

 Pregnancy
Occasionally prescribed by specialist centres. Taken close to delivery, it may cause drowsiness in the newborn baby. Discuss with your doctor.

 Breast-feeding
The drug passes into the breast milk and may affect the baby. Discuss with your doctor.

 Infants and children
Not recommended for infants under 1 year. Reduced dose necessary for older children.

 Over 60
Initial dosage is low; it may be increased if there are no adverse reactions.

 Driving and hazardous work
Avoid such activities until you have learned how chlorpromazine affects you as the drug can cause drowsiness and slowed reactions.

 Alcohol
Avoid. Alcohol may increase the sedative effects of this drug.

Surgery and general anaesthetics
Chlorpromazine may need to be stopped before you have a general anaesthetic. Discuss with your doctor or dentist.

POSSIBLE ADVERSE EFFECTS

Chlorpromazine commonly causes mild drowsiness and has an anticholinergic effect, which can cause various symptoms.

Symptom/effect	Frequency		Discuss with doctor		Stop taking drug now	Call doctor now
	Common	Rare	Only if severe	In all cases		
Drowsiness/lethargy/dry mouth	●		●			
Weight gain	●		●			
Tremor/abnormal movements	●		●			
Blurred vision	●			●		
Dizziness/fainting	●			●		
Infrequent menstrual periods		●		●		
Light-sensitive rash		●		●	●	
Jaundice		●		●	●	

INTERACTIONS

Drugs for parkinsonism Chlorpromazine may reduce the effect of these drugs.

Anticholinergic drugs These drugs may intensify the anticholinergic properties (see p.35) of chlorpromazine.

Sedatives All drugs that have a sedative effect on the central nervous system are likely to increase the sedative properties of chlorpromazine.

PROLONGED USE

If used for many years, chlorpromazine may cause tardive dyskinesia (involuntary movements of the face, jaw, and tongue), which may be irreversible. It may also cause blood abnormalities, so periodic blood tests may be performed.

CICLOSPORIN

Brand names Capimune, Deximune, Neoral, Sandimmun, Verkazia
Used in the following combined preparations None

GENERAL INFORMATION

Ciclosporin is an immunosuppressant, a drug that suppresses the body's natural defences against infection and foreign cells. This action is of particular use following organ transplants, when the recipient's immune system may reject the transplanted organ unless the immune system is controlled.

Ciclosporin is widely used after many types of transplant, such as heart, bone marrow, kidney, liver, and pancreas; its use has considerably reduced the risk of rejection. It is sometimes used to treat rheumatoid arthritis, some severe types of dermatitis, severe psoriasis, and, as eye drops, to treat a severe dry eye condition (Sjögren's syndrome).

Because ciclosporin reduces the immune system's effectiveness, it can make you more liable to infections. It can also cause kidney damage.

Different brands of ciclosporin may reach different levels in your blood. It is important to know which brand you are taking. Do not try to make dose changes on your own.

INFORMATION FOR USERS

Your drug prescription is tailored for you. Do not alter dosage without checking with your doctor.

How taken/used

Capsules, liquid, injection, eye drops.

Frequency and timing of doses
Liquid 1–2 x daily. The liquid can be mixed with water, apple juice, or orange juice just before taking. Do not mix with grapefruit juice.

Dosage range
Dosage is calculated on an individual basis according to age and weight.

Onset of effect
Within 12 hours.

Duration of action
Up to 3 days.

Diet advice
Avoid high-potassium foods, such as bananas and tomatoes; potassium supplements; and grapefruit, pomelo, and purple grape juice.

Storage
Capsules should be left in the blister pack until required. Keep in original container at room temperature out of the reach of children. Do not refrigerate.

Missed dose
Take as soon as you remember. If your dose is more than 36 hours late, consult your doctor.

Stopping the drug
Do not stop taking the drug without consulting your doctor; stopping the drug may lead to transplant rejection.

Exceeding the dose
An occasional unintentional extra dose is unlikely to cause problems. Large overdoses may cause vomiting and diarrhoea and may affect kidney function. Notify your doctor.

SPECIAL PRECAUTIONS

Ciclosporin is prescribed only under close medical supervision, taking account of your condition and medical history.

 Pregnancy
Use in pregnancy depends on condition under treatment. Discuss with your doctor.

 Breast-feeding
Not recommended. The drug passes into the breast milk and safety has not been established. Discuss with your doctor.

 Infants and children
Used only by specialist children's doctors.

 Over 60
Reduced dose may be necessary.

 Driving and hazardous work
No known problems with tablets, but eye drops may cause blurred vision.

 Alcohol
No known problems.

Sunlight and sunbeds
Avoid prolonged, unprotected exposure; apply sunscreen or sunblock.

Vaccination
Avoid vaccination with live attenuated vaccines. Discuss with your doctor.

POSSIBLE ADVERSE EFFECTS

The most common adverse effects are gum swelling, excessive hair growth, nausea and vomiting, and tremor, especially at the start of treatment. Headache and muscle cramps may also occur. Less common effects are diarrhoea, facial swelling, flushing, "pins and needles", rash, and itching. Eye pain and discharge are commonly reported with eye drops.

Symptom/effect	Frequency		Discuss with doctor		Stop taking drug now	Call doctor now
	Common	Rare	Only if severe	In all cases		
Increased body hair	●		●			
Headache	●		●			
Muscle cramps/fatigue	●		●			
Nausea	●				●	
Tremor	●				●	
Swelling of gums	●				●	

INTERACTIONS

General note Ciclosporin may interact with a large number of drugs. Check with your doctor or pharmacist before taking any new prescription or over-the-counter medications. Grapefruit juice can increase blood levels of ciclosporin. Avoid all grapefruit flesh and juice while taking ciclosporin (see Diet advice, above). St John's wort can reduce ciclosporin levels and even precipitate rejection of a transplanted organ. Avoid St John's wort completely while taking ciclosporin.

PROLONGED USE

Long-term use, especially in high doses, can affect kidney and/or liver function. It may reduce numbers of white blood cells, thus increasing susceptibility to infection. It may also cause an increase in blood pressure.

Monitoring Regular blood tests should be carried out as well as tests for liver and kidney function. Ciclosporin blood levels should also be checked regularly, and blood pressure should be monitored.

CIMETIDINE

Brand name Tagamet
Used in the following combined preparations None

GENERAL INFORMATION

Cimetidine reduces the secretion of gastric acid and pepsin (an enzyme that helps in the digestion of protein) and thereby promotes ulcer healing in the stomach and duodenum (see p.67). It is also used for reflux oesophagitis, in which acid stomach contents may flow up the oesophagus. Treatment is usually given in four- to eight-week courses, with further short courses if symptoms recur. Cimetidine also affects the actions of certain enzymes in the liver. It is therefore prescribed with caution to people taking other drugs, particularly drugs whose levels need to be carefully controlled. Since cimetidine promotes healing of the stomach lining, it may mask the symptoms of stomach cancer and delay diagnosis. It is therefore prescribed with caution to patients whose symptoms change or persist, and in middle-aged and older people.

(see p.67)

QUICK REFERENCE

Drug group Anti-ulcer drug (p.67)
Overdose danger rating Low
Dependence rating Low
Prescription needed No (some preparations)
Available as generic Yes

(p.67)

INFORMATION FOR USERS

Follow instructions on the label. Call your doctor if symptoms worsen.

How taken/used

Tablets, liquid.

Frequency and timing of doses
1–4 x daily (after meals and at bedtime).

Adult dosage range
800–1,600mg daily (occasionally increased to 2,400mg daily).

Onset of effect
Within 90 minutes.

Duration of action
2–6 hours.

Diet advice
None.

Storage
Keep in original container at room temperature out of the reach of children. Protect from light.

Missed dose
Do not take the missed dose. Take your next dose as usual.

Stopping the drug
If prescribed by your doctor, do not stop taking the drug without consulting him or her because symptoms may recur.

Exceeding the dose
An occasional unintentional extra dose is unlikely to be a cause for concern. But if you notice any unusual symptoms, or if a large overdose has been taken, notify your doctor.

SPECIAL PRECAUTIONS

Be sure to tell your doctor if:
- You have long-term liver or kidney problems.
- You are taking other medicines.

Pregnancy
Safety in pregnancy not established. Discuss with your doctor.

Breast-feeding
The drug passes into the breast milk, but at normal doses adverse effects on the baby are unlikely. Discuss with your doctor.

Infants and children
Reduced dose necessary.

Over 60
Risk of stomach cancer is higher in older people and it must be excluded before cimetidine is prescribed. The drug is also more likely to cause confusion and depression in older users.

Driving and hazardous work
Avoid such activities until you have learned how cimetidine affects you because the drug may cause dizziness and confusion.

Alcohol
Avoid. Alcohol may aggravate the underlying condition and counter the beneficial effects of cimetidine.

POSSIBLE ADVERSE EFFECTS

Adverse effects of cimetidine are uncommon. They are usually related to dosage level and almost always disappear when the drug is stopped.

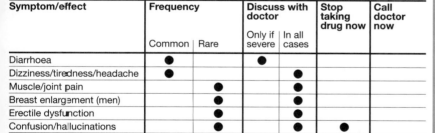

Symptom/effect	Frequency		Discuss with doctor		Stop taking drug now	Call doctor now
	Common	Rare	Only if severe	In all cases		
Diarrhoea	●		●			
Dizziness/tiredness/headache	●			●		
Muscle/joint pain		●		●		
Breast enlargement (men)		●		●		
Erectile dysfunction		●		●		
Confusion/hallucinations		●		●	●	

INTERACTIONS

Anticoagulant drugs Cimetidine may increase the effect of anticoagulants and their dose may need to be reduced.

Anticonvulsant drugs, beta blockers, anti-arrhythmic drugs, and theophylline/aminophylline Cimetidine may increase the blood levels of these drugs, and their dose may need to be reduced.

Benzodiazepines Cimetidine may increase the blood levels of some of these drugs, increasing the risk of adverse effects.

Ciclosporin and tacrolimus Cimetidine may increase the blood levels of these drugs.

Itraconazole and posaconazole Cimetidine may reduce the absorption of these drugs.

Sildenafil Cimetidine may increase the blood level of this drug.

PROLONGED USE

Courses of longer than 8 weeks are not usually necessary.

If you have bought a preparation of cimetidine over the counter for indigestion, heartburn, or acid reflux and symptoms persist for more than 2 weeks, you should consult your doctor.

CINNARIZINE

Brand names Cinarin, Cinaziere, Stugeron
Used in the following combined preparation Arlevert

GENERAL INFORMATION

Introduced in the 1970s, cinnarizine is an antihistamine used mainly to control nausea and vomiting, especially motion (travel) sickness. The drug is also used to control the symptoms (nausea and vertigo) of inner ear disorders such as labyrinthitis and Ménière's disease. Taken in high doses, cinnarizine has a vasodilator effect.

Cinnarizine has adverse effects that are similar to those of most other antihistamines. Drowsiness is the most common problem, but it is usually less severe than with other antihistamines.

QUICK REFERENCE

Drug group Antihistamine anti-emetic drug (p.46)

Overdose danger rating Medium

Dependence rating Low

Prescription needed No

Available as generic Yes

INFORMATION FOR USERS

Follow instructions on the label. Call your doctor if symptoms worsen.

How taken/used

Tablets, capsules.

Frequency and timing of doses
2–3 x daily. For the prevention of motion sickness, the first dose should be taken 2 hours before travel.

Dosage range
Adults 90mg daily (nausea/vomiting); 30mg 2 hours before travel, then 15mg every 8 hours as needed (motion sickness).
Children aged 5–12, 15mg 2 hours before travel, then 7.5mg every 8 hours as needed (motion sickness).

Onset of effect
Within 2 hours.

Duration of action
Up to 8 hours.

Diet advice
None.

Storage
Keep in original container at room temperature out of the reach of children.

Missed dose
Take as soon as you remember. If your next dose is due within 2 hours, take a single dose now and skip the next.

Stopping the drug
If you are taking cinnarizine to treat an inner ear disorder, do not stop the drug without consulting your doctor; symptoms may recur. However, when taken for motion sickness, the drug can be safely stopped as soon as you no longer need it.

Exceeding the dose
An occasional unintentional extra dose is unlikely to cause problems. Large overdoses may cause drowsiness or agitation. Notify your doctor.

SPECIAL PRECAUTIONS

Be sure to tell your doctor if:
- You have low blood pressure.
- You have Parkinson's disease.
- You have glaucoma.
- You have porphyria.
- You have an enlarged prostate.
- You are taking other medicines.

 Pregnancy
Safety in pregnancy not established. Discuss with your doctor.

 Breast-feeding
Safety not established. Discuss with your doctor.

 Infants and children
Reduced dose necessary.

 Over 60
No special problems.

 Driving and hazardous work
Avoid such activities until you have learned how cinnarizine affects you because the drug can cause drowsiness.

 Alcohol
Avoid. Alcohol may increase the sedative effects of this drug.

PROLONGED USE

Development or aggravation of extrapyramidal symptoms (abnormal movements) may occur rarely in older people after prolonged use of cinnarizine. If such symptoms develop, treatment should be discontinued.

POSSIBLE ADVERSE EFFECTS

Drowsiness is the main adverse effect of this drug. Anticholinergic effects such as blurred vision and dry mouth may also occur occasionally.

Symptom/effect	Frequency		Discuss with doctor		Stop taking drug now	Call doctor now
	Common	Rare	Only if severe	In all cases		
Drowsiness/lethargy	●		●			
Blurred vision		●	●			
Dry mouth		●	●			
Gastrointestinal problems		●	●			
Rash		●		●	●	

INTERACTIONS

General note All drugs that have a sedative effect on the central nervous system may increase the sedative properties of cinnarizine. Such drugs include sleeping drugs, antidepressants, anti-anxiety drugs, and opioid analgesics.

CIPROFLOXACIN

Brand names Cetraxal, Ciloxan, Ciproxin
Used in the following combined preparations None

GENERAL INFORMATION

Ciprofloxacin, a quinolone antibacterial drug, is used to treat bacteria resistant to other commonly used antibiotics. It is especially useful for chest, intestine, urinary tract, and eye infections. When taken by mouth, ciprofloxacin works quickly and effectively. In more severe systemic bacterial infections, however, it may be necessary to administer the drug by injection. Eye infections are usually treated with topical preparations.

The most common side effect of oral or injected ciprofloxacin is intestinal disturbance. Occasionally it may cause tendon inflammation and damage (see advice for levofloxacin, p.299). Topical eye preparations may sometimes cause eye discomfort or blurred vision.

see advice for levofloxacin, p.299

QUICK REFERENCE

Drug group Antibacterial drug (p.89)

Overdose danger rating Medium

Dependence rating Low

Prescription needed Yes

Available as generic Yes

INFORMATION FOR USERS

Your drug prescription is tailored for you. Do not alter dosage without checking with your doctor.

How taken/used

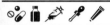

Tablets, liquid, injection, eye drops, eye ointment.

Frequency and timing of doses
2 x daily with plenty of fluids; variable with topical eye preparations.

Adult dosage range
500mg–1.5g daily (tablets); 400mg–1.2g daily (injection); variable with topical eye preparations

Onset of effect
Within a few hours, although full beneficial effect may not be felt for several days.

Duration of action
About 12 hours.

Diet advice
Do not become dehydrated. Avoid dairy products; they may reduce the drug's absorption. No special dietary precautions needed for topical eye preparations.

Storage
Keep in original container at room temperature out of the reach of children. The injection must be protected from light.

Missed dose
Take as soon as you remember, and take your next dose as usual.

Stopping the drug
Take the full course. Even if you feel better the original infection may still be present, and symptoms may recur if treatment is stopped too soon.

Exceeding the dose
An occasional unintentional extra dose is unlikely to cause problems. Large overdoses of oral or injected preparations may cause kidney problems, mental disturbance, and seizures. Notify your doctor.

SPECIAL PRECAUTIONS

Be sure to tell your doctor if:
- You have long-term liver or kidney problems.
- You have heart rhythm problems.
- You have had epileptic seizures.
- You have glucose-6-phosphate dehydrogenase (G6PD) deficiency.
- You have myasthenia gravis.
- You are taking other medicines.

 Pregnancy
Safety in pregnancy not established. Discuss with your doctor.

 Breast-feeding
The drug passes into the breast milk and may affect the baby adversely. Discuss with your doctor.

 Infants and children
Not usually recommended (oral and injected forms); reduced dose may be necessary (topical eye preparations).

 Over 60
Reduced dose may be necessary.

 Driving and hazardous work
Avoid such activities until you have learned how ciprofloxacin affects you; the drug may cause dizziness and confusion. Topical eye preparations may cause blurred vision.

 Alcohol
Avoid if using oral or injected preparations as alcohol may increase the sedative effects of this drug.

Sunlight and sunbeds
Avoid direct exposure to sunlight or sunlamps; increased risk of a photosensitivity reaction.

POSSIBLE ADVERSE EFFECTS (oral and injected forms)

Most side effects are rare, except when very high doses are given. Report painful tendons or joints to your doctor at once, discontinue treatment, and rest the affected limbs.

Symptom/effect	Frequency		Discuss with doctor		Stop taking drug now	Call doctor now
	Common	Rare	Only if severe	In all cases		
Nausea/vomiting	●		●			
Abdominal pain/diarrhoea	●		●			
Rash/itching	●			●		
Dizziness/headache		●	●			
Sleep disturbance		●	●			
Photosensitivity		●		●		
Jaundice		●		●		
Confusion		●		●		
Seizures		●		●	●	●
Painful joints/tendons		●		●	●	●

INTERACTIONS

General note A large number of drugs interact with ciprofloxacin. Do not take any over-the-counter or prescription medications without consulting your doctor or pharmacist.

Oral iron preparations and antacids containing magnesium or aluminium hydroxide interfere with absorption of ciprofloxacin. Do not take antacids within 2 hours of taking ciprofloxacin tablets.

PROLONGED USE

Ciprofloxacin is not usually prescribed for long-term use.

CISPLATIN

Brand names None
Used in the following combined preparations None

GENERAL INFORMATION

Cisplatin is an effective treatment for a wide variety of cancers including cancer of the ovaries, testes, head, neck, lung, bladder, and cervix, blood cancers, and certain children's cancers. It is usually given with other anticancer drugs and can be given alongside radiotherapy.

The most common and serious adverse effect of cisplatin is impaired kidney function. To reduce the risk of permanent damage, the drug is usually given only once every three weeks, and plenty of fluid must be taken to minimize the effect on the kidneys. Cisplatin also frequently causes severe nausea and vomiting, usually starting within an hour and lasting for up to 24 hours, but in some cases persisting for up to a week. To prevent or control these symptoms, anti-emetic drugs are usually given. Damage to hearing is uncommon; it may be more severe in children and become more apparent at the end of treatment. Cisplatin may also increase the risk of anaemia, blood clotting disorders, and infection. It is likely to reduce fertility, especially in men, so approaches to preserve sperm may be offered.

INFORMATION FOR USERS

This drug is given only under medical supervision and is not for self-administration.

How taken/used

Injection.

Frequency and timing of doses
Every 3 weeks for up to 5 days; it may be given alone or in combination with other anticancer drugs.

Adult dosage range
Dosage is determined individually according to body height, weight, and response.

Onset of effect
Some adverse effects, such as nausea and vomiting, may appear within 1 hour of starting treatment.

Duration of action
Some adverse effects may last for up to 1 week after treatment has stopped.

Diet advice
Prior to treatment it is important that the body is well hydrated. Therefore, 1–2 litres of fluid are usually given by infusion over 8–12 hours.

Storage
Not applicable. The drug is not normally kept in the home.

Missed dose
Not applicable. The drug is given only in hospital under medical supervision.

Stopping the drug
Not applicable. The drug will be stopped under medical supervision.

Exceeding the dose
Overdosage is unlikely since treatment is carefully monitored, and the drug is given intravenously only under close supervision.

POSSIBLE ADVERSE EFFECTS

Most adverse effects appear within a few hours of injection and are carefully monitored in hospital after each dose. Some effects wear off within 24 hours. Nausea and loss of appetite may last for up to a week.

Symptom/effect	Frequency		Discuss with doctor		Stop taking drug now	Call doctor now
	Common	Rare	Only if severe	In all cases		
Loss of appetite/taste	●		●			
Nausea/vomiting	●			●		
Ringing in the ears/hearing loss		●		●		
Breathing difficulties/wheezing		●		●		●
Abnormal sensations		●		●		●
Swollen face/rash		●		●		●
Reduced urine output		●		●	●	●

INTERACTIONS

General note A number of drugs (e.g. antibacterials such as gentamicin) increase the adverse effects of cisplatin. Because cisplatin is given only under close medical supervision, these interactions are carefully monitored and the dosage is adjusted accordingly.

SPECIAL PRECAUTIONS

Cisplatin is prescribed only under close medical supervision, taking account of your present condition and your medical history. However, tell your doctor if:
- You have impaired kidney function.
- You are planning to have children.
- You are taking other medicines.

Pregnancy
Not usually prescribed. Cisplatin may cause birth defects or premature birth. Discuss with your doctor.

Breast-feeding
Not advised. The drug passes into the breast milk and may affect the baby adversely. Discuss with your doctor.

Infants and children
The risk of hearing loss is increased. Reduced dose used.

Over 60
Reduced dose may be necessary. Increased risk of adverse effects.

Driving and hazardous work
No known problems.

Alcohol
No known problems.

PROLONGED USE

There is an increased risk of long-term damage to the kidneys, nerves, and bone marrow, and to hearing. The drug may also increase the risk of further cancers later in life.

Monitoring Hearing tests and blood checks to monitor kidney function and bone marrow activity are carried out regularly.

CITALOPRAM/ESCITALOPRAM

Brand names [escitalopram] Cipralex; [citalopram] Cipramil
Used in the following combined preparations None

GENERAL INFORMATION

Citalopram and escitalopram are selective serotonin re-uptake inhibitor (SSRI) antidepressant drugs used for depressive illness and panic disorder; escitalopram is also given for social and generalized anxiety disorders. They gradually improve mood, increase physical activity, and restore interest in everyday pursuits. Both are generally well tolerated, and any gastrointestinal adverse effects, such as nausea, vomiting, or diarrhoea, are dose related and usually diminish with continued use. Like other SSRIs, citalopram and escitalopram cause fewer anticholinergic side effects and are less sedating than tricyclic antidepressants. They are also less likely to be harmful in overdose, but can cause drowsiness and impair performance of tasks such as driving.

QUICK REFERENCE

Drug group Antidepressant drug (p.40)

Overdose danger rating Medium

Dependence rating Low

Prescription needed Yes

Available as generic Yes (both drugs)

INFORMATION FOR USERS

Your drug prescription is tailored for you. Do not alter dosage without checking with your doctor.

How taken/used

Tablets, oral drops.

Frequency and timing of doses
Once daily in the morning or evening.

Adult dosage range
Depressive illness 20–40mg (citalopram); 10–20mg (escitalopram).
Panic attacks 10–40mg (citalopram); 5–20mg (escitalopram).
Social anxiety disorder 5–20mg (escitalopram).
Generalized anxiety disorder 10–20mg (escitalopram).

Onset of effect
Some benefit may appear within 7 days, but full benefits may not be felt for 2–6 weeks (panic attacks may take longer to resolve).

Duration of action
Antidepressant effect may persist for some weeks following prolonged treatment.

Diet advice
None.

Storage
Keep in original container at room temperature out of the reach of children.

Missed dose
Take as soon as you remember. If your next dose is due within 8 hours, take a single dose now and skip the next.

Stopping the drug
Do not stop taking the drug without consulting your doctor. Stopping abruptly can cause withdrawal symptoms.

Exceeding the dose
An occasional unintentional extra dose is unlikely to be a cause for concern. If you notice any unusual symptoms, or if a large overdose has been taken, notify your doctor.

SPECIAL PRECAUTIONS

Be sure to tell your doctor if:
- You have epilepsy.
- You have diabetes.
- You have liver or kidney problems.
- You have had manic-depressive illness and/or suicidal thoughts.
- You have or have had heart problems, particularly heart rhythm disturbances.
- You have been taking monoamine oxidase inhibitors (MAOIs) or other antidepressants.
- You are taking other medicines.

 Pregnancy
Safety in pregnancy not established. Discuss with your doctor.

 Breast-feeding
May pass into breast milk and affect the baby. Discuss with your doctor.

 Infants and children
Not generally recommended under 18 years.

 Over 60
Reduced dose may be necessary.

 Driving and hazardous work
Avoid such activities until you have learned how the drugs affect you because they can cause drowsiness.

 Alcohol
No special problems.

POSSIBLE ADVERSE EFFECTS

Common side effects such as gastrointestinal problems usually diminish with reduced dose. If seizures, rash, or heart rate or rhythm problems occur, consult your doctor at once.

Symptom/effect	Frequency		Discuss with doctor		Stop taking drug now	Call doctor now
	Common	Rare	Only if severe	In all cases		
Nausea/vomiting/indigestion	●			●		
Diarrhoea/constipation	●			●		
Sexual dysfunction	●			●		
Anxiety/insomnia	●			●		
Headache/tremor	●			●		
Dizziness/drowsiness	●			●		
Dry mouth/sweating	●			●		
Suicidal thoughts/attempts		●		●	●	●

INTERACTIONS

Sumatriptan, other 5HT1 agonists, and lithium There is an increased risk of adverse effects when citalopram and escitalopram are taken with these drugs.

Anticoagulants The effect of these drugs may be increased by citalopram and escitalopram and bruising may occur.

St John's wort may increase the adverse effects of citalopram and escitalopram.

Monoamine oxidase inhibitors (MAOIs) may cause a severe reaction if taken with citalopram and escitalopram; avoid if MAOIs have been taken in the last 14 days.

PROLONGED USE

No problems expected in most otherwise healthy adults. However, high doses are associated with an increased risk of developing heart problems, especially in those over 65. Mild withdrawal symptoms may occur if the drug is not stopped gradually. There is also a small risk of suicidal thoughts and self-harm in children and adolescents, although the drug is rarely used for this age group.

Monitoring Any person experiencing drowsiness, confusion, muscle cramps, or seizures should be monitored for low sodium levels in the blood. Under-18s should be monitored for suicidal thoughts and self-harm.

CLARITHROMYCIN

Brand names Clarosip, Febzin XL, Klaricid, Klaricid XL, Mycifor XL
Used in the following combined preparations None

GENERAL INFORMATION

Clarithromycin is a macrolide antibiotic similar to erythromycin (p.247), from which it is derived. It has similar actions and uses to erythromycin, but is slightly more active. Clarithromycin is used for ear, nose, and throat infections, such as middle ear infections, sinusitis, and pharyngitis, and respiratory tract infections, including whooping cough, bronchitis, and pneumonia, as well as for skin and soft tissue infections. Given with antiulcer drugs (p.67) and other antibiotics, it is used to eradicate *Helicobacter pylori*, the bacterium that causes many peptic ulcers.

Prolonged use of clarithromycin is not usually necessary.

QUICK REFERENCE

Drug group Antibiotic (p.86)
Overdose danger rating Low
Dependence rating Low
Prescription needed Yes
Available as generic No

INFORMATION FOR USERS

Your drug prescription is tailored for you. Do not alter dosage without checking with your doctor.

How taken/used

Tablets, liquid, granules, injection.

Frequency and timing of doses
2 x daily, up to 14 days; 1 x daily (XL preparations).

Adult dosage range
500mg–1g daily.

Onset of effect
1–4 hours.

Duration of action
1–12 hours; 24 hours (XL preparations).

Diet advice
None.

Storage
Keep in original container at room temperature out of the reach of children. Protect from light.

Missed dose
Take as soon as you remember. If your next dose is due within 2 hours, take a single dose now and skip the next.

Stopping the drug
Take the full course. Even if you feel better, the infection may still be present and symptoms may recur if treatment is stopped too soon.

Exceeding the dose
An occasional unintentional extra dose is unlikely to be a cause for concern. But if you notice any unusual symptoms, or if a large overdose has been taken, notify your doctor.

SPECIAL PRECAUTIONS

Be sure to tell your doctor if:
- You have liver or kidney problems.
- You have had an allergic reaction to erythromycin or clarithromycin.
- You have a heart problem.
- You have porphyria.
- You are taking other medicines.

Pregnancy
Safety has not been established. Discuss with your doctor.

Breast-feeding
Clarithromycin passes into the breast milk and may affect the baby. Discuss with your doctor.

Infants and children
Reduced dose necessary.

Over 60
No special problems.

Driving and hazardous work
No known problems.

Alcohol
No known problems.

PROLONGED USE

In courses of over 14 days, there is a risk of developing antibiotic-resistant infections.

POSSIBLE ADVERSE EFFECTS

Clarithromycin is generally well tolerated. Gastrointestinal disturbances are the most common problems encountered. Hearing loss is a rare possibility, but it is usually reversible on stopping the drug.

Symptom/effect	Frequency		Discuss with doctor		Stop taking drug now	Call doctor now
	Common	Rare	Only if severe	In all cases		
Nausea/vomiting/diarrhoea	●		●			
Indigestion	●		●			
Headache	●		●			
Joint/muscle pain	●		●			
Rash	●			●	●	
Altered sense of taste/smell		●		●		
Anxiety/insomnia		●		●		
Confusion/hallucinations		●		●		
Jaundice		●		●	●	

INTERACTIONS

Warfarin, midazolam, disopyramide, lovastatin, repaglinide, rifabutin, ranolazine, ticagrelor, ciclosporin, tacrolimus, sildenafil, ergotamine, and valproate Blood levels and effects of these drugs are increased by clarithromycin.

Carbamazepine, phenytoin, theophylline, digoxin, and colchicine Blood levels and toxicity of these drugs are increased by clarithromycin.

Amiodarone, citalopram, domperidone, ondansetron, quinine, and ranolazone Avoid taking with clarithromycin as they may cause cardiac arrhythmias.

Lipid-lowering drugs whose names end in 'statin' There is a risk of rhabdomyolysis (muscle damage) with clarithromycin.

Zidovudine Blood levels of zidovudine are reduced if this drug is taken at the same time as clarithromycin.

CLINDAMYCIN

Brand names Dalacin, Dalacin C, Dalacin T, Zindaclin
Used in the following combined preparation Duac Once Daily, Treclin

GENERAL INFORMATION

Clindamycin is an effective antibiotic against a broad range of bacteria. This action, combined with the fact that the drug reaches good concentrations in the bones and skin, makes it especially useful for treating diseases such as the bone infection osteomyelitis and the skin infections erysipelas and cellulitis. Clindamycin is also effective against protozoa, such as those causing toxoplasmosis and falciparum malaria. However, it may cause proliferation of other bacteria such as *Clostridium difficile*, especially in the intestines when the drug is used in oral or intravenous forms. Clindamycin-induced *Clostridium difficile* diarrhoea is a serious and sometimes life-threatening side effect, which limits the use of this antibiotic. For this reason the drug should be used under specialist supervision and avoided in older people. Clindamycin may also be used topically for acne as well as vulval and vaginal infections.

QUICK REFERENCE

Drug group Antibiotic (p.86)
Overdose danger rating Low
Dependence rating Low
Prescription needed Yes
Available as generic Yes

INFORMATION FOR USERS

Your drug prescription is tailored for you. Do not alter dosage without checking with your doctor.

How taken/used

Capsules, injection, topical solution, vaginal cream.

Frequency and timing of doses
4 x daily with plenty of water (capsules); 2–4 x times daily (injection); 1–2 x daily (topical solution or vaginal cream).

Adult dosage range
600mg–1.8g daily (capsules); 0.6–4.8g daily in divided doses (injection); 5g daily (vaginal cream); 1 pre-prepared applicator daily (topical solution).

Onset of effect
1 hour.

Duration of action
6 hours.

Diet advice
None.

Storage
Keep in original container at room temperature out of the reach of children.

Missed dose
Take as soon as you remember, and take your next dose as usual.

Stopping the drug
Take the full course. Even if you feel better the original infection may still be present, and symptoms may recur if treatment is stopped too soon.

Exceeding the dose
An occasional unintended extra dose is unlikely to cause problems. Large overdoses may cause nausea or, in rare cases, seizures. Notify your doctor immediately.

SPECIAL PRECAUTIONS

Be sure to tell your doctor if:
- You have a history of antibiotic-associated or *Clostridium difficile* diarrhoea.
- You have gastrointestinal disease.
- You have kidney or liver problems.

 Pregnancy
Use in pregnancy only if clearly needed. Discuss with your doctor.

 Breast-feeding
The drug passes into the breast milk, but at normal doses adverse effects on the baby are unlikely. Discuss with your doctor.

 Infants and children
Reduced dose necessary.

 Over 60
Not recommended.

 Driving and hazardous work
No special problems.

 Alcohol
No special problems.

POSSIBLE ADVERSE EFFECTS

Most side effects are rare and rash/itching is the only likely adverse reaction to the topical solution or vaginal cream. Nausea and hypersensitivity reactions are possible with oral and injected forms of the drug. The most serious side effect is *Clostridium difficile* diarrhoea. Report any diarrhoea to your doctor immediately and stop taking the drug.

Symptom/effect	Frequency		Discuss with doctor		Stop taking drug now	Call doctor now
	Common	Rare	Only if severe	In all cases		
Nausea	●		●			
Rash/itching		●		●		
Jaundice		●		●	●	
Diarrhoea	●			●	●	●

PROLONGED USE

No major problems with the topical solution or vaginal cream. Oral and injected forms of the drug carry an ongoing risk of *Clostridium difficile* diarrhoea.

Monitoring Liver and renal function will need to be monitored if oral or injected treatment exceeds 10 days.

INTERACTIONS

General note Interactions are unlikely with the topical solution and vaginal cream.

Warfarin Clindamycin may alter the effectiveness of warfarin.

Muscle relaxants Clindamycin may enhance the action of neuromuscular blocking drugs.

Pyridostigmine and neostigmine Clindamycin reduces the effectiveness of these drugs.

Oral typhoid vaccine Clindamycin may make this vaccine less effective if taken at the time of vaccination.

CLOBETASOL

Brand names Clarelux, Clobaderm, Dermovate, Etrivex
Used in the following combined preparation Dermovate-NN

GENERAL INFORMATION

Clobetasol is a very potent corticosteroid drug (p.99) used for the short-term treatment of inflammatory skin conditions that have not responded to treatment with a less potent corticosteroid. Clobetasol is used to treat conditions such as resistant eczema, discoid lupus erythematosus, lichen planus, and lichen simplex.

Because clobetasol is one of the strongest topical corticosteroids, it should be applied thinly and sparingly only to affected areas, and for the shortest possible duration. This is to prevent skin damage and to avoid rare systemic side effects, which can occur from absorption of the drug through the skin. Such side effects include pituitary or adrenal gland suppression and Cushing's syndrome. In addition, clobetasol should not be used on untreated bacterial, fungal, or viral skin infections.

Treatment of psoriasis with clobetasol must only be carried out under specialist care and supervision.

INFORMATION FOR USERS

Your drug prescription is tailored for you. Do not alter dosage without checking with your doctor.

How taken/used

Cream, ointment, scalp application.

Frequency and timing of doses
1–2 x daily. For the face (only under specialist advice), use for no more than 5 days.

Dosage range
Usually limited to 50g weekly, but prescribed dose depends on the condition and its extent.

Onset of effect
12 hours. Full beneficial effect after 48 hours.

Duration of action
Up to 24 hours.

Diet advice
None.

Storage
Keep in original container at room temperature out of the reach of children.

Missed dose
Use as soon as you remember. If your next application is due within 8 hours, apply the usual amount now and skip the next application.

Stopping the drug
Do not stop using the drug without consulting your doctor, who may advise a gradual reduction in dosage to reduce the likelihood of a flare-up of symptoms.

Exceeding the dose
An occasional unintentional extra application is unlikely to cause problems. But if you notice any unusual symptoms, notify your doctor.

POSSIBLE ADVERSE EFFECTS

Most people who use clobetasol as directed do not have problems. Adverse effects mainly affect the skin. Some of these effects may not be reversible.

Symptom/effect	Frequency		Discuss with doctor		Stop taking drug now	Call doctor now
	Common	Rare	Only if severe	In all cases		
Thinning of the skin		●		●		
Stretch marks/thread veins		●		●		
Increased capillary size in skin		●		●		
Acne/dermatitis		●		●		
Loss of skin pigment	●		●			
Unwanted hair growth	●		●			

INTERACTIONS

None.

SPECIAL PRECAUTIONS

Be sure to tell your doctor if:
- You have a cold sore or chickenpox.
- You have any other infection.
- You have psoriasis.
- You have acne or rosacea.
- You are taking other medicines.

 Pregnancy
Safety in pregnancy not established. Discuss with your doctor.

 Breast-feeding
The drug passes into the breast milk and may affect the baby. Discuss with your doctor.

 Infants and children
Not recommended for infants under 1 year. Used only with great caution for short periods in older children because overuse increases the risk of side effects.

 Over 60
No special problems.

 Driving and hazardous work
No special problems.

 Alcohol
No special problems.

PROLONGED USE

Clobetasol is not normally used for more than 4 weeks. If the condition has not improved in 2 to 4 weeks, you should notify your doctor.

CLOMIFENE

Brand name Clomid
Used in the following combined preparations None

GENERAL INFORMATION

Clomifene is used for female infertility due to failure of ovulation. It stimulates ovulation by increasing production of hormones by the hypothalamus and pituitary gland. Tablets are taken within about five days of the onset of each menstrual cycle. If clomifene does not stimulate ovulation after several months, other drugs may be prescribed.

Multiple pregnancies (usually with twins) occur more commonly in women treated with clomifene. Adverse effects include an increased risk of ovarian cysts and ectopic pregnancy. Ovarian hyperstimulation syndrome (over-stimulation of the ovaries) has also been reported; symptoms include pain and swelling of the abdomen, swelling of the hands and legs, shortness of breath, weight gain, nausea, and vomiting. You should consult your doctor immediately if any of these symptoms develop.

QUICK REFERENCE

Drug group Drug for infertility (p.124)
Overdose danger rating Low
Dependence rating Low
Prescription needed Yes
Available as generic Yes

INFORMATION FOR USERS

Your drug prescription is tailored for you. Do not alter dosage without checking with your doctor.

How taken/used

Tablets.

Frequency and timing of doses
Once daily for 5 days in each menstrual cycle.

Dosage range
50mg daily initially; dose may be increased up to 100mg daily.

Onset of effect
Ovulation occurs 11–12 days after the last dose in any cycle. However, ovulation may not occur for several months.

Duration of action
5 days.

Diet advice
None.

Storage
Keep in original container at room temperature out of the reach of children. Protect from light.

Missed dose
Take as soon as you remember. If your next dose is due at this time, take the missed dose and the next scheduled dose together.

Stopping the drug
Take as directed by your doctor. Stopping the drug will reduce the chances of conception.

Exceeding the dose
An occasional unintentional extra dose is unlikely to be a cause for concern. But if you notice any unusual symptoms, or if a large overdose has been taken, notify your doctor.

POSSIBLE ADVERSE EFFECTS

Most side effects are related to the dose taken. Ovarian enlargement and cyst formation can occur. If this happens the problem usually resolves within a few weeks of stopping the drug.

Symptom/effect	Frequency Common	Frequency Rare	Discuss with doctor Only if severe	Discuss with doctor In all cases	Stop taking drug now	Call doctor now
Hot flushes	●		●			
"Breakthrough" bleeding	●		●			
Nausea/vomiting	●			●		
Abdominal discomfort/bloating	●			●		
Headache		●	●			
Breast tenderness		●		●		
Dry skin/hair loss/rash		●		●		
Dizziness		●		●		
Blurred/disturbed vision		●		●	●	
Seizures/swollen limbs		●		●	●	●
Severe pain in chest/abdomen		●		●	●	●

INTERACTIONS

None.

SPECIAL PRECAUTIONS

Be sure to tell your doctor if:
• You have a long-term liver problem.
• You are pregnant.
• You have uterine fibroids, ovarian cysts, or abnormal vaginal bleeding.
• You are taking other medicines.

 Pregnancy
Not prescribed. The drug is stopped as soon as pregnancy occurs.

 Breast-feeding
Not prescribed.

 Infants and children
Not prescribed.

 Over 60
Not prescribed.

 Driving and hazardous work
Avoid such activities until you have learned how clomifene affects you because the drug can cause blurred vision.

 Alcohol
Keep consumption low.

PROLONGED USE

Prolonged use of clomifene may cause visual impairment. Also, no more than 6 courses of treatment are recommended since this may lead to an increased risk of ovarian cancer.

Monitoring Eye tests may be recommended if symptoms of visual impairment are noticed. Monitoring of body temperature and blood or urine hormone levels, or ultrasound scans of the ovaries are performed to detect signs of ovulation and pregnancy.

CLOMIPRAMINE

Brand names Anafranil
Used in the following combined preparations None

GENERAL INFORMATION

Clomipramine belongs to the class of antidepressant drugs known as the tricyclics. It is used mainly in the long-term treatment of depression.

Clomipramine is particularly useful in the treatment of obsessive and phobic disorders. In this case, the drug has to be taken for many months to achieve its full effect. It is also used to treat cataplexy (sudden loss of muscle tone) and narcolepsy (attacks of sleepiness).

Clomipramine has similar adverse effects to other tricyclic drugs, such as drowsiness, dizziness, dry mouth, and constipation. In overdose, clomipramine may cause coma and dangerously abnormal heart rhythms.

INFORMATION FOR USERS

Your drug prescription is tailored for you. Do not alter dosage without checking with your doctor.

How taken/used

Tablets, capsules.

Frequency and timing of doses
1–3 x daily.

Adult dosage range
10–250mg daily but 30–50mg is often effective.

Onset of effect
Some effects, a few days; full antidepressant effect, up to 6 weeks; phobic and obsessional disorders, full effect up to 12 weeks.

Duration of action
During prolonged treatment antidepressant effect may last up to 2 weeks.

Diet advice
Avoid grapefruit and cranberry juice because they may interact with clomipramine and increase the drug's effects.

Storage
Keep in original container at room temperature out of the reach of children.

Missed dose
Take as soon as you remember. If your next dose is due within 3 hours, take a single dose now and skip the next.

Stopping the drug
Stopping abruptly can cause withdrawal symptoms and a recurrence of the original disorder. Consult your doctor, who will supervise a gradual reduction in dosage.

OVERDOSE ACTION

 Seek immediate medical advice in all cases. Take emergency action if palpitations are noted or consciousness is lost.

See Drug poisoning emergency guide (p.518).

POSSIBLE ADVERSE EFFECTS

The possible adverse effects of this drug are mainly the result of its anticholinergic action, and include drowsiness and dizziness, dry mouth, and constipation.

Symptom/effect	Frequency		Discuss with doctor		Stop taking drug now	Call doctor now
	Common	Rare	Only if severe	In all cases		
Drowsiness/dizziness	●		●			
Sweating/flushing	●		●			
Dry mouth	●		●			
Blurred vision	●					
Constipation	●		●			
Weight gain	●		●			
Difficulty in passing urine		●		●	●	
Palpitations		●		●	●	●

INTERACTIONS

Sedatives All drugs that have a sedative effect may intensify those of clomipramine.

Anticonvulsant drugs Clomipramine may reduce the effects of these drugs and vice versa.

Antihypertensives Clomipramine may enhance the effect of some of these drugs.

Monoamine oxidase inhibitors (MAOIs) A serious reaction may occur if these drugs are given with clomipramine.

Grapefruit and cranberry juice These may increase the effects of clomipramine.

Cigarette smoking and St. John's wort may decrease the effect of clomipramine.

SPECIAL PRECAUTIONS

Be sure to tell your doctor if:
- You have heart problems.
- You have had epileptic seizures.
- You have long-term liver or kidney problems.
- You have had glaucoma.
- You have had prostate problems.
- You have had mania or a psychotic illness.
- You are taking other medicines

 Pregnancy
Safety in pregnancy not established. Discuss with your doctor.

 Breast-feeding
The drug passes into the breast milk and may affect the baby. Discuss with your doctor.

 Infants and children
Not recommended.

 Over 60
Increased likelihood of adverse effects. Reduced dose may therefore be necessary.

 Driving and hazardous work
Avoid such activities until you have learned how clomipramine affects you because the drug may cause blurred vision, drowsiness, and dizziness.

 Alcohol
Avoid. Alcohol may increase the sedative effects of this drug.

Surgery and general anaesthetics
Clomipramine treatment may need to be stopped before you have a general anaesthetic. Discuss this with your doctor or dentist before any operation

PROLONGED USE

No problems expected.

Monitoring Regular checks on heart and liver function are recommended.

CLONAZEPAM

Brand names None
Used in the following combined preparations None

GENERAL INFORMATION

Clonazepam belongs to a group of drugs known as the benzodiazepines, which are mainly used in the treatment of anxiety and insomnia (see Anti-anxiety drugs, p.39). However, clonazepam is usually used as an anticonvulsant to prevent and treat epileptic seizures. It is particularly useful for the prevention of brief muscle spasms (myoclonus) and absence seizures (petit mal) in children, but other forms of epilepsy, such as sudden flaccidity or seizures induced by flashing lights, also respond to clonazepam treatment. Being a benzodiazepine, the drug also has sedative effects.

Clonazepam is used either alone or together with other anticonvulsant drugs. Its anticonvulsant effect may begin to wear off after some months, which often limits its long-term use.

QUICK REFERENCE

Drug group Benzodiazepine anticonvulsant drug (p.42)

Overdose danger rating Medium

Dependence rating Medium

Prescription needed Yes

Available as generic Yes

INFORMATION FOR USERS

Your drug prescription is tailored for you. Do not alter dosage without checking with your doctor.

How taken/used

Tablets, liquid.

Frequency and timing of doses
1–4 x daily.

Dosage range
Adults 1mg daily at night (starting dose), increased gradually to 4–8mg daily (maintenance dose).
Children Reduced dose according to age and weight.

Onset of effect
1–4 hours.

Duration of action
24–48 hours.

Diet advice
None.

Storage
Keep in original container at room temperature out of the reach of children.

Missed dose
No cause for concern, but take as soon as you remember. Take your next dose when it is due.

Stopping the drug
Do not stop taking the drug without consulting your doctor because symptoms may recur, and withdrawal symptoms may occur.

Exceeding the dose
An occasional unintentional extra dose is unlikely to cause problems. Larger overdoses may cause excessive drowsiness and confusion. Notify your doctor.

POSSIBLE ADVERSE EFFECTS

The principal adverse effects of this drug are related to its sedative and tranquillizing properties. These effects normally diminish after the first few days of treatment and can often be reduced by medically supervised adjustment of dosage.

Symptom/effect	Frequency		Discuss with doctor		Stop taking drug now	Call doctor now
	Common	Rare	Only if severe	In all cases		
Daytime drowsiness	●		●			
Dizziness/unsteadiness	●		●			
Altered behaviour	●			●		
Forgetfulness/confusion		●		●		
Muscle weakness		●		●		

INTERACTIONS

Sedatives All drugs that have a sedative effect on the central nervous system are likely to increase the sedative properties of clonazepam. Such drugs include anti-anxiety and sleeping drugs, antihistamines, opioid analgesics, antidepressants, and antipsychotics.

Other anticonvulsants Clonazepam may alter the effects of other anticonvulsants you are taking, or they may alter its effect. Adjustment of dosage or change of drug may be necessary.

SPECIAL PRECAUTIONS

Be sure to tell your doctor if:
- You have severe respiratory disease, including sleep apnoea.
- You have long-term liver or kidney problems.
- You have porphyria.
- You have myasthenia gravis.
- You have misused drugs or alcohol.
- You have mental health problems.
- You are taking other medicines.

Pregnancy
May cause adverse effects in the baby if used in late pregnancy or labour. Discuss with your doctor.

Breast-feeding
The drug passes into the breast milk and may affect the baby adversely. Discuss with your doctor.

Infants and children
Reduced dose necessary.

Over 60
Reduced dose may be necessary.

Driving and hazardous work
Your condition, as well as the risk of drowsiness with clonazepam, may make such activities inadvisable. Discuss with your doctor.

Alcohol
Avoid. Alcohol may increase the sedative effects of this drug.

PROLONGED USE

Both beneficial and adverse effects of clonazepam may become less marked during prolonged treatment as the body adapts. Prolonged use may also result in dependence and difficulty in withdrawing.

CLOPIDOGREL

Brand names Grepid, Plavix
Used in the following combined preparations None

GENERAL INFORMATION

Clopidogrel is an antiplatelet drug used to prevent blood clots from forming. It is prescribed to patients who have a tendency to form clots in the fast-flowing blood of the arteries and heart, or those who have had a stroke or heart attack. It is also widely used to prevent clots forming in metal stents inserted into coronary arteries. It may be used alone or in combination with aspirin.

Clopidogrel reduces the sticking together of platelets, which can lead to abnormal bleeding. You should therefore report any unusual bleeding to your doctor at once, and, if you require dental treatment, you should tell your dentist that you are taking clopidogrel.

Adverse effects are common with clopidogrel and are usually associated with bleeding.

QUICK REFERENCE

Drug group Antiplatelet drug (p.62)
Overdose danger rating Medium
Dependence rating Low
Prescription needed Yes
Available as generic Yes

INFORMATION FOR USERS

Your drug prescription is tailored for you. Do not alter dosage without checking with your doctor.

How taken/used

Tablets.

Frequency and timing of doses
Once daily.

Dosage range
75mg; up to 300mg as initial dose in hospital.

Onset of effect
1 hour.

Duration of action
Antiplatelet effect may last up to 1 week.

Diet advice
None.

Storage
Keep in original container at room temperature out of the reach of children.

Missed dose
Take as soon as you remember. If your next dose is due within 4 hours, take a single dose now and skip the next.

Stopping the drug
Do not stop taking the drug without consulting your doctor. Stopping the drug may lead to a recurrence of the original condition.

Exceeding the dose
An occasional unintentional extra dose is unlikely to be a cause for concern. But if you notice any unusual symptoms, or if a large overdose has been taken, notify your doctor.

POSSIBLE ADVERSE EFFECTS

The most frequent side effects of clopidogrel are bleeding and bruising. Nausea and diarrhoea are less common.

Symptom/effect	Frequency		Discuss with doctor		Stop taking drug now	Call doctor now
	Common	Rare	Only if severe	In all cases		
Diarrhoea/abdominal pain	●		●			
Bruising/nosebleeds	●				●	
Nausea/vomiting		●	●			
Headache/dizziness		●	●			
Constipation		●	●			
Blood in urine/faeces		●		●		
Rash/itching		●		●		
Sore throat/fever		●		●		●

INTERACTIONS

Aspirin and other non-steroidal anti-inflammatory drugs (NSAIDs)
Clopidogrel increases the effect of aspirin on platelets. The risk of gastrointestinal bleeding is increased when clopidogrel is used with these drugs.

Anticoagulant drugs (e.g. warfarin)
The risk of bleeding with these drugs is increased if they are taken with clopidogrel.

Proton pump inhibitors (especially omeprazole and esomeprazole) These may reduce the antiplatelet effect of clopidogrel and should be avoided.

SPECIAL PRECAUTIONS

Be sure to tell your doctor if:
- You have liver or kidney problems.
- You have a history of peptic ulcers.
- You have had a bleed into your gut or brain.
- You have a bleeding disorder.
- You are taking other medicines.

Pregnancy
Safety in pregnancy not established. Discuss with your doctor.

Breast-feeding
The drug passes into the breast milk and may affect the baby. Discuss with your doctor.

Infants and children
Not recommended.

Over 60
No special problems.

Driving and hazardous work
No special problems.

Alcohol
Avoid. Stomach irritation from alcohol can increase the risk of bleeding.

Surgery and general anaesthetics
Clopidogrel may need to be stopped a week before surgery. Discuss this with your doctor or dentist.

PROLONGED USE

Increased risk of bleeding from any trauma, even a minor head injury.

CLOTRIMAZOLE

Brand names Boots Thrush Cream, Canesten, Care Clotrimazole Cream
Used in the following combined preparations Canesten HC, Lotriderm

GENERAL INFORMATION

Clotrimazole is an antifungal drug that is commonly used to treat fungal and yeast infections. It is used for treating tinea (ringworm) infections of the skin, and candida (thrush) infections of the ear, mouth, vagina, or penis. The drug is applied in the form of a cream, spray, topical solution, or dusting powder to the affected area and inserted as pessaries or cream to treat vaginal conditions such as candida.

Adverse effects from clotrimazole are very rare, although some people may experience burning and irritation on the skin surface in the area where the drug has been applied.

INFORMATION FOR USERS

Your drug prescription is tailored for you. Do not alter dosage without checking with your doctor.

How taken/used

Pessaries, cream, topical solution, spray, dusting powder.

Frequency and timing of doses
2–3 x daily (skin cream, spray, solution); once daily at bedtime (pessaries); once daily at bedtime (vaginal cream). Solutions for ear infections should be continued for at least 14 days after the infection has disappeared.

Dosage range
Vaginal infections One applicatorful (5g) per dose (vaginal cream); 100–500mg per dose (pessaries).
Skin infections (skin cream, spray, solution) as directed.

Onset of effect
Within 2–3 days.

Duration of action
Up to 12 hours.

Diet advice
None.

Storage
Keep in original container at room temperature out of the reach of children.

Missed dose
No cause for concern, but make up the missed dose or application as soon as you remember.

Stopping the drug
Apply the full course. Even if symptoms disappear, the original infection may still be present and symptoms may recur if treatment is stopped too soon.

Exceeding the dose
An occasional unintentional extra dose is unlikely to cause problems. But if you notice unusual symptoms or if a large amount has been swallowed, notify your doctor.

SPECIAL PRECAUTIONS

Be sure to tell your doctor if:
- You are taking other medicines.

Pregnancy
No evidence of risk to the developing baby, but only use with the advice of your doctor.

Breast-feeding
No evidence of risk.

Infants and children
No special problems, but use of pessaries not recommended.

Over 60
No special problems.

Driving and hazardous work
No known problems.

Alcohol
No known problems.

POSSIBLE ADVERSE EFFECTS

Clotrimazole rarely causes adverse effects. Skin preparations and vaginal applications may occasionally cause localized burning and irritation.

Symptom/effect	Frequency		Discuss with doctor		Stop taking drug now	Call doctor now
	Common	Rare	Only if severe	In all cases		
Localized burning or stinging	●		●			
Skin irritation		●	●			
Rash		●	●		●	

INTERACTIONS

Latex contraceptives Damage may occur to contraceptives made from latex; additional precautions are needed during use of clotrimazole and for at least 5 days after the end of treatment.

PROLONGED USE

No problems expected.

CLOZAPINE

Brand names Clozaril, Denzapine, Zaponex
Used in the following combined preparations None

GENERAL INFORMATION

Clozapine is an atypical antipsychotic for schizophrenia and for psychosis in Parkinson's disease. The drug is given to patients who have not responded to other treatments or who have experienced intolerable side effects with other drugs. Clozapine helps to control severe resistant schizophrenia. The improvement is gradual, and relief of severe symptoms can take several weeks to months. All treatment is supervised by a consultant psychiatrist, and the patient and the pharmacist must be registered with the drug manufacturer. The drug can cause a very serious side effect: agranulocytosis (a large decrease in white blood cells). Blood tests are performed before and during treatment; the drug is supplied only if results are normal. Clozapine may also cause heart muscle problems, which must be monitored for.

INFORMATION FOR USERS

This drug is given only under strict medical supervision and continual monitoring.

How taken/used

Tablets, liquid.

Frequency and timing of doses
1–2 x daily; a larger dose may be given at night.

Adult dosage range
12.5–900mg daily.

Onset of effect
Gradual. Some effect may appear within 3–5 days, but the full beneficial effect may not be felt for some months.

Duration of action
Up to 16 hours.

Diet advice
None.

Storage
Keep in original container at room temperature out of the reach of children.

Missed dose
Take as soon as you remember. If your next dose is due within 2 hours, take a single dose now and skip the next. If you miss more than 2 days of tablets, notify your doctor because you may need to restart at a lower dose.

Stopping the drug
Do not stop the drug without consulting your doctor because symptoms may recur.

Exceeding the dose
An occasional unintentional extra dose is unlikely to cause problems. Large overdoses may cause unusual drowsiness, seizures, and agitation. Notify your doctor.

POSSIBLE ADVERSE EFFECTS

Unlike other antipsychotics, clozapine is less likely to cause parkinsonian side effects (tremor and stiffness). The most serious side effect is agranulocytosis; strict monitoring is necessary.

Symptom/effect	Frequency		Discuss with doctor		Stop taking drug now	Call doctor now
	Common	Rare	Only if severe	In all cases		
Drowsiness/tiredness	●		●			
Excess saliva	●		●			
Dry mouth	●		●			
Weight gain	●		●			
Fast heartbeat	●			●		
Dizziness/fainting	●			●		
Constipation	●			●		
Blurred vision	●			●		
Fever/sore throat		●		●		●
Seizures		●		●		●

INTERACTIONS

General note A number of drugs increase the risk of adverse effects on the blood. Do not take other medication without checking with your doctor or pharmacist. Smoking lowers clozapine levels, which may reduce its effect.

Sedatives Drugs with a sedative effect on the central nervous system are likely to increase the sedative properties of clozapine.

Anticholinergic drugs There is a risk of severe constipation or even bowel obstruction when used with clozapine.

SPECIAL PRECAUTIONS

Be sure to tell your doctor if:
- You have long-term liver or kidney problems.
- You have a history of blood disorders.
- You have had epileptic seizures.
- You have heart problems.
- You have colon problems or have had bowel surgery.
- You have diabetes.
- You have glaucoma.
- You have prostate problems.
- You are taking other medicines.

Pregnancy
Not usually prescribed. Safety not established. Discuss with your doctor.

Breast-feeding
The drug passes into the breast milk and may affect the baby adversely. Discuss with your doctor.

Infants and children
Not prescribed.

Over 60
Adverse effects are more likely. Initial dose is low and is slowly increased.

Driving and hazardous work
Avoid such activities until you know how clozapine affects you because the drug can cause blurred vision, drowsiness, and dizziness.

Alcohol
Avoid. Alcohol may increase the sedative effects of this drug.

PROLONGED USE

Agranulocytosis and heart muscle problems may occur, and occasionally liver function may be upset. Significant weight gain may also occur.

Monitoring Blood tests are carried out weekly for 18 weeks, fortnightly until the end of the first year, and, if blood counts are stable, every 4 weeks thereafter. Liver function tests, weighing, and tests for diabetes are done every 3–6 months. Heart monitoring is also carried out.

CODEINE

Used in the following combined preparations Aspirin with codeine, Co-codamol, Codafen Continus, Cuprofen Plus, Galcodine, Migraleve, Nurofen Plus, Panadol Ultra, Paracodol, Pulmo Bailly, Solpadeine, Solpadol, Syndol, Veganin, and others

GENERAL INFORMATION

Codeine is a mild opioid analgesic that is similar to, but weaker than, morphine. It has been in common medical use since the beginning of the last century, although raw opium, of which codeine is a constituent, has been used for much longer.

Codeine is prescribed primarily to relieve mild to moderate pain, and is often combined with a non-opioid analgesic such as paracetamol. It is also an effective cough suppressant and, for

this reason, is included as an ingredient in many non-prescription cough syrups and cold relief preparations.

Like the other opioid drugs, codeine is constipating, a characteristic that sometimes makes it useful in the short-term control of diarrhoea.

Although codeine is habit-forming, addiction seldom occurs if the drug is used for a limited period of time and the recommended dosage is followed.

QUICK REFERENCE

Drug group Opioid analgesic (p.37), antidiarrhoeal drug (p.68), and cough suppressant (p.52)

Overdose danger rating High

Dependence rating High

Prescription needed Yes (some preparations)

Available as generic Yes

INFORMATION FOR USERS

Your drug prescription is tailored for you. Do not alter dosage without checking with your doctor.

How taken/used

Tablets, liquid, injection.

Frequency and timing of doses
4–6 x daily (pain); 3–4 x daily when necessary (cough); every 6–8 hours when necessary (diarrhoea).

Adult dosage range
120–240mg daily (pain); 45–120mg daily (cough); 30–120mg daily (diarrhoea).

Onset of effect
30–60 minutes.

Duration of action
4–6 hours.

Diet advice
None.

Storage
Keep in original container at room temperature out of the reach of children. Protect from light.

Missed dose
Take as soon as you remember if needed for relief of symptoms. If not needed, do not take the missed dose, and return to your normal dose schedule when necessary.

Stopping the drug
Can be safely stopped as soon as you no longer need it.

OVERDOSE ACTION

 Seek immediate medical advice in all cases. Take emergency action if there are symptoms such as slow or irregular breathing, severe drowsiness, or loss of consciousness.

See Drug poisoning emergency guide (p.518).

SPECIAL PRECAUTIONS

Be sure to consult your doctor or pharmacist before taking this drug if:
- You have long-term liver, kidney, or bowel problems.
- You have a lung disorder such as asthma or bronchitis.
- You are taking other medicines.

 Pregnancy
No evidence of risk, but regular use may cause withdrawal symptoms in the baby and if used during delivery can reduce the baby's breathing.

 Breast-feeding
Should not be used during breast-feeding as the drug passes into the breast milk and may harm the baby.

 Infants and children
Not for use in children under 12 years, nor for children under 18 years having tonsillectomy or adenoidectomy for obstructive sleep apnoea. Not advised for any child with respiratory problems.

 Over 60
Reduced dose may be necessary.

 Driving and hazardous work
Avoid until you have learned how codeine affects you because the drug may cause dizziness and drowsiness.

 Alcohol
Avoid. Alcohol may increase the sedative effects of this drug.

PROLONGED USE

Codeine is normally used only for short-term relief of symptoms. It can be habit-forming if taken for extended periods, especially if higher-than-average doses are taken.

POSSIBLE ADVERSE EFFECTS

Serious adverse effects are rare with codeine. Constipation occurs especially with prolonged use, but other side effects, such as nausea, vomiting, and drowsiness, are not usually troublesome at recommended doses, and usually disappear if the dose is reduced.

Symptom/effect	Frequency		Discuss with doctor		Stop taking drug now	Call doctor now
	Common	Rare	Only if severe	In all cases		
Constipation	●		●			
Nausea/vomiting	●		●			
Drowsiness	●		●			
Dizziness	●		●			
Agitation/restlessness		●		●	●	
Rash/hives		●		●	●	●
Wheezing/breathlessness		●		●	●	

INTERACTIONS

Sedatives All drugs, including alcohol, that have a sedative effect on the central nervous system are likely to increase sedation with codeine. Such drugs include sleeping drugs, antidepressant drugs, antihistamines, and antipsychotics.

COLCHICINE

Brand names None
Used in the following combined preparations None

GENERAL INFORMATION

Colchicine, a drug originally extracted from the autumn crocus flower and later synthesized, has been used since the 18th century for gout. It has now, to an extent, been superseded by newer drugs, but is still often used to relieve joint pain and inflammation in flare-ups. It is most effective when taken at the first sign of symptoms, and almost always produces an improvement. Its use is limited by the development of side effects, such as nausea, vomiting and diarrhoea, at high doses. The drug may also be given at a lower dose during the first few months of treatment with allopurinol or probenecid (other drugs for gout), because these may at first increase the frequency of gout attacks.

Colchicine is occasionally prescribed for the relief of symptoms of familial Mediterranean fever (a rare congenital condition).

QUICK REFERENCE

Drug group Drug for gout (p.77)
Overdose danger rating High
Dependence rating Low
Prescription needed Yes
Available as generic Yes

INFORMATION FOR USERS

Your drug prescription is tailored for you. Do not alter dosage without checking with your doctor.

How taken/used

Tablets.

Frequency and timing of doses
Prevention of gout attacks Twice daily.
Relief of gout attacks Every 4 hours.

Adult dosage range
Prevention of gout attacks 0.5mg 2 x daily.
Relief of gout attacks 0.5mg 2–4 x daily, until relief of pain, vomiting, or diarrhoea occurs, or until a total dose of 6mg is reached. This course must not be repeated within 3 days.

Onset of effect
Relief of symptoms in an attack of gout may be felt in 6–24 hours. Full effect in gout prevention may not be felt for several days.

Duration of action
Up to 2 hours. Some effects may last longer.

Diet advice
Certain foods are known to make gout worse. Discuss with your doctor.

Storage
Keep in original container at room temperature out of the reach of children. Protect from light.

Missed dose
Take as soon as you remember. If your next dose is due within 30 minutes, take a single dose now and skip the next.

Stopping the drug
When taking colchicine frequently during an acute attack of gout, stop if diarrhoea or abdominal pain develop. In other cases, do not stop without consulting your doctor.

OVERDOSE ACTION

Seek immediate medical advice in all cases. Some reactions can be fatal. Take emergency action if severe nausea, vomiting, bloody diarrhoea, severe abdominal pain, or loss of consciousness occur.

See Drug poisoning emergency guide (p.518).

SPECIAL PRECAUTIONS

Be sure to tell your doctor if:
• You have long-term liver or kidney problems.
• You have heart problems.
• You have a blood disorder.
• You have stomach ulcers.
• You have chronic inflammation of the bowel.
• You are taking other medicines.

 Pregnancy
Not recommended. May cause defects in the unborn baby. Discuss with your doctor.

 Breast-feeding
The drug passes into the breast milk and may affect the baby. Discuss with your doctor.

 Infants and children
Not recommended.

 Over 60
Increased likelihood of adverse effects.

 Driving and hazardous work
No special problems.

 Alcohol
Avoid. Alcohol may increase stomach irritation caused by colchicine.

PROLONGED USE

Prolonged use of this drug may lead to hair loss, rashes, tingling in the hands and feet, muscle pain and weakness, and blood disorders.

Monitoring Periodic blood checks are usually required.

POSSIBLE ADVERSE EFFECTS

The appearance of any symptom that may be an adverse effect of the drug is a sign that you should stop the drug until you have received further medical advice.

Symptom/effect	Frequency		Discuss with doctor		Stop taking drug now	Call doctor now
	Common	Rare	Only if severe	In all cases		
Nausea/vomiting	●			●	●	
Diarrhoea/abdominal pain	●			●	●	
Numbness and tingling		●		●	●	
Unusual bleeding/bruising		●		●	●	
Rash		●		●	●	

INTERACTIONS

Ciclosporin, clarithromycin, erythromycin, itraconazole, ketoconazole, and verapamil These drugs may significantly increase the adverse effects of colchicine.

Statins Taking statins with colchicine may increase the risk of adverse effects on the muscles.

Protease inhibitors may increase the risk of colchicine toxicity.

COLESTYRAMINE

Brand names Questran, Questran Light
Used in the following combined preparations None

GENERAL INFORMATION

Colestyramine is a resin that binds bile acids in the intestine, preventing their reabsorption. Cholesterol in the body is normally converted to bile acids. Therefore, colestyramine reduces cholesterol levels in the blood. This action on the bile acids makes bowel movements bulkier, creating an antidiarrhoeal effect (hence its use in diarrhoea associated with, for example, Crohn's disease, gallbladder removal, removal of part of the intestine, or radiotherapy). Colestyramine is used to treat hyperlipidaemia (high levels of fat in the blood) in people who have not responded to dietary changes. In liver disorders such as primary biliary cirrhosis, bile salts sometimes accumulate in the bloodstream, and colestyramine may be prescribed to alleviate any accompanying itching.

Taken in large doses, colestyramine often causes bloating, mild nausea, and constipation. It may also interfere with the body's ability to absorb fat and certain fat-soluble vitamins, causing pale, bulky, foul-smelling faeces.

QUICK REFERENCE

Drug group Lipid-lowering drug (p.61)

Overdose danger rating Low

Dependence rating Low

Prescription needed Yes

Available as generic Yes

INFORMATION FOR USERS

Your drug prescription is tailored for you. Do not alter dosage without checking with your doctor.

How taken/used

Powder mixed with water, juice, or soft food.

Frequency and timing of doses
1–6 x daily before meals and at bedtime.

Adult dosage range
4–36g daily.

Onset of effect
May take several weeks to achieve full beneficial effects.

Duration of action
12–24 hours.

Diet advice
A low-fat, low-calorie diet may be advised for patients who are overweight. Use of this drug may deplete levels of certain vitamins. Supplements may be advised.

Storage
Keep in original container at room temperature out of the reach of children.

Missed dose
Take as soon as you remember.

Stopping the drug
Do not stop taking the drug without consulting your doctor.

Exceeding the dose
An occasional unintentional extra dose is unlikely to cause problems. But if you notice any unusual symptoms, or if a large overdose has been taken, notify your doctor.

POSSIBLE ADVERSE EFFECTS

Adverse effects are more likely if large doses are taken by people over 60. Minor side effects such as indigestion and abdominal discomfort are rarely a cause for concern. More serious adverse effects are usually the result of vitamin deficiency.

Symptom/effect	Frequency		Discuss with doctor		Stop taking drug now	Call doctor now
	Common	Rare	Only if severe	In all cases		
Indigestion	●		●			
Abdominal discomfort	●		●			
Nausea/vomiting	●		●			
Constipation	●		●			
Bruising/increased bleeding		●			●	
Diarrhoea (high doses)		●			●	

INTERACTIONS

General note Colestyramine reduces the body's ability to absorb other drugs. If you are taking other medicines, you should tell either your doctor or your pharmacist so that they can discuss with you the best way to take all your drugs. To avoid any problems, take other drugs at least 1 hour before, or 4–6 hours after, colestyramine. The dosage of other drugs may need to be adjusted.

SPECIAL PRECAUTIONS

Be sure to tell your doctor if:
• You have jaundice.
• You have a peptic ulcer.
• You have diabetes.
• You have haemorrhoids.
• You are taking other medicines.

Pregnancy
Safety in pregnancy not established. Discuss with your doctor.

Breast-feeding
Safety not established. The drug binds fat-soluble vitamins long term and may cause vitamin deficiency in the baby. Discuss with your doctor.

Infants and children
Not recommended under 6 years. Reduced dose necessary in older children.

Over 60
Increased likelihood of adverse effects.

Driving and hazardous work
No special problems.

Alcohol
Although this drug does not interact with alcohol, your underlying condition may make it inadvisable to take alcohol.

PROLONGED USE

As this drug reduces vitamin absorption, supplements of vitamins A, D, and K and folic acid may be advised.

Monitoring Periodic blood checks are usually required to monitor the level of cholesterol in the blood.

CONJUGATED OESTROGENS

Brand name Premarin
Used in the following combined preparations Duavive, Premique

GENERAL INFORMATION

Conjugated oestrogens are preparations of naturally occurring oestrogens. Taken by mouth, they are used to relieve menopausal symptoms such as hot flushes and sweating, but are usually only advised for short-term use around the menopause and are not normally recommended for long-term use or for treatment of osteoporosis.

As replacement therapy, conjugated oestrogens are usually taken on a cyclic dosing schedule, in conjunction with a progestogen, to simulate the hormonal changes of a normal menstrual cycle. On their own, these drugs are not recommended for women with an intact uterus. Conjugated oestrogens do not provide contraception. Pregnancy is still possible for 2 years after a woman's last period (if she is under 50 years) or 1 year after the end of menstruation (if she is over 50).

INFORMATION FOR USERS

Your drug prescription is tailored for you. Do not alter dosage without checking with your doctor.

How taken/used

Tablets.

Frequency and timing of doses
Once daily.

Adult dosage range
Replacement therapy 0.625–1.25mg daily.
Osteoporosis prevention 0.625–1.25mg daily.

Onset of effect
5–20 days.

Duration of action
1–2 days.

Diet advice
None.

Storage
Keep in original container at room temperature out of the reach of children.

Missed dose
Take as soon as you remember.

Stopping the drug
Do not stop the drug without consulting your doctor because symptoms may recur.

Exceeding the dose
An occasional unintentional extra dose is unlikely to be a cause for concern. But if you notice any unusual symptoms, or if a large overdose has been taken, notify your doctor.

SPECIAL PRECAUTIONS

Be sure to tell your doctor if:
- You have heart disease, high blood pressure, or thrombophilia (abnormal clotting) or have had blood clots or a stroke.
- You have porphyria or diabetes.
- You have a history of breast disease or breast cancer.
- You have had uterine fibroids, abnormal vaginal bleeding, or endometrial cancer.
- You have migraine or epilepsy.
- You have long-term liver or kidney problems.
- You are taking other medicines.

 Pregnancy
Not prescribed. May affect the baby adversely. Discuss with your doctor.

 Breast-feeding
Not prescribed. The drug passes into the breast milk and may inhibit its flow. Discuss with your doctor.

 Infants and children
Not prescribed.

 Over 60
No special problems.

 Driving and hazardous work
No known problems.

 Alcohol
No known problems.

Surgery and general anaesthetics
Conjugated oestrogens may need to be stopped several weeks before you have surgery. Discuss with your doctor.

POSSIBLE ADVERSE EFFECTS

The most common adverse effects are similar to symptoms that occur in early pregnancy and generally diminish or disappear after 2–3 months of treatment. Women on a cyclic schedule will have a menstrual bleed towards the end of each cycle. Sudden, sharp pain in the chest, groin, or legs may indicate a blood clot that requires urgent medical attention.

Symptom/effect	Frequency		Discuss with doctor		Stop taking drug now	Call doctor now
	Common	Rare	Only if severe	In all cases		
Nausea/vomiting	●		●			
Breast swelling/tenderness	●		●			
Increase or decrease in weight	●		●			
Bloating/abdominal pain	●		●			
Reduced sex drive		●	●			
Headache/migraine		●		●		
Depression		●		●		
Vaginal bleeding		●		●		
Pain in chest/groin/legs		●		●		●
Jaundice		●		●	●	

INTERACTIONS

General note A number of medications can alter oestrogen levels, including some antibiotics, anticonvulsants, antifungals, anti-HIV drugs, and St John's wort. Check with your doctor or pharmacist before taking any other medicines.

Tobacco smoking increases the risk of serious adverse effects on the heart and circulation with conjugated oestrogens.

Oral anticoagulants Their anticoagulant effect is reduced by conjugated oestrogens.

PROLONGED USE

Conjugated oestrogens are normally only advised for use around the menopause. Long-term use may raise the risk of breast, endometrial, or ovarian cancer, venous thrombosis, heart attack, and stroke.

Monitoring Regular physical examinations (e.g. mammograms) and blood pressure checks are advised.

CO-PHENOTROPE

Brand name Lomotil
Used in the following combined preparations None

GENERAL INFORMATION

Co-phenotrope is an antidiarrhoeal drug that contains diphenoxylate and atropine. It reduces bowel contractions and the fluidity and frequency of bowel movements. It is used to relieve sudden or recurrent bouts of diarrhoea. It may also be used to control consistency of faeces following colostomy or ileostomy. The drug is not suitable for treating diarrhoea caused by infections, poisons, or antibiotics as it may delay recovery by slowing expulsion of harmful substances from the bowel. Co-phenotrope can cause toxic megacolon, a dangerous dilation of the bowel that shuts off the blood supply to the wall of the bowel and increases the risk of perforation.

At recommended doses, serious adverse effects are rare. However, if taken in excessive amounts, the atropine will cause highly unpleasant anticholinergic effects. This drug is especially dangerous for young children and should be stored out of their reach.

INFORMATION FOR USERS

Your drug prescription is tailored for you. Do not alter dosage without checking with your doctor.

How taken/used

Tablets.

Frequency and timing of doses
3–4 x daily.

Dosage range
Adults 4 tablets (equivalent to 10mg diphenoxylate) initially, followed by 2 tablets (5mg) every 6 hours until diarrhoea is controlled. *Children* Reduced dose necessary according to age (not recommended under 4 years).

Onset of effect
Within 1 hour. Control of diarrhoea may take some hours.

Duration of action
3–4 hours (single dose).

Diet advice
Always drink plenty of water during an attack of diarrhoea.

Storage
Keep in original container at room temperature out of the reach of children. Protect from light.

Missed dose
Take as soon as you remember. If your next dose is due within 3 hours, take a single dose now and skip the next.

Stopping the drug
Can be safely stopped as soon as you no longer need it.

Exceeding the dose
An occasional unintentional extra dose is unlikely to cause problems. Large overdoses may cause unusual drowsiness, dryness of the mouth and skin, restlessness, and in extreme cases, loss of consciousness. Symptoms of overdose may be delayed. Notify your doctor urgently if you have taken a large overdose.

SPECIAL PRECAUTIONS

Be sure to tell your doctor if:
- You have long-term liver or kidney problems.
- You have severe abdominal pain.
- You have bloodstained diarrhoea.
- You have recently taken antibiotics.
- You have ulcerative colitis.
- You have prostate problems.
- You have recently travelled abroad.
- You are taking other medicines.

Pregnancy
Safety in pregnancy not established. Discuss with your doctor.

Breast-feeding
The drug passes into the breast milk and may cause drowsiness in the baby. Discuss with your doctor.

Infants and children
Not recommended under 4 years. Reduced dose necessary for older children.

Over 60
Reduced dose may be necessary.

Driving and hazardous work
Avoid such activities until you have learned how co-phenotrope affects you because the drug may cause drowsiness and dizziness.

Alcohol
Avoid. Alcohol may increase the sedative effects of this drug.

PROLONGED USE

Not usually recommended.

POSSIBLE ADVERSE EFFECTS

Side effects occur infrequently with co-phenotrope. If abdominal pain or distension, nausea, or vomiting occur, notify your doctor.

Symptom/effect	Frequency		Discuss with doctor		Stop taking drug now	Call doctor now
	Common	Rare	Only if severe	In all cases		
Drowsiness	●		●			
Restlessness		●	●			
Headache		●	●			
Skin rash/itching		●		●		
Dizziness		●		●	●	
Difficulty in passing urine		●		●	●	
Nausea/vomiting		●		●	●	●
Abdominal discomfort		●		●	●	●

INTERACTIONS

Sedatives All drugs that have a sedative effect on the central nervous system may increase co-phenotrope's sedative effect. These include anti-anxiety and sleeping drugs, antihistamines, opioid analgesics, antidepressants, and antipsychotics.

Monoamine oxidase inhibitors (MAOIs) There is a risk of a dangerous rise in blood pressure if MAOIs (a class of antidepressants; see p.40) are taken together with co-phenotrope.

CO-TRIMOXAZOLE

Brand name None
Used in the following combined preparation (Co-trimoxazole is a combination of two drugs)

GENERAL INFORMATION

Co-trimoxazole is a mixture of two antibacterial drugs: trimethoprim and sulfamethoxazole. It is prescribed for serious respiratory and urinary tract infections only when they cannot be treated with other drugs. Co-trimoxazole is also used to treat pneumocystis pneumonia, toxoplasmosis, and the bacterial infection nocardiasis. The drug may also be used for otitis media in children if no safer drug is suitable. Although co-trimoxazole was widely prescribed in the past, its use has greatly declined in recent years with the introduction of new, more effective, and safer drugs.

Rare but serious adverse effects of co-trimoxazole may occur and these include skin rashes, blood disorders, and liver or kidney damage.

INFORMATION FOR USERS

Your drug prescription is tailored for you. Do not alter dosage without checking with your doctor.

How taken/used

Tablets, liquid, injection.

Frequency and timing of doses
Normally 2 x daily, preferably with food.

Adult dosage range
Usually 4 tablets daily (each standard tablet is 480mg). Higher doses may be used for the treatment of pneumocystis pneumonia, toxoplasmosis, and nocardiasis.

Onset of effect
1–4 hours.

Duration of action
24 hours.

Diet advice
Drink plenty of fluids, particularly in warm weather.

Storage
Keep in original container at room temperature out of the reach of children. Protect from light.

Missed dose
Take as soon as you remember. If your normal dose is 480mg, double this; if it is more than 480mg, take one dose only.

Stopping the drug
Take the full course. Even if you feel better, the original infection may still be present and symptoms may recur if treatment is stopped too soon.

Exceeding the dose
An occasional unintentional extra dose is unlikely to be a cause for concern. Large overdoses may cause nausea, vomiting, dizziness, and confusion. Notify your doctor.

SPECIAL PRECAUTIONS

Be sure to tell your doctor if:
- You have long-term liver or kidney problems.
- You have a blood disorder.
- You have asthma.
- You have glucose-6-phosphate dehydrogenase (G6PD) deficiency.
- You are allergic to sulfonamide drugs.
- You have porphyria.
- You are taking other medicines.

Pregnancy
Not prescribed. May cause defects in the baby.

Breast-feeding
The drug passes into the breast milk, but at normal levels adverse effects on the baby are unlikely. Discuss with your doctor.

Infants and children
Not recommended in infants under 6 weeks old. Reduced dose necessary in older children.

Over 60
Side effects are more likely. Used only when necessary.

Driving and hazardous work
No known problems.

Alcohol
No known problems.

POSSIBLE ADVERSE EFFECTS

The most common problems are nausea, rash, and itching. Other less common reactions include diarrhoea, headache, and sore tongue.

Symptom/effect	Frequency		Discuss with doctor		Stop taking drug now	Call doctor now
	Common	Rare	Only if severe	In all cases		
Nausea	●		●			
Diarrhoea	●		●			
Headache	●		●			
Rash/itching	●			●	●	●
Mouth ulcers/sore tongue		●		●	●	●
Jaundice		●		●	●	●

PROLONGED USE

Long-term use of this drug may lead to folic acid deficiency, which can cause anaemia. Folic acid supplements may be needed.

Monitoring Regular blood tests are recommended.

INTERACTIONS

Warfarin Co-trimoxazole may increase its anticoagulant effect; the dose of warfarin may have to be reduced. Blood-clotting status may have to be checked.

Ciclosporin Taking ciclosporin with co-trimoxazole can impair kidney function.

Phenytoin Co-trimoxazole may cause a build-up of phenytoin in the body; the dose of phenytoin may have to be reduced.

Amiodarone Co-trimoxazole may increase the risk of irregular heart beats when given with amiodarone.

Methotrexate Co-trimoxazole may increase the blood level of methotrexate and regular blood tests may be necessary.

CYCLOPHOSPHAMIDE

Brand names None
Used in the following combined preparations None

GENERAL INFORMATION

Cyclophosphamide belongs to a group of anticancer drugs known as alkylating agents. It is used for a wide range of cancers, including lymphomas (lymph gland cancers), leukaemias, and solid tumours. It is commonly given together with radiotherapy or other drugs. It has also been used for autoimmune diseases, such as rheumatoid arthritis and systemic lupus erythematosus when it involves the kidneys. The drug causes nausea, vomiting, and hair loss, and can affect the heart, lungs, and liver.

It can also cause bladder damage in susceptible people because it produces a toxic substance called acrolein. To reduce toxicity, people considered to be at risk may be given a drug called mesna before and after each dose of cyclophosphamide. Also, because the drug often reduces production of blood cells, it may lead to abnormal bleeding and increased risk of infection. It may also reduce fertility in both men and women; approaches to preserve sperm are likely to be offered with treatment.

INFORMATION FOR USERS

Your drug prescription is tailored for you. Do not alter dosage without checking with your doctor.

How taken/used

Tablets, injection.

Frequency and timing of doses
Varies from once daily to every 3 weeks, depending on the condition being treated.

Dosage range
Dosage is determined individually according to the nature of the condition, body weight, and response.

Onset of effect
Some effects may appear within hours of starting treatment. Full beneficial effects may not be felt for many weeks.

Duration of action
Several weeks.

Diet advice
High fluid intake with frequent bladder emptying is recommended. This will usually prevent the drug causing bladder irritation.

Storage
Keep in original container at room temperature out of the reach of children. Protect from light.

Missed dose
Injections are given only in hospital. If you are taking tablets, take the missed dose as soon as you remember. If your next dose is due within 6 hours, take a single dose now and skip the next. Tell your doctor that you missed a dose.

Stopping the drug
The drug will be stopped under medical supervision (injection). Do not stop taking the drug without consulting your doctor (tablets); stopping the drug may lead to worsening of the underlying condition.

Exceeding the dose
An occasional unintentional extra dose is unlikely to cause problems. Large overdoses may cause nausea, vomiting, and bladder damage. Notify your doctor.

POSSIBLE ADVERSE EFFECTS

Cyclophosphamide often causes nausea and vomiting, which usually diminish as your body adjusts. Also, women often experience irregular periods. Blood in the urine may be a sign of bladder damage and requires prompt medical attention. Those thought to be at risk of bladder damage may be given mesna before and after doses of cyclophosphamide.

Symptom/effect	Frequency		Discuss with doctor		Stop taking drug now	Call doctor now
	Common	Rare	Only if severe	In all cases		
Nausea/vomiting	●		●			
Hair loss	●		●			
Irregular menstruation	●			●		
Mouth ulcers		●		●		
Breathlessness		●		●		
Bloodstained urine		●		●		●
Fever		●		●		

INTERACTIONS

General note A number of drugs reduce the effects of cyclophosphamide and increase the risk of side effects. Such drugs include allopurinol, chloramphenicol, chloroquine, imipramine, and phenothiazines (e.g. chlorpromazine).

SPECIAL PRECAUTIONS

Cyclophosphamide is given only under close medical supervision, taking account of your present condition and medical history. However, tell your doctor if:
• You have liver or kidney problems.
• You have porphyria.
• You plan to have children in the future.

 Pregnancy
Not usually prescribed. Cyclophosphamide may cause birth defects. Pregnancy should be avoided during, and for 3 months after, treatment. Discuss with your doctor.

 Breast-feeding
Not advised. The drug passes into the breast milk and may affect the baby adversely. Discuss with your doctor.

 Infants and children
Reduced dose necessary.

 Over 60
No special problems.

 Driving and hazardous work
No known problems.

 Alcohol
Cyclophosphamide may increase nausea and vomiting.

PROLONGED USE

Prolonged use of this drug may reduce the production of blood cells in the bone marrow. It may also cause pigmentation of the nails, palms, and soles of the feet.

Monitoring Periodic checks on blood composition and blood chemistry are usually required.

CYPROTERONE

Brand names Androcur, Cyprostat
Used in the following combined preparations Co-cyprindiol (Dianette)

GENERAL INFORMATION

Cyproterone reduces the action and production of androgens (male sex hormones) in the body. It is used in males for conditions due to the action of androgens, such as prostate cancer, hypersexuality, sexual deviation, and precocious puberty in boys. It is used in women to treat certain conditions due to abnormally high androgen levels, such as hirsutism, male-pattern baldness, and severe acne. For women taking cyproterone combined with an oestrogen for acne or hirsutism, it also provides contraception. Cyproterone alone is also used to facilitate hormonal male-to-female gender reassignment. Common side effects in men include reduced libido, erectile dysfunction (impotence), and infertility, which is usually reversible. Occasionally, it may disrupt liver function, and it significantly increases the risk of thrombosis.

INFORMATION FOR USERS

Your drug prescription is tailored for you. Do not alter dosage without checking with your doctor.

How taken/used

Tablets.

Frequency and timing of doses
1–3 x daily, with liquid after meals.
Oral contraceptives Once daily on certain days of the menstrual cycle.

Adult dosage range
50–300mg daily, usually in divided doses.
Oral contraceptives 2mg daily.

Onset of effect
Up to a week; longer for acne, possibly several months.

Duration of action
Several days.

Diet advice
None.

Storage
Keep at room temperature, away from heat, moisture, and direct light and out of the reach of children.

Missed dose
Take as soon as you remember and take the next dose when it is due.

Stopping the drug
Do not stop taking the drug without consulting your doctor; stopping the drug may lead to recurrence or worsening of your symptoms. If you have diabetes, stopping the drug may upset control of your blood sugar levels.

POSSIBLE ADVERSE EFFECTS

Cyproterone may cause a wide range of adverse effects, although serious ones are rare. If you develop abnormal itching, jaundice, breathlessness, chest pain, or swollen or painful calves, you should stop the drug and consult your doctor immediately.

Symptom/effect	Frequency		Discuss with doctor		Stop taking drug now	Call doctor now
	Common	Rare	Only if severe	In all cases		
Decreased libido/impotence	●		●			
Weight change/fluid retention	●		●			
Low mood/restlessness	●		●			
Breast swelling/tenderness	●		●			
Enlarged/tender breasts in men	●		●			
Hot flushes/sweating	●		●			
Hair loss/dry skin	●		●			
Persistent abdominal pain		●		●	●	
Jaundice/itching		●		●	●	●
Breathlessness/chest pain		●		●	●	●
Calf pain/swelling		●		●	●	●

INTERACTIONS

Thiazolidinedione antidiabetic drugs (e.g. pioglitazone) The dose may need to be reduced when taken with cyproterone.

Rifampicin, phenytoin, and St John's wort may reduce the level of cyproterone.

Ketoconazole, itraconazole, and clotrimazole may increase the level of cyproterone.

Statins Increased risk of muscle side effects from statins when taken with cyproterone.

SPECIAL PRECAUTIONS

Be sure to tell your doctor if:
- You have liver problems.
- You have diabetes.
- You have sickle cell anaemia.
- You have a history of depression.
- You have a family history of venous thrombosis or have had blood clots, stroke, or a heart attack.
- You have or have had a meningioma.
- You are taking other medicines.

 Pregnancy
Not prescribed. It can feminize a male fetus.

 Breast-feeding
Not prescribed.

 Infants and children
Reduced dose necessary

 Over 60
No special problems.

 Driving and hazardous work
Avoid such activities until you have learned how cyproterone affects you because the drug may cause tiredness and weakness.

 Alcohol
Avoid. Alcohol can reduce the effect of cyproterone.

PROLONGED USE

The development of meningiomas (a type of brain tumour), abnormal liver function, suppression of adrenal gland function, and, very rarely, liver tumours have been reported with prolonged use of cyproterone at high doses. Meningiomas are not a risk with co-cyprindiol (Dianette).

Monitoring Your blood count and liver function will be checked regularly, and your adrenal function may also be monitored. If you have diabetes, your blood sugar control will be monitored. Men may have their sperm count checked.

DABIGATRAN

Brand names Pradaxa
Used in the following combined preparations None

GENERAL INFORMATION

Dabigatran is an oral anticoagulant drug with a rapid onset of action. It is used to treat or prevent deep-vein thrombosis (blood clots that form in veins, such as the leg veins) and pulmonary embolism (blockage of blood vessels in the lungs by clots from elsewhere in the body). Dabigatran is also used to prevent strokes and blood clots in the arteries in patients with the heart rhythm problem atrial fibrillation. The most serious side effect is an increased risk of bleeding. Dabigatran should not be used in people with damaged or artificial heart valves, for whom warfarin is usually more suitable. In emergencies the drug Praxbind (idarucizumab) may be given to reverse the effects of dabigatran.

QUICK REFERENCE

Drug group Anticoagulant drug (p.62)

Overdose danger rating High

Dependence rating Low

Prescription needed Yes

Available as generic No

INFORMATION FOR USERS

Your drug prescription is tailored for you. Do not alter dosage without checking with your doctor.

How taken/used

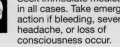

Capsules.

Frequency and timing of doses
1–2 x daily.

Dosage range
75–300mg daily.

Onset of effect
1 hour.

Duration of action
12–24 hours.

Diet advice
None.

Storage
Keep in original container at room temperature out of the reach of children.

Missed dose
Take as soon as you remember. If your next dose is due within 6 hours, take a single dose now and skip the next dose. Do not take a double dose to make up for missed individual doses.

Stopping the drug
Do not stop the drug without consulting your doctor; stopping the drug may lead to worsening of the underlying condition.

OVERDOSE ACTION

 Seek immediate medical advice in all cases. Take emergency action if bleeding, severe headache, or loss of consciousness occur.

See Drug poisoning emergency guide (p.518).

POSSIBLE ADVERSE EFFECTS

Bleeding is the most common adverse effect. If you have excessive bruising or bleeding from a minor wound, vomit blood, or pass bloody or black stools, tell your doctor immediately.

Symptom/effect	Frequency		Discuss with doctor		Stop taking drug now	Call doctor now
	Common	Rare	Only if severe	In all cases		
Bleeding/bruising	●			●		●
Abdominal pain/diarrhoea	●			●		
Nausea/vomiting	●			●		
Rash/itching		●		●		
Jaundice		●		●		●

INTERACTIONS

Other anticoagulants, antiplatelet drugs, non-steroidal anti-inflammatory drugs, and SSRI antidepressants There is an increased risk of bleeding if these are used at the same time as dabigatran.

Anticonvulsant drugs, rifampicin, and St John's wort These may lower the blood concentration of dabigatran and reduce its effectiveness.

Antibacterial drugs, antifungal drugs, amiodarone, verapamil, ciclosporin, and tacrolimus These may increase the blood concentration of dabigatran and increase the risk of bleeding.

Ciclosporin, itraconazole, dronedarone, and the fixed-dose combination glecaprevir/pibrentasvir significantly increase the risk of bleeding.

SPECIAL PRECAUTIONS

Be sure to tell your doctor if:
- You have had a stroke or a brain haemorrhage.
- You have liver or kidney problems.
- You have high blood pressure.
- You have a bleeding disorder.
- You have peptic ulcers.
- You have had recent surgery.
- You have had a metal heart valve fitted.
- You are taking other medicines.

 Pregnancy
Safety not established. Discuss with your doctor.

 Breast-feeding
Safety not established. Discuss with your doctor.

 Infants and children
Safety not established. Discuss with your doctor.

 Over 60
Reduced dose recommended in over 75s.

 Driving and hazardous work
Use caution. Even minor injuries may cause severe bruising and bleeding.

 Alcohol
Avoid excessive intake.

Surgery and general anaesthetics
Dabigatran may need to be stopped before surgery. Discuss with your doctor or dentist.

PROLONGED USE

No special problems known but the need for continued treatment should be reviewed.

Monitoring Kidney function should be monitored at least annually.

DAPAGLIFLOZIN

Brand names Forxiga
Used in the following combined preparations Qtern (with saxaglipitin), Xigduo (with metformin)

GENERAL INFORMATION

Dapagliflozin is an oral antidiabetic drug used to treat type 2 diabetes in adults if the diabetes cannot be controlled with other medicines, diet, and exercise. It reduces blood glucose levels by increasing the amount of glucose removed from the blood by the kidneys and excreted in the urine. It can be used alone or in combination with other glucose-lowering medications, including insulin. Common side effects of dapagliflozin include urinary and genital yeast infections, dehydration, low blood pressure, and, if taken with certain other diabetes medications, low blood sugar.

INFORMATION FOR USERS

Your drug prescription is tailored for you. Do not alter dosage without checking with your doctor.

How taken/used

Tablets.

Frequency and timing of doses
Once daily with half a glass of water; can be taken with or without food.

Adult dosage range
5 or 10mg daily.

Onset of effect
Within hours, but may take a week to develop full effect.

Duration of action
24 hours.

Diet advice
Your doctor will advise an individualized diet to ensure good control of your diabetes.

Storage
Keep in original container at room temperature and out of the reach of children.

Missed dose
If it is less than 12 hours until the next dose, skip the missed dose and take the next dose at the usual time. If it is more than 12 hours to the next dose, take a dose as soon as you remember.

Stopping the drug
Do not stop taking the drug without consulting your doctor; stopping the drug may lead to worsening of your diabetes control.

Exceeding the dose
An occasional unintentional extra dose is unlikely to be a cause for concern. If symptoms of low blood sugar develop, such as sweating, hunger, trembling, confusion, headache, or feeling faint, eat or drink something sugary. If a large overdose has been taken, seek immediate medical attention.

SPECIAL PRECAUTIONS

Be sure to tell your doctor if:
- You have liver or kidney problems.
- You have or have had bladder cancer.
- You get frequent urinary tract infections.
- You have a history of heart disease or stroke.
- You have low blood pressure.
- You are taking any other medicines.

 Pregnancy
Not prescribed in pregnancy. Discuss with your doctor.

 Breast-feeding
May pass into breast milk and affect the baby. Discuss with your doctor.

 Infants and children
Not recommended.

 **Over 60**
Increased risk of adverse effects. Reduced dose may be necessary.

 Driving and hazardous work
Avoid such activities if you have warning signs of low blood sugar.

 Alcohol
Avoid excessive intake as alcohol may upset blood sugar control.

Surgery and anaesthetic
Dapagliflozin should be halted before any major surgical procedure or during severe illness due to increased risk of ketoacidosis.

POSSIBLE ADVERSE EFFECTS

Urinary or genital infections and faintness or light-headedness are common side effects. Low blood sugar (resulting in dizziness, confusion, sweating, and shaking) may occur if dapagliflozin is taken with insulin or sulfonylureas. A rare but potentially serious effect is diabetic ketoacidosis: a build-up of ketones in the body, producing nausea, vomiting, stomach pain, excessive thirst, breathing problems, unusual tiredness, or confusion. Another serious side effect is Fournier's gangrene: severe swelling, pain and redness of the perineal area (between the genitals and anus), with fever or malaise. Seek immediate medical assistance if any of these symptoms develop.

Symptom/effect	Frequency		Discuss with doctor		Stop taking drug now	Call doctor now
	Common	Rare	Only if severe	In all cases		
Light-headedness/faintness	●			●	●	
Vaginal odour/itching/discharge	●			●		
Penile rash/swelling/itching/discharge	●			●		
Cloudy/smelly urine	●			●		
Increased urination	●			●		
Blood in urine		●		●		
Low blood sugar		●		●	●	
Ketoacidosis		●		●	●	●

INTERACTIONS

Diuretics When these drugs are taken with dapagliflozin, there is a risk of dehydration and low blood pressure.

PROLONGED USE

No problems expected.

Monitoring Regular checks of blood sugar control and kidney function are necessary. Urine will test positive for glucose while on dapagliflozin but this is no cause for concern unless there are other indications of poor blood sugar control. Blood cholesterol levels should be monitored as dapagliflozin may cause an increase in blood cholesterol.

DESMOPRESSIN

Brand names DDAVP, DDAVP Melt, DesmoMelt, Desmospray, Desmotabs, Noqdirna, Octim
Used in the following combined preparations None

GENERAL INFORMATION

Desmopressin is a synthetic form of the hormone vasopressin. Low levels of vasopressin in the body can lead to diabetes insipidus, which causes excess urine production and continual thirst.

Desmopressin can be used to correct the deficiency of vasopressin. It is also used to test for diabetes insipidus, to check kidney function, and to treat nocturnal enuresis (bedwetting) in both children and adults. When given by injection, it helps to boost clotting factors in haemophilia and von Willebrand's disease.

Side effects include low blood sodium and fluid retention (which sometimes requires monitoring of body weight and blood pressure to check the body's water balance). Desmopressin should not be taken during an episode of vomiting and diarrhoea because the body's fluid balance may be upset.

INFORMATION FOR USERS

Your drug prescription is tailored for you. Do not alter dosage without checking with your doctor.

How taken/used

Tablets, sublingual tablets, injection, nasal solution, nasal spray.

Frequency and timing of doses
Diabetes insipidus 3 x daily (tablets/sublingual tablets); 1–2 x daily (nasal spray/solution). *Nocturnal enuresis* At bedtime (tablets/ sublingual tablets, nasal spray/solution). Avoid fluids from 1 hour before bedtime to 8 hours afterwards.

Dosage range
Diabetes insipidus: *Adults* 300–600mcg daily (tablets/sublingual tablets); 1–4 puffs (nasal spray); 10–40mcg daily (nasal solution). *Children* 300–600mcg daily (tablets/sublingual tablets); up to 2 puffs (nasal spray); 20mcg (nasal solution).
Nocturnal enuresis: 200–400mcg for adults and children over 5 years only (tablets/sublingual tablets); 20–40mcg (nasal solution); 2–4 puffs (nasal spray).

Onset of effect
A few minutes: full effects, a few hours (injection, nasal solution/nasal spray); 30–90 minutes (tablets/ sublingual tablets).

Duration of action
Tablets/sublingual tablets 6–12 hours; injection/ nasal solutions/nasal spray 5–21 hours.

Diet advice
Your doctor may advise you to avoid excessive fluid intake.

Storage
Keep in original container at room temperature (tablets/sublingual tablets) or in a refrigerator, without freezing (nasal solution/nasal spray), out of the reach of children. Protect from light.

Missed dose
Take as soon as you remember. If your next dose is due within 2 hours, take a single dose now and skip the next.

Stopping the drug
Do not stop the drug without consulting your doctor; symptoms may recur.

Exceeding the dose
An occasional unintentional extra dose is unlikely to cause problems. Large overdoses may cause seizures. Notify your doctor without delay.

SPECIAL PRECAUTIONS

Be sure to tell your doctor if:
• You have heart problems.
• You have high blood pressure.
• You have kidney problems.
• You have cystic fibrosis.
• You have asthma or allergic rhinitis.
• You have epilepsy.
• You are taking other medicines.

 Pregnancy
Safety in pregnancy not established. Discuss with your doctor.

 Breast-feeding
The drug passes into breast milk, in small amounts, but adverse effects on the baby are unlikely.

 Infants and children
No special problems in children; infants may need monitoring to ensure that fluid balance is correct.

 Over 60
May need monitoring to ensure that fluid balance is correct.

 Driving and hazardous work
No known problems.

 Alcohol
Your doctor may advise on fluid intake.

POSSIBLE ADVERSE EFFECTS

Desmopressin can cause fluid retention and low blood sodium (in serious cases with seizures). Headache, nausea, vomiting, and nosebleeds may also occur.

Symptom/effect	Frequency		Discuss with doctor		Stop taking drug now	Call doctor now
	Common	Rare	Only if severe	In all cases		
Headache/nausea/vomiting		●	●			
Nasal congestion/nosebleeds		●	●			
Increased body weight		●		●		
Stomach pain		●		●		
Seizures		●		●	●	●

INTERACTIONS

Antidepressants, chlorpropamide, chlorpromazine, fludrocortisone, and carbamazepine These drugs may increase the effects of desmopressin.

Non-steroidal anti-inflammatory drugs (NSAIDs) may increase the body's response to desmopressin.

Loperamide This drug may significantly increase blood levels of desmopressin.

PROLONGED USE

Diabetes insipidus: no problems expected.

Nocturnal enuresis: the drug will be withdrawn for at least a week after 3 months for assessment of the need to continue treatment.

Monitoring The levels of electrolytes (such as sodium) in the blood should be monitored periodically, as well as blood pressure and the levels of electrolytes in the urine.

DESOGESTREL

Brand name Aizea, Cerazette, Cerelle, Desomono, Desorex, Feanolla, Zelleta, and others
Used in the following combined preparations Alenvona, Bimizza, Cimizt, Gedarel, Marvelon, Mercilon, Munalea, and others

GENERAL INFORMATION

Desogestrel is a synthetic hormone that is similar to the natural female sex hormone progesterone. It is used alone as a progestogen-only pill, or "POP", (p.121) and is especially helpful as contraception in women who do not tolerate oestrogens or those who are breast-feeding. Desogestrel works by thickening the mucus at the neck of the cervix, making it difficult for sperm to enter. Unlike other POPs, the drug also works by preventing ovulation (release of an egg from the ovary). In addition, it changes the quality of the endometrium (lining of the uterus), preventing implantation of a fertilized egg.

Desogestrel is also used in combination with the oestrogen drug ethinylestradiol as an oral contraceptive.

When desogestrel is taken without an oestrogen, irregular vaginal bleeding may occur in the form of slight spotting, heavier bleeding, or no bleeding at all. Desogestrel, either alone or in a combined oral contraceptive, also carries a significant risk of venous thrombosis.

INFORMATION FOR USERS

Your drug prescription is tailored for you. Do not alter dosage without checking with your doctor.

How taken/used

Tablets.

Frequency and timing of doses
One tablet at the same time each day.

Adult dosage range
75mcg daily.

Onset of effect
Within a few hours.

Duration of action
24 hours.

Diet advice
None.

Storage
Keep in original container at room temperature out of the reach of children. Protect from light.

Missed dose
If a tablet is delayed by 12 hours or more, regard it as a missed pill. See What to do if you miss a pill (p.123).

Stopping the drug
The drug can be safely stopped as soon as contraceptive protection is no longer required. For treatment of menstrual symptoms, consult your doctor before stopping the drug.

Exceeding the dose
An occasional unintentional dose is unlikely to be a cause for concern. But if you notice any unusual symptoms, or if a large overdose has been taken, notify your doctor.

SPECIAL PRECAUTIONS

Be sure to tell your doctor if:
- You have jaundice or a liver problem.
- You have diabetes.
- You have a history of breast cancer.
- You have had an ectopic pregnancy.
- You have unexplained abnormal vaginal bleeding.
- You have had epileptic seizures.
- You have had venous thrombosis or a stroke.
- You are taking other medicines.

Pregnancy
Not prescribed. May cause defects in the developing baby. Discuss with your doctor.

Breast-feeding
The drug passes into the breast milk, but at normal doses adverse effects on the baby are unlikely. Discuss with your doctor.

Infants and children
Not prescribed.

Over 60
Not prescribed.

Driving and hazardous work
No known problems.

Alcohol
No known problems.

POSSIBLE ADVERSE EFFECTS

Irregular vaginal bleeding is the most common side effect of desogestrel taken alone. If you experience heavy or prolonged bleeding, consult your doctor. If you experience vomiting within 3–4 hours of taking a tablet, absorption of the drug may be reduced and you should use additional contraceptive measures for the next 7 days.

Symptom/effect	Frequency		Discuss with doctor		Stop taking drug now	Call doctor now
	Common	Rare	Only if severe	In all cases		
Irregular vaginal bleeding	●		●			
Nausea/vomiting	●		●			
Headache	●		●			
Breast discomfort/tenderness	●		●			
Weight changes	●		●			
Acne	●		●			
Mood changes/reduced libido	●			●		
Skin pigmentation		●	●			

INTERACTIONS

General note The beneficial effects of many drugs, including oral anticoagulants, anticonvulsants, and antihypertensive and antidiabetic drugs, may be affected by desogestrel. Many other drugs may reduce the contraceptive effect of desogestrel. These include anticonvulsants, antituberculous drugs, antidepressants, and the herbal remedy St John's wort.

PROLONGED USE

There is a small increase in the risk of breast cancer in women who have used a progestogen-only pill. However, the risk is related to the age at which the pill is stopped rather than duration of use. The increased risk reduces to zero over 10 years after stopping use.

Monitoring Regular blood pressure checks may be carried out.

DEXAMETHASONE

Brand names Dexsol, Dropodex, Eythalm, Glensoludex, Martapan, Maxidex, Neofordex, Ozurdex
Used in the following combined preparations Maxitrol, Otomize, Sofradex, Tobradex, and others

GENERAL INFORMATION

Dexamethasone is a long-acting, potent corticosteroid drug used to suppress inflammatory and allergic disorders, shock, and brain swelling (as a result of injury or tumour), and to relieve the lung complications of COVID-19 coronavirus infection. It is also used in conjunction with other drugs to alleviate nausea and vomiting associated with chemotherapy.

Dexamethasone is available in different forms, including tablets, oral solution, injection, and eye and ear drops.

Low doses of dexamethasone taken for short periods rarely cause serious side effects. However, as with other corticosteroids, long-term treatment, especially with high doses, can cause significant adverse effects.

QUICK REFERENCE

Drug group Corticosteroid (p.99)
Overdose danger rating Low
Dependence rating Low
Prescription needed Yes
Available as generic Yes

INFORMATION FOR USERS

Your drug prescription is tailored for you. Do not alter dosage without checking with your doctor.

How taken/used

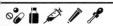

Tablets, liquid, injection, eye ointment, eye/ear drops, ear/nasal spray.

Frequency and timing of doses
1–4 x daily with food (by mouth); 1–6 hourly (eye drops); 1–4 x daily (ear drops/spray, eye ointment); 2–6 x daily (nasal spray).

Dosage range
Usually 0.5–10mg daily (by mouth).

Onset of effect
1–4 days.

Duration of action
Some effects may last several days.

Diet advice
None.

Storage
Keep in original container at room temperature out of the reach of children. Protect from light.

Missed dose
Take as soon as you remember. If your next dose is due within 2 hours, take a single dose now and skip the next.

Stopping the drug
Do not stop taking the drug without consulting your doctor. It may be necessary to withdraw the drug gradually.

Exceeding the dose
An occasional unintentional extra dose is unlikely to be a cause for concern. But if you notice any unusual symptoms, or if a large overdose has been taken, notify your doctor.

POSSIBLE ADVERSE EFFECTS

Weight gain, acne, and mood changes are common adverse effects. More serious effects only occur when high doses are taken for long periods of time. These are carefully monitored during prolonged treatment. Rarely, severe psychiatric side effects, such as depression or suicidal thoughts or behaviour, may occur. If affected, consult your doctor without delay.

Symptom/effect	Frequency		Discuss with doctor		Stop taking drug now	Call doctor now
	Common	Rare	Only if severe	In all cases		
Indigestion	●			●		
Weight gain	●			●		
Acne and other skin effects	●			●		
Fluid retention	●			●		
Muscle weakness		●			●	
Mood changes	●			●		

INTERACTIONS

Antidiabetic drugs Dexamethasone reduces the action of these drugs. Dosage may need to be adjusted accordingly to prevent abnormally high blood sugar.

Barbiturates, phenytoin, rifampicin, and carbamazepine These drugs may reduce the effectiveness of dexamethasone. The dosage may need to be adjusted accordingly.

Oral anticoagulant drugs Dexamethasone may increase the effects of these drugs.

Non-steroidal anti-inflammatory drugs These drugs may increase the likelihood of indigestion from dexamethasone.

Antacids These drugs may reduce the effectiveness of, and should be taken at least 2 hours apart from, dexamethasone.

Vaccines Dexamethasone can interact with some vaccines. Discuss with your doctor before having any vaccinations.

SPECIAL PRECAUTIONS

Be sure to tell your doctor if:
- You have had a peptic ulcer.
- You have glaucoma.
- You have high blood pressure.
- You have congestive heart failure.
- You have diabetes.
- You have epilepsy.
- You have had tuberculosis.
- You have had depression or mental illness.
- You are taking other medicines.

Pregnancy
Safety in pregnancy not established. Discuss with your doctor.

Breast-feeding
Safety not established. The drug passes into the breast milk. Discuss with your doctor.

Infants and children
Reduced dose necessary.

Over 60
No known problems.

Driving and hazardous work
No known problems, although eye drops or ointment may cause temporary visual disturbances.

Alcohol
Avoid. Alcohol may increase the risk of indigestion and peptic ulcer with this drug.

Surgery and general anaesthetics
You must tell your doctor or anaesthetist that you are taking dexamethasone; close monitoring is required during surgery.

Infection
Avoid exposure to chickenpox, shingles, and measles if you are on systemic treatment.

PROLONGED USE

Prolonged use by mouth can lead to peptic ulcers, glaucoma, fragile bones, muscle weakness, and growth retardation in children. People receiving long-term treatment are advised to carry a steroid treatment card.

DIAZEPAM/LORAZEPAM

Brand names [diazepam] Diazemuls, Diazepam Rectubes, Stesolid, Valclair; [lorazepam] Ativan
Used in the following combined preparations None

GENERAL INFORMATION

Introduced in the early 1960s, diazepam is the best known and most widely used benzodiazepine, and lorazepam is closely related to it. Benzodiazepines help to relieve tension and nervousness, relax muscles, and encourage sleep. Their actions and adverse effects are described more fully on p.39.

Diazepam and lorazepam have a wide range of uses. Besides being commonly used in the treatment of anxiety and anxiety-related insomnia, they are given in treating alcohol withdrawal, and for the relief of epileptic seizures. Diazepam is also given as a muscle relaxant. Given intravenously, they are used to sedate people undergoing certain uncomfortable medical procedures.

Diazepam and lorazepam can be habit-forming if taken regularly over a long period. Their effects may also diminish with time. For these reasons, courses of treatment are limited to two weeks whenever possible.

INFORMATION FOR USERS

Your drug prescription is tailored for you. Do not alter dosage without checking with your doctor.

How taken/used

Tablets, liquid, injection, suppositories, rectal solution.

Frequency and timing of doses
1–4 x daily.

Dosage range
Anxiety 2–30mg daily (diazepam); 1–4mg daily (lorazepam).

Onset of effect
Immediate effect (injection); 30 minutes–2 hours (other methods of administration).

Duration of action
Up to 24 hours; some effect: up to 4 days.

Diet advice
None.

Storage
Keep in original container at room temperature out of the reach of children.

Missed dose
Take as soon as you remember. If your next dose is due within 2 hours, take a single dose now and skip the next.

Stopping the drug
If you have been taking the drug for less than 2 weeks, it can be stopped as soon as no longer needed. If you have been taking it for longer, consult your doctor, who will supervise a gradual reduction in dosage. Stopping abruptly may lead to withdrawal symptoms (see p.24).

OVERDOSE ACTION

Seek immediate medical advice. Large overdoses may cause excessive drowsiness and possibly even deep coma requiring emergency action.

See Drug poisoning emergency guide (p.518).

SPECIAL PRECAUTIONS

Be sure to tell your doctor if:
- You have severe respiratory disease.
- You have long-term liver or kidney problems.
- You have had problems with alcohol or drug abuse.
- You have myasthenia gravis or muscle weakness.
- You have sleep apnoea.
- You have a marked personality disorder.
- You have porphyria.
- You are taking other medicines.

 Pregnancy
Not usually recommended; may cause adverse effects on newborn baby at the time of delivery. Discuss with your doctor.

 Breast-feeding
The drugs pass into the breast milk and may affect the baby. Discuss with your doctor.

 Infants and children
Reduced dose necessary.

 Over 60
Increased likelihood of adverse effects. Reduced dose may therefore be necessary.

 Driving and hazardous work
Avoid such activities until you have learned how diazepam or lorazepam affect you because the drugs can cause reduced alertness, slowed reactions, and increased aggression.

 Alcohol
Avoid. Alcohol may increase the sedative effects of these drugs.

POSSIBLE ADVERSE EFFECTS

The principal adverse effects of this drug are related to its sedative properties. The effects normally diminish after a few days and can often be reduced by adjustment of dosage.

Symptom/effect	Frequency		Discuss with doctor		Stop taking drug now	Call doctor now
	Common	Rare	Only if severe	In all cases		
Daytime drowsiness	●		●			
Dizziness/unsteadiness	●			●		
Forgetfulness/confusion	●			●		
Headache		●	●			
Blurred vision		●		●		

INTERACTIONS

Sedatives All drugs with a sedative effect on the central nervous system can increase the sedative properties of diazepam and lorazepam. If combined with opiates, both diazepam and lorazepam carry a risk of potentially fatal respiratory depression.

Rifampicin may reduce the effects of diazepam.

Omeprazole (diazepam), **cimetidine, isoniazid, fosamprenavir, and ritonavir** may increase blood levels of diazepam and lorazepam and the risk of adverse effects.

PROLONGED USE

Regular use of these drugs over several weeks can lead to a reduction in their effect as the body adapts. They may also be habit-forming when taken for extended periods, and severe withdrawal reactions can occur if they are stopped abruptly.

DICLOFENAC

Brand names Dicloflex, Diclomax SR, Dyloject, Fenactol, Motifene, Voltarol, and many others
Used in the following combined preparation Arthrotec (with misoprostol)

GENERAL INFORMATION

Taken as a single dose, diclofenac has analgesic properties similar to those of paracetamol. The drug is used to relieve mild to moderate headache, menstrual pain, and pain following minor surgery. When taken regularly over a long period, diclofenac has an anti-inflammatory effect, and it is used to relieve pain and stiffness associated with rheumatoid arthritis and advanced osteoarthritis. It may also be prescribed to treat acute gout attacks, and may be given as eye drops to relieve eye inflammation.

The combined preparation, Arthrotec, contains diclofenac and misoprostol (see p.330). Misoprostol helps prevent gastroduodenal ulceration, which is sometimes caused by diclofenac, and may be particularly useful in patients at risk of developing this problem.

QUICK REFERENCE

Drug group Non-steroidal anti-inflammatory drug (p.74), analgesic (p.36), and drug for gout (p.77)
Overdose danger rating Medium
Dependence rating Low
Prescription needed Yes (except for some gel formulations)
Available as generic Yes

INFORMATION FOR USERS

Your drug prescription is tailored for you. Do not alter dosage without checking with your doctor.

How taken/used

Tablets, SR tablets, dispersible tablets, capsules, SR capsules, injection, suppositories, gel, eye drops.

Frequency and timing of doses
1–3 x daily with food.

Adult dosage range
75–150mg daily.

Onset of effect
Around 1 hour (pain relief); full anti-inflammatory effect may take 2 weeks.

Duration of action
Up to 12 hours; up to 24 hours (SR preparations).

Diet advice
None.

Storage
Keep in original container at room temperature out of the reach of children.

Missed dose
Take as soon as you remember. If your next dose is due within 2 hours, take a single dose now and skip the next.

Stopping the drug
When taken for short-term pain relief, diclofenac can be safely stopped as soon as you no longer need it. If prescribed for long-term treatment (e.g. for arthritis), speak to your doctor before stopping the drug.

Exceeding the dose
An occasional unintentional extra dose is unlikely to be a cause for concern. But if you notice any unusual symptoms or if a large overdose has been taken, notify your doctor.

SPECIAL PRECAUTIONS

Be sure to tell your doctor if:
- You have long-term liver or kidney problems.
- You have a bleeding disorder.
- You have had a peptic ulcer or you have indigestion.
- You have porphyria.
- You are allergic to aspirin or other NSAIDs.
- You have asthma, heart problems, or high blood pressure.
- You are taking other medicines.

Pregnancy
The drug may increase the risks of adverse effects on the baby's heart and may prolong labour if taken in the third trimester. Discuss with your doctor.

Breast-feeding
Small amounts pass into the breast milk, but adverse effects on the baby are unlikely. Discuss with your doctor.

Infants and children
Reduced dose necessary.

Over 60
Increased risk of adverse effects. Reduced dose may be necessary.

Driving and hazardous work
Avoid such activities until you have learned how diclofenac affects you; the drug can cause dizziness, drowsiness and vertigo.

Alcohol
Avoid. Alcohol may increase the risk of stomach irritation.

Surgery and general anaesthetics
Discuss with your doctor or dentist before any surgery.

POSSIBLE ADVERSE EFFECTS

The most common adverse effects are gastrointestinal disturbances. Black or bloodstained vomit or faeces should be reported to your doctor without delay.

Symptom/effect	Frequency		Discuss with doctor		Stop taking drug now	Call doctor now
	Common	Rare	Only if severe	In all cases		
Heartburn/indigestion	●		●			
Nausea/vomiting	●		●			
Headache		●	●			
Dizziness/drowsiness		●	●			
Swollen feet or legs		●	●			
Weight gain		●	●			
Rash/itching		●		●	●	
Wheezing/breathlessness		●		●	●	●
Black/bloodstained faeces		●		●	●	●

INTERACTIONS

General note Interacts with other NSAIDs, oral anticoagulants, corticosteroids, and SSRI antidepressants to increase the risk of bleeding and/or peptic ulceration.

Ciclosporin and tacrolimus Diclofenac may increase the risk of kidney problems.

Antihypertensive drugs and diuretics The beneficial effects of these drugs may be reduced with diclofenac.

Lithium, digoxin, and methotrexate Diclofenac may increase the blood levels of these drugs to an undesirable extent.

PROLONGED USE

There is an increased risk of ulceration, perforation, or bleeding from the bowel wall with prolonged use of diclofenac. There is also a small risk of a heart attack or stroke. To minimize these risks, the lowest effective dose is given for the shortest duration.

DICYCLOVERINE (DICYCLOMINE)

Brand name None
Used in the following combined preparation Kolanticon

GENERAL INFORMATION

Dicycloverine is a mild anticholinergic drug that relieves painful abdominal cramps caused by spasms of the smooth muscle in the wall of the gastrointestinal tract. It can be used to treat irritable bowel syndrome, and colicky conditions in babies (only those over 6 months).

Because the drug has anticholinergic properties (see p.35), it is also included in some combined preparations used for flatulence, indigestion, and diarrhoea. Dicycloverine relieves the symptoms but does not cure the underlying condition. Additional treatment with other drugs and self-help measures, such as dietary changes, may be recommended by your doctor.

Side effects with dicycloverine are rare, but they include headaches, constipation, urinary difficulties, and palpitations.

QUICK REFERENCE

Drug group Drug for irritable bowel syndrome (p.68)

Overdose danger rating Medium

Dependence rating Low

Prescription needed No (doses of 10mg or less); Yes (doses of more than 10mg)

Available as generic Yes

INFORMATION FOR USERS

Follow instructions on the label. Call your doctor if symptoms worsen.

How taken/used

Tablets, liquid.

Frequency and timing of doses
3–4 x daily before or after meals.

Dosage range
Adults 30–60mg daily.
Children Reduced dose according to age and weight.

Onset of effect
Within 1–2 hours.

Duration of action
4–6 hours.

Diet advice
None.

Storage
Keep in original container at room temperature out of the reach of children. Protect from light.

Missed dose
Take as soon as you remember. If your next dose is due within 2 hours, take a single dose now and skip the next.

Stopping the drug
The drug can be stopped without causing problems when it is no longer needed.

Exceeding the dose
An occasional unintentional extra dose is unlikely to cause problems. Large overdoses may cause drowsiness, dizziness, and difficulty in swallowing. Notify your doctor.

SPECIAL PRECAUTIONS

Be sure to tell your doctor if:
- You have glaucoma.
- You have urinary problems and/or an enlarged prostate gland.
- You have a hiatus hernia or you have heartburn or acid reflux.
- You have any heart condition.
- You have myasthenia gravis.
- You are taking other medicines.

 Pregnancy
No evidence of risk.

 Breast-feeding
The drug passes into the breast milk, but at normal doses adverse effects on the baby are unlikely. Discuss with your doctor.

 Infants and children
Reduced dose necessary. Not recommended in infants under 6 months.

 Over 60
Reduced dose may be necessary. Older people are more susceptible to anticholinergic side effects.

 Driving and hazardous work
Avoid such activities until you have learned how dicycloverine affects you; the drug can cause drowsiness and blurred vision.

 Alcohol
Caution. Alcohol may increase the sedative effects of this drug.

POSSIBLE ADVERSE EFFECTS

Most people do not notice any adverse effects when taking dicycloverine. Those that do occur are related to its anticholinergic properties and include drowsiness and dry mouth. Such symptoms may be overcome by adjusting the dosage, or they may disappear after a few days of usage as your body adjusts to the drug.

Symptom/effect	Frequency		Discuss with doctor		Stop taking drug now	Call doctor now
	Common	Rare	Only if severe	In all cases		
Dry mouth		●	●			
Headache		●	●			
Blurred vision		●	●			
Constipation		●	●			
Drowsiness/dizziness		●	●			
Difficulty in passing urine		●		●		
Palpitations		●		●		

INTERACTIONS

Sedatives All drugs that have a sedative effect on the central nervous system may increase the sedative properties of dicycloverine.

Anticholinergic drugs These drugs may increase the adverse effects of dicycloverine.

PROLONGED USE

No problems expected.

DIGOXIN

Brand name Lanoxin
Used in the following combined preparations None

GENERAL INFORMATION

Digoxin is the most widely used extract of digitalis, a compound originally obtained from the leaves of the foxglove plant. It is given to treat irregular heart rhythms such as atrial fibrillation or atrial flutter; it may also sometimes be used to treat congestive heart failure.

Digoxin increases the force of the heartbeat, making it more effective in pumping blood around the body. This in turn helps to control breathlessness, fluid retention, and tiredness in people with heart failure.

The effective dose of digoxin can be close to the toxic dose and, therefore, treatment needs careful monitoring to prevent toxic doses being reached. A number of adverse effects (see below) may indicate that the toxic level is close and should be reported to your doctor.

QUICK REFERENCE

Drug group Digitalis drug (p.54)
Overdose danger rating High
Dependence rating Low
Prescription needed Yes
Available as generic Yes

INFORMATION FOR USERS

Your drug prescription is tailored for you. Do not alter dosage without checking with your doctor.

How taken/used

Tablets, liquid, injection.

Frequency and timing of doses
Up to 3 x daily (starting dose); once daily, or divided to reduce nausea (maintenance dose).

Adult dosage range
Usually 0.0625–0.25mg daily (by mouth), but doses of up to 0.5mg are occasionally used.

Onset of effect
Within a few minutes (injection); within 1–2 hours (by mouth).

Duration of action
Up to 4 days.

Diet advice
Drug may be more toxic if potassium levels are low. Include potassium-rich fruit and vegetables, such as bananas and tomatoes, in your diet.

Storage
Keep in original container at room temperature out of the reach of children. Protect from light.

Missed dose
Take as soon as you remember. If your next dose is due within 8 hours, take a dose now and skip the next.

Stopping the drug
Do not stop the drug without consulting your doctor; stopping the drug may lead to worsening of the underlying condition.

OVERDOSE ACTION

Seek immediate medical advice in all cases. Take emergency action if palpitations, severe weakness, chest pain, or loss of consciousness occur.

See Drug poisoning emergency guide (p.518).

SPECIAL PRECAUTIONS

Be sure to tell your doctor if:
- You have had previous problems with your heart rhythm.
- You have kidney problems.
- You have a thyroid disorder.
- You are taking other medicines.

 Pregnancy
No evidence of risk, but adjustment in dose may be necessary.

 Breast-feeding
The drug passes into breast milk, but at normal doses adverse effects on the baby are unlikely. Discuss with your doctor.

 Infants and children
Reduced dose necessary.

 Over 60
Increased likelihood of adverse effects. Reduced dose may therefore be necessary.

 Driving and hazardous work
Special problems are unlikely, but do not undertake these activities until you know how digoxin affects you because it can cause tiredness and visual disturbances.

 Alcohol
No special problems.

PROLONGED USE

No problems expected.

Monitoring Periodic checks on blood levels of digoxin and body salts may be advised.

POSSIBLE ADVERSE EFFECTS

The possible adverse effects of digoxin are usually due to increased levels of the drug in the blood. Any symptoms should be reported to your doctor without delay.

Symptom/effect	Frequency		Discuss with doctor		Stop taking drug now	Call doctor now
	Common	Rare	Only if severe	In all cases		
Tiredness	●		●			
Nausea/loss of appetite	●			●		
Confusion		●		●		
Visual disturbance		●		●	●	●
Palpitations		●		●	●	●

INTERACTIONS

General note Many drugs interact with digoxin. Do not take any medication without consulting your doctor or pharmacist.

Diuretics may increase the risk of adverse effects from digoxin if they lower potassium levels.

Ciclosporin and tacrolimus may increase blood levels of digoxin.

Calcium channel blockers and anti-arrhythmic drugs (e.g. amiodarone and quinidine) may increase blood levels of digoxin.

Antacids may reduce the effects of digoxin. The effect of digoxin may increase when antacids are stopped.

DIHYDROCODEINE

Brand names DF118 Forte, DHC Continus
Used in the following combined preparations Co-dydramol, Paramol

GENERAL INFORMATION

Dihydrocodeine is an opioid analgesic related to codeine and of similar potency if taken by mouth. It is used mainly for the relief of moderately severe pain but has also been used as a cough suppressant. As with codeine, side effects limit the dose that can be taken; dihydrocodeine causes constipation, nausea, and vomiting. The drug is also used in combination with paracetamol; in this way, a lower dose of the opioid can be used to give pain relief with fewer side effects. A combined preparation containing dihydrocodeine and paracetamol is available under the generic name of co-dydramol.

INFORMATION FOR USERS

Your drug prescription is tailored for you. Do not alter dosage without checking with your doctor.

How taken/used

Tablets, SR tablets, liquid, injection.

Frequency and timing of doses
2–6 x daily.

Adult dosage range
120–240mg daily.

Onset of effect
30–60 minutes (tablets, liquid); 3–4 hours (SR tablets).

Duration of action
4–6 hours (tablets, liquid); 12 hours (SR tablets).

Diet advice
None.

Storage
Keep in original container at room temperature out of the reach of children.

Missed dose
Take as soon as you remember if needed for relief of symptoms. If not needed, do not take the missed dose, and return to your normal dosage schedule when necessary.

Stopping the drug
Can usually be safely stopped as soon as you no longer need it. However, if you have been taking it for a long time or at high doses, you may experience withdrawal effects. Discuss with your doctor.

OVERDOSE ACTION

Seek immediate medical advice in all cases. Take emergency action if slow or irregular breathing, severe drowsiness, or loss of consciousness occur.

See Drug poisoning emergency guide (p.518).

SPECIAL PRECAUTIONS

Be sure to tell your doctor if:
- You have liver or kidney problems.
- You have a phaeochromocytoma.
- You have a lung disorder such as asthma or bronchitis.
- You have a problem with alcohol abuse.
- You have an enlarged prostate.
- You have low blood pressure.
- You have an underactive thyroid.
- You are taking other medicines.

 Pregnancy
Safety not established, although drug has been widely used in pregnancy for many years without obvious effect (except close to delivery).

 Breast-feeding
Safety not established. Discuss with your doctor.

Infants and children
Not recommended for children under 4 years. In children over 4 years a reduced dose is necessary.

 Over 60
Reduced dose necessary.

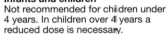 **Driving and hazardous work**
Avoid such activities until you have learned how dihydrocodeine affects you because the drug may cause drowsiness, dizziness, and confusion.

Alcohol
Avoid. Alcohol may increase the sedative effects of the drug.

PROLONGED USE

Dihydrocodeine is generally only used in the short term since it can be habit forming if used long term.

POSSIBLE ADVERSE EFFECTS

The most common adverse effects are constipation, nausea, vomiting, headache, and vertigo. Tolerance and dependence may occur.

Symptom/effect	Frequency		Discuss with doctor		Stop taking drug now	Call doctor now
	Common	Rare	Only if severe	In all cases		
Constipation	●			●		
Nausea/vomiting	●			●		
Drowsiness/dizziness	●			●		
Headache	●			●		
Abdominal pain		●		●		
Rash/itching		●	●			
Confusion/hallucinations		●	●			
Breathing difficulties		●		●	●	●

INTERACTIONS

Sedatives All drugs that have a sedative effect on the central nervous system increase dihydrocodeine's sedative properties. These include other opioid analgesics, sleeping drugs, antihistamines, antipsychotics, and antidepressants.

Monoamine oxidase inhibitors (MAOIs) may cause a dangerous rise in blood pressure. Avoid using together and for 14 days after stopping MAOI treatment.

DILTIAZEM

Brand names Adizem-SR, Dilzem SR, Dilzem XL, Slozem, Tildiem, and others
Used in the following combined preparations None

GENERAL INFORMATION

Diltiazem is a calcium channel blocker (p.59). This class of drugs interrupts the conduction of nerve signals in the muscles of the heart and blood vessels.

Diltiazem is used in the treatment of angina, and longer-acting formulations are used for high blood pressure. When taken regularly this drug reduces the frequency of angina attacks, but it does not work quickly enough to reduce the pain of an angina attack that is already in progress. Topical diltiazem is also used to treat chronic anal fissure.

Diltiazem does not adversely affect breathing and is valuable for people who suffer from asthma, for whom other anti-angina drugs may not be suitable. Different brands of sustained-release (SR) diltiazem may not be equivalent, so you should always take the same brand.

QUICK REFERENCE

Drug group Calcium channel blocker (p.59) and antihypertensive drug (p.60)

Overdose danger rating Medium

Dependence rating Low

Prescription needed Yes

Available as generic Yes

INFORMATION FOR USERS

Your drug prescription is tailored for you. Do not alter dosage without checking with your doctor.

How taken/used

Tablets, SR tablets, capsules, SR capsules, cream.

Frequency and timing of doses
3 x daily (tablets/capsules); 1–2 x daily (SR tablets/capsules); 2 x daily (cream).

Adult dosage range
Angina/high blood pressure 180–480mg daily.
Anal fissure 1 inch of cream applied to anal area twice daily for 2 months.

Onset of effect
2–3 hours.

Duration of action
6–8 hours.

Diet advice
None.

Storage
Keep in original container at room temperature out of the reach of children.

Missed dose
Take as soon as you remember. If your next dose is due within 2 hours, take a single dose now and skip the next.

Stopping the drug
Do not stop taking the drug without consulting your doctor; symptoms may recur. Stopping suddenly may worsen angina.

Exceeding the dose
Occasional unintentional extra dose is unlikely to be a problem. Large overdose may cause dizziness or collapse. Tell your doctor urgently.

SPECIAL PRECAUTIONS

Be sure to tell your doctor if:
- You have long-term liver or kidney problems.
- You have heart failure, heart block, or heart valve problems.
- You have acute porphyria.
- You are taking other medicines.

 Pregnancy
Not usually prescribed. Discuss with your doctor.

 Breast-feeding
The drug passes into the breast milk and may affect the baby. Discuss with your doctor.

 Infants and children
Not recommended.

 Over 60
Increased risk of adverse effects. Reduced dose may be necessary.

 Driving and hazardous work
Avoid such activities until you have learned how diltiazem affects you because the drug can cause dizziness due to lowered blood pressure.

 Alcohol
Avoid excessive amounts. Alcohol may lower blood pressure, causing dizziness.

POSSIBLE ADVERSE EFFECTS

Diltiazem can cause minor symptoms common to calcium channel blockers, such as nausea and headache. The most serious adverse effect is a slowed heart beat, which may cause tiredness or dizziness. These effects can sometimes be controlled by adjusting dosage.

Symptom/effect	Frequency		Discuss with doctor		Stop taking drug now	Call doctor now
	Common	Rare	Only if severe	In all cases		
Headache	●		●			
Nausea/vomiting	●		●			
Dry mouth	●		●			
Ankle swelling	●		●			
Breast/gum enlargement		●		●		
Dizziness/tiredness		●		●		
Rash		●		●		

PROLONGED USE

No problems expected.

INTERACTIONS

Antihypertensive drugs Diltiazem increases the effects of these drugs, leading to a further reduction in blood pressure.

Anticonvulsant drugs Levels of these drugs may be altered by diltiazem.

Anti-arrhythmic drugs There is a risk of side effects on the heart if these are taken with diltiazem.

Beta blockers increase the risk of the heart slowing.

Digoxin Blood levels and adverse effects of this drug may be increased if it is taken with diltiazem. The dosage of digoxin may need to be reduced.

Simvastatin Diltiazem may increase blood levels and adverse effects of this drug. The dosage of simvastatin may need to be reduced.

Theophylline/aminophylline Diltiazem may increase the levels of this drug.

DIPYRIDAMOLE

Brand names Attia, Ofcram PR, Trolactin
Used in the following combined preparation Molita (dipyridamole with aspirin)

GENERAL INFORMATION

Dipyridamole was introduced in the late 1970s as an anti-angina drug to improve the capability of people with angina to exercise. More effective drugs are now available, but dipyridamole is still prescribed as an antiplatelet drug. It acts by reducing the ability of platelets to stick to each other and to blood vessel walls, which reduces the likelihood of clots forming. This action is especially important in people who have had a stroke or transient ischaemic attacks (TIAs) or have undergone heart valve replacement surgery. Dipyridamole is usually given with other drugs such as warfarin or aspirin. The drug can also be given by injection during certain types of diagnostic test on the heart.

Side effects may occur, especially during the early days of treatment. If they persist, your doctor may advise a reduction in dosage.

QUICK REFERENCE

Drug group Antiplatelet drug (p.62)
Overdose danger rating Medium
Dependence rating Low
Prescription needed Yes
Available as generic Yes

INFORMATION FOR USERS

Your drug prescription is tailored for you. Do not alter dosage without checking with your doctor.

How taken/used

Tablets, capsules, MR capsules, liquid, injection (for diagnostic tests only).

Frequency and timing of doses
3–4 x daily, 1 hour before meals (tablets, capsules, liquid). 2 x daily with food (MR capsules).

Adult dosage range
300–600mg daily (tablets, capsules, liquid); 400mg daily (MR capsules).

Onset of effect
Within 1 hour. Full therapeutic effect may not be reached for 2–3 weeks.

Duration of action
Up to 8 hours. Up to 12 hours (MR capsules).

Diet advice
None.

Storage
Keep in original container at room temperature out of the reach of children. Protect from light.

Missed dose
Take as soon as you remember. If your next dose is due within 2 hours, take a single dose now and skip the next.

Stopping the drug
Do not stop taking the drug without consulting your doctor; withdrawal of the drug could lead to abnormal blood clotting.

Exceeding the dose
An occasional unintentional extra dose is unlikely to be a cause for concern. Large overdoses may cause dizziness or vomiting. Notify your doctor.

SPECIAL PRECAUTIONS

Be sure to tell your doctor if:
- You have low blood pressure.
- You have a blood clotting disorder.
- You have migraines.
- You have angina or heart valve problems.
- You have myasthenia gravis.
- You have had a recent heart attack.
- You are taking other medicines.

Pregnancy
Safety in pregnancy not established. Discuss with your doctor.

Breast-feeding
The drug passes into the breast milk but at normal doses adverse effects on the baby are unlikely. Discuss with your doctor.

Infants and children
Reduced dose necessary.

Over 60
No special problems.

Driving and hazardous work
Avoid such activities until you have learned how dipyridamole affects you because the drug may cause dizziness and faintness.

Alcohol
Avoid until you have learned how dipyridamole affects you because the drug may cause dizziness and faintness when taken with alcohol.

PROLONGED USE

No known problems.

POSSIBLE ADVERSE EFFECTS

Adverse effects are rare. Possible symptoms include dizziness, headache, flushing, stomach upsets including nausea, and rash. In rare cases, the drug may aggravate angina.

Symptom/effect	Frequency		Discuss with doctor		Stop taking drug now	Call doctor now
	Common	Rare	Only if severe	In all cases		
Stomach upset/nausea	●			●		
Headache	●			●		
Flushing	●			●		
Diarrhoea		●		●		
Dizziness/fainting		●		●		
Rash		●		●	●	
Breathing difficulties/swollen lips		●		●	●	●

INTERACTIONS

Anticoagulant drugs The effect of these drugs may be increased by dipyridamole, thereby increasing the risk of uncontrolled bleeding. The dosage of the anticoagulant may need to be adjusted accordingly.

Adenosine should not be given to somebody who is taking dipyridamole as the combination can cause a serious drop in blood pressure.

Antihypertensives Dipyridamole may increase the effect of these drugs.

Cholinesterase inhibitors Used to treat myasthenia gravis, the effect of these drugs may be reduced by dipyridamole.

Antacids may reduce the effectiveness of dipyridamole.

DISULFIRAM

Brand name Antabuse, Esperal
Used in the following combined preparations None

GENERAL INFORMATION

Disulfiram is used to help alcohol misusers abstain from alcohol. It does not cure alcoholism but provides a powerful deterrent to drinking.

If you are taking disulfiram and drink even a small amount of alcohol, highly unpleasant reactions follow. These are due to high levels of acetaldehyde in the body, because disulfiram prevents its breakdown. Flushing, throbbing headache, nausea, breathlessness, thirst, palpitations, dizziness, and fainting may be experienced. Such reactions may last from 30 minutes to several hours, leaving you feeling drowsy and fatigued. The reactions can also include unconsciousness, so it is wise to carry a card stating the person to be notified in an emergency.

It is important not to drink any alcohol for at least 24 hours before beginning disulfiram treatment, and for at least a week after stopping. Foods, medicines, and even toiletries that contain alcohol should also be avoided. Disulfiram treatment is usually only started by specialist services and in conjunction with social support.

INFORMATION FOR USERS

Your drug prescription is tailored for you. Do not alter dosage without checking with your doctor.

How taken/used

Tablets.

Frequency and timing of doses
Once daily.

Adult dosage range
800mg initially, gradually reduced over 5 days to 100–200mg (maintenance dose).

Onset of effect
Interaction with alcohol occurs within a few minutes of taking alcohol.

Duration of action
Interaction with alcohol can occur for up to 6 days after the last dose of disulfiram.

Diet advice
Avoid all alcoholic drinks, even in very small amounts. Food, fermented vinegar, medicines, mouthwashes, and lotions containing alcohol should also be avoided.

Storage
Keep in original container at room temperature out of the reach of children. Protect from light.

Missed dose
Take as soon as you remember. If your next dose is due within 2 hours, take a single dose now and skip the next.

Stopping the drug
Do not stop taking the drug without consulting your doctor.

Exceeding the dose
An occasional unintentional extra dose is unlikely to cause problems. Large overdoses may cause a temporary increase in adverse effects. Notify your doctor.

POSSIBLE ADVERSE EFFECTS

Adverse effects of disulfiram usually disappear when you get used to taking the drug. If they persist or become severe, the dosage may need to be adjusted.

Symptom/effect	Frequency		Discuss with doctor		Stop taking drug now	Call doctor now
	Common	Rare	Only if severe	In all cases		
Drowsiness/fatigue	●		●			
Nausea/vomiting	●		●			
Halitosis	●		●			
Reduced libido		●	●			

INTERACTIONS

General note A number of drugs can produce an adverse reaction when taken with disulfiram. You are advised to check with your doctor or pharmacist before taking any other medication.

Phenytoin Disulfiram increases the blood levels of this drug.

Anticoagulant drugs (e.g. warfarin) Disulfiram increases the effect of these drugs.

Metronidazole A severe reaction can occur if this drug is taken with disulfiram.

Theophylline Disulfiram may increase the toxic effects of this drug.

Diazepam/chlordiazepoxide Disulfiram increases the effect of these drugs.

Tricyclic antidepressants Disulfiram increases the blood levels of these drugs.

SPECIAL PRECAUTIONS

Be sure to tell your doctor if:
- You have long-term liver or kidney problems.
- You have heart problems, coronary artery disease, or high blood pressure, or have had a previous stroke.
- You have had epileptic seizures.
- You have diabetes.
- You have breathing problems.
- You have depression.
- You are taking other medicines.

Pregnancy
Safety in pregnancy not established. Discuss with your doctor.

Breast-feeding
Avoid. No information available on whether the drug passes into breast milk. Discuss with your doctor.

Infants and children
Not recommended.

Over 60
Reduced dose may be necessary.

Driving and hazardous work
Avoid such activities until you have learned how disulfiram affects you because the drug can cause drowsiness and dizziness.

Alcohol
Never drink alcohol while under treatment with disulfiram, and avoid foods, medicines, and toiletries containing alcohol. This drug may interact dangerously with alcohol.

PROLONGED USE

Not usually prescribed for longer than 6 months without review. It is wise to carry a card indicating you are taking disulfiram with instructions as to who should be notified in an emergency.

DOMPERIDONE

Brand name Motilium
Used in the following combined preparations None

GENERAL INFORMATION

Domperidone, an anti-emetic drug, was first introduced in the early 1980s. It is particularly effective for treating nausea and vomiting caused by gastroenteritis, chemotherapy, or radiotherapy. It is not effective for motion sickness or nausea caused by inner ear disorders such as Ménière's disease.

The main advantage of domperidone over other anti-emetic drugs is that it does not usually cause drowsiness or other adverse effects such as abnormal movement. Domperidone is not suitable, however, for the long-term treatment of gastrointestinal disorders, for which an alternative drug treatment is often prescribed.

Domperidone is now restricted to use in the relief of nausea and vomiting. The drug is also sometimes given in single doses to manage acute attacks of migraine by enhancing the absorption of other drugs for migraine, such as paracetamol.

INFORMATION FOR USERS

Follow instructions on the label. Call your doctor if symptoms worsen.

How taken/used

Tablets, liquid.

Frequency and timing of doses
1–3 x daily.

Adult dosage range
Up to a maximum of 30mg daily.

Onset of effect
Within 1 hour. The effects of the drug may be delayed if taken after the onset of nausea.

Duration of action
Approximately 6 hours.

Diet advice
Avoid taking domperidone with grapefruit juice because it may increase the risk of heart rhythm problems.

Storage
Keep in original container at room temperature out of the reach of children. Protect from light.

Missed dose
If your next dose is due within 4 hours, take a single dose now and skip the next. Then return to your normal dose schedule.

Stopping the drug
Can be stopped when you no longer need it.

Exceeding the dose
An occasional unintentional extra dose is unlikely to cause problems. Large overdoses may cause dizziness. Notify your doctor.

POSSIBLE ADVERSE EFFECTS

Adverse effects from this drug are rare. However, if you experience symptoms such as irregular heartbeat or fainting, you should stop taking the drug and seek immediate medical attention.

Symptom/effect	Frequency		Discuss with doctor		Stop taking drug now	Call doctor now
	Common	Rare	Only if severe	In all cases		
Breast enlargement		●		●		
Milk secretion from breast		●		●		
Muscle spasms/tremors		●		●		
Reduced libido		●		●		
Rash		●		●		
Irregular heart beat/fainting		●		●	●	●

INTERACTIONS

Anticholinergic drugs These may reduce the beneficial effects of domperidone.

Bromocriptine and cabergoline Domperidone may reduce the effects of these drugs in some people.

Ketoconazole and erythromycin These drugs should not be taken while also taking domperidone as the combination increases the risk of heart rhythm problems.

Opioid analgesics These may reduce the beneficial effects of domperidone.

SPECIAL PRECAUTIONS

Be sure to tell your doctor or pharmacist before using this drug if:
- You have a long-term kidney problem or liver disease.
- You have thyroid disease.
- You have a pituitary tumour.
- You have or have had heart disease.
- You are taking other medicines.

Pregnancy
Safety in pregnancy not established. Discuss with your doctor.

Breast-feeding
The drug may pass into the breast milk, but at normal doses adverse effects on the baby are unlikely. Discuss with your doctor.

Infants and children
Do not use in children under 16 years, except on a doctor's advice.

Over 60
Reduced dose may be necessary.

Driving and hazardous work
No special problems.

Alcohol
No special problems, but alcohol is best avoided in cases of nausea and vomiting.

PROLONGED USE

Treatment should be reviewed after one week and the need for continued treatment reassessed. In people with heart disease, there is a small increased risk of collapse or sudden death.

DONEPEZIL

Brand names Aricept, Aricept Evess
Used in the following combined preparations None

GENERAL INFORMATION

Donepezil is an inhibitor of the enzyme acetylcholinesterase. This enzyme breaks down the neurotransmitter acetylcholine (see p.35) to limit its effects. Blocking the enzyme raises levels of acetylcholine; in the brain, this increases awareness and memory. Donepezil has been found to improve symptoms of dementia in Alzheimer's disease (mild to moderate disease) and is used to slow the deterioration. It is not currently recommended for dementia due to other causes. Treatment with donepezil is initiated under specialist supervision. It is usual to assess those being treated at six-monthly intervals to decide whether the drug is helping.

Side effects may include bladder outflow obstruction and psychiatric problems, such as agitation and aggression, which may be due to the disease itself.

QUICK REFERENCE

Drug group Drug for dementia (p.43)
Overdose danger rating Medium
Dependence rating Low
Prescription needed Yes
Available as generic Yes

INFORMATION FOR USERS

Your drug prescription is tailored for you. Do not alter dosage without checking with your doctor.

How taken/used

Tablets, dispersible tablets, liquid.

Frequency and timing of doses
Once daily at bedtime.

Adult dosage range
5–10mg.

Onset of effect
1 hour. Full effects may take up to 3 months.

Duration of action
Usually 1–2 days.

Diet advice
None.

Storage
Keep in original container at room temperature out of the reach of children.

Missed dose
Take as soon as you remember. A carer should ensure that the maximum dose taken in 24 hours does not exceed 10mg.

Stopping the drug
Do not stop taking the drug without consulting your doctor; symptoms may recur.

Exceeding the dose
An occasional unintentional extra dose is unlikely to be a cause for concern. But if you notice any unusual symptoms, or if a large overdose has been taken, notify your doctor.

POSSIBLE ADVERSE EFFECTS

Adverse effects include such problems as accidents and falls, which are common in this group of people even when not treated.

Symptom/effect	Frequency		Discuss with doctor		Stop taking drug now	Call doctor now
	Common	Rare	Only if severe	In all cases		
Nausea/vomiting	●		●			
Diarrhoea	●		●			
Fatigue/insomnia	●		●			
Muscle cramps	●		●			
Urinary incontinence	●			●		
Headache		●	●			
Fainting/dizziness		●		●		
Palpitations		●		●		
Difficulty in passing urine		●		●		
Seizures		●		●	●	●

INTERACTIONS

Muscle relaxants used in surgery
Donepezil may increase the effect of some muscle relaxants, but it may also block some others

Fluoxetine, erythromycin and ketoconazole can increase the levels and adverse effects of donepezil.

SPECIAL PRECAUTIONS

Be sure to tell your doctor if:
- You have liver or kidney problems.
- You have a heart problem.
- You have asthma or respiratory problems.
- You have had a gastric or duodenal ulcer.
- You are taking a non-steroidal anti-inflammatory drug (NSAID) regularly.
- You are taking other medicines.

 Pregnancy
Not recommended. Safety in pregnancy not established.

 Breast-feeding
Not recommended.

 Infants and children
Not recommended.

 Over 60
Treatment may have to be stopped if you develop low heart rate, heart block, or unexplained fainting.

 Driving and hazardous work
Your underlying condition may make such activities inadvisable. Discuss with your doctor.

 Alcohol
Avoid. Alcohol may reduce the effect of donepezil.

Surgery and general anaesthetics
Treatment may need to be stopped before you have a general anaesthetic. Discuss with your doctor or dentist before any operation.

PROLONGED USE

May be continued for as long as there is benefit. Stopping the drug leads to a gradual loss of the improvements over several weeks.

Monitoring Periodic checks should be carried out at 6-monthly intervals to test whether the drug is still providing some benefit.

DORZOLAMIDE

Brand name Eydelto, Trusopt
Used in the following combined preparation Cosopt, Eylamdo, Tidomat

GENERAL INFORMATION

Dorzolamide is a carbonic anhydrase inhibitor (a kind of diuretic) that is used, in the form of eye drops only, to treat glaucoma. It is also used for ocular hypertension (high pressure inside the eye). The drug relieves the pressure by reducing the production of aqueous humour, the fluid in the front chamber of the eye.

Dorzolamide may be used either alone or combined with a beta blocker (see p.55) by people who are resistant to the effects of beta blockers or for whom beta blockers are not suitable.

Most side effects of dorzolamide are local to the eye, but systemic effects may occur if enough of the drug is absorbed by the body. Systemic absorption from eye drops may also result in an increase in the effects of other carbonic acid inhibitors taken orally (such as acetazolamide) if they are used concurrently.

INFORMATION FOR USERS

Your drug prescription is tailored for you. Do not alter dosage without checking with your doctor.

How taken/used

Eye drops.

Frequency and timing of doses
3 x daily (on its own); 2 x daily (combined preparation).

Adult dosage range
1 drop in the affected eye(s) or as directed. If using additional eye drops, allow 5 minutes between applying the different types of drop.

Onset of effect
15–30 minutes.

Duration of action
4–8 hours.

Diet advice
None.

Storage
Keep in original container at room temperature out of the reach of children. Protect from light. Discard eye drops 4 weeks after opening.

Missed dose
Use as soon as you remember. If your next dose is due, skip the missed dose and then go back to your normal dosing schedule.

Stopping the drug
Do not stop the drug without consulting your doctor; symptoms may recur.

Exceeding the dose
An occasional unintentional extra application is unlikely to cause problems. Excessive use may provoke side effects as described below.

SPECIAL PRECAUTIONS

Be sure to tell your doctor if:
• You have liver or kidney problems.
• You are allergic to sulfonamide drugs.
• You are allergic to benzalkonium chloride.
• You are taking other medicines.

 Pregnancy
Not prescribed. Discuss with your doctor.

 Breast-feeding
Not recommended. Discuss with your doctor.

 Infants and children
Not recommended.

 Over 60
No special problems.

 Driving and hazardous work
Avoid such activities until you have learned how dorzolamide affects you because the drug can affect your vision.

 Alcohol
No special problems.

POSSIBLE ADVERSE EFFECTS

Local side effects of dorzolamide include inflammation of the surface of the eye and the skin of the eyelids. Systemic side effects may also occur but are rare. If you develop an itchy rash, swelling of the lips or tongue, or breathing difficulties, you should consult your doctor urgently.

Symptom/effect	Frequency		Discuss with doctor		Stop taking drug now	Call doctor now
	Common	Rare	Only if severe	In all cases		
Burning/stinging eyes	●		●			
Bitter taste in the mouth	●		●			
Blurred vision/runny eyes	●		●			
Headache	●		●			
Inflamed/sore eyes	●			●		
Rash/breathing difficulties		●		●	●	●
Swollen lips/tongue		●		●	●	●

INTERACTIONS

None.

PROLONGED USE

Rarely, prolonged use of this drug may lead to development of kidney stones.

DOSULEPIN (DOTHIEPIN)

Brand name Prothiaden
Used in the following combined preparations None

GENERAL INFORMATION

Dosulepin belongs to the tricyclic class of antidepressants and is used in the long-term treatment of depression. It is particularly useful when depression is accompanied by anxiety and insomnia. The drug elevates mood, increases physical activity, improves appetite, and restores interest in everyday activities. Taken at night, dosulepin encourages sleep and helps eliminate the need for additional sleeping drugs.

Dosulepin takes several weeks to achieve its full antidepressant effect. It has adverse effects common to all tricyclics, including a risk of dangerous heart rhythms, seizures, and coma, if taken in overdose. It should not be used by anyone with a serious heart condition.

QUICK REFERENCE

Drug group Tricyclic antidepressant drug (p.40)

Overdose danger rating High

Dependence rating Low

Prescription needed Yes

Available as generic Yes

INFORMATION FOR USERS

Your drug prescription is tailored for you. Do not alter dosage without checking with your doctor.

How taken/used

Tablets, capsules.

Frequency and timing of doses
2–3 x daily or once at night.

Adult dosage range
75–150mg daily (a maximum dose of up to 225mg may be given in some circumstances).

Onset of effect
Full antidepressant effect may not be felt for 2–6 weeks, but adverse effects may be noticed within a day or two.

Duration of action
Several days.

Diet advice
None.

Storage
Keep in original container at room temperature out of the reach of children.

Missed dose
Take as soon as you remember. If your next dose is due within 2 hours, take a single dose now and skip the next.

Stopping the drug
Do not stop taking the drug without consulting your doctor, who may supervise a gradual reduction in dosage. Abrupt cessation of the drug may cause withdrawal symptoms and a recurrence of the original problem.

OVERDOSE ACTION

Seek immediate medical advice in all cases. Take emergency action if palpitations or loss of consciousness occur.

See Drug poisoning emergency guide (p.518).

POSSIBLE ADVERSE EFFECTS

The adverse effects of this drug are mainly the result of its anticholinergic action. These effects are more common in the early days of treatment. It can also affect normal heart rhythm.

Symptom/effect	Frequency		Discuss with doctor		Stop taking drug now	Call doctor now
	Common	Rare	Only if severe	In all cases		
Drowsiness	●		●			
Dry mouth	●		●			
Sweating	●		●			
Blurred vision	●			●		
Dizziness/fainting		●		●		
Difficulty in passing urine		●		●	●	
Palpitations		●		●	●	●

INTERACTIONS

Antiarrhythmic drugs Dosulepin should be avoided in patients on amiodarone, sotalol, and other medications that can affect heart rhythms.

Monoamine oxidase inhibitors (MAOIs) In the rare cases where these drugs are given with dosulepin, serious interactions may occur.

Sedatives All drugs that have a sedative effect on the central nervous system increase the sedative properties of dosulepin.

Anticonvulsant drugs Dosulepin may reduce the effectiveness of these drugs.

SPECIAL PRECAUTIONS

Be sure to tell your doctor if:
- You have heart problems.
- You have had epileptic seizures.
- You have long-term liver or kidney problems.
- You have glaucoma.
- You have had mania or a psychotic illness.
- You are taking other medicines.

Pregnancy
Safety in pregnancy not established. Discuss with your doctor.

Breast-feeding
The drug passes into the breast milk, but effects on the baby are unlikely. Discuss with your doctor.

Infants and children
Not recommended.

Over 60
Greater risk of adverse effects. Reduced dose necessary.

Driving and hazardous work
Avoid such activities until you have learned how dosulepin affects you because the drug can reduce alertness and may cause blurred vision, dizziness, and drowsiness.

Alcohol
Avoid. Alcohol may increase the sedative effects of this drug.

Surgery and general anaesthetics
Treatment with dosulepin may need to be stopped before you have a general anaesthetic. Discuss this with your doctor or dentist before any operation.

PROLONGED USE

No problems expected.

DOXAZOSIN

Brand names Cardozin, Cardura, Cardura XL, Doxadura, Raporsin, Slocinx XL
Used in the following combined preparations None

GENERAL INFORMATION

Doxazosin is an antihypertensive vasodilator that relieves hypertension (high blood pressure) by relaxing the muscles in the blood vessel walls. It may be administered together with other antihypertensive drugs, because its effects on blood pressure are increased when it is combined with most other antihypertensives.

Doxazosin can also be given to patients with an enlarged prostate gland. It relaxes the muscles around the prostate gland and bladder exit, making bladder emptying easier. However, this effect may cause incontinence when the drug is used in women.

Dizziness and fainting may occur with doxazosin. Typically, this effect occurs on standing and may improve with continued treatment but it may limit the drug's use, especially in older people. Doxazosin may be better tolerated if it is taken at night.

QUICK REFERENCE

Drug group A vasodilator (p.56), antihypertensive drug (p.60), and drug for urinary disorders (p.126)

Overdose danger rating Medium

Dependence rating Low

Prescription needed Yes

Available as generic Yes

INFORMATION FOR USERS

Your drug prescription is tailored for you. Do not alter dosage without checking with your doctor.

How taken/used

Tablets, MR tablets.

Frequency and timing of doses
1–2 x daily.

Adult dosage range
Hypertension 1mg (starting dose for tablets), increased gradually as necessary up to 16mg; or 4mg (starting dose for MR tablets) increased as necessary to 8mg.
Enlarged prostate 1mg (starting dose), increased gradually at 1–2-week intervals up to 8mg.

Onset of effect
Within 2 hours.

Duration of action
24 hours.

Diet advice
None.

Storage
Keep in original container at room temperature out of the reach of children.

Missed dose
If you forget to take a tablet, skip that dose completely but carry on as normal the following day.

Stopping the drug
Do not stop taking the drug without consulting your doctor; stopping the drug may lead to a rise in blood pressure.

Exceeding the dose
An occasional unintentional extra dose is unlikely to be a cause for concern. Larger overdoses may cause dizziness or fainting. Notify your doctor.

SPECIAL PRECAUTIONS

Be sure to tell your doctor if:
- You have long-term liver problems.
- You have heart problems.
- You have problems with urinary incontinence.
- You have attacks of fainting, especially on standing up or while urinating.
- You have had an allergic reaction to doxazosin in the past.
- You are due to have cataract surgery or another operation.
- You are taking other medicines.

 Pregnancy
Safety in pregnancy not established. Discuss with your doctor.

 Breast-feeding
Safety not established. The drug passes into the breast milk. Discuss with your doctor.

 Infants and children
Not recommended.

 Over 60
Reduced dose may be necessary. Take extra care when standing up until you have learned how the drug affects you.

 Driving and hazardous work
Avoid such activities until you have learned how doxazosin affects you because the drug can cause drowsiness, dizziness, and fainting.

 Alcohol
Avoid excessive amounts. Alcohol may increase some of the adverse effects of this drug, such as dizziness, drowsiness, and fainting.

Surgery and general anaesthetics
A general anaesthetic may increase the low blood pressure effect of doxazosin.

POSSIBLE ADVERSE EFFECTS

Nausea and weakness are common with doxazosin, but the main problem is that it may cause dizziness or fainting when you stand up, especially when first using the drug.

Symptom/effect	Frequency		Discuss with doctor		Stop taking drug now	Call doctor now
	Common	Rare	Only if severe	In all cases		
Nausea	●		●			
Weakness/drowsiness	●		●			
Swollen ankles	●		●			
Dizziness/fainting		●	●			
Stuffy/runny nose		●	●			
Sleep disturbances		●				
Incontinence (in women)		●		●		
Rash		●		●		
Palpitations/chest pain		●		●		●
Headache/sleepiness		●	●			

INTERACTIONS

General note Any drugs that can reduce blood pressure are likely to increase the blood-pressure-lowering effect of doxazosin. These include diuretics, beta blockers, ACE inhibitors, calcium channel blockers, nitrates, some antipsychotics and antidepressants, and drugs for erectile dysfunction (sildenafil and tadalafil).

PROLONGED USE

No known problems.

DOXORUBICIN

Brand names Caelyx, Myocet
Used in the following combined preparations None

GENERAL INFORMATION

Doxorubicin is one of the most effective anticancer drugs. It is prescribed to treat a wide variety of cancers, usually in conjunction with other anticancer drugs. It is used in cancer of the lymph nodes (Hodgkin's disease), lung, breast, bladder, stomach, thyroid, and reproductive organs. It is also used to treat Kaposi's sarcoma in AIDS patients.

Nausea and vomiting after injection are the most common side effects. Although these effects are unpleasant, they tend to become less severe as the body adjusts to treatment. The drug may stain the urine bright red, but this is not harmful. More seriously, because doxorubicin interferes with the production of blood cells, blood clotting disorders, anaemia, and infections may occur. Hair loss is also a common side effect. Heart rhythm disturbance and heart failure are possible, although less common, dose-dependent side effects. The heart failure is usually irreversible and is worsened by trastuzumab (Herceptin). The brand-name drugs Caelyx and Myocet are special formulations in which the doxorubicin is enclosed in fatty spheres. This makes the drug more suitable for treating certain types of cancer – for example AIDS-related Kaposi's sarcoma.

QUICK REFERENCE

Drug group Cytotoxic anticancer drug (p.112)

Overdose danger rating Medium

Dependence rating Low

Prescription needed Yes

Available as generic Yes

INFORMATION FOR USERS

This drug is given only under medical supervision and is not for self-administration.

How taken/used

Injection, bladder instillation.

Frequency and timing of doses
Every 1–3 weeks (injection); once a month (bladder instillation).

Adult dosage range
Dosage is determined individually according to body height, weight, and response.

Onset of effect
Some adverse effects may appear within 1 hour of starting treatment, but full beneficial effects may not be felt for up to 4 weeks.

Duration of action
Adverse effects can persist for up to 2 weeks after stopping treatment.

Diet advice
None.

Storage
Not applicable. The drug is not normally kept in the home.

Missed dose
The drug is administered in hospital under close medical supervision. If for some reason you miss your dose, contact your doctor as soon as you can.

Stopping the drug
Discuss with your doctor. Stopping the drug prematurely may lead to a worsening of the underlying condition.

Exceeding the dose
Overdosage is unlikely since treatment is carefully monitored and supervised.

SPECIAL PRECAUTIONS

Doxorubicin is prescribed only under close medical supervision, taking account of your present condition and medical history. Be sure to tell your doctor if:
- You have heart problems or have had a previous heart attack.
- You have kidney or liver problems.

 Pregnancy
Not usually prescribed. Doxorubicin may cause birth defects or premature birth. Discuss with your doctor.

 Breast-feeding
Not advised. The drug passes into the breast milk and may affect the baby adversely. Discuss with your doctor.

 Infants and children
Reduced dose necessary.

 Over 60
Increased risk of adverse effects. Reduced dose may be necessary.

 Driving and hazardous work
No known problems.

 Alcohol
No known problems.

POSSIBLE ADVERSE EFFECTS

Nausea and vomiting generally occur within an hour of injection. Many people also experience hair loss and loss of appetite. Palpitations may indicate an adverse effect of the drug on the heart. Since treatment is closely supervised in hospital, all adverse effects are monitored.

Symptom/effect	Frequency		Discuss with doctor		Stop taking drug now	Call doctor now
	Common	Rare	Only if severe	In all cases		
Nausea/vomiting/loss of appetite	●			●		
Hair loss	●			●		
Bruising	●			●		
Fever	●			●		●
Diarrhoea		●		●		
Mouth ulcers/skin irritation/ulcers		●		●		
Palpitations		●		●		●
Breathlessness		●		●		●

PROLONGED USE

Prolonged use of doxorubicin may suppress the activity of the bone marrow, leading to reduced production of all types of blood cell. It may also adversely affect the pumping capacity of the heart.

Monitoring Periodic checks on blood counts and liver function are required. Regular heart examinations are also carried out.

INTERACTIONS

General note A wide range of drugs can interact with doxorubicin. Consult your doctor or pharmacist before using any other medications.

DOXYCYCLINE

Brand names Doxylar, Efracea, Periostat, Vibramycin, Vibramycin-D
Used in the following combined preparations None

GENERAL INFORMATION

Doxycycline is a tetracycline antibiotic. It is used to treat infections of the urinary, respiratory, and gastrointestinal tracts. It is also prescribed for treatment of some oral and dental infections; sexually transmitted diseases; skin, eye, and prostate infections; acne; and malaria prevention (in some parts of the world, see p.95).

Doxycycline is less likely to cause diarrhoea than other tetracyclines, and milk and food do not significantly impair its absorption. It can therefore be taken with meals to reduce side effects such as nausea or indigestion. It is also safer than most other tetracyclines for people with impaired kidney function. Like other tetracyclines, it can stain developing teeth and may affect development of bone; it is therefore usually avoided for children under 12 years old and for pregnant women.

see p.95

QUICK REFERENCE

Drug group Tetracycline antibiotic (p.86)

Overdose danger rating Low

Dependence rating Low

Prescription needed Yes

Available as generic Yes

INFORMATION FOR USERS

Your drug prescription is tailored for you. Do not alter dosage without checking with your doctor.

How taken/used

Tablets, dispersible tablets, capsules.

Frequency and timing of doses
1–2 x daily with plenty of water, or with or after food, in a sitting or standing position, well before going to bed to avoid risk of throat irritation.

Dosage range
100–200mg daily.

Onset of effect
1–12 hours; several weeks (acne).

Duration of action
Up to 24 hours; several weeks (acne).

Diet advice
None.

Storage
Keep in original container at room temperature out of the reach of children.

Missed dose
Take as soon as you remember. If your next dose is due within 6 hours, take a single dose now and skip the next.

Stopping the drug
Take the full course. Even if you feel better, the original infection may still be present and symptoms may recur if treatment is stopped too soon.

Exceeding the dose
An occasional unintentional extra dose is unlikely to be a cause for concern. But if you notice any unusual symptoms, or if a large overdose has been taken, notify your doctor.

SPECIAL PRECAUTIONS

Be sure to tell your doctor if:
- You have a long-term liver problem.
- You have previously had an allergic reaction to a tetracycline antibiotic.
- You have porphyria.
- You have systemic lupus erythematosus.
- You have myasthenia gravis.
- You have a history of angioedema.
- You are taking other medicines.

 Pregnancy
Not used in pregnancy. May discolour the teeth of the developing baby.

 Breast-feeding
The drug passes into the breast milk and may lead to discoloration of the baby's teeth and may also have other adverse effects. Discuss with your doctor.

 Infants and children
Not recommended under 12 years. Reduced dose necessary for older children.

 Over 60
No special problems. Dispersible tablets should be used because they are less likely to cause oesophageal irritation or ulceration.

 Driving and hazardous work
Avoid such activities if doxycycline causes visual disturbances, such as blurred vision.

 Alcohol
Excessive amounts may decrease the effectiveness of doxycycline.

Surgery and general anaesthetics
Notify your doctor or dentist that you are taking doxycycline.

POSSIBLE ADVERSE EFFECTS

Adverse effects from doxycycline are rare, although nausea, vomiting, or diarrhoea may occur. Rash, itching, and photosensitivity of the skin are other possible adverse effects.

Symptom/effect	Frequency		Discuss with doctor		Stop taking drug now	Call doctor now
	Common	Rare	Only if severe	In all cases		
Nausea/vomiting/diarrhoea		●	●			
Rash/itching		●		●	●	
Photosensitivity		●		●	●	
Headache/visual disturbances		●		●	●	●

INTERACTIONS

Antacids and preparations containing iron, calcium, or magnesium may impair absorption of this drug. Do not take within 2–3 hours of doxycycline.

Barbiturates, carbamazepine, and phenytoin All of these drugs reduce the effectiveness of doxycycline. Doxycycline dosage may need to be increased.

Oral contraceptives There is a slight risk of doxycycline reducing the effectiveness of oral contraceptives. Discuss with your doctor.

Oral anticoagulant drugs Doxycycline may increase the anticoagulant action of these drugs.

Penicillin antibiotics Doxycycline interferes with the antibacterial action of these drugs.

Ciclosporin and lithium Doxycycline may increase levels of these drugs in the blood.

Methotrexate Doxycycline may increase the risk of methotrexate toxicity.

PROLONGED USE

Not usually prescribed long term, except for acne and a few other skin conditions including the blistering disorder bullous pemphigoid.

DULAGLUTIDE

Brand names Trulicity
Used in the following combined preparations None

GENERAL INFORMATION

Dulaglutide is a long-acting injectable antidiabetic drug used to treat type 2 diabetes mellitus together with diet, exercise, and weight control. The drug is usually combined with other diabetes medications.

Dulaglutide mimics the action of a natural hormone called GLP-1, which is produced by the gut and parts of the brain and is involved in regulating blood sugar levels. The drug works by increasing the secretion of insulin in response to high blood sugar levels and lowering the secretion of the hormone glucagon, which leads to a decreased output of glucose from the liver. It also slows emptying of the stomach, so smoothing out the rise in blood sugar after meals. Nausea, vomiting, diarrhoea, and abdominal discomfort are common side effects but often subside within a few weeks.

INFORMATION FOR USERS

Your drug prescription is tailored for you. Do not alter dosage without checking with your doctor.

How taken/used

Injection (subcutaneous) in stomach or thigh.

Frequency and timing of doses
Once a week.

Dosage range
0.75–1.5mg weekly.

Onset of effect
A few days to a few weeks.

Duration of action
At least 1 week.

Diet advice
An individualized diabetic diet must be followed for the drug to be fully effective.

Storage
Store unused injection pens in the refrigerator. After first use a pen may be stored at room temperature for up to 14 days, away from heat and light, and out of reach of children.

Missed dose
If 3 days or more until next dose, administer as soon as possible; if less than 3 days, skip missed dose.

Stopping the drug
Do not stop the drug without consulting your doctor. Stopping the drug may lead to worsening of the underlying condition.

OVERDOSE ACTION

Seek immediate medical advice. If you have nausea and vomiting and signs of low blood sugar (hunger, anxiety, slurred speech, tremor, cold sweats, blurred vision, headache), eat or drink something sugary. Take emergency action if seizures or unconsciousness occur.

See Drug poisoning emergency guide (p.518).

SPECIAL PRECAUTIONS

Be sure to tell your doctor if:
- You have type 1 diabetes mellitus.
- You have long-term kidney problems.
- You have stomach or bowel problems.
- You have a history of pancreatitis.
- You have a gallbladder disorder.
- You have a history or family history of medullary thyroid cancer or multiple endocrine neoplasia 2 (MEN 2).
- You are taking other medicines.

Pregnancy
Not prescribed. The drug may harm the baby.

Breast-feeding
Unknown if the drug passes into breast milk. Not prescribed. May have to switch to insulin.

Infants and children
Not usually prescribed.

Over 60
No special problems.

Driving and hazardous work
Usually no problem, but be aware of warning signs of low blood sugar and avoid such activities if you have these signs.

Alcohol
Avoid. Alcohol may upset diabetic control.

Diabetic ketoacidosis has occurred in patients who had their insulin doses reduced rapidly. This can present as excessive thirst, passing urine more often than normal, excessive tiredness, rapid breathing, nausea and vomiting, and "fruity" smelling breath.

POSSIBLE ADVERSE EFFECTS

Common adverse effects include nausea, fatigue, and reduced appetite. For severe, persistent abdominal pain, and localized or general allergic reactions, seek medical help.

Symptom/effect	Frequency		Discuss with doctor		Stop taking drug now	Call doctor now
	Common	Rare	Only if severe	In all cases		
Nausea/vomiting/diarrhoea	●			●		
Weight loss/low appetite	●			●		
Dizziness/headache/fatigue	●			●		
Persistent abdominal pain		●		●	●	●
Reaction at injection site		●	●			
Wheeze/itchy rash/ swollen face and lips		●		●	●	
Low blood sugar reading	●			●		

INTERACTIONS

General note Many drugs, especially other antidiabetic drugs, may interact with dulaglutide to affect blood sugar levels. The dose of diabetes medication such as insulin and sulfonylureas may have to be reduced. Check with your doctor or pharmacist before taking other medicines.

PROLONGED USE

Monitoring Regular monitoring of your diabetes control is necessary. You may also have periodic assessment of your eyes, heart, and kidneys, and of the lipids in your blood.

DYDROGESTERONE

Brand names None
Used in the following combined preparations Femoston 1/10 and 2/10, Femoston-conti

GENERAL INFORMATION

Dydrogesterone is a synthetic version of the natural female sex hormone progesterone that has more specific hormonal effects and greater potency than progesterone itself. The drug is no longer used alone but is still available together with an oestrogen as part of hormone replacement therapy (HRT) for use following the menopause. Dydrogesterone is added either to each HRT tablet (continuous combined HRT)

or only the tablets taken during the second half of each 28-day cycle (cyclical HRT). Only cyclical HRT produces regular shedding of the lining of the uterus, mimicking a period. However, both types prevent the risk of endometrial cancer in women on HRT who have an intact uterus. Dydrogesterone with estradiol may also be used to prevent osteoporosis in women with an intact uterus.

QUICK REFERENCE

Drug group Female sex hormone (p.105)
Overdose danger rating Low
Dependence rating Low
Prescription needed Yes
Available as generic No

INFORMATION FOR USERS

Your drug prescription is tailored for you. Do not alter dosage without checking with your doctor.

How taken/used

Tablets.

Frequency and timing of doses
Once daily.

Adult dosage range
5–10mg daily in combined preparations.

Onset of effect
Beneficial effects of this drug may not be felt for several months.

Duration of action
12–24 hours.

Diet advice
None.

Storage
Keep in original container at room temperature out of the reach of children. Protect from light.

Missed dose
Take as soon as you remember. If your next dose is due within 2 hours, take a single dose now and skip the next.

Stopping the drug
Take as soon as you remember. If more than 24 hours have elapsed, do not take the missed tablet and take the next tablet at the normal time. Missed doses may increase the risk of irregular bleeding or spotting.

Exceeding the dose
An occasional unintentional extra dose is unlikely to be a cause for concern. But if you notice any unusual symptoms, or if a large overdose has been taken, notify your doctor.

SPECIAL PRECAUTIONS

Be sure to tell your doctor if:
- You have long-term liver or kidney problems.
- You have heart or circulatory problems, especially a history of venous or pulmonary thrombosis.
- You have diabetes.
- You have high blood pressure.
- You have porphyria.
- You or a family member have had breast cancer.
- You are taking other medicines.

 Pregnancy
Not used. If you become pregnant, stop the drug immediately and contact your doctor.

 Breast-feeding
Not used.

 Infants and children
Not prescribed.

 Over 60
No special problems.

 Driving and hazardous work
Avoid such activities until you have learned how dydrogesterone affects you because the drug may rarely cause dizziness.

 Alcohol
No special problems.

POSSIBLE ADVERSE EFFECTS

Irregular periods and "breakthrough" bleeding are the most common adverse effects of this drug. These symptoms may be helped by dosage adjustment.

Symptom/effect	Frequency		Discuss with doctor		Stop taking drug now	Call doctor now
	Common	Rare	Only if severe	In all cases		
Swollen feet/ankles	●		●			
Rash	●		●			
Weight gain	●		●			
Irregular vaginal bleeding	●			●		
Nausea/vomiting		●	●			
Breast tenderness		●	●			
Headache/dizziness		●		●		

INTERACTIONS

Anticonvulsants Some of these drugs may reduce the effect of dydrogesterone, and dydrogesterone may reduce the effect of lamotrigine.

Ciclosporin Dydrogesterone increases the effects of this drug.

St. John's wort may reduce the effect of dydrogesterone.

PROLONGED USE

As part of HRT, dydrogesterone is usually only advised for short-term use after the menopause. It is not normally recommended for long-term use or for treating osteoporosis. HRT increases the risk of both venous thrombosis and breast cancer. This risk diminishes after stopping the drug, disappearing entirely after 10 years.

Monitoring Blood-pressure checks and physical examinations, including regular mammograms, may be performed.

EFAVIRENZ

Brand name Sustiva
Used in the following combined preparation Atripla

GENERAL INFORMATION

Efavirenz is a non-nucleoside reverse transcriptase inhibitor, which is a type of antiretroviral drug used to treat HIV infection (see p.116); it is active against HIV type 1 but not against type 2 (which is rare in the UK). Efavirenz is never used alone but is combined with other antiretrovirals – for example, two nucleoside analogues – to reduce viral replication. The aim of this treatment is to minimize viral damage to the immune system and to make the emergence of drug resistance less likely. Combination antiretroviral therapy (or ART) is not a cure for HIV, but if the drugs are taken regularly on a long-term basis, they can reduce the viral load and improve the outlook for the patient. However, the patient remains infectious and will suffer a relapse if treatment is stopped.

QUICK REFERENCE

Drug group Drug for HIV and immune deficiency (p.116)

Overdose danger rating Medium

Dependence rating Low

Prescription needed Yes

Available as generic Yes

INFORMATION FOR USERS

Your drug prescription is tailored for you. Do not alter dosage without checking with your doctor.

How taken/used

Tablets, capsules, oral solution.

Frequency and timing of doses
Once daily, usually at night to minimize adverse effects; best taken on an empty stomach.

Adult dosage range
Up to 600mg, according to body weight (tablets/capsules); for patients over 3 years, according to body weight (liquid).

Onset of effect
1 hour.

Duration of action
24 hours.

Diet advice
None.

Storage
Keep in the original container in a cool, dry place out of the reach of children.

Missed dose
Take as soon as you remember. If your next dose is due within 2 hours, take a single dose now and skip the next. It is very important not to miss doses on a regular basis as this can lead to the development of drug-resistant HIV.

Stopping the drug
Do not stop taking the drug without consulting your doctor. It may be necessary to withdraw all your drugs gradually, starting with efavirenz.

Exceeding the dose
An occasional unintentional extra dose is unlikely to cause problems. But if you notice any unusual symptoms, or if a large overdose has been taken, notify your doctor.

SPECIAL PRECAUTIONS

Be sure to tell your doctor if:
- You have liver or kidney problems.
- You have lactose or galactose intolerance.
- You have an infection such as hepatitis B or C.
- You are pregnant or planning a pregnancy.
- You have a mental health disorder.
- You have porphyria.
- You have epilepsy.
- You are taking other medicines.

Pregnancy
Should not be used during pregnancy except on strict medical advice. Pregnancy should be avoided; use barrier methods of contraception in addition to other methods.

Breast-feeding
Safety not established. Breast-feeding is not recommended for HIV-positive mothers as the virus may be passed to the baby.

Infants and children
Not prescribed to children under 3 years. Reduced dose necessary in older children.

Over 60
Reduced dose may be necessary to minimize adverse effects.

Driving and hazardous work
Avoid such activities until you have learned how efavirenz affects you because the drug can cause dizziness.

Alcohol
No known problems, although some people may find the effects of alcohol are more pronounced with efavirenz.

POSSIBLE ADVERSE EFFECTS

Gastrointestinal upset and rash are the most common adverse effects. Efavirenz can cause vivid dreams and changes in sleep patterns, but these tend to wear off with time.

Symptom/effect	Frequency		Discuss with doctor		Stop taking drug now	Call doctor now
	Common	Rare	Only if severe	In all cases		
Nausea/vomiting	●		●			
Diarrhoea	●		●			
Vivid dreams	●		●			
Rash	●			●		●
Mood changes		●		●		

INTERACTIONS

General note A wide range of drugs may interact with efavirenz, causing either an increase in adverse effects or a reduction in the effect of the antiretroviral drugs. Check with your doctor or pharmacist before taking any new drugs, including those from the dentist and supermarket, and herbal medicines.

PROLONGED USE

No known problems.

Monitoring Your doctor will take regular blood samples to check the drug's effects on the viral load. Blood will also be checked for changes in lipid, cholesterol, and sugar levels.

EMTRICITABINE

Brand name Emtriva
Used in the following combined preparations Atripla, Descovy, Genova, Ictastan, Odefsey, Stribild, Truvada

GENERAL INFORMATION

Emtricitabine is an antiviral drug used to treat (but not cure) HIV. It is a type of drug known as a nucleoside reverse transcriptase inhibitor, which blocks the enzyme reverse transcriptase that HIV needs in order to multiply. In treating HIV infection, emtricitabine is usually used in combination with other anti-HIV drugs to reduce production of new viruses before the immune system is irreversibly damaged. This combined therapy (antiretroviral therapy, or ART) reduces the viral load in people with HIV but does not completely rid the body of the virus. HIV may still be transmitted to other people, so it is important to continue taking precautions to avoid infecting others.

QUICK REFERENCE

Drug group Drug for HIV and immune deficiency (p.116)

Overdose danger rating Medium

Dependence rating Low

Prescription needed Yes

Available as generic No

INFORMATION FOR USERS

Your drug prescription is tailored for you. Do not alter dosage without checking with your doctor.

How taken/used

Capsules, oral solution.

Frequency and timing of doses
Once daily. Swallow capsules whole with water. If you vomit within 1 hour of a dose, take another one; if you vomit more than 1 hour after a dose, do not take another one.

Adult dosage range
People over 33kg: 200mg daily capsules, or 240ml daily liquid. (Reduced dose for children/people weighing under 33kg. Less frequent doses for those with renal problems.)

Onset of effect
May take from many weeks to a year before the drug reduces virus levels significantly.

Duration of action
Up to several days.

Diet advice
None.

Storage
Keep in original container at room temperature and out of the reach of children.

Missed dose
Take the missed dose as soon as you remember unless your next dose is due within 12 hours, in which case omit the missed dose and take the next dose as scheduled.

Stopping the drug
Do not stop the drug without consulting your doctor; your condition may worsen.

Exceeding the dose
An occasional unintentional extra dose is unlikely to cause problems. However, a large overdose may cause serious side effects; notify your doctor immediately.

SPECIAL PRECAUTIONS

Be sure to tell your doctor if:
- You have kidney or liver disease.
- You have had hepatitis B or C.
- You have diabetes.
- You have a high blood cholesterol level.
- You are or intend to become pregnant.
- You are taking other medicines, especially corticosteroids.

 Pregnancy
Safety not established. Discuss with your doctor. If you receive nucleoside reverse transcriptase inhibitors during pregnancy, your baby should be monitored during and after birth.

 Breast-feeding
It is not known if this drug passes into breast milk. However, HIV can be passed to the baby in breast milk so breast-feeding is not recommended.

 Infants and children
Not recommended under 4 months.

 Over 60
No known problems.

 Driving and hazardous work
Avoid such activities until you have learned how the drug affects you because it may cause dizziness.

 Alcohol
Avoid. Alcohol increases the risk of developing serious bone problems.

POSSIBLE ADVERSE EFFECTS

The most common side effects are headache, diarrhoea, nausea, and muscle aches. Used in combination therapy, the drug may affect blood sugar and cholesterol and cause redistribution of body fat. It may also cause darkening of the skin, rash, and blood abnormalities.

Symptom/effect	Frequency		Discuss with doctor		Stop taking drug now	Call doctor now
	Common	Rare	Only if severe	In all cases		
Dizziness/headache	●		●			
Nausea/diarrhoea	●		●			
Muscle aches	●		●			
Rash/darkening of skin	●		●			
Body fat redistribution	●		●			
Fever/sore throat	●				●	
Tiredness/lethargy		●			●	
Joint stiffness/pain		●			●	
Rapid breathing/drowsiness		●			●	●

PROLONGED USE

Emtricitabine as part of ART may cause redistribution of body fat and abnormal blood sugar and lipid levels. Rarely, it may also cause bone destruction, especially in the hip.

Monitoring Liver function tests are routine and people being treated for HIV will have additional regular checks of blood cell counts (including CD4 counts), viral load, blood sugar and cholesterol levels, and response to treatment.

INTERACTIONS

General note Various drugs that affect the kidneys may affect blood levels of emtricitabine. Discuss with your doctor before taking any other medications.

Lamivudine and zalcitabine should not be used with emtricitabine because all three drugs are chemically similar and there is therefore a risk of increased toxicity.

Orlistat may reduce absorption of emtricitabine.

ENALAPRIL

Brand name Innovace
Used in the following combined preparation Innozide

GENERAL INFORMATION

Enalapril belongs to the ACE inhibitor group of vasodilator drugs, which are used to treat hypertension (high blood pressure) and heart failure (reduced ability of the heart to pump blood). It is also given to patients following a heart attack. Enalapril may be given with a diuretic to increase its effect.

The first dose of enalapril may cause a sudden drop in blood pressure. For this reason, you should be resting at the time and be able to lie down for 2 to 3 hours afterwards.

The more common adverse effects, such as dizziness and headache, usually diminish with long-term treatment. Rashes can also occur but usually disappear when the drug is stopped. In some cases, they clear up on their own despite continued treatment.

QUICK REFERENCE

Drug group ACE inhibitor (p.56) and antihypertensive drug (p.60)

Overdose danger rating Medium

Dependence rating Low

Prescription needed Yes

Available as generic Yes

INFORMATION FOR USERS

Your drug prescription is tailored for you. Do not alter dosage without checking with your doctor.

How taken/used

Tablets.

Frequency and timing of doses
1–2 x daily.

Adult dosage range
2.5–5mg daily (starting dose), increased to 10–40mg daily (maintenance dose).

Onset of effect
30–60 minutes; full beneficial effect may take several weeks.

Duration of action
24 hours.

Diet advice
Your doctor may advise you to reduce your salt intake to help control your blood pressure.

Storage
Keep in original container below 25°C and out of the reach of children. Protect from light.

Missed dose
Take as soon as you remember. If your next dose is due within 8 hours, take a single dose now and skip the next.

Stopping the drug
Do not stop the drug without consulting your doctor; stopping the drug may lead to worsening of the underlying condition.

Exceeding the dose
An occasional unintentional extra dose is unlikely to be a cause for concern. Large overdoses may cause dizziness or fainting. Notify your doctor.

SPECIAL PRECAUTIONS

Be sure to tell your doctor if:
- You have kidney or liver problems.
- You have heart problems.
- You have had angioedema or a previous allergic reaction to ACE inhibitors.
- You are taking other medicines.
- You are or intend to become pregnant.

 Pregnancy
Not prescribed. There is evidence of harm to the developing fetus.

 Breast-feeding
May be taken during breast-feeding but there is a risk of low blood pressure in the baby, especially if preterm. Discuss with your doctor.

 Infants and children
Not recommended.

 Over 60
Reduced dose may be necessary.

 Driving and hazardous work
Avoid until you have learned how enalapril affects you because the drug can cause dizziness and fainting.

 Alcohol
Avoid. Alcohol may increase the blood-pressure-lowering and adverse effects of the drug.

Surgery and general anaesthetics
Enalapril may have to be stopped before you have a general anaesthetic. Discuss with your doctor or dentist before any operation.

PROLONGED USE

No problems expected.

Monitoring Periodic checks on potassium levels, white blood cell count, kidney function, and urine are usually performed.

POSSIBLE ADVERSE EFFECTS

Common adverse effects such as dizziness usually diminish with long-term treatment. Less common problems may also diminish with time, but dose adjustment may be necessary. Rashes may occur but usually disappear when the drug is stopped.

Symptom/effect	Frequency		Discuss with doctor		Stop taking drug now	Call doctor now
	Common	Rare	Only if severe	In all cases		
Rash	●			●		
Persistent dry cough	●			●		
Mouth ulcers/sore mouth		●		●		
Dizziness		●		●		
Sore throat/fever		●		●		
Swelling of mouth/lips		●		●	●	●
Breathing difficulty		●		●	●	●

INTERACTIONS

Potassium supplements and potassium-sparing diuretics Enalapril may enhance the effect of these drugs, leading to raised levels of potassium in the blood.

Non-steroidal anti-inflammatory drugs (NSAIDs) Some of these drugs may reduce the effectiveness of enalapril. There is also risk of kidney damage when they are taken with enalapril.

Vasodilators, diuretics, and other anti-hypertensives These may increase the blood-pressure-lowering effect of enalapril.

Lithium Enalapril increases the levels of lithium in the blood, and serious adverse effects from lithium excess may occur.

Ciclosporin Taken with enalapril, this drug may increase blood levels of potassium.

EPHEDRINE

Brand name None
Used in the following combined preparations None

GENERAL INFORMATION

Chemically related to amfetamine, ephedrine promotes the release of the neurotransmitter norepinephrine (noradrenaline). It was once widely prescribed to relax constricted muscles around the airways due to asthma, bronchitis, and emphysema, but more effective drugs have now replaced ephedrine for these uses. Its main use now is as a nasal decongestant. Ephedrine injections may be used to restore normal blood pressure after anaesthetic procedures, especially spinal and epidural anaesthesia.

Adverse effects are unusual from nasal drops used in moderation, but taken by mouth or injection the drug may stimulate the heart and central nervous system, causing palpitations and anxiety, and it is best avoided by people with high blood pressure.

Ephedrine was also widely used in dietary supplements and is present in the Chinese herbal medicine ma huang.

QUICK REFERENCE

Drug group Bronchodilator (p.48) and decongestant (p.51)

Overdose danger rating Medium

Dependence rating Low

Prescription needed No

Available as generic Yes

INFORMATION FOR USERS

Follow instructions on the label. Call your doctor if symptoms worsen.

How taken/used

Tablets, injection, nasal drops.

Frequency and timing of doses
By mouth 3 x daily.
Nasal drops 3–4 x daily.

Dosage range
Adults 45–180mg daily (by mouth); 1–2 drops into each nostril per dose (drops); 3–6mg every 3–4 minutes to a maximum of 30mg (injection).
Children Reduced dose according to age and weight.

Onset of effect
Within 15–60 minutes.

Duration of action
3–6 hours.

Diet advice
None.

Storage
Keep in original container at room temperature out of the reach of children. Protect from light.

Missed dose
Do not take the missed dose. Take your next dose as usual.

Stopping the drug
Can be safely stopped as soon as you no longer need it.

Exceeding the dose
An occasional unintentional extra dose is unlikely to cause problems. Large overdoses may cause shortness of breath, high fever, seizures, or loss of consciousness. Notify your doctor immediately.

SPECIAL PRECAUTIONS

Be sure to tell your doctor or pharmacist before taking this drug if:
- You have a long-term kidney problem.
- You have heart disease.
- You have high blood pressure.
- You have diabetes.
- You have an overactive thyroid gland.
- You have had glaucoma.
- You have urinary difficulties.
- You are taking other medicines, especially an MAOI antidepressant.

Pregnancy
Safety in pregnancy not established. Discuss with your doctor.

Breast-feeding
The drug passes into the breast milk and may affect the baby. Discuss with your doctor.

Infants and children
Not recommended under 6 years. Should only be used in children 6–12 years under medical supervision.

Over 60
Not usually prescribed.

Driving and hazardous work
Avoid such activities until you have learned how ephedrine affects you. No special problems with nasal drops.

Alcohol
No special problems.

Surgery and general anaesthetics
Ephedrine may need to be stopped before you have a general anaesthetic. Discuss with your doctor or dentist before surgery.

POSSIBLE ADVERSE EFFECTS

Adverse effects from ephedrine nasal drops are uncommon, although local irritation can occur. When taken by mouth, the drug may have adverse effects on the central nervous system (for example, insomnia and anxiety) and the cardiovascular system (palpitations). Taking the last dose before 4 pm may help to prevent insomnia.

Symptom/effect	Frequency		Discuss with doctor		Stop taking drug now	Call doctor now
	Common	Rare	Only if severe	In all cases		
Anxiety/restlessness	●		●			
Insomnia	●		●			
Cold extremities		●	●			
Dry mouth		●	●			
Tremor		●	●			
Urinary difficulties		●		●		
Palpitations/chest pain		●		●	●	●

INTERACTIONS

Monoamine oxidase inhibitors (MAOIs) Ephedrine may interact with these drugs to cause a dangerous rise in blood pressure.

Beta blockers Ephedrine may interact with these drugs to cause a dangerous rise in blood pressure.

Antihypertensive drugs Ephedrine may counteract the effects of some antihypertensive drugs.

Theophylline taken with ephedrine can lower potassium levels in children. The two drugs should not be given together.

PROLONGED USE

Prolonged use is not recommended. Excessive use in nasal drops leads to reduced decongestant effects and rebound congestion when stopped. Long-term use of ephedrine-containing herbal preparations is associated with stroke.

EPINEPHRINE (ADRENALINE)

Brand names Emerade, EpiPen, Jext
Used in the following combined preparations Several local anaesthetics (e.g. bupivacaine and xylocaine)

GENERAL INFORMATION

Epinephrine is a neurotransmitter (see p.34) that is produced in the centre (medulla) of the adrenal glands, hence its original name, adrenaline. Synthetic epinephrine has been made since 1900. The drug is given in an emergency to stimulate heart activity and raise low blood pressure. It also narrows blood vessels in the skin and intestine.

Epinephrine is injected to counteract cardiac arrest, or to relieve severe allergic reactions (anaphylaxis) to drugs, food, or insect stings. For patients who are at risk of anaphylactic shock (see p.520), it is provided as a pre-filled syringe for immediate self-injection into a muscle at the start of an attack.

Because it constricts blood vessels, epinephrine is used in preparations of local anaesthetics to slow the dispersal of the anaesthetic through the body and thereby prolong its effect.

INFORMATION FOR USERS

Your drug prescription is tailored for you. Do not alter dosage without checking with your doctor.

How taken/used

Self-administration Injection into thigh muscle.
Cardiac arrest Injection into vein.

Frequency and timing of doses
Self-administration As directed, in emergency.

Dosage range
Pre-filled syringe (e.g. EpiPen) Usually 300 mcg.
Hospital use 500mcg ampoules.

Onset of effect
Within 5 minutes.

Duration of action
Up to 4 hours.

Diet advice
None.

Storage
Keep in original container at room temperature out of the reach of children. Protect from light.

Missed dose
Not applicable. By itself, the drug is used for one-off emergencies.

Stopping the drug
Not applicable. By itself, the drug is used for one-off emergencies.

OVERDOSE ACTION

Seek immediate medical advice in all cases. Take emergency action if palpitations, breathing difficulties, or loss of consciousness occur.

See Drug poisoning emergency guide (p.518).

POSSIBLE ADVERSE EFFECTS

The principal adverse effects of this drug are related to its stimulant action on the heart and central nervous system. As epinephrine by itself is used in emergency situations, medical help should always be sought after its use.

Symptom/effect	Frequency		Discuss with doctor		Stop taking drug now	Call doctor now
	Common	Rare	Only if severe	In all cases		
Dry mouth	●			●		
Nervousness/restlessness	●			●		
Nausea/vomiting	●			●		
Cold extremities	●			●		
Palpitations	●			●		
Headache/blurred vision	●			●		

INTERACTIONS

General note Epinephrine may interact with a wide variety of drugs, including monoamine oxidase inhibitors (MAOIs); tricyclic antidepressants such as amitriptyline; some beta blockers, such as propranolol; and antidiabetic drugs. However, because epinephrine is usually used only to treat life-threatening medical emergencies, possible drug interactions are usually of secondary importance.

SPECIAL PRECAUTIONS

Be sure to tell your doctor if:
- You have a heart problem.
- You have an overactive thyroid gland.
- You have high blood pressure.
- You are taking other medications, especially a beta blocker.

Pregnancy
Discuss with your doctor. Although the drug may cause defects in the fetus and prolong labour, epinephrine by itself is used only for medical emergencies and its use may be life-saving.

Breast-feeding
Adverse effects on the baby are unlikely. Discuss with your doctor.

Infants and children
Reduced dose necessary.

Over 60
Increased likelihood of adverse effects. Reduced dose may therefore be necessary.

Driving and hazardous work
Not applicable. By itself, the drug is used for one-off emergencies.

Alcohol
No known problems.

Surgery and general anaesthetics
Epinephrine may interact with some general anaesthetics. If you have used or been treated with epinephrine within the past 24 hours, discuss this with your doctor or dentist before surgery.

PROLONGED USE

Epinephrine is not normally used long term.

ERGOTAMINE

Brand names None
Used in the following combined preparations Cafergot, Migril

GENERAL INFORMATION

Ergotamine is used to treat migraine attacks, but its use has largely been superseded by newer agents with fewer adverse effects. It may also be used in the prevention and treatment of cluster headaches. For migraine, its use should be restricted to occasions when other treatments are ineffective, and the drug should be taken only at the first sign of migraine (the "aura"); later use may be ineffective and cause stomach upset. Ergotamine causes temporary narrowing of blood vessels, and therefore it should not be used by people who have poor circulation. If taken too frequently, the drug can dangerously reduce circulation to the hands and feet (ergotism); it should never be taken regularly. Frequent migraine attacks may indicate the need for a drug to prevent migraine.

QUICK REFERENCE

Drug group Drug for migraine (p.45)
Overdose danger rating Medium
Dependence rating Medium
Prescription needed Yes
Available as generic Yes

INFORMATION FOR USERS

Your drug prescription is tailored for you. Do not alter dosage without checking with your doctor.

How taken/used

Tablets, suppositories.

Frequency and timing of doses
Once at the onset, repeated if needed after 30 minutes (tablets) up to the maximum dose (see below).

Adult dosage range
Varies according to product. Generally, 1–2mg per dose. Take no more than 4mg in 24 hours or 8mg in 1 week. Treatment should not be repeated within 4 days or more than twice a month.

Onset of effect
15–30 minutes.

Duration of action
Up to 24 hours.

Diet advice
Changes in diet are unlikely to affect the action of this drug, but certain foods may provoke migraine attacks in some people.

Storage
Keep in original container at room temperature out of the reach of children. Protect from light.

Missed dose
Regular doses of this drug are not necessary and may be dangerous. Take only when you have symptoms of migraine.

Stopping the drug
Can be safely stopped as soon as you no longer need it.

Exceeding the dose
An occasional unintentional extra dose is unlikely to cause problems. A large overdose may cause vomiting, thirst, diarrhoea, dizziness, seizures, or coma. Notify your doctor immediately.

SPECIAL PRECAUTIONS

Be sure to tell your doctor if:
- You have long-term liver or kidney problems.
- You have heart problems.
- You have poor circulation.
- You have high blood pressure.
- You have had a recent stroke.
- You have an overactive thyroid gland.
- You have anaemia.
- You are taking other medicines.

 Pregnancy
Not prescribed. Ergotamine can cause contractions of the uterus

 Breast-feeding
Not recommended. The drug passes into the milk and may have adverse effects on the baby. It may also reduce your milk supply.

 Infants and children
Not usually prescribed.

 Over 60
Not recommended. May aggravate existing heart or circulatory problems.

 Driving and hazardous work
Avoid such activities until you have learned how ergotamine affects you because the drug can cause dizziness.

 Alcohol
No special problems, but some spirits may provoke migraine in some people.

Surgery and general anaesthetics
Notify your doctor if you have used ergotamine within 48 hours prior to surgery.

PROLONGED USE

Reduced circulation to the hands and feet may result if doses near to the maximum are taken for too long. The recommended dosage and length of treatment should not be exceeded. Rebound headache may occur if the drug is taken too frequently. Cardiovascular complications, such as heart rhythm problems or problems with the heart valves or coronary blood vessels, may also develop with prolonged use.

POSSIBLE ADVERSE EFFECTS

Digestive disturbances and nausea (for which an anti-emetic may be given) are common with ergotamine treatment. Rare but serious adverse effects may result from arterial spasm.

Symptom/effect	Frequency		Discuss with doctor		Stop taking drug now	Call doctor now
	Common	Rare	Only if severe	In all cases		
Nausea/vomiting	●		●			
Abdominal pain	●		●			
Muscle cramps	●		●			
Diarrhoea		●	●			
Dizziness		●		●		
Muscle pain/stiffness		●		●		
Chest pain		●		●	●	●
Leg/groin pain		●		●	●	●
Cold/numb fingers/toes		●		●	●	●

INTERACTIONS

Beta blockers These drugs may increase circulatory problems with ergotamine.

Sumatriptan and related drugs There is an increased risk of adverse effects on the blood circulation if ergotamine is used with these drugs.

Erythromycin and related antibiotics and antivirals taken with ergotamine increase the likelihood of adverse effects.

Oral contraceptives There is an increased risk of blood clotting in women taking these drugs with ergotamine.

ERYTHROMYCIN

Brand names Erythrocin, Erythrolar, Erythroped
Used in the following combined preparations Aknemycin Plus, Isotrexin, Zineryt

GENERAL INFORMATION

One of the safest and most widely used antibiotics, erythromycin is effective against many bacteria. It is commonly used as an alternative in people allergic to penicillin and related antibiotics.

Erythromycin is used to treat throat, middle ear, and chest infections (including some rare types of pneumonia, such as Legionnaires' disease). It is also used for sexually transmitted diseases such as chlamydial infections, and in some forms of gastroenteritis.

Erythromycin may also be included as part of the treatment for diphtheria and is sometimes given to treat, and reduce the likelihood of infecting others with, pertussis (whooping cough).

When taken by mouth, erythromycin may sometimes cause nausea and vomiting. Other possible adverse effects include rash as well as a rare risk of liver disorders. Oral administration or topical application of the drug is sometimes helpful in treating acne.

INFORMATION FOR USERS

Your drug prescription is tailored for you. Do not alter dosage without consulting your doctor.

How taken/used

Tablets, capsules, GR capsules, liquid, injection, topical solution.

Frequency and timing of doses
Every 6–12 hours before or with meals.

Dosage range
1–4g daily.

Onset of effect
1–4 hours.

Duration of action
6–12 hours.

Diet advice
None.

Storage
Keep in original container at room temperature out of the reach of children.

Missed dose
Take as soon as you remember. If your next dose is due within 2 hours, take a single dose now and skip the next.

Stopping the drug
Take the full course. Even if you feel better, the original infection may still be present and symptoms may recur if treatment is stopped too soon.

Exceeding the dose
An occasional unintentional extra dose is unlikely to be a cause for concern. But if you notice any unusual symptoms, or if a large overdose has been taken, notify your doctor.

POSSIBLE ADVERSE EFFECTS

Nausea and vomiting are common and most likely with large doses by mouth. Fever, rash, and jaundice may be signs of a liver disorder and should be reported to your doctor.

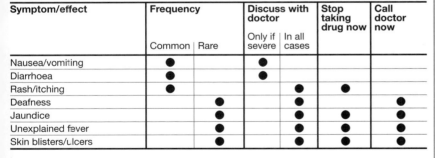

Symptom/effect	Frequency		Discuss with doctor		Stop taking drug now	Call doctor now
	Common	Rare	Only if severe	In all cases		
Nausea/vomiting	●		●			
Diarrhoea	●		●			
Rash/itching	●			●	●	
Deafness		●		●		●
Jaundice		●		●	●	●
Unexplained fever		●		●	●	●
Skin blisters/ulcers		●		●	●	●

SPECIAL PRECAUTIONS

Be sure to tell your doctor if:
- You have a long-term liver problem.
- You have had a previous allergic reaction to erythromycin.
- You have porphyria.
- You have myasthenia gravis.
- You are taking other medicines.

 Pregnancy
No evidence of risk to the developing fetus. Discuss with your doctor.

 Breast-feeding
The drug passes into the breast milk. It should be avoided in newborns under 2 weeks old, but at normal doses adverse effects on the baby are unlikely. Discuss with your doctor.

 Infants and children
Reduced dose necessary.

 Over 60
No special problems.

 Driving and hazardous work
No known problems.

 Alcohol
No known problems.

PROLONGED USE

Oral courses of longer than 14 days may increase the risk of liver damage.

INTERACTIONS

General note Erythromycin interacts with a number of other drugs, particularly:

Mizolastine Erythromycin increases the risk of adverse effects on the heart with this drug.

Warfarin Erythromycin increases the risk of bleeding with warfarin.

Carbamazepine, digoxin, and some immunosuppressants Erythromycin may increase blood levels of these drugs.

Theophylline/aminophylline Erythromycin increases the risk of adverse effects with these drugs.

Simvastatin and other "statins" Erythromycin should not be taken with simvastatin; increased risk of muscle aches and pains with other statins.

Ergotamine Erythromycin increases the risk of side effects with this drug.

ERYTHROPOIETIN

Brand names Aranesp, Binocrit, Eprex, Mircera, NeoRecormon, Retacrit
Used in the following combined preparations None

GENERAL INFORMATION

Erythropoietin is a naturally occurring hormone that is produced by the kidneys and stimulates the body to produce red blood cells. In medicine, artificially produced erythropoietin is used to treat the anaemia associated with chronic kidney disease, and with certain cancer treatments and certain dysfunctions of the bone marrow. Erythropoietin is also used to boost the level of red blood cells before surgery. In addition, it may be used as an alternative to blood transfusions in major orthopaedic (bone) surgery.

Erythropoietin has been used by athletes to enhance their performance. However, this is not a recognized use, and the drug is banned by sport governing bodies.

Erythropoietin may worsen hypertension (high blood pressure), and blood pressure should therefore be monitored during treatment with the drug.

INFORMATION FOR USERS

Your drug prescription is tailored for you. Do not alter dosage without checking with your doctor.

How taken/used

Injection.

Frequency and timing of doses
1–3 x weekly, depending on the product and condition being treated.

Dosage range
Dosage is calculated on an individual basis according to body weight. The dosage also varies depending on the product and condition being treated.

Onset of effect
Active inside the body within 4 hours, but effects may not be noted for 2–3 months.

Duration of action
Some effects may persist for several days.

Diet advice
None. However, if you have kidney failure, you may have to follow a special diet.

Storage
Store at 2–8°C, out of the reach of children. Do not freeze or shake. Protect from light.

Missed dose
Do not make up any missed doses.

Stopping the drug
Discuss with your doctor.

Exceeding the dose
A single excessive dose is unlikely to be a cause for concern. Too high a dose over a long period can increase the likelihood of adverse effects.

SPECIAL PRECAUTIONS

Be sure to tell your doctor if:
- You have high blood pressure.
- You have a long-term liver problem.
- You have previously suffered allergic reactions to any drugs.
- You have peripheral vascular disease.
- You have had epileptic seizures.
- You are taking other medicines.

Pregnancy
Not usually prescribed. Safety in pregnancy not established. Discuss with your doctor.

Breast-feeding
Safety not established. Discuss with your doctor.

Infants and children
Reduced dose necessary.

Over 60
No known problems.

Driving and hazardous work
Not applicable.

Alcohol
Follow your doctor's advice regarding alcohol.

POSSIBLE ADVERSE EFFECTS

The most common effects are increased blood pressure and problems at the site of the injection; all unusual symptoms should be discussed with your doctor immediately.

Symptom/effect	Frequency		Discuss with doctor		Stop taking drug now	Call doctor now
	Common	Rare	Only if severe	In all cases		
Increased blood pressure	●			●		
Problems at injection site	●			●		
Chest pain		●		●		
Swelling in one leg		●		●		
Flu symptoms/bone pain		●		●		
Epileptic seizures		●		●		●
Skin rash		●		●		
Headache (stabbing pain)		●		●		●

INTERACTIONS

Ciclosporin Erythropoietin may affect the blood level of ciclosporin, and more frequent monitoring of ciclosporin blood levels should therefore be carried out when erythropoietin treatment starts.

PROLONGED USE

If the level of anaemia is overcorrected, there is an increased risk of thrombosis, which is potentially fatal, hence the need for careful monitoring. Prolonged use of erythropoietin may also reduce survival in some patients with cancer.

Monitoring Regular blood tests to monitor blood composition and blood pressure monitoring are required.

ESTRADIOL

Brand names Climaval, Elleste, Estraderm, FemSeven, Oestrogel, Progynova, Zumenon, and others
Used in the following combined preparations Angeliq, Climesse, Trisequens, and others

GENERAL INFORMATION

Estradiol is a natural oestrogen (female sex hormone). It is used mainly as hormone replacement therapy (HRT) for menopausal and postmenopausal symptoms. The drug is often given with a progestogen, either separately or as a combined preparation. Estradiol alone is associated with an increased risk of cancer of the uterus, but using it with a progestogen reduces the risk; it is used alone only in women who have had a hysterectomy. HRT is usually only advised for short-term use around the menopause (see p.105) or in women with premature failure of the ovaries. Estradiol may help prevent osteoporosis in women at high risk of fractures who are intolerant to other medication.

(see p.105)

QUICK REFERENCE

Drug group Female sex hormone (p.105)

Overdose danger rating Low

Dependence rating Low

Prescription needed Yes

Available as generic Yes

(p.105)

INFORMATION FOR USERS

Your drug prescription is tailored for you. Do not alter dosage without checking with your doctor.

How taken/used

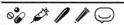

Tablets, implants, pessaries, vaginal rings, skin gel, patches.

Frequency and timing of doses
Once daily (tablets, gel); every 1–7 days (skin patches); every 4–8 months (implants); every 1–7 days (pessaries); every 3 months (vaginal ring).

Adult dosage range
1–2mg daily (tablets); as per instructions (skin gel); 25–100mcg daily (skin patches); 25–100mg per dose (implants); 25mcg per dose (pessaries); 7.5mcg daily (vaginal ring).

Onset of effect
10–20 days.

Duration of action
Up to 24 hours; some effects may be longer lasting.

Diet advice
None.

Storage
Keep in original container at room temperature out of the reach of children.

Missed dose
Take as soon as you remember. If your next daily treatment is due within 4 hours, take a single dose now and skip the next.

Stopping the drug
Do not stop the drug without consulting your doctor; symptoms may recur.

Exceeding the dose
An occasional unintentional extra dose is unlikely to be a cause for concern. But if you notice any unusual symptoms, or if a large overdose has been taken, notify your doctor.

POSSIBLE ADVERSE EFFECTS

The most common adverse effects are similar to symptoms of early pregnancy, and generally diminish with time. Sudden sharp pain in the chest, groin, or legs may indicate a blood clot.

Symptom/effect	Frequency		Discuss with doctor		Stop taking drug now	Call doctor now
	Common	Rare	Only if severe	In all cases		
Nausea/vomiting/abdominal pain	●		●			
Weight gain/fluctuation	●		●			
Fluid retention/swollen legs	●		●			
Breast swelling/tenderness	●			●		
Headache		●				
Depression/altered mood		●		●		
Pain in chest/groin/legs		●		●	●	●

INTERACTIONS

Tobacco smoking increases the risk of heart and circulatory damage with estradiol.

Anticonvulsants The effects of estradiol are reduced by topiramate, carbamazepine, phenytoin, and phenobarbital; estradiol reduces the effects of lamotrigine.

Anticoagulant drugs The effects of these drugs are reduced by estradiol.

St John's wort and rifampicin may reduce the effects of estradiol.

Lenalidomide and tranexamic acid may increase the risk of blood clots with estradiol.

Thyroxine If taken with estradiol, the dose may need to be adjusted.

SPECIAL PRECAUTIONS

Be sure to tell your doctor if:
- You have a long-term liver problem, gallstones, or raised blood triglycerides.
- You have hypertension, or heart or circulation problems.
- You have a personal or family history of blood clots or stroke.
- You have diabetes, porphyria, or lupus erythematosus.
- You have breast cancer or abnormal vaginal bleeding.
- You are a smoker.
- You have migraine or epilepsy.
- You are taking other medicines.

 Pregnancy
Not prescribed.

 Breast-feeding
Not prescribed. The drug passes into breast milk. Discuss with your doctor.

 Infants and children
Not usually prescribed.

 Over 60
No special problems.

 Driving and hazardous work
No problems expected.

 Alcohol
No known problems.

Surgery and general anaesthetics
You may need to stop estradiol before having major surgery. Discuss with your doctor.

PROLONGED USE

As part of HRT, estradiol is usually only advised for short-term use around the menopause and is not normally recommended for long-term use or for treatment of osteoporosis. Long-term use increases the risk of breast, uterine, and ovarian cancer, venous thrombosis, heart attack, and stroke.

Monitoring Blood pressure checks and physical examinations, including regular mammograms, may be performed.

ETANERCEPT

Brand names Benepali, Enbrel, Erelzi
Used in the following combined preparations None

GENERAL INFORMATION

Etanercept is a synthetic protein. One part acts like an antibody (p.92) and the other part blocks a molecule called tumour necrosis factor (TNF); in this way it alters the functioning of the immune system. As a result, etanercept reduces inflammation and improves the course of diseases such as psoriasis and rheumatological conditions including rheumatoid arthritis and juvenile idiopathic arthritis. It is given by injection once or twice weekly. The injections are often given in hospital initially but can be self-administered after you have been trained how to use them yourself.

Like many drugs that alter the immune system, etanercept increases the risk of infections, which vary from common colds and flu to more unusual ones like tuberculosis. In addition, there may be a slightly higher risk of immune system cancers and skin cancer, but these risks have to be balanced against the benefits from the treatments.

QUICK REFERENCE

Drug group Drug for psoriasis (p.138) and disease-modifying antirheumatic drug (p.75)

Overdose danger rating Low

Dependence rating Low

Prescription needed Yes

Available as generic No

INFORMATION FOR USERS

This drug is usually given under medical supervision. If you need to administer the drug yourself at home, you will be taught how to do so.

How taken/used

Subcutaneous injection.

Frequency and timing of doses
1–2 x weekly.

Adult dosage range
25–50mg weekly for up to 24 weeks.

Onset of effect
12–24 hours. Full beneficial effect may take several weeks.

Duration of action
2–8 weeks.

Diet advice
None.

Storage
Store in a refrigerator (2–8°C). Do not freeze.
Keep the pre-filled pens in the outer carton to protect from light. If you need to keep the drug at home, you will be instructed about its storage.

Missed dose
If you are administering the drug at home and forget a dose, you should inject it as soon as you remember, unless the next scheduled dose is the next day, in which case you should skip the missed dose. Then continue to inject the drug on the usual day(s). Do not take a double dose (two doses on the same day) to make up for a missed dose. If you are receiving the drug in hospital and miss your dose, contact your doctor as soon as possible.

Stopping the drug
Discuss with your doctor. Stopping the drug prematurely may lead to worsening of the underlying condition.

Exceeding the dose
Overdosage is unlikely since treatment is closely monitored and supervised. If you think you have received an overdose, tell your doctor as soon as possible.

SPECIAL PRECAUTIONS

Be sure to tell your doctor if:
- You have had or been exposed to chickenpox, shingles, hepatitis B or C, or tuberculosis.
- You have signs of infection (e.g. fever, shivering).
- You have liver or kidney problems.
- You have recently had, or are scheduled to have, a vaccination.
- You have a central nervous system disorder, such as multiple sclerosis.
- You have heart problems.
- You have diabetes.
- You are taking other medicines.

 Pregnancy
Not recommended. Women of childbearing age should avoid becoming pregnant. Discuss with your doctor.

 Breast-feeding
Not recommended. Discuss with your doctor.

 Infants and children
Reduced dose necessary.

 Over 60
No special problems.

 Driving and hazardous work
Do not undertake such activities until you have learned how etanercept affects you.

 Alcohol
No special problems.

POSSIBLE ADVERSE EFFECTS

The main side effects at the beginning of treatment are injection site reactions, such as bruising, redness, and itching. Other side effects include infections, nausea, abdominal pain, fever and headache.

Symptom/effect	Frequency		Discuss with doctor		Stop taking drug now	Call doctor now
	Common	Rare	Only if severe	In all cases		
Injection site reaction	●		●			
Fever/headache		●		●		
Chest tightness/wheezing		●		●	●	●
Sore throat		●		●	●	●
Itch/rash	●			●	●	●
Easy bruising/spontaneous bleeding		●		●	●	●

INTERACTIONS

Anakinra and abatacept should not be used together with etanercept because there is an increased risk of side effects.

Vaccines The effectiveness of some vaccines may be reduced by etanercept, and live vaccines must not be given during a course of treatment with etanercept.

PROLONGED USE

There is an increased risk of infections and of some cancers, particularly skin cancers, following etanercept treatment.

Monitoring Periodic blood tests will be carried out to monitor your response to treatment. Body temperature, heart rate, and blood pressure may be monitored when you first receive the drug.

ETHAMBUTOL

Brand names Myambutol
Used in the following combined preparations Rimstar, Voractiv

GENERAL INFORMATION

Ethambutol is an antibiotic used in the treatment of tuberculosis. It is combined with other antituberculous drugs to enhance its effect and reduce the risk of the infection becoming drug resistant. Ethambutol is not used in all cases of tuberculosis. It is more likely to be used in people with a history of tuberculosis; those with a low immune status; and in those in whom the infection may be caused by a resistant organism.

Although the drug has few common adverse effects, it may occasionally cause optic neuritis, a type of eye damage leading to blurring and fading of vision. As a result, ethambutol is not usually prescribed for children under six years of age or for other patients who are unable to communicate their symptoms adequately. Before starting treatment, a full ophthalmic examination is recommended.

QUICK REFERENCE

Drug group Antituberculous drug (p.90)

Overdose danger rating Medium

Dependence rating Low

Prescription needed Yes

Available as generic Yes

INFORMATION FOR USERS

Your drug prescription is tailored for you. Do not alter dosage without checking with your doctor.

How taken/used

Tablets.

Frequency and timing of doses
Once daily.

Adult dosage range
According to body weight.

Onset of effect
It may take several days for symptoms to improve.

Duration of action
Up to 24 hours.

Diet advice
None.

Storage
Keep in original container at room temperature out of the reach of children.

Missed dose
Take as soon as you remember. If your next dose is due within 6 hours, take a single dose now and skip the next.

Stopping the drug
Take the full course. Even if you feel better the original infection may still be present and may recur if treatment is stopped too soon.

Exceeding the dose
An occasional unintentional extra dose is unlikely to cause problems. Large overdoses may cause headache and abdominal pain. Notify your doctor.

POSSIBLE ADVERSE EFFECTS

Side effects are uncommon with this drug but are more likely after prolonged treatment at high doses. Blurred vision or eye pain require prompt medical attention.

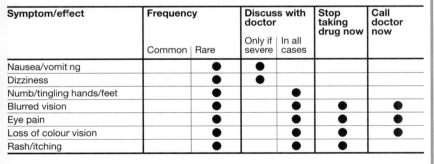

Symptom/effect	Frequency		Discuss with doctor		Stop taking drug now	Call doctor now
	Common	Rare	Only if severe	In all cases		
Nausea/vomiting		●	●			
Dizziness		●	●			
Numb/tingling hands/feet		●		●		
Blurred vision		●		●	●	●
Eye pain		●		●	●	●
Loss of colour vision		●		●	●	●
Rash/itching		●		●	●	

INTERACTIONS

Antacids Those containing aluminium salts may decrease levels of ethambutol and should be taken at least 2 hours before ethambutol or 4 hours after.

SPECIAL PRECAUTIONS

Be sure to tell your doctor if:
- You have a kidney problem.
- You have cataracts or other eye problems.
- You have gout.
- You have had a previous allergic reaction to this drug.
- You are taking other medicines.

 Pregnancy
No evidence of risk. Discuss with your doctor.

 Breast-feeding
The drug passes into the breast milk, but at normal doses adverse effects on the baby are unlikely. Discuss with your doctor.

 Infants and children
Not generally prescribed under 6 years unless the child can reliably report any vision changes.

 Over 60
Increased likelihood of adverse effects. Reduced dose may therefore be necessary.

 Driving and hazardous work
Avoid such activities until you have learned how ethambutol affects you because the drug may cause dizziness.

 Alcohol
No known problems.

PROLONGED USE

Prolonged use may increase the risk of eye damage.

Monitoring Periodic eye tests are usually necessary.

ETHINYLESTRADIOL

Used in the following combined preparations Co-cyprindiol, combined oral contraceptives (e.g. Akizza, Brevinor, Dianette, Elevin, Femodene, Katya, Loestrin, Marvelon, Mercilon, Microgynon 30, Norimin, Ovranette, Rigevidon, Yacella, Yasmin)

GENERAL INFORMATION

Ethinylestradiol is a synthetic oestrogen similar to estradiol, a natural female sex hormone. It is widely used in oral contraceptives in combination with a synthetic progestogen. These can also be used to treat an irregular menstrual cycle and for conditions in women due to high levels of androgen (male sex hormones), such as polycystic ovary syndrome and hirsutism; the drugs may also be used as HRT for the short-term relief of menopausal symptoms. Ethinylestradiol may be used to treat hypogonadism (late or absent sexual development) in women. More rarely, it may be given for osteoporosis, prostate cancer and, in combination with cyproterone, acne in women.

Oral contraceptives containing ethinylestradiol carry an increased risk of venous thrombosis. This risk is greater in overweight women and smokers.

INFORMATION FOR USERS

Your drug prescription is tailored for you. Do not alter dosage without checking with your doctor.

How taken/used

Tablets.

Frequency and timing of doses
Once daily. Often at certain times of the menstrual cycle.

Adult dosage range
Menopausal symptoms 10–20mcg daily.
Hormone deficiency 10–50mcg daily.
Combined contraceptive pills 20–40mcg daily, depending on preparation.
Acne 35mcg daily.
Prostate cancer 0.15–1.5mg daily.

Onset of effect
10–20 days. Contraceptive protection is effective after 7 days in most cases.

Duration of action
1–2 days.

Diet advice
None.

Storage
Keep in original container at room temperature out of the reach of children.

Missed dose
Take as soon as you remember. If your next dose is due within 4 hours, take a single dose now and skip the next. If you are taking the drug for contraceptive purposes, see What to do if you miss a pill (p.123).

Stopping the drug
Do not stop the drug without consulting your doctor. Contraceptive protection is lost unless an alternative is used.

Exceeding the dose
An occasional unintentional extra dose is unlikely to be a cause for concern. But if you notice any unusual symptoms, or if a large overdose has been taken, notify your doctor.

SPECIAL PRECAUTIONS

Be sure to tell your doctor if:
- You have heart failure, high blood pressure, or high blood triglyceride (lipid) levels.
- You have had venous thrombosis or a stroke.
- You have gallstones or a long-term liver or kidney problem.
- You have had breast or endometrial cancer.
- You have diabetes, porphyria, sickle cell anaemia, or lupus erythematosus.
- You are a smoker.
- You have migraines or epilepsy.
- You are taking other medicines.

Pregnancy
Not prescribed. High doses may adversely affect the baby. Discuss with your doctor.

Breast-feeding
The drug passes into the breast milk; it may also inhibit milk flow. Discuss with your doctor.

Infants and children
Not usually prescribed.

Over 60
No special problems.

Driving and hazardous work
No known problems.

Alcohol
No known problems.

Surgery and general anaesthetics
The drug may need to be stopped before major surgery. Discuss with your doctor.

POSSIBLE ADVERSE EFFECTS

The common adverse effects generally diminish with time. Sudden, sharp pain in the chest, groin, or legs may indicate an abnormal blood clot and requires urgent attention.

Symptom/effect	Frequency Common	Frequency Rare	Discuss with doctor Only if severe	Discuss with doctor In all cases	Stop taking drug now	Call doctor now
Nausea/vomiting	●		●			
Breast swelling/tenderness	●		●			
Weight gain/fluid retention	●		●			
Bleeding between periods	●		●			
Headache		●	●			
Depression		●		●		
Pain in chest/groin/legs		●		●	●	●
Sudden breathlessness		●		●	●	●
Itching/jaundice		●		●	●	●

INTERACTIONS

Tobacco smoking This increases the risk of serious adverse effects on the heart and circulation with ethinylestradiol.

Rifampicin and anticonvulsants These significantly reduce the effectiveness of oral contraceptives containing ethinylestradiol.

Antihypertensive drugs, anticoagulants, and diuretics Ethinylestradiol may reduce the effectiveness of these drugs.

Antibiotics and St John's wort may reduce the effectiveness of oral contraceptives containing ethinylestradiol.

PROLONGED USE

As part of HRT, ethinylestradiol is usually only advised for short-term use around the menopause and is not normally recommended for long-term use or for treatment of osteoporosis. Long-term use increases the risk of breast cancer, venous thrombosis, heart attack, and stroke.

Monitoring Physical examinations and blood pressure checks may be performed.

EVOLOCUMAB

Brand names Repatha, Repatha SureClick
Used in the following combined preparations None

GENERAL INFORMATION

Evolocumab (and the related drug alirocumab) is a monoclonal antibody. It belongs to a new drug class called PCSK9 inhibitors and is used to lower blood cholesterol in patients who have not responded adequately to other therapies (e.g. statins) or patients who have a genetic predisposition to high cholesterol (e.g. homozygous familial hypercholesterolaemia). It works by reducing blood levels of a protein called PCSK9, which leads to increased uptake of bad cholesterol (LDL-cholesterol) from the blood into the liver. PCSK9 inhibition is highly effective at lowering LDL-cholesterol and is generally better tolerated than statins.

The drug is given as an injection under the skin. Injection site reactions and flu-like symptoms are the most common side effects of evolocumab or alirocumab.

QUICK REFERENCE

Drug group Lipid-lowering drug (p.61)

Overdose danger rating Low

Dependence rating Low

Prescription needed Yes

Available as generic No

INFORMATION FOR USERS

Your drug prescription is tailored for you. Do not alter dosage without checking with your doctor.

How taken/used

Injection under the skin; recommended sites include the thigh, abdomen, or upper arm. Injections should not be given into areas where the skin is red, bruised, tender, or hard.

Frequency and timing of doses
Every 2–4 weeks.

Adult dosage range
140–420mg every 2 weeks.

Onset of effect
It may take weeks for blood cholesterol to be reduced. Response to treatment should be reviewed at 12 weeks.

Duration of action
Up to 4 weeks.

Diet advice
Your doctor will recommend a low-fat diet.

Storage
Store in a refrigerator (2–8°C).

Missed dose
Take as soon as you remember. Delaying by a few days is expected to have negligible effect.

Stopping the drug
Do not stop the drug without consulting your doctor; the underlying condition may worsen.

Exceeding the dose
An unintentional extra dose is unlikely to be a cause for concern. But if you notice any unusual symptoms, notify your doctor.

SPECIAL PRECAUTIONS

Be sure to tell your doctor if:
• You have long-term liver or kidney problems.

 Pregnancy
Safety in pregnancy not established. Discuss with your doctor.

 Breast-feeding
Safety not established. Discuss with your doctor.

 Infants and children
The safety and effectiveness have not been established.

 Over 60
No special problems.

 Driving and hazardous work
No special problems.

 Alcohol
No known problems.

POSSIBLE ADVERSE EFFECTS

Mild side effects are common and include nasopharyngitis, upper respiratory tract infection, back pain, joint aches, and skin reactions. Serious side effects are rare.

Symptom/effect	Frequency		Discuss with doctor		Stop taking drug now	Call doctor now
	Common	Rare	Only if severe	In all cases		
Runny/stuffy nose	●		●			
Back pain	●		●			
Joint aches	●		●			
Nausea	●		●			
Injection site reactions	●			●		
Rash	●			●		
Increased infections	●			●		

INTERACTIONS

There are no known interactions.

PROLONGED USE

Prolonged use can be associated with injection site reactions including bruising, bleeding, pain, and swelling. Rotation of the injection site, using different areas of skin, reduces this risk.

EXENATIDE

Brand names Bydureon, Byetta
Used in the following combined preparations None

GENERAL INFORMATION

Exenatide is an injected antidiabetic drug used to treat type 2 diabetes together with other antidiabetic drugs, as well as diet, exercise, and weight control. It is a synthetic protein that mimics the action of a natural hormone called GLP-1, which is involved in regulating blood sugar levels. The drug works by increasing secretion of insulin in response to high blood sugar levels and lowering the secretion of the hormone glucagon, which leads to a decreased output of glucose from the liver. It also slows emptying of the stomach, so smoothing out the rise in blood sugar after meals.

INFORMATION FOR USERS

Your drug prescription is tailored for you. Do not alter dosage without checking with your doctor.

How taken/used

Injection under the skin (see p.101).

Frequency and timing of doses
2 x daily, doses at least 6 hours apart. Take within 1 hour before a meal (do not take after a meal). Bydureon is injected once weekly, same day each week, at any time of the day.

Adult dosage range
10–20mcg daily. Bydureon: 2mg per week.

Onset of effect
Within 1 hour.

Duration of action
8–12 hours.

Diet advice
An individualized diabetic diet must be maintained for the drug to be fully effective.

Storage
Store unused injection pens in the refrigerator, protected from light. After first use, a pen may be stored at room temperature, away from heat and light, and out of reach of children.

Missed dose
Take as soon as you remember, but only if you have not yet had a meal. If you have already eaten, wait until your next scheduled dose.

Stopping the drug
Do not stop the drug without consulting your doctor. Stopping the drug may lead to worsening of the underlying condition.

OVERDOSE ACTION

Seek immediate medical help. If you have severe nausea and vomiting or warning signs of low blood sugar (e.g. faintness, dizziness, headache, confusion, sweating, or tremor), eat or drink something sugary. Take emergency action if seizures or unconsciousness occur.

See Drug poisoning emergency guide (p.518).

POSSIBLE ADVERSE EFFECTS

Gastrointestinal side effects are common but generally lessen with use. Exenatide may also cause low blood sugar (see above). Very rarely it may cause inflammation of the pancreas.

Symptom/effect	Frequency		Discuss with doctor		Stop taking drug now	Call doctor now
	Common	Rare	Only if severe	In all cases		
Nausea/vomiting/diarrhoea	●		●			
Weight loss/decreased appetite	●		●			
Dizziness/headache	●		●			
Sweating	●		●			
Severe abdominal pain		●		●	●	●
Wheezing/itchy rash		●		●	●	●
Reactions at injection site		●		●	●	●
Swelling of face/lips		●		●	●	●
Easy bleeding or bruising		●		●	●	●

INTERACTIONS

General note Many drugs, especially other antidiabetics, may interact with exenatide to affect blood sugar levels. Exenatide can affect the absorption of some drugs, so the timing of doses may need to be changed. Check with your doctor or pharmacist.

Anticoagulants (e.g. warfarin) Exenatide may increase their anticoagulant effect.

Oral contraceptives and antibiotics These should be taken at least 1 hour before exenatide to ensure adequate absorption.

SPECIAL PRECAUTIONS

Be sure to tell your doctor if:
• You have long-term kidney problems.
• You have stomach or bowel problems.
• You have a history of pancreatitis.
• You are taking other medicines.

 Pregnancy
Safety not established. Switching to insulin is safe. Discuss with your doctor.

 Breast-feeding
Safety not established. Switching to insulin is safe. Discuss with your doctor.

 Infants and children
Not prescribed.

 Over 60
No special problems.

 Driving and hazardous work
Usually no problem, but be aware of warning signs of low blood sugar and avoid such activities if you have these signs.

 Alcohol
Avoid. Alcohol may upset diabetic control.

Surgery and general anaesthetics
Notify your doctor or dentist that you have diabetes. Surgery may affect diabetic control and your diabetes treatment may need to be adjusted or, in some cases, insulin may need to be substituted.

PROLONGED USE

No problems expected.

Monitoring Regular monitoring of your diabetes control is necessary. You may also have periodic assessment of your eyes, heart, and kidneys, and of the lipids in your blood.

EZETIMIBE

Brand name Ezetrol
Used in the following combined preparation Inegy

GENERAL INFORMATION

Ezetimibe is a lipid-lowering drug that is used to treat hypercholesterolaemia (high levels of cholesterol in the blood) in people at risk of developing heart disease. It works in the small intestine to reduce the absorption of cholesterol.

Ezetimibe is prescribed in conjunction with a low-fat diet and usually in combination with a statin (a drug that blocks the action, in the liver, of an enzyme needed for the manufacture of cholesterol). It is also prescribed alone

to people in whom a statin is considered inappropriate or is not tolerated.

Common side effects of ezetimibe include headache, abdominal pain, and diarrhoea. It is important to notify your doctor if you are taking over-the-counter statins. When ezetimibe is combined with statins, it can, rarely, cause marked muscle pain, weakness, or tenderness, which should be reported to your doctor immediately. This is less likely to occur when ezetimibe is used alone.

INFORMATION FOR USERS

Your drug prescription is tailored for you. Do not alter dosage without checking with your doctor.

How taken/used

Tablets.

Frequency and timing of doses
Once daily.

Adult dosage range
10mg daily.

Onset of effect
2 weeks.

Duration of action
24 hours.

Diet advice
A low-fat diet is usually recommended.

Storage
Keep in original container at room temperature out of the reach of children.

Missed dose
Take as soon as you remember. If your next dose is due within 12 hours, do not take the missed dose, but take the next one on schedule.

Stopping the drug
Do not stop taking the drug without consulting your doctor. Stopping the drug may lead to a recurrence of the original condition.

Exceeding the dose
An occasional unintentional extra dose is unlikely to cause problems. But if you notice any unusual symptoms or if a large overdose has been taken, notify your doctor.

POSSIBLE ADVERSE EFFECTS

The most common adverse effects of ezetimibe include headache, fatigue, abdominal pain, and diarrhoea.

Symptom/effect	Frequency		Discuss with doctor		Stop taking drug now	Call doctor now
	Common	Rare	Only if severe	In all cases		
Headache	●		●			
Fatigue	●		●			
Abdominal pain/diarrhoea	●		●			
Nausea		●	●			
Joint pain		●	●			
Bleeding or bruising		●		●		
Rash/swollen face and tongue		●		●	●	●
Muscle pain/weakness		●		●	●	●

INTERACTIONS

Fibrates (e.g. gemfibrozil, bezafibrate) These drugs, which also reduce cholesterol, may raise levels of ezetimibe.

Colestyramine may reduce the effects of ezetimibe. Ezetimibe should be taken either 2 hours before or 4 hours after colestyramine.

Ciclosporin The levels of both drugs may be increased when they are taken together.

Warfarin If ezetimibe is added to warfarin the INR (International Normalized Rate, a standardized measure of blood clotting) should be closely monitored.

SPECIAL PRECAUTIONS

Be sure to tell your doctor if:
- You have liver problems.
- You are taking a statin.
- You have lactose intolerance or glucose-galactose malabsorption.
- You are taking other medicines.

Pregnancy
Not usually prescribed. Safety not established. Discuss with your doctor.

Breast-feeding
Not usually prescribed. It is not known whether the drug passes into the breast milk. Discuss with your doctor.

Infants and children
Not recommended under 10 years.

Over 60
Increased likelihood of adverse effects.

Driving and hazardous work
No special problems.

Alcohol
No special problems.

PROLONGED USE

No known problems.

Monitoring Regular blood tests to check the drug's effectiveness in reducing cholesterol levels may be performed. Blood tests of liver and muscle function may also be carried out.

FELODIPINE

Brand names Cardioplen, Felotens, Folpik, Keloc, Neofel, Parmid, Plendil, Vascalpha
Used in the following combined preparation Triapin

GENERAL INFORMATION

Felodipine belongs to a group of drugs known as calcium channel blockers. It is used either alone or with another antihypertensive, such as an ACE inhibitor or a diuretic, in the treatment of hypertension (high blood pressure). It may be used alone or with a beta blocker in the treatment of angina.

The drug works by relaxing the lining of the muscles in small blood vessels, dilating them. This enables blood to be pumped more easily throughout the body, thereby lowering blood pressure and reducing the strain on the heart.

Felodipine is not usually prescribed to people with unstable angina or uncontrolled heart failure. The drug is prescribed with caution to people whose liver function is impaired.

As with other drugs of its class, felodipine may cause the blood pressure to fall too low at the start of treatment.

QUICK REFERENCE

Drug group Anti-angina drug (p.59) and antihypertensive drug (p.60)

Overdose danger rating Medium

Dependence rating Low

Prescription needed Yes

Available as generic Yes

INFORMATION FOR USERS

Your drug prescription is tailored for you. Do not alter dosage without checking with your doctor.

How taken/used

Tablets, MR tablets.

Frequency and timing of doses
Once daily, in the morning, swallowed whole with at least half a glass of water; do not chew or crush.

Adult dosage range
Hypertension 5mg (2.5mg for older people) daily (initial dose), increased to 10mg daily (maintenance dose).
Angina 5mg daily, increased to 10mg if needed.

Onset of effect
1–2 hours.

Duration of action
24 hours.

Diet advice
Felodipine should not be taken with grapefruit juice.

Storage
Keep in original container at room temperature out of the reach of children.

Missed dose
Take as soon as you remember. Take the next dose as scheduled. Do not take an extra dose to make up.

Stopping the drug
Do not stop taking the drug without consulting your doctor. Stopping abruptly may worsen the underlying condition.

Exceeding the dose
An occasional unintentional extra dose is unlikely to cause problems. Large overdoses may cause dizziness or collapse. Notify your doctor urgently.

SPECIAL PRECAUTIONS

Be sure to tell your doctor if:
- You have liver problems.
- You have angina.
- You have had a recent heart attack.
- You have heart problems, especially aortic stenosis.
- You have lactose intolerance.
- You are taking other medicines.

Pregnancy
Not prescribed. May cause defects in the unborn baby.

Breast-feeding
Not recommended. The drug passes into the breast milk and may affect the baby adversely.

Infants and children
Not recommended. Safety not established.

Over 60
Increased likelihood of adverse effects. Reduced dose may therefore be necessary.

Driving and hazardous work
Do not undertake such activities until you have learned how felodipine affects you because the drug can cause dizziness.

Alcohol
Avoid. Alcohol may increase dizziness and the blood-pressure-lowering effect of felodipine, especially at the start of treatment.

POSSIBLE ADVERSE EFFECTS

Flushing, headache, palpitations, and fatigue are common. They are usually transient and are most likely to occur at the start of treatment or after an increase in dosage. Dizziness may be due to excessively lowered blood pressure.

Symptom/effect	Frequency		Discuss with doctor		Stop taking drug now	Call doctor now
	Common	Rare	Only if severe	In all cases		
Flushing/headache/dizziness	●			●		
Palpitations	●			●		
Fatigue		●		●		
Ankle swelling	●			●		
Worsening angina		●			●	
Gingivitis		●			●	

PROLONGED USE

No problems expected.

INTERACTIONS

Other antihypertensives may increase felodipine's blood-pressure-lowering effects.

Erythromycin, itraconazole, ketoconazole, atazanavir, and ritonavir may increase the effects of felodipine.

Anticonvulsants may reduce the effectiveness of felodipine.

Ciclosporin, tacrolimus, and theophylline/aminophylline Toxicity of these drugs may be increased with felodipine.

Grapefruit juice may block the breakdown of felodipine, increasing its effects.

FILGRASTIM

Brand names Accofil, Neupogen, Nivestim, Zarzio
Used in the following combined preparations None

GENERAL INFORMATION

Filgrastim is a synthetic form of G-CSF (granulocyte-colony stimulating factor), a naturally occurring protein responsible for the manufacture of white blood cells, which fight infection.

The drug works by stimulating bone marrow to produce white blood cells. It also causes bone marrow cells to move into the bloodstream, where they can be collected for use in the treatment of bone marrow disease, or to replace bone marrow lost during intensive cancer treatment. Filgrastim is used to treat patients with congenital neutropenia (deficiency of G-CSF from birth), some AIDS patients, and those who have recently received high doses of chemo- or radiotherapy during bone-marrow transplantation or cancer treatment. Such patients are prone to frequent and severe infections.

Bone pain is a common adverse effect, but it can be controlled using painkillers. There is an increased risk of leukaemia (cancer of white blood cells) if filgrastim is given to patients with certain rare blood disorders.

INFORMATION FOR USERS

Your drug prescription is tailored for you. Do not alter dosage without checking with your doctor.

How taken/used

Injection.

Frequency and timing of doses
Once daily.

Adult dosage range
0.1–1.2 million units/kg body weight, depending upon condition being treated and response to treatment.

Onset of effect
24 hours (increase in numbers of white blood cells); several weeks (recovery of normal numbers of white blood cells).

Duration of action
1–7 days.

Diet advice
None.

Storage
Store in a refrigerator out of the reach of children.

Missed dose
Take as soon as you remember. If your next dose is due within 6 hours, do not take the missed dose. Take the next scheduled dose as usual.

Stopping the drug
Do not stop taking the drug without consulting your doctor; stopping the drug may lead to worsening of the underlying condition.

Exceeding the dose
An occasional unintentional extra dose is unlikely to cause problems. But if you notice any unusual symptoms or if a large overdose has been taken, notify your doctor.

SPECIAL PRECAUTIONS

Be sure to tell your doctor if:
- You suffer from any blood disorders.
- You have sickle-cell disease.
- You have a history of lung problems or lung infections.
- You have osteoporosis.
- You are taking other medicines.

 Pregnancy
Safety in pregnancy not established. Discuss with your doctor.

 Breast-feeding
Safety in breast-feeding not established. Discuss with your doctor.

 Infants and children
No special problems.

 Over 60
No special problems.

 Driving and hazardous work
No known problems.

 Alcohol
No known problems.

POSSIBLE ADVERSE EFFECTS

Adverse effects resulting from short courses of filgrastim are unusual. Most common is bone pain, which is probably linked to the stimulant effect of the drug on bone marrow.

Symptom/effect	Frequency		Discuss with doctor		Stop taking drug now	Call doctor now
	Common	Rare	Only if severe	In all cases		
Bone/muscle pain	●		●			
Abdominal pain		●	●			
Skin rash		●		●		
Cough/breathlessness		●		●		
Generalized/abdominal swelling		●		●		●

INTERACTIONS

Cytotoxic chemotherapy or radiotherapy should not be administered within 24 hours of taking filgrastim because of the risk of increasing the damage these treatments inflict on the bone marrow.

PROLONGED USE

Prolonged use may lead to a slightly increased risk of certain leukaemias. Cutaneous vasculitis (inflammation of blood vessels of the skin), osteoporosis (weakening of the bones), hair thinning, enlargement of the spleen and liver, and bleeding due to reduction in platelet numbers may also occur.

Monitoring Blood checks and regular physical examinations are performed, as well as bone scans to check for bone thinning.

FINASTERIDE

Brand names Aindeem, Propecia, Proscar
Used in the following combined preparations None

GENERAL INFORMATION

Finasteride is an anti-androgen drug (see Male sex hormones, p.104) that blocks the conversion of testosterone to a more potent androgen (dihydrotestosterone) in the body. It is used to treat benign prostatic hyperplasia (BPH), in which the prostate gland enlarges, making urination difficult. The drug gradually shrinks the prostate, thus improving urine flow and other obstructive symptoms such as difficulty in starting urination.

Because finasteride is excreted in semen and can feminize a male fetus, you should use a condom if your sexual partner may be, or is likely to become, pregnant. Women of childbearing age should not handle broken or crushed tablets because small quantities of the drug are absorbed through the skin.

The symptoms of BPH are similar to those of prostate cancer, and so the drug is used only when the possibility of cancer has been ruled out.

Finasteride is also used, at a lower dose, to reverse male-pattern baldness by preventing the hair follicles from becoming inactive. Noticeable improvements may take about 3–6 months but will disappear within a year of treatment being stopped.

INFORMATION FOR USERS

Your drug prescription is tailored for you. Do not alter dosage without checking with your doctor.

How taken/used

Tablets.

Frequency and timing of doses
Once daily.

Adult dosage range
Prostate disease 5mg.
Male-pattern baldness 1mg.

Onset of effect
The drug action takes effect within 1 hour, but effects on the prostate and scalp hair may take months to appear.

Duration of action
24 hours.

Diet advice
None.

Storage
Keep in original container at room temperature out of the reach of children. Protect from light.

Missed dose
Do not take the missed dose, but take your next scheduled dose as usual.

Stopping the drug
Do not stop taking the drug without consulting your doctor; stopping the drug may lead to worsening of the underlying condition.

Exceeding the dose
An occasional unintentional extra dose is unlikely to cause problems. But if you notice any unusual symptoms, or if a large overdose has been taken, notify your doctor.

SPECIAL PRECAUTIONS

Be sure to tell your doctor if:
• You have liver problems.
• You are taking other medicines.

 Pregnancy
Not prescribed.

 Breast-feeding
Not applicable.

 Infants and children
Not prescribed.

 Over 60
No special problems.

 Driving and hazardous work
No special problems.

 Alcohol
No special problems.

POSSIBLE ADVERSE EFFECTS

Most people experience very few adverse effects when taking finasteride. However, any changes in the breast tissue, such as lumps, pain, enlargement, or nipple discharge, should be reported promptly to your doctor.

Symptom/effect	Frequency		Discuss with doctor		Stop taking drug now	Call doctor now
	Common	Rare	Only if severe	In all cases		
Impotence/decreased libido	●		●			
Reduced ejaculate volume	●		●			
Breast swelling or tenderness	●			●		
Altered mood/depression		●	●			
Testicular pain		●		●		
Rash/lip swelling/wheezing		●		●	●	●

INTERACTIONS

No drug interactions, but finasteride does interfere with the prostate specific antigen (PSA) screening test for prostate cancer.

PROLONGED USE

Treatment with finasteride for benign prostatic hyperplasia and male-pattern baldness is reviewed after about 6 months to see if it has been effective. Long-term use of the drug carries a small increase in the risk of men developing breast cancer.

FLUCLOXACILLIN

Brand names Floxapen, Fluclomix, Ladropen
Used in the following combined preparations Co-Fluampicil, Flu-Amp, Magnapen

GENERAL INFORMATION

Flucloxacillin is a penicillin antibiotic. The drug was developed to deal with staphylococci bacteria that are resistant to other antibiotics. Such bacteria make enzymes (penicillinases) that neutralize the antibiotics, but flucloxacillin is not inactivated by penicillinases and is therefore effective for treating penicillin-resistant staphylococcal infections. The drug is used to treat ear infections, pneumonia, impetigo, cellulitis, osteomyelitis, and endocarditis.

Flucloxacillin is also available combined in equal parts with ampicillin, which is known as co-fluampicil. This is used for treating mixed infections of penicillinase-producing organisms.

Staphylococci have evolved so that some strains are now resistant to flucloxacillin as well. These are the so-called methicillin-resistant *Staphylococcus aureus* infections (MRSA). Only a few antibiotics held in reserve can deal with them.

INFORMATION FOR USERS

Your drug prescription is tailored for you. Do not alter dosage without checking with your doctor.

How taken/used

Capsules, liquid, injection.

Frequency and timing of doses
4 x daily at least 30 minutes before food.

Adult dosage range
1–2g daily (oral); 1–8g daily (injection); 8–12g daily (endocarditis).

Onset of effect
30 minutes.

Duration of action
4–6 hours.

Diet advice
Make sure you keep well hydrated.

Storage
Keep in original container at room temperature out of the reach of children.

Missed dose
Take as soon as you remember. Take your next dose at the scheduled time.

Stopping the drug
Take the full course. Even if you feel better, the original infection may still be present and symptoms may recur if treatment is stopped too soon.

Exceeding the dose
An occasional unintentional extra dose is unlikely to be a cause for concern. But if you notice any unusual symptoms, or if a large overdose has been taken, notify your doctor.

SPECIAL PRECAUTIONS

Be sure to tell your doctor if:
- You are allergic to penicillin antibiotics or cephalosporin antibiotics.
- You have a history of allergy.
- You have liver problems, or have had previous liver problems with flucloxacillin.
- You are taking other medicines.

 Pregnancy
No evidence of risk.

 Breast-feeding
No evidence of risk.

 Infants and children
Reduced dose necessary.

 Over 60
No known problems.

 Driving and hazardous work
No known problems.

 Alcohol
No known problems.

POSSIBLE ADVERSE EFFECTS

The most common adverse effects are gastrointestinal. If you develop a rash, itching, wheezing or breathing difficulties, or swollen joints (signs of an allergic reaction), or jaundice, which may occur weeks or even months after finishing treatment, call your doctor.

Symptom/effect	Frequency		Discuss with doctor		Stop taking drug now	Call doctor now
	Common	Rare	Only if severe	In all cases		
Diarrhoea/nausea	●		●			
Rash	●			●		
Abdominal pain		●		●		
Bruising		●		●		
Sore throat/fever		●		●		
Itching		●		●	●	●
Breathing difficulties/wheezing		●		●	●	●
Jaundice		●		●	●	●

PROLONGED USE

Although the drug is not normally necessary for long-term use, osteomyelitis and endocarditis may require longer than usual courses of treatment.

Monitoring Regular tests of liver and kidney function will be performed if a longer course of treatment is prescribed.

INTERACTIONS

Methotrexate Flucloxacillin reduces the excretion of methotrexate, thereby increasing the risk of toxicity.

Oral typhoid vaccine Flucloxacillin inactivates the vaccine. Avoid taking flucloxacillin for 3 days before and after having the vaccine.

FLUCONAZOLE

Brand names Azocan, Azocan-P, Canesten Oral, Care Fluconazole, Diflucan
Used in the following combined preparations None

GENERAL INFORMATION

Fluconazole is an antifungal drug that is used to treat local candida infections ("thrush") affecting the vagina, mouth, and skin as well as systemic or more widespread candida infections. The drug is also used to treat some more unusual fungal infections, including cryptococcal meningitis, and it may be used to prevent fungal infections in patients with defective immunity. The dosage and length of course will depend on the condition being treated.

The drug is generally well tolerated, although side effects such as nausea and vomiting, diarrhoea, and abdominal discomfort are common.

QUICK REFERENCE

Drug group Antifungal drug (p.96)
Overdose danger rating Medium
Dependence rating Low
Prescription needed Yes (except for oral treatments for vaginal infections)
Available as generic Yes

INFORMATION FOR USERS

Your drug prescription is tailored for you. Do not alter dosage without checking with your doctor.

How taken/used

Capsules, liquid, injection.

Frequency and timing of doses
Once daily.

Adult dosage range
50–400mg daily.

Onset of effect
Within a few hours, but full beneficial effects may take several days.

Duration of action
Up to 24 hours.

Diet advice
None.

Storage
Keep in original container at room temperature out of the reach of children. Store liquid in a refrigerator (do not freeze) for no longer than 14 days.

Missed dose
Take as soon as you remember. If your next dose is due within 6 hours, take a single dose now and skip the next.

Stopping the drug
Take the full course. Even if you feel better, the original infection may still be present and may recur if treatment is stopped too soon.

Exceeding the dose
An occasional unintentional extra dose is unlikely to be a cause for concern. But if you notice any unusual symptoms, or if a large overdose has been taken, notify your doctor.

SPECIAL PRECAUTIONS

Be sure to tell your doctor if:
- You have long-term liver or kidney problems.
- You have a history of heart rhythm problems.
- You have previously had an allergic reaction to antifungal drugs.
- You have acute porphyria.
- You are taking other medicines.

 Pregnancy
May adversely affect the fetus if taken during pregnancy, and should be avoided.

 Breast-feeding
The drug passes into the breast milk, although probably too little to be harmful. Discuss with your doctor.

 Infants and children
Reduced dose necessary.

 Over 60
Normal dose used as long as kidney function is not impaired.

 Driving and hazardous work
No known problems.

 Alcohol
No known problems.

POSSIBLE ADVERSE EFFECTS

Fluconazole is generally well tolerated. Most side effects affect the gastrointestinal tract.

Rarely, a rash may occur and should be reported to your doctor.

Symptom/effect	Frequency		Discuss with doctor		Stop taking drug now	Call doctor now
	Common	Rare	Only if severe	In all cases		
Nausea/vomiting	●		●			
Abdominal discomfort	●		●			
Flatulence/diarrhoea	●		●			
Headache	●		●			
Rash		●		●	●	

INTERACTIONS

General note Interactions with other drugs relate to multiple doses of fluconazole. The relevance of a single dose is not established, but is likely to be small. As well as the drugs listed here, fluconazole also interacts with a number of other medications and can affect the breakdown of many other drugs. Consult your doctor or pharmacist before using any other drug with fluconazole.

Rifampicin The effect of fluconazole may be reduced by rifampicin. Avoid using both drugs together.

Anticoagulant drugs Fluconazole may increase the effect of oral anticoagulants such as warfarin.

Oral antidiabetic drugs Fluconazole may increase the risk of hypoglycaemia with sulfonylureas and other drugs such as nateglinide and repaglinide.

Theophylline/aminophylline, midazolam, ciclosporin, tacrolimus, zidovudine, phenytoin, and carbamazepine Fluconazole may increase blood levels of these drugs.

Bosentan, eletriptan, ergotamine, erythromycin, ivabradine, methysergide, and pimozide These drugs should not be used with fluconazole because of potentially dangerous interactions that can affect the rhythm of your heart beat.

PROLONGED USE

Fluconazole is usually given for short courses of treatment, although long-term courses may be prescribed for those with recurrent candidiasis. For prevention of relapse of cryptococcal meningitis in patients with defective immunity, it may be administered indefinitely.

FLUOROURACIL

Brand names Efudix 5% Cream
Used in the following combined preparations Actikerall

GENERAL INFORMATION

Fluorouracil (or 5-FU) is a chemotherapy drug for cancers including colon and breast cancer. It may be used on its own or combined with other chemotherapy drugs. It is thought to act by stopping the production of DNA.

The drug is usually given by injection or infusion. It can also be applied as a cream for pre-cancerous areas of sun-damaged skin, and for skin cancers called superficial basal cell carcinomas.

Patients having injections or infusions should first be screened for deficiency of an enzyme called dihydropyramidine dehydrogenase (DPD), which could lead to severe or fatal toxicity with fluorouracil.

QUICK REFERENCE

Drug group Anticancer drug (p.112)
Overdose danger rating Low
Dependence rating Low
Prescription needed Yes
Available as generic Yes

INFORMATION FOR USERS

Your drug prescription is tailored for you. Do not alter dosage without checking with your doctor.

How taken/used

Injection/infusion; cream (topical).

Frequency and timing of doses
Regime decided by doctor (injection/infusion). 1–2 x daily for 3–4 weeks (cream).

Adult dosage range
Injection/infusion dose determined by weight. For cream, maximum area of skin to be treated at one time is 500cm² (23cm x 23cm).

Onset of effect
Benefits and adverse effects of cream usually develop within 1–2 weeks.

Duration of action
Effects of cream should settle by 4–6 weeks.

Diet advice
Drink plenty of liquid before, during, and after injections or infusions.

Storage
Store cream at room temperature and out of the reach of children. The cream is flammable.

Missed dose
If you miss a dose of cream, apply as soon as possible. If it is nearly time for next dose, skip the missed dose and continue as before.

Stopping the drug
Try to complete courses of cream as your doctor has prescribed. If the skin inflammation is intolerable, seek advice from your doctor.

Exceeding the dose
Unlikely to occur but contact your doctor if you have any concerns or unusual symptoms.

SPECIAL PRECAUTIONS

Fluorouracil given by injection or infusion is prescribed under close medical supervision, taking into account your present condition and medical history. However, be sure to tell your doctor if:
- You have impaired liver function.
- You have impaired kidney function.
- You have a known personal or family history of DPD enzyme deficiency.
- You are pregnant or planning a pregnancy.
- You are breast-feeding.
- You have a known allergy to fluorouracil (cream or injection/infusion).
- You take any other medications, including over-the-counter treatments.

 Pregnancy
Strictly contraindicated in pregnant women. Women having fluorouracil by injection, infusion, or cream should avoid pregnancy during treatment and for 6 months afterwards. Men should avoid fathering a child during and for 6 months after treatment.

 Breast-feeding
Not advised. Discuss with your doctor.

 Infants and children
Safety and efficacy have not been established.

 Over 60
Dose reduction may be required.

 Driving and hazardous work
No known problems, but see how the drug affects you as it can cause nausea.

 Alcohol
Alcohol can be taken in moderation.

POSSIBLE ADVERSE EFFECTS

Side effects are common with the injections. The cream used for skin lesions may cause significant inflammatory skin reactions as well as abdominal pain and diarrhoea.

Symptom/effect	Frequency Common	Frequency Rare	Discuss with doctor Only if severe	Discuss with doctor In all cases	Stop taking drug now	Call doctor now
Infusion/injection						
Loss of appetite	●		●			
Hair loss	●		●			
Weakness/fatigue	●		●			
Nausea/vomiting/diarrhoea	●			●		
Nosebleed	●			●		
Mouth or lip ulceration	●			●		
Rash		●		●		●
Chest pain/palpitations	●			●		●
Cream						
Skin irritation	●		●			

INTERACTIONS

Cimetidine and metronidazole increase the blood level and toxicity of systemic fluorouracil.

Phenytoin Systemic fluorouracil increases the concentration of phenytoin so blood levels of phenytoin should be monitored and dose adjusted if necessary.

Live vaccines e.g. influenza should be avoided with systemic fluorouracil due to risk of generalized/life-threatening infection.

Warfarin Systemic fluorouracil increases the anticoagulant effect of warfarin.

Methotrexate may increase the risk of a severe skin reaction to topical fluorouracil.

PROLONGED USE

No specific problems, but the length of the course will be decided by your doctor.

FLUOXETINE

Brand names Olena, Prozac, Prozep
Used in the following combined preparations None

GENERAL INFORMATION

Fluoxetine belongs to the group of antidepressants called selective serotonin re-uptake inhibitors (SSRIs). These drugs tend to cause less sedation, have different side effects, and are safer if taken in overdose than older antidepressants. Fluoxetine elevates mood, increases physical activity, and restores interest in everyday pursuits.

Fluoxetine is broken down slowly and remains in the body for several weeks after treatment is stopped. The drug is used to treat depression, to reduce binge eating and purging activity (bulimia nervosa), and to treat obsessive–compulsive disorder.

INFORMATION FOR USERS

Your drug prescription is tailored for you. Do not alter dosage without checking with your doctor.

How taken/used

Capsules, dispersible tablets, liquid.

Frequency and timing of doses
Once daily in the morning.

Adult dosage range
20–60mg daily.

Onset of effect
Some benefits may appear in 14 days, but full benefits may not be felt for 6 weeks or more. Obsessive–compulsive disorder and bulimia may take longer to respond.

Duration of action
Beneficial effects may last for up to 6 weeks following prolonged treatment. Adverse effects may wear off within 1–2 weeks.

Diet advice
None.

Storage
Keep in original container at room temperature out of the reach of children.

Missed dose
Take as soon as you remember. If your next dose is due within 8 hours, take a single dose now and skip the next.

Stopping the drug
Do not stop the drug without consulting your doctor, who may supervise a gradual reduction in dosage.

Exceeding the dose
An occasional unintentional extra dose is unlikely to cause problems. Large overdoses may cause adverse effects. Notify your doctor.

SPECIAL PRECAUTIONS

Be sure to tell your doctor if:
- You have long-term liver or kidney problems.
- You have a history of mania.
- You have diabetes.
- You have had epileptic seizures.
- You have previously had an allergic reaction to fluoxetine or other SSRIs.
- You are taking other medicines.

Pregnancy
Avoid if possible. Discuss with your doctor.

Breast-feeding
The drug passes into the breast milk. Discuss with your doctor.

Infants and children
Not generally recommended under 18 years.

Over 60
Reduced dose may be necessary.

Driving and hazardous work
Avoid such activities until you have learned how fluoxetine affects you because the drug can cause drowsiness and can affect your judgement and coordination.

Alcohol
No special problems.

PROLONGED USE

No problems expected in adults. Side effects tend to decrease with time. There is a small risk of suicidal thoughts and self-harm in children and adolescents, although the drug is rarely used for this age group.

Monitoring Any person experiencing drowsiness, confusion, muscle cramps, or seizures should be monitored for low sodium levels in the blood. Under-18s should be monitored for suicidal thoughts and self-harm.

POSSIBLE ADVERSE EFFECTS

The most common adverse effects of this drug are restlessness, insomnia, and intestinal irregularities. Fluoxetine produces fewer anticholinergic side effects than the tricyclics.

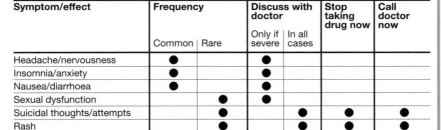

Symptom/effect	Frequency		Discuss with doctor		Stop taking drug now	Call doctor now
	Common	Rare	Only if severe	In all cases		
Headache/nervousness	●		●			
Insomnia/anxiety	●		●			
Nausea/diarrhoea	●		●			
Sexual dysfunction		●	●			
Suicidal thoughts/attempts		●		●	●	●
Rash		●		●	●	●

INTERACTIONS

Sedatives All drugs having a sedative effect may increase the sedative effects of fluoxetine.

Monoamine oxidase inhibitors (MAOIs) Fluoxetine should not be started less than 14 days after stopping an MAOI (except moclobemide) as serious adverse effects can occur. An MAOI should not be started less than 5 weeks after stopping fluoxetine.

Tricyclic antidepressants Fluoxetine reduces the breakdown of tricyclics and may increase the toxicity of these drugs.

Antipsychotics The levels and effects of some of these drugs can be increased by fluoxetine.

FLUPENTIXOL

Brand names Depixol, Fluanxol, Psytixol
Used in the following combined preparations None

GENERAL INFORMATION

Flupentixol is an antipsychotic drug that is prescribed to treat schizophrenia and similar illnesses. It is also occasionally used as an antidepressant for mild to moderate depression. The side effects are similar to those of phenothiazines, but flupentixol is less sedating. The drug is not suitable for any patients who suffer from mania because it may worsen the symptoms. Flupentixol has fewer anticholinergic effects than the phenothiazines but, because it has antidopaminergic effects, it can cause side effects such as parkinsonism.

QUICK REFERENCE

Drug group Antipsychotic drug (p.41)
Overdose danger rating Medium
Dependence rating Low
Prescription needed Yes
Available as generic No

INFORMATION FOR USERS

Your drug prescription is tailored for you. Do not alter dosage without checking with your doctor.

How taken/used

Tablets, injection.

Frequency and timing of doses
1–2 x daily no later than 4 pm (tablets); every 2–4 weeks (injection).

Adult dosage range
Schizophrenia and other psychoses 6–18mg daily (tablets); from 20mg every 4 weeks to a maximum of 400mg weekly (injection). *Depression* 1–3mg daily (tablets).

Onset of effect
10 days (side effects may appear much sooner).

Duration of action
Up to 12 hours (by mouth); 1–2 months (by depot injection).

Diet advice
None.

Storage
Store at room temperature out of the reach of children. Protect injections from light.

Missed dose
Take as soon as you remember. If your next dose is due within 2 hours, do not take the missed dose, but take your next scheduled dose as usual.

Stopping the drug
Do not stop taking the drug without consulting your doctor, who will supervise a gradual reduction in dosage. Abrupt cessation of the drug may cause withdrawal symptoms and a recurrence of the original problem.

Exceeding the dose
An occasional unintentional extra dose is unlikely to cause problems. Larger overdoses may cause severe drowsiness, seizures, low blood pressure, or shock. Notify your doctor.

SPECIAL PRECAUTIONS

Be sure to tell your doctor if:
- You have long-term liver or kidney problems.
- You have heart problems.
- You have had epileptic seizures.
- You have Parkinson's disease.
- You have glaucoma.
- You have porphyria.
- You have lactose intolerance.
- You are taking other medicines.

 Pregnancy
Not usually prescribed. May cause lethargy in the baby during labour. Discuss with your doctor.

 Breast-feeding
The drug passes into the breast milk and may affect the baby. Discuss with your doctor.

 Infants and children
Not recommended.

 Over 60
Reduced dose necessary. Increased risk of late-appearing movement disorders or confusion.

 Driving and hazardous work
Avoid such activities until you have learned how flupentixol affects you because the drug can cause drowsiness and slowed reactions.

 Alcohol
Avoid. Flupentixol enhances the sedative effect of alcohol.

Surgery and general anaesthetics
Treatment may need to be stopped before you have any surgery. Discuss this with your doctor or dentist.

POSSIBLE ADVERSE EFFECTS

Any adverse effects are mainly the result of the drug's anticholinergic and antidopaminergic actions and its blocking action on the transmission of signals through the heart.

Symptom/effect	Frequency		Discuss with doctor		Stop taking drug now	Call doctor now
	Common	Rare	Only if severe	In all cases		
Weight gain	●		●			
Nausea	●		●			
Drowsiness	●		●			
Sexual dysfunction	●		●			
Breast growth/absent periods	●		●			
Blurred vision	●			●		
Parkinsonism/tremor	●			●		
Dizziness/fainting/confusion	●			●		●
Palpitations		●		●		
Jaundice		●		●	●	

PROLONGED USE

The risk of late-appearing movement disorders increases as treatment with flupentixol continues. Blood disorders, as well as jaundice and other liver disorders, are occasionally seen.

INTERACTIONS

Anti-arrhythmic drugs and antibiotics (e.g. erythromycin and moxifloxacin) Taken with these drugs, flupentixol may increase the risk of arrhythmias.

Antihypertensive drugs Flupentixol may increase the effects of some antihypertensives.

Anticholinergic drugs Flupentixol may increase the effects of these drugs.

Antiparkinson drugs and anticonvulsants Flupentixol may reduce the effects of these drugs.

Sedatives Flupentixol enhances the effect of all sedative drugs.

FLUTAMIDE

Brand names None
Used in the following combined preparations None

GENERAL INFORMATION

Flutamide is an anti-androgen drug used in the treatment of advanced prostate cancer, often in combination with drugs such as goserelin that control the production of the male sex hormones (androgens). Both drugs are effective because the cancer is dependent on androgens for its continued development. Treatment with goserelin-type drugs causes an initial increase in release of the hormone testosterone, leading to a growth spurt of the cancer ("tumour flare"), which flutamide is prescribed to stop. Flutamide is also used to treat prostate cancer when goserelin-type drugs are not prescribed.

Flutamide may discolour the urine amber or yellow-green, but this is harmless. However, you should notify your doctor straight away if your urine becomes dark-coloured, because this may be an indication of liver damage.

INFORMATION FOR USERS

Your drug prescription is tailored for you. Do not alter dosage without checking with your doctor.

How taken/used

Tablets.

Frequency and timing of doses
3 x daily, starting 3 days before the goserelin-type drug and continuing for 3 weeks.

Adult dosage range
250mg.

Onset of effect
1 hour.

Duration of action
8 hours.

Diet advice
None.

Storage
Keep in original container at room temperature out of the reach of children.

Missed dose
Take as soon as you remember. If your next dose is due within 2 hours, take a single dose now and skip the next.

Stopping the drug
Do not stop taking the drug without consulting your doctor because the condition may worsen rapidly.

Exceeding the dose
An occasional unintentional extra dose is unlikely to be a cause for concern. But if you notice any unusual symptoms, or if a large overdose has been taken, notify your doctor.

SPECIAL PRECAUTIONS

Be sure to tell your doctor if:
- You have heart problems.
- You have had a blood clot, such as a deep vein thrombosis.
- You have liver problems.
- You are taking other medicines.

 Pregnancy
Not prescribed to women. The drug causes fetal abnormalities in animals; for safety, barrier contraception must be used by men when on flutamide, and their female partners should also use effective contraception.

 Breast-feeding
Not prescribed.

 Infants and children
Not prescribed.

 Over 60
No special problems.

 Driving and hazardous work
Do not undertake such activities until you have learned how flutamide affects you because the drug can cause blurred vision and dizziness.

 Alcohol
No special problems, but excessive consumption should be avoided.

POSSIBLE ADVERSE EFFECTS

Nausea and tiredness are common. Breast swelling and tenderness may occur if the drug is given at an effective dose; these are usually reversible when it is stopped or reduced.

Symptom/effect	Frequency		Discuss with doctor		Stop taking drug now	Call doctor now
	Common	Rare	Only if severe	In all cases		
Breast swelling/tenderness	●		●			
Nausea/vomiting/diarrhoea	●		●			
Insomnia/tiredness/headache	●		●			
Decreased libido/hot flushes	●		●			
Thirst	●		●			
Dizziness/blurred vision		●	●			
Fluid retention		●	●			
Stomach or chest pain		●		●		
Rash		●		●	●	
Jaundice/dark urine		●		●	●	●

INTERACTIONS

Warfarin Flutamide increases the anticoagulant effect of warfarin.

Theophylline Flutamide may increase blood levels of theophylline.

Idelalisib and ivacaftor severely increase flutamide levels in the body and should be avoided. Several antiretrovirals can also increase flutamide levels to a lesser degree.

Drugs that increase the risk of heart arrhythmias, which include amiodarone, sotalol, moxifloxacin, and methadone, should be used with caution when taking flutamide. ECG monitoring is advised.

PROLONGED USE

Prolonged use of flutamide may cause liver damage. Because it is an anti-androgen, the drug also reduces sperm count.

Monitoring Periodic liver-function tests are usually performed. ECG monitoring may also be performed. Bone density may be monitored annually as osteoporotic bone fractures are more likely if flutamide is used for long periods. Glucose levels/HbA1c may be monitored as the risk of diabetes is higher on combined treatment with flutamide plus GnRH agents such as goserelin.

FLUTICASONE

Brand names AirFluSal, Avamys, Combisal, Cutivate, Dymista, Flixonase, Flixotide, Nasofan, Pirinase, Sereflo, Trelegy Ellipta
Used in the following combined preparations Aerivio, Flutiform, Relvar, Seretide

GENERAL INFORMATION

Fluticasone is a corticosteroid drug used to control inflammation in asthma and allergic rhinitis. It does not produce relief immediately, so it is important to take the drug regularly. For allergic rhinitis, treatment with the nasal spray needs to begin two to three weeks before the hay fever season starts. Fluticasone should be taken regularly by inhaler to prevent asthma attacks; proper instruction is essential to ensure correct use. The drug is also prescribed in the form of an ointment or cream to treat dermatitis and eczema (see Topical corticosteroids, p.134).

Fluticasone has few serious adverse effects because it is administered directly into the lungs (by inhaler) or nasal mucosa (by nasal spray). Fungal infection causing irritation of the mouth and throat is a possible side effect of the inhaled form but can be minimized by thoroughly rinsing the mouth and gargling with water after each inhalation.

QUICK REFERENCE

Drug group Corticosteroid (p.99)

Overdose danger rating Low

Dependence rating Low

Prescription needed Yes (except for nasal spray)

Available as generic No

INFORMATION FOR USERS

Follow instructions on the label. Call your doctor if symptoms worsen.

How taken/used

Ointment, cream, inhaler, nasal spray.

Frequency and timing of doses
Allergic rhinitis 1–2 x daily; *asthma* 2 x daily

Adult dosage range
Allergic rhinitis 1–2 sprays into each nostril per dose; *asthma* 100–1,000mcg per dose.

Onset of effect
4–7 days (asthma); 3–4 days (allergic rhinitis).

Duration of action
The effects can last for several days after stopping the drug.

Diet advice
None.

Storage
Keep in original container at room temperature out of the reach of children.

Missed dose
Take as soon as you remember.

Stopping the drug
Do not stop the drug without consulting your doctor; symptoms may recur.

Exceeding the dose
An occasional unintentional extra dose is unlikely to be a cause for concern. Adverse effects may occur if the recommended dose is regularly exceeded over a prolonged period.

POSSIBLE ADVERSE EFFECTS

Adverse effects are unlikely. Nasal spray may irritate the nasal passages. Inhalers may cause fungal infection of the throat and mouth; this can be minimized by rinsing out the mouth, brushing the teeth, or gargling with water. If wheezing and breathlessness suddenly worsen after inhaler use (paradoxical bronchospasm), stop the drug and call the doctor immediately.

Symptom/effect	Frequency		Discuss with doctor		Stop taking drug now	Call doctor now
	Common	Rare	Only if severe	In all cases		
Inhaler/nasal spray						
Nasal discomfort/irritation	●		●			
Cough	●		●			
Bruising	●		●			
Sore throat/hoarseness	●			●		
Nosebleed	●			●		
Cream/ointment						
Skin changes (long-term use)	●			●		

INTERACTIONS

Atazanavir, clarithomycin, ritonavir, telaprevir, and itraconazole may increase the blood level of fluticasone and the risk of adrenal gland suppression.

Vaccines High-dose fluticasone may cause serious generalized infections if live vaccines are given with this drug. Discuss with your doctor.

Non-steroidal anti-inflammatory drugs (NSAIDs) such as ibuprofen with fluticasone can cause a small but significant increase in the risk of gastrointestinal bleeding.

SPECIAL PRECAUTIONS

Be sure to tell your doctor if:
- You have chronic sinusitis.
- You have had recent nasal ulcers or nasal surgery.
- You have had tuberculosis or another respiratory infection.
- You are taking other medicines.

 Pregnancy
Safety in pregnancy not established. Discuss with your doctor.

 Breast-feeding
Safety in breast-feeding not established. Drug unlikely to pass into breast milk; discuss with doctor.

 Infants and children
Not recommended under 4 years. Reduced dose necessary in older children. Avoid prolonged use of ointment in children.

 Over 60
No known problems.

 Driving and hazardous work
No known problems.

 Alcohol
No known problems.

PROLONGED USE

Long-term use of topical and inhaled fluticasone can lead to peptic ulcers, muscle weakness, osteoporosis, growth retardation in children, and rarely, adrenal gland suppression. Rarely, nasal spray may cause glaucoma and cataracts. The incidence of long-term side effects from inhalation can be reduced by use of a spacer. Long-term topical treatment may cause skin thinning. Patients on long-term fluticasone should carry a steroid card or wear a MedicAlert bracelet.

Monitoring Periodic checks on adrenal gland function may be required if large doses are being taken. Children should have their height monitored.

FUROSEMIDE (FRUSEMIDE)

Brand names Froop, Frusol, Lasix, and others
Used in the following combined preparations Co-Amilofruse, Frumil, Lasilactone, and others

GENERAL INFORMATION

Furosemide is a powerful, short-acting loop diuretic that has been in use for many decades. Like other diuretics, it is used to treat oedema (accumulation of fluid in tissue spaces) caused by heart failure, and certain lung, liver, and kidney disorders.

Because it is fast acting, furosemide is often used in emergencies to relieve pulmonary oedema (fluid in the lungs).

The drug is particularly useful for people who have impaired kidney function because these people do not respond well to thiazide diuretics (see p.57).

Furosemide increases potassium loss from the body, which can produce a wide variety of symptoms. For this reason, potassium supplements or a potassium-sparing diuretic may be given with the drug.

QUICK REFERENCE

Drug group Loop diuretic (p.57) and antihypertensive drug (p.60)

Overdose danger rating Low

Dependence rating Low

Prescription needed Yes

Available as generic Yes

INFORMATION FOR USERS

Your drug prescription is tailored for you. Do not alter dosage without checking with your doctor.

How taken/used

Tablets, liquid, injection.

Frequency and timing of doses
Once daily, usually in the morning; 4–6 x hourly (high-dose therapy).

Adult dosage range
20–80mg daily. Dose may be increased to a maximum of 2g daily if doctor considers it necessary.

Onset of effect
Within 1 hour (by mouth); within 5 minutes (by injection).

Duration of action
Up to 6 hours.

Diet advice
Use of this drug may reduce potassium in the body. Eat plenty of potassium-rich fresh fruits and vegetables, such as bananas and tomatoes, unless you have very impaired renal function or you are on dialysis.

Storage
Keep in original container at room temperature out of the reach of children. Protect from light.

Missed dose
No cause for concern, but take as soon as you remember. However, if it is late in the day do not take the missed dose, or you may need to get up during the night to pass urine. Take the next scheduled dose as usual.

Stopping the drug
Do not stop the drug without consulting your doctor; symptoms may recur.

Exceeding the dose
An occasional unintentional extra dose is unlikely to be a cause for concern. But if you notice any unusual symptoms, or if a large overdose has been taken, notify your doctor.

SPECIAL PRECAUTIONS

Be sure to tell your doctor if:
- You have long-term liver or kidney problems.
- You have gout.
- You have previously had an allergic reaction to furosemide or sulfonamides.
- You have prostate problems.
- You are taking other medicines.

 Pregnancy
Safety in pregnancy not established. Discuss with your doctor.

 Breast-feeding
The drug may reduce milk supply, but the amount in the milk is unlikely to affect the baby. Discuss with your doctor.

 Infants and children
Reduced dose necessary

 Over 60
Reduced dose may be necessary.

 Driving and hazardous work
Avoid such activities until you have learned how furosemide affects you because the drug may reduce mental alertness and cause dizziness.

 Alcohol
Keep consumption low. Furosemide increases the likelihood of dehydration after drinking alcohol, and alcohol can increase the blood-pressure-lowering effect of furosemide.

POSSIBLE ADVERSE EFFECTS

Adverse effects are mainly due to the rapid fluid loss from furosemide and the disturbance in body salts and water balance. These diminish as the body adjusts to the drug.

Symptom/effect	Frequency		Discuss with doctor		Stop taking drug now	Call doctor now
	Common	Rare	Only if severe	In all cases		
Dizziness/nausea	●		●			
Lethargy		●	●			
Muscle cramps		●	●			
Rash/photosensitivity		●		●	●	
Vomiting		●		●	●	

INTERACTIONS

Non-steroidal anti-inflammatory drugs (NSAIDs) Some of these drugs may reduce the diuretic effect of furosemide.

Lithium Furosemide may increase blood levels and risk of lithium poisoning.

Digoxin Loss of potassium with furosemide may lead to digoxin toxicity.

Aminoglycoside antibiotics used with furosemide may increase the risks of hearing and kidney problems.

Thiazides taken with furosemide may lead to excessive urination.

ACE inhibitors and angiotensin-2-receptor blockers with furosemide may cause severe hypotension so careful dose adjustment may be needed.

Sucralfate, cholestyramine, and colestipol can decrease the absorption of furosemide. Leave at least 2 hours between taking these drugs and furosemide.

PROLONGED USE

Serious problems are unlikely, but levels of salts, such as potassium, sodium, magnesium, and calcium, may become depleted. Low blood pressure, palpitations, headaches, problems passing urine, or muscle cramps may develop, particularly in older people.

Monitoring Periodic tests may be performed to check kidney function and levels of body salts.

GABAPENTIN

Brand name Gabapentin Zentiva, Neurontin
Used in the following combined preparations None

GENERAL INFORMATION

Gabapentin is an anticonvulsant drug (see p.42). It is used to treat partial seizures, and is often prescribed in combination with other drugs when a patient's epilepsy is not being satisfactorily controlled with the other drugs alone. Unlike some of the other anticonvulsant drugs, gabapentin does not need blood level monitoring. In addition, it does not have any significant interactions with other anticonvulsants.

Gabapentin is also used to relieve neuropathic pain, such as the pain suffered after shingles or by some people with diabetes.

Patients with impaired kidney function should be given smaller doses, and diabetic patients taking gabapentin may notice fluctuations in their blood sugar levels.

Gabapentin is a Schedule III (Class C) controlled drug (see p.13).

QUICK REFERENCE

Drug group Anticonvulsant drug (p.42)

Overdose danger rating Medium

Dependence rating Medium

Prescription needed Yes

Available as generic Yes

INFORMATION FOR USERS

Your drug prescription is tailored for you. Do not alter dosage without checking with your doctor.

How taken/used

Tablets, capsules, oral solution. Tablets should be swallowed whole; do not crush.

Frequency and timing of doses
Dose is gradually built up to 3 x daily as maintenance treatment. No more than 12 hours should elapse between doses.

Adult dosage range
900–3,600mg daily; maintenance dose reached gradually over a few days.

Onset of effect
The full anticonvulsant effect may not be seen for 48 hours.

Duration of action
6–8 hours.

Diet advice
None.

Storage
Keep in original container at room temperature out of the reach of children.

Missed dose
Take as soon as you remember. If your next dose is due within 4 hours, take a dose now and skip the next.

Stopping the drug
Gabapentin should not be stopped abruptly. Gradual withdrawal over at least 7 days is advised to reduce the risk of seizures in those being treated for epilepsy.

Exceeding the dose
An occasional unintentional extra dose is unlikely to be a cause for concern. Large overdoses may lead to dizziness, double vision, and slurred speech. Notify your doctor.

SPECIAL PRECAUTIONS

Be sure to tell your doctor if:
- You have a kidney problem.
- You have diabetes.
- You have a history of psychiatric illness.
- You have a history of substance misuse.
- You are taking other medicines.

 Pregnancy
The drug is likely to reach the fetus and its effects are unknown. Discuss with your doctor.

 Breast-feeding
The drug passes into the breast milk, and the effects on the baby are unknown. Discuss with your doctor.

 Infants and children
Rarely used in children under 6 years. Reduced doses based on body weight are required in children under 12 years.

 Over 60
Doses may have to be adjusted to allow for decreased kidney function.

 Driving and hazardous work
Avoid driving or hazardous work until you have learned how the drug affects you. Gabapentin may produce drowsiness or dizziness.

 Alcohol
Alcohol may increase the sedative effects of gabapentin.

POSSIBLE ADVERSE EFFECTS

The most common adverse effects of gabapentin are sleepiness and dizziness. Vision difficulties are less common, as are indigestion and weight gain. The most unusual adverse effects are mood changes, rash, and respiratory depression.

Symptom/effect	Frequency		Discuss with doctor		Stop taking drug now	Call doctor now
	Common	Rare	Only if severe	In all cases		
Drowsiness/dizziness/fatigue	●		●			
Muscle tremor	●			●		
Vision disturbances		●		●		
Indigestion		●		●		
Weight gain		●		●		
Mood changes/hallucinations		●		●		●
Rash		●		●		●

PROLONGED USE

No problems expected.

INTERACTIONS

Antacids containing aluminium or magnesium These may reduce the effect of gabapentin. The drug should not be taken within 2 hours of antacid preparations.

Urinary protein tests for diabetes False-positive readings have been recorded with some tests. Special procedures are required for people with diabetes who are taking gabapentin.

Morphine This may increase gabapentin blood levels and increase the risk of respiratory depression.

GENTAMICIN

Brand names Cidomycin, Gentacidin, Gentasol, Genticin, Minims gentamicin
Used in the following combined preparation Gentisone HC

GENERAL INFORMATION

Gentamicin is one of the aminoglycoside antibiotics. The injectable form is usually reserved for hospital treatment of serious lung, urinary tract, bone, joint, wound, and other infections, peritonitis, septicaemia, and meningitis. This form is also used together with a penicillin to prevent and treat heart valve infections (endocarditis). Gentamicin drops are used to treat eye and ear infections.

Gentamicin given by injection can have serious adverse effects on the ears and the kidneys. Damage to the ears may lead to deafness and problems with the balance mechanism in the inner ear. Courses of treatment are, therefore, limited to seven days when possible. Treatment is monitored by measuring blood levels of gentamicin, especially when high doses are needed or kidney function is poor. Rarely, gentamicin can be associated with histamine-related adverse reactions (see Histamine and histamine receptors, p.81).

QUICK REFERENCE

Drug group Aminoglycoside antibiotic (p.86)

Overdose danger rating Low

Dependence rating Low

Prescription needed Yes

Available as generic Yes

INFORMATION FOR USERS

Your drug prescription is tailored for you. Do not alter dosage without checking with your doctor.

How taken/used

Injection, eye/ear drops.

Frequency and timing of doses
1–3 x daily (injection); 3–4 x daily or as directed (ear drops); every 2 hours or as directed (eye drops).

Adult dosage range
According to condition and response (injection); according to your doctor's instructions (eye and ear drops).

Onset of effect
Within 1–2 hours.

Duration of action
8–12 hours.

Diet advice
None.

Storage
Keep in original container at room temperature out of the reach of children.

Missed dose
Apply eye/ear preparations as soon as you remember.

Stopping the drug
Complete the course. Even if you feel better, the original infection may still be present and may recur if treatment is stopped too soon.

Exceeding the dose
Although overdose by injection is dangerous, it is unlikely because treatment is carefully monitored. For other preparations of the drug, an occasional unintentional extra dose is unlikely to cause concern. But if you notice any unusual symptoms, notify your doctor.

SPECIAL PRECAUTIONS

Be sure to tell your doctor if:
- You have a long-term kidney problem.
- You have a hearing disorder, especially a perforated eardrum.
- You have myasthenia gravis.
- You have Parkinson's disease.
- You have previously had an allergic reaction to aminoglycosides.
- You are taking other medicines.

 Pregnancy
No evidence of risk with eye or ear drops. Injections are not prescribed, as they may cause hearing defects in the baby. Discuss with your doctor.

 Breast-feeding
No evidence of risk with eye or ear preparations. Given by injection, the drug may pass into the breast milk. Discuss with your doctor.

 Infants and children
Reduced dose necessary for injections.

 Over 60
Increased likelihood of adverse effects. Close monitoring of treatment is therefore necessary.

 Driving and hazardous work
No known problems from preparations for the eye or ear.

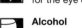 **Alcohol**
No known problems.

POSSIBLE ADVERSE EFFECTS

Adverse effects are rare, but those that occur with injections may be serious. Dizziness, loss of balance (vertigo), impaired hearing, and changes in urine should be reported promptly. If ear drops are used when the eardrum is perforated, damage to the inner ear may occur. Allergic reactions such as rash and itching may occur with all preparations. Blurred vision or eye irritation may occur with eye drops; notify your doctor if severe.

Symptom/effect	Frequency		Discuss with doctor		Stop taking drug now	Call doctor now
	Common	Rare	Only if severe	In all cases		
Nausea/vomiting		●	●			
Dizziness/vertigo		●		●	●	●
Rash/itching		●		●	●	●
Ringing in the ears		●		●	●	●
Loss of hearing		●		●	●	●
Bloody/cloudy urine		●		●	●	●
Eye irritation/blurred vision	●			●		

INTERACTIONS

General note A wide range of drugs, including furosemide, vancomycin, and cephalosporins, increase the risk of hearing loss and/or kidney failure with gentamicin given by injection.

PROLONGED USE

Not usually given for longer than 7 days. When given by injection, there is a risk of adverse effects on hearing and balance.

Monitoring Blood levels of the drug are usually checked if it is given by injection. Tests on kidney function are also usually carried out.

GLIBENCLAMIDE

Brand names Gliken, Liamide
Used in the following combined preparations None

GENERAL INFORMATION

Glibenclamide is an oral antidiabetic drug that belongs to the sulfonylurea class. Like other drugs of this type, it stimulates the production and secretion of insulin from the islet cells in the pancreas. This promotes the uptake of sugar into body cells, thereby lowering the blood sugar level.

Glibenclamide is used in the treatment of Type 2 diabetes, in conjunction with exercise and a diet that is low in sugar and fats. In conditions of severe illness, injury, or stress, however, the drug may lose its effectiveness, making insulin injections necessary.

Adverse effects are generally mild. The most common side effect is hypoglycaemia (low blood sugar).

QUICK REFERENCE

Drug group Drug for diabetes (p.100)

Overdose danger rating High

Dependence rating Low

Prescription needed Yes

Available as generic Yes

INFORMATION FOR USERS

Your drug prescription is tailored for you. Do not alter dosage without checking with your doctor.

How taken/used

Tablets.

Frequency and timing of doses
1 x daily in the morning with your first meal.

Adult dosage range
5–15mg daily.

Onset of effect
Within 3 hours.

Duration of action
10–15 hours.

Diet advice
An individualized diabetic diet must be maintained in order for the drug to be fully effective. Follow the advice of your doctor.

Storage
Keep in original container at room temperature out of the reach of children. Protect from light.

Missed dose
Take with next meal; do not double the dose to account for missed dose.

Stopping the drug
Do not stop the drug without consulting your doctor; stopping the drug may lead to worsening of your diabetes.

OVERDOSE ACTION

Seek immediate medical advice in all cases. If any warning symptoms of excessively low blood sugar (such as faintness, dizziness, headache, confusion, sweating, or tremor) occur, eat or drink something sugary. Take emergency action if seizures or loss of consciousness occur.

See Drug poisoning emergency guide (p.518).

POSSIBLE ADVERSE EFFECTS

Serious adverse effects are rare. More common symptoms, often accompanied by hunger, may be signs of low blood sugar due to lack of food or too high a dose of the drug.

Symptom/effect	Frequency		Discuss with doctor		Stop taking drug now	Call doctor now
	Common	Rare	Only if severe	In all cases		
Faintness/confusion	●			●		
Weakness/tremors	●			●		
Sweating	●			●		
Constipation/diarrhoea	●		●			
Nausea/vomiting		●		●		
Rash/itching		●		●		
Weight changes		●		●		
Jaundice		●		●		●

INTERACTIONS

General note A variety of drugs may reduce the effect of glibenclamide and so may raise blood sugar levels. These include corticosteroids, oestrogens, diuretics, and rifampicin. Others increase the risk of low blood sugar. These include warfarin, aspirin, sulfonamides and other antibacterials, antifungals, NSAIDs, and ACE inhibitors.

Beta blockers may mask hypoglycaemia symptoms, especially non-cardioselective beta blockers such as propranolol.

SPECIAL PRECAUTIONS

Be sure to tell your doctor if:
- You have long-term liver or kidney problems.
- You are allergic to sulfonylurea drugs.
- You have thyroid problems.
- You have porphyria or glucose-6-phosphate dehydrogenase (G6PD) deficiency.
- You have ever had problems with your adrenal glands.
- You are taking other medicines.

 Pregnancy
Not usually prescribed. Insulin is generally used in pregnancy because it gives better diabetic control.

 Breast-feeding
Drug passes into breast milk and may cause low blood sugar in the baby.

 Infants and children
Not prescribed.

 Over 60
Reduced dose may be necessary. Greater likelihood of low blood sugar exists when glibenclamide is used.

 Driving and hazardous work
Usually no problems, but avoid these activities if you have warning signs of low blood sugar.

 Alcohol
Avoid. Alcoholic drinks may upset diabetic control, increasing the risk of hypoglycaemia.

Surgery and general anaesthetics
Notify your doctor or dentist that you have diabetes before undergoing any surgery.

Sunlight and sunbeds
Take care with exposure to sunlight and tanning beds as the drug may increase the skin's sensitivity to ultraviolet light.

PROLONGED USE

No problems expected.

Monitoring Regular testing of blood sugar control is required. Periodic assessment of the eyes, heart, and kidneys may also be advised.

GLICLAZIDE

Brand names Bilxona, Dacadis MR, Diamicron (MR), Edicil MR, Laaglyda MR, Nazdol MR, Vamju, Ziclaseg, Zicron (PR)
Used in the following combined preparations None

GENERAL INFORMATION

Gliclazide is an oral drug for diabetes belonging to the sulfonylurea group. It stimulates the production and secretion of insulin from the islet cells in the pancreas. This promotes the uptake of sugar into body cells, and thereby lowers the level of sugar in the blood. The drug is used to treat Type 2 diabetes mellitus, in conjunction with diet, exercise, and weight loss. In conditions of severe illness, injury, stress, or surgery, the drug may lose its effectiveness, necessitating the use of insulin injections. Adverse effects of gliclazide are generally mild.

QUICK REFERENCE

Drug group Drug for diabetes (p.100)

Overdose danger rating High

Dependence rating Low

Prescription needed Yes

Available as generic Yes

INFORMATION FOR USERS

Your drug prescription is tailored for you. Do not alter dosage without checking with your doctor.

How taken/used

Tablets, MR tablets.

Frequency and timing of doses
1–2 x daily (in the morning and evening with a meal).

Dosage range
40–320mg daily (doses above 160mg are divided into two doses).

Onset of effect
Within 1 hour.

Duration of action
12–24 hours.

Diet advice
An individualized diabetic diet must be maintained for the drug to be fully effective. Follow the advice of your doctor.

Storage
Keep in original container at room temperature out of the reach of children.

Missed dose
Take with next meal; do not double the dose to account for missed dose.

Stopping the drug
Do not stop the drug without consulting your doctor; stopping the drug may lead to worsening of the underlying condition.

OVERDOSE ACTION

 Seek immediate medical advice in all cases. If any warning symptoms of excessively low blood sugar (such as faintness, dizziness, headache, confusion, sweating, or tremor) occur, eat or drink something sugary. Take emergency action if seizures or loss of consciousness occur.

See Drug poisoning emergency guide (p.518).

SPECIAL PRECAUTIONS

Be sure to tell your doctor if:
- You have long-term liver or kidney problems
- You are allergic to sulfonylurea drugs.
- You have thyroid problems.
- You have porphyria.
- You have ever had problems with your adrenal glands.
- You are taking other medicines.

 Pregnancy
Not recommended. May cause abnormally low blood sugar in the newborn baby. Insulin is generally substituted in pregnancy because it gives better diabetic control.

 Breast-feeding
The drug passes into the breast milk and may cause low blood sugar in the baby. Discuss with your doctor.

 Infants and children
Not prescribed.

 Over 60
Signs of low blood sugar may be more difficult to recognize. Reduced dose may be necessary.

 Driving and hazardous work
Avoid such activities until you have learned how gliclazide affects you because it can cause dizziness, drowsiness, and confusion.

 Alcohol
Avoid. Alcoholic drinks may upset diabetic control, increasing the risk of hypoglycaemia.

Surgery and general anaesthetics
Notify your doctor or dentist that you have diabetes before undergoing any surgery.

Sunlight and sunbeds
Avoid exposure to the sun and do not use a sunlamp or sunbed.

POSSIBLE ADVERSE EFFECTS

Serious adverse effects are rare. Dizziness, confusion, tremors, sweating, and weakness may be signs of low blood sugar due to lack of food or too high a dose of gliclazide.

Symptom/effect	Frequency		Discuss with doctor		Stop taking drug now	Call doctor now
	Common	Rare	Only if severe	In all cases		
Faintness/confusion	●			●		
Weakness/tremor	●			●		
Sweating	●			●		
Constipation/diarrhoea	●		●			
Nausea/vomiting		●		●		
Rash/itching		●		●		
Weight changes		●		●		
Jaundice		●		●		●

INTERACTIONS

General note A variety of drugs may reduce the effect of gliclazide and so may raise blood sugar levels. These include corticosteroids, oestrogens, NSAIDs, diuretics, and rifampicin. Other drugs increase the risk of low blood sugar. These include warfarin, sulfonamides and other antibacterials, aspirin, beta blockers, ACE inhibitors, and antifungals (gliclazide should not be used with miconazole in particular).

PROLONGED USE

No problems expected.

Monitoring Regular testing of blood sugar control is required. Periodic assessment of the eyes, heart, and kidneys may also be advised.

GLUCAGON

Brand name GlucaGen
Used in the following combined preparations None

GENERAL INFORMATION

Glucagon is a hormone produced by the pancreas. A synthetic form is injected as emergency treatment for low blood sugar (hypoglycaemia) in unconscious diabetic patients on insulin. In contrast to insulin, glucagon raises blood sugar by mobilizing liver stores of glycogen, which is released into the blood as glucose. It will not work when glycogen stores are depleted, as in starvation or extreme fasting, alcohol-induced hypoglycaemia, or impaired adrenal function. Glucagon blocks smooth muscle activity in the intestines so may be used to test bowel motility. It can also stimulate contraction of heart muscle so may be used to treat severe beta-blocker overdoses, and it can be used to investigate adult growth hormone deficiency.

Although it is usually given by medical personnel, some people with diabetes may receive packs for emergency use.

INFORMATION FOR USERS

Your drug prescription is tailored for you. Do not alter dosage without checking with your doctor.

How taken/used

Injection.

Frequency and timing of doses
Hypoglycaemia 1 x intramuscular or subcutaneous injection.
Bowel motility testing 1 x intravenous injection.

Adult dosage range
Hypoglycaemia 1mg.
Bowel motility testing 0.2–1.0mg.

Onset of effect
Within 10 minutes.

Duration of action
Up to 40 minutes (intramuscular/subcutaneous injection) or 20 minutes (intravenous injection).

Diet advice
If used to treat hypoglycaemia, carbohydrates should be eaten as soon as possible after the injection to prevent further hypoglycaemia.

Storage
Store at 2–8°C; do not freeze, protect from light, and keep out of the reach of children. The drug should be reconstituted from its powder form just before administration. Packs for personal use in emergencies will last up to 18 months.

Missed dose
Not applicable as the drug is for one-off use only.

Stopping the drug
Not applicable as the drug is for one-off use only.

Exceeding the dose
If the drug is used under medical supervision, overdosage is unlikely. In other situations, exceeding the dose is unlikely to cause major problems but you should consult your doctor promptly if you have nausea or vomiting.

POSSIBLE ADVERSE EFFECTS

Adverse effects of glucagon vary according to its use. If used to treat hypoglycaemia (low blood sugar) in a person with diabetes, the most common effects are nausea and vomiting. If used for diagnostic purposes, adverse effects are rare but may include symptoms of hypoglycaemia (e.g. faintness, confusion, sweating, and dizziness).

Symptom/effect	Frequency		Discuss with doctor		Stop taking drug now	Call doctor now
	Common	Rare	Only if severe	In all cases		
Used for hypoglycaemia						
Nausea	●		●			
Vomiting	●		●			
Abdominal pain		●	●			
Rash/swelling of lips/tongue		●		●	●	●
Bowel motility testing						
Hypoglycaemia		●		●	●	●
Low blood pressure		●		●	●	●
Palpitations		●		●	●	●

INTERACTIONS

Indomethacin may reduce the effectiveness of glucagon.

Warfarin Glucagon may increase the effects of warfarin.

Insulin counteracts the effects of glucagon.

Beta blockers These may cause a short-lived rise in blood pressure and heart rate after patients receive glucagon.

SPECIAL PRECAUTIONS

Be sure to tell your doctor if:
- You have heart problems.
- You have a phaeochromocytoma (a rare tumour of the adrenal gland).
- You have an insulinoma or glucagonoma (rare tumours of the pancreas).
- You are allergic to glucagon or lactose.
- You are taking other medicines.

 Pregnancy
No evidence of risk.

 Breast-feeding
No evidence of risk.

 Infants and children
Reduced dose necessary.

 Over 60
Increased likelihood of adverse effects.

 Driving and hazardous work
If the drug has been used to treat hypoglycaemia, avoid such activities until all signs of hypoglycaemia have disappeared. If the drug has been used diagnostically, avoid such activities until after carbohydrates have been consumed.

 Alcohol
Avoid until blood sugar levels are normal.

PROLONGED USE

Glucagon is not used long term.

GLYCERYL TRINITRATE

Brand names Deponit, Minitran, Nitrocine, Nitro-Dur, Nitrolingual, Nitronal, Percutol, Rectogesic, Transiderm-Nitro, and others
Used in the following combined preparations None

GENERAL INFORMATION

Glyceryl trinitrate is a type of vasodilator called a nitrate and is used to relieve the pain of angina attacks. It is available in short-acting forms (sublingual or buccal tablets, ointment, and spray) and long-acting forms (slow-release tablets and patches). The short-acting forms act very fast to relieve angina. Glyceryl trinitrate is given by injection or infusion in hospital for severe angina, heart failure, and to control high blood pressure. The drug may also be used topically to treat anal fissures.

Glyceryl trinitrate may cause a variety of minor symptoms, such as flushing and headache, most of which can be controlled by adjusting the dosage. It is best taken for the first time while sitting, as fainting may follow the drop in blood pressure caused by the drug.

QUICK REFERENCE

Drug group Anti-angina drug (p.59)

Overdose danger rating Medium

Dependence rating Low

Prescription needed No (most preparations); Yes (injection)

Available as generic Yes

INFORMATION FOR USERS

Follow instructions on the label. Call your doctor if symptoms worsen.

How taken/used

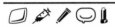

Buccal tablets, sublingual tablets, injection, infusion, ointment, gel, skin patches, spray.

Frequency and timing of doses
Angina prevention 3 x daily (buccal tablets); every 3–4 hours (ointment); once daily (patches). *Angina relief* Use buccal or sublingual tablets, ointment, or spray at the onset of an attack or immediately prior to exercise. Dose may be repeated within 5 minutes if further relief required.
Anal fissure Every 12 hours for up to 8 weeks.

Adult dosage range
Angina prevention 2–15mg daily (buccal tablets); 5–15mg daily (patches); as directed (ointment).
Angina relief 0.3–1mg per dose (sublingual tablets); 1–3mg per dose (buccal tablets); 1–2 sprays per dose (spray).
Anal fissure 3mg daily in 2 equal doses.

Onset of effect
Angina 1–3 minutes (buccal and sublingual tablets and spray); 30–60 minutes (patches and ointment).
Anal fissure 12 hours.

Duration of action
20–30 minutes (sublingual tablets and spray); 3–5 hours (buccal tablets and ointment); up to 24 hours (patches); up to 12 hours (anal fissure preparations).

Diet advice
None.

Storage
Keep sublingual tablets in an airtight glass container fitted with a foil-lined, screw-on cap in a cool, dry place out of the reach of children. Protect from light. Do not expose to heat. Discard tablets within 8 weeks of opening. Check label of other preparations for storage conditions.

Missed dose
If your next dose is due within 6 hours, skip the missed dose and take your next scheduled dose as usual (buccal tablets); take as soon as you remember, or when needed. If your next dose is due within 2 hours, take a single dose now and skip the next (other preparations).

Stopping the drug
Do not stop taking the drug without consulting your doctor.

Exceeding the dose
An occasional unintentional extra dose is unlikely to cause problems. Large overdoses may cause symptoms such as dizziness, vomiting, severe headache, sweating, seizures, or loss of consciousness. Notify your doctor.

SPECIAL PRECAUTIONS

Be sure to consult your doctor or pharmacist before taking this drug if:
- You have any other heart condition.
- You have a lung condition.
- You have long-term liver or kidney problems.
- You have any blood disorders.
- You have glaucoma.
- You have thyroid disease.
- You have low blood pressure.
- You have anaemia.
- You have a recent head injury or stroke.
- You are taking other medicines.

 Pregnancy
Safety in pregnancy not established. Discuss with your doctor.

 Breast-feeding
It is not known whether the drug passes into the breast milk. Discuss with your doctor.

 Infants and children
Not usually prescribed.

 Over 60
No special problems.

 Driving and hazardous work
Avoid such activities until you have learned how glyceryl trinitrate affects you because the drug can cause dizziness.

 Alcohol
Avoid excessive intake. Alcohol may increase the risk of lowered blood pressure, causing dizziness and fainting.

POSSIBLE ADVERSE EFFECTS

The most serious adverse effect is lowered blood pressure, which may cause fainting and collapse. Other adverse effects usually decrease in severity after regular use and can also be controlled by an adjustment in dosage.

Symptom/effect	Frequency		Discuss with doctor		Stop taking drug now	Call doctor now
	Common	Rare	Only if severe	In all cases		
Headache	●		●			
Flushing	●		●			
Dizziness	●			●		
Fainting/collapse		●		●	●	●

INTERACTIONS

Antihypertensive drugs and other anti-angina drugs These drugs increase the possibility of lowered blood pressure or fainting when taken with glyceryl trinitrate.

Sildenafil, tadalafil, and vardenafil The hypotensive effect of glyceryl trinitrate is increased significantly by these drugs; they should not be used with glyceryl trinitrate.

PROLONGED USE

The effects of the drug usually become slightly weaker during prolonged use as the body adapts. Timing of the doses may be changed to prevent this effect. Preparations for anal fissures should not be used for more than 8 weeks.

Monitoring Periodic checks on blood pressure are usually required when the drug is used for angina.

GOSERELIN

Brand names Zoladex, Zoladex LA
Used in the following combined preparations None

GENERAL INFORMATION

Goserelin is a synthetic analogue of the hormone gonadorelin (now more commonly known as gonadotrophin-releasing hormone, or GnRH). Like GnRH, it stimulates the release of other hormones from the pituitary gland, and these in turn control the production of sex hormones.

Goserelin reduces testosterone levels in men and oestrogen levels in premenopausal women, and is used to treat prostate cancer in men and breast cancer in women. At the start of treatment for prostate cancer, it is often given with an anti-androgen drug (see p.104) to control an initial growth spurt of the tumour – known as "tumour flare". The drug is also used in the management of endometriosis and fibroids in women, and assisted reproduction. The first dose is normally given during menstruation to avoid the possibility that the patient may be pregnant. Women of childbearing age are advised to use barrier methods of contraception during treatment.

Loss of bone density is an important side effect in women. Therefore, repeat courses of the drug are given only for cancerous conditions.

QUICK REFERENCE

Drug group Anticancer drug (p.112)
Overdose danger rating Low
Dependence rating Low
Prescription needed Yes
Available as generic No

INFORMATION FOR USERS

Your drug prescription is tailored for you. Do not alter dosage without checking with your doctor.

How taken/used

Implant injection, long-acting implant injection.

Frequency and timing of doses
Endometriosis Every 28 days, maximum of a single 6-month treatment course only (implant).
Fibroids Every 28 days, maximum 3 months' treatment (implant).
Breast and prostate cancer Every 28 days.
Prostate cancer Every 12 weeks (LA implant).

Adult dosage range
3.6mg (implant) every 28 days (endometriosis/fibroids/breast and prostate cancer); 10.8mg (LA implant) every 3 months.

Onset of effect
Within 24 hours (endometriosis/fibroids/breast cancer); 1–2 weeks after tumour flare (prostate).

Duration of action
28 days (implant); 12 weeks (LA implant).

Diet advice
None.

Storage
Not applicable. The drug is not for home use.

Missed dose
No cause for concern. Treatment can be resumed when possible.

Stopping the drug
Do not stop treatment without consulting your doctor.

Exceeding the dose
Overdosage is unlikely since treatment is not self-administered.

POSSIBLE ADVERSE EFFECTS

Symptoms similar to those of the menopause, such as hot flushes and changes in breast size, are common. Some women experience vaginal bleeding during the early stages of treatment. Rare adverse effects should be reported to your doctor straight away.

Symptom/effect	Frequency		Discuss with doctor		Stop taking drug now	Call doctor now
	Common	Rare	Only if severe	In all cases		
Hot flushes/sweating	●		●			
Decreased libido/impotence	●		●			
Bone pain	●		●			
Rash/wheezing		●		●		
Reaction at injection site		●		●		
Ovarian cysts		●		●		
Dizziness/fainting		●		●		
Leg weakness/numbness		●		●		●

INTERACTIONS

Antidiabetic drugs Goserelin may reduce the blood-sugar-lowering effect of these drugs.

SPECIAL PRECAUTIONS

Be sure to tell your doctor if:
- You have osteoporosis.
- You have diabetes.
- You may be pregnant.
- You have previously been treated with goserelin (or another gonadorelin analogue) for endometriosis or fibroids.
- You have polycystic ovarian disease.
- You are allergic to gonadorelin analogues.
- You are taking other medicines.

 Pregnancy
Not prescribed. Risk of harm to the fetus.

 Breast-feeding
Not recommended. Discuss with your doctor.

 Infants and children
Not recommended.

 Over 60
No special problems.

 Driving and hazardous work
No special problems.

 Alcohol
No special problems.

PROLONGED USE

Goserelin is only used in the long term for treatment of prostate or breast cancer. Bone density may be lost, and medication to counteract this may be given.

Monitoring Women are usually monitored for changes in bone density.

HALOPERIDOL

Brand name Haldol, Halkid
Used in the following combined preparations None

GENERAL INFORMATION

Introduced in the 1960s, haloperidol is an antipsychotic drug used to treat schizophrenia and other psychoses, to control mania, and to reduce agitation and violent behaviour. Haloperidol is also used in the short term to treat severe anxiety. It does not cure the underlying disorder but relieves the distressing symptoms. The drug is also used in the control of Tourette's syndrome and to treat intractable hiccups and vomiting.

The main drawback of haloperidol is that it can produce the side effect of abnormal, involuntary movements of the face and stiffness of the limbs. As a result, it is no longer recommended for first-line treatment of schizophrenia.

QUICK REFERENCE

Drug group Butyrophenone antipsychotic drug (p.41)

Overdose danger rating Medium

Dependence rating Low

Prescription needed Yes

Available as generic Yes

INFORMATION FOR USERS

Your drug prescription is tailored for you. Do not alter dosage without checking with your doctor.

How taken/used

Tablets, capsules, liquid, injection, depot injection.

Frequency and timing of doses
2–4 x daily.

Adult dosage range
Mental illness 3–10mg daily initially, up to a maximum of 20mg daily.
Severe anxiety 1mg daily.

Onset of effect
2–3 hours (by mouth); 20–30 minutes (by injection).

Duration of action
6–24 hours (by mouth); 2–4 hours (injection); up to 4 weeks (depot injection).

Diet advice
None.

Storage
Keep in original container at room temperature out of the reach of children.

Missed dose
Take as soon as you remember. If your next dose is due within 3 hours, take a single dose now and skip the next.

Stopping the drug
Do not stop the drug without consulting your doctor; symptoms may recur.

Exceeding the dose
An occasional unintentional extra dose is unlikely to cause problems. Larger overdoses may cause unusual drowsiness, muscle weakness or rigidity, and/or faintness. Notify your doctor.

SPECIAL PRECAUTIONS

Be sure to tell your doctor if:
- You have long-term liver or kidney problems
- You have heart or circulation problems or have had a stroke.
- You have had epileptic seizures.
- You have Parkinson's disease or other movement disorders.
- You are taking other medicines.

Pregnancy
Short-term nervous system problems may occur in babies when haloperidol is taken during the third trimester. The drug is occasionally used under psychiatric supervision. Discuss with your doctor.

Breast-feeding
The drug passes into the breast milk and may affect the baby. Discuss with your doctor.

Infants and children
Rarely required. Reduced dose necessary.

Over 60
Reduced dose may be necessary.

Driving and hazardous work
Avoid such activities until you have learned how haloperidol affects you because the drug may cause drowsiness and slowed reactions.

Alcohol
Avoid. Alcohol may increase the sedative effect of this drug.

POSSIBLE ADVERSE EFFECTS

Haloperidol can cause a variety of minor anticholinergic symptoms that often become less marked with time. The most significant adverse effect, abnormal movements of the face and limb stiffness (parkinsonism), may be controlled by dosage adjustment.

Symptom/effect	Frequency		Discuss with doctor		Stop taking drug now	Call doctor now
	Common	Rare	Only if severe	In all cases		
Drowsiness/lethargy/insomnia	●		●			
Sexual dysfunction	●		●			
Parkinsonism	●			●		
Abnormal movements	●			●		
Breathlessness	●			●		
Palpitations/sweating/stiffness		●		●		
High fever/confusion		●		●	●	●

INTERACTIONS

Sedatives Sedatives are likely to increase the sedative properties of haloperidol.

Rifampicin and anticonvulsants may reduce the effects of haloperidol, the dosage of which may need to be increased.

Lithium This drug may increase the risk of parkinsonism and effects on the nerves.

Methyldopa This drug may increase the risk of parkinsonism and low blood pressure.

Anticholinergic drugs Haloperidol may increase the side effects of these drugs.

Drugs that can affect heart rhythm (e.g. antidepressants, antifungals, anti-arrhythmics, antibiotics, and antihistamines) There is an increased risk of irregular heart rhythms when these drugs are used with haloperidol.

PROLONGED USE

Use of this drug for more than a few months may lead to tardive dyskinesia (abnormal, involuntary movements of the eyes, face, and tongue). Occasionally, jaundice may occur. In older people with dementia who take haloperidol, a small increase in strokes, blood clots, seizures, and death has been reported.

HEPARIN/LOW MOLECULAR WEIGHT HEPARINS

Brand names [dalteparin] Fragmin, [enoxaparin] Clexane, Inhixa, [tinzaparin] Innohep
Used in the following combined preparations None

GENERAL INFORMATION

Heparin is an anticoagulant drug used to prevent formation of blood clots and help clots disperse. Because the drug acts quickly, it is particularly useful in emergencies to prevent further clotting when a clot has already reached the lungs or the brain, for instance. People undergoing open heart surgery or kidney dialysis are given heparin to prevent clotting. A low dose is sometimes given following surgery to prevent the development of deep vein thrombosis (clots in the leg veins). Heparin is often given in conjunction with other slower-acting anticoagulants, such as warfarin. It is also used to treat unstable angina.

The most serious adverse effect, as with all anticoagulants, is excessive bleeding, so the blood's clotting ability is watched very carefully. Bruising may occur around the injection site.

Several types of heparin, called low molecular weight heparins (LMWH), do not have to be administered in hospital.

QUICK REFERENCE

Drug group Anticoagulant drug (p.62)

Overdose danger rating High

Dependence rating Low

Prescription needed Yes

Available as generic Yes (both heparin and LMWH)

INFORMATION FOR USERS

This drug is given only under medical supervision and is not for self-administration.

How taken/used

Injection, intravenous infusion.

Frequency and timing of doses
Every 8–12 hours, or continuous intravenous infusion once daily (LMWH).

Dosage range
Dosage is determined by the nature of the condition being treated or prevented.

Onset of effect
Within 15 minutes.

Duration of action
4–12 hours after treatment is stopped; 24 hours after end of treatment (LMWH).

Diet advice
None.

Storage
Keep in original container at room temperature out of the reach of children.

Missed dose
Notify your doctor.

Stopping the drug
Do not stop taking the drug without consulting your doctor. Stopping the drug may lead to clotting of blood.

OVERDOSE ACTION

Seek immediate medical advice in all cases. Take emergency action if bleeding, severe headache, or loss of consciousness occur.

See Drug poisoning emergency guide (p.518).

SPECIAL PRECAUTIONS

Be sure to tell your doctor if:
- You have long-term liver or kidney problems.
- You have high blood pressure.
- You bleed easily or are currently bleeding.
- You have any allergies.
- You have peptic ulcers.
- You have diabetes.
- You have had a previous reaction to heparin.
- You have had a recent stroke, injury, or surgery.
- You are taking other medicines.

 Pregnancy
Careful monitoring is necessary as it may cause the mother to bleed excessively if taken near delivery. Discuss with your doctor.

 Breast-feeding
No evidence of risk.

 Infants and children
Reduced dose necessary according to age and weight.

 Over 60
No special problems, but older people may be more prone to bleeding.

 Driving and hazardous work
Avoid risk of injury, since excessive bruising and bleeding may occur.

 Alcohol
No special problems.

Surgery and general anaesthetics
Heparin may need to be stopped beforehand. Discuss this with your doctor or dentist before having any surgery.

POSSIBLE ADVERSE EFFECTS

As with all anticoagulants, bleeding is the most common adverse effect of heparin, and the risk of bleeding is increased in people with impaired kidney function. The less common effects may occur during long-term treatment.

Symptom/effect	Frequency		Discuss with doctor		Stop taking drug now	Call doctor now
	Common	Rare	Only if severe	In all cases		
Bleeding/bruising	●			●		●
Hair loss		●		●		
Aching bones		●		●		
Breathing difficulties		●		●		●
Jaundice/vomiting blood		●		●		●
Rash		●		●	●	●

INTERACTIONS

Aspirin and other NSAIDs may increase the anticoagulant effect of heparin and the risk of bleeding in the intestines or joints. Do not take these drugs with heparin.

ACE inhibitors and potassium supplements taken with heparins may increase the risk of high blood potassium.

Clopidogrel, ticlopidine, and dipyridamole The anticoagulant effect of heparin may be increased when it is taken with these drugs. The dosage of heparin may need to be adjusted accordingly.

PROLONGED USE

Osteoporosis and hair loss may occur very rarely with long-term use; tolerance to heparin may also develop.

Monitoring Periodic blood and liver function tests will be required.

HYDROCHLOROTHIAZIDE

Brand names None
Used in the following combined preparations Acezide, Capozide, Co-amilozide, Cozaar Comp, Dyazide, Moduretic, and others

GENERAL INFORMATION

Hydrochlorothiazide belongs to the thiazide group of diuretic drugs, which remove excess water from the body and reduce oedema (fluid retention) in people with congestive heart failure, kidney disorders, cirrhosis of the liver, and premenstrual syndrome. It is also used in combination with other antihypertensive drugs (see p.60), to treat high blood pressure; in the UK, it is only available in combination with other antihypertensives. The drug increases potassium loss in the urine, which can cause a variety of symptoms (see p.57), and increases the likelihood of irregular heart rhythms, particularly in patients who are taking drugs such as digoxin. For this reason, potassium supplements or potassium-sparing diuretics are often given with hydrochlorothiazide.

(see p.60), (see p.57),

QUICK REFERENCE

Drug group Thiazide diuretic (p.57)
Overdose danger rating Low
Dependence rating Low
Prescription needed Yes
Available as generic No

(p.57)

INFORMATION FOR USERS

Your drug prescription is tailored for you. Do not alter dosage without checking with your doctor.

How taken/used

Tablets.

Frequency and timing of doses
Once daily, or every 2 days, early in the day.

Adult dosage range
Hypertension 25–50mg daily.
Oedema 25–100mg daily.

Onset of effect
Within 2 hours.

Duration of action
6–12 hours.

Diet advice
Use of this drug may reduce potassium in the body. Eat plenty of fresh fruit and vegetables. Discuss with your doctor the advisability of reducing your salt intake.

Storage
Keep in original container at room temperature out of the reach of children. Protect from light.

Missed dose
No cause for concern, but take as soon as you remember. However, if it is late in the day do not take the missed dose, or you may have to get up during the night to pass urine. Take the next scheduled dose as usual.

Stopping the drug
Do not stop the drug without consulting your doctor; symptoms may recur.

Exceeding the dose
An occasional unintentional extra dose is unlikely to be a cause for concern. But if you notice any unusual symptoms, or if a large overdose has been taken, notify your doctor.

SPECIAL PRECAUTIONS

Be sure to tell your doctor if:
- You have long-term liver or kidney problems.
- You have had gout.
- You have diabetes.
- You are taking other medicines.

 Pregnancy
Safety in pregnancy not established. Discuss with your doctor.

 Breast-feeding
The drug passes into the breast milk, but at normal doses adverse effects on the baby are unlikely. Discuss with your doctor.

 Infants and children
Not usually prescribed. Reduced dose necessary.

 Over 60
Increased likelihood of adverse effects.

 Driving and hazardous work
Avoid such activities until you have learned how hydrochlorothiazide affects you because the drug may reduce mental alertness and cause dizziness.

 Alcohol
Keep intake low. Hydrochlorothiazide increases the likelihood of dehydration and hangovers after consumption of alcohol.

POSSIBLE ADVERSE EFFECTS

Most effects are caused by excessive loss of potassium. This can usually be corrected by taking a potassium supplement. In rare cases, gout may occur in susceptible people, and certain forms of diabetes may become more difficult to control.

Symptom/effect	Frequency Common	Frequency Rare	Discuss with doctor Only if severe	Discuss with doctor In all cases	Stop taking drug now	Call doctor now
Muscle cramps	●		●			
Lethargy	●		●			
Dizziness/headache	●		●			
Erectile dysfunction	●		●			
Nausea/vomiting	●			●		
Constipation	●			●		
Rash	●			●	●	
New skin lesions	●			●		

INTERACTIONS

Non-steroidal anti-inflammatory drugs (NSAIDs) Some NSAIDs may reduce the diuretic effect of hydrochlorothiazide, whose dose may need to be adjusted.

Anti-arrhythmic and digitalis drugs increase the risk of toxicity from low blood potassium with hydrochlorothiazide.

Corticosteroids These drugs further increase loss of potassium from the body when taken with hydrochlorothiazide, and may reduce its diuretic effect.

Lithium Hydrochlorothiazide may increase lithium levels in the blood, leading to a risk of serious adverse effects.

PROLONGED USE

Excessive loss of potassium and imbalances of other salts may result.

Hydrochlorothiazide increases skin sensitivity to sunlight, and long-term use carries an increased risk of non-melanoma skin cancers. Patients should see their doctor if they develop any new skin lesions.

Monitoring Blood tests may be performed periodically to check kidney function and levels of potassium and other salts.

HYDROCORTISONE

Brand names Corlan, Dioderm, Efcortelan, Efcortesol, Hydrocortistab, Hydrocortone, Mildison, Solu-Cortef
Used in the following combined preparations Alphaderm, Anusol Plus HC, Xyloproct, and many others

GENERAL INFORMATION

Hydrocortisone is chemically identical to the hormone cortisol, which is produced by the adrenal glands, and is therefore prescribed to replace natural hormones in adrenal insufficiency (Addison's disease). The main use of this drug is in treating a variety of allergic and inflammatory conditions. In topical preparations, it gives prompt relief from inflammation of the skin, eye, and outer ear. It is also used orally or by injection to relieve asthma, inflammatory bowel disease, and many rheumatic and allergic disorders. Injected directly into the joints, the drug relieves pain and stiffness (see p.76).

Overuse of skin preparations can lead to permanent thinning of the skin. Taken by mouth, long-term treatment with high doses may cause serious side effects.

QUICK REFERENCE

Drug group Corticosteroid (p.99)

Overdose danger rating Low

Dependence rating Low

Prescription needed Yes (except for some topical preparations)

Available as generic Yes

INFORMATION FOR USERS

Your drug prescription is tailored for you. Do not alter dosage without checking with your doctor.

How taken/used

Tablets, lozenges, injection, rectal foam, cream, ointment, eye/ear ointment/drops.

Frequency and timing of doses
Varies according to condition and preparation.

Dosage range
Varies according to condition and preparation.

Onset of effect
Within hours. Full effect may not be felt for several days.

Duration of action
Up to 12 hours.

Diet advice
Salt intake may need to be restricted when the drug is taken by mouth. It may also be necessary to take potassium supplements.

Storage
Keep in original container at room temperature out of the reach of children.

Missed dose
Take as soon as you remember. If your next dose is due within 2 hours, take a single dose now and skip the next.

Stopping the drug
Do not stop the drug without consulting your doctor, particularly after prolonged treatment with oral hydrocortisone – sudden cessation of the drug may be harmful. Your doctor will supervise a gradual reduction in dosage.

Exceeding the dose
An occasional unintentional extra dose is unlikely to be a cause for concern. But if you notice any unusual symptoms, or if a large overdose has been taken, notify your doctor.

SPECIAL PRECAUTIONS

Be sure to tell your doctor if:
- You have liver or kidney problems.
- You have had a peptic ulcer.
- You have had a mental illness or epilepsy.
- You have glaucoma.
- You have had tuberculosis.
- You have diabetes or heart problems.
- You are taking other medicines.

 Pregnancy
No evidence of risk with topical preparations. Oral doses may adversely affect the developing baby. Discuss with your doctor.

 Breast-feeding
The drug passes into the breast milk and may affect the baby. Discuss with your doctor.

 Infants and children
Reduced dose necessary.

 Over 60
Reduced dose may be necessary.

 Driving and hazardous work
No special problems.

 Alcohol
Avoid. Alcohol may increase the risk of peptic ulcer when this drug is taken by mouth.

Surgery and general anaesthetics
Notify your doctor; you may need to have hydrocortisone by injection in hospital.

Infection
Avoid exposure to chickenpox, shingles, or measles if you are on systemic treatment.

POSSIBLE ADVERSE EFFECTS

The most serious adverse effects only occur when hydrocortisone is taken by mouth in high doses for long periods of time. These are carefully monitored during treatment.

Symptom/effect	Frequency		Discuss with doctor		Stop taking drug now	Call doctor now
	Common	Rare	Only if severe	In all cases		
Indigestion	●		●			
Weight gain	●		●			
Acne	●		●			
Fluid retention		●		●		
Muscle weakness		●		●		
Mood changes		●		●		
Menstrual irregularities		●		●		

INTERACTIONS

Barbiturates, anticonvulsants, and rifampicin These drugs reduce the effectiveness of hydrocortisone.

Antidiabetic drugs Hydrocortisone reduces the action of these drugs.

Antihypertensive drugs Hydrocortisone reduces the effects of these drugs.

Vaccines Severe reactions can occur if certain vaccines are given while taking hydrocortisone.

Aspirin and other NSAIDs Increased risk of peptic ulcer and bleeding from the stomach with hydrocortisone.

PROLONGED USE

Prolonged high dosage can lead to peptic ulcers, glaucoma, muscle weakness, osteoporosis, and growth retardation in children. People on long-term treatment should carry a steroid treatment card.

Monitoring Periodic checks on blood pressure and blood sugar levels are usually required (oral forms).

HYOSCINE

Brand names Boots Travel Calm, Buscopan, Joy-Rides, Kwells, Scopoderm TTS
Used in the following combined preparation Papaveretum and Hyoscine Injection

GENERAL INFORMATION

Originally derived from the henbane plant (*Hyoscyamus niger*), hyoscine is an anticholinergic drug (see p.35) that has both an antispasmodic effect on the intestine and a calming action on the nerve pathways that control nausea and vomiting. By its anticholinergic action, hyoscine also dilates the pupil.

The drug is produced in two forms. Hyoscine butylbromide is prescribed to reduce spasm of the gastrointestinal tract in irritable bowel syndrome, and sometimes with other drugs to treat dysmenorrhoea (painful menstruation). Hyoscine hydrobromide is used to control motion sickness and nausea and giddiness caused by disturbances of the inner ear (see Vertigo and Ménière's disease, p.46) and can be given as tablets and skin patches. Eye drops containing this form are used to dilate the pupil in eye examinations and eye surgery. It is also used as premedication to dry secretions before operations.

QUICK REFERENCE

Drug group Drug for irritable bowel syndrome (p.68), drug affecting the pupil (p.130), and anti-emetic drug (p.46)

Overdose danger rating Medium

Dependence rating Low

Prescription needed No (for most preparations)

Available as generic Yes

INFORMATION FOR USERS

Follow instructions on the label. Call your doctor if symptoms worsen.

How taken/used

Tablets, injection, skin patches.

Frequency and timing of doses
Irritable bowel syndrome Up to 4 x daily, as required, by mouth (tablets).
Motion sickness Up to 3 x daily (tablets); every 3 days as required (patches).

Adult dosage range
Irritable bowel syndrome 30–80mg daily (hyoscine butylbromide).
Motion sickness 0.3mg per dose (tablets); 1 mg over 72 hours (hyoscine hydrobromide patches).

Onset of effect
Within 1 hour.

Duration of action
Up to 6 hours (by mouth); up to 72 hours (patches).

Diet advice
None.

Storage
Keep in original container at room temperature out of the reach of children. Protect from light.

Missed dose
Take when you remember. Adjust the timing of your next dose accordingly.

Stopping the drug
Can be safely stopped as soon as you no longer need it.

Exceeding the dose
An occasional unintentional extra dose is unlikely to cause problems. Large overdoses may cause drowsiness or agitation. Notify your doctor.

SPECIAL PRECAUTIONS

Be sure to consult your doctor or pharmacist before taking this drug if:
- You have long-term liver or kidney problems.
- You have heart problems.
- You have epilepsy.
- You have megacolon or intestinal obstruction problems.
- You have had glaucoma.
- You have prostate trouble or urinary retention.
- You have porphyria.
- You are taking other medicines.

 Pregnancy
Safety not established. Discuss with your doctor.

 Breast-feeding
Safety not established. Discuss with your doctor.

 Infants and children
Not recommended under 4 years for motion sickness. Patches not recommended under 10 years. Other uses not recommended under 6 years. Reduced dose necessary in older children.

 Over 60
Reduced dose may be necessary.

 Driving and hazardous work
Avoid such activities until you have learned how hyoscine affects you because the drug can cause drowsiness and blurred vision.

 Alcohol
Avoid. Alcohol may increase the sedative effect of this drug.

POSSIBLE ADVERSE EFFECTS

Taken by mouth or by injection, hyoscine has a strong anticholinergic effect on the body, causing a variety of minor symptoms, such as dry mouth. These can sometimes be minimized by a reduction in dosage. The butylbromide form of hyoscine is less likely to cause these side effects.

Symptom/effect	Frequency		Discuss with doctor		Stop taking drug now	Call doctor now
	Common	Rare	Only if severe	In all cases		
Drowsiness	●		●			
Dry mouth	●		●			
Blurred vision	●			●		
Constipation		●	●			
Difficulty in passing urine		●		●		
Increase in heart rate		●		●		

INTERACTIONS

Anticholinergic drugs Many drugs have anticholinergic, or antimuscarinic, effects, such as dry mouth, difficulty in passing urine, and constipation. The risk of such side effects is increased with hyoscine.

Sedatives All drugs that have a sedative effect on the central nervous system are likely to increase the sedative properties of hyoscine. Such drugs include anti-anxiety and sleeping drugs, antidepressants, opioid analgesics, and antipsychotics.

Sublingual tablets Hyoscine can cause a dry mouth and may reduce the effectiveness of sublingual tablets.

PROLONGED USE

Use of this drug for longer than a few days is unlikely to be necessary.

IBUPROFEN

Brand names Anadin Ultra, Brufen, Calprofen, Fenbid, Hedex, Ibugel, Ibuleve, Ibumousse, Nurofen, and many others
Used in the following combined preparations Nurofen Plus, Nuromol, Solpadeine Migraine, and others

GENERAL INFORMATION

Ibuprofen is a non-steroidal anti-inflammatory drug (NSAID) which, like other drugs in this group, reduces pain, stiffness, fever, and inflammation. It is an effective treatment for the symptoms of osteoarthritis, rheumatoid arthritis, and gout. In the treatment of rheumatoid arthritis, ibuprofen may be prescribed with slower-acting drugs. Other uses of the drug include the relief of mild to moderate headache (including migraine), juvenile arthritis, menstrual and dental pain, ankylosing spondylitis, pain resulting from soft tissue injuries, or the pain that may follow an operation.

Ibuprofen has fewer side effects (especially at low doses) than many other NSAIDs, and a lower risk of gastrointestinal bleeding and ulceration.

Ibuprofen is also available as a cream or gel that can be applied to the skin for muscular aches and sprains.

QUICK REFERENCE

Drug group Analgesic (p.36) and non-steroidal anti-inflammatory drug (p.74)

Overdose danger rating Low

Dependence rating Low

Prescription needed No (some preparations)

Available as generic Yes

INFORMATION FOR USERS

Follow instructions on the label. Call your doctor if symptoms worsen.

How taken/used

Tablets, SR tablets, capsules, SR capsules, liquid, granules, cream, mousse, gel.

Frequency and timing of doses
1–2 x daily (SR preparations); 3–4 x daily (topical forms and other oral preparations). Take all oral preparations with or after food.

Dosage range
Adults 600mg–2.4g daily.
Children Dosage varies according to age and/or body weight.

Onset of effect
Pain relief begins in 15 minutes–2 hours. The full anti-inflammatory effect in arthritic conditions may not be felt for up to 2 weeks.

Duration of action
5–10 hours.

Diet advice
None.

Storage
Keep in original container at room temperature out of the reach of children.

Missed dose
Take as soon as you remember. If your next dose is due within 2 hours, take a single dose now and skip the next.

Stopping the drug
When taken for short-term pain relief, the drug can be safely stopped if no longer needed. If it is given for long-term treatment of arthritis, seek medical advice before stopping it.

Exceeding the dose
An occasional unintentional extra dose is unlikely to be a cause for concern. But if you notice any unusual symptoms, or if a large overdose has been taken, notify your doctor.

SPECIAL PRECAUTIONS

Be sure to consult your doctor or pharmacist before taking this drug if:
- You have long-term kidney or liver problems.
- You have high blood pressure, heart problems, or coronary artery disease, or have had a previous stroke.
- You have had a peptic ulcer, oesophagitis, or acid indigestion.
- You are allergic to aspirin or other NSAIDs.
- You have asthma.
- You are taking other medicines.

 Pregnancy
The drug may increase the risks of adverse effects on the baby's heart and may prolong labour if taken in the third trimester. Discuss with your doctor.

 Breast-feeding
The drug passes into the breast milk, but at normal doses adverse effects on the baby are unlikely. Discuss with your doctor.

 Infants and children
Reduced dose necessary.

 Over 60
Reduced dose may be necessary.

 Driving and hazardous work
No problems expected.

 Alcohol
Avoid. Alcohol may increase the risk of stomach disorders with ibuprofen.

Surgery and general anaesthetics
Ibuprofen may prolong bleeding. Discuss with your doctor or dentist before any surgery.

POSSIBLE ADVERSE EFFECTS

The most common adverse effects are the result of gastrointestinal disturbances. Black or bloodstained faeces should be reported to your doctor without delay.

Symptom/effect	Frequency		Discuss with doctor		Stop taking drug now	Call doctor now
	Common	Rare	Only if severe	In all cases		
Heartburn/indigestion	●		●			
Nausea/vomiting	●		●			
Headache		●	●			
Dizziness/drowsiness		●	●			
Swollen feet or legs		●	●			
Weight gain		●	●			
Rash/itching		●		●	●	
Wheezing/breathlessness		●		●	●	●
Black/bloodstained faeces		●		●	●	●

INTERACTIONS

General note Ibuprofen interacts with a wide range of drugs, including aspirin, other NSAIDs, oral anticoagulants, corticosteroids, and SSRI antidepressants, to increase the risk of bleeding and/or peptic ulcers.

Ciprofloxacin Ibuprofen increases risk of seizures with this and related antibiotics.

Antihypertensive drugs and diuretics The beneficial effects of these drugs may be reduced by ibuprofen; rarely, diuretics can also increase the risk of adverse effects on the kidneys.

Ciclosporin and tacrolimus increase the risk of adverse effects on the kidneys.

PROLONGED USE

There is an increased risk of bleeding from peptic ulcers and in the bowel with prolonged use of ibuprofen. There is also a small risk of a heart attack or stroke. To minimize these risks, the lowest effective dose is given for the shortest duration.

IMATINIB

Brand name Glivec
Used in the following combined preparations None

GENERAL INFORMATION

Imatinib belongs to an expanding class of anticancer drugs called tyrosine kinase inhibitors, which act by blocking a specific enzyme (tyrosine kinase) in certain cancer cells, thus halting their growth and replication. Because of this targeted action, the drugs have relatively little effect on non-cancerous cells (unlike many older anticancer drugs). Imatinib is used principally against chronic myeloid leukaemia (CML) but may also be used to treat some other bone marrow cancers and some rare gastrointestinal tumours. It can be used alone or in combination with other anticancer drugs.

Imatinib generally produces fewer adverse effects than older anticancer drugs. However, it does not usually provide a long-term cure because the cancer cells eventually mutate to become resistant to its effects.

INFORMATION FOR USERS

Your drug prescription is tailored for you. Do not alter dosage without checking with your doctor.

How taken/used

Tablets.

Frequency and timing of doses
1–2 x daily with food, at same time every day.

Adult dosage range
100–800mg daily.

Onset of effect
The drug starts inhibiting the enzyme within hours but the effect on cancer cells may take days to weeks to become detectable.

Duration of action
Several days.

Diet advice
None.

Storage
Store in original packaging below 30°C out of the reach of children.

Missed dose
Take as soon as you remember that day. If you do not remember that day, omit the missed dose and take the next dose as scheduled. Do not double your next dose.

Stopping the drug
Do not stop the drug without consulting your doctor because this may lead to a worsening of the underlying condition.

Exceeding the dose
An occasional unintentional extra dose is unlikely to cause major problems. But if you notice any unusual symptoms or if a large overdose has been taken, notify your doctor.

SPECIAL PRECAUTIONS

Be sure to tell your doctor if:
• You have liver, kidney, or heart problems.
• You have a history of hepatitis E.
• You have had your thyroid gland removed and are taking thyroxine.
• You are taking other medicines.

 Pregnancy
Safety not established. Discuss with your doctor.

 Breast-feeding
Not recommended.

 Infants and children
Used only by specialist children's doctors.

 Over 60
No special problems.

 Driving and hazardous work
Avoid until you have learned how the drug affects you. It may sometimes cause dizziness or blurred vision.

 Alcohol
No special problems.

POSSIBLE ADVERSE EFFECTS

Imatinib can cause a variety of adverse effects, commonly gastrointestinal symptoms such as nausea, vomiting, and diarrhoea. Oedema (fluid build-up) is also common. The drug may affect the blood count, which may give rise to bruising, bleeding, and signs of infection. If these symptoms occur, you should report them to your doctor.

Symptom/effect	Frequency		Discuss with doctor		Stop taking drug now	Call doctor now
	Common	Rare	Only if severe	In all cases		
Headache/muscle pain	●		●			
Dizziness/lightheadedness	●		●			
Nausea/vomiting/diarrhoea	●		●			
Rapid weight gain/oedema	●			●		
Rash/red skin/blistering	●			●		
Fever/sore throat/mouth ulcers	●			●		●
Unexpected bleeding/bruising	●			●		●
Chest pain/palpitations/cough		●		●		
Jaundice/severe abdominal pain		●		●		●

INTERACTIONS

General note A wide range of drugs (including over-the-counter and herbal remedies) may affect levels of imatinib in the body, and it is therefore important to check with your doctor or pharmacist before taking any new medication or remedy.

Thyroxine Imatinib can increase the breakdown of thyroxine so the thyroxine dose may need adjustment.

Warfarin Imatinib may affect the level of warfarin; this may require adjustment of the warfarin dose, or you may be switched to heparin.

PROLONGED USE

Imatinib tends to produce fewer adverse effects than many other anticancer drugs when used long term, but the cancer cells may become resistant to the drug's effects, in which case treatment will be stopped.

Monitoring Regular monitoring is carried out to check your blood count and the function of organs such as the liver and kidney. Blood tests are also performed to monitor the response of the cancer to imatinib. Children who are being treated with imatinib should have their growth regularly monitored.

IMIPRAMINE

Brand names None
Used in the following combined preparation None

GENERAL INFORMATION

Imipramine belongs to the tricyclic class of antidepressant drugs. The drug is used mainly in the long-term treatment of depression to elevate mood, improve appetite, increase physical activity, and restore interest in everyday life. Because imipramine is less sedating than some other tricyclic antidepressants, it is particularly useful when a depressed person has become withdrawn or apathetic. Imipramine is also prescribed to treat night-time enuresis (bedwetting) in children.

The most common adverse effects of imipramine are the result of the drug's anticholinergic action. In overdose, imipramine may cause coma and abnormal heart rhythms.

QUICK REFERENCE

Drug group Antidepressant (p.40) and drug for urinary disorders (p.126)

Overdose danger rating High

Dependence rating Low

Prescription needed Yes

Available as generic Yes

INFORMATION FOR USERS

Your drug prescription is tailored for you. Do not alter dosage without checking with your doctor.

How taken/used

Tablets, liquid.

Frequency and timing of doses
1–3 x daily.

Dosage range
Adults Usually 75–200mg daily (up to a maximum of 300mg in hospital patients). *Children* Reduced dose according to age and weight. Usual starting dose 25mg daily in children aged 6–7 years.

Onset of effect
Some benefits and effects may appear within hours, but full antidepressant effect may not be felt for 2–6 weeks.

Duration of action
Following prolonged treatment, antidepressant effect may persist for up to 6 weeks, common adverse effects for 1–2 weeks.

Diet advice
None.

Storage
Keep in original container at room temperature out of the reach of children.

Missed dose
Take as soon as you remember. If your next dose is due within 3 hours, take a single dose now and skip the next.

Stopping the drug
Do not stop taking the drug without consulting your doctor, who will supervise a gradual reduction in dosage. Stopping abruptly may cause withdrawal symptoms.

OVERDOSE ACTION

 Seek immediate medical advice in all cases. Take emergency action if palpitations are noted or consciousness is lost.

See Drug poisoning emergency guide (p.518).

SPECIAL PRECAUTIONS

Be sure to tell your doctor if:
- You have had heart problems.
- You have long-term liver or kidney problems.
- You have had epileptic seizures.
- You have porphyria.
- You have had glaucoma.
- You have prostate problems.
- You have had mania or a psychotic illness.
- You are taking other medicines.

 Pregnancy
Avoid if possible. Discuss with your doctor.

 Breast-feeding
The drug passes into the breast milk, but at normal doses adverse effects on the baby are unlikely. Discuss with your doctor.

 Infants and children
Not recommended under 6 years. Reduced dose necessary in older children.

 Over 60
Increased likelihood of adverse effects. Reduced dose may therefore be necessary.

 Driving and hazardous work
Avoid such activities until you have learned how imipramine affects you because the drug can cause reduced alertness and blurred vision.

 Alcohol
Avoid. Alcohol may increase the sedative effect of imipramine.

Surgery and general anaesthetics
Imipramine treatment may need to be stopped before you have a general anaesthetic. Discuss this with your doctor or dentist before any operation.

POSSIBLE ADVERSE EFFECTS

The possible adverse effects of this drug are mainly the result of its anticholinergic action and its effect on the normal rhythm of the heart.

Symptom/effect	Frequency		Discuss with doctor		Stop taking drug now	Call doctor now
	Common	Rare	Only if severe	In all cases		
Sweating/flushing/dry mouth	●		●			
Constipation/weight gain	●		●			
Blurred vision	●			●		
Dizziness/drowsiness	●			●		
Difficulty in passing urine		●		●	●	
Confusion		●		●	●	
Palpitations		●		●	●	●

INTERACTIONS

Anti-arrhythmic drugs increase the risk of abnormal heart rhythms.

Sedatives and warfarin Imipramine may increase the effects of these drugs.

Antihypertensives and anticonvulsants The effects of these are reduced by imipramine.

Monoamine oxidase inhibitors (MAOIs) are prescribed with imipramine only under strict supervision due to the possibility of a serious interaction.

Some selective serotonin reuptake inhibitors (SSRIs) can increase levels of imipramine.

PROLONGED USE

No problems expected. Imipramine is not usually prescribed for children as a treatment for bedwetting for longer than 3 months.

INDAPAMIDE

Brand names Alkapamid, Cardide SR, Indipam, Lorvacs XL, Natrilix, Natrilix SR, Rawel, Tensaid XL
Used in the following combined preparation Coversyl Plus

GENERAL INFORMATION

Indapamide is closely related to thiazide diuretics in its effects but is mainly used to treat hypertension (high blood pressure). The drug increases secretion of salt by the kidneys in the same way as thiazide diuretics. This causes more water to be lost from the body, which reduces the total blood volume and lowers blood pressure. Indapamide is sometimes combined with other antihypertensive drugs but not with other diuretics. Indapamide's diuretic effects are slight at low doses, but susceptible people need to have their blood levels of potassium and uric acid monitored. These include older people, those taking digitalis drugs, or those with gout or hyperaldosteronism (overproduction of the hormone aldosterone). Unlike the thiazides, indapamide does not affect control of diabetes at low doses.

INFORMATION FOR USERS

Your drug prescription is tailored for you. Do not alter dosage without checking with your doctor.

How taken/used

Tablets, SR tablets.

Frequency and timing of doses
Once daily in the morning.

Adult dosage range
1.5–2.5mg.

Onset of effect
1–2 hours, but the full effect may take several months.

Duration of action
12–24 hours.

Diet advice
None.

Storage
Keep in original container at room temperature out of the reach of children.

Missed dose
Take as soon as you remember. If your next dose is due within 4 hours, take a single dose now and skip the next.

Stopping the drug
Do not stop taking the drug without consulting your doctor; high blood pressure may return.

Exceeding the dose
An occasional unintentional extra dose is unlikely to cause problems. But if you notice any unusual symptoms, or if a large overdose has been taken, notify your doctor.

SPECIAL PRECAUTIONS

Be sure to tell your doctor if:
- You have liver or kidney problems.
- You have diabetes.
- You have gout.
- You have hyperaldosteronism or hyperparathyroidism.
- You are allergic to sulfonamide drugs.
- You are taking other medicines.

Pregnancy
Safety not established. Discuss with your doctor.

Breast-feeding
Safety not established. Discuss with your doctor.

Infants and children
Not prescribed.

Over 60
No special problems.

Driving and hazardous work
No special problems.

Alcohol
No special problems.

POSSIBLE ADVERSE EFFECTS

Indapamide usually causes few adverse effects. Rashes and mild disruptions in blood chemistry (due to loss of electrolytes such as potassium in the urine) are the most common problems.

Symptom/effect	Frequency		Discuss with doctor		Stop taking drug now	Call doctor now
	Common	Rare	Only if severe	In all cases		
Fatigue/muscle cramps	●		●			
Rash	●			●		
Headache/dizziness		●	●			
Diarrhoea/constipation/nausea		●	●			
Palpitations/fainting		●		●		
Tingling/"pins and needles"		●		●		
Erectile dysfunction		●		●		

PROLONGED USE

Long-term use of indapamide may lead to potassium loss.

Monitoring Blood potassium and uric acid levels may be checked periodically.

INTERACTIONS

Loop diuretics There is a risk of imbalance of salts in the blood if these drugs are taken with indapamide.

Lithium Blood levels of lithium are increased when it is taken with indapamide.

Anti-arrhythmic and digitalis drugs Loss of potassium with indapamide use may lead to toxicity with these drugs.

INFLIXIMAB

Brand names Flixabi, Inflectra, Remicade, Remsima, Zessly
Used in the following combined preparations None

GENERAL INFORMATION

Infliximab is a monoclonal antibody (see p.114) that can modify the activity of the immune system and thereby reduce inflammation. It reduces the activity of a substance produced by the body called tumour necrosis factor alpha (TNF-alpha), which drives a number of inflammatory conditions, such as psoriasis, rheumatoid arthritis, Crohn's disease, ankylosing spondylitis, and ulcerative colitis. The drug can therefore be used to treat these conditions by reducing TNF-alpha activity.

Infliximab is given by intravenous infusion, generally into the arm.

Infections, most often affecting the upper respiratory tract and the urinary tract, occur more commonly with infliximab treatment.

QUICK REFERENCE

Drug group Drug for inflammatory bowel disease (p.70) and disease-modifying antirheumatic drug (p.75)

Overdose danger rating Low

Dependence rating Low

Prescription needed Yes

Available as generic Yes

INFORMATION FOR USERS

The drug is given only under medical supervision and is not for self-administration.

How taken/used

Intravenous infusion.

Frequency and timing of doses
Every 6–8 weeks, although doses may be more frequent at the start of treatment. Infusion time is generally over a 2-hour period.

Adult dosage range
Dosing is based on body weight; 3mg/kg to 5mg/kg per dose.

Onset of effect
1 hour; full beneficial effect may take several weeks to develop.

Duration of action
2–8 weeks.

Diet advice
None.

Storage
Not applicable. The drug is not normally kept in the home.

Missed dose
As infliximab is dosed every 6–8 weeks, it is important to adhere to the dosing schedule arranged by your doctor. Missed doses should be rectified as soon as possible.

Stopping the drug
No adverse effects have been reported when stopping infliximab abruptly.

Exceeding the dose
Infliximab is given in hospital under close supervision so it is unlikely that the dose will be exceeded.

POSSIBLE ADVERSE EFFECTS

Infusion reactions may occur during treatment, or within 1 to 2 hours afterwards, particularly with the first or second treatment. Delayed reactions, including muscle and joint pain, fever, and rash, may occur from 3 to 12 days after infusion.

Symptom/effect	Frequency		Discuss with doctor		Stop taking drug now	Call doctor now
	Common	Rare	Only if severe	In all cases		
Nausea/vomiting/diarrhoea	●		●			
Headache	●		●			
Back pain	●		●			
Dizziness	●		●			
Infusion reactions	●			●		
Susceptibility to infection		●		●		
Swollen tongue/wheezing/rash		●		●	●	●

INTERACTIONS

Anakinra and abatacept These drugs should not be combined with infliximab because there is an increased risk of reactions and serious infections.

Vaccines Infliximab may affect the efficacy of vaccines.

SPECIAL PRECAUTIONS

Infliximab is prescribed only under close medical supervision. However, be sure to tell your doctor if:
- You have active tuberculosis or any other current infection.
- You have any signs of infection (e.g. fever, malaise, wounds, dental problems).
- You are having any surgery or dental treatment.
- You have liver or kidney problems.
- You have a central nervous system disorder such as multiple sclerosis.
- You have recently received, or are scheduled to receive, a vaccine.
- You have had heart failure.
- You are taking other medicines.

 Pregnancy
Limited clinical data on effects. Used only if essential.

 Breast-feeding
Not recommended during breast-feeding or for 6 months after last dose of the drug.

 Infants and children
Not recommended.

 Over 60
No special problems.

 Driving and hazardous work
Do not undertake such activities until you have learned how infliximab affects you because the drug can cause fatigue and dizziness.

 Alcohol
No special problems.

PROLONGED USE

There is an increased risk of infections (including tuberculosis). A rare type of lymphoma has been reported in a few patients, but no causal relationship with taking infliximab has been established.

Monitoring Periodic blood and liver-function tests may be carried out. Body temperature, heart rate, and blood pressure may be monitored during the first infusion.

INSULIN

Brand names Abasaglar (glargine), Actrapid, Apidra, Fiasp, Humalog, Human Mixtard, Humulin, Hypurin, Hypurine porcine, Insulatard, Insuman, Lantus, Levemir, Lyumjev, Novomix, NovoRapid, Suliqua, Toujeo, Tresiba, Xultophy, and others

GENERAL INFORMATION

Insulin is a hormone made by the pancreas and vital to the body's ability to use sugar. It is given by injection to supplement or replace natural insulin in treating diabetes mellitus. It is the only effective treatment in Type 1 diabetes and may also be prescribed in Type 2 diabetes. Insulin should be used with a carefully controlled diet. Illness, vomiting, or changes in diet or exercise levels may require dosage adjustment. It is available in short-, medium-, or long-acting preparations; combinations of types are often given. People using insulin should carry a warning card or tag. They should watch out for signs of hypoglycaemia (low blood sugar) and eat something sugary if these do occur.

QUICK REFERENCE

Drug group Drug for diabetes (p.100)

Overdose danger rating High

Dependence rating Low

Prescription needed Yes

Available as generic No

INFORMATION FOR USERS

Your drug prescription is tailored for you. Do not alter dosage without checking with your doctor.

How taken/used

Injection, infusion pump, pen injection.

Frequency and timing of doses
1–5 x daily injected under skin (see p.101) via insulin syringe. Usually 15–30 minutes before meals (short-acting); some forms given directly before or after eating. Exact timing of injections and longer-acting preparations tailored to individual needs; follow instructions given.

Adult dosage range
Exact timing of doses is tailored to individual needs. Follow manufacturer's instructions.

Onset of effect
10–60 minutes (short-acting); within 2 hours (medium-acting); 2–4 hours (long-acting).

Duration of action
2–8 hours (short-acting); 18–26 hours (medium-acting); 28–36 hours (long-acting).

Diet advice
A special diabetes diet is necessary. Follow your doctor's advice.

Storage
Refrigerate, but once opened may be stored at room temperature for 1 month. Do not freeze. Follow the instructions on the container.

Missed dose
Discuss with your doctor. Appropriate action depends on dose and type of insulin.

Stopping the drug
Do not stop taking the drug without consulting your doctor; confusion and coma may occur.

OVERDOSE ACTION

 Seek immediate medical advice. If warning signs of low blood sugar (e.g. faintness, dizziness, headache, confusion, sweating, or tremor) occur, have a sugary food or drink. Take emergency action if seizures or loss of consciousness occur.

See Drug poisoning emergency guide (p.518).

SPECIAL PRECAUTIONS

Be sure to tell your doctor if:
- You have had a previous allergic reaction to insulin.
- You are taking other medicines, or your other drug treatment is changed.

 Pregnancy
No evidence of risk to the developing baby from insulin, but poor control of diabetes increases the risk of birth defects. Careful monitoring is required because insulin requirements may change.

 Breast-feeding
No evidence of risk. Adjustment in dose may be necessary while breast-feeding.

 Infants and children
Reduced dose necessary.

 Over 60
No special problems.

 Driving and hazardous work
You must inform the DVLA you are taking insulin. You must check your blood sugar before driving and follow DVLA guidelines. Avoid driving or dangerous activities if you have signs of low blood sugar.

 Alcohol
Avoid. Alcoholic drinks upset diabetic control.

Surgery and general anaesthetics
Insulin requirements may increase during surgery, and blood glucose levels will need to be monitored during and after an operation. Notify your doctor or dentist that you are diabetic before any surgery.

POSSIBLE ADVERSE EFFECTS

Low blood sugar (see Overdose action, above) is the most common side effect of insulin. Serious allergic reactions (rash, swelling, and shortness of breath) are rare.

Symptom/effect	Frequency		Discuss with doctor		Stop taking drug now	Call doctor now
	Common	Rare	Only if severe	In all cases		
Injection-site irritation/lump	●			●		
Weakness/sweating	●			●		
Dimpling at injection site		●		●		
Eyesight problems		●		●		
Rash/facial swelling		●		●		●
Shortness of breath		●		●		●

INTERACTIONS

General note 1 Many drugs, including some antibiotics, monoamine oxidase inhibitors (MAOIs), and oral antidiabetic drugs, increase the risk of low blood sugar.

Corticosteroids, growth hormone, oestrogens, thyroxine, and diuretics may oppose the effect of insulin.

General note 2 Check with your doctor or pharmacist before taking any medicines; some contain sugar and may upset control of diabetes.

Beta blockers may affect insulin needs and mask signs of low blood sugar.

PROLONGED USE

Insulin can affect fat tissue under the skin, causing lumps or dimples that may affect absorption. Rotation of the injection sites within the injection area can help to prevent these reactions. No other problems expected.

Monitoring Regular monitoring of blood sugar levels is required.

INTERFERON

Brand names Avonex, Betaferon, Extavia, Flixabi, Immukin, IntronA, Pegasys, PegIntron, Rebif, Roferon-A, Viraferon
Used in the following combined preparations None

GENERAL INFORMATION

Interferons are a group of substances normally produced in cells that have been infected with viruses or stimulated by other substances. They are thought to promote resistance to several types of viral infection (p.84). Three main types of interferon (alfa, beta, and gamma) are used to treat a range of diseases. Interferon alfa is used for leukaemias, other cancers, and chronic hepatitis B and C. Interferon beta reduces the frequency and severity of relapses in multiple sclerosis. Interferon gamma is prescribed in conjunction with antibiotics for patients suffering from chronic granulomatous disease or from severe malignant osteopetrosis (a rare inherited condition in which the bones become abnormally dense).

Interferons commonly cause flu-like side effects. They may also cause more severe adverse effects (see below).

QUICK REFERENCE

Drug group Antiviral drug (p.91) and anticancer drug (p.112)

Overdose danger rating Medium

Dependence rating Low

Prescription needed Yes

Available as generic Yes

INFORMATION FOR USERS

This drug is given only under medical supervision and is not for self-administration.

How taken/used

Injection.

Frequency and timing of doses
Once daily 3 times a week, depending on product and condition being treated.

Adult dosage range
Depends on product and condition being treated. Dosage may sometimes be calculated from body surface area or weight.

Onset of effect
Active inside the body within 1 hour, but effects may not be noted for 1–2 months.

Duration of action
Immediate effects last for about 12 hours.

Diet advice
None.

Storage
Store in a refrigerator at 2–8°C. Do not let it freeze, and protect from light. Keep out of the reach of children.

Missed dose
Not applicable. This drug is usually given only in hospital under close medical supervision.

Stopping the drug
Discuss with your doctor.

Exceeding the dose
Overdosage is unlikely since treatment is carefully monitored.

SPECIAL PRECAUTIONS

Interferon is prescribed only under close medical supervision, taking account of your present condition and medical history. But be sure to tell your doctor if:
- You have long-term liver or kidney problems.
- You have heart disease.
- You have very abnormal blood lipid levels.
- You have diabetes.
- You have depression or suicidal thoughts.
- You have had epileptic seizures, asthma, eczema, psoriasis, or previous drug allergies.
- You are taking other medicines, including complementary remedies.

Pregnancy
Not usually prescribed, but some interferons may be considered if necessary. Discuss with your doctor.

Breast-feeding
Some types of interferon can be used during breast-feeding. Discuss with your doctor.

Infants and children
Not usually used in infants. Some types of interferon may be used in children.

Over 60
Increased risk of adverse effects. Reduced dose may be necessary.

Driving and hazardous work
Not applicable.

Alcohol
Avoid. Alcohol may increase the sedative effects of this drug.

POSSIBLE ADVERSE EFFECTS

The symptoms below are the most common problems; some are dose-related, and dosage reduction may be necessary. Inform your doctor of all unusual symptoms without delay.

Symptom/effect	Frequency		Discuss with doctor		Stop taking drug now	Call doctor now
	Common	Rare	Only if severe	In all cases		
Headache	●		●			
Lethargy/depression	●		●			
Dizziness/drowsiness	●			●		
Digestive disturbances	●			●		
Chills/fever/muscle aches	●			●		
Poor appetite and weight loss	●			●		
Hair loss		●		●		
Vision problems		●		●		
Shortness of breath/cough		●		●		

INTERACTIONS

General note A number of drugs increase the risk of adverse effects on the blood, heart, or nervous system. This is taken into account when prescribing an interferon with other drugs.

Vaccines Interferon may reduce the effectiveness of vaccines.

Sedatives All drugs that have a sedative effect on the central nervous system are likely to increase the sedative properties of interferon. Such drugs include opioid analgesics, anti-anxiety and sleeping drugs, antihistamines, antidepressants, and antipsychotics.

Theophylline/aminophylline The effects of this drug may be increased by interferon.

PROLONGED USE

There may be an increased risk of liver damage. Blood cell production in the bone marrow may be reduced. Repeated large doses are associated with lethargy, fatigue, collapse, and coma.

Monitoring Frequent blood tests are required to monitor blood composition and liver function. With interferon alfa, monitoring of thyroid function, blood lipids, and vision are also necessary.

IPRATROPIUM BROMIDE

Brand names Atrovent, Iprovent, Rinatec
Used in the following combined preparations Combivent, Duovent, Otrivine Extra Dual Relief

GENERAL INFORMATION

Ipratropium bromide is an anticholinergic bronchodilator that relaxes the muscles surrounding the bronchioles (the airways in the lungs). The drug is used primarily in the maintenance of airways in reversible airway disorders, particularly chronic obstructive pulmonary disease (COPD). It is given only by inhaler or via a nebulizer for these conditions. It is also used in treating acute attacks of asthma, especially severe attacks in hospital. In these cases, ipratropium

bromide is usually used together with sympathomimetic bronchodilators, such as salbutamol (see p.391). In addition, the drug is prescribed as a nasal spray for treating a continually runny nose due to allergy.

Unlike with other anticholinergic drugs, side effects are rare. Ipratropium bromide must be used with caution by people with glaucoma, but problems are unlikely at normal doses and if an inhaler or nebulizer is used correctly.

INFORMATION FOR USERS

Your drug prescription is tailored for you. Do not alter dosage without checking with your doctor.

How taken/used

Inhaler, liquid for nebulizer, nasal spray.

Frequency and timing of doses
3–4 x daily (inhaler); 2 sprays into each nostril 2–3 x daily (nasal spray).

Adult dosage range
80–320mcg daily (inhaler); 400–2,000mcg daily (nebulizer); 1–2 puffs to the affected nostril 2–3 x daily (nasal spray).

Onset of effect
3–30 minutes.

Duration of action
Up to 8 hours.

Diet advice
None.

Storage
Keep in original container at room temperature out of the reach of children. Do not puncture or burn containers.

Missed dose
Take as soon as you remember. If your next dose is due within 2 hours, take a single dose now and skip the next.

Stopping the drug
Do not stop taking the drug without consulting your doctor; symptoms may recur.

Exceeding the dose
An occasional unintentional extra dose is unlikely to be a cause for concern. But if you notice any unusual symptoms, or if a large overdose has been taken, notify your doctor.

SPECIAL PRECAUTIONS

Be sure to tell your doctor if:
- You have glaucoma.
- You have prostate problems.
- You have difficulty in passing urine.
- You have cystic fibrosis.
- You are taking other medicines.

 Pregnancy
No evidence of risk, but discuss with your doctor before using in the first 3 months of pregnancy.

 Breast-feeding
No evidence of risk, but discuss with your doctor.

 Infants and children
Reduced dose necessary.

 Over 60
No special problems.

 Driving and hazardous work
Avoid such activities until you know how the drug affects you because it may cause blurred vision or dizziness, especially if administered by nebulizer.

 Alcohol
No known problems.

PROLONGED USE

No special problems.

POSSIBLE ADVERSE EFFECTS

Side effects are rare; the most common adverse effects are dry mouth or throat and nausea and headache. Eye problems may occur if the drug comes into contact with the eyes during use with an inhaler or nebulizer.

Rarely, wheezing or breathlessness may worsen immediately after inhaler use (paradoxical bronchospasm); if this happens, stop using the drug and contact your doctor immediately.

Symptom/effect	Frequency		Discuss with doctor		Stop taking drug now	Call doctor now
	Common	Rare	Only if severe	In all cases		
Dry mouth/throat	●		●			
Nausea/headache	●		●			
Cough	●		●			
Constipation		●	●			
Difficulty in passing urine		●		●		
Fast heart rate/palpitations		●		●		
Skin rash/facial swelling		●		●	●	
Worsening breathlessness		●		●	●	●
Eye pain/altered vision		●		●	●	●

INTERACTIONS

Pasireotide may increase the risk of bradycardia (abnormally slow heart

rate) when used with ipratropium bromide.

IRBESARTAN

Brand name Aprovel, Ifirmasta
Used in the following combined preparation CoAprovel

GENERAL INFORMATION

Irbesartan is a member of the group of vasodilators (drugs that widen blood vessels) called angiotensin II blockers (p.56) and is used to treat hypertension (high blood pressure). It is also used to protect the kidneys in people with Type 2 diabetes who have hypertension and impaired kidney function.

Unlike ACE inhibitors, irbesartan does not cause a persistent dry cough. Irbesartan is also available in combination with a diuretic (CoAprovel), which may increase its blood-pressure-lowering effect.

QUICK REFERENCE

Drug group Vasodilator (p.56) and antihypertensive drug (p.60)

Overdose danger rating Medium

Dependence rating Low

Prescription needed Yes

Available as generic No

INFORMATION FOR USERS

Your drug prescription is tailored for you. Do not alter dosage without checking with your doctor.

How taken/used

Tablets.

Frequency and timing of doses
Once daily.

Adult dosage range
150mg (maintenance dose), increased to 300mg if needed; 75mg may be used in people over 75 years and those on haemodialysis.

Onset of effect
Within 1 hour. Blood pressure is lowered within 1–2 weeks, and maximum beneficial effect occurs 4–6 weeks from start of treatment.

Duration of action
24 hours.

Diet advice
None.

Storage
Keep in original container at room temperature out of the reach of children.

Missed dose
Take as soon as you remember. If your next dose is due within 8 hours, take a single dose now and skip the next.

Stopping the drug
Do not stop the drug without consulting your doctor. Stopping the drug may lead to worsening of the underlying condition.

Exceeding the dose
An occasional unintentional extra dose is unlikely to be a cause for concern. A large overdose may cause dizziness, fainting, and a faint pulse or slow heart rate. Call your doctor.

SPECIAL PRECAUTIONS

Be sure to tell your doctor if:
- You have heart problems, including heart failure.
- You have kidney problems or stenosis of the kidney's arteries.
- You have lactose/galactose intolerance or glucose/galactose malabsorption.
- You are taking other medicines.

 Pregnancy
Not prescribed. If you become pregnant during treatment, consult your doctor without delay.

 Breast-feeding
Safety not established. Discuss with your doctor.

 Infants and children
Not prescribed.

 Over 60
Increased risk of adverse effects. Reduced dose may therefore be necessary.

 Driving and hazardous work
Avoid such activities until you have learned how irbesartan affects you because the drug can cause dizziness and fatigue.

 Alcohol
Regular intake of excessive alcohol may raise the blood pressure and reduce the effectiveness of irbesartan.

POSSIBLE ADVERSE EFFECTS

Adverse effects are usually mild and transient. However, an exaggerated drop in blood pressure may occur if you take the drug when you are dehydrated.

Symptom/effect	Frequency		Discuss with doctor		Stop taking drug now	Call doctor now
	Common	Rare	Only if severe	In all cases		
Dizziness/fatigue	●		●			
Flushing	●		●			
Nausea	●		●			
Headache		●	●			
Muscle or joint pains		●	●			
Rash		●		●		
Swollen face or lips		●		●	●	●

PROLONGED USE

No special problems.

Monitoring Periodic checks on blood potassium levels and kidney function may be performed.

INTERACTIONS

Diuretics There is a risk of a sudden fall in blood pressure if these drugs are being taken when irbesartan treatment is started. They may also affect sodium and potassium levels in the blood.

Potassium supplements, potassium-sparing diuretics, and ciclosporin Used with irbesartan, these drugs may raise levels of potassium in the blood.

Antihypertensives increase the effects of irbesartan.

Lithium Irbesartan increases the blood levels and toxicity of lithium.

NSAIDs (p.74) Some of these drugs may reduce the blood-pressure-lowering effects of irbesartan, and there is a risk that they may worsen kidney function.

ACE inhibitors (e.g. enalapril, captopril, lisinopril, or ramipril) and potassium salts may increase potassium levels when taken with irbesartan. However, these drugs are not routinely prescribed with irbesartan.

ISONIAZID

Brand names Cemidon, Tebesium [solutions for injection]
Used in the following combined preparations Rifater, Rifinah, Rimstar, Voractiv

GENERAL INFORMATION

Isoniazid (also known as INAH or INH) has been in use since the 1950s and is still an effective drug for tuberculosis. It is given alone to prevent tuberculosis and in combination with other drugs for the treatment of the disease. Treatment usually lasts for six months. However, courses lasting nine months or a year may sometimes be prescribed.

Although isoniazid usually causes few adverse effects, one of its side effects is the increased loss of pyridoxine (vitamin B_6) from the body. This effect, which is more likely with high doses, is rare in children but common among people with poor nutrition. Since pyridoxine deficiency can lead to irreversible nerve damage, supplements are usually given.

INFORMATION FOR USERS

Your drug prescription is tailored for you. Do not alter dosage without checking with your doctor.

How taken/used

Tablets, injection.

Frequency and timing of doses
Normally once daily.

Dosage range
Adults 300mg daily.
Children According to age and weight.

Onset of effect
Over 2–3 days.

Duration of action
Up to 24 hours.

Diet advice
Take 30 minutes before food because food decreases absorption of isoniazid.

Storage
Keep in original container at room temperature out of the reach of children. Protect from light.

Missed dose
Take as soon as you remember. If your next dose is scheduled within 8 hours, take a single dose now and skip the next.

Stopping the drug
Take the full course. Even if you feel better the infection may still be present and may recur if treatment is stopped too soon.

OVERDOSE ACTION

Seek immediate medical advice in all cases. Take emergency action if breathing difficulties, seizures, or loss of consciousness occur.

See Drug poisoning emergency guide (p.518).

SPECIAL PRECAUTIONS

Be sure to tell your doctor if:
- You have long-term liver or kidney problems.
- You have had liver damage following isoniazid treatment in the past.
- You have problems with drug or alcohol abuse.
- You have diabetes.
- You have porphyria.
- You have HIV infection.
- You have had epileptic seizures.
- You are taking other medicines.

Pregnancy
No evidence of risk. Discuss with your doctor.

Breast-feeding
The drug passes into the breast milk and may affect the baby. The infant should be monitored for signs of toxic effects. Discuss with your doctor.

Infants and children
Reduced dose necessary.

Over 60
Increased likelihood of adverse effects.

Driving and hazardous work
No special problems.

Alcohol
Avoid excessive amounts.

POSSIBLE ADVERSE EFFECTS

Although serious problems are uncommon, all adverse effects of this drug should receive prompt medical attention because of the possibility of nerve or liver damage. Signs of liver toxicity include fatigue, malaise, nausea, and jaundice.

Symptom/effect	Frequency		Discuss with doctor		Stop taking drug now	Call doctor now
	Common	Rare	Only if severe	In all cases		
Nausea/vomiting	●		●			
Fatigue/weakness	●			●		
Numbness/tingling	●			●		
Rash	●			●		
Mood changes	●			●		
Blurred vision	●			●	●	
Jaundice	●			●	●	●
Twitching/muscle weakness	●			●	●	●

INTERACTIONS

Alcohol and rifampicin Large quantities of alcohol may reduce the effectiveness of isoniazid. If the two are taken together, the likelihood of liver damage is increased; if rifampicin is also being taken, the risk of liver damage is increased further.

Theophylline Isoniazid may increase levels and effects of theophylline.

Anticonvulsants The effects of these drugs may be increased with isoniazid.

Antacids These drugs may reduce the absorption of isoniazid.

Ketoconazole Isoniazid reduces the blood concentration of ketoconazole.

PROLONGED USE

Pyridoxine (vitamin B_6) deficiency may occur with prolonged use and lead to nerve damage. Supplements are usually prescribed. There is also a risk of serious liver damage.

Monitoring Periodic blood tests are usually performed to monitor liver function.

ISOSORBIDE DINITRATE/MONONITRATE

Brand names [dinitrate] Isoket Retard; [mononitrate] Chemydur, Elantan, Imdur, Isib, Ismo, Isodur, Isotard, Modisal, Monomax, Monomil XL, Monosorb XL, Zemon
Used in the following combined preparations None

GENERAL INFORMATION

Isosorbide dinitrate and isosorbide mononitrate are vasodilator drugs similar to glyceryl trinitrate (see p.272). They are usually used to treat patients who have angina, and are also used in some cases of heart failure.

Unlike glyceryl trinitrate, however, both of these drugs are stable and can be stored for long periods without losing their effectiveness.

Headache, flushing, and dizziness are common side effects during the early stages of treatment; small doses of the drug given in the initial stages can help to minimize these symptoms. The effectiveness of isosorbide dinitrate and isosorbide mononitrate are reduced if the drugs are taken continuously. To minimize this, formulations are often designed to give a drug-free period when taken once daily.

similar to glyceryl trinitrate (see p.272).

QUICK REFERENCE

Drug group Nitrate vasodilator (p.56) and anti-angina drug (p.59)

Overdose danger rating Medium

Dependence rating Low

Prescription needed No (some preparations); yes (other preparations and injection)

Available as generic Yes

INFORMATION FOR USERS

Follow instructions on the label. Call your doctor if symptoms worsen.

How taken/used

Dinitrate Tablets, SR tablets, injection, spray.
Mononitrate Tablets, SR tablets, SR capsules.

Frequency and timing of doses
Relief of angina attacks As required (spray).
Heart failure/prevention of angina 2–4 x daily; 1–2 x daily (SR tablets, capsules).

Adult dosage range
Prevention of angina 30–120mg daily (in divided doses).
Treatment of angina 1–3 doses under the tongue (spray).
Heart failure 40–240mg daily (in divided doses).

Onset of effect
2–3 minutes (spray); 20–30 minutes (SR tablets, capsules).

Duration of action
4–6 hours (dinitrate tablets); 8–10 hours (mononitrate tablets); up to 17 hours (SR tablets); up to 10 hours (SR capsules); 1–2 hours (spray).

Diet advice
None.

Storage
Keep in original container at room temperature out of the reach of children. Protect from light.

Missed dose
Take as soon as you remember. If your next dose is due within 2 hours, take a single dose now and skip the next.

Stopping the drug
Do not stop taking the drug without consulting your doctor; stopping the drug may lead to worsening of the underlying condition.

Exceeding the dose
An occasional unintentional extra dose is unlikely to cause problems. Large doses may cause dizziness, headache, or shortness of breath. Notify your doctor.

SPECIAL PRECAUTIONS

Be sure to consult your doctor or pharmacist before taking this drug if:
- You have long-term liver or kidney problems.
- You have any blood disorders or anaemia.
- You have glaucoma.
- You have low blood pressure.
- You have ever had a heart attack.
- You have an underactive thyroid.
- You have glucose-6-phosphate dehydrogenase (G6PD) deficiency.
- You have had a recent head injury.
- You are taking other medicines.

 Pregnancy
Safety in pregnancy not established. Discuss with your doctor.

 Breast-feeding
Safety not established. Discuss with your doctor.

 Infants and children
Not usually prescribed.

 Over 60
No special problems.

 Driving and hazardous work
Avoid such activities until you have learned how isosorbide dinitrate or mononitrate affects you because these drugs can cause dizziness.

 Alcohol
Avoid. Alcohol may further lower blood pressure, depressing the heart and causing dizziness and fainting.

PROLONGED USE

The initial adverse effects may disappear with prolonged use. The effects of the drug become weaker as the body adapts. This may be overcome by a change in the dose to allow a drug-free period during each day.

POSSIBLE ADVERSE EFFECTS

The most serious adverse effect is excessively lowered blood pressure, and this may need to be monitored on a regular basis. Other adverse effects of both forms of the drug usually improve after regular use; dose adjustment may help.

Symptom/effect	Frequency		Discuss with doctor		Stop taking drug now	Call doctor now
	Common	Rare	Only if severe	In all cases		
Headache	●		●			
Flushing	●		●			
Dizziness	●			●		
Fainting/weakness		●		●		
Fast or slow heart rate		●		●		

INTERACTIONS

Sildenafil, tadalafil, and vardenafil The blood-pressure-lowering effect of nitrates is significantly enhanced by these drugs; they should not be used together.

Antihypertensives A further lowering of blood pressure occurs when such drugs are taken with nitrates.

ISOTRETINOIN

Brand names Reticutan, Roaccutane
Used in the following combined preparation None

GENERAL INFORMATION

Isotretinoin, a drug that is chemically related to vitamin A, is prescribed for the treatment of severe acne that has failed to respond to other treatments.

The drug reduces production of the skin's natural oils (sebum) and of the horny protein (keratin) in the skin's outer layers, making it useful in conditions such as ichthyosis, in which the skin thickens abnormally, causing scaling.

A single 16-week course of treatment often clears the acne. The skin may be very dry, flaky, and itchy at first, but this usually improves with continued use. Serious adverse effects include liver damage and bowel inflammation.

QUICK REFERENCE

Drug group Drug for acne (p.137)
Overdose danger rating Medium
Dependence rating Low
Prescription needed Yes
Available as generic Yes

INFORMATION FOR USERS

Your drug prescription is tailored for you. Do not alter dosage without checking with your doctor.

How taken/used

Capsules.

Frequency and timing of doses
1–2 x daily (take with food or milk).

Adult dosage range
Dosage is determined individually.

Onset of effect
2–4 weeks. Acne may worsen initially in some people but usually improves in 7–10 days.

Duration of action
Effects persist for several weeks after the drug is stopped. Acne is usually completely cleared.

Diet advice
None.

Storage
Keep in original container at room temperature out of the reach of children. Protect from light.

Missed dose
Take as soon as you remember. If your next dose is due within 4 hours, take a single dose now and skip the next.

Stopping the drug
Can be safely stopped as soon as you no longer need it, but best results are achieved when the course of treatment is completed as prescribed.

Exceeding the dose
An occasional unintentional extra dose is unlikely to cause problems. Large overdoses may cause headaches, vomiting, abdominal pain, facial flushing, incoordination, and dizziness. Notify your doctor.

SPECIAL PRECAUTIONS

Do not donate blood during or after taking isotretinoin. Be sure to tell your doctor if:
- You have long-term liver or kidney problems.
- You have diabetes, arthritis, or gout.
- You have a history of depression.
- You have fructose intolerance or are allergic to soya or peanuts.
- You have high blood fat levels.
- You wear contact lenses.
- You are pregnant or planning a pregnancy.
- You are taking other medicines.

 Pregnancy
Must not be prescribed. The drug causes fetal abnormalities. Women of childbearing age must use at least one user-independent hormonal form of contraception or two barrier methods for 1 month before, during, and 1 month after treatment.

 Breast-feeding
Not recommended. Likely to pass into the breast milk and affect the baby.

 Infants and children
Not prescribed to children under 12 years.

 Over 60
Not usually prescribed.

 Driving and hazardous work
Avoid such activities until you know how the drug affects you because it can cause vision problems in dim light.

Alcohol
Regular heavy drinking may raise blood fat levels and increase the risk of hepatitis with isotretinoin.

Sunlight, sunbeds, and skin care
To avoid skin damage, use a sunscreen or sunblock; do not use a sunlamp or sunbed. Avoid wax depilation, laser treatment, and dermabrasion for 6 months after treatment.

POSSIBLE ADVERSE EFFECTS

Dryness of the nose, mouth, and eyes, inflammation of the lips, and flaking of the skin occur in most cases. Temporary loss or increase of hair may also occur. If headache, along with nausea, vomiting, abdominal pain with diarrhoea, blood in the faeces, or visual impairment develop, consult your doctor promptly.

Symptom/effect	Frequency		Discuss with doctor		Stop taking drug now	Call doctor now
	Common	Rare	Only if severe	In all cases		
Dry skin and lips/nosebleeds	●		●			
Muscle/joint pain	●		●			
Eye dryness/inflammation	●			●		
Skin pigmentation changes		●	●			
Mood changes		●		●		
Headache/nausea/vomiting		●		●		
Impaired vision		●		●		
Skin rash or bruising		●		●		
Abdominal pain/diarrhoea		●		●	●	●

INTERACTIONS

Tetracycline antibiotics increase the risk of high pressure in the skull, leading to headaches, nausea, and vomiting.

Skin-drying preparations Medicated cosmetics, soaps, and toiletries, and anti-acne or abrasive skin preparations increase the likelihood of dryness and irritation of the skin with isotretinoin.

Vitamin A supplements increase the risk of adverse effects from isotretinoin and should be avoided.

Progestogen-only contraceptive pills work poorly during isotretinoin treatment. Women should use an alternative method of contraception (see right) for 1 month before, during, and for 1 month after treatment.

PROLONGED USE

Treatment rarely exceeds 16 weeks. Prolonged use may raise blood fat levels and increase the risk of heart and blood vessel disease. Bone changes may occur.

Monitoring Liver function tests and checks on blood fat levels are performed.

KETOCONAZOLE

Brand names Boots Anti-Dandruff Ketoconazole Shampoo, Daktarin Gold, Dandrazol, Nizoral
Used in the following combined preparations None

GENERAL INFORMATION

Ketoconazole was previously used to treat severe, internal systemic fungal infections by mouth, but this application has been discontinued because of the risk of severe liver damage. However, the drug is still available as a topical cream to treat fungal skin and vaginal infections, and as a shampoo for the treatment of scalp infections and seborrhoeic dermatitis. Used in this way, ketoconazole is extremely safe because very little of this drug is absorbed into the blood – so little, in fact, that blood levels of the drug are usually undetectably low.

Side effects of ketoconazole are uncommon. However, the drug may occasionally alter the colour of the hair or cause itching, skin rashes, or in rare cases, hair loss.

INFORMATION FOR USERS

Your drug prescription is tailored for you. Do not alter dosage without checking with your doctor.

How taken/used

Cream, shampoo.

Frequency and timing of doses
1–2 x daily (cream); 1–2 times weekly (shampoo for seborrhoeic dermatitis); 1 x daily for 5 days (shampoo for tinea versicolor).

Dosage range
As directed.

Onset of effect
Within a few hours; full beneficial effect may take several days (or weeks in severe infections).

Duration of action
Up to 24 hours.

Diet advice
None.

Storage
Keep in original container at room temperature out of the reach of children.

Missed dose
No cause for concern, but apply the missed application as soon as you remember.

Stopping the drug
Apply the full course. Even if you feel better, the original infection may still be present and may recur if treatment is stopped too soon.

Exceeding the dose
An occasional unintentional extra application is unlikely to be a cause for concern.

POSSIBLE ADVERSE EFFECTS

Applied to the skin or hair, ketoconazole is extremely safe, although it may affect hair colour, cause skin rashes, or, rarely, cause hair loss (alopecia).

Symptom/effect	Frequency		Discuss with doctor		Stop taking drug now	Call doctor now
	Common	Rare	Only if severe	In all cases		
Changes to hair colour	●		●			
Itching/rash	●			●	●	
Hair loss	●			●	●	

INTERACTIONS

None known.

SPECIAL PRECAUTIONS

Be sure to consult your doctor or pharmacist before taking this drug if:
- You have previously had an allergic reaction to antifungal drugs.
- You are taking other medicines.

Pregnancy
No evidence of risk.

Breast-feeding
No evidence of risk. The drug does not pass into the breast milk in detectable amounts.

Infants and children
No special problems.

Over 60
No special problems.

Driving and hazardous work
No special problems.

Alcohol
No known problems.

PROLONGED USE

No problems expected. However, the drug is usually used only until the infection has cleared up.

KETOPROFEN

Brand names Orudis, Oruvail, Powergel, Valket, and many others
Used in the following combined preparations None

GENERAL INFORMATION

Ketoprofen is a non-steroidal anti-inflammatory (NSAID) drug. Like other NSAIDs, it relieves pain and reduces inflammation and stiffness in rheumatoid arthritis, osteoarthritis, and ankylosing spondylitis. The drug does not cure the underlying disease, however.

Ketoprofen is also given to relieve mild to moderate pain associated with menstruation and soft tissue injuries, and to ease the pain that occurs following operations.

The most common adverse reactions to ketoprofen, as with all NSAIDs, are gastrointestinal disturbances such as nausea and indigestion. Switching to another NSAID may be recommended by your doctor if unwanted effects are persistent or troublesome.

QUICK REFERENCE

Drug group Non-steroidal anti-inflammatory drug (p.74)

Overdose danger rating Medium

Dependence rating Low

Prescription needed Yes (except for some topical preparations)

Available as generic Yes

INFORMATION FOR USERS

Follow instructions on the label. Call your doctor if symptoms worsen.

How taken/used

Capsules, SR capsules, suppositories, gel.

Frequency and timing of doses
Once daily (SR capsules) or 2–4 x daily (capsules) with food; 4 x daily for up to 3 days (injection); 2 x daily (suppositories).

Adult dosage range
100–200mg daily.

Onset of effect
Pain relief may be felt in 30 minutes to 2 hours. Full anti-inflammatory effect may not be felt for up to 2 weeks.

Duration of action
Up to 8–12 hours.

Diet advice
None.

Storage
Keep in original container at room temperature out of the reach of children.

Missed dose
Take as soon as you remember. If your next dose is due within 4 hours, take a single dose now and skip the next.

Stopping the drug
Seek medical advice before stopping the drug.

Exceeding the dose
An occasional unintentional extra dose is unlikely to be a cause for concern. Large overdoses may cause vomiting, confusion, or irritability. Notify your doctor.

SPECIAL PRECAUTIONS

Be sure to consult your doctor or pharmacist before taking this drug if:
- You have long-term liver or kidney problems.
- You have heart problems.
- You have high blood pressure.
- You have asthma.
- You have had a peptic ulcer, oesophagitis, or acid indigestion.
- You have bleeding problems.
- You are allergic to aspirin or other NSAIDs.
- You are taking other medicines.

Pregnancy
The drug may increase the risk of adverse effects on the baby's heart and may prolong labour if taken in the third trimester. Discuss with your doctor.

Breast-feeding
The drug passes into the breast milk and may affect the baby. Discuss with your doctor.

Infants and children
Not recommended for children under 12 years.

Over 60
Increased likelihood of adverse effects. Reduced dose may therefore be necessary.

Driving and hazardous work
Avoid such activities until you have learned how ketoprofen affects you because the drug can cause dizziness and drowsiness.

Alcohol
Avoid. Alcohol may increase the risk of stomach disorders with ketoprofen.

Surgery and general anaesthetics
Ketoprofen may prolong bleeding. Discuss with your doctor or dentist before any surgery.

POSSIBLE ADVERSE EFFECTS

Gastrointestinal disturbances are common with oral forms; suppositories may cause rectal irritation. Black or bloodstained faeces should be reported promptly. Topical forms may cause photosensitivity, and treated areas should be protected from sunlight.

Symptom/effect	Frequency		Discuss with doctor		Stop taking drug now	Call doctor now
	Common	Rare	Only if severe	In all cases		
Heartburn/indigestion	●		●			
Nausea/vomiting	●		●			
Headache		●	●			
Dizziness/drowsiness		●	●			
Swollen feet or legs		●	●			
Weight gain		●	●			
Rash/itching		●		●	●	
Wheezing/breathlessness		●		●	●	●
Black/bloodstained faeces		●		●	●	●

INTERACTIONS

General note Ketoprofen interacts with a wide range of drugs, such as aspirin and other NSAIDs, oral anticoagulants, and corticosteroids, to increase the risk of bleeding and/or stomach ulcers.

Lithium, digoxin, and methotrexate Ketoprofen may raise blood levels of these drugs to an undesirable extent.

Phenytoin Ketoprofen may enhance the effects of phenytoin.

Quinolone antibiotics Ketoprofen may increase the risk of seizures if taken with these drugs.

Antihypertensive drugs Ketoprofen may reduce the beneficial effects of these drugs.

PROLONGED USE

There is an increased risk of bleeding from peptic ulcers and in the bowel with prolonged use of ketoprofen. There is also a small risk of a heart attack or stroke. To minimize these risks, the lowest effective dose is given for the shortest duration.

LACTULOSE

Brand names Duphalac, Lactugal
Used in the following combined preparations None

GENERAL INFORMATION

Lactulose is an effective laxative that softens faeces by increasing the amount of water in the large intestine. It is used for the relief of constipation and faecal impaction, especially in older people. This drug is less likely than some other laxatives to disrupt normal bowel action.

Lactulose is also used for preventing and treating a form of brain disturbance associated with liver failure, a condition known as hepatic encephalopathy.

Because lactulose acts locally in the large intestine and is not absorbed into the body, it is safer than many other laxatives. However, the drug can cause stomach cramps and flatulence, especially at the start of treatment.

INFORMATION FOR USERS

Follow instructions on the label. Call your doctor if symptoms worsen.

How taken/used

Liquid, powder.

Frequency and timing of doses
Chronic constipation 2 x daily.
Liver failure 3–4 x daily.

Adult dosage range
Chronic constipation 15–30ml daily.
Liver failure 90–150ml daily.

Onset of effect
24–48 hours.

Duration of action
6–18 hours.

Diet advice
It is important to maintain an adequate intake of fluid – up to 8 glasses of water daily.

Storage
Keep in original container at room temperature out of the reach of children. Do not store after diluting. Do not refrigerate or freeze.

Missed dose
Take as soon as you remember. If your next dose is due within 3 hours, take a single dose now and skip the next.

Stopping the drug
In the treatment of constipation, the drug can be safely stopped as soon as you no longer need it.

Exceeding the dose
An occasional unintentional extra dose is unlikely to be a cause for concern. But if you notice any unusual symptoms, or if a large overdose has been taken, notify your doctor.

POSSIBLE ADVERSE EFFECTS

Adverse effects are rarely serious and often disappear when your body adjusts to the medicine. Diarrhoea may indicate that the dosage of lactulose is too high and needs to be adjusted. Consult your doctor.

Symptom/effect	Frequency		Discuss with doctor		Stop taking drug now	Call doctor now
	Common	Rare	Only if severe	In all cases		
Flatulence/belching	●		●			
Stomach cramps	●		●			
Diarrhoea	●				●	
Nausea/vomiting		●	●			
Abdominal distension		●		●		

INTERACTIONS

Other laxatives Lactulose combined with other laxative drugs increases the risk of diarrhoea.

SPECIAL PRECAUTIONS

Be sure to consult your doctor or pharmacist before taking this drug if:
• You have severe abdominal pain.
• You have diabetes.
• You suffer from lactose intolerance or galactosaemia.
• You are taking other medicines.

Pregnancy
No evidence of risk. Discuss with your doctor.

Breast-feeding
No evidence of risk.

Infants and children
Reduced dose necessary.

Over 60
No special problems.

Driving and hazardous work
No known problems.

Alcohol
No known problems.

PROLONGED USE

Prolonged use, overuse, or too high a dosage of lactulose may lead to diarrhoea and disturbances in the balance of body salts. In children, prolonged use may contribute to the development of dental caries (tooth decay).

LAMOTRIGINE

Brand name Lamictal
Used in the following combined preparations None

GENERAL INFORMATION

Lamotrigine is an anticonvulsant drug that is prescribed, either alone or in combination with other anticonvulsant drugs, for the treatment of epilepsy. The drug acts by restoring the balance between excitatory and inhibitory neurotransmitters (see p.34) in the brain. Lamotrigine may be less sedating than older anticonvulsants, and there is no need for blood tests to determine the level of the drug in the blood.

Lamotrigine may cause a number of minor adverse effects (see below), most of which will respond to an adjustment in dosage.

Lamotrigine is also occasionally used in specialist centres to treat bipolar affective disorder (manic depression).

(see p.34)

QUICK REFERENCE

Drug group Anticonvulsant drug (p.42)

Overdose danger rating Medium

Dependence rating Low

Prescription needed Yes

Available as generic Yes

(p.42)

INFORMATION FOR USERS

Your drug prescription is tailored for you. Do not alter dosage without checking with your doctor.

How taken/used

Tablets, chewable tablets, dispersible tablets.

Frequency and timing of doses
1–2 x daily.

Adult dosage range
100–500mg daily (maintenance) (100–200mg with sodium valproate). Smaller doses are used at start of treatment. Dose may vary if other anticonvulsant drugs are being taken.

Onset of effect
Approximately 5 days at a constant dose.

Duration of action
Up to 24 hours.

Diet advice
None.

Storage
Keep in original container at room temperature out of the reach of children.

Missed dose
Take as soon as you remember. If your next dose is due within 2 hours, take a single dose now and skip the next.

Stopping the drug
Do not stop taking the drug without consulting your doctor, who will supervise a gradual reduction in dosage. Abrupt cessation increases the risk of rebound seizures.

Exceeding the dose
An occasional unintentional extra dose is unlikely to be a cause for concern. Large overdoses may cause sedation, double vision, loss of muscular coordination, nausea, and vomiting. Contact your doctor immediately.

SPECIAL PRECAUTIONS

Be sure to tell your doctor if:
- You have long-term liver or kidney problems.
- You have any blood disorder.
- You are taking other medicines.

Pregnancy
Safety in pregnancy not established. Discuss with your doctor.

Breast-feeding
The drug passes into the breast milk and may affect the baby. Discuss with your doctor.

Infants and children
Not recommended under 2 years. Not recommended as a single therapy under 12 years. Doses may be relatively higher than adult doses due to increased metabolism.

Over 60
No special problems.

Driving and hazardous work
Your underlying condition, in addition to the possibility of sedation, dizziness, and vision disturbances while taking lamotrigine, may make such activities inadvisable. Discuss with your doctor.

Alcohol
Alcohol may increase the adverse effects of this drug.

PROLONGED USE

No special problems.

POSSIBLE ADVERSE EFFECTS

Serious adverse effects are rare. The most common side effects are skin rash, nausea, headache, tiredness, insomnia, blurred or double vision, dizziness, and poor muscle coordination. Although common, a rash may indicate a serious hypersensitivity reaction, especially when accompanied by mouth ulcers; call your doctor immediately. If sore throat, flu-like symptoms, or unusual bruising or bleeding occur, call your doctor immediately.

Symptom/effect	Frequency		Discuss with doctor		Stop taking drug now	Call doctor now
	Common	Rare	Only if severe	In all cases		
Headache	●		●			
Blurred vision/double vision	●			●		
Tremor/incoordination	●			●		
Rash	●			●		●
Nausea		●	●			
Flu-like symptoms		●		●		●
Sore throat/bruising		●		●		●
Swelling around the face		●		●		●

INTERACTIONS

Sodium valproate increases and prolongs the effectiveness of lamotrigine. A reduced dose of lamotrigine will be used.

Antidepressants, antipsychotics, rifampicin, mefloquine, and chloroquine may counteract the anticonvulsant effect of lamotrigine.

Carbamazepine may reduce lamotrigine blood levels, but lamotrigine may increase the side effects of carbamazepine.

Phenytoin and phenobarbital may decrease blood levels of lamotrigine so a higher dose of lamotrigine may be needed.

LANSOPRAZOLE

Brand names Zoton FasTab
Used in the following combined preparations None

GENERAL INFORMATION

Lansoprazole belongs to a group of drugs called proton pump inhibitors (see p.67). It is used to treat gastro-oesophageal reflux (rising of stomach acid into the oesophagus), to treat Zollinger-Ellison syndrome (production of large quantities of stomach acid, leading to ulceration), and to prevent or treat peptic ulcers. It works by reducing the amount of acid that the stomach produces. Lansoprazole may be given in combination with antibiotics to eradicate *Helicobacter pylori* bacteria, the main cause of peptic ulcers. Because lansoprazole may mask the symptoms of stomach cancer, it is prescribed only when the possibility of this disease has been ruled out.

QUICK REFERENCE

Drug group Anti-ulcer drug (p.67)
Overdose danger rating Low
Dependence rating Low
Prescription needed Yes
Available as generic Yes

INFORMATION FOR USERS

Your drug prescription is tailored for you. Do not alter dosage without checking with your doctor.

How taken/used

Capsules, dispersible tablets, liquid (suspension).

Frequency and timing of doses
Usually once, sometimes twice, daily before food in the morning.

Dosage range
Peptic ulcer/gastro-oesophageal reflux 30mg daily.
NSAID-induced ulcer 15–30mg daily.
Acid-related dyspepsia 15–30mg daily.
Zollinger-Ellison syndrome 60mg daily initially, adjusted according to response.
H. pylori-associated ulcer 60mg daily, half the dose in the morning and half in the evening.

Onset of effect
1–2 hours.

Duration of action
24 hours.

Diet advice
None, although spicy foods and alcohol may exacerbate the condition being treated.

Storage
Keep in original container at room temperature out of the reach of children. Do not refrigerate.

Missed dose
Take as soon as you remember. If your next dose is due within 8 hours, take a single dose now and skip the next.

Stopping the drug
Do not stop taking the drug without consulting your doctor; symptoms may recur.

Exceeding the dose
An occasional unintentional extra dose is unlikely to be a cause for concern. But if you notice any unusual symptoms, or if a large overdose has been taken, notify your doctor.

SPECIAL PRECAUTIONS

Be sure to tell your doctor if:
• You have liver problems.
• You are taking other medicines.

Pregnancy
Safety not established. Discuss with your doctor.

Breast-feeding
Safety not established. Discuss with your doctor.

Infants and children
Not recommended.

Over 60
No special problems.

Driving and hazardous work
No special problems.

Alcohol
Avoid. Alcohol irritates the stomach.

PROLONGED USE

Long-term use of lansoprazole may increase the risk of certain intestinal infections (such as *Salmonella* and *Clostridium difficile* infections) because of the loss of natural protection against such infections provided by stomach acid. Prolonged use also increases the risk of fractures and may increase the risk of low levels of magnesium in the blood.

POSSIBLE ADVERSE EFFECTS

Common side effects include headache, indigestion, and diarrhoea. A sore throat, mouth, or tongue are very rare but should be reported to your doctor at once.

Symptom/effect	Frequency		Discuss with doctor		Stop taking drug now	Call doctor now
	Common	Rare	Only if severe	In all cases		
Headache/dizziness	●			●		
Diarrhoea/constipation	●			●		
Flatulence/abdominal pain	●			●		
Nausea/vomiting	●			●		
Fatigue/malaise		●		●		
Rash/itching		●			●	●
Sore throat/mouth/tongue		●			●	●

INTERACTIONS

Antifungals (ketoconazole and fluconazole) and theophylline Lansoprazole may reduce the effect of these drugs.

Antacids and sucralfate may reduce the absorption of lansoprazole, and should not be taken within an hour of the drug.

Digoxin Lansoprazole may increase blood levels of digoxin.

Cilostazol Lansoprazole may increase the effect of cilostazol; the two drugs should not be taken together.

Tacrolimus Lansoprazole may increase blood levels of tacrolimus.

Atazanavir Lansoprazole may decrease the effect of atazanavir; the two drugs should not be taken together.

LATANOPROST

Brand names Fixapost, Medizol, Monopost, Xalatan
Used in the following combined preparation Xalacom

GENERAL INFORMATION

Latanoprost is a synthetic derivative of the prostaglandin dinoprost, which constricts the smooth muscle lining the blood vessels and airways. Latanoprost is used as eye drops to reduce pressure inside the eye in open-angle (chronic) glaucoma (p.128) and to relieve ocular hypertension by increasing the outflow of fluid from the eye. The drug is used when patients have not responded to or cannot tolerate the drug of first choice, usually a beta blocker (such as timolol, p.418). Sometimes, combined eye drops of latanoprost and timolol may be prescribed when timolol alone is not adequately controlling the pressure.

Latanoprost eye drops can gradually increase the amount of brown pigment in the eye, darkening the iris. This will be particularly noticeable if only one eye needs treatment. Irises of mixed coloration are especially susceptible; pure blue eyes do not seem to be affected. Latanoprost has also been reported to cause darkening, thickening, and lengthening of eyelashes.

INFORMATION FOR USERS

Your drug prescription is tailored for you. Do not alter dosage without checking with your doctor.

How taken/used

Eye drops.

Frequency and timing of doses
1 x daily, in the evening.

Adult dosage range
1 drop per eye, daily.

Onset of effect
3–4 hours.

Duration of action
24 hours.

Diet advice
None.

Storage
Keep the eye drops in the outer cardboard package to protect from light. Store at room temperature, out of the reach of children. Discard any unused solution 4 weeks after opening.

Missed dose
Use the next dose as normal.

Stopping the drug
Do not stop taking the drug without consulting your doctor; symptoms may recur.

Exceeding the dose
An occasional unintentional extra application is unlikely to cause problems. Excessive use may irritate the eye and produce adverse effects in other parts of the body. Notify your doctor.

POSSIBLE ADVERSE EFFECTS

Darkening of the iris is very common. Changes to the eyelashes occur almost as often.

Irritation of the eye is also a very common adverse effect.

Symptom/effect	Frequency		Discuss with doctor		Stop taking drug now	Call doctor now
	Common	Rare	Only if severe	In all cases		
Darkening of iris	●		●			
Eye irritation	●		●			
Eyelash changes	●		●			
Blurred vision	●		●			
Eye pain	●			●		
Bloodshot eye	●			●		
Inflamed eyelids	●			●		
Eye/facial swelling		●		●		
Chest pains		●		●	●	
Wheeziness/breathing difficulty		●		●	●	

INTERACTIONS

Other eye drops should not be used within 5 minutes of using latanoprost.

SPECIAL PRECAUTIONS

Be sure to tell your doctor if:
- You wear contact lenses.
- You may have an eye infection.
- You are allergic to latanoprost or any of the ingredients in the formulation.
- You have heart problems.
- You have asthma.
- You are taking other medicines.

Pregnancy
Safety not established. Prostaglandins may affect the fetus. Discuss with your doctor.

Breast-feeding
The drug may pass into the breast milk and may affect the baby. Discuss with your doctor.

Infants and children
Not recommended. Safety not established.

Over 60
No special problems.

Driving and hazardous work
The eye drops may cause temporary blurring of vision. Avoid driving and hazardous work until vision has returned to normal.

Alcohol
No known problems.

PROLONGED USE

No known problems apart from changes to iris pigment and eyelashes. These changes do not affect vision, but they may not diminish once treatment has been stopped.

Monitoring Although there should be no problems with long-term use, your doctor will continue to monitor eye pigmentation as well as control of the glaucoma.

LEVETIRACETAM

Brand names Desitrend, Keppra
Used in the following combined preparations None

GENERAL INFORMATION

Levetiracetam is given for the treatment of some forms of epilepsy as it reduces the likelihood of seizures caused by abnormal nerve signals in the brain. It may be used alone or in combination with other anticonvulsant drugs. It is chemically different from other anticonvulsants, and the precise way in which it works is not fully understood.

Compared to other anticonvulsant drugs, levetiracetam usually produces relatively few adverse effects, most commonly headache, dizziness, drowsiness, and gastrointestinal disturbances such as nausea, vomiting, and indigestion. In addition, it does not interact with other anticonvulsants, which is a significant advantage and has led to it becoming increasingly commonly prescribed. As with all anticonvulsant drugs, it is important that levetiracetam is not stopped abruptly without medical advice as this can precipitate an epileptic seizure.

QUICK REFERENCE

Drug group Anticonvulsant drug (p.42)

Overdose danger rating Medium

Dependence rating Low

Prescription needed Yes

Available as generic Yes

INFORMATION FOR USERS

Your drug prescription is tailored for you. Do not alter dosage without checking with your doctor.

How taken/used

Tablets, liquid, injection.

Frequency and timing of doses
1–2 x daily.

Adult dosage range
Initially 250mg once daily, increased after 1–2 weeks to 250mg twice daily. If necessary, dosage can be further increased up to a maximum of 1.5g twice daily.

Onset of effect
Up to 48 hours.

Duration of action
12 hours.

Diet advice
None.

Storage
Store in original container at room temperature out of reach of children.

Missed dose
Take as soon as you remember. If your next dose is due within 4 hours, take a single dose now and skip the next.

Stopping the drug
Do not stop the drug without consulting your doctor; symptoms may recur.

Exceeding the dose
An occasional unintentional extra dose is unlikely to cause problems. Large overdoses may cause agitation, impaired consciousness, and coma. Notify your doctor immediately.

SPECIAL PRECAUTIONS

Be sure to tell your doctor if:
- You have long-term liver or kidney problems.
- You have a psychotic illness.
- You have a depressive illness.
- You are taking other medicines.

 Pregnancy
Safety not established. Discuss with your doctor.

 Breast-feeding
Safety not established. The drug passes into the breast milk. Discuss with your doctor.

 Infants and children
Reduced dose necessary.

 Over 60
No special problems.

 Driving and hazardous work
Avoid such activities until you have learned how levetiracetam affects you because the drug can cause drowsiness in some people.

 Alcohol
Avoid. Alcohol may worsen any drowsiness caused by levetiracetam.

PROLONGED USE

Usually no problems, although very rarely it can cause depression, other mood changes, personality changes, and suicidal thoughts.

POSSIBLE ADVERSE EFFECTS

Most people experience few adverse effects with this drug; the most common are headache, dizziness, drowsiness, and gastrointestinal problems. In rare cases, levetiracetam may cause thoughts of suicide; if this occurs, consult your doctor immediately.

Symptom/effect	Frequency		Discuss with doctor		Stop taking drug now	Call doctor now
	Common	Rare	Only if severe	In all cases		
Dizziness/headache	●		●			
Drowsiness	●		●			
Nausea/vomiting	●		●			
Indigestion/abdominal pain	●					
Itching/rash	●			●		
Cough		●	●			
Mood changes/depression		●		●		
Suicidal thoughts		●		●		●

INTERACTIONS

Antidepressant drugs (MAOIs, tricyclics and SSRIs) and mefloquine may reduce the anticonvulsant effect of levetiracetam.

St John's wort may reduce the anticonvulsant effect of levetiracetam.

LEVODOPA/CO-BENELDOPA/CO-CARELDOPA

Brand names None
Used in the following combined preparations Caramet CR, Duodopa, Madopar, Madopar CR, Sinemet, Sinemet CR, Stalevo

GENERAL INFORMATION

The treatment of Parkinson's disease underwent dramatic change in the 1960s with the introduction of levodopa. Since the body can transform levodopa into dopamine, a chemical messenger in the brain the absence or shortage of which causes Parkinson's disease (see p.43), rapid improvements in control were obtained. These improvements were not a cure but a marked relief of symptoms.

It was found, however, that, while levodopa was effective, it produced severe side effects, such as nausea, dizziness, and palpitations. Even when treatment was initiated gradually, it was difficult to balance the benefits against the adverse reactions.

Today levodopa is prescribed in a combined form with carbidopa (as co-careldopa) or benserazide (as co-beneldopa); both of these enhance the effects of levodopa in the brain, as well as helping to reduce the side effects of levodopa. The drug is taken by mouth and, in severe cases, can be given in the form of intestinal gel.

QUICK REFERENCE

Drug group Drug for parkinsonism (p.43)

Overdose danger rating Medium

Dependence rating Low

Prescription needed Yes

Available as generic Yes

INFORMATION FOR USERS

Your drug prescription is tailored for you. Do not alter dosage without checking with your doctor.

How taken/used

Tablets, MR tablets, dispersible tablets, capsules, intestinal gel.

Frequency and timing of doses
2–6 x daily with food or milk.

Adult dosage range
125–500mg initially, increased until benefits and side effects are balanced.

Onset of effect
Within 1 hour.

Duration of action
2–12 hours.

Diet advice
None.

Storage
Keep in original container at room temperature out of the reach of children. Store intestinal gel in a refrigerator. Protect from light.

Missed dose
Take as soon as you remember. If your next dose is due within 2 hours, take a single dose now and skip the next.

Stopping the drug
Do not stop taking the drug without consulting your doctor; stopping the drug may lead to severe worsening of the underlying condition.

Exceeding the dose
An occasional unintentional extra dose is unlikely to cause problems. Larger overdoses may cause vomiting or drowsiness. Notify your doctor.

SPECIAL PRECAUTIONS

Be sure to tell your doctor if:
- You have heart problems.
- You have long-term liver or kidney problems.
- You have epilepsy.
- You have had glaucoma.
- You have a peptic ulcer.
- You have diabetes or any other endocrine disorder.
- You have any serious mental illness.
- You are taking other medicines.

 Pregnancy
Unlikely to be required. Safety not established. Discuss with your doctor.

 Breast-feeding
Unlikely to be required. May suppress milk production. Discuss with your doctor.

 Infants and children
Not normally used in children (and rarely given to patients under 25 years).

 Over 60
No special problems.

 Driving and hazardous work
Your underlying condition, as well as the possibility of levodopa causing fainting, dizziness, and sudden sleep episodes, may make such activities inadvisable. Discuss with your doctor.

 Alcohol
No known problems, although levodopa may enhance the sedative effects of alcohol.

PROLONGED USE

Effectiveness usually declines with time, necessitating increased dosage. Also, the adverse effects become severe at the end of one dose and the onset of another, so that the dosage, frequency, or formulation must be fine-tuned for each individual. Ultimately, other antiparkinsonian drugs may need to be substituted.

POSSIBLE ADVERSE EFFECTS

Adverse effects of levodopa are related to dosage levels. At the start of treatment, on a low dosage, unwanted effects are likely to be mild. Such effects may increase in severity as dosage is increased. All adverse effects should be discussed with your doctor.

Symptom/effect	Frequency		Discuss with doctor		Stop taking drug now	Call doctor now
	Common	Rare	Only if severe	In all cases		
Dark urine	●		●			
Digestive disturbance	●			●		
Abnormal movement	●			●		
Nervousness/agitation	●			●		
Hallucinations/confusion	●			●		
Dizziness/fainting		●		●		
Fatigue/sudden sleep		●		●		
Compulsive behaviour		●		●		

INTERACTIONS

Antidepressant drugs Levodopa may interact with monoamine oxidase inhibitors (MAOIs) to cause a dangerous rise in blood pressure. It may also interact with tricyclic antidepressants.

Iron Absorption of levodopa may be reduced by iron.

Antipsychotic drugs Some of these drugs may reduce the effect of levodopa.

LEVOFLOXACIN

Brand names Evoxil, Oftaquix, Quinsair, Tavanic
Used in the following combined preparations None

GENERAL INFORMATION

Levofloxacin is a quinolone antibacterial drug used for soft-tissue and respiratory and urinary tract infections that have not responded to other antibiotics. It is usually prescribed as tablets, but may be given by intravenous infusion to people with serious systemic infections or to those who cannot take drugs by mouth. It may also be given by nebulizer for respiratory infections.

Like other quinolones, levofloxacin may occasionally cause inflammation and damage of tendons, especially in older people, those with rheumatoid arthritis, and those on corticosteroids. Report any tendon pain or inflammation to your doctor immediately and stop taking the drug. Rest the affected limbs until symptoms have subsided.

Levofloxacin may also be given as eye drops to treat eye infections. The most common side effects are eye discomfort and blurred vision; there is no risk of tendon problems.

QUICK REFERENCE

Drug group Antibacterial drug (p.89)

Overdose danger rating Medium

Dependence rating Low

Prescription needed Yes

Available as generic Yes

INFORMATION FOR USERS

Your drug prescription is tailored for you. Do not alter dosage without checking with your doctor.

How taken/used

Tablets, intravenous infusion, liquid for nebulizer, eye drops.

Frequency and timing of doses
1 x 2 times daily for 7–14 days depending on infection (tablets); variable with other forms.

Adult dosage range
250–1,000mg daily; variable with eye drops.

Onset of effect
1 hour.

Duration of action
12–24 hours.

Diet advice
None.

Storage
Keep in original container at room temperature out of the reach of children.

Missed dose
Take as soon as you remember, then take your next dose when it is due.

Stopping the drug
Take the full course. Even if you feel better, the original infection may still be present, and symptoms may recur if treatment is stopped too soon.

Exceeding the dose
An occasional unintentional extra dose is unlikely to cause problems. Large overdoses of oral, infused, or inhaled preparations may cause mental disturbances and seizures. Notify your doctor.

SPECIAL PRECAUTIONS

Be sure to tell your doctor if:
- You have kidney problems.
- You have epilepsy.
- You have porphyria.
- You have myasthenia gravis.
- You have a history of psychotic illness.
- You have had a previous allergic reaction to a quinolone antibacterial.
- You have had a previous tendon problem with a quinolone.
- You are taking other medicines.

Pregnancy
Safety not established. Discuss with your doctor.

Breast-feeding
Safety not established. Discuss with your doctor.

Infants and children
Not recommended.

Over 60
No special problems, except that tendon damage is more likely over the age of 60.

Driving and hazardous work
Avoid such activities until you have learned how levofloxacin affects you because the drug can cause dizziness, drowsiness, visual disturbances, and hallucinations.

Alcohol
Avoid. Alcohol may increase the sedative effects of levofloxacin.

Sunlight and sunbeds
Avoid exposure to strong sunlight or artificial ultraviolet rays because photosensitization may occur.

POSSIBLE ADVERSE EFFECTS (oral/infused/inhaled forms)

Infused or inhaled forms may cause palpitations and a fall in blood pressure; oral forms most commonly cause nausea and vomiting. Aortic aneurysm or dissection have occurred in rare cases; for any sudden onset of chest, back, or abdominal pain, seek urgent medical help.

Symptom/effect	Frequency		Discuss with doctor		Stop taking drug now	Call doctor now
	Common	Rare	Only if severe	In all cases		
Nausea/vomiting	●		●			
Diarrhoea/abdominal pain	●					
Headache/dizziness		●	●			
Drowsiness/restlessness		●	●			
Skin rash/itching/jaundice		●		●	●	
Fever/allergic reaction		●		●	●	
Confusion/seizures		●		●	●	●
Painful or inflamed tendons		●		●	●	●

INTERACTIONS (oral/infused/inhaled forms)

Anticoagulants The effect of these drugs may be increased by levofloxacin.

Oral iron preparations and antacids containing magnesium or aluminium hydroxide interfere with absorption of levofloxacin. Do not take antacids within 2 hours of taking levofloxacin tablets.

Ciclosporin used with levofloxacin carries an increased risk of kidney damage.

NSAIDs (p.74) and theophylline increase the risk of seizures if taken with levofloxacin.

Corticosteroids may increase the risk of tendon rupture with levofloxacin.

PROLONGED USE

Levofloxacin is not usually prescribed for long-term use.

LEVONORGESTREL

Brand names Emerres, Kyleena, Levonelle 1500, Levonelle One Step, Levosert, Logynon, Mirena, Norgeston, Upostelle
Used in the following combined preparations Logynon ED, Microgynon 30, Ovranette, Rigevidon, and others

GENERAL INFORMATION

Levonorgestrel is a synthetic hormone similar to progesterone, a natural female sex hormone. Its primary use is in oral contraceptives. It performs this function by thickening the mucus at the neck of the uterus (cervix), thereby making it difficult for sperm to enter the uterus.

The drug is available in combined oral contraceptives (COCs) with an oestrogen drug. It is given in a higher dose as a progestogen-only preparation (POP) for emergency postcoital contraception and can be obtained over the counter by women over 16 years. It is also combined with an oestrogen drug in hormone replacement therapy (HRT) for the short-term treatment of menopausal symptoms (see p.105).

It rarely causes serious adverse effects, but when used alone, menstrual irregularities, especially mid-cycle, or "breakthrough" bleeding, may occur.

INFORMATION FOR USERS

Your drug prescription is tailored for you. Do not alter dosage without checking with your doctor.

How taken/used

Tablets, intrauterine device (IUD), patches.

Frequency and timing of doses
Once daily, at the same time each day (tablets).

Adult dosage range
Progestogen-only contraceptive 30mcg daily.
Postcoital contraceptive 1.5mg as a single dose as soon as possible, within 12 hours, but no later than after 72 hours.
HRT and combined oral contraceptive Dosage varies according to preparation used.

Onset of effect
Within 4 hours, but contraceptive protection may not be fully effective for 14 days, depending on day of cycle tablets are started.

Duration of action
24 hours. Some effects, not including contraception, may persist for up to 3 months after levonorgestrel is stopped.

Diet advice
None.

Storage
Keep in original container at room temperature out of the reach of children.

Missed dose
Progestogen-only contraceptive: If a tablet is delayed by 3 hours or more, regard it as a missed dose. See What to do if you miss a pill (p.123). *Postcoital contraceptive*: If vomiting occurs within 3 hours, take another tablet immediately. If problem persists speak to your doctor or pharmacist without delay. *Combined oral contraceptive*: Depends on preparation used. See What to do if you miss a pill (p.123).

Stopping the drug
The drug can be safely stopped as soon as contraceptive protection is no longer required. For treatment of menopausal symptoms, consult your doctor before stopping the drug.

Exceeding the dose
An occasional unintentional extra dose is unlikely to be a cause for concern. But if you notice any unusual symptoms, or if a large overdose has been taken, notify your doctor.

SPECIAL PRECAUTIONS

Be sure to tell your doctor if:
- You have a personal or family history of breast cancer.
- You have liver or kidney problems, heart failure, high blood pressure, diabetes, asthma, epilepsy, porphyria, or sickle cell anaemia.
- You have abnormal vaginal bleeding.
- You have ever had migraines, severe headaches, blood clots, or a stroke.
- You have a history of depression.
- You are taking other medicines.

 Pregnancy
Not prescribed. May cause abnormalities in the developing baby. Discuss with your doctor.

 Breast-feeding
The drug passes into the breast milk, but at normal doses adverse effects on the baby are unlikely. Discuss with your doctor.

 Infants and children
Not prescribed.

 Over 60
Not prescribed.

 Driving and hazardous work
No known problems.

 Alcohol
No known problems.

Surgery and general anaesthetics
The drug should be stopped before surgery.

POSSIBLE ADVERSE EFFECTS

Menstrual irregularities (blood spotting between menstrual periods or absence of menstruation) are the most common side effects of levonorgestrel alone. Pain in the lower abdomen is rare but may indicate pregnancy; consult your doctor promptly.

Symptom/effect	Frequency		Discuss with doctor		Stop taking drug now	Call doctor now
	Common	Rare	Only if severe	In all cases		
Swollen feet/ankles	●		●			
Weight gain	●		●			
Irregular vaginal bleeding	●			●		
Nausea/vomiting		●	●			
Breast tenderness		●	●			
Depression/headache		●		●		
Lower abdominal pain		●		●		●

INTERACTIONS

General note A number of drugs can reduce blood levels of levonorgestrel and hence its contraceptive protection. These include phenytoin, carbamazepine, rifampicin, some HIV drugs, and herbal remedies such as St John's wort. Consult your doctor or pharmacist before taking other medications.

PROLONGED USE

In a COC, levonorgestrel increases the thrombosis and breast cancer risk but reduces the endometrial and ovarian cancer risk. In a POP, it carries a small increased risk of breast cancer. In HRT, it increases the risk of thrombosis and breast cancer. HRT is advised only for short-term use around the menopause.

Monitoring Blood pressure checks, physical examination, and mammograms may be performed.

LEVOTHYROXINE

Brand name Eltroxin
Used in the following combined preparations None

GENERAL INFORMATION

Levothyroxine is the main hormone produced by the thyroid gland. A deficiency of this hormone causes hypothyroidism, which is associated with symptoms such as weight gain and slowing of body functions. A synthetic preparation is given to replace the natural hormone when it is deficient. It is sometimes given in combination with carbimazole or propylthiouracil in the treatment of an overactive thyroid gland (Graves' disease). Levothyroxine is also given (in higher doses) to people who have had thyroid cancer. Doses are usually increased gradually to help prevent adverse effects, and particular care is required in patients with heart problems such as angina.

INFORMATION FOR USERS

Your drug prescription is tailored for you. Do not alter dosage without checking with your doctor.

How taken/used

Tablets, liquid.

Frequency and timing of doses
1 x daily, ideally before breakfast or first meal.

Dosage range
Adults Doses of 25–150mcg daily, increased at 3–4-week intervals as required. The usual maximum dose is 200mcg daily.

Onset of effect
Within 48 hours. Full beneficial effects may not be felt for several weeks.

Duration of action
1–3 weeks.

Diet advice
None.

Storage
Keep in original container at room temperature out of the reach of children. Protect from light.

Missed dose
Take as soon as you remember. If your next dose is due within 8 hours, take a single dose now and skip the next.

Stopping the drug
Do not stop the drug without consulting your doctor; symptoms may recur.

Exceeding the dose
An occasional unintentional extra dose is unlikely to cause problems. Large overdoses may cause palpitations in next few days. Notify your doctor.

SPECIAL PRECAUTIONS

Be sure to tell your doctor if:
- You have high blood pressure.
- You have heart problems, such as angina, heart rhythm problems, or heart failure.
- You have diabetes.
- You have an adrenal gland disorder.
- You are taking other medicines.

 Pregnancy
No evidence of risk, but dosage adjustment may be necessary.

 Breast-feeding
The drug passes into the breast milk, but at normal doses adverse effects on the baby are unlikely. Discuss with your doctor.

 Infants and children
Dosage depends on age and weight.

 Over 60
Reduced dose usually necessary, together with careful dose escalation.

 Driving and hazardous work
No known problems.

 Alcohol
No known problems.

POSSIBLE ADVERSE EFFECTS

Adverse effects are rare with levothyroxine and are usually the result of overdosage causing thyroid overactivity. These effects diminish as the dose is lowered. Too low a dose may cause signs of hormone deficiency, such as weight gain, constipation, and altered periods.

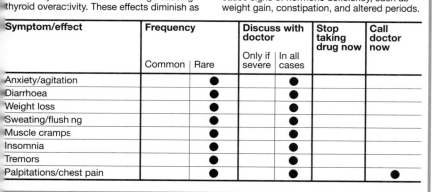

Symptom/effect	Frequency		Discuss with doctor		Stop taking drug now	Call doctor now
	Common	Rare	Only if severe	In all cases		
Anxiety/agitation	●			●		
Diarrhoea	●			●		
Weight loss	●			●		
Sweating/flushing	●			●		
Muscle cramps	●			●		
Insomnia	●			●		
Tremors	●			●		
Palpitations/chest pain	●			●		●

PROLONGED USE

No special problems.

Monitoring Periodic tests of thyroid function are required.

INTERACTIONS

Oral anticoagulants Levothyroxine may increase the effect of these drugs.

Colestyramine This drug may reduce the absorption of levothyroxine.

Amiodarone may affect thyroid activity; levothyroxine dosage may need adjustment.

Antidiabetic agents The doses of these drugs may need increasing once levothyroxine treatment is started.

Anticonvulsant drugs These drugs may reduce the effect of levothyroxine.

Calcium/iron preparations and sucralfate may reduce levothyroxine absorption unless the drugs are taken several hours apart.

Antidepressants Levothyroxine may enhance effects of tricyclic antidepressants.

Oral contraceptives may increase levothyroxine requirements.

LISINOPRIL

Brand names Carace, Zestril
Used in the following combined preparations Carace Plus, Lisoretic, Zestoretic

GENERAL INFORMATION

Lisinopril is an ACE inhibitor drug used in the treatment of high blood pressure, diabetic nephropathy (kidney disease), heart failure, and following a heart attack. It works by relaxing the muscles in blood vessel walls, allowing them to dilate (widen), thereby easing blood flow. After a heart attack, it reduces the risk of heart failure if taken long term.

Lisinopril can initially cause a rapid fall in blood pressure, especially when taken with a diuretic drug. Therefore, treatment for heart failure is usually started under close medical supervision, in hospital in severe cases. The first dose is usually very small, and should be taken while lying down, preferably at bedtime.

QUICK REFERENCE

Drug group ACE inhibitor (p.56) and antihypertensive drug (p.60)

Overdose danger rating Medium

Dependence rating Low

Prescription needed Yes

Available as generic Yes

INFORMATION FOR USERS

Your drug prescription is tailored for you. Do not alter dosage without checking with your doctor.

How taken/used

Tablets, oral solution.

Frequency and timing of doses
1 x daily.

Adult dosage range
Hypertension 2.5–10mg (starting dose) up to 80mg.
Heart failure 2.5mg (starting dose) up to 35mg.
Prevention of further heart attacks 2.5–5mg (starting dose) up to 10mg.
Diabetic nephropathy 2.5–20mg.

Onset of effect
1–2 hours; full beneficial effect may take several weeks.

Duration of action
12–24 hours.

Diet advice
Your doctor may advise you to reduce your salt intake to help control your blood pressure.

Storage
Keep in original container at room temperature out of the reach of children.

Missed dose
Take as soon as you remember. If your next dose is due within 8 hours, take a single dose now and skip the next.

Stopping the drug
Do not stop taking the drug without consulting your doctor. Stopping the drug may lead to worsening of the underlying condition.

Exceeding the dose
An occasional unintentional extra dose is unlikely to be a cause for concern. Larger overdoses may cause dizziness or fainting. Notify your doctor.

POSSIBLE ADVERSE EFFECTS

Lisinopril may cause various minor adverse effects, most commonly a rash and a persistent dry cough. A reduction of dosage may minimize these effects.

Symptom/effect	Frequency		Discuss with doctor		Stop taking drug now	Call doctor now
	Common	Rare	Only if severe	In all cases		
Rash	●			●		
Persistent dry cough	●			●		
Mouth ulcers/sore mouth		●		●		
Dizziness		●		●		
Sore throat/fever		●		●		
Swelling of mouth/lips		●		●	●	●
Breathing difficulty		●		●	●	●

INTERACTIONS

Potassium supplements, potassium-sparing diuretics, and ciclosporin Taken with lisinopril, these drugs increase the risk of high blood potassium levels.

Non-steroidal anti-inflammatory drugs (NSAIDs) Some may reduce the effect of lisinopril. Increased risk of kidney damage.

Immunosuppressants and allopurinol may increase risk of reduced white cell counts.

Vasodilators, diuretics, and other drugs for hypertension These drugs may increase the blood-pressure-lowering effect of lisinopril.

Lithium Lisinopril may increase blood levels.

Insulin and antidiabetic drugs Lisinopril may increase the effect of these drugs.

mTOR inhibitors such as sirolimus with lisinopril may increase risk of angioedema.

SPECIAL PRECAUTIONS

Be sure to tell your doctor if:
- You have long-term kidney or liver problems.
- You have heart problems.
- You have had angioedema or a previous allergic reaction to ACE inhibitors.
- You are pregnant or intend to become pregnant.
- You are taking other medicines.

Pregnancy
Not prescribed. There is evidence of harm to the developing fetus.

Breast-feeding
Safety not established. Discuss with your doctor.

Infants and children
Not recommended.

Over 60
Reduced dose may be necessary.

Driving and hazardous work
Avoid such activities until you have learned how lisinopril affects you because the drug can cause dizziness and fainting.

Alcohol
Avoid. Alcohol may increase the blood-pressure-lowering and adverse effects of the drug.

Surgery and general anaesthetics
Lisinopril may have to be stopped before you have a general anaesthetic. Discuss with your doctor or dentist before any operation.

PROLONGED USE

No problems expected.

Monitoring Periodic checks on potassium levels, white blood cell count, kidney function, and urine are usually performed.

LITHIUM

Brand names Camcolit, Li-liquid, Liskonum, Priadel
Used in the following combined preparations None

GENERAL INFORMATION

Lithium, the lightest known metal, has been used since the 1940s to treat manic depression (bipolar affective disorder). It decreases the intensity and frequency of the swings from extreme excitement to deep depression that characterize the disorder. The drug is sometimes used together with an antidepressant for depression that has not responded to an antidepressant

alone. Lithium is also sometimes used to control aggressive or self-harming behaviour. High levels of lithium can cause serious adverse effects, so blood levels must be carefully monitored. Any apparent benefit may take two to three weeks to appear; an antipsychotic drug is often given with lithium until it takes effect. Lithium cards, with details of side effects, are available from pharmacies.

QUICK REFERENCE

Drug group Antimanic drug (p.41)
Overdose danger rating High
Dependence rating Low
Prescription needed Yes
Available as generic Yes

INFORMATION FOR USERS

Your drug prescription is tailored for you. Do not alter dosage without checking with your doctor.

How taken/used

Tablets, SR tablets, liquid.

Frequency and timing of doses
1–2 x daily with meals. Always take the same brand of lithium to ensure a consistent effect; change of brand must be closely supervised.

Adult dosage range
0.3–1.6g daily. Dosage may vary according to individual response and blood levels.

Onset of effect
Effects may be noticed in 3–5 days, but the full preventative effect may take 6–12 months.

Duration of action
18–36 hours. Some effects may last for several days.

Diet advice
Lithium levels in the blood are affected by the amount of salt in the body, so do not

suddenly alter the amount of salt in your diet. Be sure to drink plenty of fluids, especially in hot weather.

Storage
Keep in original container at room temperature out of the reach of children.

Missed dose
Take as soon as you remember. If your next dose is due within 4 hours, take a single dose now and skip the next.

Stopping the drug
Do not stop the drug without consulting your doctor; symptoms may recur.

OVERDOSE ACTION

Seek immediate medical advice in all cases. Take emergency action if seizures or loss of consciousness occur.

See Drug poisoning emergency guide (p.518).

SPECIAL PRECAUTIONS

Be sure to tell your doctor if:
- You have long-term liver or kidney problems.
- You have heart or circulation problems.
- You have an overactive thyroid gland.
- You have Addison's disease.
- You are taking other medicines.

Pregnancy
Not usually prescribed. May cause defects in the unborn baby. Discuss with your doctor.

Breast-feeding
The drug passes into the breast milk and may affect the baby. Discuss with your doctor.

Infants and children
Not recommended.

Over 60
Increased likelihood of adverse effects. Reduced dose may therefore be necessary.

Driving and hazardous work
Avoid such activities until you have learned how lithium affects you because the drug can cause reduced alertness.

Alcohol
Avoid. Alcohol may increase the sedative effects of this drug.

PROLONGED USE

Prolonged lithium use may lead to kidney and thyroid problems. Treatment for periods of longer than 5 years is not normally advised unless the benefits are significant and tests show no sign of reduced kidney function. When the decision is taken to stop lithium, it should be reduced gradually over a few weeks.

Monitoring Once stabilized, lithium levels should be checked every 3 months. Thyroid function should be checked every 6–12 months. Kidney function should also be monitored regularly.

POSSIBLE ADVERSE EFFECTS

Many of the symptoms below are signs of a high lithium level in the blood. Stop taking the

drug and seek medical advice promptly if you notice any of these symptoms.

Symptom/effect	Frequency		Discuss with doctor		Stop taking drug now	Call doctor now
	Common	Rare	Only if severe	In all cases		
Increase in urine/thirst	●		●			
Nausea/vomiting/diarrhoea	●			●		
Tremor	●			●		
Weight gain		●	●			
Drowsiness/lethargy		●		●	●	
Blurred vision		●		●	●	
Unsteadiness/slurred speech		●		●	●	

INTERACTIONS

General note Many drugs interact with lithium. Do not take any over-the-counter or prescription drugs without consulting your doctor or pharmacist. Paracetamol should be used in preference to other analgesics for everyday pain relief.

Diuretics, aspirin, and non-steroidal anti-inflammatory drugs (NSAIDs) can increase lithium to a dangerous level. Blood levels of lithium should be monitored closely.

LOFEPRAMINE

Brand names None
Used in the following combined preparations None

GENERAL INFORMATION

Lofepramine is a tricyclic antidepressant used primarily in long-term treatment of depression. It works to elevate the mood, improve appetite, increase physical activity, and restore interest in everyday pursuits. Less sedating than some other tricyclic antidepressants, lofepramine is particularly useful when depression is accompanied by lethargy.

The main advantage of lofepramine over other similar drugs is that it seems to have a weaker anticholinergic action (see p.35) and therefore has milder side effects. In overdose, it is thought to be less harmful than other tricyclic antidepressants. However, like other tricyclic antidepressants, lofepramine lowers the threshold for seizures.

QUICK REFERENCE

Drug group Tricyclic antidepressant drug (p.40)

Overdose danger rating Medium

Dependence rating Low

Prescription needed Yes

Available as generic Yes

INFORMATION FOR USERS

Your drug prescription is tailored for you. Do not alter dosage without checking with your doctor.

How taken/used

Tablets, liquid.

Frequency and timing of doses
2–3 x daily.

Adult dosage range
140–210mg daily.

Onset of effect
Sedation can occur within hours; full antidepressant effect may not be felt for 2–6 weeks.

Duration of action
Antidepressant effect: may last for 6 weeks. Common adverse effects: for first 1–2 weeks.

Diet advice
None.

Storage
Keep in original container at room temperature out of the reach of children. Protect from light.

Missed dose
Take as soon as you remember. If your next dose is due within 3 hours, take a single dose now and skip the next.

Stopping the drug
An abrupt stop can cause withdrawal symptoms and a recurrence of the original problem. Consult your doctor, who may supervise a gradual reduction in dosage over at least 4 weeks.

Exceeding the dose
An occasional unintentional extra dose is unlikely to be a cause for concern. But if you notice any unusual symptoms, or if a large overdose has been taken, notify your doctor.

SPECIAL PRECAUTIONS

Be sure to tell your doctor if:
- You have heart problems.
- You have had epileptic seizures.
- You have long-term liver or kidney problems.
- You have glaucoma.
- You have an overactive thyroid gland.
- You have prostate trouble.
- You have porphyria.
- You are taking other medicines.

Pregnancy
Safety in pregnancy not established. Discuss with your doctor.

Breast-feeding
The drug passes into the breast milk and may affect the baby. Discuss with your doctor.

Infants and children
Not recommended.

Over 60
Reduced dose may be necessary as older patients are more sensitive to adverse reactions.

Driving and hazardous work
Avoid such activities until you have learned how lofepramine affects you because the drug may cause blurred vision and reduced alertness.

Alcohol
Avoid. Alcohol may increase the sedative effects of this drug.

Surgery and general anaesthetics
Lofepramine may need to be stopped. Discuss with your doctor or dentist before you have any surgery.

POSSIBLE ADVERSE EFFECTS

The possible adverse effects of this drug are mainly the result of its mild anticholinergic action and its blocking action on the transmission of signals though the heart.

Symptom/effect	Frequency		Discuss with doctor		Stop taking drug now	Call doctor now
	Common	Rare	Only if severe	In all cases		
Sweating/flushing	●		●			
Drowsiness	●		●			
Constipation		●	●			
Dry mouth		●	●			
Blurred vision		●		●		
Difficulty in passing urine		●		●		
Dizziness/fainting		●		●	●	
Palpitations		●		●	●	●

PROLONGED USE

No problems expected.

INTERACTIONS

Sedatives All drugs that have sedative effects may intensify those of lofepramine.

Anti-arrhythmic drugs and sotalol These drugs may increase the risk of abnormal heart rhythms.

Warfarin Lofepramine may, rarely, increase the effects of warfarin.

Monoamine oxidase inhibitors (MAOIs) Serious interactions are possible. These drugs are only prescribed together under close specialist medical supervision.

Selective serotonin re-uptake inhibitors (SSRIs) Some SSRIs can increase the amount of lofepramine in the body, leading to more marked adverse effects.

LOPERAMIDE

Brand names Arret, Boots Diareze, Diocalm Ultra, Imodium
Used in the following combined preparations Diocalm Plus, Imodium Plus

GENERAL INFORMATION

Loperamide is an antidiarrhoeal drug available as tablets, capsules, or liquid. It reduces the loss of water and salts from the bowel and slows bowel activity, resulting in the passage of firmer bowel movements at less frequent intervals.

A fast-acting drug, loperamide is widely prescribed for both sudden and recurrent bouts of diarrhoea. However, it is not generally recommended for diarrhoea caused by infection or poisons because it may delay the expulsion of harmful substances from the bowel. The drug is often prescribed for people who have had a colostomy or an ileostomy, to reduce fluid loss from the stoma (outlet).

Adverse effects are rare. There is no risk of abuse, as there may be with the opium-based antidiarrhoeals, because loperamide is only minimally absorbed from the gut. It can be purchased over the counter in a pharmacy.

QUICK REFERENCE

Drug group Antidiarrhoeal drug (p.68)

Overdose danger rating Medium

Dependence rating Low

Prescription needed No (most preparations)

Available as generic Yes

INFORMATION FOR USERS

Follow instructions on the label. Call your doctor if symptoms worsen.

How taken/used

Tablets, capsules, liquid.

Frequency and timing of doses
Acute diarrhoea Take a double dose at start of treatment, then a single dose after each loose bowel movement, up to maximum daily dose. *Chronic diarrhoea* 2 x daily.

Adult dosage range
Acute diarrhoea 4mg (starting dose), then 2mg after each loose bowel movement (12–16mg daily); usual dose 6–8mg daily. Use for up to 5 days only (3 days only for children 4–8 years), then consult your doctor. *Chronic diarrhoea* 4–8mg daily (up to 16mg daily).

Onset of effect
Within 1–2 hours.

Duration of action
6–18 hours.

Diet advice
Ensure adequate fluid, sugar, and salt intake during a diarrhoeal illness.

Storage
Keep in original container at room temperature out of the reach of children.

Missed dose
Do not take the missed dose. Take your next dose if needed.

Stopping the drug
Can be safely stopped as soon as you no longer need it.

Exceeding the dose
An occasional unintentional extra dose is unlikely to be a cause for concern. Large overdoses may cause constipation, vomiting, or drowsiness, and affect breathing. Notify your doctor.

POSSIBLE ADVERSE EFFECTS

Most adverse effects are rare with loperamide and often difficult to distinguish from the effects of the diarrhoea it is used to treat.

If symptoms such as bloating, abdominal pain, or fever persist or worsen during treatment with loperamide, consult your doctor.

Symptom/effect	Frequency		Discuss with doctor		Stop taking drug now	Call doctor now
	Common	Rare	Only if severe	In all cases		
Headache	●		●			
Bloating		●	●			
Abdominal pain		●	●			
Dry mouth		●	●			
Drowsiness or dizziness		●	●		●	
Constipation		●	●		●	
Itching skin		●		●		
Rash		●		●		●

INTERACTIONS

None.

SPECIAL PRECAUTIONS

Be sure to consult your doctor or pharmacist before taking this drug if:
- You have long-term liver or kidney problems.
- You have had recent abdominal surgery.
- You have an infection or blockage in the intestine, pseudomembranous colitis, or ulcerative colitis.
- You are taking other medicines.

 Pregnancy
Safety in pregnancy not established. Discuss with your doctor.

 Breast-feeding
The drug passes into the breast milk and may affect the baby. Discuss with your doctor.

 Infants and children
Not to be given to children under 4 years. Reduced dose necessary in older children. Children can be very sensitive to the effects of this drug so it should only be used in children under 12 on medical advice.

 Over 60
No special problems.

 Driving and hazardous work
Avoid such activities until you have learned how loperamide affects you because the drug can cause dizziness or drowsiness.

 Alcohol
No known problems.

PROLONGED USE

Although this drug is not usually taken for prolonged periods (except by those with a medically diagnosed long-term gastrointestinal condition), special problems are not expected during long-term use.

LOPINAVIR/RITONAVIR

Brand name Kaletra
Used in the following combined preparations None

GENERAL INFORMATION

Lopinavir and ritonavir are both antiretroviral drugs from the same class of drugs, known as protease inhibitors. Combined together as a single drug, they are used in the treatment of HIV infection. The drugs work by interfering with an enzyme used by the virus to produce genetic material (see p.116).

The combination drug is prescribed with other antiretroviral drugs, usually two nucleoside analogues, which together slow down the production of HIV. The aim of this combination therapy is to reduce the damage done to the immune system by the virus.

Combination antiretroviral therapy is not a cure for HIV. Taken regularly on a long-term basis, it can reduce the level of the virus in the body and improve the outlook for a person who has HIV. However, the person will remain infectious and will experience a relapse if the treatment is stopped.

QUICK REFERENCE

Drug group Drug for HIV and immune deficiency (p.116)
Overdose danger rating Medium
Dependence rating Low
Prescription needed Yes
Available as generic No

INFORMATION FOR USERS

Your drug prescription is tailored for you. Do not alter dosage without checking with your doctor.

How taken/used

Tablets, oral liquid.

Frequency and timing of doses
Every 12 hours, with food.

Adult dosage range
400mg lopinavir with 100mg ritonavir 2 x daily; alternatively 800/200mg 1 x daily (tablets); 5ml (400mg lopinavir with 100mg ritanovir) 2 x daily (liquid).

Onset of effect
Within 1 hour.

Duration of action
12 hours.

Diet advice
None.

Storage
Keep in original container at room temperature (tablets), or refrigerator (liquid) out of the reach of children.

Missed dose
Take as soon as you remember. If your next dose is due within 2 hours, take a single dose now and skip the next. It is very important not to miss doses on a regular basis as this can lead to the development of drug-resistant HIV.

Stopping the drug
Do not stop taking the drug without consulting your doctor.

Exceeding the dose
An occasional unintentional extra dose is unlikely to cause problems. But if you notice any unusual symptoms, or if a large overdose has been taken, notify your doctor.

SPECIAL PRECAUTIONS

Be sure to tell your doctor if:
- You have long-term liver or kidney problems.
- You have heart problems.
- You take recreational drugs.
- You have acute porphyria.
- You have haemophilia.
- You are taking other medicines.

 Pregnancy
Tablets can be used during pregnancy if clinically needed. The oral solution is not recommended. Discuss with your doctor.

 Breast-feeding
Safety not established. Breast-feeding is not recommended for HIV-positive mothers as the virus may be passed to the baby.

 Infants and children
Not recommended in children under 2 years. Reduced dose recommended in children over 2 years.

 Over 60
Reduced dose may be necessary to minimize adverse effects.

 Driving and hazardous work
No known problems.

 Alcohol
The liquid drug contains a small amount of alcohol, so care should be taken with alcohol consumption.

POSSIBLE ADVERSE EFFECTS

Gastrointestinal upset is the most common adverse effect. Other problems, which are more likely to occur with prolonged use, include changes in body shape. These effects should be discussed with your doctor.

Symptom/effect	Frequency		Discuss with doctor		Stop taking drug now	Call doctor now
	Common	Rare	Only if severe	In all cases		
Nausea/vomiting/diarrhoea	●			●		
Loss of appetite	●			●		
Fatigue	●			●		
Body shape changes		●		●		
Severe abdominal pain		●		●		●

PROLONGED USE

Changes in body shape may occur, including redistribution of body fat from the arms and/or legs to the abdomen and back of the neck.

Monitoring Your doctor will take regular blood samples to check the effect of the drugs on the virus. Blood will also be checked for changes in lipids, liver function, cholesterol, and sugar levels.

INTERACTIONS

General note A wide range of drugs may interact with lopinavir and ritonavir, causing either an increase in adverse effects or a reduction in the effect of the antiretroviral drugs. Check with your doctor or pharmacist before taking any new drugs, including those from the dentist and supermarket, and herbal medicines. Ritonavir is known to interact with some recreational drugs, including ecstasy, and it is essential that you discuss the use of such drugs with your doctor or pharmacist.

LORATADINE/DESLORATADINE

Brand names [loratadine] Boots Hayfever and Allergy Relief All Day, Clarityn, Clarityn Allergy; [desloratadine] NeoClarityn
Used in the following combined preparations None

GENERAL INFORMATION

Loratadine, a long-acting antihistamine drug, is used for the relief of symptoms associated with allergic rhinitis, such as sneezing, nasal discharge, and itching and burning of the eyes. Symptoms are normally relieved within an hour of oral administration. Loratadine is also used to treat allergic skin conditions such as chronic urticaria (itching). An advantage of loratadine over older antihistamines, such as chlorphenamine, is that it has fewer sedative and anticholinergic effects, so this drug is less likely to cause drowsiness.

Desloratadine is the active breakdown product of loratadine. This drug is available as a separate product (NeoClarityn) but offers no advantages over loratadine itself.

Loratadine and desloratadine should be discontinued about four days prior to skin testing for allergy as they may decrease or prevent the detection of positive results.

QUICK REFERENCE

Drug group Antihistamine (p.82)

Overdose danger rating Low

Dependence rating Low

Prescription needed No (loratadine); yes (desloratadine)

Available as generic Yes

INFORMATION FOR USERS

Follow instructions on the label. Call your doctor if symptoms worsen.

How taken/used

Tablets, liquid.

Frequency and timing of doses
Once daily.

Adult dosage range
10mg daily (loratadine); 5mg daily (desloratadine).

Onset of effect
Usually within 1 hour.

Duration of action
Up to 24 hours.

Diet advice
None.

Storage
Keep in original container at room temperature out of the reach of children.

Missed dose
Take as soon as you remember. If your next dose is due within 6 hours, take a single dose now and skip the next.

Stopping the drug
Can be safely stopped as soon as you no longer need it.

Exceeding the dose
An occasional unintentional extra dose is unlikely to be a cause for concern. But if you notice any unusual symptoms, or if a large overdose has been taken, notify your doctor.

POSSIBLE ADVERSE EFFECTS

The incidence of adverse effects with loratadine/desloratadine is low.

Symptom/effect	Frequency		Discuss with doctor		Stop taking drug now	Call doctor now
	Common	Rare	Only if severe	In all cases		
Drowsiness		●	●			
Fatigue		●	●			
Nausea		●	●			
Headache		●	●			
Dry mouth		●	●			
Palpitations		●		●		
Fainting		●		●		

INTERACTIONS

Cimetidine, clarithromycin, erythromycin, ketoconazole, fluoxetine, fluconazole, quinidine, and fosamprenavir These drugs may increase the blood levels and effects of loratadine and desloratadine, but this has not been found to cause problems.

SPECIAL PRECAUTIONS

Be sure to consult your doctor or pharmacist before taking this drug if:
- You have liver disease.
- You are taking other medicines.

 Pregnancy
Safety in pregnancy not established. Discuss with your doctor.

 Breast-feeding
Safety not established. The drug passes into the breast milk. Discuss with your doctor.

 Infants and children
Not recommended under 2 years (loratadine). Not recommended under 1 year (desloratadine).

 Over 60
No problems expected.

 Driving and hazardous work
Problems are unlikely, but you need to be aware of how the drug affects you before driving or carrying out hazardous work.

 Alcohol
Alcohol will increase any sedative effects of loratadine/desloratadine.

PROLONGED USE

No problems expected.

LOSARTAN

Brand name Cozaar
Used in the following combined preparation Cozaar-Comp

GENERAL INFORMATION

Losartan is a member of the group of vasodilator drugs called angiotensin II blockers. Used to treat hypertension (high blood pressure), the drug works by blocking the action of angiotensin II, a naturally occurring substance that constricts blood vessels. This action causes the blood vessel walls to relax, thereby easing blood pressure. Losartan may also be used for the treatment of heart failure and for treating kidney disease associated with diabetes and hypertension. Unlike ACE inhibitors, losartan does not cause a persistent dry cough.

Adverse effects, which include diarrhoea, dizziness, and headache, do not commonly occur.

QUICK REFERENCE

Drug group Vasodilator (p.56) and antihypertensive drug (p.60)

Overdose danger rating Medium

Dependence rating Low

Prescription needed Yes

Available as generic Yes

INFORMATION FOR USERS

Your drug prescription is tailored for you. Do not alter dosage without checking with your doctor.

How taken/used

Tablets, liquid.

Frequency and timing of doses
Once daily.

Adult dosage range
50–100mg. People over 75 years, and other groups that are especially sensitive to the drug's effects, may start on 25mg.

Onset of effect
Blood pressure 1–2 weeks, with maximum effect in 3–6 weeks from start of treatment.
Other conditions Within 1 hour.

Duration of action
12–24 hours.

Diet advice
None.

Storage
Keep in original container at room temperature out of the reach of children.

Missed dose
Take as soon as you remember. If your next dose is due within 8 hours, take a single dose now and skip the next.

Stopping the drug
Do not stop the drug without consulting your doctor. Stopping the drug may lead to worsening of the underlying condition.

Exceeding the dose
An occasional unintentional extra dose is unlikely to cause problems. Large overdoses may cause dizziness and fainting. Notify your doctor.

SPECIAL PRECAUTIONS

Be sure to tell your doctor if:
- You have stenosis of the kidney arteries.
- You have liver or kidney problems.
- You have experienced angioedema.
- You have galactose intolerance.
- You are taking other medicines.

 Pregnancy
Not prescribed. There is evidence of harm to the developing fetus.

 Breast-feeding
Not prescribed. Safety not established.

 Infants and children
Not prescribed. Safety not established.

 Over 60
Reduced dose may be necessary for people over 75 years.

 Driving and hazardous work
Do not undertake such activities until you have learned how losartan affects you because the drug can cause dizziness.

 Alcohol
Avoid. Alcohol may increase the blood-pressure-lowering and adverse effects of losartan.

POSSIBLE ADVERSE EFFECTS

Side effects, of which dizziness, headache, and diarrhoea are the most common, are usually mild. If wheezing or swelling of the lips or tongue occur, stop taking the drug and contact your doctor immediately.

Symptom/effect	Frequency		Discuss with doctor		Stop taking drug now	Call doctor now
	Common	Rare	Only if severe	In all cases		
Dizziness	●		●			
Headache		●	●			
Diarrhoea		●	●			
Muscle, joint, or back pain		●		●		
Cough		●		●		
Wheezing/swollen lips or tongue		●		●	●	●

INTERACTIONS

Vasodilators, diuretics, and other antihypertensives may increase the blood-pressure-lowering effect of losartan.

Potassium supplements, potassium-sparing diuretics, and ciclosporin Losartan increases the effect of these drugs, leading to raised levels of potassium in the blood.

Lithium Losartan may increase the levels and toxicity of lithium.

Non-steroidal anti-inflammatory drugs (NSAIDs) Certain NSAIDs may reduce the blood-pressure-lowering effect of losartan and may also increase the risk of kidney problems when taken with losartan.

Fluconazole and rifampicin may significantly reduce the blood level of the active form of losartan.

PROLONGED USE

No special problems.

Monitoring Periodic checks on blood potassium levels and kidney function may be performed.

MAGNESIUM HYDROXIDE

Brand names Cream of Magnesia, Milk of Magnesia
Used in the following combined preparations Carbellon, Maalox, Milpar, Mucogel, and others

GENERAL INFORMATION

Magnesium hydroxide is a fast-acting antacid given to neutralize stomach acid. The drug is available in a number of over-the-counter preparations for the treatment of indigestion and heartburn. Magnesium hydroxide also prevents pain caused by stomach and duodenal ulcers, gastritis, and reflux oesophagitis, although other drugs are normally used for these problems nowadays. It is also used as a laxative; it works by drawing salt and water from the wall of the bowel to soften the faeces.

Magnesium hydroxide is not often used alone as an antacid because of its laxative effect. However, this effect is countered when the drug is used in combination with aluminium hydroxide, which can cause constipation.

INFORMATION FOR USERS

Follow instructions on the label. Call your doctor if symptoms worsen.

How taken/used

Tablets, liquid, powder.

Frequency and timing of doses
Antacid 1–4 x daily as needed with water, preferably an hour after food and at bedtime. *Laxative* Once daily, at bedtime.

Adult dosage range
Antacid 1–2c per dose (tablets); 5–10ml per dose (liquid). *Laxative* 30–45ml per dose (liquid).

Onset of effect
Antacid within 15 minutes. *Laxative* 2–8 hours.

Duration of action
2–4 hours.

Diet advice
None.

Storage
Keep in original container at room temperature out of the reach of children.

Missed dose
Take as soon as you remember.

Stopping the drug
When used as an antacid, the drug can be safely stopped as soon as you no longer need it. When given as ulcer treatment, follow your doctor's advice.

Exceeding the dose
An occasional unintentional extra dose is unlikely to be a cause for concern. But if you notice any unusual symptoms, or if a large overdose has been taken, notify your doctor.

SPECIAL PRECAUTIONS

Be sure to consult your doctor or pharmacist before taking this drug if:
- You have a long-term kidney problem.
- You have liver problems.
- You have a bowel disorder.
- You are taking other medicines.

 Pregnancy
No evidence of risk, but discuss the most appropriate treatment with your doctor.

 Breast-feeding
No evidence of risk, but discuss the most appropriate treatment with your doctor.

 Infants and children
Not recommended under 3 years except on the advice of a doctor. Reduced dose necessary for older children.

 Over 60
No special problems.

 Driving and hazardous work
No known problems.

 Alcohol
Avoid excessive alcohol as it irritates the stomach and may reduce the benefits of the drug.

POSSIBLE ADVERSE EFFECTS

Diarrhoea is the only common adverse effect. Dizziness and muscle weakness due to the body's absorption of excess magnesium may occur in people with poor kidney function.

Symptom/effect	Frequency		Discuss with doctor		Stop taking drug now	Call doctor now
	Common	Rare	Only if severe	In all cases		
Diarrhoea	●			●		

INTERACTIONS

General note Magnesium hydroxide interferes with the absorption of a wide range of drugs taken by mouth, including tetracycline antibiotics, iron supplements, diflunisal, phenytoin, gabapentin, and penicillamine; therefore, you should allow 1–2 hours between magnesium hydroxide and other medications.

Enteric-coated tablets As with other antacids, magnesium hydroxide may allow break-up of the enteric coating of tablets, sometimes leading to stomach irritation.

PROLONGED USE

Magnesium hydroxide is for occasional use and should not be taken for prolonged periods without consulting your doctor, especially if you experience persistent abdominal pain while taking the drug. If you are over 40 years of age and are experiencing long-term indigestion or heartburn, your doctor will probably refer you to a specialist. Prolonged use in people with kidney damage may cause drowsiness, dizziness, and weakness, resulting from accumulation of magnesium in the body.

MALATHION

Brand names Derbac-M
Used in the following combined preparations None

GENERAL INFORMATION

Malathion is an organophosphate insecticide used in the treatment of lice and mite infestations. The drug kills parasites by interfering with their nervous system function, causing paralysis and death.

Malathion is applied topically as a shampoo or a lotion. The lotion is more convenient to use than shampoo, requiring only a single application. It is also more effective because shampoo is diluted in use. Lotions with a high alcohol content are unsuitable for small children or people with asthma, who may be affected by the solvent, or for treating crab lice in the genital area, but the water-based liquid is suitable. Care should be taken to avoid contact of the drug with the eyes or broken skin.

If resistance occurs during a course of treatment, your practitioner will recommend an alternative insecticide such as permethrin. Treatment with malathion will not prevent infestation.

QUICK REFERENCE

Drug group Drug to treat skin parasites (p.136)

Overdose danger rating Low (medium if swallowed)

Dependence rating Low

Prescription needed No

Available as generic No

INFORMATION FOR USERS

Follow instructions on the label. Call your doctor if symptoms worsen.

How taken/used

Topical liquid, lotion, shampoo.

Frequency and timing of doses
Scabies 2 doses, 7 days apart (lotion or topical liquid).
Lice 3 applications, 3 days apart (shampoo); 2 doses, 7 days apart (lotion or topical liquid).

Adult dosage range
As directed. Family members and close contacts should also be treated.

Onset of effect
Lotion or topical liquid Leave on for 12 hours (lice), or 24 hours (scabies), before washing off. For treatment of scabies, if hands are washed with soap within 24 hours of an application, another dose should be applied.
Shampoo Leave on for 5 minutes, rinse off, repeat, then use a fine-toothed comb.

Duration of action
Until washed off.

Diet advice
None.

Storage
Keep in original container at room temperature out of the reach of children. Protect from light.

Missed dose
When a repeat application of the shampoo has been missed, it should be carried out as soon as is practicable.

Stopping the drug
Malathion should be applied as a single application or as a short course of treatment.

Exceeding the dose
An extra application is unlikely to cause problems. Take emergency action if the insecticide has been swallowed.

SPECIAL PRECAUTIONS

Be sure to consult your doctor or pharmacist before taking this drug if:
• You have severe asthma or eczema.

Pregnancy
No evidence of risk. It is unlikely that enough malathion would be absorbed after occasional application to affect the developing fetus.

Breast-feeding
No evidence of risk. It is unlikely that enough malathion would be absorbed after occasional application to affect the baby.

Infants and children
No special problems, but seek medical advice for infants under 6 months.

Over 60
No special problems.

Driving and hazardous work
No special problems.

Alcohol
No special problems.

POSSIBLE ADVERSE EFFECTS

Used correctly, malathion preparations are unlikely to produce adverse effects, although the alcoholic fumes given off by some lotions may cause wheezing in people with asthma.

Symptom/effect	Frequency		Discuss with doctor		Stop taking drug now	Call doctor now
	Common	Rare	Only if severe	In all cases		
Skin irritation		●	●			

INTERACTIONS

None.

PROLONGED USE

Malathion is intended for intermittent use only. The lotion should not be used more than once a week for 3 weeks at a time. If there is a need to use malathion more frequently, it is possible that resistance has built up; seek your doctor's advice.

MEBENDAZOLE

Brand names Boots Threadworm Tablets, Ovex, Vermox
Used in the following combined preparations None

GENERAL INFORMATION

Mebendazole is used to treat various intestinal worm infestations, including threadworms, roundworms, hookworms, and whipworms. Only threadworm infection is common in the UK, but the others can be acquired during travel to countries with poor sanitation. The drug works by paralysing the worms, which are then passed out in the faeces. However, mebendazole does not kill threadworm eggs, which are deposited on the skin around the anus by adult worms, and reinfection may occur by transfer of the eggs from the anus to the mouth. To prevent reinfection, the drug must be combined with hygiene measures (see below), and all members of the family should be treated at the same time. Side effects of mebendazole are uncommon and tend to be mainly gastrointestinal. More serious side effects are rare.

QUICK REFERENCE

Drug group Anthelmintic drug (p.97)

Overdose danger rating Low

Dependence rating Low

Prescription needed No (threadworm infection) Yes (other worm infections)

Available as generic Yes

INFORMATION FOR USERS

Follow instructions on the label and follow hygiene measures for at least 6 weeks. Call your doctor if symptoms do not improve in a few days or if treatment is unsuccessful.

How taken/used

Tablets, oral suspension.

Frequency and timing of doses
Threadworm Single dose; can be repeated after 2 weeks if reinfection occurs.
Other worms 2 x daily for 3 days.

Adult dosage range
Threadworm 100mg.
Other worms 200mg daily.

Onset of effect
Within a few hours.

Duration of action
12–24 hours.

Diet advice
None.

Storage
Keep in original container at room temperature out of the reach of children.

Missed dose
Threadworm Take as soon as you remember.
Other worms Take as soon as you remember, but no more than 2 tablets or 10ml of liquid in 24 hours.

Stopping the drug
Threadworm The drug is taken as a single dose, repeated only if necessary. It can safely be stopped when no longer needed.
Other worms The 3-day course should be completed to ensure effective eradication.

Exceeding the dose
A larger than recommended dose is unlikely to cause harm. A very large dose may cause dizziness, abdominal discomfort, or diarrhoea in adults. In infants, it may cause seizures. Notify your doctor.

Hygiene measures
To prevent threadworm reinfection, wash the hands thoroughly and scrub the nails frequently, especially after going to the toilet and before eating; keep the nails short; avoid biting the nails and sucking the fingers; wash bed linen and towels to kill the eggs; do not share towels, flannels, or sponges; bathe or shower every morning; change underwear every morning; regularly vacuum and clean the house to remove any infective eggs. Oro-anal contact during sex can also cause infection or reinfection and should therefore be avoided.

SPECIAL PRECAUTIONS

Be sure to consult your doctor or pharmacist before taking this drug if:
• You have fructose intolerance.

Pregnancy
Safety in pregnancy not established. Discuss with your doctor.

Breast-feeding
It is not known if the drug passes into the breast milk, so breast-feeding is not recommended. Discuss with your doctor.

Infants and children
Not recommended under 2 years.

Over 60
No special problems.

Driving and hazardous work
No special problems.

Alcohol
No special problems.

PROLONGED USE

Mebendazole is not used long term.

POSSIBLE ADVERSE EFFECTS

The most common side effects are gastrointestinal symptoms, and these are most likely to occur when the infestation level is very high. Rashes and seizures are rare.

Symptom/effect	Frequency		Discuss with doctor		Stop taking drug now	Call doctor now
	Common	Rare	Only if severe	In all cases		
Abdominal pain	●		●			
Diarrhoea	●		●			
Seizures		●		●	●	●
Rash		●		●	●	●

INTERACTIONS

Cimetidine may increase the blood level of mebendazole and should be avoided.

Metronidazole may increase the risk of serious skin rashes when used with mebendazole. The two drugs should not be used together.

MEBEVERINE

Brand names Aurobeverine, Boots IBS Relief, Colofac IBS, Colofac MR
Used in the following combined preparation Fybogel Mebeverine

GENERAL INFORMATION

Mebeverine is an antispasmodic drug used to relieve painful spasms of the intestine (known as colic), such as those resulting from irritable bowel syndrome and diverticular disease. It has a direct relaxing effect on the muscle in the bowel wall, and may also have an anticholinergic action (see p.35), which reduces the transmission of nerve signals to the smooth muscle of the bowel wall and thereby prevents spasm. It does not have serious side effects.

In addition to being available on its own, mebeverine is also produced in a combined form with ispaghula husk to provide roughage in an easily assimilable formulation. Both the drug on its own and the combined form are commonly used to control symptoms of irritable bowel syndrome.

INFORMATION FOR USERS

Follow instructions on the label. Call your doctor if symptoms worsen.

How taken/used

Tablets, SR capsules, liquid, granules.

Frequency and timing of doses
2–3 x daily, 20 minutes before meals. Combined preparations that contain ispaghula should not be taken immediately before going to bed.

Adult dosage range
300–450mg daily.

Onset of effect
30–60 minutes.

Duration of action
6–8 hours.

Diet advice
Combined preparations that contain ispaghula should be taken with plenty of water.

Storage
Keep in original container at room temperature out of the reach of children. Protect from light.

Missed dose
Take as soon as you remember, then return to your normal dosing schedule.

Stopping the drug
The drug can be stopped as soon as you no longer need it.

Exceeding the dose
An occasional unintentional extra dose is unlikely to be a cause for concern. Larger overdoses will probably cause constipation, and may cause central nervous system excitability.

SPECIAL PRECAUTIONS

Be sure to consult your doctor or pharmacist before taking this drug if:
• You have cystic fibrosis.
• You have porphyria.

 Pregnancy
Safety in pregnancy not established. Discuss with your doctor.

 Breast-feeding
Safety in breast-feeding not established. Discuss with your doctor.

 Infants and children
Not used in infants and children under 18 years.

 Over 60
No special problems.

 Driving and hazardous work
No special problems.

 Alcohol
No special problems.

POSSIBLE ADVERSE EFFECTS

Mebeverine rarely produces side effects.

Symptom/effect	Frequency		Discuss with doctor		Stop taking drug now	Call doctor now
	Common	Rare	Only if severe	In all cases		
Constipation		●	●			
Rash/lip swelling		●		●	●	

INTERACTIONS

None.

PROLONGED USE

No problems expected.

MEDROXYPROGESTERONE

Brand names Climanor, Depo-Provera, Provera, Syana
Used in the following combined preparations Indivina, Premique, Tridestra

GENERAL INFORMATION

Medroxyprogesterone is a progestogen, a synthetic female sex hormone similar to the natural hormone progesterone. This drug is used as part of hormone replacement therapy (HRT, p.105) for women who have a uterus and need progesterone in addition to their long-term oestrogen. Medroxyprogesterone is often used to treat endometriosis, in which there is abnormal growth of the uterine-lining tissue in the pelvic cavity. It may also be used to treat certain menstrual disorders, such as secondary amenorrhoea and abnormal bleeding. Depot injections of the drug are used as a contraceptive. However, since they may cause serious side effects, such as persistent uterine bleeding, amenorrhoea, and prolonged infertility, their use is controversial. They are recommended only under special circumstances.

Medroxyprogesterone may be used to treat some types of cancer, such as cancer of the breast, uterus, or kidney.

QUICK REFERENCE

Drug group Female sex hormone (p.105)

Overdose danger rating Low

Dependence rating Low

Prescription needed Yes

Available as generic No

INFORMATION FOR USERS

Your drug prescription is tailored for you. Do not alter dosage without checking with your doctor.

How taken/used

Tablets, injection.

Frequency and timing of doses
1–3 x daily with plenty of water (by mouth); tablets may need to be taken at certain times during your cycle; follow the instructions you have been given. Every 3 months (depot injection and intramuscular injection).

Adult dosage range
Menstrual disorders 2.5–10mg daily.
Endometriosis 30mg daily.
Cancer 100–1,500mg daily.
Contraception 150mg 12-weekly injection.

Onset of effect
1–2 months (cancer); 1–2 weeks (other conditions).

Duration of action
1–2 days (by mouth); up to some months (depot injection).

Diet advice
None.

Storage
Keep in original container at room temperature out of the reach of children.

Missed dose
Take as soon as you remember. If your next dose is due within 3 hours, take a single dose now and skip the next.

Stopping the drug
Do not stop the drug without consulting your doctor; symptoms may recur.

Exceeding the dose
An occasional unintentional extra dose is unlikely to be a cause for concern. But if you notice any unusual symptoms, or if a large overdose has been taken, notify your doctor.

SPECIAL PRECAUTIONS

Be sure to tell your doctor if:
- You have high blood pressure.
- You have had venous thrombosis, a heart attack, or a stroke.
- You have long-term liver or kidney problems.
- You have porphyria.
- You have epilepsy or a history of depression.
- You have breast cancer.
- You have a history of gallstones, migraines, or lupus.
- You have a history of osteoporosis.
- You are taking other medicines.

 Pregnancy
Not prescribed. May cause defects in the fetus. Discuss with your doctor.

 Breast-feeding
The drug passes into breast milk, but normal doses are unlikely to harm the baby. Discuss with your doctor.

 Infants and children
Not usually prescribed.

 Over 60
No special problems.

 Driving and hazardous work
No known problems.

 Alcohol
No known problems.

POSSIBLE ADVERSE EFFECTS

Medroxyprogesterone rarely causes serious adverse effects. Fluid retention may lead to weight gain, swollen feet or ankles, and breast tenderness.

Symptom/effect	Frequency		Discuss with doctor		Stop taking drug now	Call doctor now
	Common	Rare	Only if severe	In all cases		
Weight gain/swollen ankles	●		●			
Headache	●		●			
Breast tenderness		●	●			
Nausea	●		●			
Fatigue/depression/altered sleep		●		●		
Irregular menstruation		●		●		
Rash/itching/acne		●		●	●	
Jaundice		●		●	●	

INTERACTIONS

Ciclosporin The effects of this drug may be increased by medroxyprogesterone.

Anticoagulants Medroxyprogesterone may reduce the effects of these drugs.

Rifamycin antibiotics, St John's wort, anticonvulsants, griseofulvin, terbinafine, and barbiturates may reduce the effects of medroxyprogesterone.

PROLONGED USE

Long-term use may slightly increase the risk of venous thrombosis in the legs, and of osteoporosis and bone fractures. Bone loss is greatest in the first 2–3 years, then stabilizes. Adequate calcium and vitamin D intake should be ensured throughout treatment. Irregular menstrual bleeding or spotting between periods may also occur.

Monitoring Checks on blood pressure, yearly cervical smear tests, and breast examinations are usually required. Bone density and lipids may also be monitored.

MEFENAMIC ACID

Brand name Ponstan, Ponstan Forte
Used in the following combined preparations None

GENERAL INFORMATION

Mefenamic acid, introduced in 1963, is a non-steroidal anti-inflammatory drug (NSAID). Like other NSAIDs, it relieves pain and inflammation. The drug is an effective painkiller and is used to treat headache, toothache, and menstrual pains (dysmenorrhoea), as well as to reduce excessive menstrual bleeding (menorrhagia). Mefenamic acid is also prescribed for long-term relief of pain and stiffness in rheumatoid arthritis and osteoarthritis.

The most common side effects of mefenamic acid are gastrointestinal: abdominal pain, nausea and vomiting, and indigestion. Other, more serious effects include kidney problems and blood disorders.

INFORMATION FOR USERS

Your drug prescription is tailored for you. Do not alter dosage without checking with your doctor.

How taken/used

Tablets, capsules, liquid.

Frequency and timing of doses
3 x daily with or after food.

Adult dosage range
1,500mg daily.

Onset of effect
1–2 hours.

Duration of action
Up to 8 hours.

Diet advice
None.

Storage
Keep in original container at room temperature out of the reach of children.

Missed dose
Take as soon as you remember. If your next dose is due within 2 hours, take a single dose now and skip the next.

Stopping the drug
Can be safely stopped as soon as you no longer need it.

Exceeding the dose
An occasional unintentional extra dose is unlikely to be a cause for concern. Large overdoses may cause poor coordination, muscle twitching, or seizures. Notify your doctor.

POSSIBLE ADVERSE EFFECTS

Gastrointestinal disturbances are the most common side effects. The drug should be stopped if diarrhoea or a rash occur, and not used again. Black or bloodstained bowel movements and wheezing and breathlessness should be reported to your doctor promptly.

Symptom/effect	Frequency		Discuss with doctor		Stop taking drug now	Call doctor now
	Common	Rare	Only if severe	In all cases		
Indigestion	●		●			
Diarrhoea	●			●	●	
Dizziness/drowsiness		●	●			
Nausea/vomiting		●		●		
Abdominal pain		●	●			
Rash		●		●	●	
Wheezing/breathlessness		●		●	●	●
Black/bloodstained faeces		●		●	●	●

INTERACTIONS

General note Mefenamic acid interacts with a wide range of drugs to increase the risk of bleeding and/or peptic ulcers. These include other non-steroidal anti-inflammatory drugs (NSAIDs) such as aspirin, as well as oral anticoagulant drugs, such as warfarin, certain antidepressants, and corticosteroids.

Lithium, digoxin, phenytoin, and methotrexate Mefenamic acid may raise blood levels of these drugs to an undesirable extent.

Antihypertensive drugs and diuretics The beneficial effects of these drugs may be reduced by mefenamic acid.

Oral antidiabetic drugs Mefenamic acid may increase the blood-sugar-lowering effect of these drugs.

Ciprofloxacin The risk of seizures with this drug and related antibiotics may be increased by mefenamic acid.

SPECIAL PRECAUTIONS

Be sure to tell your doctor if:
- You have liver or kidney problems.
- You have had a peptic ulcer, oesophagitis, or acid indigestion.
- You have inflammatory bowel disease.
- You have asthma.
- You have high blood pressure.
- You are allergic to aspirin.
- You have any heart problems.
- You are taking other medicines.

Pregnancy
Not usually prescribed. May cause defects in the unborn baby and, taken in late pregnancy, may affect the baby's cardiovascular system. Discuss with your doctor.

Breast-feeding
Not recommended. The drug passes into the breast milk. Discuss with your doctor.

Infants and children
Reduced dose necessary.

Over 60
Increased likelihood of adverse effects.

Driving and hazardous work
Avoid such activities until you have learned how mefenamic acid affects you because the drug can cause drowsiness and dizziness.

Alcohol
Avoid. Alcohol may increase the risk of stomach irritation with mefenamic acid.

Surgery and general anaesthetics
The drug may prolong bleeding. Discuss with your doctor or dentist before any surgery.

PROLONGED USE

There is an increased risk of bleeding from peptic ulcers and in the bowel with prolonged use of mefenamic acid. There is also a small risk of a heart attack or stroke. To minimize these risks, the lowest effective dose is given for the shortest duration.

MEFLOQUINE

Brand name Lariam
Used in the following combined preparations None

GENERAL INFORMATION

Mefloquine is used for the prevention and treatment of malaria. It is principally recommended for use in areas where malaria is resistant to other drugs.

However, the use of mefloquine is limited by the fact that it can cause serious side effects in some patients, such as depression, suicidal tendencies, anxiety, panic, confusion, hallucinations, paranoid delusions, and seizures.

As with all antimalarials, the use of mosquito repellents and a mosquito net at night are as important in preventing malaria as taking the drug itself.

QUICK REFERENCE

Drug group Antimalarial drug (p.95)
Overdose danger rating High
Dependence rating Low
Prescription needed Yes
Available as generic No

INFORMATION FOR USERS

Your drug prescription is tailored for you. Do not alter dosage without checking with your doctor.

How taken/used

Tablets.

Frequency and timing of doses
Prevention Once weekly, starting 2–3 weeks before entering endemic area, and continuing until 4 weeks after leaving.
Treatment Up to 3 x daily every 6–8 hours, after food and with plenty of water.

Adult dosage range
Prevention 137.5–250mg once weekly.
Treatment 20–25mg/kg body weight up to a maximum dose of 1.5g.

Onset of effect
2–3 days.

Duration of action
Over 1 week. Low levels of the drug and any adverse effects may persist for several months.

Diet advice
None.

Storage
Keep in original container at room temperature out of the reach of children.

Missed dose
Take as soon as you remember. If your next dose is due within 48 hours (if taken once weekly for prevention), take a single dose now and skip the next. If vomiting occurs, within 30 minutes of taking a dose, take another.

Stopping the drug
If you feel it necessary to stop taking the drug, consult your doctor about alternative treatment before the next dose is due.

OVERDOSE ACTION

Seek immediate medical advice in all cases. Take emergency action if collapse or loss of consciousness occurs.

See Drug poisoning emergency guide (p.518).

POSSIBLE ADVERSE EFFECTS

Mefloquine commonly causes dizziness, vertigo, nausea, vomiting, and headache. In rare cases, serious adverse effects on the nervous system can occur, including anxiety or panic attacks, depression, hallucinations, and paranoid delusions.

Symptom/effect	Frequency		Discuss with doctor		Stop taking drug now	Call doctor now
	Common	Rare	Only if severe	In all cases		
Dizziness/vertigo	●		●			
Nausea/vomiting	●		●			
Headache	●		●			
Abdominal pain	●		●			
Depression		●		●	●	
Anxiety/panic attacks		●		●	●	
Hallucinations/delusions		●		●	●	
Hearing disorders		●		●	●	
Palpitations		●		●	●	

INTERACTIONS

General note Mefloquine may increase the effects on the heart of drugs such as beta blockers, calcium channel blockers, and digitalis drugs. It may also affect live-vaccine immunization, which should be completed at least 3 days before the first dose of mefloquine.

Anticonvulsant drugs Mefloquine may decrease the effect of these drugs.

Other antimalarial drugs Mefloquine may increase the risk of adverse effects when taken with these drugs.

SPECIAL PRECAUTIONS

Be sure to tell your doctor if:
- You have long-term liver or kidney problems.
- You have had epileptic seizures.
- You have had depression or other psychiatric illness.
- You have had a previous allergic reaction to mefloquine or quinine.
- You have heart problems.
- You are taking other medicines.

 Pregnancy
Not usually prescribed. If unavoidable, the drug is given only after the first trimester. Pregnancy must be avoided during and for 3 months after mefloquine use.

 Breast-feeding
Not prescribed. The drug passes into the breast milk.

 Infants and children
Not used in infants under 3 months old. Reduced dose necessary in older children.

 Over 60
Careful monitoring is necessary if liver or kidney problems or heart disease are present.

 Driving and hazardous work
Avoid such activities when taking mefloquine for prevention until you know how the drug affects you. Also avoid during treatment and for 3 weeks afterwards as the drug can cause dizziness or disturb balance.

 Alcohol
Keep consumption low.

PROLONGED USE

May be taken for prevention of malaria for up to 1 year.

MERCAPTOPURINE

Brand names Hanixol, Puri-Nethol, Xaluprine
Used in the following combined preparations None

GENERAL INFORMATION

Mercaptopurine is an anticancer drug that is widely used in the treatment of certain forms of leukaemia. It is usually given in combination with other anticancer drugs.

Nausea and vomiting, mouth ulcers, and loss of appetite are the most common side effects of mercaptopurine. Such symptoms tend to be milder than those caused by other cytotoxic drugs, and often disappear as the body adjusts to the drug.

More seriously, mercaptopurine can interfere with blood cell production, resulting in blood clotting disorders and anaemia, and can also cause liver damage. The frequency and severity of infections is also increased.

INFORMATION FOR USERS

Your drug prescription is tailored for you. Do not alter dosage without checking with your doctor.

How taken/used

Tablets.

Frequency and timing of doses
Once daily.

Dosage range
Dosage is determined individually according to body weight and response.

Onset of effect
1–2 weeks.

Duration of action
Side effects may persist for several weeks after stopping treatment.

Diet advice
The drug can be taken with food or on an empty stomach, but this should be kept consistent each day. Dairy products should be avoided for at least 2 hours before taking the tablets to 1 hour after.

Storage
Keep in original container at room temperature out of the reach of children. Protect from light.

Missed dose
If your next dose is due within 6 hours, take a single dose now and skip the next. Tell your doctor that you missed a dose.

Stopping the drug
Do not stop taking the drug without consulting your doctor; stopping the drug may lead to worsening of your underlying condition.

Exceeding the dose
An occasional unintentional extra dose is unlikely to cause problems. Large overdoses may cause nausea and vomiting. Notify your doctor.

SPECIAL PRECAUTIONS

Be sure to tell your doctor if:
- You have long-term liver or kidney problems.
- You have gout.
- You have recently had any infection.
- You are taking other medicines.

 Pregnancy
Not usually prescribed. Discuss with your doctor.

 Breast-feeding
Not advised. The drug passes into the breast milk and may affect the baby adversely. Discuss with your doctor.

 Infants and children
No special problems.

 Over 60
Reduced dose may be necessary. Increased risk of adverse effects.

 Driving and hazardous work
No known problems.

 Alcohol
Avoid. Alcohol may increase the adverse effects of this drug.

POSSIBLE ADVERSE EFFECTS

The most common adverse effects are nausea, vomiting, and loss of appetite. Because mercaptopurine interferes with the production of blood cells, it may cause anaemia and blood clotting disorders; in addition, infections are more likely.

Symptom/effect	Frequency		Discuss with doctor		Stop taking drug now	Call doctor now
	Common	Rare	Only if severe	In all cases		
Nausea/vomiting/loss of appetite	●		●			
Mouth ulcers	●			●		●
Abdominal pain		●	●			
Easy bruising/bleeding		●		●	●	●
Sore throat/fever/jaundice		●		●		●

INTERACTIONS

Allopurinol This drug increases blood levels of mercaptopurine, and the dosages of both drugs should be adjusted.

Warfarin The effects of warfarin may be decreased by mercaptopurine.

Febuxostat This drug should not be used with mercaptopurine; the combination may lead to reduced levels of white blood cells.

Methotrexate This drug increases blood levels of mercaptopurine. Reduced dose of mercaptopurine may be needed.

Ribavirin Increased risk of drug toxicity when ribavirin is used with mercaptopurine. The two drugs should not be used together.

Co-trimoxazole, trimethoprim, mesalazine, olsalazine, and sulfasalazine These drugs increase the risk of blood problems with mercaptopurine.

Vaccines Mercaptopurine may affect your response to live vaccines. Discuss with your doctor before having a vaccine.

PROLONGED USE

Prolonged use of this drug may reduce bone marrow activity, leading to a reduction of all types of blood cell. Some people have a genetic susceptibility to this effect. There is also a small increase in the risk of developing certain cancers, such as skin cancer, sarcoma, and lymphoma.

Monitoring Regular blood checks, including tests on liver function, are required.

MESALAZINE

Brand names Asacol, Mesren MR, Mezavant XL, Octasa, Pentasa, Salofalk, Zintasa
Used in the following combined preparations None

GENERAL INFORMATION

Mesalazine is prescribed for patients with ulcerative colitis and is sometimes used for Crohn's disease, which affects the ileum and large intestine. The drug is given to relieve symptoms in an acute attack and is also taken as a preventive measure. When mesalazine is used to treat severe cases, it is often taken with other drugs such as corticosteroids.

When the drug is taken as tablets, the active component is released in the large intestine, where its local effect relieves the inflamed mucosa. Always stick to the same brand of tablet. Enemas and suppositories are also available and are particularly useful when the disease affects the rectum and lower colon.

This drug produces fewer side effects than some older treatments, such as sulfasalazine. Patients unable to tolerate sulfasalazine may be able to take mesalazine with no problem. Anyone hypersensitive to salicylates, such as aspirin, should not take mesalazine.

INFORMATION FOR USERS

Your drug prescription is tailored for you. Do not alter dosage without checking with your doctor.

How taken/used

Tablets, SR tablets, granules, suppositories, enema (foam or liquid).

Frequency and timing of doses
3 x daily, swallowed whole and not chewed (tablets); 3 x daily (suppositories); once daily at bedtime (enema).

Adult dosage range
2.4–4.8g daily (acute attack); 1.2–2.4g daily (maintenance dose). Dose varies with brand used.

Onset of effect
Adverse effects may be noticed within a few days, but full beneficial effects may not be felt for a couple of weeks.

Duration of action
Up to 12 hours.

Diet advice
Your doctor may advise you, taking account of the condition affecting you.

Storage
Keep in original container at room temperature out of the reach of children. Protect from light. Keep aerosol container out of direct sunlight.

Missed dose
Take as soon as you remember. If your next dose is due within 2 hours, take a single dose now and skip the next.

Stopping the drug
Do not stop taking the drug without consulting your doctor; symptoms may recur.

Exceeding the dose
An occasional unintentional extra dose is unlikely to be a cause for concern. But if you notice any unusual symptoms, or if a large overdose has been taken, notify your doctor.

SPECIAL PRECAUTIONS

Be sure to tell your doctor if:
- You have long-term liver or kidney problems.
- You have a blood disorder.
- You are allergic to aspirin.
- You are taking other medicines.

 Pregnancy
Negligible amounts of the drug cross the placenta. However, safety in pregnancy is not established. Discuss with your doctor.

 Breast-feeding
Negligible amounts of the drug pass into the breast milk. However, safety is not established. Discuss with your doctor.

 Infants and children
Not recommended for children under 5 years.

 Over 60
Dosage reduction not normally necessary unless there is kidney impairment.

 Driving and hazardous work
No special problems.

 Alcohol
No special problems.

PROLONGED USE

No problems expected.

Monitoring Regular blood tests and checks on kidney function are usually required.

POSSIBLE ADVERSE EFFECTS

The common side effects of mesalazine affect the gastrointestinal tract. Other problems rarely occur. However, unexplained bleeding, bruising, sore throat, fever, or malaise should be reported to your doctor, who will carry out a blood test to eliminate blood disorders.

Symptom/effect	Frequency		Discuss with doctor		Stop taking drug now	Call doctor now
	Common	Rare	Only if severe	In all cases		
Nausea	●		●			
Abdominal pain	●		●			
Diarrhoea	●		●			
Colitis worsening		●		●	●	
Rash		●		●	●	
Fever/wheezing		●		●	●	●
Spontaneous bleeding/bruising		●		●	●	●
Sore throat/malaise		●		●	●	●

INTERACTIONS

Lactulose The release of mesalazine at its site of action may be reduced by lactulose.

Warfarin Mesalazine may reduce the effect of warfarin.

Azathioprine and mercaptopurine may increase the risk of blood problems with mesalazine.

METFORMIN

Brand names Bolamyn SR, Diagemet XL, Glucient SR, Glucophage SR, Meijumet, Metabet SR, Sukkarto SR, Yaltormin SR
Used in the following combined preparations Competact, Eucreas, Janumet, Jentadueto, Komboglyze, Synjardy, Vipdomet, Vokanamet, Xigduo

GENERAL INFORMATION

Metformin is an antidiabetic drug that is commonly used to treat Type 2 diabetes, in which some insulin is still produced by the pancreas. The drug lowers blood sugar levels by delaying absorption of glucose, reducing glucose production in the liver, and helping your body respond better to its own insulin so that the cells will take up glucose more effectively from the blood.

Metformin is used in conjunction with diet, weight management, and exercise. It can be given with insulin or other antidiabetics but is often used alone to treat people with Type 2 diabetes who are obese. Metformin is also used in the treatment of polycystic ovary syndrome.

The drug often causes abdominal upset when first started, but this usually subsides over time.

INFORMATION FOR USERS

Your drug prescription is tailored for you. Do not alter dosage without checking with your doctor.

How taken/used

Tablets.

Frequency and timing of doses
2–3 x daily with food.

Adult dosage range
500mg–3000mg daily with a low dose at the start of the treatment.

Onset of effect
Within 2 hours. It may take 2 weeks to achieve control of diabetes.

Duration of action
8–12 hours.

Diet advice
An individualized low-fat, low-sugar diet must be maintained in order for the drug to be fully effective. Follow your doctor's advice.

Storage
Keep in original container at room temperature out of the reach of children.

Missed dose
Take as soon as you remember. If your next dose is due within 2 hours, take a single dose now and skip the next.

Stopping the drug
Do not stop taking the drug without consulting your doctor; stopping the drug may lead to worsening of the underlying condition.

OVERDOSE ACTION

 Seek immediate medical advice in all cases. Take emergency action if seizures or loss of consciousness occur.

See Drug poisoning emergency guide (p.518).

SPECIAL PRECAUTIONS

Be sure to tell your doctor if:
- You have long-term liver or kidney problems.
- You have heart failure.
- You are a heavy drinker.
- You are taking other medicines.

 Pregnancy
Not usually prescribed. Insulin is usually substituted because it provides better diabetic control during pregnancy. Discuss with your doctor.

 Breast-feeding
Safety not established. Discuss with your doctor.

 Infants and children
Not recommended under 10 years.

 Over 60
Increased likelihood of adverse effects. Reduced dose may therefore be necessary.

 Driving and hazardous work
Usually no problems. Avoid such activities if you have warning signs of low blood sugar.

 Alcohol
Avoid. Alcohol increases the risk of low blood sugar, and can cause coma by increasing the acidity of the blood.

Surgery and general anaesthetics
Surgery may reduce the response to this drug. Notify your doctor that you are diabetic before any surgery; insulin treatment may need to be substituted. Tell your doctor if you are to have a contrast X-ray; metformin should be stopped before the procedure.

POSSIBLE ADVERSE EFFECTS

Minor gastrointestinal symptoms, such as nausea, are often helped by taking the drug with food. Diarrhoea usually settles after a few days of treatment. The most serious side effect is a potentially fatal build-up of lactic acid in the blood. This is very rare and usually occurs only in people with diabetes who have impaired kidney function.

Symptom/effect	Frequency		Discuss with doctor		Stop taking drug now	Call doctor now
	Common	Rare	Only if severe	In all cases		
Loss of appetite/metallic taste	●		●			
Nausea/vomiting	●		●			
Diarrhoea	●			●		
Dizziness/confusion		●		●		
Weakness/sweating		●		●		
Rash		●		●		

INTERACTIONS

General note A number of drugs reduce the effects of metformin. These include corticosteroids, oestrogens, and diuretics. Other drugs, notably monoamine oxidase inhibitors (MAOIs) and beta blockers, increase its effects.

Warfarin Metformin may increase the effect of this anticoagulant drug. The dosage of warfarin may need to be adjusted accordingly.

PROLONGED USE

Prolonged treatment with metformin can deplete reserves of vitamin B_{12} and this may rarely cause anaemia.

Monitoring Regular checks on kidney function and on blood sugar control are usually required. Vitamin B_{12} levels may also be checked annually.

METHADONE

Brand names Methadose, Metharose, Physeptone
Used in the following combined preparations None

GENERAL INFORMATION

Methadone is a synthetic drug belonging to the opioid analgesic group. It is used in the control of severe pain, and as a cough suppressant in terminal illness, but it is more widely used to replace morphine or heroin in the treatment of dependence. For this, methadone can be given once daily to prevent withdrawal symptoms. In some cases, dosage can be reduced until the drug is no longer needed.

Tolerance to methadone is marked. Although the initial dose for a person not used to opioids is very low, the dose needed by someone who is dependent could be fatal for a non-user.

QUICK REFERENCE

Drug group Opioid analgesic (p.37)
Overdose danger rating High
Dependence rating High
Prescription needed Yes
Available as generic Yes

INFORMATION FOR USERS

Your drug prescription is tailored for you. Do not alter dosage without checking with your doctor.

How taken/used

Tablets, liquid, injection.

Frequency and timing of doses
Pain 3–4 x daily; 2 x daily (prolonged use).
Cough 4–6 x daily (starting dose); 2 x daily (prolonged use).
Opioid addiction Once daily.

Adult dosage range
Pain 5–10mg per dose initially, adjusted according to response.
Cough 1–2mg per dose.
Opioid addiction 10–20mg (starting dose); 40–60mg daily (maintenance dose).

Onset of effect
15–60 minutes.

Duration of action
36–48 hours.

Diet advice
None.

Storage
Keep in original container at room temperature out of the reach of children. Protect injections and liquids from light.

Missed dose
Take as soon as you remember and return to your normal dosing schedule as soon as possible. If you missed the dose because it caused you to vomit, or if you cannot swallow, consult your doctor.

Stopping the drug
If the reason for taking methadone no longer exists, the drug can be slowly reduced and safely stopped. Discuss with your doctor.

OVERDOSE ACTION

Seek immediate medical advice in all cases. Take emergency action if symptoms such as slow or irregular breathing, severe drowsiness, or loss of consciousness occur.

See Drug poisoning emergency guide (p.518).

POSSIBLE ADVERSE EFFECTS

Drowsiness and nausea are the most common side effects of methadone, but these diminish as the body adapts to the drug. Constipation is also common and may be longer lasting.

Symptom/effect	Frequency		Discuss with doctor		Stop taking drug now	Call doctor now
	Common	Rare	Only if severe	In all cases		
Nausea/vomiting	●		●			
Drowsiness	●		●			
Constipation	●		●			
Dizziness/confusion	●			●		●
Loss of consciousness		●		●	●	●
Slow, difficult breathing		●		●	●	●

INTERACTIONS

Phenytoin, carbamazepine, rifampicin, and ritonavir may reduce the effects of methadone.

Monoamine oxidase inhibitors (MAOIs) and selegiline Taken with methadone, these drugs may produce a dangerous rise or fall in blood pressure.

Erythromycin, clarithromycin, fluconazole, cimetidine, and ranitidine may increase the effects of methadone.

Sedatives The effects of all drugs that have a sedative effect on the central nervous system are likely to be increased by methadone.

SPECIAL PRECAUTIONS

Be sure to tell your doctor if:
- You have heart or circulatory problems.
- You have liver or kidney problems.
- You have lung problems such as asthma or bronchitis.
- You have thyroid disease.
- You have a history of epileptic seizures.
- You have a phaeochromocytoma (a type of adrenal gland tumour).
- You have problems with alcohol misuse.
- You are taking other medicines.

 Pregnancy
Not prescribed in pregnancy if possible. May cause breathing difficulties in the newborn baby. Discuss with your doctor.

 Breast-feeding
Safety not established. The drug passes into breast milk and may affect the baby adversely. Discuss with your doctor.

 Infants and children
Not recommended.

 Over 60
Reduced dose necessary.

 Driving and hazardous work
Your underlying condition or side effects of the medication itself, such as drowsiness, may make such activities inadvisable. Discuss with your doctor.

 Alcohol
Avoid. Alcohol increases the sedative effects of the drug and may depress breathing.

PROLONGED USE

Treatment with methadone is always closely monitored. If the drug is being taken long term, the dose must be carefully reduced before the drug is stopped.

METHOTREXATE

Brand names Jylamvo, Maxtrex, Methofill, Metoject, Nordimet, Zlatal
Used in the following combined preparations None

GENERAL INFORMATION

Methotrexate is an anticancer drug used, together with other anticancer drugs, in the treatment of leukaemia, lymphoma, and solid cancers such as those of the breast, bladder, head, and neck. It is also used alone to treat inflammatory conditions such as severe uncontrolled psoriasis, rheumatoid arthritis, and Crohn's disease.

As with most anticancer drugs, methotrexate affects both healthy and cancerous cells, so that its usefulness is limited by its adverse effects and toxicity. Folic acid supplements may reduce its toxicity; when methotrexate is given in high doses, it is usually given with folinic acid to prevent it from destroying bone marrow cells. Because of its toxicity and adverse effects it is very important that you do not take methotrexate more often than prescribed by your doctor.

INFORMATION FOR USERS

Your drug prescription is tailored for you. Do not alter dosage without checking with your doctor.

How taken/used

Tablets, injection, liquid.

Frequency and timing of doses
Cancer Single dose once weekly or every 3 weeks.
Other conditions Single dose once weekly.

Adult dosage range
Cancer Dosage is determined individually according to the nature of the condition, body weight, and response.
Rheumatoid arthritis 7.5-20mg weekly.
Psoriasis 10-25mg weekly.

Onset of effect
30–60 minutes.

Duration of action
Short-term effects last up to 24 hours.

Diet advice
None.

Storage
Keep in original container at room temperature out of the reach of children. Wash your hands after handling the tablets.

Missed dose
Take as soon as you remember and consult your doctor.

Stopping the drug
Do not stop taking the drug without consulting your doctor. Stopping the drug may lead to worsening of the underlying condition.

OVERDOSE ACTION

Seek immediate medical advice in all cases. Take emergency action if breathing problems or loss of consciousness occur.

See Drug poisoning emergency guide (p.518).

SPECIAL PRECAUTIONS

Be sure to tell your doctor if:
- You have liver or kidney problems.
- You have porphyria.
- You have a problem with alcohol misuse.
- You have a peptic or other digestive-tract ulcer.
- You are taking other medicines especially NSAIDs or antibiotics.

 Pregnancy
Not prescribed. Methotrexate may cause birth defects in the unborn baby.

 Breast-feeding
Not advised. The drug passes into the breast milk and may affect the baby adversely.

 Infants and children
For cancer treatment only. Reduced dose necessary.

 Over 60
Increased likelihood of adverse effects. Reduced doses necessary.

 Driving and hazardous work
No special problems.

 Alcohol
Avoid. Alcohol may increase the adverse effects of methotrexate.

POSSIBLE ADVERSE EFFECTS

Nausea and vomiting may occur within a few hours of taking methotrexate. Diarrhoea and mouth ulcers are also common side effects occurring a few days after starting treatment.

Symptom/effect	Frequency		Discuss with doctor		Stop taking drug now	Call doctor now
	Common	Rare	Only if severe	In all cases		
Dry cough/chest pain	●		●			
Nausea/vomiting	●			●		
Diarrhoea	●			●		
Mouth/gum ulcers/inflammation	●			●	●	●
Mood changes/confusion		●		●		
Rash		●		●	●	
Jaundice		●		●	●	●
Sore throat/fever		●		●	●	●
Easy bruising/bleeding		●		●	●	●
Breathlessness		●		●	●	●

PROLONGED USE

Long-term treatment may be needed for rheumatoid arthritis. Once the condition is controlled, the drug is reduced as much as possible to the lowest effective dose. Long-term methotrexate treatment may occasionally lead to breathing problems due to scarring of the lungs or, rarely, unusual respiratory infections, such as pneumocystis pneumonia.

Monitoring Full blood counts and kidney and liver function tests will be performed before treatment starts and at intervals during treatment.

INTERACTIONS

General note Many drugs, including NSAIDs (see p.74), diuretics, ciclosporin, phenytoin, and probenecid, may increase blood levels and toxicity of methotrexate.

Co-trimoxazole, trimethoprim, and certain antimalarial drugs These drugs may enhance the effects of methotrexate.

METHYLCELLULOSE

Brand name Celevac
Used in the following combined preparations None

GENERAL INFORMATION

Methylcellulose is a laxative used for the treatment of constipation, diverticular disease, and irritable bowel syndrome. Taken by mouth, methylcellulose is not absorbed into the bloodstream but remains in the intestine. It absorbs up to 25 times its volume of water, thereby softening faeces and increasing their volume. It s also used to reduce the frequency and increase the firmness of faeces in chronic watery diarrhoea, and to control the consistency of faeces after colostomies and ileostomies.

Methylcellulose preparations are used with appropriate dieting in some cases of obesity. The bulking agent swells to give the user a feeling of fullness, thereby encouraging adherence to a reducing diet.

QUICK REFERENCE

Drug group Laxative (p.69) and antidiarrhoeal drug (p.68)

Overdose danger rating Low

Dependence rating Low

Prescription needed No

Available as generic No

INFORMATION FOR USERS

Follow instructions on the label. Call your doctor if symptoms worsen.

How taken/used

Tablets.

Frequency and timing of doses
3–6 tablets 2 x daily. If used as laxative, unless otherwise instructed, break in mouth and swallow with full glass of water; do not take at bedtime.

Adult dosage range
1.5–6g daily.

Onset of effect
Within 24 hours.

Duration of action
Up to 3 days.

Diet advice
If taken as a laxative, drink plenty of fluids, and drink at least 300ml with each dose. If taken for diarrhoea, avoid liquids for 30 minutes before and after each dose.

Storage
Keep in original container at room temperature out of the reach of children.

Missed dose
Take as soon as you remember. Take the next dose as scheduled.

Stopping the drug
Can be safely stopped as soon as you no longer need it.

Exceeding the dose
An occasional unintentional extra dose is unlikely to be a cause for concern. But if you notice any unusual symptoms, or if a large overdose has been taken, notify your doctor.

SPECIAL PRECAUTIONS

Be sure to consult your doctor or pharmacist before taking this drug if:
- You have severe constipation and/or abdominal pain.
- You have unexplained rectal bleeding.
- You have difficulty in swallowing.
- You vomit readily.
- You are taking other medicines.

 Pregnancy
No evidence of risk to developing baby, but discuss with your doctor.

 Breast-feeding
No evidence of risk.

 Infants and children
Reduced dose necessary, but discuss with your doctor.

 Over 60
No special problems.

 Driving and hazardous work
No known problems.

 Alcohol
No known problems.

POSSIBLE ADVERSE EFFECTS

When taken by mouth, the drug may cause bloating and excess wind. Insufficient fluid intake may cause blockage of the oesophagus (gullet) or intestine. Consult your doctor if you experience severe abdominal pain or if you have no bowel movement for 2 days after taking methylcellulose.

Symptom/effect	Frequency		Discuss with doctor		Stop taking drug now	Call doctor now
	Common	Rare	Only if severe	In all cases		
Abdominal distension		●	●			
Flatulence		●	●			
Abdominal pain		●		●		

INTERACTIONS

None.

PROLONGED USE

No problems expected.

METHYLPHENIDATE

Brand names Concerta XL, Delmosart, Equasym XL, Matoride, Medikinet XL, Ritalin, Tranquilyn, Xaggitin XL, Xenidate XL
Used in the following combined preparations None

GENERAL INFORMATION

Methylphenidate is related to amfetamine and shares similar stimulant properties. Paradoxically, however, methylphenidate is used, under specialist supervision, to treat overactivity in children with severe, persistent attention deficit hyperactivity disorder (ADHD). Children with moderate ADHD should only receive it when psychological treatments have been unsuccessful. In all cases, the drug should be part of an overall treatment programme for ADHD. Growth may be retarded in children receiving the drug, and should be closely monitored. However, in affected children it often returns to normal once the drug is stopped. Methylphenidate is also used to treat narcolepsy in adults and children.

INFORMATION FOR USERS

Your drug prescription is tailored for you. Do not alter dosage without checking with your doctor.

How taken/used

Tablets, XL tablets, XL capsules.

Frequency and timing of doses
1 or 2 x daily (an extra bedtime dose may be needed) whole, not chewed, before meals.

Dosage range
ADHD 2.5–60mg (children), up to 100mg (adults) daily.
Narcolepsy 10–60mg daily.

Onset of effect
1–2 hours.

Duration of action
3–6 hours (up to 9 hours for XL preparations).

Diet advice
None.

Storage
Keep in original container at room temperature out of the reach of children.

Missed dose
Take next dose at the usual time. Do not take a double dose.

Stopping the drug
Do not stop the drug without consulting your doctor; symptoms may recur.

OVERDOSE ACTION

Seek immediate medical advice. Although an occasional unintended dose is unlikely to be a cause for concern, a large overdose can be extremely dangerous. Take emergency action if a seizure occurs.

See Drug poisoning emergency guide (p.518).

SPECIAL PRECAUTIONS

Be sure to tell your doctor if:
- You have a history of heart problems.
- You have a family history of Tourette's syndrome.
- You have a drug dependency.
- You have epilepsy.
- You have a psychiatric illness.

 Pregnancy
Safety in pregnancy not established. Discuss with your doctor.

 Breast-feeding
Safety in breast-feeding not established. Discuss with your doctor.

 Infants and children
Dose varies according to age.

 Over 60
Not usually prescribed.

 Driving and hazardous work
Avoid such activities until you have learned how methylphenidate affects you.

 Alcohol
Avoid. Effects of methylphenidate may be enhanced by alcohol.

PROLONGED USE

No problems expected in adults. Methylphenidate may retard growth in children if used for prolonged periods.

Monitoring Regular monitoring of growth should be carried out when methylphenidate is used for prolonged periods in children.

POSSIBLE ADVERSE EFFECTS

Adverse effects from methylphenidate are common but rarely serious. In some cases, side effects may be difficult to interpret due to pre-existing behavioural problems. In each case a careful assessment should be made by a specialist at regular intervals.

Symptom/effect	Frequency		Discuss with doctor		Stop taking drug now	Call doctor now
	Common	Rare	Only if severe	In all cases		
Nausea	●		●			
Abdominal discomfort	●		●			
Dry mouth	●		●			
Irritability/agitation/aggression	●			●		
Rash	●			●		
Palpitations	●			●		
Depression		●		●		

INTERACTIONS

SSRI and tricyclic antidepressants Methylphenidate can increase blood levels of these drugs. Reduced doses may be required.

MAOI antidepressants When taken with methylphenidate, there is a risk of an extreme rise in blood pressure. Concomitant use of these drugs should be avoided.

Phenytoin Methylphenidate increases blood levels of phenytoin. Reduced dose of phenytoin may be required.

Oral anticoagulants (e.g. warfarin) The anticoagulant effect of these drugs is increased by methylphenidate.

METOCLOPRAMIDE

Brand names Maxolon, Maxolon High Dose, Maxolon SR, Primperan
Used in the following combined preparation MigraMax, Paramax

GENERAL INFORMATION

Metoclopramide has a direct action on the gastrointestinal tract. It is used for conditions in which there is a need to encourage normal propulsion of food through the stomach and intestine.

The drug has powerful anti-emetic properties, and its most common use is in preventing and treating nausea and vomiting. It is particularly effective for the relief of the nausea that sometimes accompanies migraine headaches, and the nausea caused by treatment with anticancer drugs. It is also prescribed to alleviate symptoms of heartburn caused by acid reflux into the oesophagus.

One side effect of metoclopramide, muscle spasm of the head and neck, is more likely to occur in children and young adults under 20 years. Other side effects are not usually troublesome.

INFORMATION FOR USERS

Your drug prescription is tailored for you. Do not alter dosage without checking with your doctor.

How taken/used

Tablets, powder, liquid, injection.

Frequency and timing of doses
Usually 3 x daily; 2 x daily (SR preparations).

Adult dosage range
Usually 15–30mg daily; may be higher for nausea caused by anticancer drugs.

Onset of effect
Within 1 hour.

Duration of action
6–8 hours.

Diet advice
Fatty and spicy foods and alcohol are best avoided if nausea is a problem.

Storage
Keep in original container at room temperature out of the reach of children.

Missed dose
Take as soon as you remember. If your next dose is due within 3 hours, take a single dose now and skip the next.

Stopping the drug
Can be safely stopped as soon as you no longer need it.

Exceeding the dose
An occasional unintentional extra dose is unlikely to be a cause for concern. Large overdoses may cause drowsiness and muscle spasms. Notify your doctor.

SPECIAL PRECAUTIONS

Be sure to tell your doctor if:
- You have long-term liver or kidney problems.
- You have epilepsy.
- You have Parkinson's disease.
- You have porphyria.
- You have phaeochromocytoma.
- You have had recent gastrointestinal illness or surgery.
- You are taking other medicines.

 Pregnancy
Safety in pregnancy not established. Discuss with your doctor.

 Breast-feeding
The drug passes into the breast milk but at normal doses adverse effects on the baby are unlikely. Discuss with your doctor.

 Infants and children
Reduced dose necessary. Restricted use in patients younger than 20 years.

 Over 60
Reduced dose may be necessary.

 Driving and hazardous work
Avoid such activities until you have learned how the drug affects you because it can cause drowsiness.

 Alcohol
Avoid. Alcohol may oppose the beneficial effects and increase the sedative effects of this drug.

POSSIBLE ADVERSE EFFECTS

The main adverse effects of metoclopramide are drowsiness and, even less commonly, uncontrolled muscle spasm. Other symptoms rarely occur.

Symptom/effect	Frequency		Discuss with doctor		Stop taking drug now	Call doctor now
	Common	Rare	Only if severe	In all cases		
Drowsiness		●	●			
Restlessness		●		●		
Diarrhoea		●		●		
Muscle tremor/rigidity		●		●		
Muscle spasm of head/neck		●		●	●	●
Rash		●		●	●	●

PROLONGED USE

Not normally used long term, except under specialist supervision for certain gastrointestinal disorders.

INTERACTIONS

Sedatives The sedative properties of metoclopramide are increased by all drugs that have a sedative effect on the central nervous system. These include benzodiazepines, antihistamines, antidepressants, and opioid analgesics.

Lithium Metoclopramide increases the risk of central nervous system side effects.

Drugs for parkinsonism There is an increased risk of adverse effects if these drugs are taken with metoclopramide.

Ciclosporin Metoclopramide may increase the blood levels of this drug.

Antipsychotics Metoclopramide increases the risk of adverse effects from these drugs.

Opioid analgesics and anticholinergic drugs These drugs oppose the gastrointestinal effects of metoclopramide.

Aspirin and paracetamol Metoclopramide increases the rate of absorption of these drugs.

METOPROLOL

Brand names Betaloc, Betaloc-SA, Lopresor, Lopresor SR
Used in the following combined preparations None

GENERAL INFORMATION

Metoprolol is a cardioselective beta blocker that is used to prevent the heart from beating too quickly in conditions such as angina, arrhythmias, and hyperthyroidism. It is also used to prevent migraine attacks and protect the heart from further damage after a heart attack. The drug is used to treat hypertension (high blood pressure) but is not usually used to initiate treatment. It is less likely than non-cardioselective beta blockers to provoke breathing difficulties. However, it should be avoided in people with asthma. It may slow the body's response to low blood sugar in diabetic people on insulin.

INFORMATION FOR USERS

Your drug prescription is tailored for you. Do not alter dosage without checking with your doctor.

How taken/used

Tablets, SR tablets, injection.

Frequency and timing of doses
1–2 x daily (hypertension); 2–3 x daily (angina/arrhythmias); 4 x daily for 2 days, then 2 x daily (heart attack prevention); 2 x daily (migraine prevention); 4 x daily (hyperthyroidism).

Adult dosage range
100–200mg daily.

Onset of effect
1–2 hours.

Duration of action
3–7 hours.

Diet advice
None.

Storage
Keep in original container at room temperature out of the reach of children.

Missed dose
Take as soon as you remember. If your next dose is due within 2 hours, take a single dose now and skip the next.

Stopping the drug
Do not stop taking the drug without consulting your doctor. Stopping suddenly may lead to worsening of the underlying condition.

OVERDOSE ACTION

Seek immediate medical advice in all cases. Take emergency action if breathing difficulties, collapse, or loss of consciousness occur.

See Drug poisoning emergency guide (p.518).

POSSIBLE ADVERSE EFFECTS

Metoprolol's adverse effects are common to most beta blockers and tend to diminish with long-term use. Fainting may be a sign that the drug has slowed the heart beat excessively.

Symptom/effect	Frequency		Discuss with doctor		Stop taking drug now	Call doctor now
	Common	Rare	Only if severe	In all cases		
Lethargy/fatigue	●			●		
Cold hands and feet	●			●		
Nausea/vomiting		●		●		
Nightmares/vivid dreams		●		●	●	
Rash/dry eyes		●		●	●	
Visual disturbances		●		●	●	
Fainting/palpitations		●		●	●	●
Breathlessness/wheeze		●		●	●	●

INTERACTIONS

Antihypertensive drugs Metoprolol may enhance the blood-pressure-lowering effect.

Calcium channel blockers may cause low blood pressure, a slow heartbeat, and heart failure if used with metoprolol.

Non-steroidal anti-inflammatory drugs (NSAIDs) may reduce the antihypertensive effect of metoprolol.

Cardiac glycosides (e.g. digoxin) may increase the heart-slowing effect of metoprolol.

Antidiabetic drugs Taken with metoprolol, these drugs may increase the risk of low blood sugar or mask its symptoms.

Antacids may increase the effects of metoprolol.

SPECIAL PRECAUTIONS

Be sure to tell your doctor if:
- You have liver or kidney problems.
- You have asthma, bronchitis, or emphysema.
- You have heart problems.
- You have diabetes.
- You have psoriasis.
- You have phaeochromocytoma (a type of adrenal gland tumour).
- You are taking other medicines.

Pregnancy
Not usually prescribed. May affect the baby. Discuss with your doctor.

Breast-feeding
The drug passes into the breast milk, but at normal doses adverse effects on the baby are unlikely. Discuss with your doctor.

Infants and children
Not recommended.

Over 60
Reduced doses necessary. There may be an increased risk of adverse effects.

Driving and hazardous work
Avoid such activities until you have learned how metoprolol affects you because the drug can cause fatigue, dizziness, and drowsiness.

Alcohol
Avoid excessive intake. Alcohol may increase the blood-pressure-lowering effects of metoprolol.

Surgery and general anaesthetics
Occasionally, metoprolol may need to be stopped before you have a general anaesthetic; but only do this after discussion with your doctor or dentist.

PROLONGED USE

No special problems.

In very rare cases, use of metoprolol is associated with Peyronie's disease (growth of abnormal fibrous tissue in the penis) and with retroperitoneal fibrosis (growth of abnormal fibrous tissue around the abdominal organs).

METRONIDAZOLE

Brand names Acea, Anabact, Flagyl, Metrogel, Metrosa, Rosiced, Rozex, Zidoval, Zyomet
Used in the following combined preparations None

GENERAL INFORMATION

Metronidazole is prescribed to treat both protozoal infections and a variety of bacterial infections.

It is widely used in the treatment of trichomonas infection of the vagina. Because the organism responsible for this disorder is sexually transmitted and may not cause any symptoms, a simultaneous course of treatment is usually advised for the sexual partner.

Certain infections of the abdomen, pelvis, and gums also respond well to metronidazole. The drug is used to treat septicaemia and infected leg ulcers and pressure sores. It is also used to treat *Clostridium difficile* infections occurring with antibiotic use. Metronidazole may be given to prevent or treat infections after surgery. Because high doses can penetrate the brain, it is prescribed to treat abscesses occurring there.

Metronidazole is also prescribed for amoebic dysentery and giardiasis, a protozoal infection.

QUICK REFERENCE

Drug group Antibacterial drug (p.89) and antiprotozoal drug (p.94)

Overdose danger rating Low

Dependence rating Low

Prescription needed Yes

Available as generic Yes

INFORMATION FOR USERS

Your drug prescription is tailored for you. Do not alter dosage without checking with your doctor.

How taken/used

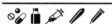

Tablets, liquid, injection, suppositories, gel, cream.

Frequency and timing of doses
3 x daily for 5–10 days, depending on condition being treated. Sometimes a single large dose is prescribed. Tablets should be taken after meals and swallowed whole with plenty of water. 1–2 x daily (topical preparations).

Adult dosage range
600–2,000mg daily (by mouth); 3g daily (suppositories); 1.5g daily (injection).

Onset of effect
The drug starts to work within an hour or so, but beneficial effects may not be felt for 1–2 days.

Duration of action
6–12 hours.

Diet advice
None.

Storage
Keep in original container at room temperature out of the reach of children. Protect from light.

Missed dose
Take as soon as you remember. If your next dose is due within 2 hours, take a single dose now and skip the next.

Stopping the drug
Take the full course. Even if you feel better the infection may still be present and symptoms may recur if treatment is stopped too soon.

Exceeding the dose
An occasional unintentional extra dose is unlikely to be a cause for concern. But if you notice unusual symptoms, especially numbness or tingling, or if a large overdose has been taken, notify your doctor.

SPECIAL PRECAUTIONS

Be sure to tell your doctor if:
• You have long-term liver or kidney problems.
• You have porphyria.
• You are taking other medicines.

 Pregnancy
Safety in pregnancy not established. Discuss with your doctor.

 Breast-feeding
The drug passes into the breast milk, but at normal doses adverse effects on the baby are unlikely. However, metronidazole may give the milk a bitter taste. Discuss with your doctor.

 Infants and children
Reduced dose necessary.

 Over 60
No special problems.

 Driving and hazardous work
Avoid such activities until you have learned how metronidazole affects you because the drug can cause drowsiness.

 Alcohol
Avoid. Taken with metronidazole, alcohol may cause flushing, nausea, vomiting, abdominal pain, and headache.

POSSIBLE ADVERSE EFFECTS

Various minor gastrointestinal disturbances are common but tend to diminish with time. The drug may cause a darkening of the urine, which is of no concern. More serious adverse effects on the nervous system, causing numbness or tingling, are extremely rare.

Symptom/effect	Frequency		Discuss with doctor		Stop taking drug now	Call doctor now
	Common	Rare	Only if severe	In all cases		
Nausea/loss of appetite	●			●		
Dark urine	●			●		
Dry mouth/metallic taste		●		●		
Headache/dizziness		●		●		
Numbness/tingling		●			●	

INTERACTIONS

Oral anticoagulants, ciclosporin, phenytoin, and fluorouracil Metronidazole may increase the effects of these drugs.

Lithium Metronidazole increases the levels of lithium and the risk of kidney damage.

Cimetidine This drug may increase the levels of metronidazole in the body.

Phenobarbital This drug may reduce the effects of metronidazole.

PROLONGED USE

Not usually prescribed for longer than 10 days. Prolonged treatment may cause loss of sensation in the hands and feet (usually temporary), and may also reduce production of white blood cells.

Monitoring Monitoring of blood counts and liver function may be considered if treatment is given for more than 10 days.

MICONAZOLE

Brand names Daktarin, Gyno-Daktarin, Loramyc
Used in the following combined preparation Daktacort

GENERAL INFORMATION

Miconazole is an antifungal drug used to treat candida (yeast) infections of the mouth, candida and bacterial infections of the vagina and gut, and a range of other fungal infections affecting the skin.

The drug is available as a treatment for oral infections in the form of a gel to be used on dentures. Cream, dusting powder, or ointment are used for skin

infections, and a variety of vaginal preparations is available.

Side effects usually only occur with oral preparations, because miconazole is absorbed in only very small quantities following topical or vaginal application.

The pessaries, vaginal capsules, and vaginal cream damage latex condoms and diaphragms.

INFORMATION FOR USERS

Follow instructions on the label. Call your doctor if symptoms worsen.

How taken/used

Buccal tablets, pessaries, vaginal cream, vaginal capsules, cream, ointment, oral gel, spray powder.

Frequency and timing of doses
1 x daily in morning (buccal tablets); 4 x daily after food (oral gel); 1–2 x daily (vaginal/skin preparations).

Adult dosage range
Vaginal infections 1 x 5g applicatorful (cream); 1 x 100mg pessary; 1 x 1.2g vaginal capsule. *Oral/skin infections* As directed.

Onset of effect
2–3 days.

Duration of action
Up to 12 hours.

Diet advice
None.

Storage
Keep in original container at room temperature out of the reach of children.

Missed dose
No cause for concern, but apply missed dose or application as soon as you remember.

Stopping the drug
Apply the full course. Even if you feel better, the original infection may still be present and may recur if treatment is stopped too soon.

Exceeding the dose
An occasional unintentional extra dose is unlikely to cause problems. But if you notice any unusual symptoms or if a large amount has been swallowed, notify your doctor.

SPECIAL PRECAUTIONS

Be sure to consult your doctor or pharmacist before taking this drug if:
- You have porphyria.
- You have liver problems.
- You are taking other medicines.

Pregnancy
No evidence of risk with topical preparations. Safety not established for other preparations. Discuss with your doctor.

Breast-feeding
Safety not established. Discuss with your doctor.

Infants and children
Reduced dose necessary (oral gel).

Over 60
No special problems.

Driving and hazardous work
No special problems.

Alcohol
No special problems.

POSSIBLE ADVERSE EFFECTS

Adverse effects are rare with miconazole and usually only occur with oral use.

Symptom/effect	Frequency		Discuss with doctor		Stop taking drug now	Call doctor now
	Common	Rare	Only if severe	In all cases		
Skin irritation/rash		●	●			
Nausea/vomiting		●	●			
Vaginal irritation		●		●		

PROLONGED USE

No problems expected. Most types of miconazole are not usually prescribed long term, but oral gel may cause diarrhoea if used for a long time.

INTERACTIONS

Oral anticoagulants, ciclosporin, phenytoin, antidiabetics, quinidine, and pimozide Miconazole oral gel and buccal tablets may increase the effects and toxicity of these drugs.

Carbamazepine, phenytoin, calcium channel blockers, sirolimus, and tacrolimus Miconazole oral gel and buccal tablets may increase the effects and toxicity of these drugs.

Simvastatin There is an increased risk of muscle damage if this drug is taken with miconazole. Avoid using together.

MINOCYCLINE

Brand names Aknemin, Dexcel Acnamino, Minocin MR, Sebomin MR
Used in the following combined preparations None

GENERAL INFORMATION

Minocycline is a tetracycline antibiotic but has a longer duration of action than tetracycline itself. The drug is most commonly used to treat acne. It may also be given to treat pneumonia or to prevent infection in people with chronic bronchitis, and to treat sexually transmitted infections such as gonorrhoea and non-gonococcal urethritis. Minocycline is also used to treat chronic gum disease in adults. The drug's most frequent side effects are nausea, vomiting, and diarrhoea. It also interferes with the balance mechanism in the ear, with resultant nausea, dizziness, and unsteadiness, but these generally disappear after the drug is stopped. Minocycline is safer to use than other tetracyclines in people with poor kidney function.

QUICK REFERENCE

Drug group Tetracycline antibiotic (p.86)

Overdose danger rating Low

Dependence rating Low

Prescription needed Yes

Available as generic Yes

INFORMATION FOR USERS

Your drug prescription is tailored for you. Do not alter dosage without checking with your doctor.

How taken/used

Tablets, capsules, MR capsules, gel.

Frequency and timing of doses
1–2 x daily.

Dosage range
Adults 100–200mg daily.
Children Reduced dose according to age and weight.

Onset of effect
4–12 hours.

Duration of action
Up to 24 hours.

Diet advice
Milk products may impair absorption; avoid from 1 hour before to 2 hours after dosage.

Storage
Keep in original container at room temperature out of the reach of children.

Missed dose
Take as soon as you remember. If your next dose is due within 4 hours, take a single dose now and skip the next.

Stopping the drug
Use the full course. Even if you feel better, the original infection may still be present and symptoms may recur if treatment is stopped too soon.

Exceeding the dose
An occasional unintentional extra dose is unlikely to be a cause for concern. But if you notice any unusual symptoms, or if a large overdose has been taken, notify your doctor.

SPECIAL PRECAUTIONS

Be sure to tell your doctor if:
- You have liver or kidney problems.
- You have previously had an allergic reaction to a tetracycline antibiotic.
- You have myasthenia gravis, acute porphyria, or systemic lupus erythematosus.
- You are taking other medicines.

Pregnancy
Not prescribed. May cause birth defects and may damage the teeth and bones of the developing baby, as well as the mother's liver. Discuss with your doctor.

Breast-feeding
Not recommended. The drug passes into the breast milk and may damage developing bones and discolour the baby's teeth. Discuss with your doctor.

Infants and children
Not recommended under 12 years. Reduced dose necessary in older children. May discolour developing teeth.

Over 60
No special problems.

Driving and hazardous work
Avoid such activities until you have learned how minocycline affects you because the drug can cause dizziness.

Alcohol
No known problems.

How to take your tablets
To prevent minocycline from sticking in your throat, take a small amount of water before, and a full glass of water after, each dose. Take this medication while sitting or standing and do not lie down immediately afterwards.

POSSIBLE ADVERSE EFFECTS

Minocycline may occasionally cause nausea, vomiting, or diarrhoea. Other less common adverse effects are rashes, an increased sensitivity of the skin to sunlight, and, in some cases, dizziness and loss of balance (vertigo).

Symptom/effect	Frequency		Discuss with doctor		Stop taking drug now	Call doctor now
	Common	Rare	Only if severe	In all cases		
Nausea/vomiting/diarrhoea	●		●			
Dizziness/vertigo	●			●	●	
Rash/itching		●		●	●	
Light-sensitive rash		●		●	●	
Headache/blurred vision		●		●	●	

INTERACTIONS

Oral anticoagulants Minocycline may increase the anticoagulant action of these drugs.

Retinoids with minocycline may increase the risk of benign intracranial hypertension (high pressure in the skull) leading to headaches, nausea, and vomiting.

Oral contraceptives Minocycline can reduce the effectiveness of these drugs.

Penicillin antibiotics Minocycline interferes with the antibacterial action of these drugs.

Iron may interfere with the absorption of minocycline and may reduce its effectiveness.

Antacids, zinc preparations, and milk interfere with absorption of minocycline and may reduce its effectiveness. Doses should be separated by 1–2 hours.

Strontium ranelate may reduce the absorption of minocycline. The two drugs should not be used together.

PROLONGED USE

Prolonged use may occasionally cause skin darkening and discoloration of the teeth. Very rarely, it may cause systemic lupus erythematosus.

Monitoring Regular blood tests should be carried out to assess liver function, especially if treatment lasts over 6 months.

MINOXIDIL

Brand names Boots Hair Loss Treatment, Loniten, Regaine
Used in the following combined preparations None

GENERAL INFORMATION

Minoxidil is a vasodilator drug (p.56) that works by relaxing the muscles of artery walls and dilating blood vessels. It is effective in controlling dangerously high blood pressure that is rising very rapidly. Because minoxidil is stronger-acting than many other antihypertensive drugs, it is particularly useful for people whose blood pressure is not controlled by other treatment.

Because minoxidil causes significant fluid retention and increased heart rate, the drug should be prescribed together with a diuretic and a beta blocker to increase effectiveness and to counteract its side effects.

Unlike many other drugs in the antihypertensive group, minoxidil rarely causes dizziness and fainting. Its major drawback is that, if it is taken for more than two months, it increases hair growth, especially on the face. Although this effect can be controlled by shaving or depilatories, some people find the abnormal growth distressing. This effect is put to use, however, to treat baldness in men and women, and for this purpose minoxidil is applied locally as a solution.

QUICK REFERENCE

Drug group Antihypertensive drug (p.60) and treatment for hair loss (p.140)

Overdose danger rating Medium

Dependence rating Low

Prescription needed Yes (except for scalp lotions)

Available as generic No

INFORMATION FOR USERS

Your drug prescription is tailored for you. Do not alter dosage without checking with your doctor.

How taken/used

Tablets, topical solution.

Frequency and timing of doses
Once or twice daily.

Adult dosage range
5mg daily initially, increasing gradually to a maximum of 100mg daily.

Onset of effect
Blood pressure Within 1 hour (tablets).
Hair growth Up to 1 year (solution).

Duration of action
Up to 24 hours. Some effect may last for 2–5 days after stopping the drug.

Diet advice
None.

Storage
Keep in original container at room temperature out of the reach of children.

Missed dose
Take as soon as you remember (tablets). If your next dose is due within 5 hours, take a single dose now and skip the next. If used topically for baldness, any regained hair will be lost when the drug is stopped.

Stopping the drug
Do not stop the drug without consulting your doctor; stopping the drug may lead to worsening of the underlying condition.

Exceeding the dose
An occasional unintentional extra dose is unlikely to cause problems. Large overdoses may cause nausea, vomiting, palpitations, or dizziness. Notify your doctor.

SPECIAL PRECAUTIONS

Be sure to tell your doctor if:
- You have a long-term kidney problem.
- You have heart problems.
- You have porphyria.
- You are taking other medicines.

 Pregnancy
Safety in pregnancy not established. Discuss with your doctor.

 Breast-feeding
The drug passes into the breast milk, but normal doses are unlikely to harm the baby. Discuss with your doctor.

 Infants and children
Reduced dose necessary.

 Over 60
Reduced dose may be necessary.

 Driving and hazardous work
Avoid such activities until you have learned how minoxidil affects you because the drug can cause dizziness and lightheadedness.

 Alcohol
Avoid. Alcohol may further reduce blood pressure.

Surgery and general anaesthetics
Minoxidil treatment may need to be stopped before you have a general anaesthetic. Discuss this with your doctor or dentist before any surgery.

POSSIBLE ADVERSE EFFECTS

Fluid retention is a common adverse effect of minoxidil, which may lead to an increase in weight. Diuretics are often prescribed to control this adverse effect. Allergic and irritant dermatitis may occur with minoxidil lotion.

Symptom/effect	Frequency		Discuss with doctor		Stop taking drug now	Call doctor now
	Common	Rare	Only if severe	In all cases		
Increased hair growth	●			●		
Fluid retention/ankle swelling	●			●		
Nausea		●		●		
Breast tenderness		●		●		
Dizziness/lightheadedness		●		●		
Rash		●		●		
Palpitations		●		●	●	●

PROLONGED USE

Prolonged use of this drug may lead to swelling of the ankles and increased hair growth.

INTERACTIONS

Antidepressant drugs The hypotensive effects of minoxidil may be enhanced by antidepressant drugs.

Other antihypertensives These drugs may increase the effects of minoxidil.

Oestrogens and progestogens (including those in some contraceptive pills) may reduce the effects of minoxidil.

MIRTAZAPINE

Brand name Zispin Soltab
Used in the following combined preparations None

GENERAL INFORMATION

Mirtazapine is an antidepressant drug that works by increasing two naturally occurring chemicals in the brain: serotonin and noradrenaline. It is used in the treatment of major depression, the symptoms of which may include feelings of worthlessness, anxiety, and increased or decreased appetite.

Mirtazapine may be given at a low dose initially and increased gradually according to the response of the individual. If there is no response to mirtazapine at the maximum dose within 2 to 4 weeks, the treatment may be discontinued.

Mirtazapine is available as tablets, orosoluble tablets (which are placed on the tongue and allowed to dissolve), and an oral solution. Because the drug has little anticholinergic action, it is better tolerated than tricyclic antidepressants.

QUICK REFERENCE

Drug group Antidepressant drug (p.40)

Overdose danger rating Medium

Dependence rating Low

Prescription needed Yes

Available as generic Yes

INFORMATION FOR USERS

Your drug prescription is tailored for you. Do not alter dosage without checking with your doctor.

How taken/used

Tablets, orosoluble tablets, liquid (oral solution).

Frequency and timing of doses
Usually once daily at bedtime.

Adult dosage range
15mg (initial dose), increased gradually to 45mg, according to response.

Onset of effect
Within 1–2 weeks, but full beneficial effect may not be felt for 2–4 weeks.

Duration of action
At least 24 hours.

Diet advice
None.

Storage
Keep in original container at room temperature out of the reach of children.

Missed dose
Take as soon as you remember, then return to your normal dosing schedule. Do not take an extra dose to make up.

Stopping the drug
Do not stop taking the drug without consulting your doctor, who will supervise a gradual reduction in dosage. Stopping abruptly can lead to withdrawal symptoms.

Exceeding the dose
An occasional unintentional extra dose is unlikely to cause problems. Larger overdoses may cause drowsiness and disorientation. Notify your doctor.

SPECIAL PRECAUTIONS

Be sure to tell your doctor if:
- You have epilepsy.
- You have liver or kidney problems.
- You have angina or have had a recent heart attack.
- You have hypertension.
- You have diabetes.
- You have a psychiatric illness or bipolar disorder.
- You have any eye disease such as glaucoma.
- You have had a previous allergic reaction to mirtazapine.
- You are taking other medicines.

 Pregnancy
Not recommended. Safety not established. Discuss with your doctor.

 Breast-feeding
Small amounts of the drug pass into the breast milk, but safety not established. Discuss with your doctor.

 Infants and children
Not recommended.

 Over 60
Not recommended.

 Driving and hazardous work
Do not undertake such activities until you have learned how mirtazapine affects you because the drug can cause initial sedation and impaired alertness and concentration.

 Alcohol
Avoid. Mirtazapine may increase the sedative effects of alcohol.

POSSIBLE ADVERSE EFFECTS

A number of the effects of mirtazapine are similar to symptoms of the illness. The drug has few anticholinergic effects, but causes sedation at the start of treatment.

Symptom/effect	Frequency		Discuss with doctor		Stop taking drug now	Call doctor now
	Common	Rare	Only if severe	In all cases		
Increased appetite/weight gain	●		●			
Drowsiness/sedation/fatigue	●		●			
Swollen ankles/feet (oedema)	●			●		
Restlessness		●	●			
Dizziness	●		●			
Headache		●	●			
Nightmares/vivid dreams		●	●			
Jaundice		●		●	●	●
Fever/sore throat		●		●	●	●

INTERACTIONS

Monoamine oxidase inhibitors (MAOIs) should not be taken with, or within 2 weeks of stopping, mirtazapine, and vice versa.

Warfarin Mirtazapine increases the anticoagulant effect of warfarin.

Antimalarials (artemether with lumefantrine) should not be taken with mirtazapine.

Carbamazepine and phenytoin may reduce blood levels of mirtazapine.

PROLONGED USE

No known problems.

Monitoring Periodic tests of liver function are usually carried out.

MISOPROSTOL

Brand name Cytotec, Mysodelle, Topogyne
Used in the following combined preparations Arthrotec, Napratec

GENERAL INFORMATION

Misoprostol reduces acid secretion in the stomach and promotes the healing of gastric and duodenal ulcers. These types of ulcer may be caused by aspirin (see p.162) and by non-steroidal anti-inflammatory drugs (NSAIDs, p.74) which block the body's synthesis of naturally occurring chemicals called prostaglandins. Misoprostol is a synthetic prostaglandin that acts as a substitute for some of the natural prostaglandins produced by the gut wall to prevent ulceration of the lining.

Treatment with misoprostol usually causes ulcers to heal in a few weeks, although it has been largely superseded by proton-pump inhibitors in this role. In some cases, misoprostol is given during treatment with aspirin or NSAIDs as a preventative measure, and combined preparations are available that reduce the likelihood of ulcers occurring.

The most common adverse effects of misoprostol are diarrhoea and indigestion; if these symptoms are severe, it may be necessary to stop taking the drug.

Misoprostol also causes the uterus to contract. This may cause premature labour, and so the drug must not be used during pregnancy. However, because of this effect, misoprostol may be used in medical terminations of pregnancy. The information below relates only to the anti-ulcer use of the drug.

see p.162, p.74

QUICK REFERENCE

Drug group Anti-ulcer drug (p.67)
Overdose danger rating Low
Dependence rating Low
Prescription needed Yes
Available as generic No

(p.67)

INFORMATION FOR USERS

Your drug prescription is tailored for you. Do not alter dosage without checking with your doctor.

How taken/used

Tablets.

Frequency and timing of doses
2–4 x daily, with or after food.

Adult dosage range
400–800mcg daily.

Onset of effect
Within 24 hours.

Duration of action
Up to 24 hours; some effects may be longer lasting.

Diet advice
None.

Storage
Keep in original container at room temperature out of the reach of children.

Missed dose
Take as soon as you remember. If your next dose is due within 3 hours, take a single dose now and skip the next.

Stopping the drug
Do not stop the drug without consulting your doctor; symptoms may recur.

Exceeding the dose
An occasional unintentional extra dose is unlikely to be a cause for concern. But if you notice any unusual symptoms, or if a large overdose has been taken, notify your doctor.

SPECIAL PRECAUTIONS

Be sure to tell your doctor if:
- You are or plan to become pregnant.
- You have had a stroke.
- You have heart problems.
- You have high blood pressure.
- You have bowel problems.
- You are taking other medicines.

Pregnancy
Misoprostol should not be taken by women of childbearing age. In exceptional cases, it may be prescribed on the condition that effective contraception is used. If taken during pregnancy, the drug can cause the uterus to contract before the baby is due.

Breast-feeding
Safety not established. Discuss with your doctor.

Infants and children
Not recommended.

Over 60
No special problems.

Driving and hazardous work
Avoid such activities until you have learned how misoprostol affects you because the drug can cause dizziness.

Alcohol
No problems expected, but excessive amounts may undermine the desired effect of the drug.

POSSIBLE ADVERSE EFFECTS

Adverse effects on the gastrointestinal tract can occur. These effects may be reduced by spreading the doses out during the day. Taking the drug with food may be recommended.

Symptom/effect	Frequency		Discuss with doctor		Stop taking drug now	Call doctor now
	Common	Rare	Only if severe	In all cases		
Diarrhoea	●		●			
Indigestion	●		●			
Nausea/vomiting		●	●			
Vaginal/intermenstrual bleeding		●		●		
Abdominal pain		●		●		
Dizziness		●		●		
Skin rashes		●		●	●	

INTERACTIONS

Magnesium-containing antacids These may increase the severity of any diarrhoea caused by misoprostol.

PROLONGED USE

No problems expected, but the drug is rarely required long term.

MODAFINIL

Brand name Provigil
Used in the following combined preparations None

GENERAL INFORMATION

Modafinil is a nervous system stimulant used to relieve the excessive sleepiness associated with narcolepsy, obstructive sleep apnoea, and chronic shift work. Modafinil has some features in common with the stimulant amfetamine (p.449), including a potential for dependence and abuse, but the risk of these issues is much lower with modafinil than with amfetamine itself. However, treatment with modafinil should be initiated by a doctor with a specialist interest in sleep disorders and only after other efforts have been made to treat the underlying condition. The drug should not be given to people who have severe or poorly controlled high blood pressure or heart disease.

QUICK REFERENCE

Drug group Nervous system stimulant (p.44)

Overdose danger rating Medium

Dependence rating Medium

Prescription needed Yes

Available as generic No

INFORMATION FOR USERS

Your drug prescription is tailored for you. Do not alter dosage without checking with your doctor.

How taken/used

Tablets.

Frequency and timing of doses
Single dose in the morning; or twice daily, in the morning and at midday.

Adult dosage range
200–400 mg daily.

Onset of effect
Within a few hours.

Duration of action
12–24 hours.

Diet advice
None.

Storage
Keep in original container at room temperature out of the reach of children.

Missed dose
Take as soon as you remember if needed for relief of symptoms. If not needed, do not take the missed dose, and return to your normal dose schedule when necessary.

Stopping the drug
Do not stop the drug without consulting your doctor; symptoms may recur.

Exceeding the dose
An occasional unintentional extra dose is unlikely to cause problems. Large overdoses may cause insomnia, restlessness, confusion, high blood pressure, and fast heart rate. Notify your doctor immediately.

SPECIAL PRECAUTIONS

Be sure to tell your doctor if:
- You have a liver or kidney problem.
- You have high blood pressure.
- You have a heart problem.
- You have had a psychiatric illness.
- You have a history of alcohol or illicit substance misuse.
- You are taking any other medicine.

Pregnancy
Not prescribed in pregnancy as the drug may cause birth defects. Discuss with your doctor.

Breast-feeding
Safety not established. Discuss with your doctor.

Infants and children
Not prescribed for children under 18 years.

Over 60
Increased risk of adverse effects. Reduced dose may be necessary.

Driving and hazardous work
Discuss with your doctor. Your underlying condition, as well as the possibility of side effects such as blurred vision or dizziness, may make such activities inadvisable.

Alcohol
No special problems.

POSSIBLE ADVERSE EFFECTS

Modafinil may cause a wide range of side effects. The most common is headache. There is also a risk of developing new mental health problems, or worsening existing ones, such as anxiety, depression (including suicidal thoughts), aggressive behaviour, or psychosis.

Symptom/effect	Frequency		Discuss with doctor		Stop taking drug now	Call doctor now
	Common	Rare	Only if severe	In all cases		
Headache	●		●			
Fast heart rate/palpitations	●		●			
Dizziness/blurred vision	●		●			
Nausea/abdominal pain	●		●			
Decreased appetite	●		●			
Nervousness/insomnia	●		●			
Abnormal thinking/depression	●			●		
Chest pain	●			●		
Rash		●		●	●	
Suicidal thoughts		●		●	●	●

PROLONGED USE

No special problems.

Monitoring If you have high blood pressure, regular blood pressure monitoring may be carried out.

INTERACTIONS

Oral contraceptives Modafinil reduces the effectiveness of oestrogen-containing contraceptive pills; additional contraceptive methods should be used during treatment and for 2 months afterwards.

Antidepressants Modafinil may increase blood levels of antidepressants, so a lower dose of antidepressant may be required.

Ciclosporin Modafinil reduces blood levels of ciclosporin.

Phenytoin Modafinil may increase blood levels of phenytoin.

Warfarin Modafinil may increase the effects of warfarin, so a lower dose of warfarin may be required.

MOMETASONE

Brand names Asmanex, Elocon, Nasonex
Used in the following combined preparations None

GENERAL INFORMATION

Mometasone is a corticosteroid drug used as an inhaler to prevent asthma attacks and as a nasal spray to relieve the symptoms of allergic rhinitis. It is also used topically for the treatment of severe inflammatory skin disorders and in conditions such as eczema that have not responded to other corticosteroids (see Topical corticosteroids, p.134).

Serious adverse effects are rare if the drug is used for short periods or in small amounts, but prolonged or excessive topical use may cause local side effects such as thin skin, and systemic side effects such as osteoporosis, muscle weakness, and peptic ulcers.

Fungal infections causing irritation of the mouth and throat are a possible side effect of inhaling mometasone. These can be avoided to some degree by rinsing the mouth and gargling with water after each inhalation.

INFORMATION FOR USERS

Your drug prescription is tailored for you. Do not alter dosage without checking with your doctor.

How taken/used

Cream, ointment, scalp lotion, inhaler, powder for inhalation, nasal spray.

Frequency and timing of doses
1 x 2 times daily (inhaler); once daily (other forms).

Adult dosage range
Inhaler 200–800mcg.
Nasal spray 100mcg (2 puffs) into each nostril.
Topical preparations As directed, applied thinly.

Onset of effect
12 hours. Full beneficial effect after 48 hours.

Duration of action
24 hours. Effects can last for several days after the drug is stopped.

Diet advice
None.

Storage
Keep in original container at room temperature out of the reach of children.

Missed dose
Take as soon as you remember. If your next dose/application is due within 8 hours, take a single dose or apply the usual amount now and skip the next.

Stopping the drug
Do not stop the drug without consulting your doctor; symptoms may recur.

Exceeding the dose
An occasional unintentional extra dose/application may not be a cause for concern, but if you notice any unusual symptoms, notify your doctor.

SPECIAL PRECAUTIONS

Be sure to tell your doctor if:
- You have had tuberculosis or another respiratory infection.
- You have any other nasal or skin infection.
- You have had recent nasal ulcers or nasal surgery.

 Pregnancy
Safety not established. Discuss with your doctor.

 Breast-feeding
No evidence of risk. Discuss with your doctor.

 Infants and children
Only used for very short courses in children.

 Over 60
No special problems.

 Driving and hazardous work
No special problems.

 Alcohol
No special problems.

POSSIBLE ADVERSE EFFECTS

Serious adverse effects are unlikely when the drug is used at low doses and/or for short periods. The most common side effects are irritation of the nasal lining and sometimes bleeding from the nose. More serious side effects, such as permanent skin changes, may occur with the cream or ointment, which should not normally be used on the face.

Symptom/effect	Frequency		Discuss with doctor		Stop taking drug now	Call doctor now
	Common	Rare	Only if severe	In all cases		
Inhaler/nasal spray						
Nasal discomfort/ irritation	●		●			
Cough	●		●			
Bruising	●		●			
Sore throat/hoarseness	●			●		
Nosebleed	●			●		
Cream/ointment						
Skin changes (long-term use)	●			●		

PROLONGED USE

Long-term use can lead to peptic ulcers, glaucoma, muscle weakness, osteoporosis, growth retardation in children, and, rarely, adrenal gland suppression. Prolonged use of topical treatment may also lead to skin thinning. Patients on long-term treatment should carry a steroid card or wear a MedicAlert bracelet.

Monitoring Periodic checks on adrenal gland function may be required if large doses are being taken. Children should have their height monitored.

INTERACTIONS

Ketoconazole and itraconazole may increase mometasone's systemic effect.

HIV protease inhibitors may increase the effect of mometasone.

Macrolides (clarithromycin) may increase the effect of mometasone.

Desmopressin with mometasone may increase the risk of low sodium levels.

MONTELUKAST

Brand name Singulair
Used in the following combined preparations None

GENERAL INFORMATION

Montelukast belongs to the leukotriene receptor antagonist (blocker) group of anti-allergy drugs and is used in the prevention of asthma and allergic rhinitis. It is thought that stimulation of leukotriene receptors by naturally occurring leukotrienes from the mast cells (see p.81) plays a part in causing asthma. Montelukast works by blocking these receptors.

The drug is given as an additional medication for asthma when combined treatment with corticosteroids and bronchodilators does not give adequate control. It is given by mouth as chewable tablets or granules.

Montelukast is not a bronchodilator, and cannot be used to treat an acute attack of asthma.

(see p.81)

QUICK REFERENCE

Drug group Anti-allergy drug (p.82)
Overdose danger rating Low
Dependence rating Low
Prescription needed Yes
Available as generic Yes

Anti-allergy drug (p.82)

INFORMATION FOR USERS

Your drug prescription is tailored for you. Do not alter dosage without checking with your doctor.

How taken/used

Chewable tablets, granules.

Frequency and timing of doses
Once daily at bedtime.

Adult dosage range
10mg.

Onset of effect
2 hours.

Duration of action
24 hours.

Diet advice
None.

Storage
Keep in original container at room temperature out of the reach of children. Protect from light.

Missed dose
Take as soon as you remember. If your next dose is due within 8 hours, take a single dose now and skip the next.

Stopping the drug
Do not stop the drug without consulting your doctor, as symptoms may recur.

Exceeding the dose
An occasional unintentional extra dose is unlikely to be a cause for concern. But if you notice any unusual symptoms, or if a large overdose has been taken, notify your doctor.

SPECIAL PRECAUTIONS

Be sure to tell your doctor if:
- You have phenylketonuria.
- You have galactose intolerance.
- You have lactose intolerance.
- You are taking other medicines.

 Pregnancy
Safety not established. Discuss with your doctor.

 Breast-feeding
Safety not established. Discuss with your doctor.

 Infants and children
Reduced dose necessary.

 Over 60
No special problems.

 Driving and hazardous work
Avoid such activities until you have learned how montelukast affects you because the drug can cause dizziness and drowsiness.

 Alcohol
No special problems.

PROLONGED USE

No special problems.

POSSIBLE ADVERSE EFFECTS

The most common adverse effects are abdominal pain and headache. Severe effects are very rare, but neuropsychiatric reactions including speech impairment and obsessive-compulsive symptoms have been reported.

Very rarely, patients on montelukast have developed features of an inflammatory condition called Churg-Strauss syndrome, which can mimic asthma.

Symptom/effect	Frequency		Discuss with doctor		Stop taking drug now	Call doctor now
	Common	Rare	Only if severe	In all cases		
Abdominal pain	●		●			
Headache	●		●			
Nausea/diarrhoea/vomiting	●		●			
Rash	●			●		
Dizziness/agitation		●	●			
Weakness		●	●			
Fever	●			●		
Flu-like symptoms	●			●		
Productive cough		●		●		
Worsening chest symptoms		●		●		
Numbness/tingling		●		●		

INTERACTIONS

Phenytoin, rifampicin, carbamazepine, and phenobarbital reduce blood levels of montelukast.

Clopidogrel, gemfibrozil, and leflunomide increase blood levels of montelukast.

MORPHINE/DIAMORPHINE

Brand names Filnarine SR, Morphgesic SR, MST Continus, MXL, Oramorph, Oramorph SR, Sevredol, Zomorph
Used in the following combined preparations Cyclimorph, J. Collis Browne's Mixture, Kaolin and Morphine Mixture

GENERAL INFORMATION

Morphine and diamorphine are opioid analgesics used to relieve the severe pain that can be caused by heart attack, injury, surgery, or chronic diseases such as cancer. They are also sometimes given as premedication before surgery, or to help treat breathlessness in patients with pulmonary oedema (fluid on the lungs) or who are terminally ill.

The drugs' painkilling effect wears off quickly, and they may be given in a slow-release (long-acting) form to relieve continuous severe pain. These drugs are habit-forming, and dependence and addiction can occur. However, most patients who take them for pain relief over brief periods of time do not become dependent and are able to stop taking them without difficulty.

Morphine is also included in very small amounts in some over-the-counter medicines for treating diarrhoea and suppressing coughs. These are not covered in the information given below.

INFORMATION FOR USERS

Your drug prescription is tailored for you. Do not alter your dosage without checking with your doctor.

How taken/used

Tablets, SR tablets, capsules, SR capsules, liquid, SR granules, injection, suppositories, SR suppositories.

Frequency and timing of doses
Every 4 hours; every 12–24 hours (SR preparations).

Adult dosage range
2.5–25mg per dose; however, some patients may need 75mg or more per dose. Doses vary considerably for each individual.

Onset of effect
Within 1 hour; within 4 hours (SR preparations).

Duration of action
4 hours; up to 24 hours (SR preparations).

Diet advice
None.

Storage
Keep in original container at room temperature out of the reach of children.

Missed dose
Take as soon as you remember. Return to your normal dosing schedule as soon as possible.

Stopping the drug
If the reason for taking the drug no longer exists, you may stop and notify your doctor.

OVERDOSE ACTION

 Seek immediate medical advice in all cases. Take emergency action if symptoms such as slow or irregular breathing, severe drowsiness, or loss of consciousness occur.

See Drug poisoning emergency guide (p.518).

SPECIAL PRECAUTIONS

Be sure to tell your doctor if:
- You have long-term liver or kidney problems.
- You have heart or circulatory problems.
- You have a lung disorder such as asthma or bronchitis.
- You have thyroid disease.
- You have a history of epileptic seizures.
- You have a history of prostate or urinary problems.
- You are taking other medicines.

 Pregnancy
Not usually prescribed. May cause breathing difficulties in the newborn baby. Discuss with your doctor.

 Breast-feeding
The drug passes into the breast milk, but low doses are unlikely to harm the baby. Discuss with your doctor.

 Infants and children
Reduced dose necessary.

 Over 60
Increased risk of adverse effects. Reduced dose may be necessary.

 Driving and hazardous work
People on morphine treatment are unlikely to be well enough to undertake such activities.

 Alcohol
Avoid. Alcohol may increase the sedative effects of these drugs.

POSSIBLE ADVERSE EFFECTS

Nausea, vomiting, and constipation are common, especially with high doses.

Anti-nausea drugs or laxatives may be needed to counteract these symptoms.

Symptom/effect	Frequency		Discuss with doctor		Stop taking drug now	Call doctor now
	Common	Rare	Only if severe	In all cases		
Drowsiness	●		●			
Nausea/vomiting/constipation	●		●			
Dizziness/headache	●			●		
Confusion	●			●		
Itching	●			●		
Breathing difficulties		●		●	●	●
Impaired consciousness		●		●	●	●

INTERACTIONS

Monoamine oxidase inhibitors (MAOIs) may produce a severe rise in blood pressure when taken with morphine and diamorphine.

Esmolol The effects of esmolol may be increased by morphine and diamorphine.

Sedatives Morphine and diamorphine increase the risk of respiratory depression with alcohol, antidepressants, sleeping drugs, antipsychotics, and antihistamines.

Buprenorphine and pentazocine increase risk of opiate withdrawal with these drugs.

PROLONGED USE

The effects of these drugs usually become weaker during prolonged use as the body adapts. Dependence may occur if they are taken for extended periods although this is unusual in patients taking the correct dose for pain relief.

MOXONIDINE

Brand name Physiotens
Used in the following combined preparations None

GENERAL INFORMATION

Moxonidine is an antihypertensive drug that is related to clonidine but is more selective and may therefore have fewer side effects. It works by stimulating alpha-receptors (see p.35) within the central nervous system, reducing the signals that constrict the blood vessels. Moxonidine also reduces resistance to blood flow in the peripheral blood vessels.

The drug is less likely than clonidine to cause dry mouth, and, unlike clonidine, has no effect on blood fat levels or glucose. However, other side effects, such as headache and dizziness, may still occur.

INFORMATION FOR USERS

Your drug prescription is tailored for you. Do not alter dosage without checking with your doctor.

How taken/used

Tablets.

Frequency and timing of doses
Once daily in the morning (initially); 1–2 x daily.

Adult dosage range
200mcg daily initially; increasing after 3 weeks to 400mcg daily, if necessary; increasing again after a further 3 weeks to maximum of 600mcg daily in 2 divided doses if necessary.

Onset of effect
30–180 minutes.

Duration of action
12 hours.

Diet advice
None.

Storage
Keep in original container at room temperature out of the reach of children.

Missed dose
Take as soon as you remember. If your next dose is due within 4 hours, take a single dose now and skip the next.

Stopping the drug
Do not stop taking the drug without consulting your doctor, who will supervise a gradual reduction in dosage over a period of 2 weeks.

Exceeding the dose
An occasional unintentional extra dose is unlikely to cause problems. Large overdoses may cause drowsiness and a fall in blood pressure.

SPECIAL PRECAUTIONS

Be sure to tell your doctor if:
- You have liver or kidney problems.
- You have heart problems, especially affecting your heart rhythm.
- You are taking other medicines.

 Pregnancy
Safety not established. Discuss with your doctor.

 Breast-feeding
Safety in breast-feeding not established. Discuss with your doctor.

 Infants and children
Not recommended.

 Over 60
No special problems.

 Driving and hazardous work
Avoid such activities until you have learned how moxonidine affects you because the drug can cause drowsiness and dizziness.

 Alcohol
Avoid. Alcohol may increase the sedative effects of this drug.

PROLONGED USE

No special problems.

POSSIBLE ADVERSE EFFECTS

Side effects that appear at the start of treatment with moxonidine often decrease in frequency and intensity during the course of treatment.

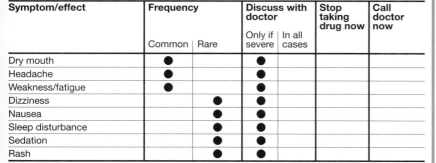

Symptom/effect	Frequency		Discuss with doctor		Stop taking drug now	Call doctor now
	Common	Rare	Only if severe	In all cases		
Dry mouth	●		●			
Headache	●		●			
Weakness/fatigue	●		●			
Dizziness		●	●			
Nausea		●	●			
Sleep disturbance		●	●			
Sedation		●	●			
Rash		●	●			

INTERACTIONS

Other antihypertensives, thymoxamine, moxisylyte, and muscle relaxants These drugs may increase the blood-pressure-lowering effect of moxonidine.

Sedatives and hypnotics The effects of these drugs may be increased by moxonidine.

Tricyclic antidepressants The effects of these drugs may be increased by moxonidine.

NAFTIDROFURYL

Brand name Praxilene
Used in the following combined preparations None

GENERAL INFORMATION

Naftidrofuryl is a vasodilator drug used in the treatment of peripheral circulatory disorders such as Raynaud's syndrome or intermittent claudication (cramp-like pain). Most of these conditions are caused by blockage of blood vessels due to spasms or sclerosis (hardening) of the vessel walls.

Naftidrofuryl may improve symptoms and mobility in these conditions, but it is not known if it has any influence on their progress. Lifestyle changes such as giving up smoking and taking exercise (and keeping warm in the case of Raynaud's) are often helpful.

Naftidrofuryl has also been used for treating night cramps, but it is not known how the drug works to reduce them. It has also been tried for circulatory disorders in the brain.

QUICK REFERENCE

Drug group Vasodilator (p.56)
Overdose danger rating Medium
Dependence rating Low
Prescription needed Yes
Available as generic Yes

INFORMATION FOR USERS

Your drug prescription is tailored for you. Do not alter dosage without checking with your doctor.

How taken/used

Capsules.

Frequency and timing of doses
3 x daily with meals, swallowed whole with at least one glass of water.

Adult dosage range
300–600mg daily.

Onset of effect
1 hour.

Duration of action
8 hours.

Diet advice
Drink plenty of water during treatment.

Storage
Keep in original container at room temperature out of the reach of children.

Missed dose
Take when you remember. If your next dose is due within 2 hours, take a single dose now and skip the next.

Stopping the drug
Do not stop taking the drug without consulting your doctor; symptoms may recur.

Exceeding the dose
An occasional unintentional extra dose is unlikely to cause problems. Large overdoses may cause heart problems and seizures. Notify your doctor immediately.

SPECIAL PRECAUTIONS

Be sure to tell your doctor if:
- You have liver or kidney problems.
- You are taking other medicines.

 Pregnancy
Safety not established. Discuss with your doctor.

 Breast-feeding
Safety not established. Discuss with your doctor.

 Infants and children
Not recommended.

 Over 60
No special problems.

 Driving and hazardous work
No special problems.

 Alcohol
No special problems.

POSSIBLE ADVERSE EFFECTS

Naftidrofuryl is generally well tolerated.

Symptom/effect	Frequency		Discuss with doctor		Stop taking drug now	Call doctor now
	Common	Rare	Only if severe	In all cases		
Nausea	●		●			
Chest pain		●		●		
Skin rash		●		●		
Jaundice		●		●	●	
Seizures		●		●	●	

PROLONGED USE

Treatment should be reviewed after 3 months to see if the condition is improving, or if the drug should be stopped.

INTERACTIONS

None known.

NAPROXEN

Brand names Feminax, Naprosyn, Nexocin, Stirlescent, and others
Used in the following combined preparation Vimovo (with esomeprazole)

GENERAL INFORMATION

Naproxen, one of the non-steroidal anti-inflammatory drugs (NSAIDs), is used to reduce pain, stiffness, and inflammation. The drug relieves the symptoms of adult and juvenile rheumatoid arthritis, ankylosing spondylitis, and osteoarthritis, although it does not cure the underlying disease.

Naproxen is also used to treat acute attacks of gout, and may sometimes be prescribed for the relief of migraine and pain following orthopaedic surgery, dental treatment, strains, and sprains. It is also effective for treating painful menstrual cramps.

Gastrointestinal side effects are fairly common, and there is an increased risk of bleeding. Hence, for long-term use, naproxen is often prescribed with a gastro-protective drug.

QUICK REFERENCE

Drug group Non-steroidal anti-inflammatory drug (p.74) and drug for gout (p.77)

Overdose danger rating Medium

Dependence rating Low

Prescription needed Yes

Available as generic Yes

INFORMATION FOR USERS

Your drug prescription is tailored for you. Do not alter dosage without checking with your doctor.

How taken/used

Tablets, liquid.

Frequency and timing of doses
Every 6–8 hours as required (general pain relief); 1–2 x daily (arthritis); every 6–8 hours (gout). All doses should be taken with or after food.

Adult dosage range
Mild to moderate pain, menstrual cramps 500mg (starting dose), then 250mg every 6–8 hours as required.
Arthritis 500–1,000mg daily.
Gout 750mg (starting dose), then 250mg every 8 hours until attack has subsided.

Onset of effect
Pain relief begins within 1 hour. Full anti-inflammatory effect may take 2 weeks.

Duration of action
Up to 12 hours.

Diet advice
None.

Storage
Keep in original container at room temperature out of the reach of children. Protect from light.

Missed dose
Take as soon as you remember. If your next dose is due within 4 hours, take a single dose now and skip the next.

Stopping the drug
When taken for short-term pain relief, naproxen can be safely stopped as soon as you no longer need it. If prescribed for long-term treatment, however, you should seek medical advice before stopping the drug.

Exceeding the dose
An occasional unintentional extra dose is unlikely to be a cause for concern. But if you notice any unusual symptoms, or if a large overdose has been taken, notify your doctor.

SPECIAL PRECAUTIONS

Be sure to tell your doctor if:
- You have long-term liver or kidney problems.
- You have heart problems or high blood pressure.
- You have a bleeding disorder.
- You have had a peptic ulcer, oesophagitis, or acid indigestion.
- You are allergic to aspirin or other NSAIDs.
- You have asthma.
- You are taking other medicines.

 Pregnancy
The drug may increase the risks of adverse effects on the baby's heart and may prolong labour if taken in the third trimester. Discuss with your doctor.

 Breast-feeding
The drug passes into the breast milk, but at normal doses adverse effects on the baby are unlikely. Discuss with your doctor.

 Infants and children
Prescribed only to treat juvenile arthritis. Reduced dose necessary.

 Over 60
Increased likelihood of adverse effects. Reduced dose may therefore be necessary.

 Driving and hazardous work
Avoid such activities until you have learned how naproxen affects you because the drug may reduce your ability to concentrate.

Alcohol
Avoid. Alcohol may increase the risk of stomach irritation with naproxen.

Surgery and general anaesthetics
Naproxen may prolong bleeding. Discuss with your doctor or dentist before surgery.

POSSIBLE ADVERSE EFFECTS

Most adverse effects are not serious and may diminish with time. Black or bloodstained bowel movements or vomiting blood (which may look like coffee grounds) should be reported to your doctor without delay.

Symptom/effect	Frequency		Discuss with doctor		Stop taking drug now	Call doctor now
	Common	Rare	Only if severe	In all cases		
Heartburn/indigestion	●			●		
Nausea/vomiting	●			●		
Headache		●		●		
Dizziness/drowsiness		●		●		
Swollen feet or legs/weight gain		●		●		
Rash/itching		●			●	●
Wheezing/breathlessness		●			●	●	●
Black/bloodstained faeces		●			●	●	●
Vomiting blood/"coffee grounds"		●			●	●	●

INTERACTIONS

General note Naproxen interacts with a wide range of drugs to increase the risk of bleeding and/or peptic ulcers. It may also increase the blood levels of lithium, methotrexate, and digoxin.

Antihypertensives and diuretics The benefit of these drugs may be reduced by naproxen and the risk of kidney damage increased.

Ciclosporin Naproxen increases the risk of kidney impairment with this drug.

PROLONGED USE

There is an increased risk of bleeding from peptic ulcers and in the bowel with prolonged use of naproxen. There is also a small risk of a heart attack or stroke. To minimize these risks, the lowest effective dose is given for the shortest duration.

NICORANDIL

Brand name Ikorel
Used in the following combined preparations None

GENERAL INFORMATION

Nicorandil is the only generally available member of a group of drugs known as potassium channel openers. It is used to treat angina pectoris.

The symptoms of angina result from the failure of narrowed coronary blood vessels to deliver sufficient oxygen to the heart. Nicorandil acts by widening blood vessels by a different mechanism to other anti-angina drugs, and is notable because it widens both veins and arteries. As a result of this, more oxygen-carrying blood reaches the heart muscle and the heart's workload is reduced since the resistance against which it has to pump is decreased.

Nicorandil is as effective as other drugs used to treat angina, and when used in combination with others may add to their effects.

INFORMATION FOR USERS

Your drug prescription is tailored for you. Do not alter dosage without checking with your doctor.

How taken/used

Tablets.

Frequency and timing of doses
2 x daily.

Adult dosage range
10–80mg daily.

Onset of effect
Within 1 hour.

Duration of action
Approximately 12 hours.

Diet advice
None.

Storage
Keep in original container at room temperature out of the reach of children.

Missed dose
Take as soon as you remember. If your next dose is due within 4 hours, take a single dose now and skip the next.

Stopping the drug
Do not stop taking the drug without consulting your doctor; stopping the drug may lead to worsening of the underlying condition.

Exceeding the dose
An occasional unintentional extra dose is unlikely to cause problems. Large overdoses may cause unusual dizziness and dangerously low blood pressure. Notify your doctor.

SPECIAL PRECAUTIONS

Be sure to tell your doctor if:
- You have low blood pressure.
- You have other heart problems.
- You have a history of angioedema.
- You are taking other medicines.

 Pregnancy
Safety in pregnancy not established. Discuss with your doctor.

 Breast-feeding
Safety not established. Discuss with your doctor.

 Infants and children
Not recommended.

 Over 60
Reduced dose may be necessary.

 Driving and hazardous work
Avoid such activities until you have learned how nicorandil affects you because the drug can cause dizziness as a result of lowered blood pressure.

 Alcohol
Avoid until you are accustomed to the effect of nicorandil. Alcohol may further reduce blood pressure, causing dizziness or other symptoms.

POSSIBLE ADVERSE EFFECTS

Adverse effects of nicorandil are generally minor. They usually wear off with continued treatment, but may necessitate a dose reduction in some cases.

Symptom/effect	Frequency		Discuss with doctor		Stop taking drug now	Call doctor now
	Common	Rare	Only if severe	In all cases		
Headache	●		●			
Flushing	●		●			
Nausea/vomiting	●		●			
Mouth/genital/anal ulcers		●		●		
Dizziness/weakness		●		●		
Jaundice		●		●		
Facial swelling		●		●		
Rash		●		●	●	
Palpitations		●		●	●	●

INTERACTIONS

Antihypertensive drugs Nicorandil may increase the effects of these drugs.

Sildenafil, tadalafil, and vardenafil increase the effects of nicorandil on blood pressure and should not be used with nicorandil.

MAOI and tricyclic antidepressant drugs may increase the effects of nicorandil on blood pressure, resulting in dizziness.

PROLONGED USE

No problems expected.

NICOTINE

Brand names NicAssist, Nicorette, Nicotinell, NiQuitin
Used in the following combined preparations None

GENERAL INFORMATION

Smoking is a difficult habit to stop due to the addiction to nicotine and the psychological aspects of smoking. Taking nicotine in a different form can help the smoker deal with both aspects. Nicotine comes as chewing gum, nasal spray, sublingual tablets, skin patches, lozenges, and inhalator for the relief of withdrawal symptoms.

Patches should be applied every 24 hours to unbroken, dry, and non-hairy skin on the trunk or the upper arm. Replacement patches should be placed on a different area, and the previous area of application avoided for several days. The strength of the patch is gradually reduced until abstinence is achieved. The lozenges, chewing gum, nasal spray, and inhalator are used when the urge to smoke occurs.

Electronic cigarettes (e-cigarettes) containing nicotine are also available, and there is evidence that they can help you stop smoking. However, there are none that are licensed as medicines in the UK, so they are not covered below.

INFORMATION FOR USERS

Follow instructions on the label.

How taken/used

Sublingual tablets, lozenges, chewing gum, skin patches, nasal spray, inhalator.

Frequency and timing of doses
Hourly (tablets and lozenges); every 24 hours, removing the patch after 16 hours (patches); when the urge to smoke is felt (gum, inhalator, or spray).

Adult dosage range
Will depend upon your previous smoking habits. 7–22mg per day (patches); 1 x 2mg piece to 15 x 4mg pieces per day (gum); up to 64 x 0.5mg puffs (spray).

Onset of effect
A few hours (patches); within minutes (other forms).

Duration of action
Up to 24 hours (patches); 30 minutes (other forms).

Diet advice
None.

Storage
Keep in original container at room temperature out of the reach of children.

Missed dose
Change your patch as soon as you remember, and keep the new patch on for the required amount of time before removing it.

Stopping the drug
The dose of nicotine is normally reduced gradually.

Exceeding the dose
Application of several nicotine patches at the same time could result in serious overdosage. Remove the patches and seek immediate medical help. Overdosage with the tablets, lozenges, gum, or spray can occur only if tablets or lozenges are taken more often than every hour, if many pieces of gum are chewed simultaneously, or if the spray is used more than 4 times an hour. Seek immediate medical help.

POSSIBLE ADVERSE EFFECTS

Any skin reaction to patches usually disappears in a couple of days. Chewing gum and nasal spray may irritate the throat or nose, affect your taste, and cause a dry mouth.

Symptom/effect	Frequency		Discuss with doctor		Stop taking drug now	Call doctor now
	Common	Rare	Only if severe	In all cases		
Local irritation	●		●			
Headache/dizziness	●		●			
Nausea/indigestion	●		●			
Cold/flu-like symptoms	●		●			
Insomnia	●		●			
Chest pains/palpitations		●		●		●

INTERACTIONS

General note Stopping smoking may increase blood levels of some drugs (such as warfarin, theophylline/aminophylline, and antipsychotics). Discuss with your doctor or pharmacist.

Nicotine patches, chewing gums, and nasal spray should not be used with other nicotine-containing products, including cigarettes and e-cigarettes.

SPECIAL PRECAUTIONS

Be sure to consult your doctor or pharmacist before taking this drug if:
- You have long-term liver or kidney problems.
- You have diabetes mellitus.
- You have thyroid disease.
- You have or have had any heart problems, including hypertension and stroke.
- You have a history of peptic ulcers.
- You have phaeochromocytoma.
- You are taking other medicines.

Pregnancy
Nicotine should be avoided altogether in pregnancy, but tobacco withdrawal using nicotine replacement may be recommended for pregnant smokers unable to quit.

Breast-feeding
Nicotine is found in breast milk but using nicotine replacement to stop smoking is less hazardous than continuing to smoke while breast-feeding.

Infants and children
Nicotine is extremely toxic to small children and may even sometimes be fatal. They should therefore not be exposed to it, and nicotine replacement products should be disposed of very carefully.

Over 60
No special problems.

Driving and hazardous work
Usually no problems.

Alcohol
No special problems.

PROLONGED USE

Nicotine replacement therapy should not normally be used for more than 3 to 6 months.

NIFEDIPINE

Brand names Adalat, Adipine, Coracten, Fortipine LA, Hypolar Retard 20, Nifedipress MR, Tensipine MR, Valni, and others
Used in the following combined preparations Beta-Adalat, Tenif

GENERAL INFORMATION

Nifedipine belongs to a group of drugs known as calcium channel blockers. Their main effect is to relax smooth muscle in the arteries supplying the heart muscle and other parts of the body. This improves blood supply to the heart and lowers blood pressure.

Nifedipine is given on a regular basis to help prevent angina attacks but is not used to treat acute attacks. The drug can be used safely by people with asthma, unlike some other anti-angina drugs (such as beta blockers). It is also widely used to reduce high blood pressure and is often helpful in improving circulation to the limbs in disorders such as Raynaud's disease.

Like other drugs of its class, it may cause blood pressure to fall too low, and occasionally causes disturbances of heart rhythm. In rare cases, it may cause angina to worsen.

QUICK REFERENCE

Drug group Anti-angina drug (p.59) and antihypertensive drug (p.60)

Overdose danger rating Medium

Dependence rating Low

Prescription needed Yes

Available as generic Yes

INFORMATION FOR USERS

Your drug prescription is tailored for you. Do not alter dosage without checking with your doctor.

How taken/used

Tablets, capsules, SR tablets, SR capsules.

Frequency and timing of doses
3 x daily; 1–2 x daily (SR preparations).

Adult dosage range
15–90mg daily.

Onset of effect
20–60 minutes.

Duration of action
6–24 hours.

Diet advice
Nifedipine should not be taken with grapefruit juice.

Storage
Keep in original container at room temperature out of the reach of children. Protect from light.

Missed dose
Take as soon as you remember, or when needed. If your next dose is due within 3 hours, take a single dose now and skip the next.

Stopping the drug
Do not stop taking the drug without consulting your doctor; sudden withdrawal may make angina worse.

Exceeding the dose
An occasional unintentional extra dose is unlikely to cause problems. Large overdoses may cause dizziness. Notify your doctor.

SPECIAL PRECAUTIONS

Be sure to tell your doctor if:
- You have liver or kidney problems.
- You have heart failure.
- You have had a recent heart attack.
- You have aortic stenosis or obstructive hypertrophic cardiomyopathy.
- You have diabetes.
- You have porphyria.
- You are taking other medicines.

Pregnancy
May inhibit labour, but the small risk to the baby has to be weighed against the risk to the mother of uncontrolled hypertension. Discuss with your doctor.

Breast-feeding
The drug passes into the breast milk but only in amounts that are probably too small to harm your baby. Discuss with your doctor.

Infants and children
Not recommended.

Over 60
Increased risk of adverse effects. Reduced dose may be necessary.

Driving and hazardous work
Avoid such activities until you have learned how nifedipine affects you because the drug can cause dizziness as a result of lowered blood pressure.

Alcohol
Avoid. Alcohol may increase the blood-pressure-lowering effects of nifedipine.

Surgery and general anaesthetics
Nifedipine may interact with some general anaesthetics, causing a fall in blood pressure. Discuss this with your doctor or dentist before any surgery.

POSSIBLE ADVERSE EFFECTS

Nifedipine can cause various minor adverse effects. Dizziness, especially on rising, may be due to reduced blood pressure. The severity or frequency of angina attacks may increase. If this happens, tell your doctor; you may need an adjustment in dosage or a change of drug.

Symptom/effect	Frequency		Discuss with doctor		Stop taking drug now	Call doctor now
	Common	Rare	Only if severe	In all cases		
Headache/flushing	●		●			
Dizziness/fatigue	●		●			
Ankle swelling	●		●			
Palpitations	●		●			
Heartburn/nausea	●		●			
Diarrhoea/bloating		●	●			
Frequency in passing urine		●	●			
Rash		●	●			
Increased angina		●		●	●	●

INTERACTIONS

General note Nifedipine may interfere with the beneficial effects of drugs such as carbamazepine, ciclosporin, magnesium (by injection), tacrolimus, and theophylline.

Antihypertensive drugs Nifedipine may increase the effects of these drugs.

Phenytoin and rifampicin These drugs may reduce the effects of nifedipine.

Digoxin Nifedipine may increase the effects and toxicity of digoxin.

Erythromycin, fluoxetine, certain anti-HIV drugs, and antifungals may increase levels of nifedipine.

Grapefruit juice may block breakdown of nifedipine, increasing its effects.

PROLONGED USE

No problems expected.

NITRAZEPAM

Brand names Mogadon
Used in the following combined preparations None

GENERAL INFORMATION

Nitrazepam is a benzodiazepine drug used for the short-term treatment of insomnia. Benzodiazepines relieve tension and nervousness, relax muscles, and encourage sleep.

Nitrazepam is long-acting, so when it is taken at night, it often produces "hangover" effects the next day. When taken every night, its effects steadily accumulate. Therefore, short courses of one or two weeks are usually prescribed. Long-term use leads to daytime sedation, tolerance, and dependence.

Stopping nitrazepam after prolonged use produces rebound insomnia, anxiety, and a withdrawal syndrome that may include confusion, toxic psychosis, and seizures. In this situation, the dosage may need to be tapered off over a period of many weeks.

It is recommended that any benzodiazepines should be used to treat insomnia only when the problem is short-term and severe, disabling, or very distressing.

INFORMATION FOR USERS

Your drug prescription is tailored for you. Do not alter dosage without checking with your doctor.

How taken/used

Tablets, liquid.

Frequency and timing of doses
Once daily, at bedtime.

Adult dosage range
5–10mg daily.

Onset of effect
1–2 hours.

Duration of action
24 hours or more.

Diet advice
None.

Storage
Keep in original container at room temperature out of the reach of children.

Missed dose
If you fall asleep without having taken a dose and wake some hours later, do not take the missed dose. If necessary, return to your normal dose schedule the following night.

Stopping the drug
If you have taken the drug for 2 weeks or less, it can be safely stopped. If you have been taking the drug for longer, consult your doctor, who may supervise a gradual reduction in dosage. Stopping abruptly may lead to withdrawal symptoms.

Exceeding the dose
An occasional unintentional extra dose is unlikely to be a cause for concern. Large overdoses may cause unusual drowsiness. Notify your doctor.

POSSIBLE ADVERSE EFFECTS

The main adverse effects (e.g. drowsiness, confusion) are related primarily to the sedative and tranquillizing properties of nitrazepam.

Symptom/effect	Frequency		Discuss with doctor		Stop taking drug now	Call doctor now
	Common	Rare	Only if severe	In all cases		
Drowsiness next day	●		●			
Confusion/forgetfulness	●		●			
Uncoordinated walking	●		●			
Dizziness/double vision	●		●			
Headache/vertigo		●	●			
Mood changes/restlessness		●		●		

INTERACTIONS

Sedatives All drugs that have a sedative effect on the central nervous system are likely to increase the sedative properties and risk of respiratory depression with nitrazepam. Such drugs include alcohol, other sleeping drugs, anti-anxiety drugs, antihistamines, opioid analgesics, antidepressants, and antipsychotics.

Rifampicin reduces the effect of nitrazepam.

Anticonvulsants The side effects and toxicity of these drugs may be increased by nitrazepam.

Ritonavir may increase the blood level of nitrazepam.

SPECIAL PRECAUTIONS

Be sure to tell your doctor if:
- You have severe respiratory disease.
- You have kidney or liver problems.
- You have myasthenia gravis.
- You suffer from sleep apnoea.
- You have acute porphyria.
- You are taking other medicines.

 Pregnancy
Safety not established. Known to affect the developing fetus. The baby may be born with dependence and have withdrawal symptoms. Discuss with your doctor.

 Breast-feeding
Avoid. Nitrazepam passes into the breast milk.

 Infants and children
Not recommended.

 Over 60
Older people are more likely to suffer adverse effects. Reduced dose and treatment duration are necessary.

 Driving and hazardous work
Do not drive. Nitrazepam's effects are still present during the day after taking a dose. It reduces alertness, slows reactions, impairs concentration, and causes drowsiness.

 Alcohol
Avoid. Alcohol will add to the sedative effects.

PROLONGED USE

Not recommended. Produces tolerance and dependence.

NORETHISTERONE

Brand names Micronor, Noriday, Noristerat, Primolut N, Utovlan
Used in the following combined preparations Brevinor, Climagest, Elleste Duet, Loestrin, Norinyl, Synphase, and others

GENERAL INFORMATION

Norethisterone is a synthetic hormone similar to the natural female sex hormone progesterone. The drug has various uses, including postponing menstruation and treating menstrual disorders such as endometriosis and dysmenorrhoea (p.120). When used for these disorders, it is taken only on certain days of the menstrual cycle. In combination with oestrogens, it is also prescribed as hormone replacement therapy (HRT; see p.105), and in the treatment of certain breast cancers.

A major use of the drug is as an oral contraceptive; it may be used either on its own or with an oestrogen. It is also available as an injectable contraceptive. Adverse effects are rare, but oral contraceptives may cause breakthrough bleeding (p.121).

QUICK REFERENCE

Drug group Female sex hormone (p.105)

Overdose danger rating Low

Dependence rating Low

Prescription needed Yes

Available as generic Yes

INFORMATION FOR USERS

Your drug prescription is tailored for you. Do not alter dosage without checking with your doctor.

How taken/used

Tablets, injection, skin patch.

Frequency and timing of doses
1–3 x daily (tablets); once every 8 weeks (injection); 2 x weekly (skin patch).

Adult dosage range
10–15mg daily (menstrual disorders); 15mg daily (postponing menstruation); 350mcg daily (progestogen-only contraceptives); 700mcg–1mg daily (HRT); 30–60mg daily (cancer).

Onset of effect
The drug starts to act within a few hours.

Duration of action
24 hours (tablets); about 3.5 days (patch); 8 weeks (injection).

Diet advice
None.

Storage
Keep in original container at room temperature out of the reach of children. Protect from light.

Missed dose
Take as soon as you remember. If you are taking the drug for contraception, see What to do if you miss a pill (p.123).

Stopping the drug
The drug can be safely stopped as soon as contraceptive protection is no longer required. If prescribed for an underlying disorder, do not stop taking the drug without consulting your doctor. When the drug is used to treat menstrual disorders, a normal period should occur 2 to 3 days after it is stopped.

Exceeding the dose
An occasional unintentional extra dose is unlikely to be a cause for concern. But if you notice any unusual symptoms, or if a large overdose has been taken, notify your doctor.

SPECIAL PRECAUTIONS

Be sure to tell your doctor if:
- You have liver or kidney problems.
- You have diabetes.
- You have had epileptic seizures.
- You have migraine.
- You have acute porphyria.
- You have heart or circulatory problems, especially a history of venous thrombosis.
- You are taking other medicines.

 Pregnancy
Not usually prescribed. May cause defects in the baby. Discuss with your doctor.

 Breast-feeding
The drug passes into the breast milk, but at normal doses adverse effects on the baby are unlikely. Discuss with your doctor.

 Infants and children
Not prescribed.

 Over 60
Not usually prescribed.

 Driving and hazardous work
No special problems.

 Alcohol
No special problems.

Surgery and general anaesthetics
Inform your doctor or dentist that you are taking norethisterone. They will tell you when to stop taking it prior to any surgery.

POSSIBLE ADVERSE EFFECTS

Adverse effects of norethisterone are rarely troublesome and are generally typical of drugs of this type. Prolonged treatment may cause jaundice due to liver damage.

Symptom/effect	Frequency		Discuss with doctor		Stop taking drug now	Call doctor now
	Common	Rare	Only if severe	In all cases		
Breakthrough bleeding	●			●		
Swollen feet/ankles/weight gain		●	●			
Breast tenderness		●	●			
Acne/skin discoloration		●	●			
Depression/headache		●		●		
Jaundice		●		●	●	
Pain or tightness in chest		●		●		●
Visual or hearing disturbances		●		●	●	●

INTERACTIONS

General note Norethisterone may interfere with the beneficial effects of many drugs, including oral anticoagulants, anticonvulsants, antihypertensives, and antidiabetic drugs. Many other drugs may reduce the contraceptive effect of norethisterone-containing pills. These include anticonvulsants, antituberculous drugs, certain antivirals, antibiotics, and St John's wort. Be sure to inform your doctor that you are taking norethisterone before taking additional prescribed medication.

Ciclosporin Levels of ciclosporin may be raised by norethisterone.

PROLONGED USE

As part of HRT, norethisterone is usually only advised for short-term use around the menopause. It is not normally recommended for long-term use or for treating osteoporosis. HRT increases the risk of venous thrombosis and breast cancer. The breast cancer risk reduces after stopping the drug, disappearing entirely after 10 years.

Monitoring Blood-pressure checks and physical examination, including regular mammograms, may be performed.

NYSTATIN

Brand name Nystan
Used in the following combined preparations Nystaform HC, Timodine

GENERAL INFORMATION

Nystatin is an antifungal drug named after the New York State Institute of Health, where it was developed in the early 1950s.

The drug has been used effectively against candidiasis (thrush), an infection caused by the candida yeast. Available in a variety of dosage forms, it is given to treat infections of the skin, mouth, throat, oesophagus, and intestinal tract. However, because it is poorly absorbed into the bloodstream from the digestive tract, it is ineffective against systemic infections. It is not given by injection as it would be too toxic in this form.

Nystatin rarely causes adverse effects and can be used during pregnancy to treat candidiasis.

QUICK REFERENCE

Drug group Antifungal drug (p.96)
Overdose danger rating Low
Dependence rating Low
Prescription needed Yes
Available as generic Yes

INFORMATION FOR USERS

Your drug prescription is tailored for you. Do not alter dosage without checking with your doctor.

How taken/used

Liquid, cream, ointment.

Frequency and timing of doses
Mouth or throat infections 4 x daily. Take after food and hold in the mouth for several minutes before swallowing (liquid).
Intestinal infections 4 x daily.
Skin infections 2–4 x daily.

Adult dosage range
2–4 million units daily (by mouth); as directed (skin preparations).

Onset of effect
Full beneficial effect may not be felt for 7–14 days.

Duration of action
Up to 6 hours.

Diet advice
None.

Storage
Keep in original container at room temperature out of the reach of children. Protect from light.

Missed dose
Take as soon as you remember. Take your next dose as usual.

Stopping the drug
Take the full course, and continue treatment for at least 48 hours after symptoms have disappeared. Even if the affected area seems to be cured, the original infection may still be present, and symptoms may recur if treatment is stopped too soon.

Exceeding the dose
An occasional unintentional extra dose is unlikely to be a cause for concern. But if you notice any unusual symptoms, or if a large overdose has been taken, notify your doctor.

SPECIAL PRECAUTIONS

Be sure to tell your doctor if:
• You are taking other medicines.

Pregnancy
No evidence of risk to the developing fetus.

Breast-feeding
No evidence of risk.

Infants and children
Reduced dose necessary.

Over 60
No special problems.

Driving and hazardous work
No known problems.

Alcohol
No known problems.

PROLONGED USE

No problems expected. Usually given as a course of treatment until the infection is cured.

POSSIBLE ADVERSE EFFECTS

Adverse effects are uncommon, and are usually mild and transient. Nausea and vomiting may occur when high doses of the drug are taken by mouth.

Symptom/effect	Frequency		Discuss with doctor		Stop taking drug now	Call doctor now
	Common	Rare	Only if severe	In all cases		
Diarrhoea		●	●			
Nausea/vomiting		●	●			
Rash		●		●		

INTERACTIONS

None.

OLANZAPINE

Brand names Zalasta, ZypAdhera, Zyprexa, Zyprexa Velotab
Used in the following combined preparations None

GENERAL INFORMATION

Olanzapine is an atypical antipsychotic drug prescribed for the treatment of schizophrenia and mania and for long-term treatment of bipolar disorder. It works by blocking several different chemical transmitters in the brain (see p.34), including dopamine, histamine, and serotonin.

In schizophrenia, the drug can be used to treat both "positive" symptoms (delusions, hallucinations, and thought disorders) and "negative" symptoms (blunted affect, emotional and social withdrawal). In mania, olanzapine can be used alone or in combination with other drugs.

Olanzapine by injection is used short term for its calming effects in agitation associated with schizophrenia or mania.

QUICK REFERENCE

Drug group Antipsychotic drug (p.41)

Overdose danger rating Medium

Dependence rating Low

Prescription needed Yes

Available as generic Yes

INFORMATION FOR USERS

Your drug prescription is tailored for you. Do not alter dosage without checking with your doctor.

How taken/used

Tablets, dispersible tablets, injection.

Frequency and timing of doses
Once daily (tablets); 1–2 x daily (injection).

Adult dosage range
Schizophrenia 10mg (starting dose). *Mania* 15mg if used alone or 10mg if used in combination with other drugs (starting dose). For all conditions, the dose can be adjusted between 5mg and 20mg daily (tablets) and 5mg and 10mg daily (injection).

Onset of effect
4–8 hours (tablets); 15–45 minutes (injection).

Duration of action
30–38 hours.

Diet advice
None.

Storage
Keep in original container at room temperature out of the reach of children. Protect from light.

Missed dose
Take as soon as you remember. If your next dose is due within 8 hours, take a single dose now and skip the next.

Stopping the drug
Do not stop the drug without consulting your doctor; symptoms may recur.

Exceeding the dose
An occasional unintentional extra dose is unlikely to cause problems. Large overdoses may cause unusual drowsiness, depressed breathing, and low blood pressure, or agitation, a rapid pulse, altered speech, and abnormal movements. Notify your doctor.

SPECIAL PRECAUTIONS

Be sure to tell your doctor if:
- You have kidney or liver problems.
- You have diabetes.
- You have glaucoma.
- You have epilepsy.
- You have Parkinson's disease or dementia.
- You have had, or are at risk of having, a stroke.
- You are taking other medicines

Pregnancy
Safety not established. Discuss with your doctor.

Breast-feeding
Safety not established. The drug passes into the breast milk and may affect your baby. Discuss with your doctor.

Infants and children
Not recommended.

Over 60
Reduced dose may be necessary. Increased risk of stroke with long-term use.

Driving and hazardous work
Avoid such activities until you have learned how olanzapine affects you because the drug can cause unusual drowsiness.

Alcohol
Avoid. Alcohol increases the sedative effects of this drug.

POSSIBLE ADVERSE EFFECTS

Unusual drowsiness and weight gain are the most common adverse effects of olanzapine.

Symptom/effect	Frequency		Discuss with doctor		Stop taking drug now	Call doctor now
	Common	Rare	Only if severe	In all cases		
Unusual drowsiness	●		●			
Increased appetite/weight gain	●		●			
Dry mouth	●		●			
Reduced libido/erectile dysfunction	●		●			
Dizziness/fainting	●			●		
Rash	●			●		
Difficulty urinating		●		●		
Breast tenderness/discharge		●		●		

INTERACTIONS

Sedatives All drugs that have a sedative effect on the central nervous system may increase the sedative effects of olanzapine.

Carbamazepine and smoking These can reduce the effects of olanzapine.

Diabetic medication Olanzapine can affect diabetic control. Dosage of diabetic medications may need to be adjusted.

Ciprofloxacin This can increase the effects of olanzapine.

PROLONGED USE

Prolonged use of olanzapine may rarely cause tardive dyskinesia, in which there are involuntary movements of the tongue and face. There is also an increased risk of raised blood lipid levels, or of developing diabetes or worsening existing diabetes. With long-term use in older patients, olanzapine also carries a greater risk of stroke than some other antipsychotic drugs.

Monitoring Blood count, blood sugar and lipid levels, heart function (ECG), and liver function may be regularly monitored.

OLAPARIB

Brand names Lynparza
Used in the following combined preparations None

GENERAL INFORMATION

Olaparib is a type of "targeted therapy" for cancer. It is part of an expanding class of drugs called PARP (poly ADP ribose polymerase) inhibitors. PARP is involved in DNA repair, so when it is inhibited by olaparib, cancer cells cannot easily repair the DNA damage that occurs normally in dividing cells. This action is even more critical on cancer cells with a faulty BRCA gene, a common genetic cause of cancer risk. BRCA genes also act in DNA repair, so if both repair mechanisms are impaired, the cancer cells are very likely to die.

The drug is used in metastatic cancers such as ovarian, breast, pancreatic and prostate, especially those with faulty BRCA genes. Side effects range from nausea and fatigue to rare but serious lung and white blood cell disorders.

INFORMATION FOR USERS

Your drug prescription is tailored for you. Do not alter dosage without checking with your doctor.

How taken/used

Tablets, capsules.

Frequency and timing of doses
2 x daily. Manufacturer recommends taking the capsules at least 1 hour after food and avoiding food for 2 hours after dose. Tablets are not affected by having or not having food.

Adult dosage range
150–400mg (capsules); 100–300mg (tablets).

Onset of effect
PARP inhibition may begin within hours, but both the beneficial effects and side effects tend to take weeks to become apparent.

Duration of action
Adverse effects may last for several weeks after drug cessation.

Diet advice
Avoid Seville orange, grapefruit, and grapefruit juice; they may increase exposure to olaparib.

Storage
Store in the original package to protect from moisture. Keep out of the reach of children. No special temperature requirements.

Missed dose
If you miss a dose, take your next normal dose at its scheduled time.

Stopping the drug
Do not stop without direction from your cancer doctor. Stopping the drug without an alternative therapy can lead to cancer growth.

Exceeding the dose
An occasional unintentional extra dose is unlikely to cause major problems. But if you notice any unusual symptoms or if a large overdose has been taken, notify your doctor.

POSSIBLE ADVERSE EFFECTS

Common side effects include gastrointestinal problems, upper abdominal pain, low white blood cell count, low red blood cell count (anaemia), and low energy. Severe side effects are rare but can be life-threatening. They include forms of white blood cell cancer, severe lung inflammation, and blood clots in the lung (pulmonary embolism).

Symptom/effect	Frequency		Discuss with doctor		Stop taking drug now	Call doctor now
	Common	Rare	Only if severe	In all cases		
Fatigue/headache	●		●			
Decreased appetite/nausea	●		●			
Cough/dizziness	●		●			
Rash	●			●		
Bleeding		●		●		●
Shortness of breath/chest pain		●		●		●
Fever		●		●		●

INTERACTIONS

General note Many drugs, over-the-counter treatments, and herbal remedies (such as St John's wort) can affect levels of olaparib. Check with your doctor or pharmacist.

Calcium antagonists Diltiazem and verapamil may both increase olaparib levels.

Antimicrobials Itraconazole, clarithromycin, erythromycin, and fluconazole can raise olaparib levels; rifampicin can reduce them.

Anticonvulsants Carbamazepine, phenytoin, and phenobarbital may reduce blood levels and effectiveness of olaparib.

SPECIAL PRECAUTIONS

Be sure to tell your doctor if:
- You have kidney or liver problems.
- You have lung or breathing problems.
- You have abnormal white blood cell or red blood cell counts.
- You have had previous lymphoma or leukaemia.
- You are taking other medicines.

Pregnancy
Olaparib should not be used in pregnancy. Two complementary forms of contraception are recommended during therapy and for 3 months after finishing. Discuss with your doctor.

Breast-feeding
Do not breast-feed while on olaparib or until at least 1 month after end of treatment. Discuss with your doctor.

Infants and children
The effects of the drug in children are not known. Olaparib could be used by specialist children's doctors.

Over 60
No special problems.

Driving and hazardous work
Avoid until you have learned how the drug affects you. It may sometimes cause dizziness or malaise.

Alcohol
No special problems.

PROLONGED USE

Long-term use can be associated with both white blood cell and red blood cell abnormalities. Hence, full blood counts are usually performed periodically. Long-term use is also associated with changes in kidney function, so this should also be monitored regularly during treatment with olaparib.

OMEPRAZOLE

Brand names Losec, Losec MUPS, Mepradec, Mezzopram
Used in the following combined preparation None

GENERAL INFORMATION

Omeprazole belongs to a group of drugs called proton pump inhibitors (see p.67), which reduce stomach acid secretion by blocking the stomach's acid-pumping mechanism. It is used to treat stomach and duodenal ulcers, reflux oesophagitis (in which stomach acid rises into the oesophagus), and Zollinger-Ellison syndrome (in which digestive system tumours cause excess production of stomach acid). Treatment for an ulcer is usually given for four to eight weeks, although it may last much longer to prevent ulcers in high-risk patients, such as those taking long-term non-steroidal anti-inflammatory drugs (NSAIDs). Omeprazole may also be given with antibiotics to eradicate the *Helicobacter pylori* bacteria that can cause peptic ulcers. Reflux oesophagitis may be treated for 4–12 weeks. In addition to being a prescription drug, omeprazole is available over the counter for short-term relief of acid reflux symptoms such as heartburn in adults over 18 years old.

Omeprazole causes few serious side effects. As with other anti-ulcer drugs, it may mask signs of stomach cancer, so it is prescribed only when the possibility of this disease has been ruled out.

INFORMATION FOR USERS

Your drug prescription is tailored for you. Do not alter dosage without checking with your doctor. For over-the-counter preparations, follow the instructions and call your doctor if symptoms worsen.

How taken/used

Tablets, capsules, injection, intravenous infusion.

Frequency and timing of doses
1–2 x daily (2 x daily for doses above 80mg).

Adult dosage range
10–40mg daily and sometimes up to 120mg daily.

Onset of effect
2–5 hours.

Duration of action
Up to 24 hours.

Diet advice
None, although spicy foods and alcohol may exacerbate the underlying condition.

Storage
Keep in original container at room temperature out of the reach of children. Omeprazole is very sensitive to moisture. It must not be transferred to another container and must be used within 3 months of opening.

Missed dose
Take as soon as you remember. If your next dose is due within 8 hours, take a single dose now and skip the next.

Stopping the drug
Do not stop the drug without consulting your doctor; symptoms may recur.

Exceeding the dose
An occasional unintentional extra dose is unlikely to be a cause for concern. But if you notice any unusual symptoms, or if a large overdose has been taken, notify your doctor.

POSSIBLE ADVERSE EFFECTS

Adverse effects such as headache and diarrhoea are usually mild, and often diminish with continued use of the drug. If you develop a rash, however, you should notify your doctor.

Symptom/effect	Frequency		Discuss with doctor		Stop taking drug now	Call doctor now
	Common	Rare	Only if severe	In all cases		
Headache	●			●		
Diarrhoea	●			●		
Nausea/constipation		●		●		
Rash		●			●	●

INTERACTIONS

Ciclosporin and tacrolimus Blood levels of these drugs are raised by omeprazole.

Atazanavir The effects of this drug are reduced by omeprazole.

Ketoconazole and itraconazole Blood levels of these drugs may be reduced by omeprazole.

Warfarin The effects of warfarin may be increased by omeprazole.

Phenytoin The effects of phenytoin may be increased by omeprazole.

Clopidogrel The antiplatelet effect of clopidogrel is reduced by omeprazole.

SPECIAL PRECAUTIONS

Be sure to consult your doctor or pharmacist before taking this drug if:
- You have a long-term liver problem.
- You are taking other medicines.

Pregnancy
No evidence of risk, but discuss with your doctor.

Breast-feeding
The drug may pass into the breast milk. Safety in breast-feeding not established. Discuss with your doctor.

Infants and children
Not usually recommended under 1 year. Reduced dose necessary in older children.

Over 60
No special problems.

Driving and hazardous work
No special problems.

Alcohol
Avoid. Alcohol irritates the stomach, which can lead to ulceration and acid reflux.

PROLONGED USE

Long-term use of omeprazole may increase the risk of certain intestinal infections (such as *Salmonella* and *Clostridium difficile* infections) because of the loss of the natural protection against such infections that is provided by stomach acid. Prolonged use also increases the risk of hip fractures in postmenopausal women, and may reduce absorption of vitamin B_{12} and magnesium in the intestine.

ONDANSETRON

Brand names Demorem, Ondemet, Setofilm, Zofran, Zofran Flexi-amp, Zofran Melt
Used in the following combined preparations None

GENERAL INFORMATION

Ondansetron, an anti-emetic, is used especially for treating the nausea and vomiting associated with radiotherapy and anticancer drugs. It may also be prescribed for the nausea and vomiting that occur after surgery.

The dose given and the frequency will depend on which anticancer drug you are having and its dose. In most instances, you will receive ondansetron, either by mouth or injection, before infusion of the anticancer agent, then tablets for up to five days after treatment has finished. The drug is less effective against the delayed nausea and vomiting that occur several days after chemotherapy than against symptoms that occur soon after treatment. For nausea and vomiting after surgery, one dose is usually given before the surgery, and two doses after.

To enhance the effectiveness of ondansetron, it is usually taken with other drugs, such as dexamethasone. Serious adverse effects are unlikely to occur.

QUICK REFERENCE

Drug group Anti-emetic drug (p.46)
Overdose danger rating Low
Dependence rating Low
Prescription needed Yes
Available as generic Yes

INFORMATION FOR USERS

Your drug prescription is tailored for you. Do not alter dosage without checking with your doctor.

How taken/used

Tablets, liquid, injection, suppositories.

Frequency and timing of doses
Normally 2 x daily but the frequency will depend on the reason for which the drug is being used.

Adult dosage range
4–32mg daily depending on the reason for which it is being used.

Onset of effect
Within 1 hour.

Duration of action
Approximately 12 hours.

Diet advice
None.

Storage
Keep in original container at room temperature out of the reach of children. Protect from light.

Missed dose
Take as soon as you remember. If your next dose is due within 2 hours, take a single dose now and skip the next.

Stopping the drug
Can be safely stopped as soon as you no longer need it.

Exceeding the dose
An occasional unintentional extra dose is unlikely to be a cause for concern. But if you notice any unusual symptoms, or if a large overdose has been taken, notify your doctor.

SPECIAL PRECAUTIONS

Be sure to tell your doctor if:
- You have a long-term liver problem.
- You have bowel problems.
- You have heart rhythm problems.
- You are taking other medicines.

 Pregnancy
Safety in pregnancy not established. Discuss with your doctor.

 Breast-feeding
The drug may pass into the breast milk. Discuss with your doctor.

 Infants and children
Reduced dose necessary.

 Over 60
No special problems.

 Driving and hazardous work
No problems expected.

 Alcohol
No known problems.

PROLONGED USE

Not generally prescribed for long-term treatment.

POSSIBLE ADVERSE EFFECTS

Ondansetron is considered to be safe and is generally well tolerated. It does not cause sedation or abnormal muscle movements – adverse effects of some other anti-emetics.

Symptom/effect	Frequency		Discuss with doctor		Stop taking drug now	Call doctor now
	Common	Rare	Only if severe	In all cases		
Constipation	●		●			
Headache	●		●			
Warm feeling in head or stomach	●		●			
Palpitations/chest pain		●		●		
Seizures/muscle stiffness		●		●		
Wheezing/itchy rash		●		●	●	●
Swollen eyelids/face/lips		●		●	●	●

INTERACTIONS

Carbamazepine, phenytoin, and rifampicin These drugs may accelerate the breakdown of ondansetron and reduce its effect.

Apomorphine may cause a drop in blood pressure when used with ondansetron; the two drugs should not be taken together.

Vandetanib may increase the risk of heart rhythm abnormalities when used with ondansetron; the two drugs should not be taken together.

Tramadol The effect of this drug may be reduced by ondansetron.

ORLISTAT

Brand names Alli, Beacita, Xenical
Used in the following combined preparations None

GENERAL INFORMATION

Orlistat blocks the action of stomach and pancreatic enzymes (lipases) that digest fats; hence, less dietary fat is absorbed and more passes out in the faeces. This leads to reduced calorie uptake and helps to produce weight loss. The effectiveness of orlistat varies from person to person, and it should only be used in conjunction with healthy lifestyle measures. The increased fat content makes faeces become oily, and this can cause flatulence. As fat absorption is reduced, there is a danger of fat-soluble vitamins being lost to the body, and a multivitamin supplement may be needed to compensate (see Diet advice, below).

QUICK REFERENCE

Drug group Anti-obesity drug
Overdose danger rating Low
Dependence rating Low
Prescription needed No
Available as generic No

INFORMATION FOR USERS

Follow instructions on the label. Call your doctor if symptoms worsen.

How taken/used

Capsules.

Frequency and timing of doses
Just before, during, or up to 1 hour after each main meal (up to 3 x daily). If a meal is omitted or contains no fat, do not take the dose of orlistat.

Adult dosage range
Up to 360mg daily.

Onset of effect
30 minutes; excretion of excess faecal fat begins about 24–48 hours after the first dose.

Duration of action
Orlistat is not absorbed from the gut, and potentially continues to work as it passes through the bowel. If you stop taking the drug, faecal fat returns to normal in 48–72 hours.

Diet advice
Eat a nutritionally balanced diet that does not contain quite enough calories, and that provides about 30 percent of the calories as fat. Eat lots of fruit and vegetables. The intake of fat, carbohydrate, and protein should be distributed over the three main meals. If a multivitamin supplement is needed, it should be taken at least 2 hours before an orlistat dose or at bedtime.

Storage
Keep in original container at room temperature out of the reach of children.

Missed dose
No cause for concern. Take the next dose with the next meal.

Stopping the drug
The drug can be safely stopped as soon as it is no longer needed.

Exceeding the dose
An occasional unintentional extra dose is unlikely to be a cause for concern. But if you notice any unusual symptoms, or if a large overdose has been taken, notify your doctor.

SPECIAL PRECAUTIONS

Be sure to consult your doctor or pharmacist before taking this drug if:
- You have diabetes.
- You have chronic malabsorption syndrome.
- You have gallbladder, kidney, or liver problems.
- You are taking lipid-lowering drugs.
- You are taking other medicines.

 Pregnancy
Safety not established. Discuss with your doctor.

 Breast-feeding
Safety not established. Discuss with your doctor.

 Infants and children
Should not be used in under-18s except on specialist advice.

 Over 60
No special problems.

 Driving and hazardous work
No special problems.

 Alcohol
No special problems.

POSSIBLE ADVERSE EFFECTS

Most of the side effects depend on how much fat is eaten, as well as the dose of orlistat.

Symptom/effect	Frequency		Discuss with doctor		Stop taking drug now	Call doctor now
	Common	Rare	Only if severe	In all cases		
Liquid, oily stools/flatulence	●			●		
Faecal urgency	●			●		
Abdominal/rectal pain	●			●		
Menstrual irregularities	●			●		
Anxiety/fatigue/nausea/headache	●			●		
Infections (e.g. influenza)	●			●		
Hypoglycaemia	●			●		
Rectal bleeding		●		●		

PROLONGED USE

Orlistat treatment should be stopped after 12 weeks if you have not lost 5 percent of your body weight since the start of treatment. It should also be stopped if you have lost less than 10 percent of your body weight over the first 6 months. If you have lost more than 10 percent, then the drug may be continued, for up to a maximum of 2 years, until your target weight is approached.

When orlistat treatment is stopped, there may be gradual weight gain.

INTERACTIONS

General note Orlistat reduces absorption of fat-soluble vitamins (A, D, E, and K) so that a multivitamin supplement may be needed. This is particularly important in growing teenagers.

Oral anticoagulants, amiodarone, anticonvulsants, ciclosporin, and antiretrovirals Orlistat may reduce the effects of these drugs.

Oral contraceptives Absorption may be reduced by orlistat; an additional method of contraception is advisable.

Acarbose Avoid using orlistat if taking acarbose.

Levothyroxine Dosage and timing of doses may need to be adjusted.

ORPHENADRINE

Brand names None
Used in the following combined preparations None

GENERAL INFORMATION

Orphenadrine is an anticholinergic drug that is prescribed to treat all forms of Parkinson's disease. However, it is less effective against the idiopathic form of the disease than other drugs (such as levodopa) and can cause confusion. Orphenadrine is particularly valuable for relieving the tremor and muscle rigidity that often occur with Parkinson's disease; it is less helpful for improving the slowing of movement that also commonly affects sufferers. It also helps reduce the excessive salivation or dribbling that can occur with Parkinson's disease and is widely used to treat the parkinson-like side effects of antipsychotic drugs. The effects of orphenadrine may become less noticeable after it has been taken for a long time.

Orphenadrine also possesses muscle-relaxant properties and is occasionally used to treat muscle pain and restless leg syndrome.

INFORMATION FOR USERS

Your drug prescription is tailored for you. Do not alter dosage without checking with your doctor.

How taken/used

Liquid.

Frequency and timing of doses
2–3 x daily.

Adult dosage range
150–400mg daily.

Onset of effect
Within 60 minutes.

Duration of action
8–12 hours.

Diet advice
None.

Storage
Keep in original container at room temperature out of the reach of children. Protect from light.

Missed dose
Take as soon as you remember. If your next dose is due within 2 hours, take a single dose now and skip the next.

Stopping the drug
Do not stop the drug without consulting your doctor; symptoms may recur.

OVERDOSE ACTION

Seek immediate medical advice in all cases. Take emergency action if palpitations, seizures, or loss of consciousness occur.

See Drug poisoning emergency guide (p.518).

SPECIAL PRECAUTIONS

Be sure to tell your doctor if:
- You have long-term liver or kidney problems.
- You have heart problems.
- You have had glaucoma.
- You have difficulty in passing urine and have an enlarged prostate.
- You are taking other medicines.

 Pregnancy
Safety not established. Discuss with your doctor.

 Breast-feeding
Safety not established. Discuss with your doctor.

 Infants and children
Not usually prescribed.

 Over 60
Increased likelihood of adverse effects. Reduced dose may therefore be necessary.

 Driving and hazardous work
Avoid such activities until you have learned how orphenadrine affects you because the drug can cause dizziness, lightheadedness, and blurred vision.

 Alcohol
Avoid. Alcohol can worsen some of the adverse effects of orphenadrine.

PROLONGED USE

No problems expected. Effectiveness in treating Parkinson's disease may diminish with time.

POSSIBLE ADVERSE EFFECTS

The adverse effects of orphenadrine are similar to those of other anticholinergic drugs. The more common symptoms, such as dryness of the mouth and blurred vision, can often be overcome by a reduction in dosage.

Symptom/effect	Frequency		Discuss with doctor		Stop taking drug now	Call doctor now
	Common	Rare	Only if severe	In all cases		
Dry mouth/skin	●		●			
Difficulty in passing urine	●		●			
Constipation	●		●			
Dizziness	●		●			
Blurred vision	●			●		
Confusion/agitation		●		●		
Palpitations		●		●	●	●

INTERACTIONS

General note Orphenadrine reduces gastric motility (spontaneous stomach movements that move stomach contents into the intestine) and so may affect the absorption of other oral drugs.

Anticholinergic drugs (e.g. tiotropium, chlorphenamine, oxybutynin) The anticholinergic effects of orphenadrine are likely to be increased by these drugs.

OSELTAMIVIR

Brand name Tamiflu
Used in the following combined preparations None

GENERAL INFORMATION

Oseltamivir is an antiviral drug that is used to prevent or treat influenza (flu), a virus that infects and multiplies within the lungs. As well as being given for regular seasonal flu, it is also effective against the avian (bird) flu and swine flu strains of the influenza virus. Oseltamivir works by blocking the entry of the virus into cells, where it normally multiplies before spreading throughout the body. This prevents or alleviates the typical symptoms of flu, which include sudden onset of fever, sweating and shivering, cough, runny or stuffy nose, headache, aching muscles, and extreme fatigue. The drug should be taken within 48 hours of the onset of these symptoms. It may reduce the duration of symptoms by 1–2 days.

Oseltamivir is not a substitute for seasonal flu vaccination and is not recommended for prevention of seasonal flu. However, because it does not alter the flu vaccine's effectiveness, it can be taken even if you have been vaccinated.

QUICK REFERENCE

Drug group Antiviral drug (p.91)
Overdose danger rating Low
Dependence rating Low
Prescription needed Yes
Available as generic No

INFORMATION FOR USERS

Your drug prescription is tailored for you. Do not alter dosage without checking with your doctor.

How taken/used

Capsules, liquid (suspension).

Frequency and timing of doses
Once daily (prevention); 2 x daily (treatment).

Dosage range
Adults and adolescents over 13 years 75mg daily (prevention); 150mg daily (treatment). *Children 1–13 years* 30–75mg daily according to body weight (prevention); 60–150mg daily according to body weight (treatment).

Onset of effect
Within 24 hours.

Duration of action
12–24 hours.

Diet advice
None.

Storage
Keep in original container at room temperature out of the reach of children.

Missed dose
Take as soon as you remember. If your next dose is due within 2 hours, take a single dose now and skip the next.

Stopping the drug
Do not stop taking the drug without consulting your doctor; symptoms may recur.

Exceeding the dose
An occasional unintentional extra dose is unlikely to cause problems. However, if you notice any unusual symptoms, or if a large overdose has been taken, notify your doctor.

SPECIAL PRECAUTIONS

Be sure to tell your doctor if:
- You have kidney problems.
- You have ever had an allergic reaction to oseltamivir.
- You are taking other medicines.

 Pregnancy
Safety in pregnancy not established. Discuss with your doctor.

 Breast-feeding
Safety in breast-feeding not established. Discuss with your doctor.

 Infants and children
No problems expected.

 Over 60
No special problems.

 Driving and hazardous work
No known problems.

 Alcohol
No known problems.

POSSIBLE ADVERSE EFFECTS

The most common side effects mostly occur following the first dose and usually subside as treatment continues. Taking oseltamivir with food helps to reduce these effects, but you should consult your doctor if they persist.

Symptom/effect	Frequency		Discuss with doctor		Stop taking drug now	Call doctor now
	Common	Rare	Only if severe	In all cases		
Nausea	●		●			
Vomiting	●		●			
Abdominal pain	●		●			
Rash		●		●	●	
Hallucinations/psychosis		●		●	●	●

INTERACTIONS

Leflunomide and teriflunomide may increase the exposure to (increase the blood level of) oseltamivir.

PROLONGED USE

No problems expected. The drug is not usually prescribed for longer than 5 days (children), 7 days (adults), or 6 weeks (adults, during an epidemic).

OXYBUTYNIN

Brand names Ditropan, Kentera, Lyrinel XL
Used in the following combined preparations None

GENERAL INFORMATION

Oxybutynin is an anticholinergic and antispasmodic drug used to treat urinary incontinence and frequency in adults and bedwetting in children. It works by reducing bladder contraction, allowing the bladder to hold more urine. The drug stops bladder spasms and delays the desire to empty the bladder. It also has some local anaesthetic effect. However, its usefulness is limited to some extent by its side effects, especially in children and older adults. It can aggravate conditions such as an enlarged prostate or coronary heart disease in older adults. Children are more susceptible to effects on the central nervous system (CNS), such as restlessness, disorientation, hallucinations, and seizures.

INFORMATION FOR USERS

Your drug prescription is tailored for you. Do not alter dosage without checking with your doctor.

How taken/used

Tablets, MR tablets, liquid, patches.

Frequency and timing of doses
2–4 x daily (tablets, liquid); 1–2 x weekly (patch).

Adult dosage range
10–20mg daily (tablets, liquid); 36mg twice weekly (patch).

Onset of effect
1 hour (tablets, liquid); 24–48 hours (patch).

Duration of action
Up to 10 hours (tablets, liquid); 96 hours (patch).

Diet advice
None.

Storage
Keep in original container at room temperature out of the reach of children. Protect liquid from light.

Missed dose
Take as soon as you remember. If your next dose is due within 2 hours, take a single dose now and skip the next (tablets and liquid). Apply when you remember (patches).

Stopping the drug
Do not stop taking the drug without consulting your doctor; symptoms may recur.

OVERDOSE ACTION

 Seek immediate medical advice in all cases. Take emergency action if symptoms such as breathing difficulty, seizures, or loss of consciousness occur.

See Drug poisoning emergency guide (p.518).

SPECIAL PRECAUTIONS

Be sure to tell your doctor if:
- You have liver or kidney problems.
- You have heart problems.
- You have an enlarged prostate.
- You have hiatus hernia.
- You have ulcerative colitis.
- You have glaucoma.
- You are taking other medicines.

 Pregnancy
Safety not established. Discuss with your doctor.

 Breast-feeding
The drug passes into breast milk and its safety in breast-feeding has not been established. Discuss with your doctor.

 Infants and children
Not recommended under 5 years. Reduced dose necessary in older children.

 Over 60
Reduced dose necessary.

 Driving and hazardous work
Avoid such activities until you have learned how oxybutynin affects you because the drug can cause drowsiness, disorientation, and blurred vision.

 Alcohol
Avoid. Alcohol increases the sedative effects of oxybutynin.

POSSIBLE ADVERSE EFFECTS

An adjustment in dosage is necessary in children and older adults to minimize the adverse effects of oxybutynin. The drug can also trigger glaucoma.

Symptom/effect	Frequency		Discuss with doctor		Stop taking drug now	Call doctor now
	Common	Rare	Only if severe	In all cases		
Dry mouth	●		●			
Constipation	●		●			
Nausea	●		●			
Facial flushing	●		●			
Difficulty in passing urine	●		●			
Blurred vision/eye pain		●	●			
Headache/confusion		●	●			
Dry skin		●		●		
Rash		●		●	●	

INTERACTIONS

General note Oxybutynin reduces gastric motility (spontaneous stomach movements that move stomach contents into the intestine) and so may affect the absorption of other oral drugs.

Other anticholinergic drugs If oxybutynin is taken with other drugs that have anticholinergic effects, the risk of anticholinergic side effects is increased.

PROLONGED USE

No special problems. The need for continued treatment may be reviewed after 6 months.

Monitoring Periodic eye tests for glaucoma may be performed.

PARACETAMOL

Brand names Alvedon, Anadin Paracetamol, Calpol, Disprol, Hedex, Mandanol, Panadol, Perfalgan, and many others
Used in the following combined preparations Anadin Extra, Codipar, Kapake, Midrid, Migraleve, Panadeine, Paracodol, Paradote, Paramax, Solpadol, Tramacet, Tylex, Zapain, and many others

GENERAL INFORMATION

One of a group of drugs known as the non-opioid analgesics, paracetamol is commonly kept in the home to relieve mild pain and to reduce fever. It is suitable for children as well as adults.

One of the primary advantages of paracetamol is that it does not cause stomach upset or bleeding problems. This makes it a particularly useful alternative for people who have peptic ulcers or those who cannot tolerate aspirin. Paracetamol is also safe for occasional use by those who are being treated with anticoagulants.

Although safe when used as directed, paracetamol is dangerous in overdose, and is capable of causing serious damage to the liver and kidneys. Even a small excess dose may be toxic in frail, older people, patients with liver damage, those with an eating disorder, or those who are malnourished.

INFORMATION FOR USERS

Follow instructions on the label. Call your doctor if symptoms worsen.

How taken/used

Tablets, capsules, liquid, suppositories, injection (administered in hospital).

Frequency and timing of doses
Every 4–6 hours as necessary, but not more than 4 doses per 24 hours in children.

Dosage range
Adults 500mg–1g per dose up to 4g daily. *Children* 60mg (3–6 months; 2–3 months for fever after immunization, and for other causes of pain and fever in infants weighing more than 4kg and who were born after 37 weeks – 2 doses only); 120mg per dose (6–24 months); 180mg per dose (2–4 years); 240mg per dose (4–6 years); 250mg per dose (6–8 years); 375mg per dose (8–10 years); 500mg per dose (10–12 years); 500–750mg per dose (12–16 years).

Onset of effect
Within 15–60 minutes.

Duration of action
Up to 6 hours.

Diet advice
None.

Storage
Keep in original container at room temperature out of the reach of children.

Missed dose
Take as soon as you remember if required to relieve pain. Otherwise do not take the missed dose, and take a further dose only when you are in pain.

Stopping the drug
Can be safely stopped as soon as you no longer need it.

OVERDOSE ACTION

Seek immediate medical advice in all cases. Take emergency action if nausea, vomiting, or stomach pain occur.

See Drug poisoning emergency guide (p.518).

SPECIAL PRECAUTIONS

Be sure to consult your doctor or pharmacist before using this drug if:
- You have liver or kidney problems.
- You have cystic fibrosis.
- You have an eating disorder.
- You are taking other medicines

 Pregnancy
Not known to be harmful.

 Breast-feeding
The drug passes into the breast milk but only in amounts too small to be harmful.

 Infants and children
Not suitable for infants under 2 months old. For older infants and children, reduced dose necessary up to 16 years of age (see dosage information, left).

 Over 60
No special problems.

 Driving and hazardous work
No special problems.

 Alcohol
Small amounts of alcohol are probably safe but regularly exceeding your daily alcohol allowance can increase the risk of liver damage from paracetamol.

PROLONGED USE

Do not take paracetamol for longer than 48 hours except on the advice of your doctor. If the drug is taken long term as recommended, there is relatively little evidence of harm.

POSSIBLE ADVERSE EFFECTS

Paracetamol has rarely been found to produce any side effects when taken as recommended. The drug should be stopped and your doctor notified if a rash occurs.

Symptom/effect	Frequency		Discuss with doctor		Stop taking drug now	Call doctor now
	Common	Rare	Only if severe	In all cases		
Nausea		●	●			
Rash		●		●	●	

INTERACTIONS

Anticoagulants such as warfarin may need dose adjustment if taken with regular high doses of paracetamol.

Carbamazepine may increase the rate at which paracetamol is metabolized.

Metoclopramide and domperidone These drugs increase the rate at which paracetamol is absorbed by the body.

Imatinib Paracetamol should be used at a reduced dosage or avoided with imatinib.

Colestyramine reduces the absorption and possibly effectiveness of paracetamol.

Anticonvulsants (e.g. carbamazepine, phenytoin, barbiturates) increase the rate at which paracetamol is metabolized. This can reduce its effects but raise the risk of toxicity.

PAROXETINE

Brand name Seroxat
Used in the following combined preparations None

GENERAL INFORMATION

Paroxetine belongs to the selective serotonin re-uptake inhibitor (SSRI) class of antidepressants. It is used in the treatment of depression, and helps to control the anxiety that often accompanies it. It is also used to treat generalized anxiety disorder, social phobia, panic disorder, obsessive–compulsive disorders, and post-traumatic stress disorder. Paroxetine is sometimes given to treat severe premenstrual syndrome.

It is less likely than the older tricyclic antidepressants to cause anticholinergic side effects such as dry mouth, blurred vision, and difficulty in passing urine, and is much less dangerous in overdose.

The most common adverse effects include nausea, diarrhoea, insomnia, and sexual problems, such as lack of orgasm. Withdrawal symptoms can occur if the drug is not stopped gradually over several weeks.

QUICK REFERENCE

Drug group Antidepressant drug (p.40)

Overdose danger rating Low

Dependence rating Low

Prescription needed Yes

Available as generic Yes

INFORMATION FOR USERS

Your drug prescription is tailored for you. Do not alter dosage without checking with your doctor.

How taken/used

Tablets, liquid.

Frequency and timing of doses
Once daily, in the morning.

Dosage range
10–40mg daily.

Onset of effect
Onset of therapeutic response usually occurs within 14 days; full antidepressant effect may not be felt for 6 weeks (or longer for anxiety disorders).

Duration of action
Antidepressant effect may last for some time following prolonged use.

Diet advice
None.

Storage
Keep in original container at room temperature out of the reach of children.

Missed dose
Take as soon as you remember.

Stopping the drug
Do not stop the drug without consulting your doctor. Stopping abruptly can cause withdrawal symptoms.

Exceeding the dose
An occasional unintentional extra dose is unlikely to be a cause for concern. Large doses may cause unusual drowsiness. Notify your doctor immediately.

SPECIAL PRECAUTIONS

Be sure to tell your doctor if:
- You have long-term liver or kidney problems.
- You have heart problems or bleeding disorders.
- You have glaucoma.
- You have a history of mania, or a history or family history of epilepsy.
- You have had problems withdrawing from other antidepressants.
- You are taking other medicines.

 Pregnancy
Safety in pregnancy not established. Discuss with your doctor.

 Breast-feeding
The drug passes into the breast milk. Discuss with your doctor.

 Infants and children
Not generally recommended under 18 years.

 Over 60
Increased likelihood of adverse effects. Reduced dose may be necessary.

 Driving and hazardous work
Avoid until you have learned how paroxetine affects you because the drug can cause drowsiness.

 Alcohol
Avoid. Alcohol may increase the sedative effects of this drug.

POSSIBLE ADVERSE EFFECTS

Common adverse effects include nausea, diarrhoea, drowsiness, sweating, tremor, weakness, insomnia, and sexual dysfunction (lack of orgasm, male ejaculation problems).

Symptom/effect	Frequency		Discuss with doctor		Stop taking drug now	Call doctor now
	Common	Rare	Only if severe	In all cases		
Nausea/diarrhoea	●		●			
Sweating	●		●			
Drowsiness/dizziness	●		●			
Sexual dysfunction (both sexes)	●		●			
Abnormal dreams	●		●			
Nervousness/anxiety/agitation		●	●			
Suicidal thoughts or attempts		●		●	●	●

INTERACTIONS

General note Any drug that affects the breakdown of others in the liver may alter blood levels of paroxetine or vice versa.

Anticoagulants Paroxetine may increase the effects of these drugs.

Antipsychotics and tricyclic antidepressants Paroxetine may increase the levels and toxicity of these drugs.

Monoamine oxidase inhibitors (MAOIs) Avoid paroxetine during or within 14 days of MAOIs as serious reactions may occur.

Aspirin and NSAIDS (p.74) There is an increased risk of gastric bleeding when these drugs are used with paroxetine.

Serotonergics increase the risk of serotonin syndrome with paroxetine. This can be fatal.

PROLONGED USE

Withdrawal symptoms may occur if the drug is not stopped gradually over at least 4 weeks. Such symptoms include dizziness, electric shock sensations, anxiety, nausea, and insomnia. These rarely last for more than 1–2 weeks. There is also a small risk of suicidal thoughts and self-harm in children and adolescents, although the drug is rarely used for this age group.

Monitoring Any person experiencing drowsiness, confusion, muscle cramps, or seizures should be monitored for low sodium levels in the blood. Under-18s should be monitored for suicidal thoughts and self-harm.

PERINDOPRIL

Brand name Coversyl
Used in the following combined preparation Coversyl Plus

GENERAL INFORMATION

Perindopril is an ACE inhibitor, one of a group of drugs used to treat high blood pressure and heart failure, and to reduce the risk of cardiac events such as heart attack in certain heart conditions. Perindopril relaxes the muscles in the blood-vessel walls, allowing the vessels to dilate, thereby easing blood flow. It lowers blood pressure promptly, but may need to be taken for several weeks to achieve maximum effect. For heart failure, it is usually combined with a diuretic. This can give dramatic improvement, relaxing the muscle in blood vessel walls and reducing the heart's workload.

At the start of treatment, ACE inhibitors can cause a very rapid fall in blood pressure. Therefore, the first dose is usually low and taken at bedtime so that the patient can stay lying down.

Perindopril can cause a persistent dry cough; this adverse effect may occur in up to 20 percent of patients.

QUICK REFERENCE

Drug group ACE inhibitor (p.56) and antihypertensive drug (p.60)
Overdose danger rating Medium
Dependence rating Low
Prescription needed Yes
Available as generic Yes

INFORMATION FOR USERS

Your drug prescription is tailored for you. Do not alter dosage without checking with your doctor.

How taken/used

Tablets.

Frequency and timing of doses
Once daily, 30 minutes before food, usually in the morning.

Adult dosage range
4mg initially, then 4–8mg daily.

Onset of effect
30–60 minutes; full beneficial effect may take several weeks.

Duration of action
24 hours.

Diet advice
Your doctor may advise you to reduce your salt intake to help control your blood pressure.

Storage
Keep in original container at room temperature out of the reach of children.

Missed dose
Take as soon as you remember. If your next dose is due within the next 8 hours, take a single dose now, and skip the next.

Stopping the drug
Do not stop the drug without consulting your doctor; stopping the drug may lead to worsening of the underlying condition.

Exceeding the dose
An occasional unintentional extra dose is unlikely to cause problems, but large overdoses may cause dizziness or fainting. Notify your doctor.

SPECIAL PRECAUTIONS

Be sure to tell your doctor if:
- You have long-term kidney or liver problems.
- You have heart problems.
- You have had angioedema or a previous allergic reaction to ACE inhibitors.
- You are taking other medicines.
- You are pregnant or intend to become pregnant.

Pregnancy
Not prescribed. There is evidence of harm to the developing fetus.

Breast-feeding
Safety not established. Discuss with your doctor.

Infants and children
Not recommended.

Over 60
Reduced dose may be necessary.

Driving and hazardous work
Avoid such activities until you have learned how perindopril affects you because the drug can cause dizziness and fainting.

Alcohol
Avoid. Alcohol may increase the blood-pressure-lowering and adverse effects of the drug.

Surgery and general anaesthetics
Perindopril may have to be stopped before you have a general anaesthetic. Discuss with your doctor or dentist before any operation.

POSSIBLE ADVERSE EFFECTS

Perindopril may cause a variety of adverse effects, but these are usually mild and often disappear soon after treatment has started. It may also cause kidney impairment.

Symptom/effect	Frequency		Discuss with doctor		Stop taking drug now	Call doctor now
	Common	Rare	Only if severe	In all cases		
Rash	●			●		
Persistent dry cough	●			●		
Mouth ulcers/sore mouth		●		●		
Dizziness		●		●		
Sore throat/fever		●		●		
Swelling of mouth/lips		●		●	●	●
Breathing difficulty		●		●	●	●

INTERACTIONS

Ciclosporin, potassium salts, and potassium-sparing diuretics increase the risk of high blood potassium levels with perindopril and should be avoided.

Non-steroidal anti-inflammatory drugs (NSAIDs) may reduce the effects of perindopril. There is also a risk of kidney damage when they are taken together.

Lithium Blood levels and toxicity of this drug may be raised by perindopril.

Vasodilators, diuretics, and other antihypertensives These drugs may increase the blood-pressure-lowering effect of perindopril.

PROLONGED USE

No problems expected.

Monitoring Periodic checks on potassium levels, white blood cell count, kidney function, and urine are usually performed.

PERMETHRIN

Brand name Lyclear
Used in the following combined preparations None

GENERAL INFORMATION

Permethrin is an insecticide used to treat pubic lice (but not head lice) and scabies infestations. The drug works by interfering with the nervous system of the parasites, causing paralysis and death in them. Permethrin is less toxic to humans than some of the other types of insecticide, although it is toxic to some animals, such as cats.

Permethrin is applied topically as a cream to treat pubic lice and scabies infestations. It should not be used on broken or infested skin. In children and older adults, the entire body surface, including the face, scalp, neck, and ears, may have to be covered; adults are treated from the neck downwards.

For pubic lice, the entire body should be treated and the permethrin left on overnight. A second treatment seven days later is needed. For both pubic lice and scabies, all family members should be treated at the same time, to prevent recontamination, and the process repeated after a week.

There are signs that the parasites are developing resistance to permethrin. If the drug does not work for you, your pharmacist should be able to suggest an alternative treatment (e.g. malathion).

Permethrin is also an ingredient of some insect repellents used to impregnate clothing and mosquito nets in malarial regions.

INFORMATION FOR USERS

Follow instructions on the label. Call your doctor if symptoms worsen.

How taken/used

Cream.

Frequency and timing of doses
Once only, repeating after 7 days (2 years and over); under specialist supervision only (infants and children under 2 years). Avoid contact with eyes and broken or infected skin.

Dosage range
As directed.

Onset of effect
Pubic lice Wash off after 12–24 hours.
Scabies Wash off after 8–12 hours.

Duration of action
Until washed off.

Diet advice
None.

Storage
Keep in original container at room temperature out of the reach of children. Protect from light.

Missed dose
Timing of the second application is not rigid; use as soon as you remember.

Stopping the drug
Not applicable.

Exceeding the dose
An occasional extra application is unlikely to cause problems. If the drug is accidentally swallowed, take emergency action.

SPECIAL PRECAUTIONS

Be sure to tell your doctor if:
- You are taking other medicines.

 Pregnancy
Safety not established. Discuss with your doctor.

 Breast-feeding
Safety not established. Discuss with your doctor.

 Infants and children
Under specialist supervision only under 2 years. No special problems in older children.

 Over 60
No special problems, but consult your doctor or a health professional.

 Driving and hazardous work
No special problems.

 Alcohol
No special problems.

Safety hazard
There is a risk of burns if treated skin or contaminated clothing is exposed to open flames, owing to the alcohol content of the preparations.

POSSIBLE ADVERSE EFFECTS

In general, permethrin is well tolerated on the skin, although mild skin irritation is common.

Symptom/effect	Frequency		Discuss with doctor		Stop taking drug now	Call doctor now
	Common	Rare	Only if severe	In all cases		
Itching	●		●			
Reddened skin/stinging	●		●			
Rash		●	●			

INTERACTIONS

Corticosteroids Any eczema-like reactions to permethrin should not be treated with corticosteroid drugs, as these drugs may lower the immune response to the mites.

PROLONGED USE

Permethrin should not be used topically for prolonged periods; it is intended for intermittent use only. Prolonged use of permethrin to impregnate clothing and netting is not known to cause serious toxic effects.

PHENELZINE

Brand name Nardil
Used in the following combined preparations None

GENERAL INFORMATION

Phenelzine is a monoamine oxidase inhibitor (MAOI) antidepressant. It works by blocking the enzyme monoamine oxidase, which normally breaks down neurotransmitters (mainly serotonin and noradrenaline) in the brain and other parts of the body (see p.34). Low levels of these neurotransmitters in the brain are a causative factor in depression, and the effect of MAOIs is to increase their levels. Due to its potentially serious adverse effects and interactions with other drugs and foods (see Diet advice, below), use of phenelzine is reserved for people for whom other antidepressants have been ineffective or those whose depression occurs together with anxiety, phobia, hysteria, or hypochondria.

INFORMATION FOR USERS

Your drug prescription is tailored for you. Do not alter dosage without checking with your doctor.

How taken/used

Tablets.

Frequency and timing of doses
Initially, 3–4 x daily. After satisfactory response has been achieved, dose may be gradually reduced to once daily or once every other day.

Adult dosage range
15–60mg daily. Patients receiving hospital treatment may be given up to 90mg daily.

Onset of effect
Effectiveness may not be felt for up to 4 weeks.

Duration of action
Antidepressant effect may last for some months or longer following prolonged use.

Diet advice
Avoid foods containing tyramine, such as cheese, meat or yeast extracts, fermented soya bean extracts, pickled herrings, hung game, and alcoholic (including low-alcohol) drinks. Discuss with your doctor.

Storage
Store between 2–8°C in a refrigerator. Keep out of the reach of children.

Missed dose
Take as soon as you remember. If your next dose is due within 12 hours, skip the missed dose and take the next dose as scheduled.

Stopping the drug
Do not stop the drug without consulting your doctor. Stopping abruptly may cause withdrawal symptoms and a recurrence of depression.

OVERDOSE ACTION

Seek immediate medical advice in all cases. An overdose may be fatal. Take emergency action if breathing problems or loss of consciousness occur.

See Drug poisoning emergency guide (p.518).

SPECIAL PRECAUTIONS

Be sure to tell your doctor if:
- You have high blood pressure or heart disease.
- You have had a stroke.
- You have liver disease.
- You have a blood disorder.
- You have diabetes.
- You have epilepsy.
- You have porphyria.
- You have phaeochromocytoma.
- You are taking any other medicines, including over-the-counter cough or cold remedies, or illicit drugs.

 Pregnancy
Safety not established. Discuss with your doctor.

 Breast-feeding
Safety not established. Discuss with your doctor.

 Infants and children
Not recommended for children under 16 years old.

 Over 60
Increased risk of adverse effects. Reduced dose may be necessary.

 Driving and hazardous work
Avoid until you have learned how phenelzine affects you because the drug may cause dizziness, drowsiness, and blurred vision.

 Alcohol
Avoid. Many alcoholic drinks contain tyramine, which may interact with phenelzine. The drug also enhances the effects of alcohol.

Surgery and general anaesthetics
Due to a potentially dangerous interaction with general anaesthetics, phenelzine should be withdrawn 2 weeks before any surgery or dentistry requiring general anaesthesia. Discuss with your doctor or dentist.

POSSIBLE ADVERSE EFFECTS

Side effects are common, and some are potentially serious. Consult your doctor immediately if you develop fever, jaundice, tightness in the muscles, or suicidal thoughts.

Symptom/effect	Frequency		Discuss with doctor		Stop taking drug now	Call doctor now
	Common	Rare	Only if severe	In all cases		
Dizziness/drowsiness	●		●			
Nausea/vomiting/constipation	●		●			
Sleep disturbance	●		●			
Blurred vision	●		●			
Twitching/jerking	●		●			
Rash		●	●			●
Fever/muscle tightness		●		●	●	●
Jaundice		●		●	●	●
Suicidal thoughts		●		●	●	●

INTERACTIONS

General note Phenelzine interacts with a wide range of drugs, and some interactions may be dangerous. Consult your doctor before taking any other medication.

Tyramine Phenelzine interacts with tyramine-containing food and drinks (see Diet advice, above) to cause a potentially life-threatening rise in blood pressure.

PROLONGED USE

Withdrawal symptoms may occur if the drug is not stopped gradually over at least 4 weeks. Such symptoms include nausea, vomiting, malaise, nightmares, and agitation.

PHENOBARBITAL (PHENOBARBITONE)

Brand names None
Used in the following combined preparations None

GENERAL INFORMATION

Phenobarbital belongs to the group of drugs called barbiturates. It is used mainly in treating epilepsy, although this use is steadily declining. It was also used as a sleeping drug and sedative before the development of safer drugs. In treating epilepsy, phenobarbital is usually given together with another anticonvulsant drug such as phenytoin.

The main disadvantage of the drug is that it often causes unwanted sedation. However, tolerance develops within a week or two, and most patients have no problem in long-term use. In children and older adults, it may occasionally cause over-excitement. Because of their sedative effect, phenobarbital and other barbiturates are sometimes misused.

QUICK REFERENCE

Drug group Barbiturate anticonvulsant drug (p.42)

Overdose danger rating High

Dependence rating High

Prescription needed Yes

Available as generic Yes

INFORMATION FOR USERS

Your drug prescription is tailored for you. Do not alter dosage without checking with your doctor.

How taken/used

Tablets, liquid, injection.

Frequency and timing of doses
Once daily, usually at night.

Dosage range
Adults 60–180mg daily.

Onset of effect
30–60 minutes (by mouth).

Duration of action
24–48 hours (some effect may persist for up to 6 days).

Diet advice
People taking the drug long term should eat plenty of fresh green vegetables to prevent possible deficiency of vitamins A, D, K, and folic acid.

Storage
Keep in original container at room temperature out of the reach of children.

Missed dose
Take as soon as you remember. If the next dose is due within 10 hours, take a single dose now and skip the next.

Stopping the drug
Do not stop taking the drug without consulting your doctor, who may supervise a gradual reduction in dosage. Stopping abruptly may cause seizures or lead to restlessness, trembling, and insomnia.

OVERDOSE ACTION

Seek immediate medical advice in all cases. Take emergency action if unsteadiness, severe weakness, confusion, or loss of consciousness occur.

See Drug poisoning emergency guide (p.518).

POSSIBLE ADVERSE EFFECTS

Most of the adverse effects of phenobarbital are the result of its sedative effect. They can sometimes be minimized by a medically supervised reduction of dosage. Rarely, the drug may cause suicidal thoughts; if this occurs, seek immediate medical help.

Symptom/effect	Frequency		Discuss with doctor		Stop taking drug now	Call doctor now
	Common	Rare	Only if severe	In all cases		
Drowsiness	●		●			
Clumsiness/unsteadiness	●		●			
Dizziness/faintness	●		●			
Mood changes/impaired memory/confusion		●		●		
Rash/localized swellings		●		●	●	●
Mouth ulcers		●		●	●	●

INTERACTIONS

General note Phenobarbital interacts with a wide range of other drugs. Consult your doctor or pharmacist before taking any new drugs, including herbal remedies.

Sedatives All such drugs are likely to increase the sedative properties of phenobarbital.

Anticoagulants, corticosteroids, oral contraceptives, protease inhibitors Their effect may be decreased by phenobarbital.

Antipsychotics, antidepressants, mefloquine, chloroquine, and St John's wort may reduce the anticonvulsant effect of phenobarbital.

SPECIAL PRECAUTIONS

Be sure to tell your doctor if:
- You have long-term liver or kidney problems.
- You have heart problems.
- You have poor circulation.
- You have porphyria.
- You have breathing problems.
- You have depression.
- You are taking other medicines.

Pregnancy
The drug may affect the fetus and increase the tendency of bleeding in newborn babies. Discuss with your doctor.

Breast-feeding
The drug passes into the breast milk and could cause drowsiness in the baby. Discuss with your doctor.

Infants and children
Reduced dose necessary.

Over 60
Increased likelihood of confusion. Reduced dose may be necessary.

Driving and hazardous work
Your underlying condition, in addition to the possibility of reduced alertness while taking phenobarbital, may make such activities inadvisable. Discuss with your doctor.

Alcohol
Never drink alcohol while under treatment with phenobarbital. Alcohol may interact dangerously with this drug.

PROLONGED USE

With prolonged use, tolerance to the drug's sedative effects may develop. Dependence may also result, and withdrawal symptoms may occur if the drug is stopped suddenly. Long-term use may also lead to deficiency of vitamins A, D, K, and folic acid.

Monitoring Blood samples may be taken periodically to test blood levels of the drug.

PHENOXYMETHYLPENICILLIN

Brand names None
Used in the following combined preparations None

GENERAL INFORMATION

Phenoxymethylpenicillin, also known as penicillin V, is a synthetic penicillin-type antibiotic that is prescribed for a wide range of infections. It is only given by mouth and was the first orally active penicillin to be synthesized.

Various commonly occurring respiratory tract infections, such as some types of tonsillitis and pharyngitis, as well as ear infections, often respond well to this drug.

Phenoxymethylpenicillin is also used to treat less common infections caused by the *Streptococcus* bacterium, such as scarlet fever and erysipelas (a skin infection). It is prescribed long term to prevent the recurrence of rheumatic fever, a rare but potentially serious condition. It is also used long term to prevent infections following removal of the spleen or in sickle cell disease.

As with other penicillin antibiotics, the most serious adverse effect that may rarely occur is an allergic reaction that may cause collapse, wheezing, and a rash in susceptible people.

QUICK REFERENCE

Drug group Penicillin antibiotic (p.86)

Overdose danger rating Low

Dependence rating Low

Prescription needed Yes

Available as generic Yes

INFORMATION FOR USERS

Your drug prescription is tailored for you. Do not alter dosage without checking with your doctor.

How taken/used

Tablets, liquid.

Frequency and timing of doses
4 x daily, at least 30 minutes before food.

Dosage range
Adults 2–4g daily.
Children Reduced dose according to age.

Onset of effect
Within a few hours.

Duration of action
Up to 12 hours.

Diet advice
None.

Storage
Keep in original container at room temperature out of the reach of children.

Missed dose
Take as soon as you remember. If your next dose is due within 2 hours, take a single dose now and skip the next.

Stopping the drug
Take the full course. Even if you feel better, the original infection may still be present and may recur if the treatment is stopped too soon.

Exceeding the dose
An occasional unintentional extra dose is unlikely to be a cause for concern. But if you notice any unusual symptoms, or if a large overdose has been taken, notify your doctor.

SPECIAL PRECAUTIONS

Be sure to tell your doctor if:
- You have a long-term kidney problem.
- You have had a previous allergic reaction to a penicillin or cephalosporin antibiotic.
- You are taking other medicines.

 Pregnancy
No evidence of risk.

 Breast-feeding
The drug passes into the breast milk, but at normal doses adverse effects on the baby are unlikely. Discuss with your doctor.

 Infants and children
Reduced dose necessary.

 Over 60
No special problems.

 Driving and hazardous work
No known problems.

 Alcohol
No known problems.

PROLONGED USE

Prolonged use may increase the risk of *Candida* infections and diarrhoea.

POSSIBLE ADVERSE EFFECTS

Common adverse effects of this drug are diarrhoea, rash, and itching. However, phenoxymethylpenicillin may rarely provoke a severe allergic reaction in susceptible people.

Symptom/effect	Frequency		Discuss with doctor		Stop taking drug now	Call doctor now
	Common	Rare	Only if severe	In all cases		
Nausea/vomiting	●		●			
Diarrhoea		●	●			
Rash/itching		●		●	●	●
Breathing difficulties		●		●	●	●

INTERACTIONS

Warfarin Phenoxymethylpenicillin potentially alters the anticoagulant effect of warfarin.

Typhoid vaccine Penicillins may inactivate oral typhoid vaccine if they are ingested concomitantly with the vaccine.

Probenecid increases the level of phenoxymethylpenicillin in the blood.

Neomycin reduces the level of phenoxymethylpenicillin in the blood.

Methotrexate Excretion of this drug may be greatly reduced by phenoxymethyl-penicillin, leading to toxicity.

PHENYTOIN/FOSPHENYTOIN

Brand names [phenytoin] Epanutin; [fosphenytoin] Pro-Epanutin
Used in the following combined preparations None

GENERAL INFORMATION

Phenytoin is used to treat epilepsy. It decreases the likelihood of convulsions by reducing abnormal electrical activity in the brain. Fosphenytoin is given by injection for severe seizures. Phenytoin has also been used for other disorders, such as migraine, trigeminal neuralgia, and certain abnormal heart rhythms.

The dose must be adjusted according to blood levels of the drug. Patients are advised to keep to one brand. Some of the adverse effects are more severe in children, so other options are preferred. Phenytoin powerfully activates liver enzymes that metabolize other drugs so can often trigger significant interactions.

INFORMATION FOR USERS

Your drug prescription is tailored for you. Do not alter dosage without checking with your doctor.

How taken/used

Tablets, chewable tablets, capsules, liquid, injection.

Frequency and timing of doses
1–2 x daily with food or plenty of water.

Dosage range
Adults 200–500mg daily (usually as a single dose).
Children According to age and weight.
Note: a small increase in the dose can cause a disproportionately high drug level in the blood.

Onset of effect
Full anticonvulsant effect may not be felt for 7–10 days.

Duration of action
24 hours.

Diet advice
Folic acid and vitamin D deficiency may occasionally occur. Make sure you eat a balanced diet containing fresh, green vegetables and dairy products.

Storage
Keep in original container at room temperature out of the reach of children.

Missed dose
Take as soon as you remember.

Stopping the drug
Do not stop the drug without consulting your doctor; seizures may recur.

OVERDOSE ACTION

Seek immediate medical advice in all cases. Take emergency action if unsteadiness, severe weakness, confusion, or loss of consciousness occur.

See Drug poisoning emergency guide (p.518).

POSSIBLE ADVERSE EFFECTS

Phenytoin has a number of adverse effects, many of which appear only after prolonged use. If they become severe, your doctor may prescribe a different anticonvulsant.

Symptom/effect	Frequency		Discuss with doctor		Stop taking drug now	Call doctor now
	Common	Rare	Only if severe	In all cases		
Dizziness/headache	●		●			
Nausea/vomiting	●		●			
Insomnia	●		●			
Increased body hair		●	●			
Overgrowth of gums		●	●			
Confusion/unsteadiness		●		●		●
Rash		●		●		●
Fever/sore throat/mouth ulcers		●		●		●

INTERACTIONS

General note Many drugs may interact with phenytoin, causing either an increase or a reduction in the phenytoin blood level. The dosage of phenytoin may need to be adjusted. Consult your doctor or pharmacist.

Oral contraceptives Phenytoin may reduce their effectiveness.

Warfarin The anticoagulant effect of this drug may be altered. An adjustment in its dosage may be necessary.

Antidepressants, antipsychotics, mefloquine, chloroquine, and St John's wort These preparations may reduce the effect of phenytoin.

SPECIAL PRECAUTIONS

Be sure to tell your doctor if:
- You have long-term liver or kidney problems.
- You have heart problems.
- You have diabetes.
- You have porphyria.
- You are taking other medicines.

 Pregnancy
The drug may be associated with malformation and a tendency to bleeding in the newborn baby. Folic acid supplements should be taken by the mother. Discuss with your doctor.

 Breast-feeding
The drug passes into the breast milk, but at normal doses adverse effects on the baby are unlikely. Discuss with your doctor.

 Infants and children
Reduced dose necessary. Increased likelihood of overgrowth of the gums and excessive growth of body hair.

 Over 60
Reduced dose may be necessary.

 Driving and hazardous work
Your underlying condition, as well the effects of phenytoin, may make such activities inadvisable. Discuss with your doctor.

 Alcohol
Avoid. Alcohol increases the sedative effects of this drug.

PROLONGED USE

There is a slight risk that blood abnormalities may occur. Prolonged use may also lead to adverse effects on skin, gums, and bones. It may also disrupt control of diabetes.

Patients of Han Chinese ethnic origin are particularly prone to toxic side effects.

Monitoring Periodic blood tests are performed to monitor levels of the drug in the body and composition of the blood cells and blood chemistry, as well as blood levels of vitamin D.

PILOCARPINE

Brand names Minims Pilocarpine, Salagen
Used in the following combined preparations None

GENERAL INFORMATION

Pilocarpine is a miotic drug that is used to treat chronic glaucoma and severe glaucoma prior to surgery. The eye drops are quick-acting, but have to be reapplied every four to eight hours. Pilocarpine frequently causes blurred vision; and spasm of the eye muscles may cause headaches, particularly at the start of treatment. However, serious adverse effects are rare.

Pilocarpine tablets are also used to treat dry mouth following radiotherapy to the head and neck, and dry mouth and eyes due to Sjögren's syndrome (an autoimmune disease).

INFORMATION FOR USERS

Your drug prescription is tailored for you. Do not alter dosage without checking with your doctor.

How taken/used

Tablets, eye drops.

Frequency and timing of doses
Eye drops 4 x daily (chronic glaucoma); 5-minute intervals until condition is controlled (acute glaucoma).
Tablets 3–4 x daily after food with plenty of water.

Adult dosage range
According to formulation and condition. In general, 1–2 eye drops are used per application.
Tablets 15–30mg daily.

Onset of effect
15–30 minutes.

Duration of action
4–8 weeks for maximum effect (tablets); 3–8 hours (eye drops).

Diet advice
None.

Storage
Keep in original container at room temperature out of the reach of children (tablets/eye drops). Discard eye drops 1 month after opening.

Missed dose
Use as soon as you remember. If not remembered until 2 hours before your next dose, skip the missed dose and take the next dose now.

Stopping the drug
Do not stop the drug without consulting your doctor; symptoms may recur.

Exceeding the dose
An occasional unintentional extra application is unlikely to cause problems. Excessive use may cause facial flushing, an increase in the flow of saliva, and sweating. If accidentally swallowed, seek medical help immediately.

POSSIBLE ADVERSE EFFECTS

Alteration in vision is common. Brow ache and eye pain are common at the start of treatment, but usually wear off after a few days.

Symptom/effect	Frequency		Discuss with doctor		Stop taking drug now	Call doctor now
	Common	Rare	Only if severe	In all cases		
Eye drops						
Blurred vision/poor night vision	●		●			
Headache/brow ache	●		●			
Sweating/chills	●		●			
Eye pain/irritation	●			●		●
Red, watery eyes		●	●			
Twitching eyelids		●				
Tablets						
Nausea/ diarrhoea	●		●			
Blurred vision/dizziness/headache	●		●			
Urinary frequency	●		●			
Wheezing		●		●	●	●

INTERACTIONS

General note A wide range of drugs may enhance the effects of pilocarpine tablets, including antihistamines (e.g. chlorphenamine), tricyclic antidepressants, and phenothiazines (e.g. chlorpromazine).

Beta blockers These drugs may reduce the effects of pilocarpine and make conduction disturbances in the heart more likely.

Calcium channel blockers may increase the systemic effect of pilocarpine.

SPECIAL PRECAUTIONS

Be sure to tell your doctor if:
- You have asthma.
- You have inflamed eyes.
- You wear contact lenses.
- You have heart, liver, or gastrointestinal problems.
- You are taking other medicines.

 Pregnancy
Avoid unless the potential benefit outweighs the risk. Safety of tablets and eye drops in pregnancy not established. Discuss with your doctor.

 Breast-feeding
It is not known whether pilocarpine is excreted into breast milk, and safety has not been established. Discuss with your doctor.

 Infants and children
Information is limited; however, no significant safety issues have been reported in children.

 Over 60
Reduced night vision is particularly noticeable; no dosage adjustment required.

 Driving and hazardous work
Avoid, especially in poor light, until you have learned how pilocarpine affects you because it may cause short sight and poor night vision.

 Alcohol
No known problems.

PROLONGED USE

The effect of the drug may occasionally wear off with prolonged use as the body adapts, but may be restored by changing temporarily to another drug.

Monitoring Pressure inside the eye and the visual fields should be monitored in patients with glaucoma who are using pilocarpine.

PIOGLITAZONE

Brand names Actos, Glidipion
Used in the following combined preparation Competact

GENERAL INFORMATION

Pioglitazone is an oral antidiabetic drug of the thiazolidinedione type, used for Type 2 diabetes. It works by reducing insulin resistance in body tissues, which leads to a reduction of blood glucose levels. The effects appear gradually and reach their full extent in about 8 weeks. Pioglitazone may be used alone but is often used with metformin and/or a sulfonylurea; it is available as a combined preparation with metformin. Pioglitazone works better in obese people with diabetes, although it often causes weight gain. It may also be used with insulin in people with Type 2 diabetes, although this may increase the risk of heart failure. Bone fractures are another possible adverse effect.

INFORMATION FOR USERS

Your drug prescription is tailored for you. Do not alter dosage without checking with your doctor.

How taken/used

Tablets.

Frequency and timing of doses
1 x daily.

Adult dosage range
15–45mg daily.

Onset of effect
60 minutes; it can take 8 weeks for full effects to appear.

Duration of action
12–24 hours.

Diet advice
An individualized diabetic diet must be maintained for the drug to be fully effective. Follow your doctor's advice.

Storage
Keep in original container at room temperature out of the reach of children.

Missed dose
Take as soon as you remember. If your next dose is due within 2 hours, take a single dose now and skip the next.

Stopping the drug
Do not stop the drug without consulting your doctor as your condition could worsen.

OVERDOSE ACTION

Seek immediate medical help. If you have warning signs of low blood sugar (such as faintness, dizziness, headache, confusion, sweating, tremor), eat something sugary. Take emergency action if loss of consciousness occurs.

See Drug poisoning emergency guide (p.518).

SPECIAL PRECAUTIONS

Be sure to tell your doctor if:
- You have liver problems.
- You are anaemic.
- You have a history of heart failure, angina, heart attack, or stroke.
- You are passing blood in your urine or have a history of bladder cancer.
- You have severe kidney failure.
- You have osteoporosis.
- You are taking other medicines.

Pregnancy
Safety not established. Discuss with your doctor.

Breast-feeding
Safety not established. Discuss with your doctor.

Infants and children
Not recommended.

Over 60
No special problems, but older people may be more susceptible to side effects of the drug.

Driving and hazardous work
No known problems.

Alcohol
Avoid excessive intake. Alcohol can increase the effect of pioglitazone.

POSSIBLE ADVERSE EFFECTS

Fatigue and weakness (due to anaemia) and weight gain (even on a strict diabetic diet) are common side effects. Less commonly, the drug has been associated with heart failure.

Symptom/effect	Frequency		Discuss with doctor		Stop taking drug now	Call doctor now
	Common	Rare	Only if severe	In all cases		
Indigestion/flatulence	●		●			
Nausea/abdominal pain	●			●		
Fatigue/weakness/headache	●			●		
Weight gain	●			●		
Dark urine		●		●		
Dizziness/pins and needles		●		●		
Bone pain in arms/hand/feet		●		●		
Oedema (water retention)		●		●		
Breathlessness/cough		●		●		
Jaundice		●		●	●	●

INTERACTIONS

Diazoxide, corticosteroids, diuretics, and progesterones may reduce the effects of pioglitazone.

Gemfibrozil reduces the metabolism of pioglitazone, so a reduced dose may be necessary.

Non-steroidal anti-inflammatory drugs (NSAIDs) may increase the risk of fluid retention.

Rifampicin reduces the blood level of pioglitazone, so an increased dose may be necessary.

PROLONGED USE

Pioglitazone, like other antidiabetic drugs, can be used indefinitely but should be discontinued if there is no evidence of an adequate response.

Heart failure signs are more common in patients on pioglitazone, but not mortality from heart failure. Long-term use increases the risk of bone fractures in the arms, hands, and feet, and there is a small risk of developing bladder cancer.

Monitoring Initial and periodic blood tests of liver function will be performed. Weight will be measured at intervals. Blood sugar levels should be monitored regularly. You should tell your doctor if you pass blood in your urine while taking the drug.

PIROXICAM

Brand names Feldene, Feldene Melt
Used in the following combined preparations None

GENERAL INFORMATION

Piroxicam is a non-steroidal anti-inflammatory drug (NSAID) that, like others in this group, reduces pain, stiffness, and inflammation. It is used for osteoarthritis, rheumatoid arthritis, acute attacks of gout, and ankylosing spondylitis. It gives relief from the symptoms of arthritis, although it does not cure the disease. Piroxicam is sometimes prescribed in conjunction with slow-acting drugs in rheumatoid arthritis to relieve pain and inflammation while these drugs take effect. It may also be given for pain relief after sports injuries, for conditions such as tendinitis and bursitis, and after minor surgery.

Blood levels of piroxicam remain high for many hours after an oral dose, so it needs to be taken only once daily. Among the NSAIDs, piroxicam is one of the most likely to cause gastrointestinal side effects.

INFORMATION FOR USERS

Your drug prescription is tailored for you. Do not alter dosage without checking with your doctor.

How taken/used

Tablets, capsules, melts, gel.

Frequency and timing of doses
1–3 x daily with food or plenty of water (oral doses). 3-4 x daily (gel).

Adult dosage range
10–20mg daily.

Onset of effect
3–4 hours (pain relief); full effect develops over 2–4 weeks (arthritis) or 4–5 days (gout).

Duration of action
Up to 2 days; 7–10 days after treatment stops.

Diet advice
None.

Storage
Keep in original container at room temperature out of the reach of children. Protect from light.

Missed dose
Take as soon as you remember. If your next dose is due within 4 hours, take a single dose now and skip the next.

Stopping the drug
When taken for short-term pain relief, the drug can be safely stopped as soon as you no longer need it. If prescribed for the long-term treatment of arthritis, however, you should seek medical advice before stopping the drug.

Exceeding the dose
An occasional unintentional extra dose is unlikely to be a cause for concern. Large overdoses may cause nausea and vomiting. Notify your doctor.

POSSIBLE ADVERSE EFFECTS

Gastrointestinal side effects, dizziness, and headache are not generally serious. Black or bloodstained bowel movements should be reported to your doctor immediately.

Symptom/effect	Frequency		Discuss with doctor		Stop taking drug now	Call doctor now
	Common	Rare	Only if severe	In all cases		
Heartburn/indigestion	●		●			
Nausea/vomiting	●		●			
Headache		●	●			
Dizziness/drowsiness		●	●			
Swollen feet or legs		●	●			
Weight gain		●	●			
Rash/itching		●		●	●	
Wheezing/breathlessness		●		●	●	●
Black/bloodstained faeces		●		●	●	●

INTERACTIONS

General note Piroxicam interacts with a wide range of drugs, including other NSAIDs, corticosteroids, and oral anticoagulant drugs, to increase the risk of bleeding and/or peptic ulcers.

Antihypertensive drugs and diuretics The beneficial effects of these drugs may be reduced by piroxicam.

Ciprofloxacin, norfloxacin, and ofloxacin Piroxicam may increase the risk of seizures when taken with these drugs.

Ritonavir This drug increases blood levels of piroxicam.

Lithium and methotrexate Piroxicam may raise blood levels of these drugs.

SPECIAL PRECAUTIONS

Be sure to tell your doctor if:
- You have liver or kidney problems.
- You have heart problems or high blood pressure.
- You have had a peptic ulcer, oesophagitis, or acid indigestion.
- You have porphyria.
- You have asthma.
- You are allergic to aspirin or other NSAIDs.
- You are taking other medicines.

Pregnancy
The drug may increase the risks of adverse effects on the baby's heart and may prolong labour if taken in the third trimester. Discuss with your doctor.

Breast-feeding
The drug passes into the breast milk but at normal doses adverse effects are unlikely. Discuss with your doctor.

Infants and children
Not recommended under 6 years. Reduced dose necessary.

Over 60
Increased likelihood of adverse effects. Reduced dose may therefore be necessary.

Driving and hazardous work
Avoid such activities until you have learned how piroxicam affects you; the drug can cause dizziness.

Alcohol
Avoid. Alcohol may increase the risk of stomach disorders with piroxicam.

Surgery and general anaesthetics
Piroxicam may prolong bleeding. Discuss with your doctor or dentist before any surgery.

PROLONGED USE

There is an increased risk of bleeding from peptic ulcers and in the bowel with prolonged use of piroxicam. There is also a small risk of a heart attack or stroke. To minimize these risks, the lowest effective dose is given for the shortest duration.

PIZOTIFEN

Brand name None
Used in the following combined preparations None

GENERAL INFORMATION

Pizotifen is an antihistamine drug with a chemical structure similar to that of the tricyclic antidepressants (p.40), and has similar anticholinergic effects. It is thought to work by blocking histamine and serotonin, chemicals that act on blood vessels in the brain. The drug is prescribed for the prevention of migraine headaches in people who experience frequent, disabling attacks. It is not effective in relieving migraine attacks once they have started.

The main disadvantage with prolonged use of pizotifen is that it stimulates the appetite and, as a result, often causes weight gain. It is usually prescribed only for people in whom other measures for migraine prevention, such as avoidance of trigger factors, have failed.

The sweetener used in the liquid medication is hydrogenated glucose syrup, and this may affect levels of blood sugar.

INFORMATION FOR USERS

Your drug prescription is tailored for you. Do not alter dosage without checking with your doctor.

How taken/used

Tablets, liquid (available only by special order).

Frequency and timing of doses
Once a day (at night) or 3 x daily.

Adult dosage range
1.5–4.5mg daily. Maximum single dose 3mg.

Onset of effect
Full beneficial effects may not be felt for several days.

Duration of action
Effects of this drug may last for several weeks.

Diet advice
Migraine sufferers may be advised to avoid foods that trigger headaches in their case.

Storage
Keep in original container at room temperature out of the reach of children. Protect from light.

Missed dose
Take as soon as you remember. If your next dose is due within 4 hours, take a single dose now and skip the next.

Stopping the drug
Do not stop the drug without consulting your doctor; symptoms may recur.

Exceeding the dose
An occasional unintentional extra dose is unlikely to cause problems, but large overdoses may cause drowsiness, nausea, palpitations, seizures, and coma. Notify your doctor.

POSSIBLE ADVERSE EFFECTS

Drowsiness is a common adverse effect that can often be minimized by starting treatment with a low dose that is gradually increased.

Symptom/effect	Frequency		Discuss with doctor		Stop taking drug now	Call doctor now
	Common	Rare	Only if severe	In all cases		
Weight gain/increased appetite	●		●			
Drowsiness	●		●			
Fatigue	●		●			
Nausea/dizziness	●		●			
Muscle pains		●	●			
Dry mouth		●	●			
Blurred vision		●	●			
Depression/anxiety		●		●		

INTERACTIONS

Anticholinergic drugs The weak anticholinergic effects of pizotifen may be increased by other anticholinergic drugs, including tricyclic antidepressants.

Antihypertensive drugs The blood-pressure-lowering effects of guanethidine and debrisoquine are reduced by pizotifen.

Sedatives All drugs that have a sedative effect on the central nervous system are likely to increase the sedative properties of pizotifen. These include alcohol, sleeping drugs, anti-anxiety drugs, opioid analgesics, and antihistamines.

SPECIAL PRECAUTIONS

Be sure to tell your doctor if:
- You have a long-term kidney problem.
- You have glaucoma.
- You have urinary retention.
- You have prostate problems.
- You have galactose intolerance.
- You have epilepsy.
- You are taking other medicines.

 Pregnancy
Safety in pregnancy not established. Discuss with your doctor.

 Breast-feeding
The drug passes into the breast milk, but at normal doses adverse effects on the baby are unlikely. Discuss with your doctor.

 Infants and children
Reduced dose usually necessary. Not recommended under 5 years.

 Over 60
No special problems.

 Driving and hazardous work
Avoid such activities until you have learned how pizotifen affects you because the drug can cause drowsiness and blurred vision.

 Alcohol
Avoid. Alcohol may increase the sedative effects of this drug.

PROLONGED USE

Pizotifen often causes weight gain during long-term use. Treatment is usually reviewed every 6 months.

PRAVASTATIN

Brand name Lipostat
Used in the following combined preparations None

GENERAL INFORMATION

Pravastatin belongs to the statin group of lipid-lowering drugs. It may be used for people with hypercholesterolaemia (high levels of cholesterol in the blood) who have not responded to other treatments, such as a special diet, and who are at risk of developing heart disease or stroke. However, it has been largely superseded by newer, more potent statins, such as atorvastatin and rosuvastatin. Pravastatin works by blocking the action of an enzyme that is needed for the manufacture of cholesterol, mainly in the liver. As a result, blood levels of cholesterol are lowered, which can help to prevent heart disease and stroke.

Side effects are usually mild and often wear off over time. Pravastatin is concentrated in the liver and it may raise levels of liver enzymes, but this does not usually indicate serious liver damage. Rarely, it may cause muscle damage; any unexpected muscle tenderness, pain, or weakness should be reported to your doctor.

QUICK REFERENCE

Drug group Lipid-lowering drug (p.61)

Overdose danger rating Medium

Dependence rating Low

Prescription needed Yes

Available as generic Yes

INFORMATION FOR USERS

Your drug prescription is tailored for you. Do not alter dosage without checking with your doctor.

How taken/used

Tablets.

Frequency and timing of doses
Once daily at night.

Adult dosage range
10–40mg daily, changed after intervals of at least 4 weeks.

Onset of effect
Within 2 weeks. Full beneficial effect may be felt within 4 weeks.

Duration of action
24 hours.

Diet advice
A low-fat diet is usually recommended.

Storage
Keep in original container at room temperature out of the reach of children. Protect from light.

Missed dose
Take as soon as you remember. If your next dose is due within 8 hours, do not take the missed dose, but take the next dose as usual.

Stopping the drug
Do not stop taking the drug without consulting your doctor; stopping the drug may lead to worsening of the underlying condition.

Exceeding the dose
An occasional unintentional extra dose is unlikely to cause problems. Large overdoses may cause liver problems. Notify your doctor.

SPECIAL PRECAUTIONS

Be sure to tell your doctor if:
- You have had liver or kidney problems.
- You have had side effects on your muscles from any other lipid-lowering drugs.
- You have an underactive thyroid.
- You have galactose intolerance.
- You are taking other medicines

 Pregnancy
Not recommended. May affect fetal development. Inform your doctor if you are or plan to become pregnant.

 Breast-feeding
The drug passes into the breast milk and may affect the baby. Discuss with your doctor.

 Infants and children
Not recommended under 5 years. Reduced dose necessary in older children, under specialist advice.

 Over 60
No special problems.

 Driving and hazardous work
No special problems.

 Alcohol
Avoid excessive amounts. Alcohol may increase the risk of developing liver problems with this drug.

POSSIBLE ADVERSE EFFECTS

Most adverse effects are mild and usually disappear with time. You should report any muscle pains, tenderness, or weakness to your doctor straight away.

Symptom/effect	Frequency		Discuss with doctor		Stop taking drug now	Call doctor now
	Common	Rare	Only if severe	In all cases		
Abdominal pain	●		●			
Constipation/diarrhoea	●		●			
Nausea/flatulence	●		●			
Sleep disturbance/headache	●		●			
Rash		●		●	●	
Muscle pain/weakness		●		●	●	●
Jaundice		●		●	●	●

PROLONGED USE

Long-term use of pravastatin can affect liver function.

Monitoring Regular blood tests to check liver and muscle function are usually required.

INTERACTIONS

Antifungal drugs Taken with pravastatin, itraconazole, ketoconazole, and possibly other antifungal drugs may increase the risk of muscle damage.

Orlistat This drug increases the blood levels and toxicity of pravastatin.

Clarithromycin and erythromycin These drugs increase blood levels of pravastatin.

Other lipid-lowering drugs (fibrates) Taken with pravastatin, these drugs may increase the risk of muscle damage.

Ciclosporin and other immuno-suppressant drugs There is an increased risk of muscle damage if pravastatin is taken with these drugs. They are not usually prescribed together.

PREDNISOLONE

Brand names Deltacortril, Minims Prednisolone, Pevanti, Pred Forte, and others
Used in the following combined preparations Scheriproct

GENERAL INFORMATION

Prednisolone, a powerful corticosteroid, is used for a wide range of conditions, including some skin diseases, rheumatic disorders, allergic states, and certain blood disorders. It is used as eye drops to reduce inflammation in conjunctivitis or iritis, and may be given as an enema to treat inflammatory bowel disease. It is also prescribed with fludrocortisone for pituitary or adrenal gland disorders.

Prednisolone taken short term either by mouth or topically rarely causes serious side effects. However, long-term treatment with high doses can cause systemic effects, such as osteoporosis, fluid retention, indigestion, diabetes, hypertension, and acne. Enteric-coated tablets reduce the local effects of the drug on the stomach but not these systemic effects.

INFORMATION FOR USERS

Your drug prescription is tailored for you. Do not alter dosage without checking with your doctor.

How taken/used

Tablets, injection, suppositories, enema, foam, eye and ear drops.

Frequency and timing of doses
Tablets Usually once daily or on alternate days with food.
Eye/ear drops 2–4 x daily; more often initially.

Adult dosage range
Considerable variation. Follow your doctor's instructions.

Onset of effect
2–4 days.

Duration of action
12–72 hours.

Diet advice
A low-sodium diet may be recommended when the oral form of the drug is prescribed for extended periods. Follow the advice of your doctor.

Storage
Keep in original container at room temperature out of the reach of children. Protect from light.

Missed dose
Take as soon as you remember. If your next dose is due within 6 hours, take a single dose now and skip the next.

Stopping the drug
Do not stop the drug without consulting your doctor. Abrupt cessation of long-term treatment by mouth may be dangerous.

Exceeding the dose
An occasional unintentional extra dose is unlikely to be a cause for concern. But if you notice any unusual symptoms, or if a large overdose has been taken, notify your doctor.

POSSIBLE ADVERSE EFFECTS

Weight gain and mood changes or depression are common adverse effects. More serious effects occur only when high doses are taken by mouth for long periods; the risk increases with dose and duration of treatment. If taking regular tablets, you should avoid close contact with chickenpox, shingles, and measles and seek urgent medical attention if exposed.

Symptom/effect	Frequency		Discuss with doctor		Stop taking drug now	Call doctor now
	Common	Rare	Only if severe	In all cases		
Indigestion	●			●		
Acne	●			●		
Weight gain	●		●			
Muscle weakness		●		●		
Mood changes/depression	●			●		
Black/bloodstained faeces		●		●	●	●

INTERACTIONS

Anticonvulsant drugs Carbamazepine, phenytoin, and phenobarbital can reduce the effects of prednisolone.

Vaccines Serious reactions can occur if live vaccines are given with this drug. Discuss with your doctor.

Antihypertensive and antidiabetic drugs and insulin Larger doses may be needed when taken with prednisolone.

Ciclosporin and tacrolimus may reduce the dose of prednisolone required.

Non-steroidal anti-inflammatory drugs (NSAIDs) There is an increased risk of peptic ulcers when these drugs are taken with prednisolone.

SPECIAL PRECAUTIONS

Be sure to tell your doctor if:
- You have had a peptic ulcer.
- You have glaucoma.
- You have depression or a psychiatric illness.
- You have any infection or have had tuberculosis.
- You have diabetes or osteoporosis.
- You have high blood pressure.
- You have liver or kidney disease.
- You are taking other medicines.

 Pregnancy
No evidence of risk with eye or ear drops. Taken as tablets in low doses, harm to the fetus is unlikely. Discuss with your doctor.

 Breast-feeding
No evidence of risk with eye or ear drops. Taken by mouth, it passes into the breast milk, but at low doses adverse effects on the baby are unlikely. Discuss with your doctor.

 Infants and children
Only given when essential. Alternate-day dosing preferred to prevent growth retardation.

 Over 60
Increased likelihood of adverse effects. Reduced dose may be necessary.

 Driving and hazardous work
No known problems.

 Alcohol
Keep consumption low. Alcohol may increase the risk of peptic ulcers with prednisolone taken by mouth or injection.

Infection
Avoid exposure to chickenpox, shingles, or measles if you are on systemic treatment.

PROLONGED USE

Prolonged use by mouth can lead to diabetes, peptic ulcers, glaucoma, muscle weakness, osteoporosis, and growth retardation in children. Prolonged topical use may also lead to skin thinning. People on long-term treatment should carry a steroid card.

PROCHLORPERAZINE

Brand names Buccastem, Stemetil
Used in the following combined preparations None

GENERAL INFORMATION

Prochlorperazine was introduced in the late 1950s and belongs to a group of drugs called the phenothiazines, which act on the central nervous system.

In small doses, prochlorperazine controls nausea and vomiting, especially when they occur as the side effects of medical treatment by drugs or radiation, or of anaesthesia. It is available over the counter for nausea and vomiting associated with migraine. The drug is also used to treat the nausea that occurs with inner ear disorders such as vertigo. In large doses, it is sometimes used as an antipsychotic to reduce aggressiveness and suppress abnormal behaviour (see p.41). It thus minimizes and controls the abnormal behaviour of schizophrenia, mania, and other mental disorders. Prochlorperazine does not cure any of these diseases, but it helps to relieve symptoms.

INFORMATION FOR USERS

Your drug prescription is tailored for you. Do not alter the dosage without checking with your doctor.

How taken/used

Tablets, buccal tablets, liquid, injection.

Frequency and timing of doses
2–3 x daily.

Adult dosage range
Nausea and vomiting 20mg initially, then 5–10mg per dose (tablets); 12.5mg per dose (injection).
Mental illness 25–100mg daily. Larger doses may be given.

Onset of effect
Within 60 minutes (by mouth); 10–20 minutes (by injection).

Duration of action
3–6 hours.

Diet advice
None.

Storage
Keep in original container at room temperature out of the reach of children. Protect from light.

Missed dose
Take as soon as you remember. If your next dose is due within 2 hours, take a single dose now and skip the next.

Stopping the drug
Do not stop the drug without consulting your doctor; symptoms may recur.

Exceeding the dose
An occasional unintentional extra dose is unlikely to be a cause for concern. Large overdoses may cause unusual drowsiness and may affect the heart. Notify your doctor.

SPECIAL PRECAUTIONS

Be sure to tell your doctor if:
- You have heart problems.
- You have liver or kidney problems.
- You have had epileptic seizures.
- You have Parkinson's disease.
- You have dementia.
- You have prostate problems.
- You have glaucoma.
- You are taking other medicines.

Pregnancy
Safety in pregnancy not established. Discuss with your doctor.

Breast-feeding
The drug passes into the breast milk and may affect the baby. Discuss with your doctor.

Infants and children
Not recommended in infants weighing less than 10kg and young children. Reduced dose necessary in older children due to increased risk of adverse effects.

Over 60
Increased likelihood of adverse effects. Reduced dose may therefore be necessary.

Driving and hazardous work
Avoid such activities until you have learned how prochlorperazine affects you because it can cause drowsiness and reduced alertness.

Alcohol
Avoid. Alcohol may increase and prolong the sedative effects of this drug.

POSSIBLE ADVERSE EFFECTS

Prochlorperazine has a strong anticholinergic effect, which can cause a variety of minor symptoms that often become less marked with time. The most significant adverse effect with high doses is tremor and muscle rigidity of the face and limbs (parkinsonism) caused by changes in the balance of brain chemicals.

Symptom/effect	Frequency		Discuss with doctor		Stop taking drug now	Call doctor now
	Common	Rare	Only if severe	In all cases		
Drowsiness/lethargy	●		●			
Dry mouth/constipation	●		●			
Dizziness/fainting	●			●		
Parkinsonism	●			●		
Rash		●		●	●	
Jaundice		●		●	●	
Abnormal facial/eye movements		●		●	●	●

INTERACTIONS

Sedatives All drugs with a sedative effect are likely to increase the sedative effects of prochlorperazine.

Drugs for Parkinson's disease Prochlorperazine may block the beneficial effect of these drugs.

Anticholinergic drugs Prochlorperazine may increase the side effects of these drugs.

Antihypertensive drugs Prochlorperazine can increase the effects of these drugs, especially doxazosin.

PROLONGED USE

Use of this drug for more than a few months may lead to the development of involuntary, potentially irreversible, eye, mouth, and tongue movements (tardive dyskinesia). Occasionally, jaundice may occur.

Monitoring Periodic blood tests may be performed.

PROCYCLIDINE

Brand names Arpicolin, Kemadrin
Used in the following combined preparations None

GENERAL INFORMATION

Introduced in the 1950s, procyclidine is an anticholinergic drug used to treat Parkinson's disease. It is especially helpful in the early stages of the disorder for treating muscle tremor. It also helps to reduce excess salivation. However, procyclidine has little effect on the shuffling gait and slow muscle movements that characterize

Parkinson's disease. Procyclidine is also often used to treat drug-induced parkinsonism resulting from treatment with antipsychotic drugs.

The drug may cause various adverse effects (see below). However, these are rarely serious enough to warrant stopping the treatment.

QUICK REFERENCE

Drug group Drug for parkinsonism (p.43)

Overdose danger rating High

Dependence rating Low

Prescription needed Yes

Available as generic Yes

INFORMATION FOR USERS

Your drug prescription is tailored for you. Do not alter dosage without checking with your doctor.

How taken/used

Tablets, liquid, injection.

Frequency and timing of doses
2–3 x daily, preferably after meals. A further dose may be added at bedtime.

Adult dosage range
7.5–30mg daily, exceptionally up to 60mg daily. Dosage is determined individually in order to find the best balance between effective relief of symptoms and the occurrence of adverse effects.

Onset of effect
Within 30 minutes.

Duration of action
8–12 hours.

Diet advice
None.

Storage
Keep in original container at room temperature out of the reach of children.

Missed dose
Take as soon as you remember. If your next dose is due within 2 hours, take a single dose now and skip the next.

Stopping the drug
Do not stop the drug without consulting your doctor; symptoms may recur.

OVERDOSE ACTION

Seek immediate medical advice in all cases. Take emergency action if palpitations, seizures, or unconsciousness occur.

See Drug poisoning emergency guide (p.518).

POSSIBLE ADVERSE EFFECTS

The possible adverse effects of procyclidine are mainly the result of its anticholinergic action. Some of the more common symptoms, such as dry mouth, constipation, and blurred vision, may be overcome by adjustment in dosage. Nausea and vomiting, nervousness, and rash have occasionally been reported.

Symptom/effect	Frequency		Discuss with doctor		Stop taking drug now	Call doctor now
	Common	Rare	Only if severe	In all cases		
Dry mouth	●		●			
Constipation	●		●			
Drowsiness/dizziness	●		●			
Blurred vision	●			●		
Difficulty in passing urine	●			●		●
Nervousness/anxiety		●	●			
Confusion		●		●		
Rash		●	●			

INTERACTIONS

Anticholinergic and antihistamine drugs These drugs may increase the adverse effects of procyclidine.

Tricyclic antidepressants, paroxetine (but not other SSRI antidepressants), and antipsychotic drugs These drugs may increase the side effects of procyclidine.

SPECIAL PRECAUTIONS

Be sure to tell your doctor if:
- You have long-term liver or kidney problems.
- You have a personal or family history of glaucoma.
- You have high blood pressure.
- You have constipation.
- You have prostate or urinary tract problems.
- You are taking other medicines.

 Pregnancy
Safety in pregnancy not established. Discuss with your doctor.

 Breast-feeding
Safety in breast-feeding not established. Discuss with your doctor.

 Infants and children
Not recommended.

 Over 60
Increased risk of adverse effects. Reduced dose may be necessary.

 Driving and hazardous work
Avoid such activities until you have learned how procyclidine affects you because the drug can cause drowsiness, blurred vision, and mild confusion.

 Alcohol
Avoid. Alcohol may increase the sedative effect of this drug.

PROLONGED USE

Prolonged use of this drug may provoke the onset of glaucoma.

Monitoring Periodic eye examinations are usually advised.

PROGUANIL WITH ATOVAQUONE

Brand name Malarone, MaloffProtect
Used in the following combined preparation Not applicable

GENERAL INFORMATION

Proguanil is an antimalarial drug given to prevent the development of malaria. Microbial resistance to its effects can occur, and this has led to it being used in combination with other drugs.

Atovaquone is an antiprotozoal drug that is also active against the fungus *Pneumocystis jirovecii* (a cause of pneumonia in people who have poor immunity). Atovaquone is less useful on its own for malaria, but when it is combined with proguanil it rapidly treats the infection. The combination is also used for the prevention of malaria,

especially in areas where resistance to other drugs is present.

For prevention, you should start taking proguanil with atovaquone a day or two before travelling. Continue during your stay and for 7 days after you return. It is important to take other precautions, such as using an insect repellent at all times and a mosquito net at night. If you develop an illness or fever in the year after your return from a malarial zone, and especially in the first three months, go to your doctor immediately and tell the doctor where you have been.

QUICK REFERENCE

Drug group Antimalarial drug (p.95)
Overdose danger rating Medium
Dependence rating Low
Prescription needed Yes
Available as generic Yes

INFORMATION FOR USERS

Your drug prescription is tailored for you. Do not alter dosage without checking with your doctor.

How taken/used

Tablets.

Frequency and timing of doses
Prevention Once daily with food or a milky drink, at the same time each day. Start 1–2 days before travel and continue for period of stay (which should not exceed 28 days) and for 7 days after return.
Treatment Once daily for 3 days, with food or a milky drink.

Adult dosage range
Prevention 1 tablet.
Treatment 4 tablets.

Onset of effect
After 24 hours.

Duration of action
24–48 hours.

Diet advice
None.

Storage
Keep in original container at room temperature out of the reach of children.

Missed dose
Take as soon as you remember. If your next dose is due at this time, take both doses together.

Stopping the drug
Do not stop taking the drug for 1 week after leaving a malaria-infected area, otherwise there is a risk that you may develop the disease.

Exceeding the dose
An occasional unintentional extra dose is unlikely to cause problems. Large overdoses may cause abdominal pain and vomiting. Notify your doctor.

SPECIAL PRECAUTIONS

Be sure to tell your doctor if:
- You have a long-term kidney problem.
- You have a liver problem.
- You currently have diarrhoea and vomiting.
- You are taking other medicines.

Pregnancy
Safety in pregnancy not established, although benefits are generally considered to outweigh risks. Folic acid supplements must be taken. Discuss with your doctor.

Breast-feeding
The drug passes into breast milk and may affect the baby. Breast-feeding is not recommended while you are taking the drug; it will not protect your baby from malaria. Discuss with your doctor.

Infants and children
Reduced dose necessary.

Over 60
No known problems.

Driving and hazardous work
Avoid such activities until you know how the drug affects you because it may cause dizziness.

Alcohol
No special problems.

PROLONGED USE

No known problems.

POSSIBLE ADVERSE EFFECTS

Adverse effects are generally fairly mild. The most frequent effects are headache, nausea, vomiting, and abdominal pain.

Symptom/effect	Frequency		Discuss with doctor		Stop taking drug now	Call doctor now
	Common	Rare	Only if severe	In all cases		
Diarrhoea	●		●			
Nausea/vomiting		●	●			
Abdominal pain/indigestion		●	●			
Mouth ulcers		●	●			
Hair loss		●		●		
Jaundice		●		●		
Rash	●			●		
Sore throat/fever		●		●		●

INTERACTIONS

Warfarin The effects of warfarin may be enhanced by proguanil with atovaquone.

Antacids The absorption of proguanil with atovaquone may be reduced by antacids.

Rifampicin, metoclopramide, and tetracycline antibiotics These drugs reduce the effect of proguanil with atovaquone.

PROMAZINE

Brand names None
Used in the following combined preparations None

GENERAL INFORMATION

Promazine, introduced in the late 1950s, belongs to a group of drugs called phenothiazines, which act on the brain to regulate abnormal behaviour.

The principal use of promazine is to calm agitated and restless behaviour. The drug is also given as a sedative for the short-term treatment of severe anxiety, especially anxiety occurring in older people and in those who have a terminal illness.

Promazine is less likely to cause the unpleasant side effects that are experienced with other phenothiazine drugs, particularly abnormal movements and shaking of the arms and legs (parkinsonism). The most common adverse effect of promazine is sedation.

INFORMATION FOR USERS

Your drug prescription is tailored for you. Do not alter dosage without checking with your doctor.

How taken/used

Tablets, liquid.

Frequency and timing of doses
4 x daily.

Adult dosage range
100–800mg daily (tablets).

Onset of effect
30 minutes–1 hour.

Duration of action
4–6 hours.

Diet advice
None.

Storage
Keep in original container at room temperature out of the reach of children. Protect from light.

Missed dose
Take as soon as you remember. If your next dose is due within 2 hours, take a single dose now and skip the next.

Stopping the drug
Do not stop the drug without consulting your doctor; symptoms may recur.

Exceeding the dose
An occasional unintentional extra dose is unlikely to be a cause for concern. Large overdoses may cause drowsiness, dizziness, unsteadiness, seizures, and coma. Notify your doctor.

POSSIBLE ADVERSE EFFECTS

The more common adverse effects of promazine, such as drowsiness, dry mouth, and blurred vision, may be helped by a reduction in dosage. Promazine may, rarely, affect the body's ability to regulate temperature (especially in older people).

Symptom/effect	Frequency		Discuss with doctor		Stop taking drug now	Call doctor now
	Common	Rare	Only if severe	In all cases		
Drowsiness/lethargy	●		●			
Dry mouth	●		●			
Constipation	●		●			
Blurred vision	●			●		
Mood changes		●	●			
Palpitations		●		●		
Parkinsonism		●		●		
Jaundice		●		●	●	

SPECIAL PRECAUTIONS

Be sure to tell your doctor if:
- You have heart problems.
- You have long-term liver or kidney problems.
- You have had epileptic seizures.
- You have prostate problems.
- You have glaucoma.
- You have Parkinson's disease.
- You have myasthenia gravis.
- You have phaeochromocytoma (a tumour of the adrenal glands).
- You are taking other medicines.

 Pregnancy
Safety in pregnancy not established. Discuss with your doctor.

 Breast-feeding
Safety in breast-feeding not established. Discuss with your doctor.

 Infants and children
Not recommended.

 Over 60
Increased likelihood of adverse effects. Reduced dose may therefore be necessary.

 Driving and hazardous work
Avoid such activities until you have learned how promazine affects you because the drug can cause drowsiness and reduced alertness.

 Alcohol
Avoid. Alcohol may increase the sedative effect of this drug.

Sunlight and sunbeds
Avoid exposure to strong sunlight because, rarely, skin reactions may occur.

INTERACTIONS

Sedatives All drugs that have a sedative effect are likely to increase the sedative properties of promazine.

Drugs for parkinsonism Promazine may reduce the effectiveness of these drugs and increase the risk of side effects when used together.

Sotalol increases the risk of heart rhythm abnormalities when used with promazine.

Lithium increases the risk of side effects when used with promazine.

Other antipsychotic drugs There is an increased risk of adverse effects when used with promazine; concurrent use should be avoided.

PROLONGED USE

Use of this drug for more than a few months may be associated with jaundice and abnormal movements. Sometimes a reduction in dose may be recommended.

Monitoring Periodic blood tests for liver function and a full blood count should be performed.

PROMETHAZINE

Brand names Avomine, Phenergan, Sominex
Used in the following combined preparations Night Nurse, Tixylix

GENERAL INFORMATION

Promethazine is one of a class of drugs known as the phenothiazines, which were developed in the 1950s for their beneficial effect on abnormal behaviour arising from mental illnesses (see Antipsychotics, p.41). However, it was found to have effects more like the antihistamines used to treat allergies (see p.82) and some types of nausea and vomiting (see Anti-emetics, p.46). The drug is widely used to reduce itching in a variety of skin conditions, including urticaria (hives), chickenpox, and eczema. It can also relieve nausea and vomiting caused by inner ear disturbances such as Ménière's disease and motion sickness. Due to its sedative effect, promethazine is sometimes used for short periods to induce sleep; it is also used to reduce agitation and is given as premedication before surgery.

Promethazine is used in combined preparations with opioid cough suppressants to relieve coughs and nasal congestion, and it is given at night for its sedative effect.

INFORMATION FOR USERS

Follow instructions on the label. Call your doctor if symptoms worsen.

How taken/used

Tablets, liquid, injection.

Frequency and timing of doses
Allergy 1–3 x daily or as a single dose at night. *Motion sickness* Bedtime on night before travelling, repeating following morning if necessary, then every 6–8 hours as necessary. *Nausea and vomiting* Every 4–6 hours as necessary.

Dosage range
Adults 25–100mg per dose depending on preparation and use. Allergy: usually 10mg. *Children* Reduced dose according to age.

Onset of effect
Within 1 hour. If dose is taken after nausea has started, the onset of effect is delayed.

Duration of action
8–16 hours.

Diet advice
None.

Storage
Keep in original container at room temperature out of the reach of children. Protect from light.

Missed dose
No cause for concern, but take as soon as you remember. Adjust the timing of your next dose accordingly.

Stopping the drug
Can be safely stopped as soon as symptoms disappear.

Exceeding the dose
An occasional unintentional extra dose is unlikely to cause problems. Large overdoses may cause drowsiness or agitation, seizures, hallucinations, unsteadiness, and coma. Notify your doctor.

POSSIBLE ADVERSE EFFECTS

Side effects are usually minor. More serious effects often occur only with long-term use or very high doses. They include photosensitivity; avoid bright sunlight while taking the drug.

Symptom/effect	Frequency		Discuss with doctor		Stop taking drug now	Call doctor now
	Common	Rare	Only if severe	In all cases		
Drowsiness/lethargy	●		●			
Dry mouth/blurred vision	●		●			
Urinary retention	●			●		
Palpitations		●		●		
Light-sensitive rash		●		●	●	
Swollen mouth/severe dizziness		●		●	●	●
Abnormal movements		●		●	●	

INTERACTIONS

Pregnancy urine test Promethazine may interfere with this test, giving a false result.

Skin-prick allergen tests Promethazine should be stopped a week before skin-prick testing with allergen extracts as it may produce a false result.

Sedatives All drugs that have a sedative effect are likely to increase the sedative properties of promethazine. Such drugs include alcohol, other antihistamines, benzodiazepines, opioid analgesics, and antipsychotics.

SPECIAL PRECAUTIONS

Be sure to consult your doctor or pharmacist before taking this drug if:
- You have liver or kidney problems.
- You have had epileptic seizures.
- You have heart disease.
- You have glaucoma.
- You have prostate problems.
- You have difficulty in passing urine.
- You are taking other medicines.

Pregnancy
The drug is probably safe in pregnancy, although safety has not been definitively established. Discuss with your doctor.

Breast-feeding
The drug passes into the breast milk, but at normal doses adverse effects on the baby are unlikely. Discuss with your doctor.

Infants and children
Not recommended for children under 6 years. Reduced dose necessary for older children.

Over 60
Reduced dose may be necessary.

Driving and hazardous work
Avoid such activities until you have learned how promethazine affects you because the drug can cause drowsiness.

Alcohol
Avoid. Alcohol may increase the sedative effects of this drug.

PROLONGED USE

Use of this drug for long periods is rarely necessary. There is also a risk that abnormal movements (extrapyramidal effects, tic-type movements, spasms) will develop with long-term use. Discuss with your doctor in all cases.

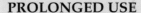

PROPRANOLOL

Brand name Bedranol
Used in the following combined preparations None

GENERAL INFORMATION

Propranolol, a non-cardioselective beta blocker, is mainly used to treat angina and abnormal heart rhythms and is helpful in controlling the symptoms of an overactive thyroid gland. It also helps to reduce the palpitations, sweating, and tremor of severe anxiety and to prevent migraine. The drug is also used to treat hypertension (high blood pressure) but this use is declining as more selective beta blockers are now available. Propranolol is not given to people with respiratory diseases (especially asthma) because it can cause breathing difficulties. It should be used with caution by people with diabetes because it affects the body's response to low blood sugar.

INFORMATION FOR USERS

Your drug prescription is tailored for you. Do not alter dosage without checking with your doctor.

How taken/used

Tablets, SR capsules, liquid, injection.

Frequency and timing of doses
2–4 x daily. Once daily (SR capsules).

Adult dosage range
Abnormal heart rhythms 30–160mg daily.
Angina 80–240mg daily.
Hypertension 160–320mg daily.
Migraine prevention; anxiety 40–160mg daily.

Onset of effect
1–2 hours (tablets); after 4 hours (SR capsules). In hypertension and migraine, it may be several weeks before full benefits are felt.

Duration of action
6–12 hours (tablets); up to 24 hours (SR capsules).

Diet advice
None.

Storage
Keep in original container at room temperature out of the reach of children. Protect from light.

Missed dose
Take as soon as you remember. If your next dose is due within 2 hours (tablets) or 12 hours (SR capsules), take a single dose now and skip the next.

Stopping the drug
Do not stop the drug without consulting your doctor. Stopping abruptly may lead to worsening of the underlying condition.

OVERDOSE ACTION

Seek immediate medical advice. Take emergency action if breathing difficulties, collapse, or loss of consciousness occur.

See Drug poisoning emergency guide (p.518).

SPECIAL PRECAUTIONS

Be sure to tell your doctor if:
- You have long-term liver or kidney problems.
- You have a breathing disorder such as asthma, bronchitis, or emphysema.
- You have heart problems.
- You have diabetes.
- You have psoriasis.
- You have poor circulation in the legs.
- You are taking other medicines.

 Pregnancy
May affect the baby. Discuss with your doctor.

 Breast-feeding
The drug passes into the breast milk, but at normal doses adverse effects on the baby are unlikely. Discuss with your doctor.

 Infants and children
Reduced dose necessary.

 Over 60
Increased risk of adverse effects. Reduced starting dose will therefore be necessary.

 Driving and hazardous work
Avoid such activities until you have learned how the drug affects you because it can cause dizziness.

 Alcohol
Avoid excessive intake. Alcohol may increase the blood-pressure-lowering effect of propranolol.

Surgery and general anaesthetics
Occasionally, propranolol may need to be stopped before you have a general anaesthetic but only do this after discussion with your doctor or dentist.

POSSIBLE ADVERSE EFFECTS

Propranolol's adverse effects are common to most beta blockers and tend to diminish with long-term use. Fainting may be a sign that the drug has slowed the heart beat excessively.

Symptom/effect	Frequency		Discuss with doctor		Stop taking drug now	Call doctor now
	Common	Rare	Only if severe	In all cases		
Lethargy/fatigue	●			●		
Cold hands and feet	●			●		
Nausea/vomiting		●		●		
Nightmares/vivid dreams		●		●		
Visual disturbances		●		●	●	
Fainting/palpitations		●		●	●	●
Breathlessness/wheeze		●		●	●	●

INTERACTIONS

Calcium channel blockers may cause low blood pressure, a slow heart beat, and heart failure if used with propranolol.

Non-steroidal anti-inflammatory drugs (NSAIDs) (e.g. indometacin) may reduce the antihypertensive effect of propranolol.

Theophylline/aminophylline Propranolol may increase blood levels of these drugs.

Antihypertensive drugs Propranolol may enhance the blood-pressure-lowering effect.

Cimetidine may increase the effects of propranolol.

Cardiac glycosides may increase the heart-slowing effect of propranolol.

PROLONGED USE

No problems expected.

PROPYLTHIOURACIL

Brand names None
Used in the following combined preparations None

GENERAL INFORMATION

Propylthiouracil is an antithyroid drug that suppresses formation of thyroid hormones and is used to manage overactivity of the thyroid gland (hyperthyroidism). In Graves' disease (the most common cause of hyperthyroidism) a course of propylthiouracil alone or combined with thyroxine ("block and replace" therapy) – usually given for 6–18 months – may cure the disorder. In other conditions, propylthiouracil is given until other treatments, such as surgery or radioiodine, take effect. If other treatments are not possible or are declined by the patient,

propylthiouracil can be given long term. It is the treatment of choice for hyperthyroidism in the first trimester of pregnancy. The full effect of the drug may take several weeks, and beta blockers may be given during this period to control symptoms.

The most important adverse effect is a reduction in white blood cells (agranulocytosis), increasing the risk of infection. Although this is rare, if you develop a sore throat, mouth ulcers, or a fever, you should see your doctor immediately to have your white blood cell count checked.

QUICK REFERENCE

Drug group Drug for thyroid disorders (p.102)
Overdose danger rating Medium
Dependence rating Low
Prescription needed Yes
Available as generic Yes

INFORMATION FOR USERS

Your drug prescription is tailored for you. Do not alter dosage without consulting your doctor.

How taken/used

Tablets.

Frequency and timing of doses
1–3 x daily.

Dosage range
Initially 200–400mg daily. Usually the dose can be reduced to 50–150mg daily.

Onset of effect
10–20 days. Full beneficial effects may not be felt for 6–10 weeks.

Duration of action
6–8 hours.

Diet advice
Your doctor may advise you to avoid foods that are high in iodine (see p.437).

Storage
Keep in original container at room temperature out of the reach of children. Protect from light.

Missed dose
Take as soon as you remember. If your next dose is due within 3 hours, take a single dose now and skip the next.

Stopping the drug
Do not stop the drug without consulting your doctor; stopping the drug may lead to a recurrence of hyperthyroidism.

Exceeding the dose
An occasional unintentional extra dose is unlikely to cause problems. Large overdoses may cause nausea, vomiting, and headache. Notify your doctor.

SPECIAL PRECAUTIONS

Be sure to tell your doctor if:
- You have long-term liver or kidney problems.
- You are pregnant.
- You are taking other medicines.

Pregnancy
Prescribed with caution. Risk of goitre and thyroid hormone deficiency (hypothyroidism) in the newborn infant if too high a dose is used. Discuss with your doctor.

Breast-feeding
The drug passes into the breast milk and may affect the baby. Discuss with your doctor.

Infants and children
Not recommended under 6 years. Reduced dose necessary in older children.

Over 60
No special problems.

Driving and hazardous work
No problems expected.

Alcohol
No known problems.

POSSIBLE ADVERSE EFFECTS

The most important side effect is a rare life-threatening reduction in white blood cells (agranulocytosis). This may be indicated by a sore throat or fever and should be reported to your doctor immediately.

Symptom/effect	Frequency		Discuss with doctor		Stop taking drug now	Call doctor now
	Common	Rare	Only if severe	In all cases		
Nausea/vomiting	●		●			
Joint pain	●			●		
Headache	●			●		
Rash	●			●		
Unusual bruising/bleeding		●		●		
Jaundice/dark urine/light faeces		●		●	●	●
Sore throat/fever/mouth ulcers		●		●	●	●

INTERACTIONS

Anticoagulants Propylthiouracil may reduce the effects of oral anticoagulants.

PROLONGED USE

Propylthiouracil may rarely cause a reduction in the number of white blood cells. There is also a small risk of liver failure, so a blood count may be done and liver function may be checked before starting treatment. A blood count and blood clotting tests may also be carried out before any surgical procedure.

Monitoring Periodic tests of thyroid function are usually required. If you have a sore throat, fever, or mouth ulcers, your white blood cell count must be checked.

PYRIDOSTIGMINE

Brand name Mestinon
Used in the following combined preparations None

GENERAL INFORMATION

Pyridostigmine is used in the treatment of myasthenia gravis (see p.79), an autoimmune disease involving faulty transmission of nerve impulses to the muscles. Pyridostigmine improves muscle strength by prolonging nerve signals, although it does not cure the disease. In severe cases, it may be prescribed with corticosteroids or other drugs. Pyridostigmine may also be used to reverse temporary paralysis of the bowel and urinary retention following surgical operations.

Cholinergic side effects (see p.35), such as nausea, abdominal cramps, increased salivation, sweating, and diarrhoea, usually disappear after reducing the dosage of pyridostigmine, although occasionally an anticholinergic drug such as propantheline is needed to counteract these effects.

QUICK REFERENCE

Drug group Drug for myasthenia gravis (p.79)

Overdose danger rating High

Dependence rating Low

Prescription needed Yes

Available as generic Yes

INFORMATION FOR USERS

Your drug prescription is tailored for you. Do not alter dosage without checking with your doctor.

How taken/used

Tablets.

Frequency and timing of doses
Every 3–4 hours initially. Thereafter, according to the needs of the individual.

Dosage range
Adults 300mg–1.2g daily (by mouth) according to response and side effects.
Children Reduced dose necessary according to age and weight.

Onset of effect
30–60 minutes.

Duration of action
3–6 hours.

Diet advice
None.

Storage
Keep in original container at room temperature out of the reach of children. Protect from light.

Missed dose
Take as soon as you remember. If your next dose is due within 2 hours, take a single dose now and skip the next.

Stopping the drug
Do not stop the drug without consulting your doctor; symptoms may recur.

OVERDOSE ACTION

Seek immediate medical advice in all cases. You may experience severe abdominal cramps, vomiting, weakness, and tremor. Take emergency action if troubled breathing, unusually slow heart beat, seizures, or loss of consciousness occur.

See Drug poisoning emergency guide (p.518).

SPECIAL PRECAUTIONS

Be sure to tell your doctor if:
- You have asthma.
- You have a long-term kidney problem.
- You have heart problems.
- You have an overactive thyroid gland.
- You have had epileptic seizures.
- You have difficulty in passing urine.
- You have a peptic ulcer.
- You have Parkinson's disease.
- You are taking other medicines.

 Pregnancy
No evidence of risk to the developing fetus in the first 6 months. Large doses near the time of delivery may cause premature labour and temporary muscle weakness in the baby. Discuss with your doctor.

 Breast-feeding
No evidence of risk, but the baby should be monitored for signs of muscle weakness.

 Infants and children
Reduced dose necessary, calculated according to age and weight.

 Over 60
Reduced dose may need to be given. Increased likelihood of adverse effects.

 Driving and hazardous work
Your underlying condition may make such activities inadvisable. Discuss with your doctor.

 Alcohol
No special problems.

Surgery and general anaesthetics
Pyridostigmine interacts with some anaesthetics. Discuss with your doctor, dentist, or anaesthetist before any surgery.

POSSIBLE ADVERSE EFFECTS

Adverse effects of pyridostigmine are usually dose-related and can be avoided by adjusting the dose. Too large a dose can, paradoxically, increase muscle weakness. In rare cases, hypersensitivity may occur, leading to an allergic skin rash.

Symptom/effect	Frequency		Discuss with doctor		Stop taking drug now	Call doctor now
	Common	Rare	Only if severe	In all cases		
Nausea/vomiting	●		●			
Increased salivation	●		●			
Sweating	●		●			
Abdominal cramps/diarrhoea	●			●		
Watering eyes/small pupils		●		●		
Muscle twitching/weakness		●		●		●
Rash		●		●		

INTERACTIONS

General note Drugs that suppress the transmission of nerve signals may oppose the effect of pyridostigmine. Such drugs include aminoglycoside antibiotics, clindamycin, digoxin, procainamide, quinidine, lithium, and chloroquine.

Propranolol may decrease the effectiveness of pyridostigmine.

PROLONGED USE

Pyridostigmine has been implicated in "Gulf War syndrome" when taken for long periods. However, there is no evidence of this occurring when the drug is used in people with myasthenia gravis.

PYRIMETHAMINE

Brand name Daraprim
Used in the following combined preparation Fansidar

GENERAL INFORMATION

Pyrimethamine is a drug used to treat protozoal infections, which include malaria. Because malaria parasites have developed resistance to pyrimethamine, the drug is now always given combined with the antibacterial drug sulfadoxine (Fansidar) and artesunate for the treatment of falciparum malaria. The activity of the combination greatly exceeds that of any of the drugs used alone. Pyrimethamine is not used for the prevention of malaria. Pyrimethamine is also given with another drug, sulfadiazine, to treat toxoplasmosis in people who have lowered immunity. Such treatment must be supervised by an expert.

Blood disorders can sometimes arise during prolonged treatment with pyrimethamine, and, because of this, blood counts are monitored regularly and vitamin supplements are given.

QUICK REFERENCE

Drug group Antiprotozoal drug (p.94) and antimalarial drug p.95)

Overdose danger rating Medium

Dependence rating Low

Prescription needed Yes

Available as generic No

INFORMATION FOR USERS

Your drug prescription is tailored for you. Do not alter dosage without checking with your doctor.

How taken/used

Tablets.

Frequency and timing of doses
Once only, daily, or weekly, depending on condition being treated.

Dosage range
Adults Depends on condition being treated.
Children Reduced dose according to age.

Onset of effect
24 hours.

Duration of action
Up to 1 week.

Diet advice
Ensure adequate fluid intake with the drug.

Storage
Keep in original container at room temperature out of the reach of children. Protect from light.

Missed dose
If you are being treated for toxoplasmosis, take as soon as you remember. If your next dose is due within 24 hours, take a single dose now and alter the dosing day so that your next dose is 1 week later.

Stopping the drug
Do not stop taking the drug without discussing it with your doctor.

Exceeding the dose
An occasional unintentional extra dose is unlikely to cause problems. Large overdoses may cause trembling, breathing difficulty, seizures, blood disorders, and vomiting. Notify your doctor.

POSSIBLE ADVERSE EFFECTS

Pyrimethamine can cause blood disorders, signs of which include tiredness, weakness, bleeding, bruising, and sore throat. Notify your doctor promptly if these occur. Breathing difficulties or signs of chest infection should be reported to your doctor immediately.

Symptom/effect	Frequency		Discuss with doctor		Stop taking drug now	Call doctor now
	Common	Rare	Only if severe	In all cases		
Headache	●		●			
Loss of appetite		●	●			
Insomnia		●	●			
Gastric irritation		●		●		
Rash		●		●		
Unusual bleeding/bruising		●		●		●
Sore throat/fever		●		●		●
Breathing problems		●		●		●
Seizures		●		●	●	●

INTERACTIONS

General note Drugs that suppress the bone marrow or cause folic acid deficiency may increase the risk of serious blood disorders if taken with pyrimethamine. These include anticancer drugs, antirheumatics, phenytoin, sulfasalazine, methotrexate, co-trimoxazole, trimethoprim, and phenylbutazone.

Lorazepam may cause liver damage when taken with pyrimethamine.

Alemtuzumab and anakinra can both increase the risk of bone marrow suppression with pyrimethamine.

SPECIAL PRECAUTIONS

Be sure to tell your doctor if:
- You have long-term liver or kidney problems.
- You have had epileptic seizures
- You have anaemia.
- You are allergic to sulfonamides.
- You have glucose-6-phosphate dehydrogenase (G6PD) deficiency.
- You are taking other medicines.

Pregnancy
Pyrimethamine may cause folic acid deficiency in the fetus, and its use is therefore generally avoided in the first trimester. Pregnant women receiving this drug should take a folic acid supplement. Discuss with your doctor.

Breast-feeding
The drug enters the breast milk and should be avoided with breast-feeding, especially if combined with sulfonamide drugs.

Infants and children
Reduced dose necessary.

Over 60
No special problems.

Driving and hazardous work
Problems are unlikely, but the drug may sometimes cause dizziness. If it does so, driving and hazardous activities should be avoided.

Alcohol
No known problems.

Sunlight and sunbeds
Avoid excessive exposure to sunlight.

PROLONGED USE

Prolonged use may cause folic acid deficiency, leading to serious blood disorders. Folic acid supplements may be recommended (in the form of folinic acid).

Monitoring Regular blood cell counts are required during high-dose or long-term treatment.

QUETIAPINE

Brand names Alaquet, Atrolak, Biquelle, Brancico, Mintreleq, Psyquet, Qethartic, Seroquel
Used in the following combined preparations None

GENERAL INFORMATION

Quetiapine is an atypical antipsychotic drug prescribed for the treatment of schizophrenia as well as for mania and depression in bipolar affective disorder (manic-depression). It can be used to treat both "positive" symptoms (thought disorders, delusions, and hallucinations) and "negative" symptoms (blunted affect and emotional and social withdrawal in schizophrenia).

Older people excrete the drug up to 50 per cent more slowly than the usual adult rate. For this reason, they need to be prescribed much lower doses in order to avoid adverse effects.

INFORMATION FOR USERS

Your drug prescription is tailored for you. Do not alter dosage without checking with your doctor.

How taken/used

Tablets.

Frequency and timing of doses
2 x daily, or 1 x daily with slow-release tablets.

Adult dosage range
Schizophrenia 50mg daily (starting dose)
Mania 100mg daily (starting dose).
The dose is increased over several days (both). Usual range is 300–450mg daily, maximum 750mg daily (schizophrenia); 800mg (mania).

Onset of effect
1–7 days.

Duration of action
Up to 12 hours.

Diet advice
Avoid grapefruit juice, because it may increase the drug's effects (see Interactions, below).

Storage
Keep in original container at room temperature out of the reach of children.

Missed dose
Take as soon as you remember. If your next dose is due within 4 hours, take a single dose now and skip the next.

Stopping the drug
Do not stop the drug without consulting your doctor; symptoms may recur.

Exceeding the dose
An occasional unintentional extra dose is unlikely to cause problems. Large overdoses may cause unusual drowsiness, palpitations, and low blood pressure. Notify your doctor.

POSSIBLE ADVERSE EFFECTS

Unusual drowsiness and weight gain are common adverse effects of quetiapine.

Constipation, dry mouth, urinary retention, and erectile dysfunction are also common.

Symptom/effect	Frequency		Discuss with doctor		Stop taking drug now	Call doctor now
	Common	Rare	Only if severe	In all cases		
Unusual drowsiness	●		●			
Weight gain/increased appetite	●		●			
Indigestion/constipation	●		●			
Dizziness/fainting	●			●		
Restlessness		●	●			
Stuffy nose/sore throat		●		●		
Breast swelling/irregular periods		●		●		
Palpitations		●		●		

INTERACTIONS

Anticonvulsants Quetiapine may oppose the effect of these drugs. However, phenytoin and carbamazepine may also reduce the effects of quetiapine.

Sedatives All drugs that have a sedative effect on the central nervous system, including alcohol, are likely to increase the sedative properties of quetiapine.

Erythromycin, clarithromycin, ketoconazole, and fluconazole These drugs may increase the effects of quetiapine.

Grapefruit juice may increase the blood levels and thus the effects of quetiapine.

Protease inhibitors These drugs for HIV/AIDS may increase the blood levels and effects of quetiapine.

SPECIAL PRECAUTIONS

Be sure to tell your doctor if:
- You have epilepsy.
- You have diabetes.
- You have liver or kidney problems.
- You have heart problems.
- You have low blood pressure.
- You have bladder problems.
- You have suicidal thoughts.
- You are taking other medicines.

Pregnancy
Safety not established. Discuss with your doctor.

Breast-feeding
Safety not established. Discuss with your doctor.

Infants and children
Not recommended.

Over 60
Reduced doses necessary. Older people eliminate quetiapine more slowly than younger adults.

Driving and hazardous work
Avoid such activities until you have learned how quetiapine affects you; the drug can cause drowsiness.

Alcohol
Avoid. Alcohol increases the sedative effects of this drug.

PROLONGED USE

Prolonged use of quetiapine may rarely cause tardive dyskinesia, in which there are involuntary movements of the tongue and face. There is also an increased risk of significant weight gain, developing diabetes, and raised blood lipid levels. With long-term use in older patients, quetiapine also carries a greater risk of stroke than some other antipsychotic drugs.

QUININE

Brand name None
Used in the following combined preparations None

GENERAL INFORMATION

Quinine was the earliest antimalarial drug. It often causes side effects but is still given for cases of malaria that are resistant to safer treatments. Due to the resistance of malaria parasites to some of the newer antimalarials, quinine remains the mainstay of treatment, but it is not used as a preventative. It is sometimes given together with an additional drug such as doxycycline or clindamycin for malaria. At the high doses used to treat malaria, quinine may cause ringing in the ears, headaches, nausea, hearing loss, and blurred vision: a group of symptoms known as cinchonism. In rare cases, it may cause bleeding problems.

Quinine is also occasionally used to treat night-time leg cramps, although its effectiveness is limited.

INFORMATION FOR USERS

Your drug prescription is tailored for you. Do not alter dosage without checking with your doctor.

How taken/used

Tablets, oral suspension, injection.

Frequency and timing of doses
Malaria Every 8 hours for 7 days.
Muscle cramps Once daily at bedtime.

Adult dosage range
Malaria 1.8g daily.
Muscle cramps 200–300mg daily.

Onset of effect
1–2 days (malaria); up to 4 weeks (cramps).

Duration of action
Up to 24 hours.

Diet advice
None.

Storage
Keep in original container at room temperature out of the reach of children. Protect from light.

Missed dose
Take as soon as you remember. If your next dose is due within 4 hours, skip the missed one and return to your normal dosing schedule thereafter.

Stopping the drug
If prescribed for malaria, take the full course. Even if you feel better, the original infection may still be present and may recur if treatment is stopped too soon. If taken for muscle cramps, the drug can safely be stopped as soon as you no longer need it.

OVERDOSE ACTION

 Seek immediate medical advice in all cases. Take emergency action if breathing problems, seizures, or loss of consciousness occur.

See Drug poisoning emergency guide (p.518).

POSSIBLE ADVERSE EFFECTS

Adverse effects are unlikely with low doses. At antimalarial doses, hearing disturbances, headache, and blurred vision are more common. Nausea and diarrhoea may occur.

Symptom/effect	Frequency		Discuss with doctor		Stop taking drug now	Call doctor now
	Common	Rare	Only if severe	In all cases		
Nausea/vomiting/diarrhoea	●			●		
Headache	●			●		
Ringing in ears/giddiness	●			●		
Rash/itching	●			●	●	●
Loss of hearing/blurred vision	●			●	●	●
Bruising/excessive bleeding	●			●	●	●

INTERACTIONS

Digoxin and flecainide Quinine increases blood levels of these drugs; the dose of digoxin should be reduced. Discuss with your doctor.

Ciclosporin Quinine may reduce the blood level of this drug. Discuss with your doctor.

Cimetidine This drug increases the blood levels of quinine.

Amiodarone and moxifloxacin These drugs should not be used with quinine as this can lead to heart rhythm irregularities.

SPECIAL PRECAUTIONS

Be sure to consult your doctor if:
- You have heart problems, especially rhythm disturbances.
- You have a long-term kidney problem.
- You have tinnitus (ringing in the ears).
- You have optic neuritis.
- You have myasthenia gravis.
- You have glucose-6-phosphate dehydrogenase (G6PD) deficiency.
- You have diabetes.
- You are taking other medicines.

 Pregnancy
Not usually prescribed. May cause defects in the unborn baby. Discuss with your doctor.

 Breast-feeding
The drug passes into the breast milk, but at normal doses adverse effects on the baby are unlikely. Discuss with your doctor.

 Infants and children
Reduced dose necessary.

 Over 60
No special problems.

 Driving and hazardous work
Avoid these activities until you know how quinine affects you because the drug may cause side effects such as visual disturbances and vertigo.

Alcohol
No known problems.

PROLONGED USE

Prolonged use of quinine can cause blood disorders. When quinine is used for night cramps, treatment should be reviewed after 4 weeks and stopped if the drug is producing no improvement. If the drug is continued, treatment should be reviewed every 3 months.

RABEPRAZOLE

Brand name Pariet
Used in the following combined preparations None

GENERAL INFORMATION

Rabeprazole belongs to a class of anti-ulcer drugs known as proton pump inhibitors (see p.67). Because the drug inhibits the secretion of gastric acid, it is used to treat gastro-oesophageal reflux disease (GORD), also called heartburn, and to help prevent it from recurring. It can also be used in the treatment of Zollinger-Ellison syndrome (a condition in which the stomach produces extremely large amounts of acid).

Rabeprazole is used to treat active duodenal and peptic ulcers by protecting them from the action of stomach acid, allowing them to heal. The drug is also used in combination with antibiotics to eradicate the *Helicobacter pylori* bacterium in patients with peptic ulcer disease. Rabeprazole is occasionally prescribed to people who experience the gastrointestinal adverse effects associated with non-steroidal anti-inflammatory drugs (NSAIDs) but need to continue NSAID treatment.

INFORMATION FOR USERS

Your drug prescription is tailored for you. Do not alter dosage without checking with your doctor.

How taken/used

Tablets.

Frequency and timing of doses
Once daily, generally in the morning, before food. Swallow whole; do not crush or chew.

Adult dosage range
Adult dosage 10–20mg.
Zollinger-Ellison syndrome 60–120mg.

Onset of effect
2–3 hours. Pain should improve in 2–3 days.

Duration of action
Up to 48 hours.

Diet advice
None, although spicy foods and alcohol may exacerbate the condition being treated.

Storage
Keep in original container at room temperature out of the reach of children.

Missed dose
Take as soon as you remember, then return to your normal dosing schedule. Do not take an extra dose to make up.

Stopping the drug
The drug can be safely stopped as soon as you no longer need it.

Exceeding the dose
An occasional unintentional extra dose is unlikely to be a cause for concern. However, if you notice any unusual symptoms, or if a large overdose has been taken, notify your doctor.

POSSIBLE ADVERSE EFFECTS

Most common adverse effects of rabeprazole are mild and usually clear up without the need to discontinue treatment.

Symptom/effect	Frequency		Discuss with doctor		Stop taking drug now	Call doctor now
	Common	Rare	Only if severe	In all cases		
Headache	●		●			
Diarrhoea	●		●			
Abdominal pain	●		●			
Flatulence	●		●			
Insomnia	●		●			
Cough/bronchitis/sinusitis	●			●		

INTERACTIONS

Itraconazole and ketoconazole Rabeprazole reduces the effects of these drugs.

Digoxin Rabeprazole may increase the effects of digoxin.

Clopidogrel The antiplatelet effect of clopidogrel may be reduced by rabeprazole.

Warfarin Rabeprazole may increase the anticoagulant effect of warfarin.

Atazanavir Rabeprazole can reduce the blood levels of atazanavir, and the two drugs should not be used together.

SPECIAL PRECAUTIONS

Be sure to tell your doctor if:
- You are allergic to other proton pump inhibitors.
- You think you might be pregnant or you are breast-feeding.
- You have a history of liver disease.
- You are taking other medicines.

 Pregnancy
Not prescribed. Safety not established.

 Breast-feeding
Not recommended. It is not known whether the drug passes into the breast milk. Discuss with your doctor.

 Infants and children
Not recommended.

 Over 60
No special problems.

 Driving and hazardous work
Do not undertake such activities until you have learned how rabeprazole affects you because the drug can cause drowsiness.

 Alcohol
Avoid. Alcohol irritates the stomach, which can lead to ulceration and acid reflux.

PROLONGED USE

Long-term use of rabeprazole may increase the risk of certain intestinal infections (such as *Salmonella* and *Clostridium difficile* infections) because of the loss of the natural protection against such infections provided by stomach acid. Prolonged use also increases the risk of hip fractures in women.

RALOXIFENE

Brand name Evista
Used in the following combined preparations None

GENERAL INFORMATION

Raloxifene is a non-steroidal anti-oestrogen drug (oestrogen is a naturally occurring female sex hormone, see p.105) that is related to clomifene and tamoxifen. It is prescribed to prevent bone fractures in postmenopausal women who are at increased risk of osteoporosis. It is not a first choice, but is recommended for women who cannot take other drugs for bone disorders.

Raloxifene has no beneficial effect on other menopausal problems such as hot flushes. It is not prescribed to women who might become pregnant because it may harm the unborn baby, and it is not prescribed to men.

There is an increased risk of a thrombosis (blood clot) developing in a vein in the leg, but the risk is similar to that from HRT (p.105). However, because of this risk, raloxifene is usually stopped if the woman taking it becomes immobile or bed-bound, when clots are more likely to form. Treatment is re-started when full activity is resumed.

INFORMATION FOR USERS

Your drug prescription is tailored for you. Do not alter dosage without checking with your doctor.

How taken/used

Tablets.

Frequency and timing of doses
Once daily.

Adult dosage range
60mg daily.

Onset of effect
1–4 hours.

Duration of action
24–48 hours.

Diet advice
Calcium supplements are recommended if dietary calcium is low.

Storage
Keep in original container at room temperature out of the reach of children. Protect from light.

Missed dose
Take as soon as you remember. If your next dose is due within 8 hours, take a single dose now and skip the next.

Stopping the drug
Do not stop the drug without consulting your doctor except under conditions specified in advance, such as immobility, which increases the risk of blood clots forming.

Exceeding the dose
An occasional unintentional extra dose is unlikely to be a cause for concern. But if you notice any unusual symptoms, or if a large overdose has been taken, notify your doctor.

SPECIAL PRECAUTIONS

Be sure to tell your doctor if:
- You have had a blood clot in a vein or a pulmonary embolism.
- You have vaginal bleeding.
- You have liver or kidney problems.
- You are taking other medicines.

 Pregnancy
Not prescribed to premenopausal women.

 Breast-feeding
Not prescribed to premenopausal women.

 Infants and children
Not prescribed.

 Over 60
No special problems.

 Driving and hazardous work
No special problems.

 Alcohol
No special problems.

POSSIBLE ADVERSE EFFECTS

Some adverse effects of raloxifene are indications of a thrombosis (blood clot) in a vein in the leg. If a clot occurs somewhere else in the body, there might not be any obvious symptoms.

Symptom/effect	Frequency		Discuss with doctor		Stop taking drug now	Call doctor now
	Common	Rare	Only if severe	In all cases		
Hot flushes	●		●			
Leg cramps	●		●			
Swollen ankles/feet	●		●			
Flu-like symptoms	●		●			
Headache		●		●		
Rash		●		●	●	
Leg pain/tenderness/swelling		●		●	●	●
Leg discoloration/ulceration		●		●	●	●

PROLONGED USE

Raloxifene is not normally used for longer than 5 years. It reduces the risk of some types of breast cancer, but this benefit has to be weighed against the increased risk of stroke and venous thrombosis.

Monitoring Liver function tests may be performed periodically.

INTERACTIONS

Anticoagulants Raloxifene reduces the effect of warfarin and acenocoumarol (nicoumalone).

Colestyramine This drug reduces the absorption of raloxifene by the body.

RAMIPRIL

Brand name Tritace
Used in the following combined preparations Triapin, Triapin mite

GENERAL INFORMATION

Ramipril belongs to the group of drugs known as ACE inhibitors. It works by reducing the production of substances that raise blood pressure, making the blood vessels relax and making it easier for the heart to pump blood. The drug is used to treat high blood pressure (p.60), to reduce strain on the heart in patients with heart failure after a heart attack, and to prevent future strokes and heart attacks in patients with established cardiovascular disease. It is also used to treat heart failure from other causes and to preserve kidney function in conditions such as diabetes mellitus. The first dose of an ACE inhibitor can cause blood pressure to drop suddenly, so a few hours' bed rest afterwards is advisable.

Side effects are usually mild. Like all ACE inhibitors, ramipril can cause the body to retain potassium. It can also cause a persistent dry cough.

INFORMATION FOR USERS

Your drug prescription is tailored for you. Do not alter dosage without checking with your doctor.

How taken/used

Tablets, capsules, oral solution.

Frequency and timing of doses
High blood pressure Usually once daily.
Heart failure or after heart attack 1–2 x daily

Adult dosage range
High blood pressure, heart failure, or after a heart attack 1.25–10mg daily.

Onset of effect
Within 2 hours; full beneficial effect may take several weeks.

Duration of action
Up to 24 hours.

Diet advice
Your doctor may advise you to decrease your salt intake to help control your blood pressure.

Storage
Keep in original container at room temperature out of the reach of children.

Missed dose
Take as soon as you remember. If your next dose is due within 6 hours, take a single dose now and skip the next. Subsequently, continue with your usual routine.

Stopping the drug
Do not stop taking the drug without consulting your doctor. Treatment of hypertension and heart failure is normally lifelong, so it may be necessary to substitute alternative therapy.

Exceeding the dose
If you notice any unusual symptoms or if a large overdose has been taken, notify your doctor.

POSSIBLE ADVERSE EFFECTS

Ramipril can cause a variety of side effects, but most are mild and transient. However, an irritating dry cough may persist and necessitate withdrawal of the drug. Rarely, ramipril may cause deterioration of kidney function, digestive tract disturbance, severe rash, or severe swelling of the face accompanied by breathing difficulties.

Symptom/effect	Frequency		Discuss with doctor		Stop taking drug now	Call doctor now
	Common	Rare	Only if severe	In all cases		
Rash	●			●		
Persistent dry cough	●			●		
Mouth ulcers/sore mouth		●		●		
Dizziness		●		●		
Sore throat/fever		●		●		
Swelling of mouth/lips		●		●	●	●
Breathing difficulty		●		●	●	●

INTERACTIONS

Non-steroidal anti-inflammatory drugs (NSAIDs) may reduce the blood-pressure-lowering effect of ramipril and increase the risk of kidney damage.

Potassium supplements and potassium-sparing diuretics may cause excess levels of potassium in the body.

Ciclosporin and tacrolimus increase the risk of high potassium levels in the blood.

Lithium Ramipril may cause raised blood lithium levels and toxicity.

Vasodilators, diuretics, and other antihypertensives may increase the blood-pressure-lowering effect of ramipril.

SPECIAL PRECAUTIONS

Be sure to tell your doctor if:
- You have long-term liver or kidney problems.
- You have heart problems.
- You have had angioedema or a previous allergic reaction to ACE inhibitors.
- You are taking other medicines.
- You are pregnant or intend to become pregnant.

 Pregnancy
Not prescribed. There is evidence of harm to the developing fetus.

 Breast-feeding
Safety not established. Discuss with your doctor.

 Infants and children
Not recommended.

 Over 60
Reduced dose may be necessary.

 Driving and hazardous work
Avoid such activities until you have learned how ramipril affects you because the drug can cause dizziness and fainting.

 Alcohol
Avoid. Alcohol may increase the blood-pressure-lowering and adverse effects of the drug.

Surgery and general anaesthetics
Ramipril may have to be stopped before you have a general anaesthetic. Discuss with your doctor or dentist before any operation.

PROLONGED USE

No problems expected.

Monitoring Periodic checks on potassium levels, white blood cell count, kidney function, and urine are usually performed.

RANITIDINE

Brand names Boots Heartburn Relief Tablets, Gavilast, Ranicalm, Zantac
Used in the following combined preparations None

GENERAL INFORMATION

Ranitidine is an anti-ulcer drug of the antihistamine (H$_2$) antagonist type (known as H$_2$ blockers). It reduces acid production by the stomach, allowing ulcers to heal, and is usually given in courses lasting four to eight weeks, with further courses if symptoms recur. In combination with antibiotics, ranitidine may be used for ulcers caused by *Helicobacter pylori* infection. It may also be used to protect against ulcers in people taking NSAIDs (see p.74), and to reduce the discomfort and ulceration of oesophagitis. In medical practice, ranitidine has been largely replaced by newer proton pump inhibitor anti-ulcer drugs, such as omeprazole. It is available over the counter for the short-term treatment of heartburn and indigestion in those over 16 years old.

Unlike the similar drug cimetidine, ranitidine does not increase blood levels of other drugs such as anticoagulants and anticonvulsants. Most people experience no serious side effects during treatment. As ranitidine promotes healing of the stomach lining, there is a risk that it might mask stomach cancer. It is therefore prescribed only when this possibility has been ruled out.

INFORMATION FOR USERS

Your drug prescription is tailored for you. Do not alter dosage without checking with your doctor. For over-the-counter preparations, follow the instructions and call your doctor if symptoms worsen.

How taken/used

Tablets, effervescent tablets, liquid, injection.

Frequency and timing of doses
Once daily at bedtime or 2–4 x daily.

Adult dosage range
150–600mg daily, depending on the condition being treated. Usual dose is 150mg twice daily.

Onset of effect
Within 1 hour.

Duration of action
12 hours.

Diet advice
None.

Storage
Keep in original container at room temperature out of the reach of children. Protect from light.

Missed dose
Take as soon as you remember. If your next dose is due within 3 hours, take a single dose now and skip the next.

Stopping the drug
Do not stop the drug without consulting your doctor; symptoms may recur.

Exceeding the dose
An occasional unintentional extra dose is unlikely to be a cause for concern. But if you notice any unusual symptoms, or if a large overdose has been taken, notify your doctor.

SPECIAL PRECAUTIONS

Be sure to consult your doctor or pharmacist before taking this drug if:
- You have long-term liver or kidney problems.
- You have porphyria.
- You are taking other medicines.

Pregnancy
Safety in pregnancy established over several decades of use. May be used in labour and during Caesarian section. Discuss with your doctor.

Breast-feeding
The drug passes into the breast milk, but there is no evidence that this is harmful to the baby.

Infants and children
Reduced dose necessary.

Over 60
In older and immunocompromised people, ranitidine may increase the risk of pneumonia.

Driving and hazardous work
Usually no problems. Dizziness can occur in a minority of patients.

Alcohol
Avoid. Alcohol may aggravate your underlying condition and reduce the beneficial effects of this drug.

POSSIBLE ADVERSE EFFECTS

The adverse effects of ranitidine, of which headache is the most common, are usually related to dosage level and almost always disappear when treatment finishes.

Symptom/effect	Frequency		Discuss with doctor		Stop taking drug now	Call doctor now
	Common	Rare	Only if severe	In all cases		
Headache/dizziness	●		●			
Nausea/vomiting		●	●			
Constipation		●	●			
Diarrhoea		●	●			
Jaundice		●		●		
Mental problems/agitation		●		●		
Sore throat/fever		●		●		●

PROLONGED USE

Long-term suppression of stomach acid secretion may increase the risk of some types of intestinal infection, such as with *Salmonella* and *Clostridium difficile*.

INTERACTIONS

Ketoconazole Ranitidine may reduce the absorption of ketoconazole. Ranitidine should be taken at least 2 hours after ketoconazole.

Glipizide Ranitidine may increase the absorption of glipizide.

Sucralfate High doses (2g) of sucralfate may reduce the absorption of ranitidine. Sucralfate should be taken at least 2 hours after ranitidine.

Theophylline/aminophylline Ranitidine may increase blood levels of these drugs.

REPAGLINIDE

Brand name Enyglid, Prandin
Used in the following combined preparations None

GENERAL INFORMATION

Repaglinide is a drug used to treat Type 2 diabetes that cannot be adequately controlled by diet and exercise alone. It acts in a similar manner to sulfonylurea drugs by stimulating the release of insulin from the pancreas. Therefore, some of the pancreatic cells need to be functioning in order for it to be effective.

Repaglinide is fast acting, but its effects last for only about four hours. The drug is sometimes given with metformin if that drug is not providing adequate diabetic control.

Repaglinide is best taken just before a meal in order for the insulin that is released to cope with the food. If a meal is likely to be missed, the dose of repaglinide should not be taken. If a tablet has been taken and a meal is not forthcoming, some carbohydrate (as specified by your doctor or dietitian) should be eaten as soon as possible.

QUICK REFERENCE

Drug group Drug for diabetes (p.100)

Overdose danger rating Medium

Dependence rating Low

Prescription needed Yes

Available as generic Yes

INFORMATION FOR USERS

Your drug prescription is tailored for you. Do not alter dosage without checking with your doctor.

How taken/used

Tablets.

Frequency and timing of doses
1–4 x daily (up to 30 minutes before a meal, and up to 4 meals a day). If you are going to miss a meal, do not take the tablet.

Adult dosage range
500mcg (starting dose), increased at intervals of 1–2 weeks according to response; 4–16mg daily (maintenance dose).

Onset of effect
15–30 minutes.

Duration of action
4–6 hours.

Diet advice
Follow the diet advised by your doctor or dietitian.

Storage
Keep in original container at room temperature out of the reach of children.

Missed dose
Do not take tablets between meals. Discuss with your doctor.

Stopping the drug
Do not stop taking the drug without consulting your doctor.

Exceeding the dose
An overdose will cause low blood sugar with faintness, dizziness, headache, confusion, sweating, or tremor. Notify your doctor.

SPECIAL PRECAUTIONS

Be sure to tell your doctor if:
- You have liver or kidney problems.
- You are taking other medicines.

 Pregnancy
Safety not established. Discuss with your doctor.

 Breast-feeding
Safety not established. Discuss with your doctor.

 Infants and children
Not recommended.

 Over 60
No special problems, but safety not established over 75 years.

 Driving and hazardous work
Avoid if low blood sugar without warning signs is likely.

 Alcohol
Avoid. Alcohol may upset diabetic control and may increase and prolong the effects of repaglinide.

POSSIBLE ADVERSE EFFECTS

Intestinal problems are common at the start of treatment with repaglinide. However, such adverse effects tend to become less troublesome as treatment continues.

Symptom/effect	Frequency		Discuss with doctor		Stop taking drug now	Call doctor now
	Common	Rare	Only if severe	In all cases		
Nausea/vomiting	●		●			
Abdominal pain	●		●			
Diarrhoea/constipation	●		●			
Hypoglycaemia	●		●			
Rash/itching		●			●	

PROLONGED USE

Repaglinide is usually prescribed indefinitely. No special problems.

Monitoring Periodic monitoring of control of blood glucose levels is necessary.

INTERACTIONS

Clarithromycin, itraconazole, ketoconazole, monoamine oxidase inhibitors (MAOIs), trimethoprim, gemfibrozil, ACE inhibitors, salicylates, non-steroidal anti-inflammatory drugs (NSAIDs), and ciclosporin These drugs may enhance and/or prolong the hypoglycaemic effect of repaglinide.

Beta blockers The symptoms of hypoglycaemia may be masked by these drugs, especially by non-cardioselective beta blockers (e.g. propranolol).

Oral contraceptives, thiazide diuretics, corticosteroids, thyroid hormones, danazol, sympathomimetics, rifampicin, barbiturates, and carbamazepine These drugs may decrease the effect of repaglinide.

RIFAMPICIN

Brand names Rifadin, Rimactane
Used in the following combined preparations Rifater, Rifinah, Voractiv

GENERAL INFORMATION

Rifampicin is an antibacterial drug that is highly effective for tuberculosis. Taken by mouth, it is widely distributed through body tissues including the brain. As a result, it is particularly useful in the treatment of tuberculous meningitis.

The drug is also used to treat leprosy and other serious infections, including brucellosis, Legionnaires' disease, and infections of the bone (osteomyelitis) and of the heart (endocarditis). In addition, it is given to anyone in close contact with meningococcal meningitis, to prevent infection. Rifampicin is always prescribed with other antibiotics or antituberculous drugs because of rapid resistance in some bacteria.

It significantly increases the liver's capacity to break down some drugs, and so reduces their effectiveness.

It may impart a harmless red-orange colour to urine, saliva, and tears, and soft contact lenses may become permanently stained.

QUICK REFERENCE

Drug group Antituberculous drug (p.90)

Overdose danger rating Medium

Dependence rating Low

Prescription needed Yes

Available as generic Yes

INFORMATION FOR USERS

Your drug prescription is tailored for you. Do not alter dosage without checking with your doctor.

How taken/used

Tablets, capsules, liquid, injection.

Frequency and timing of doses
1 x daily, 30 minutes before breakfast (leprosy, tuberculosis) or once a month (leprosy); 2 x daily (prevention of meningococcal meningitis); 2–4 x daily, 30 minutes before or 2 hours after meals (other serious infections).

Adult dosage range
According to weight; usually 450–600mg daily (tuberculosis, leprosy) or 600mg once a month (leprosy); 600mg–1.2g daily (other serious infections); 1.2g daily for 2 days (meningococcal meningitis).

Onset of effect
Over several days.

Duration of action
Up to 24 hours.

Diet advice
None.

Storage
Keep in original container at room temperature out of the reach of children. Protect from light.

Missed dose
Take as soon as you remember. If your next dose is due within 6 hours, take a single dose now, then return to normal dosing schedule.

Stopping the drug
Take the full course. Even if you feel better, the original infection may still be present and symptoms may recur if treatment is stopped too soon. In rare cases stopping the drug suddenly after high-dose treatment can lead to a severe flu-like illness.

Exceeding the dose
An occasional unintentional extra dose is unlikely to cause problems. Large overdoses may cause liver damage, nausea, vomiting, and lethargy. Notify your doctor immediately.

SPECIAL PRECAUTIONS

Be sure to tell your doctor if:
- You have a long-term liver or kidney problem.
- You have porphyria.
- You wear contact lenses.
- You are taking other medicines.

Pregnancy
Safety in pregnancy not established. Discuss with your doctor

Breast-feeding
The drug passes into the breast milk, but at normal doses adverse effects on the baby are unlikely. Discuss with your doctor.

Infants and children
Reduced dose necessary.

Over 60
Increased risk of adverse effects. Reduced dose may be necessary.

Driving and hazardous work
No problems expected.

Alcohol
Avoid excessive amounts. Heavy alcohol consumption may increase the risk of liver damage.

POSSIBLE ADVERSE EFFECTS

A harmless red-orange discoloration of body fluids normally occurs. Serious adverse effects are rare, but any jaundice should be reported to your doctor. Headache and breathing difficulties may occur after stopping high-dose treatment.

Symptom/effect	Frequency		Discuss with doctor		Stop taking drug now	Call doctor now
	Common	Rare	Only if severe	In all cases		
Nausea/vomiting/diarrhoea		●	●			
Muscle cramps/aches		●		●		
Rash/itching		●		●		
Jaundice		●		●		●
Flu-like illness		●		●	●	●
Easy bruising/bleeding		●		●	●	●

PROLONGED USE

Prolonged use of rifampicin may cause liver damage.

Monitoring Periodic blood tests may be performed to monitor liver function.

INTERACTIONS

General note Rifampicin may reduce the effectiveness of a wide variety of drugs, including oral contraceptives (in which case alternative contraceptive methods may be necessary), phenytoin, corticosteroids, oral antidiabetics, anti-arrhythmics, and warfarin-like anticoagulants. Dosage adjustment of these drugs may be necessary at the start or end of treatment with rifampicin. Consult your doctor or pharmacist for advice.

RISEDRONATE

Brand names Actonel, Actonel Once a Week
Used in the following combined preparation Actonel Combi

GENERAL INFORMATION

Risedronate belongs to a group of drugs called bisphosphonates. Used in the treatment of bone disorders such as Paget's disease, the drug works directly on the bones by increasing the amount of calcium they absorb, thereby making them stronger.

Risedronate is also used to prevent or treat osteoporosis in postmenopausal women. Taken as either a daily or a weekly dose, it reduces the risk of fractures of the hip or vertebrae. In addition, the drug is used to treat or prevent corticosteroid-induced osteoporosis.

To reduce the risk of gastrointestinal adverse effects, you should take risedronate first thing in the morning, on an empty stomach and in a standing position, and remain upright for at least 30 minutes afterwards. Risedronate should not be taken at bedtime.

QUICK REFERENCE

Drug group Drug for bone disorders (p.80)

Overdose danger rating Medium

Dependence rating Low

Prescription needed Yes

Available as generic Yes

INFORMATION FOR USERS

Your drug prescription is tailored for you. Do not alter dosage without checking with your doctor.

How taken/used

Tablets.

Frequency and timing of doses
Paget's disease Once daily (30mg dose).
Osteoporosis Once daily (5mg dose); once weekly, on the same day (35mg dose). Swallow whole with water, on rising and before food; or avoid food or drink for at least two hours before and after dose.

Adult dosage range
Paget's disease 30mg daily.
Osteoporosis 5mg daily; 35mg weekly.

Onset of effect
Within 1 month.

Duration of action
Some effects may persist for several weeks or months.

Diet advice
Avoid calcium-containing products (e.g. milk), vitamin and mineral supplements, and antacids for at least two hours before and after dose.

Storage
Keep in original container at room temperature out of the reach of children.

Missed dose
Take as soon as you remember. Then return to your original dosing schedule. Do not make up for the missed dose (weekly).

Stopping the drug
The drug can be safely stopped as soon as you no longer need it.

Exceeding the dose
An occasional unintentional dose is unlikely to cause problems. However, if you notice any unusual symptoms, or if a large overdose has been taken, drink a large glass of milk and notify your doctor.

SPECIAL PRECAUTIONS

Be sure to tell your doctor if:
- You have kidney problems.
- You have a history of peptic ulcers or stomach problems.
- You have low calcium levels in your blood.
- You are/may be pregnant or are planning a pregnancy.
- You are breast-feeding.
- You are unable to sit or stand upright for at least 30 minutes.
- You have had pain/difficulty in swallowing, or problems with your oesophagus.
- You are taking other medicines.

 Pregnancy
Not recommended.

 Breast-feeding
Not recommended.

 Infants and children
Not recommended.

 Over 60
No special problems.

 Driving and hazardous work
No special problems.

 Alcohol
Avoid. May cause further stomach irritation.

PROLONGED USE

In patients with Paget's disease, courses of treatment longer than 2 months are not usually prescribed but repeat courses may be required. When used to treat or prevent osteoporosis, risedronate may be taken safely long term.

Monitoring Your doctor may monitor your bone mineral density. Blood and urine tests may be carried out at intervals.

POSSIBLE ADVERSE EFFECTS

Most adverse effects of risedronate are mild to moderate and do not usually require the treatment to be stopped.

Symptom/effect	Frequency		Discuss with doctor		Stop taking drug now	Call doctor now
	Common	Rare	Only if severe	In all cases		
Nausea	●		●			
Diarrhoea/constipation	●		●			
Muscle pain	●		●			
Headache	●		●			
Abdominal pain	●			●		
New or worsening heartburn	●			●		
Jaw pain		●		●		
Difficulty/pain on swallowing		●		●	●	
Jaundice		●		●	●	
Allergic rash/itch/facial swelling		●		●	●	●

INTERACTIONS

Antacids, and products containing calcium or iron These reduce the absorption of risedronate and should be taken at a different time of day.

RISPERIDONE

Brand names Risperdal, Risperdal Consta, Risperdal Quicklet
Used in the following combined preparations None

GENERAL INFORMATION

Risperidone is used to treat people with acute psychiatric disorders and long-term psychotic illnesses, such as schizophrenia and mania. By blocking dopamine receptors in the brain, it helps to alleviate, although not cure, "positive" symptoms (such as hallucinations, thought disturbances, and hostility) and "negative" symptoms (such as emotional and social withdrawal). It may also help with the depression and anxiety that may occur with schizophrenia. Risperidone is an atypical antipsychotic drug. It is less likely than some other antipsychotics to cause sedation or movement disorders as a side effect. The drug can also be used for short-term treatment of severe aggression in people with dementia, and may be helpful in autism or Asperger's syndrome.

QUICK REFERENCE

Drug group Antipsychotic drug (p.41)

Overdose danger rating Medium

Dependence rating Low

Prescription needed Yes

Available as generic Yes

INFORMATION FOR USERS

Your drug prescription is tailored for you. Do not alter dosage without checking with your doctor.

How taken/used

Tablets, dispersible tablets, liquid, injection.

Frequency and timing of doses
1–2 x daily (tablets, liquid).

Adult dosage range
Tablets 2mg daily (starting dose) increasing to 4-6mg daily (usual maintenance dose); maximum 16mg daily.
Injection 25mg every 2 weeks (starting dose) increasing to 50mg every two weeks (maximum maintenance dose).

Onset of effect
Tablets Within 2–3 days, but may take up to 6 weeks before maximum effect is seen.
Injection Up to 3 weeks before onset of effect.

Duration of action
Approximately 2 days.

Diet advice
None.

Storage
Keep in original container at room temperature (tablets) or in a refrigerator (injection) out of the reach of children. Protect from light.

Missed dose
Take as soon as you remember. If your next dose is due within 3 hours, take a single dose now and skip the next.

Stopping the drug
Do not stop taking the drug without consulting your doctor; symptoms may recur.

Exceeding the dose
An occasional unintentional extra dose is unlikely to cause problems. If larger doses have been taken, notify your doctor.

SPECIAL PRECAUTIONS

Be sure to tell your doctor if:
- You have liver, kidney, or bladder problems.
- You have heart or circulation problems.
- You have diabetes or high blood lipid levels.
- You have had a stroke, deep vein thrombosis, or pulmonary embolism.
- You have epilepsy.
- You have Parkinson's disease.
- You have dementia.
- You are taking other medicines

Pregnancy
Short-term nervous system problems may occur in babies when the drug is taken in the third trimester. Discuss with your doctor.

Breast-feeding
The drug probably passes into breast milk. Discuss with your doctor.

Infants and children
Not recommended under 15 years.

Over 60
Reduced dose may be necessary.

Driving and hazardous work
Avoid such activities until you have learned how risperidone affects you because the drug may cause difficulty in concentrating and slowed reactions.

Alcohol
Avoid. Alcohol may increase the sedative effects of this drug.

PROLONGED USE

If used long term, permanent movement disorders (tardive dyskinesia) may occur, although they are less likely than with many other antipsychotic drugs. In patients with dementia, there may be an increased risk of stroke and death when taking risperidone. Risperidone may also lead to high levels of prolactin, which may stimulate breast tissue and change the pattern of menstrual periods.

POSSIBLE ADVERSE EFFECTS

Risperidone is generally well tolerated, with a low incidence of movement disorders. This drug is less sedating than some of the other antipsychotics.

Symptom/effect	Frequency		Discuss with doctor		Stop taking drug now	Call doctor now
	Common	Rare	Only if severe	In all cases		
Insomnia/anxiety/agitation	●		●			
Headache	●		●			
Difficulty in concentrating	●		●			
Weight gain	●		●			
Shakiness/tremor	●			●		
Sexual dysfunction		●	●			
Dizziness/drowsiness		●		●		
Fever/rigid muscles/confusion		●		●	●	●

INTERACTIONS

Sedatives All drugs that have a sedative effect on the central nervous system are likely to increase any sedative effect of risperidone.

Lithium increases the risk of nerve toxicity when used with risperidone.

Drugs for parkinsonism Risperidone may reduce the effect of these drugs.

Fluoxetine, paroxetine, and verapamil These drugs increase the blood levels of risperidone and the risk of side effects.

Carbamazepine and rifampicin These drugs reduce the effects of risperidone. Other liver-enzyme-inducing drugs (e.g. phenytoin) may have the same effect.

RITUXIMAB

Brand name MabThera, Rixathon, Ruxience, Truxima
Used in the following combined preparations None

GENERAL INFORMATION

Rituximab is a monoclonal antibody (see p.113) that suppresses the immune system and reduces inflammation. It works by reducing the number of B-lymphocytes (a type of white blood cell involved in the production of antibodies by the immune system). It is used with chemotherapy to treat some types of lymphoid cancer, especially B-cell lymphomas and chronic lymphocytic leukaemia, and in combination with methotrexate to treat severe rheumatoid arthritis. It may also be used to treat systemic lupus erythematosus, autoimmune anaemias and platelet disorders, vasculitis, and some skin conditions, such as pemphigus. In addition, it is used to treat acute graft rejection in transplant patients.

Because rituximab suppresses the immune system, serious infections can occur or reactivate with its use. It is important that you tell your doctor if you have previously had hepatitis B or tuberculosis as these disorders may reactivate with rituximab treatment.

QUICK REFERENCE

Drug group Anticancer drug (p.112)
Overdose danger rating Low
Dependence rating Low
Prescription needed Yes
Available as generic Yes

INFORMATION FOR USERS

This drug is given only under medical supervision and is not for self-administration.

How taken/used

Intravenous infusion.

Frequency and timing of doses
Usually 4–8 treatment courses over a period of up to 2 years, but the precise dosing schedule depends on the condition being treated.

Adult dosage range
Each dose: 375–500mg/m^2 of body surface area, depending on condition being treated.

Onset of effect
Response to rituximab is often evident only about 6 weeks after the start of treatment.

Duration of action
6–9 months.

Diet advice
None.

Storage
Not applicable. The drug is not normally kept at home.

Missed dose
The drug is administered in hospital under close medical supervision. If you miss your dose, contact your doctor as soon as possible.

Stopping the drug
Discuss with your doctor. Stopping the drug prematurely may lead to worsening of the underlying condition.

Exceeding the dose
Overdosage is unlikely since treatment is carefully monitored and supervised.

POSSIBLE ADVERSE EFFECTS

Fever, chills, shivering, nausea or vomiting, and flushing may occur during the first infusion. Less commonly, allergic reactions (e.g. wheezing, tongue swelling, itchiness, or rash) may also occur. People with angina may have worsening of their symptoms. Tell the person giving you the infusion immediately if you develop any of these symptoms.

Symptom/effect	Frequency		Discuss with doctor		Stop taking drug now	Call doctor now
	Common	Rare	Only if severe	In all cases		
Infections	●			●		
Wheezing	●			●		
Rash	●			●		
Palpitations	●			●		
Nausea/vomiting/diarrhoea	●			●		
Abdominal pain	●			●		
Forgetfulness/confusion/ paralysis		●		●		

INTERACTIONS

Vaccines Rituximab suppresses the immune system, so live vaccines should not be used while undergoing rituximab treatment. The drug may also make attenuated vaccines less effective. Discuss with your doctor.

Antihypertensive drugs The blood-pressure-lowering effect of these drugs may be enhanced when they are taken together with rituximab.

SPECIAL PRECAUTIONS

Be sure to tell your doctor if:
- You have an infection, wound, dental problem, or have had recent surgery.
- You have previously had tuberculosis or hepatitis B.
- You have angina or other heart problems.
- You are, may be, or intend to become pregnant.
- You have recently been vaccinated or are due to be vaccinated.
- You are taking any other medications, especially for high blood pressure.

Pregnancy
Safety not established. Discuss with your doctor.

Breast-feeding
Not recommended during treatment with rituximab and for 12 months following end of treatment.

Infants and children
Not recommended

Over 60
No special problems.

Driving and hazardous work
No known problems.

Alcohol
No special problems.

PROLONGED USE

Rituximab increases susceptibility to infection, and any infection that develops should be treated promptly. Very rarely, a serious brain infection may develop; you should tell your doctor immediately if you develop memory problems, confusion, difficulty walking, or vision problems.

Monitoring Periodic blood tests may be carried out. Body temperature, blood pressure, and heart rate may be monitored during rituximab infusions.

RIVAROXABAN

Brand name Xarelto
Used in the following combination preparations None

GENERAL INFORMATION

Rivaroxaban is an oral anticoagulant drug with a rapid onset of action. It is used to treat or prevent deep-vein thrombosis (blood clots in the leg veins) and pulmonary embolism (blockage of blood vessels in the lungs from clots that have travelled from elsewhere in the body). It is used to prevent strokes and blood clots in the arteries in patients with the heart rhythm problem atrial fibrillation. Combined with antiplatelet drugs, rivaroxaban is also used to prevent coronary thrombosis after a heart attack or severe angina. The most serious side effect is an increased risk of bleeding. It should not be used in people with damaged or artificial heart valves or those with antiphospholipid syndrome.

INFORMATION FOR USERS

Your drug prescription is tailored for you. Do not alter dosage without checking with your doctor.

How taken/used

Tablets.

Frequency and timing of doses
1–2 x daily, with food; tablets may be crushed.

Dosage range:
2.5–15mg twice daily, or 20mg once a day.

Onset of effect
1 hour.

Duration of action
12–24 hours.

Diet advice
None.

Storage
Keep in the original container at room temperature out of the reach of children.

Missed dose
Take as soon as you remember. Make up the total daily dose during the day, regardless of gap between dosing (e.g. if on a twice-daily regimen, both doses can be taken at once). However, do not take more than the indicated daily dose.

Stopping the drug
Do not stop the drug without consulting your doctor; stopping the drug may lead to worsening of the underlying condition.

OVERDOSE ACTION

Seek immediate medical advice in all cases. Take emergency action if bleeding or loss of consciousness occur.

See Drug Poisoning emergency guide (p.518).

POSSIBLE ADVERSE EFFECTS

Bleeding is the most common adverse effect of rivaroxaban. If you notice excessive bruising or prolonged bleeding from a minor wound, consult your doctor immediately.

Symptom/effect	Frequency		Discuss with doctor		Stop taking drug now	Call doctor now
	Common	Rare	Only if severe	In all cases		
Bleeding/bruising	●			●		●
Abdominal pain	●			●		
Faintness/dizziness	●			●		
Nausea/vomiting	●			●		
Rash/itching	●			●		●
Jaundice		●		●	●	●
Swollen mouth/tongue		●		●	●	●

INTERACTIONS

Other anticoagulants, antiplatelet drugs, non-steroidal anti-inflammatory drugs, antibacterial drugs, antifungal drugs, and antiviral drugs There is an increased risk of bleeding if these are used with rivaroxaban.

Anticonvulsant drugs, rifampicin, and St John's wort These may lower the blood level of rivaroxaban and reduce its effectiveness.

SPECIAL PRECAUTIONS

Be sure to tell your doctor if:
- You have liver or kidney problems.
- You have high blood pressure.
- You have a bleeding disorder.
- You have peptic ulcers.
- You have had a brain haemorrhage.
- You have had recent surgery.
- You are taking other medicines.

Pregnancy
Safety not established. Discuss with your doctor.

Breast-feeding
Safety not established. Discuss with your doctor.

Infants and children
Safety not established. Discuss with your doctor.

Over 60
No special problems.

Driving and hazardous work
Use caution. Even minor injuries may cause serious bruising and bleeding.

Alcohol
Avoid excessive intake.

Surgery and general anaesthetics
Rivaroxaban may need to be stopped before surgery. Discuss with your doctor or dentist.

PROLONGED USE

No special problems known, but the need for continued treatment should be reviewed. Rivaroxaban is usually used long term only in people with recurrent deep-vein thrombosis or pulmonary embolism.

RIVASTIGMINE

Brand names Alzest, Eluden, Exelon, Kerstipon, Nimvastid, Prometax, Rivatev, Voleze
Used in the following combined preparations None

GENERAL INFORMATION

Rivastigmine is an inhibitor of anti-cholinesterase. This enzyme breaks down the naturally occurring neurotransmitter acetylcholine (see p.35) to limit its effects. Blocking the enzyme raises the levels of acetylcholine; in the brain, the effect is to increase alertness, awareness, and memory. Rivastigmine improves the symptoms of dementia in Alzheimer's disease, and is used to slow the rate of deterioration in that disease. The drug is not recommended for dementia due to other causes.

Treatment with rivastigmine is initiated under specialist supervision. It is usual to assess those having the treatment at 6-monthly intervals to decide whether the drug is helping. As the disease progresses, however, the benefit obtained may diminish.

Side effects may include slow heart rate, collapse, agitation, confusion, and depression. The latter three effects are also possible symptoms of Alzheimer's disease, so may be hard to distinguish from the effects of the disease itself.

INFORMATION FOR USERS

Your drug prescription is tailored for you. Do not alter dosage without checking with your doctor.

How taken/used

Capsules, liquid, transdermal patch.

Frequency and timing of doses
2 x daily.

Adult dosage range
3mg daily (starting dose); 6–12mg daily (maintenance dose); 4.6–13.3mg every 24 hours (transdermal patch).

Onset of effect
30–60 minutes. Full effect may take up to 3 months.

Duration of action
9–12 hours.

Diet advice
None.

Storage
Keep in original container at room temperature out of the reach of children.

Missed dose
Take as soon as you remember. If your next dose is due within 4 hours, take a single dose now and skip the next. A carer should oversee the taking of tablets.

Stopping the drug
Do not stop the drug without consulting your doctor; symptoms may recur.

Exceeding the dose
An occasional unintentional extra dose is unlikely to be a problem. Large overdoses may cause nausea, vomiting, and diarrhoea. Notify your doctor.

SPECIAL PRECAUTIONS

Be sure to tell your doctor if:
- You have a heart problem.
- You have liver or kidney problems.
- You have asthma or respiratory problems.
- You have a history of peptic ulcers.
- You have had an epileptic seizure.
- You are taking other medicines.

 Pregnancy
Not recommended. Safety in pregnancy not established.

 Breast-feeding
Not recommended.

 Infants and children
Not recommended.

 Over 60
Particular risk of heart problems, low heart rate, and collapse.

 Driving and hazardous work
Your underlying condition may make such activities inadvisable. Discuss with your doctor.

 Alcohol
Avoid. Alcohol increases the sedative effects of rivastigmine.

Surgery and general anaesthetics
Treatment with rivastigmine may need to be stopped before you have a general anaesthetic. Discuss this with your doctor or dentist before any operation.

POSSIBLE ADVERSE EFFECTS

Adverse effects include mental changes and intestinal problems. Although common, these effects are usually quite mild. However, women may be more susceptible to nausea, vomiting, and weight loss.

Symptom/effect	Frequency		Discuss with doctor		Stop taking drug now	Call doctor now
	Common	Rare	Only if severe	In all cases		
Drowsiness/dizziness	●		●			
Weakness/trembling	●		●			
Reduced appetite/weight loss	●			●		
Nausea/abdominal pain	●			●		
Agitation/confusion	●			●		
Urinary incontinence/infection	●			●		
Collapse		●		●	●	●
Seizures		●		●	●	●

INTERACTIONS

Muscle relaxants used in surgery
Rivastigmine may increase the effects of some muscle relaxants, but it may also block the effects of some others.

PROLONGED USE

May be continued for as long as there is benefit. Stopping the drug leads to a gradual loss of the improvements.

Monitoring Checks at 6-monthly intervals may be performed to test whether the drug is still providing some benefit.

ROPINIROLE

Brand names Adartrel (restless legs only), Aimpart XL, Ralnea XL, Repinex XL, Requip, Requip XL
Used in the following combined preparations None

GENERAL INFORMATION

Ropinirole mimics the neurotransmitter dopamine in the brain. It is used to treat Parkinson's disease, in which there is a lack of dopamine in the brain. It may be used either alone or in combination with levodopa. Patients taking levodopa alone over several years may experience extremes of activity: overactivity after taking levodopa ("on effect") and underactivity ("off effect") before the next dose of levodopa is due. When used with levodopa, ropinirole helps to reduce these on-off fluctuations. Unlike some other drugs for Parkinson's disease, ropinirole does not cause fibrosis (thickening of connective tissue) of the abdomen or heart. However, the drug may cause excessive sleepiness and a tendency to lower blood pressure on standing (postural hypotension). It may also be used for restless legs syndrome (Ekbom's disease).

INFORMATION FOR USERS

Your drug prescription is tailored for you. Do not alter dosage without checking with your doctor.

How taken/used

Tablets, MR tablets.

Frequency and timing of doses
Parkinson's 3 x daily (tablets) or 1 x daily (MR tablets).
Restless legs 1 x daily at night (tablets).
In all cases, doses should be taken with or after food.

Adult dosage range
Parkinson's 750mcg–3mg daily (tablets), 750mcg–24mg (MR tablets). Initially a low dose is given; this is increased until there is a satisfactory response. If given with levodopa, the dose of ropinirole may be reduced.
Restless legs 250mcg each night, increasing slowly to 4mg maximum.

Onset of effect
1–2 hours.

Duration of action
6–12 hours.

Diet advice
None.

Storage
Keep in original container at room temperature out of the reach of children.

Missed dose
Take as soon as you remember. If your next dose is due within two hours, take a single dose now and skip the next.

Stopping the drug
Do not stop the drug without consulting your doctor; symptoms may recur.

Exceeding the dose
An occasional unintended extra dose is unlikely to be a cause for concern. If you notice any unusual symptoms, or if a large overdose has been taken, notify your doctor.

SPECIAL PRECAUTIONS

Be sure to tell your doctor if:
- You have postural hypotension or dizziness on standing.
- You have changed or intend to change your smoking habit.
- You have long-standing kidney or liver problems.
- You have had a psychotic illness.

Pregnancy
Safety in pregnancy not established. Discuss with your doctor.

Breast-feeding
Safety not established, and the drug may suppress lactation. Discuss with your doctor.

Infants and children
Unlikely to be required.

Over 60
Reduced dose may be necessary.

Driving and hazardous work
Avoid such activities until you have learned how ropinirole affects you as this drug may cause dizziness and severe drowsiness.

Alcohol
No known problems, although ropinirole may enhance the sedative effects of alcohol.

PROLONGED USE

No special problems.

POSSIBLE ADVERSE EFFECTS

Nausea, drowsiness, and dizziness on standing are common side effects. In some cases, the drowsiness can be severe, with sudden onset of sleep during the day. Starting with small doses that are gradually increased helps to reduce the likelihood of side effects. Rarely, ropinirole can cause increased sexuality and compulsive behaviours, such as compulsive gambling.

Symptom/effect	Frequency		Discuss with doctor		Stop taking drug now	Call doctor now
	Common	Rare	Only if severe	In all cases		
Nausea	●		●			
Dizziness on standing	●		●			
Drowsiness	●		●			
Confusion		●		●		
Hallucinations		●		●		
Compulsive behaviours		●		●		

INTERACTIONS

Ciprofloxacin The effect of ropinirole may be increased, necessitating dose reduction of ropinirole or use of an alternative antibiotic.

Memantine May enhance the effects of ropinirole. Dose reduction of ropinirole may be required.

Metoclopramide and antipsychotics These drugs reduce the effect of ropinirole and may worsen symptoms.

Smoking reduces blood levels of ropinirole, so stopping smoking may produce side effects due to a significant rise in blood levels of ropinirole.

ROSUVASTATIN

Brand name Crestor
Used in the following combined preparations None

GENERAL INFORMATION

Rosuvastatin is a statin: a lipid-lowering drug that is used in the treatment of hypercholesterolaemia (high blood cholesterol levels). Cholesterol is a lipid (fat) that is produced in the body and is necessary for the production of many other body chemicals. Rosuvastatin works by inhibiting an enzyme involved in the manufacture of cholesterol in the liver. It is more potent than other statins so can produce lower cholesterol levels than the other statins. It is prescribed to people who have not responded to other forms of therapy, such as a special diet or less potent statins, and who have, or are at risk of developing, coronary artery disease or stroke.

Adverse effects are usually mild and wear off with time, but any unexplained aches or pains or muscle weakness should be reported to your doctor immediately. People of Asian origin are given lower starting doses because the drug works more potently in them.

INFORMATION FOR USERS

Your drug prescription is tailored for you. Do not alter dosage without checking with your doctor.

How taken/used

Tablets.

Frequency and timing of doses
Once daily at night.

Adult dosage range
5–40mg (5–20mg for patients of Asian origin); 10mg (initial dose), increased to 20mg after 4 weeks, if necessary; a maximum dose of 40mg may be given for severe hypercholesterolaemia.

Onset of effect
2–4 weeks.

Duration of action
24 hours.

Diet advice
A low-fat diet is usually recommended.

Storage
Keep in original container at room temperature, out of the reach of children.

Missed dose
Do not take the missed dose. Take the next scheduled dose as usual.

Stopping the drug
Do not stop taking the drug without consulting your doctor. Symptoms may recur.

Exceeding the dose
An occasional unintentional extra dose is unlikely to be a cause for concern. However, if you notice any unusual symptoms, or if a large overdose has been taken, notify your doctor.

SPECIAL PRECAUTIONS

Be sure to tell your doctor if:
- You have liver or kidney problems.
- You have a personal or family history of muscle problems.
- You have porphyria.
- You are of Asian origin.
- You are taking other medicines.

 Pregnancy
Not recommended. May affect fetal development. Discuss with your doctor if you are pregnant or intend to become pregnant.

 Breast-feeding
Not recommended. Safety not established. Discuss with your doctor.

 Infants and children
Not recommended.

 Over 60
Reduced initial dose. Discuss with your doctor.

 Driving and hazardous work
No special problems.

 Alcohol
Avoid excessive amounts. Alcohol may increase the risk of developing liver problems with this drug.

POSSIBLE ADVERSE EFFECTS

Most adverse effects are usually mild and transient. However, if you develop muscle tenderness, pain, or weakness, consult your doctor at once.

Symptom/effect	Frequency		Discuss with doctor		Stop taking drug now	Call doctor now
	Common	Rare	Only if severe	In all cases		
Abdominal pain	●		●			
Constipation/diarrhoea	●		●			
Nausea/flatulence	●		●			
Sleep disturbance/headache	●		●			
Rash		●		●	●	
Muscle pain/weakness		●		●	●	●
Jaundice		●		●	●	●

INTERACTIONS

Ciclosporin increases blood levels of rosuvastatin.

Warfarin Rosuvastatin may enhance the effects of warfarin. The level of anticoagulation (INR) should be monitored.

Erythromycin reduces the effectiveness of rosuvastatin.

Oestrogens Rosuvastatin increases blood levels of some of these drugs.

Gemfibrozil and other lipid-lowering drugs There is an increased risk of adverse effects when these drugs are taken with rosuvastatin.

Antacids may reduce the effectiveness of rosuvastatin.

Anti-HIV drugs may increase the risk of muscle damage when taken with rosuvastatin.

PROLONGED USE

Prolonged treatment with rosuvastatin can adversely affect liver function and may unmask type 2 diabetes.

Monitoring Periodic blood tests to test for muscle toxicity and assess liver function are recommended. If high doses are taken, regular blood tests may also be done to assess renal function.

SACUBITRIL/VALSARTAN

Brand names Entresto
Used in the following combined preparations None

GENERAL INFORMATION

Sacubitril/valsartan is a new drug that has been approved for the long-term management of heart failure. It is a combination tablet consisting of sacubitril (an inhibitor of the enzyme neprilysin, which affects the pumping action of the heart) and valsartan (an angiotensin II receptor blocker, or ARB, for lowering blood pressure; see p.60).

Sacubitril/valsartan reduces the strain on the heart in addition to improving the structure and function of the heart.

Studies show that it provides long-term benefit in patients with symptoms of heart failure. It is administered in conjunction with other therapies for heart failure and in place of other angiotensin II receptor blockers or ACE inhibitors.

Low blood pressure may occur when taking sacubitril/valsartan. Therefore, if you experience light-headedness, dizziness, or headache, you should inform your doctor.

INFORMATION FOR USERS

Your drug prescription is tailored for you. Do not alter dosage without checking with your doctor.

How taken/used

Tablets.

Frequency and timing of doses
2 x daily.

Dosage range
Adult starting dose either 24/26mg 2 x daily or 49/51mg 2 x daily. Dose may be increased every 2–4 weeks to maximum 97/103mg 2 x daily depending upon response.

Onset of effect
Effect on blood pressure develops within a few hours. Full beneficial effect on heart failure may take weeks to develop.

Duration of action
12 hours.

Diet advice
None.

Storage
Keep in original container at room temperature out of the reach of children.

Missed dose
Take as soon as you remember. If your next dose is within 6 hours, take a single dose now and skip the next. Continue usual schedule.

Stopping the drug
Do not stop the drug without consulting your doctor. Stopping the drug may lead to worsening of the underlying condition.

Exceeding the dose
An occasional unintentional extra dose is unlikely to cause problems. Large overdoses may cause dizziness, fainting, and a faint pulse. Notify your doctor.

SPECIAL PRECAUTIONS

Be sure to tell your doctor if:
- You have heart problems, including heart failure.
- You have had angioedema or a previous allergic reaction to an ACE inhibitor or ARB.
- You have long-term liver or kidney problems or stenosis of the kidney's arteries.
- You are or intend to become pregnant.
- You are taking other medicines.

 Pregnancy
Not prescribed. Discuss with your doctor.

 Breast-feeding
Safety not established. Discuss with your doctor.

 Infants and children
Not prescribed.

 Over 60
Reduced dose may be necessary.

 Driving and hazardous work
Avoid such activities until you have learned how sacubitril/valsartan affects you because the drug can cause dizziness, fatigue, and fainting.

 Alcohol
Avoid. Alcohol may increase the blood-pressure-lowering and adverse effects of the drug.

Surgery and general anaesthetics
Sacubitril/valsartan may have to be stopped before you have a general anaesthetic. Discuss with your doctor or dentist.

PROLONGED USE

No special problems. However, periodic checks on serum potassium levels and kidney function are usually performed. Haemoglobin and liver tests may also be carried out.

POSSIBLE ADVERSE EFFECTS

Most effects are minor and disappear soon after treatment starts. However, if you have wheezing or swollen lips or tongue, stop the drug and contact your doctor immediately.

Symptom/effect	Frequency		Discuss with doctor		Stop taking drug now	Call doctor now
	Common	Rare	Only if severe	In all cases		
Diarrhoea	●			●		
Headache	●			●		
Cough	●			●		
Nausea	●			●		
Dizziness/fatigue	●			●		
Rash		●		●		
Breathing difficulty		●		●	●	●
Swelling of mouth/lips		●		●	●	●

INTERACTIONS

Potassium supplements (including some salt substitutes), potassium-sparing diuretics, and ciclosporin May raise levels of potassium in the blood.

Statins Blood levels of some statins may increase, making their side effects more likely, especially at higher doses.

Lithium Sacubitril/valsartan may cause raised blood lithium levels and toxicity.

Vasodilators, diuretics, and other antihypertensives May increase the drug's blood-pressure-lowering effect.

NSAIDs (p.74) Some may increase the risk of kidney damage with sacubitril/valsartan.

SALBUTAMOL

Brand names Airomir, Airsalb, Salamol, Salbulin, Ventmax, Ventolin, and others
Used in the following combined preparations Combivent

GENERAL INFORMATION

Salbutamol is a sympathomimetic bronchodilator used to treat conditions such as asthma, chronic obstructive pulmonary disease (COPD), and bronchospasm, in which the airways become constricted. Although it can be taken by mouth, inhalation is more effective because the drug is delivered directly to the airways, thus giving rapid relief, allowing smaller doses, and causing fewer side effects. If you need to use inhaled salbutamol more than twice a week, or have to use it at night, you will probably also be prescribed an inhaled corticosteroid to improve control of your asthma.

Compared to some similar drugs, salbutamol has little stimulant effect on the heart rate and blood pressure, making it safer for people with heart problems or high blood pressure. Because salbutamol relaxes the muscle of the uterus, it is also used to prevent premature labour.

QUICK REFERENCE

Drug group Bronchodilator (p.48), drug to treat asthma (p.49), and drug used in premature labour (p.125)

Overdose danger rating Low

Dependence rating Low

Prescription needed Yes

Available as generic Yes

INFORMATION FOR USERS

Your drug prescription is tailored for you. Do not alter dosage without checking with your doctor.

How taken/used

Tablets, SR tablets, SR capsules, liquid, injection, inhaler, nebules for nebulizer, powder for inhalation.

Frequency and timing of doses
3–4 x daily (tablets/liquid); 2 x daily (SR preparations); 1–2 inhalations 3–4 x daily (inhaler); up to 4 x daily (nebules).

Dosage range
8–16mg daily (by mouth); 400–800mcg daily (inhaler); 2.5–20mg daily (nebules).

Onset of effect
Within 30–60 minutes (by mouth); within 5–15 minutes (inhaler/nebules).

Duration of action
Up to 8 hours (tablets); up to 6 hours (inhaler); up to 12 hours (SR preparations).

Diet advice
None.

Storage
Keep in original container at room temperature out of the reach of children. Protect from light. Do not puncture or burn inhalers.

Missed dose
Take as soon as you remember if you need it. If your next dose is due within 2 hours, take a single dose now and skip the next.

Stopping the drug
Do not stop the drug without consulting your doctor; symptoms may recur.

Exceeding the dose
An occasional unintentional extra dose is unlikely to be a cause for concern. But if you notice any unusual symptoms, or if a large overdose has been taken, notify your doctor.

SPECIAL PRECAUTIONS

Be sure to tell your doctor if:
- You have heart problems.
- You have high blood pressure.
- You have diabetes.
- You have a tendency towards low potassium levels.
- You have an overactive thyroid gland.
- You are taking other medicines.

Pregnancy
No evidence of risk when used to treat asthma, or to treat or prevent premature labour. Discuss with your doctor.

Breast-feeding
The drug passes into the breast milk, but at normal doses adverse effects on the baby are unlikely. Discuss with your doctor.

Infants and children
Reduced dose necessary.

Over 60
Increased likelihood of adverse effects. Reduced dose may therefore be necessary.

Driving and hazardous work
Avoid such activities until you have learned how salbutamol affects you because the drug can cause tremors.

Alcohol
No known problems.

POSSIBLE ADVERSE EFFECTS

Muscle tremor, which particularly affects the hands, anxiety, and restlessness are the most common adverse effects. Rarely, wheezing or breathlessness may worsen immediately after inhaler use (paradoxical bronchospasm); if this happens, stop using the drug and contact your doctor immediately.

Symptom/effect	Frequency		Discuss with doctor		Stop taking drug now	Call doctor now
	Common	Rare	Only if severe	In all cases		
Anxiety/nervous tension	●		●			
Muscle tremor	●		●			
Restlessness	●		●			
Headache	●			●		
Muscle cramps		●		●		
Palpitations	●			●	●	
Worsening breathlessness		●		●	●	●

INTERACTIONS

Theophylline, corticosteroids, and diuretics There is a risk of low potassium levels in the blood if this drug is taken with salbutamol.

Other sympathomimetic drugs may increase the effects of salbutamol, thereby also increasing the risk of adverse effects.

Digoxin Salbutamol may cause low potassium levels, increasing the risk of digoxin toxicity. Salbutamol by mouth or injection can reduce digoxin levels.

Beta blockers Drugs in this group may reduce the action of salbutamol.

PROLONGED USE

No problems expected. However, you should contact your doctor if you find you need to use your salbutamol inhaler more than usual. Failure to respond to the drug may be a result of worsening asthma that requires urgent medical attention.

Monitoring Periodic blood tests for potassium may be needed in people on high-dose treatment with salbutamol combined with other asthma drugs and/or diuretics.

SALMETEROL

Brand name Neovent, Sereflo, Serevent, Soltel
Used in the following combined preparation AirFluSal, Combisal, Fusacomb, Seretide, Sirdupla, Stalplex

GENERAL INFORMATION

Salmeterol is a sympathomimetic bronchodilator used to treat conditions, such as asthma, chronic obstructive pulmonary disease (COPD) and bronchospasm, in which the airways become constricted. The advantage of this drug over salbutamol (see p.391) is that it is longer acting.

Salmeterol relaxes the muscle surrounding the airways in the lungs but, because of its slow onset of effect,

it is not used for immediate relief of symptoms of asthma. It is prescribed to prevent attacks, however, and can be helpful in preventing night-time asthma.

Salmeterol should always be used in combination with inhaled or oral corticosteroids. Taken by inhalation, the drug is delivered directly to the airways. This allows smaller doses to be administered and reduces the risk of adverse effects.

QUICK REFERENCE

Drug group Bronchodilator (p.48), drug to treat asthma (p.49), and drug used in premature labour (p.125)

Overdose danger rating Low

Dependence rating Low

Prescription needed Yes

Available as generic Yes

INFORMATION FOR USERS

Your drug prescription is tailored for you. Do not alter dosage without checking with your doctor.

How taken/used

Inhaler, powder for inhalation.

Frequency and timing of doses
2 x daily.

Dosage range
100–200mcg daily.

Onset of effect
10–20 minutes.

Duration of action
12 hours.

Diet advice
None.

Storage
Keep in original container at room temperature out of the reach of children.

Missed dose
Take as soon as you remember. If your next dose is due within 4 hours, take a single dose now and skip the next.

Stopping the drug
Do not stop the drug without consulting your doctor; symptoms may recur.

Exceeding the dose
An occasional unintentional extra dose is unlikely to be a cause for concern. But if you notice any unusual symptoms, or if a large overdose has been taken, notify your doctor.

SPECIAL PRECAUTIONS

Be sure to tell your doctor if:
• You have heart problems.
• You have high blood pressure.
• You have an overactive thyroid gland.
• You have diabetes.
• You have a tendency towards low potassium levels.
• You are taking other medicines.

 Pregnancy
No evidence of risk when used to treat asthma. Benefits of treatment usually outweigh risk that mother's worsening asthma has on developing baby. Discuss with your doctor.

 Breast-feeding
The drug passes into the breast milk, but at normal doses adverse effects on the baby are unlikely. Discuss with your doctor.

 Infants and children
Reduced dose necessary. Not recommended for children under 4 years.

 Over 60
No special problems.

 Driving and hazardous work
No special problems.

 Alcohol
No known problems.

POSSIBLE ADVERSE EFFECTS

Side effects are usually mild. If wheezing and breathlessness suddenly worsen after using the inhaler (paradoxical bronchospasm), stop the drug and contact your doctor immediately.

Symptom/effect	Frequency		Discuss with doctor		Stop taking drug now	Call doctor now
	Common	Rare	Only if severe	In all cases		
Tremor	●		●			
Palpitations	●			●		
Headache		●		●		
Muscle cramps	●			●		
Worsening breathlessness		●		●	●	●

INTERACTIONS

Corticosteroids, theophylline, and diuretics There is an increased risk of low blood potassium levels when high doses of salmeterol are taken with these drugs.

Other sympathomimetics may increase the effects of salmeterol, thereby also increasing the risk of adverse effects.

Triazole antifungals (e.g. itraconazole and voriconazole) increase the body's exposure to salmeterol.

Digoxin Salmeterol may cause low potassium levels in the blood, which increases the risk of digoxin toxicity.

Protease inhibitors (e.g. ritonavir, saquinavir, and telaprevir) increase the risk of abnormal heart rhythms when used with salmeterol.

PROLONGED USE

Salmeterol is intended to be used long term together with an inhaled corticosteroid. The main problem comes from using combinations of anti-asthma drugs, with or without diuretics, leading to low blood potassium levels.

Monitoring Periodic blood tests are usually carried out to monitor potassium levels.

SERTRALINE

Brand name Lustral
Used in the following combined preparations None

GENERAL INFORMATION

Sertraline is a member of the group of antidepressants called selective serotonin re-uptake inhibitors (SSRIs). These drugs tend to cause less sedation than older types of antidepressant, and have different side effects.

Sertraline elevates mood, increases physical activity, and restores interest in everyday activities. It is used to treat depression, including accompanying anxiety, and obsessive–compulsive disorder (OCD). Sertraline is also prescribed for post-traumatic stress disorder (PTSD).

Treatment is usually stopped gradually over at least four weeks, because symptoms such as headache, nausea, and dizziness may occur if the drug is withdrawn suddenly.

QUICK REFERENCE

Drug group Antidepressant drug (p.40)

Overdose danger rating Low

Dependence rating Low

Prescription needed Yes

Available as generic Yes

INFORMATION FOR USERS

Your drug prescription is tailored for you. Do not alter dosage without checking with your doctor.

How taken/used

Tablets.

Frequency and timing of doses
Once daily, usually in the morning.

Adult dosage range
25–200mg daily.

Onset of effect
Some benefits may appear within 14 days, but full effects may take another 6 weeks; anxiety disorders may take longer.

Duration of action
Antidepressant effect may continue for some weeks following prolonged use.

Diet advice
None.

Storage
Keep in original container at room temperature out of the reach of children.

Missed dose
Take as soon as you remember. If your next dose is due within 8 hours, take a single dose now and skip the next.

Stopping the drug
Do not stop the drug without consulting your doctor, who may supervise a gradual reduction in dosage.

Exceeding the dose
An occasional unintentional extra dose is unlikely to cause problems. Large overdoses may cause adverse effects. Notify your doctor.

SPECIAL PRECAUTIONS

Be sure to tell your doctor if:
- You have long-term liver or kidney problems.
- You have had epileptic seizures.
- You have heart problems.
- You have a history of bleeding disorders.
- You have a history of mania.
- You are taking other medicines.

 Pregnancy
Safety not established. Discuss with your doctor.

 Breast-feeding
Safety not established. Discuss with your doctor.

 Infants and children
Not generally recommended under 18 years.

 Over 60
No special problems.

 Driving and hazardous work
Avoid such activities until you know how sertraline affects you because the drug can cause drowsiness and visual disturbances.

 Alcohol
Avoid excessive intake. SSRIs may increase the sedative effects of alcohol.

POSSIBLE ADVERSE EFFECTS

The most common side effects caused by sertraline are restlessness, insomnia, and gastrointestinal problems.

Symptom/effect	Frequency		Discuss with doctor		Stop taking drug now	Call doctor now
	Common	Rare	Only if severe	In all cases		
Nausea/indigestion	●		●			
Diarrhoea/loose stools	●		●			
Insomnia/sleepiness/anxiety	●		●			
Sexual dysfunction	●		●			
Suicidal thoughts/attempts		●		●	●	●
Rash/itching/skin eruptions		●		●	●	●

INTERACTIONS

St John's wort There is a danger of increasing the side effects of both substances.

Monoamine oxidase inhibitors (MAOIs) Sertraline's effects and toxicity are greatly increased by MAOIs.

Antipsychotics Sertraline may increase the levels and effects of some antipsychotics.

Tramadol and 5HT₁ agonists (e.g. sumatriptan) There is an increased risk of adverse effects if these drugs are taken with sertraline.

Anticoagulants The effects of these drugs may be increased by sertraline.

PROLONGED USE

No known problems in adults. There is a small risk of suicidal thoughts and self-harm in children and adolescents, although the drug is rarely used for this age group.

Monitoring Any person experiencing drowsiness, confusion, muscle cramps, or seizures should be monitored for low sodium levels in the blood. Under-18s should be monitored for suicidal thoughts and self-harm.

SILDENAFIL/TADALAFIL

Brand names [sildenafil] Aronix, Granpidam, Mysildecard, Nipatra, Revatio, Viagra, Vizarsin; [tadalafil] Adcirca, Cialis
Used in the following combined preparations None

GENERAL INFORMATION

Sildenafil and tadalafil are used to treat erectile dysfunction. They do not directly cause an erection, but they prevent the muscle walls of the blood-filled chambers in the penis from relaxing. The drugs are taken only before sexual activity. Sildenafil is also occasionally used for pulmonary hypertension (high blood pressure in the arteries supplying the lungs) and Raynaud's disease. Tadalafil may also be used to treat non-cancerous prostate enlargement. Because both drugs are vasodilators, they can lower blood pressure and may increase the effects of antihypertensive drugs. They should not be taken if you are using a nitrate (see p.56) because they greatly increase its effects.

Viagra (one brand of sildenafil) is available over the counter to men aged 40–65 who pass a medical check by the pharmacist.

INFORMATION FOR USERS

Your drug prescription is tailored for you. Do not alter dosage without checking with your doctor.

How taken/used

Tablets, intravenous injection.

Frequency and timing of doses
Erectile dysfunction As needed; maximum one dose daily, 1 hour before sexual activity.
Pulmonary hypertension 3 x daily.

Adult dosage range
Erectile dysfunction (sildenafil) 25–100mg per dose; (tadalafil) 10–20mg per dose.
Pulmonary hypertension (sildenafil) 60mg daily (tablets); 30mg (injection).

Onset of effect
30 minutes.

Duration of action
4 hours (sildenafil); up to 36 hours (tadalafil).

Diet advice
None, although the drugs take longer to work after a meal, especially a high-fat meal. Grapefruit juice may increase sildenafil levels.

Storage
Keep in original container at room temperature out of the reach of children.

Missed dose
For erectile dysfunction, use only as needed. For pulmonary hypertension, take as soon as you remember; take next dose as scheduled.

Stopping the drug
For erectile dysfunction, the drugs can be stopped if no longer needed. For pulmonary hypertension, do not stop without consulting your doctor; your condition may worsen.

Exceeding the dose
An occasional unintentional extra dose is unlikely to cause problems. Large overdoses may cause headache, dizziness, flushing, and altered vision. Notify your doctor.

POSSIBLE ADVERSE EFFECTS

Side effects are common but usually minor. However, for persistent, painful erection lasting more than 4 hours, or chest pain, stop the drug and seek immediate medical help.

Symptom/effect	Frequency		Discuss with doctor		Stop taking drug now	Call doctor now
	Common	Rare	Only if severe	In all cases		
Headache/dizziness	●		●			
Flushing	●		●			
Indigestion	●		●			
Nasal congestion	●		●			
Altered colour vision/blurring	●		●			
Back pain	●		●			
Persistent erection (priapism)		●		●	●	●
Chest pain		●		●	●	●

INTERACTIONS

Nitrates The effects of these drugs are greatly increased by sildenafil and tadalafil so they are not prescribed together.

Cimetidine, erythromycin, nicorandil, ketoconazole (oral), and antivirals These drugs increase the blood levels and toxicity of sildenafil and tadalafil.

Antihypertensive drugs Sildenafil and tadalafil may enhance the blood-pressure-lowering effect of these drugs.

SPECIAL PRECAUTIONS

Be sure to tell your doctor if:
- You have heart problems.
- You have had a stroke or heart attack.
- You have liver or kidney problems.
- You have low or high blood pressure.
- You have sickle cell anaemia, leukaemia, or myeloma.
- You have an inherited eye problem.
- You have an abnormality of the penis.
- You are taking other medicines, especially a nitrate drug.

 Pregnancy
Not prescribed.

 Breast-feeding
Not prescribed.

 Infants and children
Not prescribed under 18 years, except rarely for pulmonary hypertension on specialist advice.

 Over 60
Reduced dose may be necessary.

 Driving and hazardous work
Avoid such activities until you have learned how sildenafil or tadalafil affects you because they can cause dizziness and altered vision.

 Alcohol
No special problems.

PROLONGED USE

No problems expected.

SIMVASTATIN

Brand names Simvador, Zocor
Used in the following combined preparations Cholib, Inegy

GENERAL INFORMATION

One of the statin group of lipid-lowering drugs, simvastatin blocks the action of an enzyme involved in the manufacture of cholesterol in the liver, resulting in lowered blood levels of cholesterol. The drug is prescribed for people with hypercholesterolaemia (high blood cholesterol) who have not responded to other forms of therapy (e.g. a special diet) and who are at risk of developing or have existing coronary heart disease or stroke. Low-dose simvastatin is available over the counter. Side effects are usually mild and wear off with time. In the body, simvastatin is found mainly in the liver, and it may raise the levels of liver enzymes but this does not usually indicate serious liver damage. Rarely, it may cause muscle damage (especially with higher doses), and any unexpected muscle tenderness, pain, or weakness should be reported to your doctor.

INFORMATION FOR USERS

Your drug prescription is tailored for you. Do not alter dosage without checking with your doctor.

How taken/used

Tablets.

Frequency and timing of doses
Once daily at night.

Adult dosage range
10–80mg daily.

Onset of effect
Within 2 weeks; full beneficial effects may not be reached for 4–6 weeks.

Duration of action
Up to 24 hours.

Diet advice
A low-fat diet is usually recommended. Avoid grapefruit juice.

Storage
Keep in original container at room temperature out of the reach of children. Protect from light.

Missed dose
Take as soon as you remember. If your next dose is due within 8 hours, do not take the missed dose, but take the next dose on schedule.

Stopping the drug
Do not stop taking the drug without consulting your doctor. Stopping the drug may lead to worsening of the underlying condition.

Exceeding the dose
An occasional unintentional extra dose is unlikely to cause problems. Large overdoses may cause liver problems. Notify your doctor.

POSSIBLE ADVERSE EFFECTS

Adverse effects are usually mild and do not last long. The most common are those affecting the gastrointestinal system. Rarely, simvastatin may cause muscle problems; any muscle pain, tenderness, or weakness should be reported to your doctor at once.

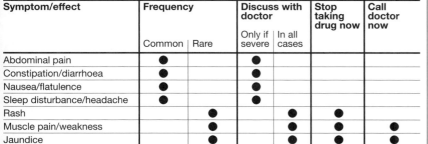

Symptom/effect	Frequency		Discuss with doctor		Stop taking drug now	Call doctor now
	Common	Rare	Only if severe	In all cases		
Abdominal pain	●		●			
Constipation/diarrhoea	●		●			
Nausea/flatulence	●		●			
Sleep disturbance/headache	●		●			
Rash		●		●	●	
Muscle pain/weakness		●		●	●	●
Jaundice		●		●	●	●

INTERACTIONS

Ciclosporin, danazol, fibrates, nicotinic acid, amiodarone, amlodipine, verapamil, diltiazem, ranolazine, itraconazole, ketoconazole, HIV protease inhibitors, macrolide antibiotics, and nefazodone Used with simvastatin, these drugs increase the risk of muscle toxicity. If they are required, simvastatin is withheld temporarily or the dose reduced.

St John's wort reduces blood levels of simvastatin.

Anticoagulants (e.g. warfarin) Simvastatin may increase the effect of these drugs. The level of anticoagulation (INR) should be monitored.

Carbamazepine reduces blood levels of simvastatin. The dose of simvastatin may need to be increased.

Grapefruit juice increases blood levels of simvastatin; regular consumption should be avoided.

SPECIAL PRECAUTIONS

Be sure to consult your doctor or pharmacist before taking this drug if:
- You have liver or kidney problems.
- You have a personal or family history of muscle problems.
- You have porphyria.
- You are taking other medicines.

 Pregnancy
Not recommended. May affect fetal development. Discuss with your doctor if you are pregnant or intend to become pregnant.

 Breast-feeding
The drug passes into the breast milk and may affect the baby. Discuss with your doctor.

 Infants and children
Not recommended under 5 years. Reduced dose necessary in older children, under specialist advice.

 Over 60
No special problems.

 Driving and hazardous work
No special problems.

 Alcohol
Avoid excessive amounts. Alcohol may increase the risk of developing liver problems with this drug.

PROLONGED USE

Prolonged treatment can adversely affect liver function.

Monitoring Periodic blood tests to test for muscle toxicity and assess liver function are recommended.

SITAGLIPTIN

Brand name Januvia
Used in the following combined preparation Janumet (with metformin)

GENERAL INFORMATION

Sitagliptin is used to treat Type 2 diabetes in combination with diet, exercise, weight control, and often other antidiabetic drugs. It is one of a new class of oral antidiabetics, known as DPP-4 inhibitors or gliptins, which block the breakdown of hormones called incretins. Incretins help to increase insulin production, but only when it is needed, such as after a meal. Gliptins increase the incretin level after a meal,

resulting in an increased insulin level, which helps to prevent a blood sugar "high" after eating.

Gliptins are less likely to cause abnormally low blood sugar levels (hypoglycaemia) than other antidiabetics if used alone. Unlike the sulfonylureas, gliptins do not cause weight gain. Sitagliptin can be used on its own or in combination with other antidiabetic drugs such as metformin or insulin.

QUICK REFERENCE

Drug group Drug for diabetes (p.100)

Overdose danger rating High

Dependence rating Low

Prescription needed Yes

Available as generic No

INFORMATION FOR USERS

Your drug prescription is tailored for you. Do not alter dosage without checking with your doctor.

How taken/used

Tablets.

Frequency and timing of doses
Once daily; can be taken with or without food.

Adult dosage range
100mg daily.

Onset of effect
Within 1 hour.

Duration of action
Up to 24 hours.

Diet advice
An individualized diabetic diet must be maintained for the drug to be fully effective. Follow the advice of your doctor.

Storage
Store at room temperature away from

moisture, heat, and light and out of the reach of children.

Missed dose
Take as soon as you remember. Do not take a double dose on the same day.

Stopping the drug
Do not stop taking the drug without consulting your doctor; stopping the drug may lead to worsening of your diabetes control.

OVERDOSE ACTION

 The drug is usually safe, but seek immediate medical help if you have warning signs of low blood sugar (such as faintness, dizziness, headache, confusion, sweating, or tremor), and eat or drink something sugary. Take emergency action if seizures or loss of consciousness occur.

See Drug poisoning emergency guide (p.518).

SPECIAL PRECAUTIONS

Be sure to tell your doctor if:
• You have long-term kidney problems.
• You have a history of pancreatitis.
• You are taking other medicines

 Pregnancy
Safety not established. Discuss with your doctor.

 Breast-feeding
Present in breast milk. Safety not established. Discuss with your doctor.

 Infants and children
Not prescribed.

 Over 60
No special problems.

 Driving and hazardous work
Avoid such activities if you have warning signs of low blood sugar.

 Alcohol
Avoid. Alcohol may upset diabetic control.

Surgery and general anaesthetics
Notify your doctor or dentist that you have diabetes. Your diabetes medication may need to be altered, and sometimes insulin may need to be substituted.

POSSIBLE ADVERSE EFFECTS

Serious side effects are rare. Symptoms such as sweating, tremor, dizziness, faintness, and confusion may indicate low blood sugar levels and are more likely when sitagliptin is used in combination with other antidiabetic drugs.

Symptom/effect	Frequency		Discuss with doctor		Stop taking drug now	Call doctor now
	Common	Rare	Only if severe	In all cases		
Stomach discomfort/diarrhoea	●		●			
Headache		●	●			
Faintness/dizziness/confusion		●	●			
Weakness/tremor		●	●			
Sweating		●	●			
Severe rash/skin blistering		●		●	●	
Severe abdominal pain/vomiting		●		●	●	●

PROLONGED USE

There is a small increased risk of upper respiratory tract and urinary infections when taking sitagliptin long term.

Monitoring Regular monitoring of your diabetes control is necessary. You may also have periodic assessment of the eyes, heart, and kidneys.

INTERACTIONS

General note Many drugs may interact with sitagliptin to affect blood sugar levels. Some medicines contain sugar and may upset diabetic control. Consult your doctor or pharmacist before taking other medicines.

Beta blockers may mask symptoms of low blood sugar when taken with sitagliptin.

Digoxin Sitagliptin may increase the blood level of digoxin.

SODIUM CROMOGLICATE

Brand names Intal, Nalcrom, Opticrom, Vividrin, and others
Used in the following combined preparations None

GENERAL INFORMATION

Sodium cromoglicate, introduced in the 1970s, is used primarily to prevent asthma and allergic conditions.

When taken by inhaler as a powder (Spinhaler) or spray, it is commonly used to reduce the frequency and severity of asthma attacks, and is also effective in helping to prevent attacks induced by exercise or cold air. The drug has a slow onset of action, and it may be up to six weeks before its full anti-asthmatic effect is felt. It is not effective for the relief of an asthma attack.

Sodium cromoglicate is also given as eye drops to prevent or treat allergic conjunctivitis. Taken as a nasal spray, it is used to prevent or treat allergic rhinitis (hay fever). It is also given, in the form of capsules, for food allergy.

Side effects are mild. Coughing and wheezing occurring on inhalation of the drug may be prevented by using a sympathomimetic bronchodilator (p.48) first. Hoarseness and throat irritation can be avoided by rinsing the mouth with water after inhalation.

QUICK REFERENCE

Drug group Anti-allergy drug (p.82)
Overdose danger rating Low
Dependence rating Low
Prescription needed No (some preparations)
Available as generic Yes

INFORMATION FOR USERS

Follow instructions on the label. Call your doctor if symptoms worsen.

How taken/used

Capsules, inhaler (various types), eye drops, nasal spray.

Frequency and timing of doses
Capsules 4 x daily before meals, swallowed whole or dissolved in water.
Inhaler, nasal spray 4–6 x daily.
Eye preparations 4 x daily (drops).

Adult dosage range
800mg daily (capsules); as directed (inhaler); apply to each nostril as directed (nasal spray); 1–2 drops in each eye per dose (eye drops).

Onset of effect
Varies with dosage, form, and condition being treated. Eye conditions and allergic rhinitis may respond after a few days' treatment with drops, while asthma and chronic allergic rhinitis may take 2–6 weeks to show improvement.

Duration of action
4–6 hours. Some effect persists for several days after treatment is stopped.

Diet advice
With capsules you may be advised to avoid certain foods. Follow your doctor's advice.

Storage
Keep in original container at room temperature out of the reach of children. Protect from light.

Missed dose
Take as soon as you remember. If your next dose is due within 2 hours, take a single dose now and skip the next.

Stopping the drug
Do not stop the drug without consulting your doctor; symptoms may recur.

Exceeding the dose
An occasional unintentional extra dose is unlikely to be a cause for concern. But if you notice any unusual symptoms, or if a large overdose has been taken, notify your doctor.

SPECIAL PRECAUTIONS

Be sure to tell your doctor or pharmacist before taking this drug if:
- You are taking other medicines.

 Pregnancy
No evidence of risk.

 Breast-feeding
It is not known whether the drug passes into the breast milk. Discuss with your doctor.

 Infants and children
Reduced dose necessary.

 Over 60
No special problems.

 Driving and hazardous work
No known problems.

 Alcohol
No known problems.

PROLONGED USE

No problems expected.

POSSIBLE ADVERSE EFFECTS

Coughing and hoarseness are common with inhalation. Nasal spray may cause sneezing. Eye drops may cause eye stinging. These effects usually diminish with continued use.

If wheezing or breathlessness worsens just after inhaler use (paradoxical bronchospasm), stop using the drug and contact your doctor immediately.

Symptom/effect	Frequency		Discuss with doctor		Stop taking drug now	Call doctor now
	Common	Rare	Only if severe	In all cases		
Coughing/hoarseness	●		●			
Local irritation	●		●			
Headache/dizziness		●	●			
Nausea/vomiting (capsules)		●		●		
Joint pain (capsules)		●		●		
Wheezing/breathlessness		●		●		
Rash (capsules)		●		●		●

INTERACTIONS

None known.

SODIUM VALPROATE (VALPROATE)

Brand names Convulex (valproic acid), Depakim, Depakote, Epilim, Epilim Chrono, Epilim Chronosphere, Episenta, Epival
Used in the following combined preparations None

GENERAL INFORMATION

Sodium valproate is an anticonvulsant drug that is effective in treating all forms of epilepsy. The action of sodium valproate is similar to that of other anticonvulsants – reducing electrical discharges in the brain to prevent the excessive build-up of discharges that can lead to epileptic seizures.

The drug is beneficial in long-term treatment and does not usually have a sedative effect. This makes it particularly suitable for children who have either atonic epilepsy (the sudden relaxing of the muscles throughout the body) or absence seizures (during which the person appears to be daydreaming). However, care should be taken if changing from one preparation to a different one.

Sodium valproate is also sometimes used in manic episodes, bipolar disorder, and migraine prevention.

QUICK REFERENCE

Drug group Anticonvulsant drug (p.42)

Overdose danger rating Medium

Dependence rating Low

Prescription needed Yes

Available as generic Yes

INFORMATION FOR USERS

Your drug prescription is tailored for you. Do not alter dosage without checking with your doctor.

How taken/used

Tablets, MR tablets, capsules, liquid, injection.

Frequency and timing of doses
1–2 x daily, after food.

Dosage range
600mg–2.5g daily, adjusted as necessary.

Onset of effect
Within 60 minutes.

Duration of action
12 hours or more.

Diet advice
None.

Storage
Keep in original container at room temperature out of the reach of children. Protect from light.

Missed dose
Take as soon as you remember. If your next dose is due within 2 hours, take a single dose now and skip the next.

Stopping the drug
Do not stop the drug without consulting your doctor, who will supervise a gradual reduction in dosage. Abrupt withdrawal may lead to a recurrence of symptoms.

Exceeding the dose
An occasional unintentional extra dose is unlikely to cause problems. Large overdoses may lead to coma. Notify your doctor.

SPECIAL PRECAUTIONS

Be sure to tell your doctor if:
- You have long-term liver or kidney problems.
- You have porphyria.
- You have any blood disorders.
- You are pregnant or intend to become pregnant.
- You are taking other medicines.

 Pregnancy
Not recommended. May cause abnormalities in the unborn baby. If sodium valproate is essential, extra folic acid supplements must also be taken. Discuss with your doctor.

 Breast-feeding
The drug passes into the breast milk, but at normal doses adverse effects on the baby are unlikely. Discuss with your doctor.

 Infants and children
Reduced dose necessary. The dose is often based on the weight of the child.

 Over 60
Reduced dose may be necessary.

 Driving and hazardous work
Your underlying condition, as well as the possibility of reduced alertness while taking sodium valproate, may make such activities inadvisable. Discuss with your doctor.

 Alcohol
Avoid. Alcohol may increase the sedative effects of this drug.

POSSIBLE ADVERSE EFFECTS

Most of the adverse effects seen with sodium valproate are uncommon, and the most serious ones are rare. They include liver failure, and platelet and bleeding abnormalities. Menstrual periods may become irregular or may cease altogether.

Symptom/effect	Frequency		Discuss with doctor		Stop taking drug now	Call doctor now
	Common	Rare	Only if severe	In all cases		
Temporary loss of hair	●		●			
Weight gain	●		●			
Nausea/indigestion	●		●			
Rash		●		●		●
Drowsiness		●		●		●
Jaundice		●		●		●
Bruising/bleeding		●		●		●

INTERACTIONS

Other anticonvulsant drugs may reduce blood levels of sodium valproate.

Zidovudine When zidovudine and sodium valproate are taken together, the blood levels of zidovudine may increase, leading to increased adverse effects.

Lamotrigine Sodium valproate increases levels of lamotrigine and may lead to increased adverse effects.

Carbapenems These antibacterial drugs reduce the blood level of sodium valproate; concomitant use should be avoided.

Antidepressants, antipsychotics, mefloquine, and chloroquine may reduce the effectiveness of sodium valproate to prevent seizures.

Clarithromycin and erythromycin may increase the effects of sodium valproate.

PROLONGED USE

Use of this drug can, very rarely, cause liver damage, which is more likely in the first 6 months of use.

Monitoring Periodic blood tests of liver function and blood composition may be carried out.

SOTALOL

Brand names Beta-Cardone, Sotacor
Used in the following combined preparations None

GENERAL INFORMATION

Sotalol is a non-cardioselective beta blocker (p.55) used in the prevention and treatment of heart rhythm problems, notably ventricular and supraventricular arrhythmias (p.58). It has an additional anti-arrhythmic action to other beta blockers. Sotalol is no longer prescribed for the other conditions for which beta blockers are used (e.g. hypertension). This is due to the risk of a serious but infrequent side effect called "torsades de pointes", a kind of ventricular arrhythmia that can cause loss of consciousness or even sudden death. For this reason, anyone prescribed sotalol will be carefully monitored.

INFORMATION FOR USERS

Your drug prescription is tailored for you. Do not alter dosage without checking with your doctor.

How taken/used

Tablets.

Frequency and timing of doses
2 x daily.

Adult dosage range
80mg daily initially, increased at 2–3-day intervals to 160–320mg daily. Higher doses of 480–640mg only under specialist supervision.

Onset of effect
12 hours.

Duration of action
12 hours.

Diet advice
None.

Storage
Keep in original container at room temperature out of the reach of children. Protect from light.

Missed dose
Take as soon as you remember. If your next dose is due within 3 hours, take a single dose now and skip the next.

Stopping the drug
Do not stop the drug without consulting your doctor, who will supervise a gradual reduction in dosage. Sudden withdrawal may lead to worsening of your condition.

OVERDOSE ACTION

Seek immediate medical advice in all cases of overdose by mouth. Take emergency action if breathing difficulties, palpitations, collapse, or loss of consciousness occur.

See Drug poisoning emergency guide (p.518).

POSSIBLE ADVERSE EFFECTS

A very fast heart rate with palpitations could be a symptom of torsades de pointes; if you experience this you should notify your doctor immediately.

Symptom/effect	Frequency		Discuss with doctor		Stop taking drug now	Call doctor now
	Common	Rare	Only if severe	In all cases		
Lethargy/fatigue	●			●		
Cold hands and feet	●			●		
Nightmares/vivid dreams		●		●	●	
Rash/dry eyes		●		●	●	
Visual disturbances		●		●	●	
Fainting/palpitations		●		●	●	●
Breathlessness/wheeze		●		●	●	●

SPECIAL PRECAUTIONS

Be sure to tell your doctor if:
- You have liver or kidney problems.
- You have a breathing disorder such as asthma, bronchitis, or emphysema.
- You have heart or heart rhythm problems.
- You have diabetes.
- You have psoriasis.
- You have poor circulation in the legs.
- You have lactose intolerance.
- You are taking other medicines.

Pregnancy
Not usually prescribed. May affect the developing baby. Discuss with your doctor.

Breast-feeding
The drug passes into the breast milk and may affect the baby. Discuss with your doctor.

Infants and children
Not prescribed.

Over 60
Reduced dose may be necessary.

Driving and hazardous work
Do not undertake such activities until you have learned how sotalol affects you because the drug can cause dizziness and fatigue.

Alcohol
Avoid excessive intake. Alcohol may increase the blood-pressure-lowering effect of sotalol.

Surgery and general anaesthetics
Occasionally, sotalol may need to be stopped before you have a general anaesthetic, but only do this after discussion with your doctor or dentist.

INTERACTIONS

Calcium channel blockers These may cause low blood pressure, a slow heart beat, and heart failure if taken with sotalol.

Diuretics, amphotericin, corticosteroids, and some laxatives These may lower blood potassium levels, increasing the risk of torsades de pointes.

Anti-arrhythmics Taking any of these drugs with sotalol may slow the heart rate and affect heart function.

Cardiac glycosides (e.g. digoxin) These may increase the heart-slowing effect of sotalol.

Antihypertensives Sotalol may enhance the blood-pressure-lowering effect of these drugs.

Phenothiazines, antidepressants, astemizole, moxifloxacin, mizolastine, ivabradine, antipsychotics, and erythromycin These drugs increase the risk of torsades de pointes with sotalol.

PROLONGED USE

Sotalol may be taken indefinitely for prevention of ventricular arrhythmias.

Monitoring Periodic blood tests are usually performed to monitor levels of potassium and magnesium. The heartbeat is usually monitored for the risk of development of torsades de pointes.

SPIRONOLACTONE

Brand name Aldactone
Used in the following combined preparations Aldactide, Lasilactone

GENERAL INFORMATION

Spironolactone belongs to the class of drugs known as potassium-sparing diuretics. It is used either alone or in combination with thiazide or loop diuretics to treat oedema (fluid retention) resulting from congestive heart failure, cirrhosis of the liver, and nephrotic syndrome (a kidney disorder). The drug is also used to reduce blood pressure, especially in people with Conn's syndrome, a condition caused by a benign adrenal gland tumour.

Spironolactone is relatively slow to act, and its effects may appear only after several days of treatment. As with other potassium-sparing diuretics, there is a risk of unusually high levels of potassium in the blood if the kidneys are functioning abnormally. For this reason, the drug is prescribed with caution to people with kidney failure.

Spironolactone does not worsen gout or diabetes, as do some other diuretics. The major adverse effect is nausea, but abnormal breast enlargement (gynaecomastia) may occur in men.

INFORMATION FOR USERS

Your drug prescription is tailored for you. Do not alter dosage without checking with your doctor.

How taken/used

Tablets, capsules, liquid.

Frequency and timing of doses
Once daily, usually in the morning.

Adult dosage range
25–400mg daily.

Onset of effect
Within 1–3 days, but full effect may take up to 2 weeks.

Duration of action
2–3 days.

Diet advice
Avoid foods that are high in potassium: for example, dried fruit and salt substitutes.

Storage
Keep in original container at room temperature out of the reach of children. Protect from light.

Missed dose
Take as soon as you remember.

Stopping the drug
Do not stop the drug without consulting your doctor; symptoms may recur.

Exceeding the dose
An occasional unintentional extra dose is unlikely to be a cause for concern. But if you notice any unusual symptoms, or if a large overdose has been taken, notify your doctor.

SPECIAL PRECAUTIONS

Be sure to tell your doctor if:
- You have long-term liver or kidney problems.
- You have porphyria.
- You have Addison's disease.
- You have a metabolic disorder.
- You are taking other medicines.

Pregnancy
Not usually prescribed. May have adverse effects on the baby. Discuss with your doctor.

Breast-feeding
The drug passes into the breast milk, but at normal doses adverse effects on the baby are unlikely. Discuss with your doctor.

Infants and children
Reduced dose necessary.

Over 60
Increased likelihood of adverse effects. Reduced dose may therefore be necessary.

Driving and hazardous work
Avoid such activities until you have learned how spironolactone affects you because the drug may occasionally cause drowsiness.

Alcohol
No known problems.

POSSIBLE ADVERSE EFFECTS

Spironolactone has few common adverse effects; the main problem is the possibility that potassium may be retained by the body, causing muscle weakness and numbness.

Symptom/effect	Frequency		Discuss with doctor		Stop taking drug now	Call doctor now
	Common	Rare	Only if severe	In all cases		
Nausea/vomiting	●		●			
Headache		●	●			
Lethargy/drowsiness		●	●			
Irregular menstruation		●	●			
Breast enlargement (both sexes)		●		●		
Erectile dysfunction		●		●		
Rash		●		●	●	●

INTERACTIONS

ACE inhibitors, NSAIDs (see p.74), angiotensin II blockers, ciclosporin, tacrolimus, and potassium salts
These drugs may increase the risk of raised blood levels of potassium, and can enhance the lowering of blood pressure caused by spironolactone.

Lithium Spironolactone may increase the blood levels of lithium, leading to an increased risk of lithium toxicity.

Digoxin Adverse effects may result from increased digoxin levels.

PROLONGED USE

Long-term use in young people is avoided if possible due to the endocrine effects of the drug; for young patients, eplerenone may be a better alternative.

Monitoring Blood tests may be performed to check on kidney function and levels of body salts.

STRONTIUM RANELATE

Brand name None
Used in the following combined preparations None

GENERAL INFORMATION

Strontium ranelate is used to treat severe osteoporosis, to reduce the risk of fractures. The active ingredient is derived from a naturally occurring element, strontium, which acts on cells in the bone to increase bone formation and reduce bone resorption, leading to a rebalance of bone turnover in favour of bone formation.

Because strontium ranelate has been associated with heart disorders, it is used, under specialist supervision, only for those with severe osteoporosis for whom there are no suitable alternative treatments. Apart from the risk of heart disorders and a small increase in the risk of deep vein thrombosis (blood clots in the legs and lungs), strontium ranelate generally causes few adverse reactions in those who are prescribed the drug. Very rarely, some people may develop a serious allergic reaction to the drug, which may affect other organs in the body.

QUICK REFERENCE

Drug group Drug for bone disorders (p.80)

Overdose danger rating Low

Dependence rating Low

Prescription needed Yes

Available as generic Yes

INFORMATION FOR USERS

Your drug prescription is tailored for you. Do not alter dosage without checking with your doctor.

How taken/used

Granules dissolved in water.

Frequency and timing of doses
Once daily, usually at night.

Adult dosage range
2g daily.

Onset of effect
3–5 hours. Beneficial effects may take several months to be felt.

Duration of action
Up to a week.

Diet advice
Food, milk, milk products, and calcium reduce absorption of strontium ranelate. You should take the drug at bedtime or between meals and allow at least 2 hours before or after food, milk, or milk products or calcium supplements.

Storage
Keep in original container below 30°C out of the reach of children. Protect from light.

Missed dose
Take the next dose at the time it is due. Do not take a double dose to make up for a missed dose.

Stopping the drug
Do not stop the drug without consulting your doctor. Stopping the drug may lead to a worsening of the underlying condition.

Exceeding the dose
An occasional unintentional extra dose is unlikely to cause problems. If a large overdose has been taken, notify your doctor.

SPECIAL PRECAUTIONS

Be sure to tell your doctor if:
- You have ever had a previous adverse reaction to strontium ranelate.
- You have long-term kidney problems.
- You have or have had heart problems.
- You have had a stroke or disease affecting the blood vessels in the brain.
- You have high blood pressure.
- You are being treated or have been treated for blood clots in your legs or lungs.
- You are confined to bed or are due to have surgery.
- You have phenylketonuria.
- You are taking other medicines.

 Pregnancy
Not prescribed. In women, the drug is used only after the menopause.

 Breast-feeding
Not prescribed. In women, the drug is used only after the menopause.

 Infants and children
Not prescribed. The drug is for use in postmenopausal women only.

 Over 60
No special problems.

 Driving and hazardous work
No specific problems.

 Alcohol
No special problems.

POSSIBLE ADVERSE EFFECTS

In general, people prescribed strontium ranelate experience few adverse effects. The common side effects of nausea and diarrhoea are mild and often settle with continued use.

Very rarely, the drug may cause a serious allergic reaction. If you develop a skin rash while taking it, you should stop the drug and consult your doctor immediately.

Symptom/effect	Frequency		Discuss with doctor		Stop taking drug now	Call doctor now
	Common	Rare	Only if severe	In all cases		
Headache/drowsiness	●		●			
Nausea/diarrhoea	●		●			
Swollen or painful leg		●		●		
Skin rash/fever/swollen glands		●		●	●	●

INTERACTIONS

Tetracycline and quinolone antibiotics (e.g. tetracycline and ciprofloxacin) Strontium ranelate may reduce absorption of these drugs. It should be stopped when taking a course of these antibiotics.

Antacids and products containing calcium, magnesium, or aluminium These can reduce the absorption of strontium ranelate so should be given at least 2 hours before or after the drug.

PROLONGED USE

The long-term safety of strontium ranelate is uncertain, especially regarding the risk of heart disorders. For this reason, it is prescribed only under specialist supervision and when there are no suitable alternatives.

Monitoring Blood and other tests may be carried out to monitor your bone density. Strontium ranelate can interfere with the blood tests used to measure calcium level.

SUCRALFATE

Brand name None
Used in the following combined preparations None

GENERAL INFORMATION

Sucralfate, a drug partly derived from aluminium, is prescribed to treat gastric and duodenal ulcers. It is particularly used to prevent stress-induced ulcers in patients who are seriously ill. The drug does not neutralize stomach acid, but it forms a protective barrier over the ulcer that protects it from attack by digestive juices, giving it time to heal.

If it is necessary during treatment to take antacids to relieve pain, they should be taken at least half an hour before or after taking sucralfate.

There are a few reports of seriously ill patients developing bezoars (balls of indigestible material) in their stomachs while on sucralfate. The safety of the drug for long-term use has not yet been confirmed. Therefore, courses of more than 12 weeks are not recommended.

INFORMATION FOR USERS

Your drug prescription is tailored for you. Do not alter dosage without checking with your doctor.

How taken/used

Tablets, liquid.

Frequency and timing of doses
2–6 x daily, 1 hour before each meal and at bedtime, at least 2 hours after food. The tablets may be dispersed in a little water before swallowing.

Dosage range
4–8g daily.

Onset of effect
Some improvement may be noted after one or two doses, but it takes a few weeks for an ulcer to heal.

Duration of action
Up to 5 hours.

Diet advice
Your doctor will advise if supplements are needed.

Storage
Keep in original container at room temperature out of the reach of children.

Missed dose
Do not make up the dose you missed. Take your next dose on your original schedule.

Stopping the drug
Do not stop the drug without consulting your doctor; symptoms may recur.

Exceeding the dose
An occasional unintentional extra dose is unlikely to be a cause for concern. But if you notice any unusual symptoms, or if a large overdose has been taken, notify your doctor.

SPECIAL PRECAUTIONS

Be sure to tell your doctor if:
- You have a long-term kidney problem.
- You are taking other medicines.

 Pregnancy
Safety in pregnancy not established, although so little is absorbed into the body that it is probably safe. Discuss with your doctor.

 Breast-feeding
It is not known whether the drug passes into breast milk. Discuss with your doctor.

 Infants and children
Not usually prescribed.

 Over 60
No special problems.

 Driving and hazardous work
Usually no problems, but sucralfate may cause dizziness in some people.

 Alcohol
Avoid. Alcohol may counteract the beneficial effect of this drug.

POSSIBLE ADVERSE EFFECTS

Most people do not experience any adverse effects while they are taking sucralfate. The most common is constipation, which will diminish as your body adjusts to the drug.

Symptom/effect	Frequency		Discuss with doctor		Stop taking drug now	Call doctor now
	Common	Rare	Only if severe	In all cases		
Indigestion	●		●			
Constipation	●		●			
Diarrhoea		●	●			
Dry mouth		●	●			
Nausea		●		●		
Rash/itching		●		●		
Dizziness/vertigo		●		●		
Headache		●	●			

INTERACTIONS

General note Sucralfate may reduce the absorption and effect of a range of drugs, including ranitidine, digoxin, phenytoin, warfarin, levothyroxine, and antibacterials. Take these and other medications at least 30 minutes before or 2 hours after sucralfate.

Antacids and other indigestion remedies These reduce the effectiveness of sucralfate and should be taken at least 30 minutes before or after sucralfate.

PROLONGED USE

Not usually prescribed for periods longer than 12 weeks at a time. Prolonged use may lead to deficiencies of vitamins A, D, E, and K.

SULFASALAZINE

Brand names Salazopyrin, Sulazine EC
Used in the following combined preparations None

GENERAL INFORMATION

Sulfasalazine, a chemical combination of a sulfonamide and a salicylate, is used to treat the inflammatory bowel disorders ulcerative colitis (which mainly affects the large intestine) and Crohn's disease (which usually affects the small intestine). It is also used to modify, halt, or slow the underlying disease process in severe rheumatoid arthritis.

Adverse effects such as nausea, loss of appetite, and general discomfort are more likely when higher doses are taken. Side effects caused by stomach irritation may be avoided by using a specially coated tablet form of the drug. Allergic reactions such as fever and skin rash may be avoided or minimized by low initial doses of the drug, followed by gradual increases. Maintenance of adequate fluid intake is important while taking this drug. In rare cases among men, temporary sterility may occur.

INFORMATION FOR USERS

Your drug prescription is tailored for you. Do not alter dosage without checking with your doctor.

How taken/used

Tablets, liquid, suppositories.

Frequency and timing of doses
2–4 x daily after meals with a glass of water (tablets); 2 x daily (suppositories).

Adult dosage range
4–8g daily in acute attacks; up to 2g daily for maintenance therapy (Crohn's disease/ulcerative colitis). 500mg–3g daily (rheumatoid arthritis).

Onset of effect
Adverse effects may occur within a few days, but full beneficial effects may take 1–3 weeks, depending on the severity of the condition.

Duration of action
Up to 24 hours.

Diet advice
It is important to drink plenty of liquids (at least 1.5 litres a day) during treatment. Sulfasalazine may reduce the absorption of folic acid from the intestine, leading to a deficiency of this vitamin. Eat plenty of green vegetables. Your doctor may also recommend folic acid supplements.

Storage
Keep in original container at room temperature out of the reach of children.

Missed dose
Take as soon as you remember. If your next dose is due within 2 hours, take a single dose now and skip the next.

Stopping the drug
Do not stop the drug without consulting your doctor; symptoms may recur.

Exceeding the dose
An occasional unintentional extra dose is unlikely to be a cause for concern. But if you notice any unusual symptoms, or if a large overdose has been taken, notify your doctor.

SPECIAL PRECAUTIONS

Be sure to tell your doctor if:
- You have long-term liver or kidney problems.
- You have asthma or severe allergies.
- You have glucose-6-phosphate dehydrogenase (G6PD) deficiency.
- You have a blood disorder.
- You have porphyria.
- You are allergic to sulfonamides or salicylates.
- You wear soft contact lenses.
- You are taking other medicines.

 Pregnancy
No evidence of risk to developing fetus. Folic acid supplements may be required. Discuss with your doctor.

 Breast-feeding
The drug passes into the breast milk and may affect the baby. Discuss with your doctor.

 Infants and children
Not recommended under 2 years. Reduced dose necessary for older children, according to body weight.

 Over 60
No special problems.

 Driving and hazardous work
No special problems.

 Alcohol
No known problems.

POSSIBLE ADVERSE EFFECTS

Adverse effects are common with high doses, but may disappear with a reduction in the dose. Symptoms such as nausea and vomiting may be helped by taking the drug with food. Orange or yellow discoloration of the urine may occur but is no cause for alarm.

Symptom/effect	Frequency		Discuss with doctor		Stop taking drug now	Call doctor now
	Common	Rare	Only if severe	In all cases		
Nausea/vomiting	●		●			
Malaise/loss of appetite	●		●			
Insomnia/mood changes	●		●			
Headache	●			●		
Joint pain	●			●		
Ringing in the ears		●	●			
Fever/rash		●		●		●
Bleeding/bruising		●		●		●

PROLONGED USE

Blood disorders may occur with prolonged use of this drug. Maintenance dosage is usually continued indefinitely.

Monitoring Periodic tests of blood composition and liver function are usually required as well as periodic urine tests.

INTERACTIONS

General note 1 Sulfasalazine may increase the effects of some drugs, including mercaptopurine and azathioprine. With azathioprine, there is also an increased risk of blood count abnormalities.

General note 2 Sulfasalazine reduces the absorption and effect of some drugs, including digoxin, folic acid, and iron.

SUMATRIPTAN

Brand names Imigran, Imigran Subject
Used in the following combined preparations None

GENERAL INFORMATION

Sumatriptan is a highly effective drug for migraine, usually given when people fail to respond to analgesics (such as aspirin and paracetamol). The drug is of considerable value in the treatment of acute migraine attacks, whether or not they are preceded by an aura, but is not meant to be taken regularly to prevent attacks. Sumatriptan is also used for the acute treatment of cluster headache (a form of migraine headache). It should be taken as soon as possible after the onset of the attack, although, unlike other drugs used in migraine, it will still be of benefit at whatever stage of the attack it is taken.

QUICK REFERENCE

Drug group Drug for migraine (p.45)

Overdose danger rating Medium

Dependence rating Low

Prescription needed Yes (injection and nasal spray) No (others)

Available as generic Yes

INFORMATION FOR USERS

Your drug prescription is tailored for you. Do not alter dosage without checking with your doctor.

How taken/used

Tablets, injection, nasal spray.

Frequency and timing of doses
Should be taken as soon as possible after the onset of an attack, but it is equally effective at any stage. Do not take a second dose for the same attack, or within 2 hours if migraine recurs.

Adult dosage range
Tablets 50–100mg per attack, up to maximum of 300mg in 24 hours if another attack occurs. Do not take a second dose for the same attack, or within 2 hours if migraine recurs. *Injection* 6mg per attack, up to maximum of 12mg (two injections) in 24 hours if another attack occurs. Do not take a second dose for the same attack, or within 1 hour if migraine recurs. *Nasal spray* Adults: 1x 20mg puff into one nostril per attack, to maximum of 40mg (2 puffs) in 24 hours if another attack occurs.

Age 12 to 17 years: 1x 10mg puff into one nostril per attack, to maximum of 20mg (2 puffs) in 24 hours if another attack occurs.

Onset of effect
30–45 minutes (tablets); 10–15 minutes (injection); 15 minutes (nasal spray).

Duration of action
Tablets 2–4 hours.
Injection 1½–2 hours.
Nasal spray 1–3 hours.

Diet advice
None, unless otherwise advised.

Storage
Keep in original container at room temperature out of the reach of children. Protect from light.

Missed dose
Not applicable, as it is taken only to treat a migraine attack.

Stopping the drug
Taken only to treat a migraine attack.

Exceeding the dose
An occasional unintentional extra tablet or injection is unlikely to cause problems. But if you notice any unusual symptoms, or if a large overdose has been taken, notify your doctor.

SPECIAL PRECAUTIONS

Be sure to consult your doctor or pharmacist before taking this drug if:
• You have liver or kidney problems.
• You have heart problems.
• You have high blood pressure.
• You have had a heart attack.
• You have had a stroke.
• You have angina.
• You are allergic to some medicines.
• You are taking other medicines.

 Pregnancy
Safety in pregnancy not established. Discuss with your doctor.

 Breast-feeding
Safety not established. Discuss with your doctor.

 Infants and children
Not recommended under 12 years.

 Over 60
Not recommended for patients over 65 years.

 Driving and hazardous work
Avoid such activities until you have learned how sumatriptan affects you because the drug can cause drowsiness.

 Alcohol
No special problems, but some drinks may provoke migraine in some people.

Surgery and general anaesthetics
Notify your doctor or dentist if you have used sumatriptan within 48 hours prior to surgery.

PROLONGED USE

Sumatriptan should not be used continuously to prevent migraine but only to treat migraine attacks.

POSSIBLE ADVERSE EFFECTS

Many of the adverse effects will disappear after about 1 hour as your body becomes adjusted to the medicine. If the symptoms persist or are severe, contact your doctor.

Symptom/effect	Frequency		Discuss with doctor		Stop taking drug now	Call doctor now
	Common	Rare	Only if severe	In all cases		
Pain at injection site	●		●			
Feeling of tingling/heat	●		●			
Flushing	●		●			
Feeling of heaviness/weakness	●		●			
Dizziness		●	●			
Fatigue/drowsiness		●	●			
Palpitations/chest pain		●		●	●	●

INTERACTIONS

Antidepressants Monoamine oxidase inhibitors (MAOIs) and some other antidepressants, such as fluvoxamine, fluoxetine, paroxetine, sertraline, and St John's wort, increase the risk of adverse effects with sumatriptan.

Lithium High risk of adverse effects if these drugs are taken together.

Ergotamine must be taken at least 6 hours after sumatriptan, and sumatriptan must be taken at least 24 hours after ergotamine.

TACROLIMUS

Brand names Adoport, Advagraf, Dailiport, Envarsus, Modigraf, Perixis, Prograf, Protopic
Used in the following combined preparations None

GENERAL INFORMATION

Tacrolimus is an immunosuppressant drug used in many types of organ transplant to help prevent rejection. It is usually used in combination with other immunosuppressants. It may also be used topically to treat skin conditions such as eczema and psoriasis when other drugs are inappropriate or have been unsuccessful. As tacrolimus suppresses the immune system when taken by mouth or injected, it increases susceptibility to infection and it can also cause kidney damage. The drug should not be taken by people who are allergic to any macrolide antibiotic. If you are taking oral tacrolimus, it is important to use the same formulation every time as they are not all interchangeable.

INFORMATION FOR USERS

Your drug prescription is tailored for you. Do not alter dosage without checking with your doctor.

How taken/used

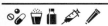

Capsules, SR capsules, granules, liquid, injection, ointment.

Frequency and timing of doses
Oral and injected preparations 1–2 x daily. Oral preparations should be taken on an empty stomach or 2–3 hours after a meal.
Topical preparation Initially 1–2 x daily; reduced to 2 x weekly when eczema improves.

Dosage range
Oral and injected preparations Dosage is calculated on an individual basis.
Topical preparation 0.1% or 0.03% ointment (adults); 0.03% ointment (children).

Onset of effect
Within 12 hours (oral and injection).1–2 weeks (ointment).

Duration of action
2–4 days.

Diet advice
If taking tacrolimus orally, avoid high-potassium foods and grapefruit juice. No special restrictions for other preparations.

Storage
Store at room temperature and protect from moisture. Keep out of the reach of children.

Missed dose
Take as soon as you remember, unless your next dose is due within 12 hours, in which case omit the missed dose and take the next dose as scheduled. Do not double your next dose.

Stopping the drug
Do not stop the drug without consulting your doctor. If it is being taken after a transplant, stopping may lead to organ rejection. If the drug is being used for eczema, stopping may lead to recurrence or worsening of symptoms.

Exceeding the dose
An occasional unintentional dose is unlikely to cause major problems. Large oral overdoses may cause tremor, headache, vomiting, and kidney damage. Notify your doctor.

POSSIBLE ADVERSE EFFECTS

Used topically, the drug may cause local irritation, rash, or paraesthesia (pins-and-needles). Taken orally, common side effects include nausea, diarrhoea, headache, and paraesthesia. It may also increase the risk of diabetes or worsen diabetic control.

Symptom/effect	Frequency		Discuss with doctor		Stop taking drug now	Call doctor now
	Common	Rare	Only if severe	In all cases		
Nausea	●		●			
Difficulty sleeping/drowsiness	●		●			
Diarrhoea/headache	●			●		
Pins-and-needles/tremor	●			●		
Spontaneous bruising/bleeding		●		●		●
Fever/sore throat		●		●		●
Confusion/seizures		●		●		●

INTERACTIONS

General note Many drugs may affect the level of tacrolimus. Check with your doctor before taking a new medication or stopping or changing current medication.

Grapefruit juice and St John's wort can affect blood levels of tacrolimus and should be avoided if taking the drug orally or by injection. If tacrolimus is being taken after a transplant, the interaction with St John's wort can cause organ rejection.

Vaccines Tacrolimus may affect your response to vaccines. Discuss with your doctor before having a vaccine.

SPECIAL PRECAUTIONS

Tacrolimus is prescribed only under medical supervision, but tell your doctor if:
• You have long-term kidney or liver problems.
• You have heart disease or high blood pressure.
• You have lactose intolerance.
• You suffer from peanut or soya allergy.
• You are pregnant or planning a pregnancy.
• You are taking other medicines.

Pregnancy
Safety not established. Discuss with your doctor.

Breast-feeding
Safety not established. Discuss with your doctor.

Infants and children
Used only by specialist children's doctors.

Over 60
No special problems.

Driving and hazardous work
If taking tacrolimus orally, avoid such activities until you know how the drug affects you. It may cause drowsiness. No known problems with topical use.

Alcohol
Avoid. Alcohol may increase drowsiness (oral tacrolimus), or cause skin irritation (topical tacrolimus).

Sunlight and sunbeds
Avoid prolonged, unprotected exposure as this can increase the risk of skin cancer.

PROLONGED USE

Long-term oral or injected tacrolimus can affect kidney and/or liver function, increases susceptibility to infection, and is linked to an increased risk of some skin and lymphoid cancers. Prolonged use may also increase the risk of high blood pressure or diabetes. Topically, the drug is associated with herpes skin infections (e.g. cold sores); there may also be an increased risk of skin cancer.

Monitoring For oral or injected forms, regular blood tests, kidney and liver function tests, blood pressure checks, and tests for diabetes should be done.

TAMOXIFEN

Brand name Soltamox
Used in the following combined preparations None

GENERAL INFORMATION

Tamoxifen is an anti-oestrogen drug (oestrogen is a naturally occurring female sex hormone; see p.105). It is used for two conditions: infertility and breast cancer.

When given as treatment of certain types of infertility, the drug is taken only on certain days of the menstrual cycle. Used as an anticancer drug for breast cancer, tamoxifen works by blocking the effect of natural oestrogens that stimulate the growth of tumours with oestrogen receptors (oestrogen-receptor-positive tumours). This reduces the risk of tumours recurring after surgical removal of the tumour.

As its effect is specific, tamoxifen has fewer adverse effects than most other drugs used for breast cancer. However, it may cause eye damage if high doses are taken for long periods.

INFORMATION FOR USERS

Your drug prescription is tailored for you. Do not alter dosage without checking with your doctor.

How taken/used

Tablets, liquid.

Frequency and timing of doses
1–2 x daily.

Adult dosage range
Breast cancer 20mg daily.
Infertility 20–80mg daily.

Onset of effect
Side effects may be felt within days, but beneficial effects may take 4–10 weeks.

Duration of action
Effects may be felt for several weeks after stopping the drug.

Diet advice
None.

Storage
Keep in original container at room temperature out of the reach of children. Protect from light.

Missed dose
Take as soon as you remember. If your next dose is due within 2 hours, take a single dose now and skip the next.

Stopping the drug
Do not stop the drug without consulting your doctor; stopping the drug may lead to worsening of your underlying condition.

Exceeding the dose
An occasional unintentional extra dose is unlikely to be a cause for concern. But if you notice any unusual symptoms, or if a large overdose has been taken, notify your doctor.

SPECIAL PRECAUTIONS

Be sure to tell your doctor if:
- You are pregnant or are planning a pregnancy.
- You have cataracts or poor eyesight.
- You suffer from porphyria.
- You have a history of venous thrombosis.
- You are taking other medicines.

Pregnancy
Not usually prescribed. May have effects on the developing baby. Discuss with your doctor.

Breast-feeding
Not usually prescribed. Discuss with your doctor.

Infants and children
Not prescribed.

Over 60
No special problems.

Driving and hazardous work
Do not drive until you have learned how tamoxifen affects you because the drug can cause dizziness and blurred vision.

Alcohol
No known problems.

Surgery and general anaesthetics
Tell your doctor or anaesthetist that you are taking tamoxifen before you have any surgery. You may be advised to stop taking it 6 weeks beforehand.

POSSIBLE ADVERSE EFFECTS

These are rarely serious and do not usually require treatment to be stopped. Nausea, vomiting, and hot flushes are the most common reactions. There is a small risk of endometrial cancer (cancer of the uterine lining) developing, so you should notify your doctor of any symptoms such as irregular vaginal bleeding as soon as possible.

Symptom/effect	Frequency		Discuss with doctor		Stop taking drug now	Call doctor now
	Common	Rare	Only if severe	In all cases		
Nausea/vomiting	●		●			
Hot flushes/hair loss	●		●			
Irregular vaginal bleeding	●			●		●
Irregular vaginal discharge	●			●		●
Bone and tumour pain		●		●		
Rash/itching		●		●		
Blurred/reduced vision		●		●		
Calf pain/swelling		●		●		●

INTERACTIONS

Anticoagulants People treated with anticoagulants such as warfarin usually need a lower dose of the anticoagulant.

SSRI antidepressants These may reduce the effectiveness of tamoxifen.

Anticancer medicines Cytotoxic medicines taken with tamoxifen may increase the risk of side effects, especially the risk of venous thrombosis.

PROLONGED USE

There is a risk of damage to the eye with long-term, high-dose treatment. There is also a small increased risk of endometrial cancer and venous thrombosis with long-term tamoxifen treatment, but these risks are outweighed by the benefit of preventing recurrence of breast cancer.

Monitoring Eyesight may be tested periodically.

TAMSULOSIN

Brand names Contiflo XL, Diffundox XL, Faramsil, Flomaxtra XL, Losinate MR, Tabphyn MR, Tamurex, and many others
Used in the following combined preparations Combodart (with dutasteride), Vesomni (with solifenacin)

GENERAL INFORMATION

Tamsulosin is a selective alpha blocker drug used to treat urinary retention due to benign prostatic hypertrophy, or BPH (enlarged prostate gland). The drug, as it passes through the prostate, relaxes the muscle in the wall of the urethra, thereby increasing urine flow.

Tamsulosin is available over the counter for men aged 45–74 years with symptoms of BPH. If symptoms have not improved (or have got worse) within two weeks, the drug should be stopped and you should consult your doctor. If symptoms have improved with the drug, you should still see your doctor within six weeks to confirm your symptoms are due to BPH.

Like other alpha blockers, tamsulosin may lower blood pressure rapidly after the first dose. For this reason, the first dose should be taken at home so that, if dizziness or weakness occur, you can lie down until they have disappeared.

QUICK REFERENCE

Drug group Drug for urinary disorders (p.126)

Overdose danger rating Medium

Dependence rating Low

Prescription needed Yes (most preparations)

Available as generic Yes

INFORMATION FOR USERS

Your drug prescription is tailored for you. Do not alter dosage without checking with your doctor. If taking an over-the-counter preparation, follow the instructions and consult your doctor if symptoms do not improve or worsen.

How taken/used

Tablets, MR tablets, capsules, MR capsules.

Frequency and timing of doses
Once daily, swallowed whole, after breakfast.

Adult dosage range
400mcg.

Onset of effect
1–2 hours.

Duration of action
24 hours.

Diet advice
None.

Storage
Keep in original container at room temperature out of the reach of children.

Missed dose
Take as soon as you remember. If your next dose is due within 4 hours, take a single dose now and skip the next.

Stopping the drug
Do not stop taking the drug without consulting your doctor; stopping suddenly may lead to a rise in blood pressure.

Exceeding the dose
An occasional unintentional extra dose is unlikely to cause problems. Large overdoses may produce sedation, dizziness, low blood pressure, and rapid pulse. Notify your doctor immediately.

POSSIBLE ADVERSE EFFECTS

Dizziness seems to be the most common adverse effect, but this usually improves after the first few doses of the drug.

Symptom/effect	Frequency		Discuss with doctor		Stop taking drug now	Call doctor now
	Common	Rare	Only if severe	In all cases		
Dizziness/weakness/fainting	●		●			
Ejaculatory problems	●		●			
Headache	●		●			
Drowsiness	●		●			
Palpitations	●		●			
Nausea/vomiting		●	●			
Diarrhoea/constipation		●	●			
Rash/itching		●		●		

INTERACTIONS

Antidepressants, beta blockers, calcium channel blockers, diuretics, and thymoxamine These drugs are likely to increase the blood-pressure-lowering effect of tamsulosin.

SPECIAL PRECAUTIONS

Be sure to consult your doctor or pharmacist before taking this drug if:
• You have had low blood pressure.
• You have liver or kidney problems.
• You have heart failure.
• You have a history of depression.
• You are taking drugs for high blood pressure.
• You collapse after passing urine.
• You are taking other medicines.
• You have cataract surgery planned.

Pregnancy
Not prescribed.

Breast-feeding
Not prescribed.

Infants and children
Not prescribed.

Over 60
No special problems.

Driving and hazardous work
Avoid until you have learned how the drug affects you because it can cause drowsiness and dizziness.

Alcohol
Avoid until you know how tamsulosin affects you because alcohol can further lower blood pressure.

Surgery and general anaesthetics
Tamsulosin may need to be stopped before you have any surgery. Discuss with your doctor or dentist.

PROLONGED USE

No special problems.

TEMAZEPAM

Brand names None
Used in the following combined preparations None

GENERAL INFORMATION

Temazepam belongs to a group of drugs known as the benzodiazepines. The actions and adverse effects of this group of drugs are described more fully under Anti-anxiety drugs (p.39).

Temazepam is used in the short-term treatment of insomnia. Because it is short-acting compared with other benzodiazepines, the drug is less likely to cause drowsiness and/or lightheadedness the following day. Temazepam is not usually effective in preventing early morning waking.

Like other benzodiazepine drugs, temazepam can be habit-forming if taken regularly over a long period. Its effects also grow weaker with time. For these reasons, treatment with temazepam is usually only continued for a few days at a time.

QUICK REFERENCE

Drug group Benzodiazepine sleeping drug (p.38)

Overdose danger rating Medium

Dependence rating High

Prescription needed Yes

Available as generic Yes

INFORMATION FOR USERS

Your drug prescription is tailored for you. Do not alter dosage without checking with your doctor.

How taken/used

Tablets, liquid.

Frequency and timing of doses
Once daily, 30 minutes before bedtime.

Adult dosage range
10–40mg.

Onset of effect
15–40 minutes, or longer.

Duration of action
6–8 hours.

Diet advice
None.

Storage
Keep in original container at room temperature out of the reach of children. Protect from light.

Missed dose
If you fall asleep without having taken a dose and wake some hours later, do not take the missed dose. If necessary, return to your normal dose schedule the following night.

Stopping the drug
If you have been taking the drug continuously for less than 2 weeks, it can be safely stopped as soon as you no longer need it. If you have been taking the drug for longer, consult your doctor, who may supervise a gradual reduction in dosage. Stopping abruptly may lead to withdrawal symptoms (see p.38).

Exceeding the dose
An occasional unintentional extra dose is unlikely to be a problem. Large overdoses may cause severe drowsiness and breathing problems. Consult your doctor immediately.

SPECIAL PRECAUTIONS

Be sure to tell your doctor if:
- You have severe respiratory disease.
- You have porphyria.
- You have liver or kidney problems.
- You have myasthenia gravis.
- You have had problems with alcohol or drug misuse.
- You are taking other medicines.

Pregnancy
Not usually recommended; may cause adverse effects on the newborn baby at the time of delivery. Discuss with your doctor.

Breast-feeding
The drug passes into the breast milk, and should be avoided during breast-feeding if possible. Discuss with your doctor.

Infants and children
Not recommended.

Over 60
Reduced dose may be necessary. Increased likelihood of adverse effects.

Driving and hazardous work
Avoid such activities until you have learned how temazepam affects you because the drug can cause reduced alertness and slowed reactions.

Alcohol
Avoid. Alcohol may increase the sedative effect of this drug.

POSSIBLE ADVERSE EFFECTS

The main adverse effects are related to the sedative and tranquillizing properties of temazepam and normally diminish after the first few days. However, some people experience a paradoxical increase in impulsivity, anxiety, and hostility.

Symptom/effect	Frequency		Discuss with doctor		Stop taking drug now	Call doctor now
	Common	Rare	Only if severe	In all cases		
Daytime drowsiness	●		●			
Headache	●		●			
Dizziness/unsteadiness		●		●		
Vivid dreams/nightmares		●		●		
Forgetfulness/confusion	●			●	●	

INTERACTIONS

Sedatives All drugs that have a sedative effect on the central nervous system are likely to increase the sedative properties of temazepam, which may potentially be fatal. Such drugs include alcohol and other anti-anxiety and sleeping drugs, opioid analgesics, antidepressants, antihistamines, and antipsychotics.

PROLONGED USE

Regular use of this drug over several weeks can lead to a reduction in its effect as the body adapts. It may also be habit-forming when taken for extended periods, and withdrawal symptoms may occur when the drug is stopped. Temazepam should not normally be used for longer than 1–2 weeks.

TENOFOVIR

Brand name Viread
Used in the following combined preparations Atripla, Eviplera, Stribild, Truvada

GENERAL INFORMATION

Tenofovir is an antiviral drug used to treat (although not cure) HIV and hepatitis B infection. It is a nucleotide reverse transcriptase inhibitor, which blocks an enzyme, reverse transcriptase, that viruses need to replicate. In treating HIV infection, tenofovir is usually used in combination with other anti-HIV drugs to reduce production of new viruses before the immune system is irreversibly damaged. This combined therapy is known as antiretroviral therapy, or ART. Tenofovir may also be used on its own to treat some cases of chronic hepatitis B infection.

Although tenofovir reduces the viral load in people with HIV or hepatitis B, it does not completely rid the body of these viruses. They may still be transmitted to other people and so it is important to continue taking precautions to avoid infecting others.

QUICK REFERENCE

Drug group Drug for HIV and immune deficiency (p.116) and antiviral drug (p.91)

Overdose danger rating Medium

Dependence rating Low

Prescription needed Yes

Available as generic No

INFORMATION FOR USERS

Your drug prescription is tailored for you. Do not alter dosage without checking with your doctor.

How taken/used

Tablets, granules.

Frequency and timing of doses
Once daily, with food or liquid, at the same time every day. If you vomit within 1 hour of taking a tablet, take another; if more than 1 hour afterwards, do not take another. Granules should be mixed with soft food, swallowed without chewing, and not mixed with liquids.

Adult dosage range
245mg daily (1 tablet, or granules as directed).

Onset of effect
May take from many weeks to a year before the drug reduces virus levels significantly.

Duration of action
Up to several days.

Diet advice
None.

Storage
Keep in original container at room temperature and out of the reach of children.

Missed dose
Take the dose as soon as you remember unless your next dose is due within 12 hours, in which case omit the missed dose and take the next dose as scheduled.

Stopping the drug
Do not stop the drug without consulting your doctor; your condition may worsen.

Exceeding the dose
An occasional unintentional extra dose is unlikely to cause problems. However, a large overdose may cause serious side effects; notify your doctor immediately.

POSSIBLE ADVERSE EFFECTS

Gastrointestinal side effects are common with tenofovir. When used in ART, the drug may also affect blood sugar and cholesterol levels and cause redistribution of body fat.

Symptom/effect	Frequency		Discuss with doctor		Stop taking drug now	Call doctor now
	Common	Rare	Only if severe	In all cases		
Dizziness/headache	●			●		
Nausea/diarrhoea	●			●		
Rash	●			●		
Muscle pain/weakness	●			●		
Tiredness/lethargy	●			●		
Body fat redistribution	●			●		
Joint stiffness/pain	●			●		
Severe upper abdominal pain		●		●	●	●

INTERACTIONS

General note Various drugs that affect the kidneys may affect blood levels of tenofovir, necessitating adjustment of its dose. These include antibacterials (e.g. aminoglycosides, pentamidine, and vancomycin); antifungals (e.g. amphotericin B); antivirals (e.g. foscarnet, ganciclovir, adefovir, and cidofovir); immunosuppressants (e.g. tacrolimus); and some anticancer drugs (e.g. interleukin-2).

Other anti-HIV drugs Tenofovir may interact with anti-HIV drugs containing didanosine to increase blood levels of didanosine and reduce CD_4 white blood cell counts, which may result in severe inflammation of the pancreas and may sometimes be fatal.

SPECIAL PRECAUTIONS

Be sure to tell your doctor if:
- You have kidney or liver disease.
- You have diabetes.
- You have a high blood cholesterol level.
- You have lactose intolerance.
- You are or plan to become pregnant.
- You are taking other medicines, especially corticosteroids.

Pregnancy
Safety not established. Discuss with your doctor.

Breast-feeding
It is not known if this drug passes into breast milk. However, the HIV and hepatitis B viruses can be passed to the baby in breast milk so breast-feeding is not recommended.

Infants and children
Not recommended.

Over 60
No known problems.

Driving and hazardous work
Avoid such activities until you have learned how the drug affects you because it may cause dizziness.

Alcohol
Avoid. Alcohol increases the risk of developing serious bone problems.

PROLONGED USE

Long-term use may cause loss of bone density and inflammation of the pancreas. In people with both HIV and hepatitis B or C, tenofovir may cause potentially fatal liver problems. ART including tenofovir may cause redistribution of body fat and abnormal blood sugar and lipid levels.

Monitoring Liver function tests are routine and people being treated for HIV will have regular checks of blood cell counts (including CD_4 counts), viral load, blood sugar and cholesterol levels, and response to treatment.

TERBINAFINE

Brand names Lamisil AT 1% Cream/Gel/Spray, Lamisil Cream, Lamisil Once, Lamisil Tablets
Used in the following combined preparations None

GENERAL INFORMATION

Terbinafine is an antifungal drug used to treat fungal infections of the skin and nails, particularly tinea (ringworm). It is also used as a cream for candida (yeast) infections.

Terbinafine has largely replaced older drugs such as griseofulvin because it is more easily absorbed and is therefore more effective.

Skin infections are treated in two to six weeks, but treatment of nail infections may take up to six months.

Rare adverse effects of terbinafine include a sore mouth and/or throat, jaundice, a severe skin rash, and bruising and/or bleeding in the mouth. All of these should be reported to your doctor without delay.

QUICK REFERENCE

Drug group Antifungal drug (p.96)
Overdose danger rating Low
Dependence rating Low
Prescription needed Yes (except for some skin preparations)
Available as generic Yes

INFORMATION FOR USERS

Your drug prescription is tailored for you. Do not alter dosage without checking with your doctor.

How taken/used

Tablets, spray, cream, gel, skin solution.

Frequency and timing of doses
Once daily (tablets); 1–2 x daily (cream or gel); once only (solution).

Adult dosage range
Tinea infections 250mg (tablets or gel).
Candida infections As directed (cream).

Onset of effect
Depends on the type and severity of infection.

Duration of action
24 hours.

Diet advice
None.

Storage
Keep in original container at room temperature out of the reach of children. Protect from light.

Missed dose
Take as soon as you remember. If your next dose is due within 4 hours, take a single dose now and skip the next.

Stopping the drug
Take the full course. Even if you feel better, the original infection may still be present and may recur if treatment is stopped too soon.

Exceeding the dose
An occasional unintentional extra dose is unlikely to be a cause for concern. But if you notice any unusual symptoms, or if a large overdose has been taken, notify your doctor.

SPECIAL PRECAUTIONS

Be sure to consult your doctor or pharmacist before taking this drug if:
- You have liver or kidney problems.
- You have psoriasis.
- You have an autoimmune disorder (e.g. systemic lupus erythematosus).
- You are taking other medicines.

Pregnancy
Safety in pregnancy not established. Discuss with your doctor.

Breast-feeding
Safety not established. Discuss with your doctor.

Infants and children
Safety not established. Discuss with your doctor.

Over 60
No special problems.

Driving and hazardous work
Avoid such activities until you know how terbinafine affects you because the drug can cause dizziness.

Alcohol
No known problems.

PROLONGED USE

Long-term use of oral terbinafine may rarely cause severe liver damage.

Monitoring Periodic blood tests are usually performed to check the effect of the drug on the liver.

POSSIBLE ADVERSE EFFECTS

Side effects of terbinafine are generally mild and transient. However, in rare cases it can cause serious toxicity affecting the skin, liver, and bone marrow.

Symptom/effect	Frequency		Discuss with doctor		Stop taking drug now	Call doctor now
	Common	Rare	Only if severe	In all cases		
Nausea/indigestion/bloating	●		●			
Abdominal pain/diarrhoea	●		●			
Headache	●		●			
Taste disturbance/loss		●	●			
Dizziness/tiredness		●	●			
Pins and needles		●	●			
Muscle or joint pain		●		●		
Severe skin rash		●		●	●	●
Sore mouth/throat		●		●	●	●
Bruising/bleeding in mouth		●		●	●	●
Jaundice		●		●	●	●
Dark urine/pale faeces		●		●	●	●

INTERACTIONS

Rifampicin This drug may reduce the blood level and effect of terbinafine.

Cimetidine This drug may increase the blood level of terbinafine.

Oral contraceptives Breakthrough bleeding may occur when these drugs are taken together with terbinafine.

Ciclosporin Terbinafine may reduce the blood level of ciclosporin.

TERBUTALINE

Brand name Bricanyl
Used in the following combined preparations None

GENERAL INFORMATION

Terbutaline is a sympathomimetic bronchodilator used to treat conditions such as asthma, chronic obstructive pulmonary disease (COPD), and bronchospasm, in which the airways become constricted. Terbutaline is also used to delay premature labour.

Muscle tremor, especially of the hands, is common with terbutaline and usually disappears on reduction of the dose or with continued use as the body adapts to the drug. In common with the other sympathomimetic drugs (see p.35), it may also produce nervousness and restlessness.

see p.35

(p.48)

QUICK REFERENCE

Drug group Bronchodilator (p.48)
Overdose danger rating Low
Dependence rating Low
Prescription needed Yes
Available as generic Yes

INFORMATION FOR USERS

Your drug prescription is tailored for you. Do not alter dosage without checking with your doctor.

How taken/used

Tablets, liquid (syrup), injection, inhaler, nebules for nebulizer.

Frequency and timing of doses
3 x daily (tablets/syrup); as necessary (inhaler).

Dosage range
Adults 7.5–15mg daily (tablets/syrup); 0.5mg when required, up to 2mg daily (inhaler); as directed by doctor (nebules).
Children Reduced dose according to age and weight.

Onset of effect
Within a few minutes (inhaler); within 1–2 hours (tablets/syrup).

Duration of action
7–8 hours (tablets/syrup).

Diet advice
None.

Storage
Keep in original container at room temperature out of the reach of children. Protect from light. Do not puncture or burn aerosol containers.

Missed dose
Do not take the missed dose. Take your next dose as usual.

Stopping the drug
Do not stop the drug without consulting your doctor; symptoms may recur.

Exceeding the dose
An occasional unintentional extra dose is unlikely to be a cause for concern. But if you notice any unusual symptoms, or if a large overdose has been taken, notify your doctor.

SPECIAL PRECAUTIONS

Be sure to tell your doctor if:
- You have heart problems.
- You have high blood pressure.
- You have an overactive thyroid.
- You have diabetes.
- You are taking other medicines.

 Pregnancy
Safety in early pregnancy not established, although drug is used in late pregnancy to prevent premature labour. Discuss with your doctor.

 Breast-feeding
The drug passes into the breast milk but in amounts too small to affect the baby.

 Infants and children
Reduced dose necessary.

 Over 60
Increased risk of adverse effects. Reduced dose may be necessary.

 Driving and hazardous work
Avoid such activities until you have learned how terbutaline affects you because the drug can cause tremor of the hands.

 Alcohol
No special problems.

PROLONGED USE

No problems expected. However, you should contact your doctor if you find you are needing to use your terbutaline inhaler more than usual. Failure to respond to the drug may be a result of worsening asthma that requires urgent medical attention.

Monitoring Periodic blood tests for potassium may be needed in people on high-dose treatment with terbutaline combined with other asthma drugs.

POSSIBLE ADVERSE EFFECTS

Muscle tremor (particularly affecting the hands), anxiety, and restlessness are the most common adverse effects. Rarely, wheezing or breathlessness may worsen immediately after inhaler use (paradoxical bronchospasm); if this happens, stop using the drug and contact your doctor immediately.

Symptom/effect	Frequency		Discuss with doctor		Stop taking drug now	Call doctor now
	Common	Rare	Only if severe	In all cases		
Anxiety/nervous tension	●		●			
Muscle tremor	●		●			
Restlessness	●		●			
Headache	●			●		
Muscle cramps		●		●		
Palpitations	●			●	●	
Worsening breathlessness		●		●	●	●

INTERACTIONS

Other sympathomimetics may add to the effects of terbutaline and vice versa, so increasing the risk of adverse effects.

Monoamine oxidase inhibitors (MAOIs) Terbutaline may interact with these drugs to cause a dangerous rise in blood pressure.

Diuretics, corticosteroids, and theophylline taken with terbutaline may reduce blood levels of potassium, causing muscle weakness.

Beta blockers may reduce the beneficial effects of terbutaline.

TESTOSTERONE

Brand names Nebido, Restandol Testocaps, Sustanon, Testavan, Testim, Testogel, Tostran
Used in the following combined preparations None

GENERAL INFORMATION

Testosterone is a male sex hormone produced by the testes and, in small quantities, by the ovaries in women. The hormone encourages bone and muscle growth in both men and women and stimulates sexual development in men.

The drug is used to treat testosterone deficiency (hypogonadism) due to pituitary or testicular disorders. It is also used to initiate puberty in male adolescents if it has been delayed due to deficiency of the natural hormone.

Testosterone can interfere with growth or cause overly rapid sexual development in adolescents. High doses may cause deepening of the voice, excessive hair growth, or hair loss in women.

INFORMATION FOR USERS

Your drug prescription is tailored for you. Do not alter dosage without checking with your doctor.

How taken/used

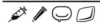

Injection, implanted pellets, gel, patch, oral and buccal preparations.

Frequency and timing of doses
Varies according to preparation and condition being treated (injection); 5g daily, according to response, to maximum of 10g daily (gel); every 6 months (implant); once daily (patch).

Dosage range
Varies with method of administration and the condition being treated.

Onset of effect
2–3 days. Full effect may take several months.

Duration of action
1 week to more than 3 months (injection); approximately 6 months (implant).

Diet advice
None.

Storage
Keep in original container at room temperature out of the reach of children. Protect from light.

Missed dose
No cause for concern, but take as soon as you remember.

Stopping the drug
Do not stop taking the drug without consulting your doctor.

Exceeding the dose
An occasional unintentional extra dose is unlikely to be a cause for concern. But if you notice unusual symptoms, or if a large overdose was taken, notify your doctor.

POSSIBLE ADVERSE EFFECTS

Most of the more serious adverse effects are likely to occur only with long-term treatment and may be helped by a reduction in dosage. Close contact with gel application sites can transfer significant amounts of the hormone to other people; pregnant women and young children are particularly at risk.

Symptom/effect	Frequency		Discuss with doctor		Stop taking drug now	Call doctor now
	Common	Rare	Only if severe	In all cases		
Acne	●		●			
Skin irritation (gel/patch)	●		●			
Hair loss/mood changes		●	●			
Water retention		●	●			
Jaundice		●		●	●	
Men only						
Abnormal erection	●				●	
Breast development		●	●			
Difficulty in passing urine		●		●		
Women only						
Unusual hair growth/loss		●	●			
Voice changes		●		●		
Enlarged clitoris		●		●		

INTERACTIONS

Anticoagulants Testosterone may increase the effect of warfarin-like anticoagulants, requiring adjustment of their dosage.

Antidiabetics Testosterone enhances their effects, requiring reduction of their dosage.

SPECIAL PRECAUTIONS

Be sure to tell your doctor if:
- You have long-term liver or kidney problems.
- You have heart problems.
- You have prostate problems.
- You have high blood pressure.
- You have epilepsy or migraine headaches.
- You have diabetes.
- You are taking other medicines.

 Pregnancy
Not prescribed. Avoid skin-to-skin transfer of testosterone from other people.

 Breast-feeding
Not prescribed. Avoid skin-to-skin transfer of testosterone from other people.

 Infants and children
Not prescribed for infants and young children. Reduced dose necessary in adolescents.

 Over 60
Rarely required. Increased risk of prostate problems in older men. Reduced dose may therefore be necessary.

 Driving and hazardous work
No special problems.

 Alcohol
No special problems.

PROLONGED USE

Prolonged use of this drug may lead to reduced growth in adolescents. In older men, it may accelerate prostate disease.

Monitoring Regular blood tests for the effects of testosterone treatment are necessary, such as red blood cell count, electrolyte levels, liver function tests, and PSA (prostate-specific antigen) levels.

TETRACYCLINE/LYMECYCLINE

Brand name Tetralysal 300
Used in the following combined preparation Deteclo

GENERAL INFORMATION

Tetracycline and lymecycline are both tetracyclines. This was once a widely used class of antibiotics, but the rise of drug-resistant bacteria has reduced their effectiveness in many types of infection. Tetracycline and lymecycline are commonly used for acne, rosacea, and diabetic diarrhoea, and to eradicate *Helicobacter pylori* infection, and are still used to treat chronic bronchitis, destructive forms of dental disease, and certain chest and genital infections due to mycoplasma organisms. They remain the treatment of choice for infections due to *Chlamydia* and *Rickettsia*.

Taken by mouth, these drugs can sometimes cause nausea, vomiting, and diarrhoea. Tetracyclines may discolour developing teeth if taken by children or by the mother during pregnancy. People with poor kidney function are not prescribed tetracycline/lymecycline because the drugs can cause further deterioration.

INFORMATION FOR USERS

Your drug prescription is tailored for you. Do not alter your dosage without checking with your doctor.

How taken/used

Tablets, capsules.

Frequency and timing of doses
By mouth 2–4 x daily, at least 1 hour before or 2 hours after meals (tetracycline); 1–2 x daily (lymecycline). Always swallow with water.

Adult dosage range
Infections 1–2g daily (tetracycline); 916–1,032mg daily (lymecycline).
Acne 1g daily (tetracycline); 408mg daily (lymecycline).

Onset of effect
4–12 hours. Improvement in acne may not be noticed for up to 4 weeks.

Duration of action
Up to 6 hours.

Diet advice
Milk products should be avoided for 1 hour before and 2 hours after taking the drug.

Storage
Keep in original container at room temperature out of the reach of children.

Missed dose
Take as soon as you remember. If your next dose is due within 2 hours, take a single dose now and skip the next.

Stopping the drug
Take the full course. Even if you feel better, the original infection may still be present and may recur if treatment is stopped too soon.

Exceeding the dose
An occasional unintentional extra dose is unlikely to be a cause for concern. But if you notice any unusual symptoms, or if a large overdose has been taken, notify your doctor.

POSSIBLE ADVERSE EFFECTS

Swallowing difficulties and/or oesophageal irritation may occur if the dose is taken with insufficient water. Do not take a dose prior to lying down.

Symptom/effect	Frequency		Discuss with doctor		Stop taking drug now	Call doctor now
	Common	Rare	Only if severe	In all cases		
Nausea/vomiting	●		●			
Diarrhoea	●		●			
Light-sensitive rash		●		●	●	
Rash/itching		●		●	●	
Jaundice		●		●	●	●
Headache/visual disturbance		●		●	●	

INTERACTIONS

Iron may reduce the effectiveness of tetracycline/lymecycline.

Oral anticoagulants Tetracycline/lymecycline may increase the action of these drugs.

Retinoids may increase the adverse effects of tetracycline/lymecycline.

Diuretics These should not be used with lymecycline.

Oral contraceptives Tetracycline/lymecycline may reduce the effectiveness of oral contraceptives.

Antacids and milk These interfere with the absorption of tetracycline/lymecycline and may reduce their effectiveness. Doses should be separated by 1–2 hours.

Methotrexate Tetracycline may increase the risk of methotrexate toxicity.

SPECIAL PRECAUTIONS

Be sure to tell your doctor if:
- You have long-term liver or kidney problems.
- You have previously suffered an allergic reaction to a tetracycline antibiotic.
- You have myasthenia gravis, acute porphyria, or systemic lupus erythematosus.
- You are taking other medicines.

Pregnancy
Not prescribed. May cause birth defects and may damage the teeth and bones of the developing baby as well as the mother's liver. Discuss with your doctor.

Breast-feeding
Not recommended. The drugs pass into the breast milk and may damage developing bones and discolour the baby's teeth. Discuss with your doctor.

Infants and children
Not recommended under 12 years. Reduced dose necessary in older children. May discolour developing teeth.

Over 60
No special problems.

Driving and hazardous work
No known problems.

Alcohol
No known problems.

Taking your tablets
To prevent the medication from sticking in your throat, take a small amount of water before and a full glass of water after each dose. Take the dose while sitting or standing and do not lie down immediately afterwards.

PROLONGED USE

No problems expected.

TEZACAFTOR/IVACAFTOR

Brand name Symkevi
Used in the following combined preparations None

GENERAL INFORMATION

Tezacaftor and ivacaftor are drugs used to treat cystic fibrosis. In this genetic disorder, the protein that regulates the flow of fluid in and out of cells lining the lungs (and other organs) is defective due to inherited mutations in the gene containing the code for this protein. The defect causes a build-up of sticky mucus in these organs, which leads to lung infections and affects other organs such as the pancreas. Tezacaftor and ivacaftor are designed to work in tandem to improve the function of the defective protein. This action leads to improved lung function and reduces the aggravated symptoms caused by repeated airway infections.

Tezacaftor and ivacaftor (Symkevi) are licensed for the specific gene mutations that cause the defective protein. The treatment is indicated in a combination regimen with ivacaftor tablets and can only be prescribed by a cystic fibrosis specialist.

INFORMATION FOR USERS

Follow instructions on the label. Call your doctor if symptoms worsen.

How taken/used

Tablets.

Frequency and timing of doses
1 Symkevi (tezacaftor and ivacaftor) tablet in the morning, 1 ivacaftor tablet in the evening, approximately 12 hours apart.

Adult dosage range
Symkevi tablet: tezacaftor 100mg/ivacaftor 150mg; ivacaftor tablet: 150mg.

Onset of effect
15 days; full effects may take weeks to appear.

Duration of action
Tezacaftor 6–7 days; ivacaftor 9 hours.

Diet advice
Take with food containing fats. Avoid food or drink containing grapefruit or Seville oranges during treatment.

Storage
Keep in original container at room temperature out of the reach of children. Protect from light.

Missed dose
If it is 6 hours or less since a missed morning or evening dose, take the dose as soon as possible and continue the usual schedule. If more than 6 hours have passed, do not take the missed dose but take the next scheduled dose at the usual time. Do not take more than one dose of either tablet at the same time.

Stopping the drug
Do not stop taking the drug without consulting your doctor. Stopping the drug may lead to worsening of the underlying condition.

Exceeding the dose
An occasional unintentional extra dose is unlikely to be a cause for concern. But if you notice any unusual symptoms, or if a large overdose has been taken, notify your doctor.

SPECIAL PRECAUTIONS

Be sure to tell your doctor if:
- You have long-term kidney or liver problems.
- You are taking other medicines

Pregnancy
Safety in pregnancy not established. Discuss with your doctor.

Breast-feeding
It is not known whether tezacaftor or ivacaftor, or substances produced by their metabolism in the body, pass into the breast milk. Discuss with your doctor.

Infants and children
Not recommended under 12 years.

Over 60
Limited information on the drug. No known problems.

Driving and hazardous work
No known problems.

Alcohol
No known problems.

PROLONGED USE

Monitoring Regular blood tests will be carried out to monitor your liver function.

POSSIBLE ADVERSE EFFECTS

Headache, nausea, and sinus congestion are all frequently reported.

Symptom/effect	Frequency		Discuss with doctor		Stop taking drug now	Call doctor now
	Common	Rare	Only if severe	In all cases		
Nasal/throat irritation	●			●		
Sinus congestion/ear problems	●			●		
Headache/dizziness	●			●		
Rash	●			●		
Nausea/abdominal pain	●			●		
Diarrhoea	●			●		
Breast mass/problems		●		●		
Cataracts		●		●		

INTERACTIONS

Rifampicin, rifabutin, phenobarbital, carbamazepine, phenytoin, St. John's wort, and grapefruit may reduce blood levels of tezacaftor and ivacaftor.

Warfarin Increased anticoagulant effect with ivacaftor.

Ketoconazole, itraconazole, posaconazole, voriconazole, fluconazole, telithromycin, clarithromycin, and erythromycin may increase blood levels of tezacaftor and ivacaftor.

THALIDOMIDE

Brand name Celgene
Used in the following combined preparations None

GENERAL INFORMATION

Thalidomide was originally introduced in the 1950s as a sedative and became popular for treating morning sickness in pregnancy. By 1961, though, it was clear that the drug caused severe birth defects and it was withdrawn.

Thalidomide was later found to be effective in treating leprosy (also known as Hansen's disease) and in blocking the growth of blood vessels to tumours. Currently in the UK there are strict controls on prescribing the drug; it is used only to treat multiple myeloma (a type of bone marrow cancer) in combination with other drugs, and, very rarely, for leprosy. Because it can cause severe birth defects when taken during pregnancy and can also be present in semen, women of childbearing age and men must ensure reliable contraception is used. Thalidomide also increases the risk of peripheral nerve damage and venous thromboembolism (deep vein thrombosis and pulmonary embolism).

QUICK REFERENCE

Drug group Drug for leprosy (p.89) and multiple myeloma

Overdose danger rating Medium

Dependence rating Low

Prescription needed Yes

Available as generic No

INFORMATION FOR USERS

Follow instructions on the label. Your drug prescription is tailored for you. Do not alter dosage without checking with your doctor.

How taken/used

Capsules.

Frequency and timing of doses
Once daily at bedtime for up to 72 weeks.

Adult dosage range
200mg daily.

Onset of effect
2–5 hours.

Duration of action
7–8 hours.

Diet advice
None.

Storage
Keep in original container out of the reach of children.

Missed dose
Take the missed dose as soon as you remember unless your next dose is due within 12 hours, in which case omit the missed dose and take the next dose as scheduled.

Stopping the drug
Do not stop the drug without consulting your doctor; your condition may worsen.

Exceeding the dose
An occasional unintentional extra dose is unlikely to cause problems. However, a large overdose may cause serious side effects; consult your doctor or go to hospital immediately.

POSSIBLE ADVERSE EFFECTS

Thalidomide often causes drowsiness and nerve damage. The latter may be mild, causing numbness or tingling in the hands or feet, or more severe and painful; in some cases, nerve damage may be irreversible. There is also a significant risk of venous thromboembolism.

Symptom/effect	Frequency		Discuss with doctor		Stop taking drug now	Call doctor now
	Common	Rare	Only if severe	In all cases		
Constipation	●		●			
Dizziness/sleepiness	●		●			
Numbness/tingling/headache	●			●		
Blurred vision	●			●	●	
Bruising/bleeding	●			●	●	●
Rash/blisters/mouth ulcers		●		●	●	●
Leg pain/swelling	●			●	●	●
Chest pain/breathlessness		●		●	●	●
Palpitations/collapse		●		●	●	●
Cessation of menstruation		●		●	●	●

INTERACTIONS

Sedative drugs Thalidomide increases the drowsiness caused by other sedative drugs, such as antihistamines, anticholinergics, opioids, benzodiazepines, and alcohol.

Beta blockers There is an increased risk of an abnormally low heart rate when beta blockers are used with thalidomide.

SPECIAL PRECAUTIONS

Be sure to tell your doctor if:
- You are sexually active, pregnant, or intend to become pregnant.
- You have lactose intolerance.
- You have kidney or liver problems.
- You have a history of thromboembolism or heart disease.
- You have problems with sensation in your hands or feet.
- You are taking other medicines.

Pregnancy
Must not be used; it causes severe birth defects. Women of childbearing age must use contraception. The drug is present in semen; men taking it must ensure that they and/or their partner use contraception. Women who think they may have become pregnant should stop the drug and consult their doctor immediately.

Breast-feeding
Avoid as it is not known whether thalidomide passes into breast milk.

Infants and children
Not recommended under 18 years.

Over 60
Older people are at increased risk of potentially serious adverse effects. Discuss with your doctor.

Driving and hazardous work
Avoid such activities if you have side effects such as dizziness, tiredness, sleepiness, or blurred vision.

Alcohol
Avoid. Alcohol increases the sedative effect of thalidomide.

PROLONGED USE

Prolonged use increases the risk of nerve damage and venous thromboembolism. If you are at high risk of thromboembolism, you may be prescribed preventative drugs.

Monitoring You will have regular blood tests and checks of your reflexes and nerve function.

THEOPHYLLINE/AMINOPHYLLINE

Brand names [theophylline] Uniphyllin; [aminophylline] Phyllocontin
Used in the following combined preparations None

GENERAL INFORMATION

Theophylline (and aminophylline, which breaks down to theophylline in the body) is used to treat bronchospasm (constriction of the air passages). It improves breathing in patients with asthma, bronchitis, and emphysema. It is usually taken continuously for prevention, but aminophylline injections are sometimes used for acute attacks.

Slow-release formulations of the drugs produce beneficial effects lasting for up to 12 hours. These preparations may be prescribed twice daily, but they are also useful as a single dose taken at night to prevent night-time asthma and early-morning wheezing.

Treatment with theophylline must be monitored because the effective dose is very close to the toxic dose. Some adverse effects, such as indigestion, nausea, headache, and agitation, can be controlled by regulating the dosage and checking blood levels of the drug.

QUICK REFERENCE

Drug group Bronchodilator (p.48)

Overdose danger rating High

Dependence rating Low

Prescription needed No (except for injection)

Available as generic Yes

INFORMATION FOR USERS

Follow instructions on the label. Call your doctor if symptoms worsen.

How taken/used

MR tablets, injection.

Frequency and timing of doses
1–2 x MR tablets every 12–24 hours. Take at the same time each day.

Dosage range
Adults 400–800mg daily, depending on which product is used.

Onset of effect
Within 90 minutes (MR tablets).

Duration of action
1–2 hours.

Diet advice
None.

Storage
Keep in original container at room temperature out of the reach of children.

Missed dose
Take as soon as you remember. If your next dose is due within 2 hours, take half the dose now (short-acting preparations) or forget about the missed dose and take your next dose now (SR preparations). Return to your normal dose schedule thereafter.

Stopping the drug
Do not stop taking the drug without consulting your doctor; stopping the drug may lead to worsening of the underlying condition.

OVERDOSE ACTION

 Seek immediate medical advice in all cases. Take emergency action if chest pain, confusion, or loss of consciousness occur.

See Drug poisoning emergency guide (p.518).

SPECIAL PRECAUTIONS

Be sure to tell your doctor if:
- You have a liver problem.
- You have angina or irregular heart beat.
- You have high blood pressure.
- You have epilepsy.
- You have hyperthyroidism.
- You have porphyria.
- You have peptic ulcers.
- You have an exacerbation of lung disease, fever, or a viral infection.
- You have prostate enlargement.
- You smoke.
- You are taking other medicines.

 Pregnancy
Safety in pregnancy not established. Discuss with your doctor.

 Breast-feeding
Drug passes into breast milk and may affect baby. Discuss with your doctor.

 Infants and children
Reduced dose necessary according to age and weight.

 Over 60
Reduced dose may be necessary.

 Driving and hazardous work
No known problems.

 Alcohol
Avoid excess as this may alter levels of the drug and may increase gastrointestinal symptoms.

Taking your tablets
Factors such as drug interactions, certain medical conditions (e.g. heart or liver failure), and smoking can affect theophylline levels. Levels also vary from brand to brand. For this reason, you must always use the same brand.

POSSIBLE ADVERSE EFFECTS

Most adverse effects relate to blood levels of the drug. The most common effects are on the gastrointestinal system and central nervous system (such as agitation and insomnia).

Symptom/effect	Frequency		Discuss with doctor		Stop taking drug now	Call doctor now
	Common	Rare	Only if severe	In all cases		
Nausea/vomiting	●		●			
Insomnia	●		●			
Headache	●			●		
Agitation		●		●		
Diarrhoea/abdominal pain		●	●			
Palpitations		●		●	●	●

INTERACTIONS

General note Many drugs interact with theophylline. Some antibiotics, antidepressants, and anticonvulsants increase the effect of theophylline by increasing its blood level. Taken with theophylline, high doses of beta 2 agonists such as salbutamol increase the risk of low blood potassium levels. Discuss with your doctor.

PROLONGED USE

No problems expected.

Monitoring Periodic checks on blood levels of drug and on risk of heart rhythm disorders are usually required.

TIMOLOL

Brand names Eysano, Timoptol, Timoptol LA, Tiopex, Travoprost
Used in the following combined preparations Azarga, Combigan, Cosopt, DuoTrav, Ganfort, Taptiqom, Xalacom

GENERAL INFORMATION

Timolol is a non-cardioselective beta blocker (p.55) used for angina. It may be given after a heart attack to prevent further damage to the heart. It is also used to treat hypertension (high blood pressure) but is not usually used to initiate treatment. The drug is commonly given as eye drops to people with some types of glaucoma and is occasionally given to prevent migraine. Timolol can occasionally cause breathing difficulties, especially in people with respiratory diseases; this is more likely with the tablets, but it can also occur with the eye drops. Timolol may also mask the body's response to low blood sugar and, for that reason, is prescribed with caution to diabetic people on insulin.

QUICK REFERENCE

Drug group Beta blocker (p.55) and drug for glaucoma (p.128)

Overdose danger rating High

Dependence rating Low

Prescription needed Yes

Available as generic Yes

INFORMATION FOR USERS

Your drug prescription is tailored for you. Do not alter dosage without checking with your doctor.

How taken/used

Tablets, eye drops.

Frequency and timing of doses
1–3 x daily.

Adult dosage range
By mouth 10–60mg daily (hypertension); 10–60mg daily (angina/hypertension); 10–20mg daily (after a heart attack); 10–20mg daily (migraine prevention).

Onset of effect
Within 30 minutes (by mouth); 15–20 minutes (eye drops).

Duration of action
Up to 24 hours.

Diet advice
None.

Storage
Keep in original container at room temperature out of the reach of children.

Missed dose
Take as soon as you remember. If your next dose is due within 3 hours, take a single dose now and skip the next.

Stopping the drug
Do not stop taking the drug without consulting your doctor; stopping the drug may lead to worsening of the underlying condition.

OVERDOSE ACTION

Seek immediate medical advice in all cases of overdose by mouth. Take emergency action if breathing difficulties, palpitations, or loss of consciousness occur.

See Drug poisoning emergency guide (p.518).

POSSIBLE ADVERSE EFFECTS

Timolol by mouth can occasionally provoke or worsen heart problems and asthma. Fainting may be a sign that the drug has slowed the heart beat or lowered blood pressure excessively. Eye drops cause these problems only rarely; eye irritation is more likely.

Symptom/effect	Frequency		Discuss with doctor		Stop taking drug now	Call doctor now
	Common	Rare	Only if severe	In all cases		
Eye irritation (eye drops)	●		●			
Lethargy/fatigue	●			●		
Cold hands and feet	●			●		
Nausea/vomiting		●		●		
Nightmares/vivid dreams		●		●	●	
Rash/dry eyes		●		●	●	
Visual disturbances		●		●	●	
Fainting/palpitations		●		●	●	●
Breathlessness/wheeze		●		●	●	●

INTERACTIONS

Calcium channel blockers may cause low blood pressure, a slow heart beat, and heart failure if used with timolol.

Cardiac glycosides (e.g. digoxin) may increase the heart-slowing effect of timolol.

Antihypertensive drugs Timolol may enhance the blood-pressure-lowering effect.

Drugs for asthma (e.g. salbutamol, salmeterol, and other beta agonists) The effects of these drugs may be reduced by timolol.

SPECIAL PRECAUTIONS

Be sure to tell your doctor if:
- You have heart problems.
- You have kidney or liver problems.
- You have a lung disorder such as asthma, bronchitis, or emphysema.
- You have diabetes.
- You have psoriasis.
- You have an overactive thyroid gland.
- You are taking other medicines.

Pregnancy
Safety in pregnancy not established. Discuss with your doctor.

Breast-feeding
The drug passes into the breast milk, but at normal doses adverse effects on the baby are unlikely. Discuss with your doctor.

Infants and children
Not usually prescribed.

Over 60
Reduced dose may be necessary.

Driving and hazardous work
Avoid until you have learned how timolol affects you because tablets may cause dizziness or fatigue, and eye drops may cause blurred vision.

Alcohol
Avoid excessive intake. Alcohol may increase the blood-pressure-lowering effects of timolol.

Surgery and general anaesthetics
Occasionally, timolol eye drops may need to be stopped before you have a general anaesthetic, but only do this after discussion with your doctor or dentist.

PROLONGED USE

No problems expected.

TIOTROPIUM

Brand names Braltus, Spiriva, Spiriva Respimat
Used in the following combined preparations Spiolto, Yanimo

GENERAL INFORMATION

Tiotropium is a long-acting anticholinergic bronchodilator that relaxes the muscles surrounding the bronchioles (airways in the lung). It is used in the maintenance treatment of chronic obstructive lung disorders, such as chronic bronchitis. The drug is not suitable for acute attacks of wheezing or in the emergency treatment of asthma, when salbutamol (see p.391) should be used and urgent medical help sought. Tiotropium is taken by inhalation of a powder or solution, and it acts directly and locally on the inner surface of the lungs and not via the blood. The most common side effect is a dry mouth.

see p.391

QUICK REFERENCE

Drug group Bronchodilator (p.48)
Overdose danger rating Low
Dependence rating Low
Prescription needed Yes
Available as generic No

INFORMATION FOR USERS

Your drug prescription is tailored for you. Do not alter dosage without checking with your doctor.

How taken/used

Powder in capsules for inhaler, solution for inhalation.

Frequency and timing of doses
1 capsule daily for inhaled powder; 2 puffs daily for inhalation solution. Use at the same time each day.

Adult dosage range
Spiriva: 18mcg; Braltus: 10mcg (powder). Spiriva Respimat: 5mcg (solution).

Onset of effect
5–30 minutes.

Duration of action
24 hours.

Diet advice
None.

Storage
Keep in original container at room temperature out of the reach of children.

Missed dose
Take as soon as you remember. If your next dose is due within 8 hours, take a single dose now and skip the next.

Stopping the drug
Do not stop the drug without consulting your doctor; symptoms may recur.

Exceeding the dose
An occasional unintentional extra dose is unlikely to be a cause for concern. But if you notice any unusual symptoms, or if a large overdose has been taken, notify your doctor.

SPECIAL PRECAUTIONS

Be sure to tell your doctor if:
- You are allergic to atropine or ipratropium.
- You have prostate problems.
- You have urinary retention.
- You have glaucoma.
- You have kidney problems.
- You have heart disease.
- You are taking other medicines.

Pregnancy
Safety not established. Discuss with your doctor.

Breast-feeding
Safety not established, but the amount present in breast milk is unlikely to harm your baby. Discuss with your doctor.

Infants and children
Not recommended under 18 years.

Over 60
No known problems.

Driving and hazardous work
Avoid until you have learned how the drug affects you as it can cause dizziness, blurred vision, or headache.

Alcohol
No known problems.

Protecting your eyes
Take care to avoid getting the drug into the eyes as it could trigger glaucoma or worsen existing glaucoma. If you develop eye or vision problems, call your doctor immediately.

PROLONGED USE

No known problems.

POSSIBLE ADVERSE EFFECTS

Dry mouth is the most common side effect. If you get the drug in your eyes, it could trigger or worsen glaucoma; if this happens you should call your doctor immediately. If wheezing and breathlessness suddenly worsen after using the inhaler (paradoxical bronchospasm), stop taking the drug and contact your doctor immediately.

Symptom/effect	Frequency		Discuss with doctor		Stop taking drug now	Call doctor now
	Common	Rare	Only if severe	In all cases		
Dry mouth/sore throat/cough	●		●			
Nosebleeds		●		●		
Altered sense of taste		●		●		
Change in voice		●		●		
Fast heartbeat/palpitations		●		●		
Difficulty in passing urine		●		●		
Rash		●		●		
Wheezing after inhalation		●		●		
Eye pain/blurred vision		●		●		●
Visual haloes		●		●		●

INTERACTIONS

Anticholinergic drugs (e.g. atropine and ipratropium) The effects and toxicity of tiotropium are likely to be increased if it is used at the same time as these drugs.

TOLBUTAMIDE

Brand names None
Used in the following combined preparations None

GENERAL INFORMATION

Tolbutamide is a sulfonylurea drug, but is shorter-acting than many others in this group. It is used to treat Type 2 diabetes, and acts by stimulating the beta cells in the pancreas to release insulin, so it will only work if functioning cells remain. For this reason, it is not effective in Type 1 diabetes, in which functioning cells are lacking. It may also be given to people with impaired kidney function because it is less likely to build up in the body and excessively lower blood sugar. If additional control of blood glucose is needed, other oral antidiabetic drugs, such as metformin or acarbose, can be added to tolbutamide.

As with other oral antidiabetics, the drug may need to be replaced with insulin during serious illnesses, injury, or surgery, when diabetic control is lost.

INFORMATION FOR USERS

Your drug prescription is tailored for you. Do not alter dosage without checking with your doctor.

How taken/used

Tablets.

Frequency and timing of doses
Taken with meals either once daily in the morning, or 2 x daily in the morning and evening.

Adult dosage range
500mg–2g daily.

Onset of effect
Within 1 hour.

Duration of action
6–24 hours.

Diet advice
An individualized diabetic diet must be maintained for the drug to be fully effective. Follow the advice of your doctor.

Storage
Keep in original container at room temperature out of the reach of children. Protect from light.

Missed dose
Take as soon as you remember. If your next dose is due within 2 hours, take a single dose now and skip the next.

Stopping the drug
Do not stop the drug without consulting your doctor; stopping the drug may lead to worsening of the underlying condition.

OVERDOSE ACTION

 Seek immediate medical advice in all cases. If you have warning signs of low blood sugar (e.g. faintness, dizziness, headache, confusion, sweating, or tremor), have something sugary. Take emergency action if seizures or loss of consciousness occur.

See Drug poisoning emergency guide (p.518).

SPECIAL PRECAUTIONS

Be sure to tell your doctor if:
- You have long-term liver or kidney problems.
- You are allergic to sulfonamides.
- You have thyroid problems.
- You have porphyria or glucose-6-phosphate dehydrogenase (G6PD) deficiency.
- You are taking other medicines.

 Pregnancy
Not prescribed. Insulin is usually substituted. May cause birth defects if taken in the first 3 months of pregnancy. Discuss with your doctor.

 Breast-feeding
The drug passes into the breast milk and may affect the baby. Discuss with your doctor.

 Infants and children
Not prescribed.

 Over 60
Risk of low blood sugar. Reduced dose may therefore be necessary.

 Driving and hazardous work
Usually no problem. Avoid these activities if you have warning signs of low blood sugar (see left).

 Alcohol
Keep consumption low. Alcohol may upset diabetic control and cause flushing, nausea, vomiting, and signs of low blood sugar (see left).

Surgery and general anaesthetics
Notify your doctor that you have diabetes before any surgery; insulin treatment may need to be substituted.

PROLONGED USE

No problems expected, but tolbutamide may lose its effect if pancreatic function grows worse.

Monitoring Periodic monitoring of control of blood glucose levels is necessary.

POSSIBLE ADVERSE EFFECTS

Serious adverse effects are rare with this drug. Symptoms such as dizziness, sweating, shaking, blurred vision, weakness, and confusion may indicate low blood sugar levels.

Symptom/effect	Frequency		Discuss with doctor		Stop taking drug now	Call doctor now
	Common	Rare	Only if severe	In all cases		
Dizziness/confusion	●			●		
Weakness/sweating	●			●		
Headache/ringing in the ears		●	●			
Weight gain		●	●			
Nausea/indigestion/diarrhoea	●			●		
Jaundice		●		●	●	●
Fever/rash/easy bruising		●		●	●	●
Sore throat		●		●	●	●

INTERACTIONS

General note A variety of drugs, including corticosteroids, oestrogens, diuretics, and rifampicin, may oppose the effect of tolbutamide and raise blood sugar levels. Others increase the risk of low blood sugar; these include sulfonamides, warfarin, chloramphenicol, aspirin and other NSAIDs (p.74), antidepressants, cimetidine, and some antibiotics and antifungals.

Beta blockers may mask the signs of low blood sugar, especially non-cardioselective beta blockers such as propranolol.

TOLTERODINE

Brand names Blerone XL, Detrusitol, Detrusitol XL, Inconex XL, Mariosea XL, Neditol XL, Preblacon XL, Tolterma XL, Tolthen XL
Used in the following combined preparations None

GENERAL INFORMATION

Tolterodine is an anticholinergic and antispasmodic drug that is similar to atropine (see p.165). It is used to treat urinary frequency and incontinence in adults. It works by reducing contraction of the bladder, allowing it to expand and hold more. It also stops spasms and delays the desire to empty the bladder. Tolterodine's usefulness is limited to some extent by its side effects, and dosage needs to be reduced in older adults. Children are more susceptible than adults to the drug's anticholinergic effects (see p.35). Tolterodine can also trigger glaucoma.

INFORMATION FOR USERS

Your drug prescription is tailored for you. Do not alter dosage without checking with your doctor.

How taken/used

Tablets, SR capsules.

Frequency and timing of doses
1–2 x daily.

Dosage range
4mg daily, reduced to 2mg daily, if necessary, to minimize side effects.

Onset of effect
1 hour.

Duration of action
12 hours.

Diet advice
None.

Storage
Keep in original container at room temperature out of the reach of children.

Missed dose
Take as soon as you remember. If your next dose is due within 2 hours, take a single dose now and skip the next.

Stopping the drug
Do not stop taking the drug without consulting your doctor; symptoms may recur.

OVERDOSE ACTION

Seek immediate medical advice in all cases. Take emergency action if symptoms such as breathing difficulty, seizures, or loss of consciousness occur.

See Drug poisoning emergency guide (p.518).

SPECIAL PRECAUTIONS

Be sure to tell your doctor if:
- You have liver or kidney problems.
- You have thyroid problems.
- You have heart problems, especially rhythm disturbances.
- You have hiatus hernia.
- You have prostate problems or urinary retention.
- You have ulcerative colitis.
- You have glaucoma.
- You have myasthenia gravis.
- You are taking other medicines.

 Pregnancy
Safety in pregnancy not established. May harm the unborn baby. Discuss with your doctor.

 Breast-feeding
Safety not established. Discuss with your doctor.

 Infants and children
Not recommended. Safety not established.

 Over 60
Increased likelihood of side effects. Reduced dose may be required.

 Driving and hazardous work
Avoid. Tolterodine may cause drowsiness, disorientation, and blurred vision.

 Alcohol
Avoid. Alcohol increases the drug's sedative effects.

POSSIBLE ADVERSE EFFECTS

The most common side effects, such as dry mouth, digestive upset, and dry eyes, are the result of the drug's anticholinergic action.

Symptom/effect	Frequency		Discuss with doctor		Stop taking drug now	Call doctor now
	Common	Rare	Only if severe	In all cases		
Dry mouth/digestive upset	●		●			
Constipation/abdominal pain	●		●			
Headache	●		●			
Dry eyes/blurred vision	●		●			
Drowsiness/nervousness	●			●		
Chest pain		●		●		
Confusion		●		●		
Urinary difficulties		●		●		
Unexplained collapse		●		●	●	●

INTERACTIONS

General note All drugs that have an anticholinergic effect will have increased side effects when taken with tolterodine.

Domperidone and metoclopramide The effects of these drugs may be decreased by tolterodine.

Erythromycin, clarithromycin, itraconazole, ketoconazole, and miconazole These drugs may increase blood levels of tolterodine.

PROLONGED USE

No special problems. Effectiveness of the drug, and continuing clinical need for it, are usually reviewed after 3–6 months.

Monitoring Periodic eye tests for glaucoma may be performed

TRAMADOL

Brand names Brimisol PR, Invodol SR, Mabron, Maneo, Marol, Maxitram SR, Tilodol SR, Tradorec XL, Tramquel SR, Tramulief, Zamadol, Zeridame SR, Zydol
Used in the following combined preparation Skudexa, Tramacet

GENERAL INFORMATION

Tramadol is a synthetic opioid analgesic that also acts on serotonin levels in the brain to relieve moderate to severe pain, either acute or chronic. The painkilling effect wears off after about 4 hours, but a modified-release (long-acting) form can provide relief for up to 24 hours. Rarely, tramadol can be habit-forming and dependence may occur, but most people who take it for a short period do not become dependent and are able to stop taking it without difficulty. Side effects of tramadol include a dry mouth, nausea, dizziness, and vomiting. Unlike morphine-like opioids, tramadol tends not to cause constipation.

INFORMATION FOR USERS

Your drug prescription is tailored for you. Do not alter dosage without checking with your doctor.

How taken/used

Tablets, MR/SR tablets, soluble tablets, capsules, MR/SR capsules, powder in sachets, injection.

Frequency and timing of doses
Usually 1 x daily (MR/SR preparations) or up to 6 x daily (other preparations).

Adult dosage range
Up to 400mg daily (by mouth); 600mg daily (injection).

Onset of effect
30–60 minutes (short-acting forms by mouth); at least 2 hours (SR preparations by mouth); 15–30 minutes (injection).

Duration of action
4 hours (short-acting); 12 or 24 hours (long-acting).

Diet advice
None.

Storage
Keep in original container at room temperature out of the reach of children.

Missed dose
Take as soon as you remember, and return to your normal schedule as soon as possible.

Stopping the drug
If the reason for taking tramadol no longer exists, you may stop taking the drug and notify your doctor, who will advise you on how to stop taking it gradually. If you have been taking it for a long time, you may experience withdrawal effects.

OVERDOSE ACTION

 Seek immediate medical advice in all cases. Take emergency action if breathing difficulties, severe drowsiness, seizures, or loss of consciousness occur.

See Drug poisoning emergency guide (p.518).

SPECIAL PRECAUTIONS

Be sure to tell your doctor if:
- You have had a head injury.
- You have liver or kidney problems.
- You have heart or circulatory problems.
- You have a lung disorder such as asthma or bronchitis.
- You have thyroid disease.
- You have a history of epileptic seizures.
- You are taking other medicines.

 Pregnancy
Safety not established. Discuss with your doctor.

 Breast-feeding
The drug passes into the breast milk and may make the baby drowsy. Discuss with your doctor.

 Infants and children
Not recommended under 12 years.

 Over 60
Reduced dose may be necessary.

 Driving and hazardous work
Avoid. Tramadol can cause drowsiness.

 Alcohol
Avoid. Alcohol increases the sedative effects of tramadol.

PROLONGED USE

Dependence may occur if tramadol is taken for long periods.

POSSIBLE ADVERSE EFFECTS

Adverse effects such as drowsiness seem more common than with some other opioids.

Symptom/effect	Frequency		Discuss with doctor		Stop taking drug now	Call doctor now
	Common	Rare	Only if severe	In all cases		
Nausea/vomiting	●		●			
Dry mouth	●		●			
Tiredness/drowsiness	●		●			
Dizziness/headache	●		●			
Constipation		●	●			
Confusion/hallucinations		●		●		
Seizures		●		●	●	●
Wheezing/breathlessness		●		●	●	●

INTERACTIONS

Antidepressants Tramadol may increase the risk of seizures if taken with antidepressants and antipsychotics.

Carbamazepine This drug may reduce blood levels and effects of tramadol.

Sedatives All drugs with a sedative effect are likely to increase the sedative effects of tramadol. These include antidepressants, antipsychotics, antihistamines, alcohol, benzodiazepines, and sleeping drugs.

TRASTUZUMAB

Brand name Herceptin, Herzuma, Kanjinti, Ontruzant, Trazimera
Used in the following combined preparation Kadcyla

GENERAL INFORMATION

Trastuzumab belongs to a group of drugs known as monoclonal antibodies (p.114) and is used in the treatment of early and advanced breast cancer and some stomach cancers. Produced synthetically, it is similar to antibodies that occur naturally to fight infection and attacks cancer cells in a similar way.

Around one breast cancer in five involves cancer cells with excessive amounts of a protein called HER2 on their surface. HER2 stimulates the growth of these cancer cells, making the tumours aggressive and fast growing.

Trastuzumab blocks the HER2 protein on the cancer cells, destroying them. Therefore, to see whether treatment would be appropriate, it is necessary for tests to be carried out to confirm the presence of HER2.

Trastuzumab may be given on its own or in combination with other treatments. It is given by intravenous infusion, either weekly or every three weeks.

QUICK REFERENCE

Drug group Anticancer drug (p.112)
Overdose danger rating Low
Dependence rating Low
Prescription needed Yes
Available as generic No

INFORMATION FOR USERS

Trastuzumab is prescribed only under close medical supervision, taking account of your present condition and medical history.

How taken/used

Intravenous infusion, subcutaneous injection.

Frequency and timing of doses
Every 1–3 weeks. Infusions are usually given over a 90-minute period.

Adult dosage range
As advised by doctors, according to your bodyweight.

Onset of effect
Not known.

Duration of action
Up to 24 weeks.

Diet advice
None.

Storage
Not applicable. The drug is not normally kept in the home.

Missed dose
The drug is administered in hospital under close medical supervision. If for some reason you miss your dose, contact your doctor as soon as possible.

Stopping the drug
Discuss with your doctor. Stopping the drug prematurely may lead to worsening of the underlying condition.

Exceeding the dose
Overdosage is unlikely since treatment is carefully monitored and supervised.

SPECIAL PRECAUTIONS

Be sure to tell your doctor if:
- You are allergic to trastuzumab.
- You have breathing difficulties.
- You have had heart failure, coronary artery disease, or high blood pressure.
- You have ever had chemotherapy before, especially with doxorubicin.
- You are or plan to become pregnant.
- You are taking other medicines.

 Pregnancy
Not recommended.

 Breast-feeding
Not advised during treatment with trastuzumab and for six months after stopping.

 Infants and children
Not recommended under 18 years. Safety not established.

 Over 60
No special problems.

 Driving and hazardous work
Trastuzumab can cause dizziness and drowsiness during treatment. If these symptoms occur, avoid hazardous activities until they have stopped.

 Alcohol
No known problems.

PROLONGED USE

Serious problems are rare.

Monitoring Treatment is carried out under specialist supervision. Patients are usually observed for at least 6 hours after the start of trastuzumab treatment and for 2 hours after subsequent treatments. Heart function should be assessed regularly with echocardiograms and ECGs during treatment.

POSSIBLE ADVERSE EFFECTS

Infusion reactions are common, especially with the first infusion. Other common effects include diarrhoea, weakness, abdominal pain, and joint and muscle pain. Trastuzumab may also cause heart failure.

Symptom/effect	Frequency		Discuss with doctor		Stop taking drug now	Call doctor now
	Common	Rare	Only if severe	In all cases		
Fever/shivering	●		●			
Nausea/diarrhoea/vomiting	●		●			
Joint pain/muscle pain		●	●			
Breathlessness/cough		●		●		
Palpitations/chest pain		●		●		●
Dizziness		●		●		●
Flu-like symptoms		●		●		●
Swelling of face or lips		●		●	●	●
Itchy rash		●		●	●	●
Wheezing		●		●	●	●

INTERACTIONS

Doxorubicin and other anticancer drugs
There is an increased risk of heart failure when these are given with trastuzumab.

TRIAMTERENE

Brand name Dytac
Used in the following combined preparations Dyazide (co-triamterzide), Frusene, Kalspare, Triam-Co

GENERAL INFORMATION

Triamterene belongs to a class of drugs known as potassium-sparing diuretics. In combination with thiazide or loop diuretics, it is given to treat hypertension and oedema (fluid retention). The drug may be used, either on its own or, more commonly, with a thiazide diuretic such as hydrochlorothiazide (see p.276) as co-triamterzide, to treat oedema as a complication of heart failure, nephrotic syndrome, or cirrhosis of the liver.

Triamterene has a mild effect on urine flow, which is apparent in 1–2 hours. For this reason, you should avoid taking the drug after about 4 pm. As with other potassium-sparing diuretics, unusually high levels of potassium may build up in the blood if the kidneys are functioning abnormally. Therefore, triamterene is prescribed with caution to people who have kidney failure.

INFORMATION FOR USERS

Your drug prescription is tailored for you. Do not alter dosage without checking with your doctor.

How taken/used

Tablets, capsules.

Frequency and timing of doses
1–2 x daily after meals or on alternate days.

Adult dosage range
50–250mg daily.

Onset of effect
1–2 hours.

Duration of action
9–12 hours.

Diet advice
Consume only small amounts of foods that are high in potassium, such as bananas, tomatoes, dried fruit, and "low salt" salt substitutes.

Storage
Keep in original container at room temperature out of the reach of children.

Missed dose
Take as soon as you remember. However, if it is late in the day, do not take the missed dose, or you may need to get up at night to pass urine. Take the next scheduled dose as usual.

Stopping the drug
Do not stop the drug without consulting your doctor; symptoms may recur.

Exceeding the dose
An occasional unintentional extra dose is unlikely to be a cause for concern. But if you notice any unusual symptoms, or if a large overdose has been taken, notify your doctor.

POSSIBLE ADVERSE EFFECTS

Triamterene has few adverse effects; the main problem is the possibility of potassium being retained by the body, causing muscle weakness and heart rhythm problems. Triamterene may colour your urine blue, but this is not a cause for concern.

Symptom/effect	Frequency		Discuss with doctor		Stop taking drug now	Call doctor now
	Common	Rare	Only if severe	In all cases		
Digestive disturbance		●	●			
Headache		●	●			
Muscle weakness		●		●	●	
Rash		●		●	●	
Dry mouth/thirst		●		●	●	

INTERACTIONS

Lithium Triamterene may increase the blood levels of lithium, leading to an increased risk of lithium toxicity.

Non-steroidal anti-inflammatory drugs (NSAIDs) may increase the risk of raised blood levels of potassium.

ACE inhibitors and angiotensin II blockers These drugs increase the risk of raised blood levels of potassium with triamterene.

Ciclosporin and tacrolimus These drugs may increase blood levels of potassium with triamterene.

SPECIAL PRECAUTIONS

Be sure to tell your doctor if:
- You have long-term liver or kidney problems.
- You have had kidney stones.
- You have gout.
- You are taking other medicines.

 Pregnancy
Not usually prescribed. May cause a reduction in the blood supply to the developing fetus. Discuss with your doctor.

 Breast-feeding
The drug passes into breast milk and may affect the baby. It could also reduce your milk supply. Discuss with your doctor.

 Infants and children
Not recommended.

 Over 60
Increased likelihood of adverse effects. Reduced dose may therefore be necessary.

 Driving and hazardous work
No special problems.

 Alcohol
No known problems.

PROLONGED USE

Serious problems are unlikely, but levels of salts such as sodium and potassium may occasionally become abnormal during prolonged use.

Monitoring Blood tests may be performed to check on kidney function and levels of body salts.

TRIMETHOPRIM

Brand names None
Used in the following combined preparation [co-trimoxazole] Septrin

GENERAL INFORMATION

Trimethoprim is an antibacterial drug that became popular in the 1970s for prevention and treatment of infections of the urinary and respiratory tracts. The drug has been used for many years in combination with another antibacterial, sulfamethoxazole, in a preparation known as co-trimoxazole (see p.216). Trimethoprim, however, has fewer adverse effects than co-trimoxazole and is equally effective in treating many conditions.

Although side effects of trimethoprim are not usually troublesome, tests to monitor blood composition are often advised when the drug is taken for prolonged periods.

QUICK REFERENCE

Drug group Antibacterial drug (p.89)

Overdose danger rating Low

Dependence rating Low

Prescription needed Yes

Available as generic Yes

INFORMATION FOR USERS

Your drug prescription is tailored for you. Do not alter dosage without checking with your doctor.

How taken/used

Tablets, liquid.

Frequency and timing of doses
1–2 x daily.

Adult dosage range
400mg daily (treatment); 100mg daily (prevention).

Onset of effect
1–4 hours.

Duration of action
Up to 24 hours.

Diet advice
None.

Storage
Keep in original container at room temperature out of the reach of children. Protect from light.

Missed dose
Take as soon as you remember.

Stopping the drug
Take the full course. Even if you feel better, the original infection may still be present and symptoms may recur if treatment is stopped too soon.

Exceeding the dose
An occasional unintentional extra dose is unlikely to be a cause for concern. But if you notice any unusual symptoms, or if a large overdose has been taken, notify your doctor.

POSSIBLE ADVERSE EFFECTS

Trimethoprim taken on its own rarely causes side effects. However, additional adverse effects may occur when trimethoprim is taken in combination with sulfamethoxazole.

Symptom/effect	Frequency		Discuss with doctor		Stop taking drug now	Call doctor now
	Common	Rare	Only if severe	In all cases		
Nausea/vomiting		●	●			
Rash/itching		●		●	●	
Sore throat/fever		●		●	●	
Spontaneous bleeding		●		●	●	
Easy bruising		●		●	●	

INTERACTIONS

Cytotoxic drugs Trimethoprim increases the risk of blood problems if taken with azathioprine or mercaptopurine. Taken with methotrexate, there is an increased risk of folate deficiency.

Ciclosporin Trimethoprim increases the risk of this drug causing kidney damage.

Phenytoin Taken with trimethoprim, this drug may increase the risk of folic acid deficiency, resulting in blood abnormalities. Trimethoprim may also increase the time taken for phenytoin to be eliminated from the body.

Warfarin Trimethoprim may increase the anticoagulant effect of warfarin.

Antimalarials containing pyrimethamine Drugs such as fansidar or maloprim may increase the risk of folic acid deficiency, resulting in blood abnormalities, if they are taken with trimethoprim.

ACE inhibitors and angiotensin II blockers Trimethoprim increases the risk of high potassium levels in the blood when used with these drugs.

Digoxin Trimethoprim may increase the time taken for digoxin to be eliminated from the body.

SPECIAL PRECAUTIONS

Be sure to tell your doctor if:
- You have long-term liver or kidney problems.
- You have a blood disorder.
- You have porphyria.
- You are taking other medicines.

 Pregnancy
Not prescribed. May cause defects in the baby.

 Breast-feeding
The drug passes into the breast milk, but at normal doses adverse effects on the baby are unlikely. Discuss with your doctor.

 Infants and children
Reduced dose necessary.

 Over 60
Increased likelihood of adverse effects. Reduced dose may be required.

 Driving and hazardous work
No known problems.

 Alcohol
No known problems.

PROLONGED USE

Long-term use of this drug may lead to folate deficiency, which, in turn, may lead to blood abnormalities. Folate supplements may be prescribed.

Monitoring Periodic blood tests to monitor blood composition are usually advised.

ULIPRISTAL

Brand names EllaOne
Used in the following combined preparations None

GENERAL INFORMATION

Ulipristal is a synthetic progesterone used as an emergency contraceptive after unprotected sexual intercourse. It works by blocking the action of naturally produced progesterone, thereby inhibiting or delaying ovulation.

Ulipristal is only effective if taken within 120 hours (5 days) of intercourse and is solely for occasional use; the drug should not be used instead of regular contraception. You can use it while taking other oral contraceptives,

but this may reduce their effectiveness. Ulipristal does not prevent pregnancy in every case: up to 2 per cent of women still become pregnant after using it. If after using ulipristal your next period is more than 7 days late or you have abnormal bleeding at the expected date of your period, the drug may have failed and you should have a pregnancy test. If the test is positive, you should see your doctor to check for the possibility of an ectopic pregnancy.

QUICK REFERENCE

Drug group Oral contraceptive (p.121)

Overdose danger rating Low

Dependence rating Low

Prescription needed Yes, but available for emergency use from a pharmacy without prescription

Available as generic No

INFORMATION FOR USERS

Your drug prescription is tailored for you. Do not alter dosage without checking with your doctor.

How taken/used

Tablets.

Frequency and timing of doses
One tablet as soon as possible but within 120 hours (5 days) of unprotected intercourse. If vomiting occurs within 3 hours, take another tablet immediately.

Adult dosage range
30mg per tablet.

Onset of effect
2 hours.

Duration of action
Up to 120 hours.

Diet advice
None.

Storage
Keep at room temperature in original packaging to protect from light. Keep out of reach of children.

Missed dose
Not applicable as treatment is one dose.

Stopping the drug
Not applicable as treatment is one dose.

Exceeding the dose
An occasional unintentional extra dose is unlikely to be a cause for concern. However, if you notice any unusual symptoms, notify your doctor.

POSSIBLE ADVERSE EFFECTS

Ulipristal generally causes few serious adverse effects, although nausea, vomiting, and dizziness are common. If you have signs of

pregnancy after taking the drug, you must consult your doctor immediately to check for the possibility of an ectopic pregnancy.

Symptom/effect	Frequency		Discuss with doctor		Stop taking drug now	Call doctor now
	Common	Rare	Only if severe	In all cases		
Nausea/vomiting	●		●			
Upper abdominal pain/discomfort	●		●			
Headache/dizziness	●		●			
Tiredness/mood swings	●		●			
Muscle aches	●		●			
Breast tenderness	●		●			
Lower abdominal/back pain		●		●		●

INTERACTIONS

General note Numerous drugs can interact with ulipristal to reduce its effectiveness, including phenytoin, phenobarbital, carbamazepine, rifampicin, ritonavir, antacids, H₂ blockers (e.g. cimetidine), proton pump inhibitors (e.g. omeprazole), and St John's wort. If you have used any of these drugs with ulipristal, you should use a barrier contraceptive until your next menstrual period.

Oral contraceptives Ulipristal may reduce the effectiveness of oral contraceptives, so you should use a reliable barrier method of contraception until your next period.

Antifungals and antibiotics Certain antifungals (e.g. ketoconazole and itraconazole) and antibiotics (e.g. telithromycin and clarithromycin) may increase the activity of ulipristal, and concomitant use should be avoided.

SPECIAL PRECAUTIONS

Be sure to tell your doctor if:
- You are definitely already pregnant.
- You have severe asthma.
- You have liver disease.
- You have lactose intolerance.
- You are taking or have recently taken any other medicines, including over-the-counter medicines and herbal remedies.

 Pregnancy
Should not be taken if you are definitely already pregnant.

 Breast-feeding
Breast-feeding is not recommended in the 36 hours after use of ulipristal.

 Infants and children
Not recommended under age 16 years.

 Over 60
Not needed for postmenopausal women.

 Driving and hazardous work
Avoid until you know how the drug has affected you. It may sometimes cause dizziness, drowsiness, blurred vision, and difficulty concentrating.

 Alcohol
No known problems.

PROLONGED USE

Ulipristal is intended for one-off use only for emergency postcoital contraception. Repeated use in the same menstrual cycle is not recommended as its safety and effectiveness are unknown.

Ulipristal is no longer licensed for long-term use in women with fibroids because of the risk of rare but severe liver injury.

VARENICLINE

Brand name Champix
Used in the following combined preparations None

GENERAL INFORMATION

Varenicline is an effective aid to stopping smoking in adults. It works in a similar way to nicotine in the body and helps reduce tobacco cravings. It has been shown to be more effective than nicotine replacement therapy or bupropion, and, like these, is also more likely to be successful in motivated individuals who are given additional expert advice and specialist support.

Treatment with varenicline is usually started 1–2 weeks before stopping smoking (the target stop date) and continued for a period of 12 weeks in total. The course may be repeated in people who have successfully given up but are at risk of relapsing. Adverse effects are common but not usually serious. Rarely, it may cause suicidal behaviour. You should discontinue treatment and seek immediate medical advice if you become agitated or depressed, or have suicidal thoughts, while taking varenicline.

QUICK REFERENCE

Drug group Smoking cessation aid
Overdose danger rating Medium
Dependence rating Low
Prescription needed Yes
Available as generic No

INFORMATION FOR USERS

Your drug prescription is tailored for you. Do not alter dosage without checking with your doctor.

How taken/used

Tablets.

Frequency and timing of doses
Treatment started 1–2 weeks before target stop date. Initially 0.5mg once daily for 3 days, increased to 0.5mg 2 x daily for 4 days, then 1mg 2 x daily for 11 weeks (reduce to 0.5mg 2 x daily if higher dose not tolerated). Take doses at same time every day.

Adult dosage range
0.5–2mg daily.

Onset of effect
3–4 hours but may take weeks for full effect to be noticeable.

Duration of action
24 hours.

Diet advice
None.

Storage
Keep in original container at room temperature and out of reach of children.

Missed dose
Take as soon as you remember unless your next dose is due within 12 hours, in which case omit the missed dose and take the next one as scheduled. Do not take a double dose to make up for a missed one.

Stopping the drug
The drug can be stopped safely when no longer needed. However, stopping before the end of the course may increase the likelihood of a relapse.

Exceeding the dose
An occasional unintentional extra dose is unlikely to cause problems, although an overdose may cause vomiting. Notify your doctor.

SPECIAL PRECAUTIONS

Be sure to tell your doctor if:
- You have a history of psychiatric problems.
- You have had a head injury or have a history of seizures or epilepsy.
- You have severe kidney disease.
- You are pregnant or planning a pregnancy.
- You are taking other medicines

 Pregnancy
Avoid. Safety in pregnancy not established. Discuss with your doctor.

 Breast-feeding
The drug passes into breast milk. Safety not established. Discuss with your doctor.

 Infants and children
Not recommended.

 Over 60
No special problems.

 Driving and hazardous work
Avoid such activities until you have learned how varenicline affects you. The drug may cause dizziness and sleepiness.

 Alcohol
Avoid. Alcohol may increase the sedative effect of varenicline.

POSSIBLE ADVERSE EFFECTS

Headache, nausea, vomiting, and sleep disturbances are common adverse effects. If you become agitated or depressed, or have suicidal thoughts, while taking varenicline, you must stop taking the drug and consult your doctor immediately.

Symptom/effect	Frequency		Discuss with doctor		Stop taking drug now	Call doctor now
	Common	Rare	Only if severe	In all cases		
Headache	●		●			
Nausea/vomiting	●		●			
Sleepiness/tiredness	●		●			
Insomnia/strange dreams	●		●			
Hallucinations/agitation		●		●	●	●
Depression/suicidal thoughts		●		●	●	●

PROLONGED USE

A course of varenicline lasts 12 weeks. If necessary, the course may be repeated in those who have stopped smoking if they are likely to relapse.

INTERACTIONS

General note Stopping smoking, with or without varenicline, may alter the effects of a wide range of drugs, sometimes necessitating a dose adjustment; important examples include insulin, theophylline, and warfarin. Consult your doctor or pharmacist if you are on other medications or before you take a new medication.

VENLAFAXINE

Brand names Alventa XL, Depefex XL, Efexor XL, Politid XL, Suveniz XL, Venaxx XL, Venlalic XL, ViePax, and others
Used in the following combined preparations None

GENERAL INFORMATION

Venlafaxine is an antidepressant with a chemical structure unlike any other available antidepressant. It combines the therapeutic properties of both the tricyclic antidepressants and selective serotonin re-uptake inhibitors (SSRIs), without anticholinergic adverse effects. Venlafaxine is used in the treatment of depression and generalized anxiety disorder. It acts to elevate mood, increase physical activity, and restore interest in everyday activities.

Nausea, dizziness, drowsiness or insomnia, and restlessness are common adverse effects. At high doses, the drug can elevate blood pressure.

QUICK REFERENCE

Drug group Antidepressant drug (p.40)

Overdose danger rating High

Dependence rating Low

Prescription needed Yes

Available as generic Yes

INFORMATION FOR USERS

Your drug prescription is tailored for you. Do not alter dosage without checking with your doctor.

How taken/used

Tablets, XL preparations (MR tablets and capsules).

Frequency and timing of doses
2 x daily (tablets); 1 x daily (XL preparations). The drug should be taken with food.

Dosage range
75–150mg daily for outpatients; up to 375mg daily in severely depressed patients.

Onset of effect
Can appear within days, although full antidepressant effect may not be felt for 2–6 weeks. Anxiety may take longer to respond.

Duration of action
About 8–12 hours (tablets); 24 hours (XL preparations) Antidepressant effects may persist for up to 6 weeks following prolonged treatment.

Diet advice
None.

Storage
Keep in original container at room temperature out of the reach of children.

Missed dose
Do not make up for a missed dose. Just take your next regularly scheduled dose.

Stopping the drug
Do not stop the drug without consulting your doctor. Stopping abruptly can cause withdrawal symptoms.

OVERDOSE ACTION

Seek immediate medical advice in all cases. Take emergency action if seizures, slow or irregular pulse, or loss of consciousness occur.

See Drug poisoning emergency guide (p.518).

SPECIAL PRECAUTIONS

Be sure to tell your doctor if:
- You have had an adverse reaction to any other antidepressants.
- You have long-term liver or kidney problems.
- You have diabetes.
- You have a heart problem, raised blood pressure, or a history of bleeding disorders.
- You have a history of epilepsy or mania.
- You have glaucoma.
- You have had problems with alcohol or drug misuse.
- You are taking other medicines.

 Pregnancy
Safety in pregnancy not established. Discuss with your doctor.

 Breast-feeding
Not recommended. Discuss with your doctor.

 Infants and children
Not recommended under 18 years.

 Over 60
Increased likelihood of adverse effects. Reduced dose may therefore be necessary.

 Driving and hazardous work
Avoid such activities until you have learned how venlafaxine affects you; it can cause dizziness, drowsiness, and blurred vision.

 Alcohol
Avoid. Alcohol may increase the sedative effects of this drug.

POSSIBLE ADVERSE EFFECTS

The most common adverse effects are weakness, nausea, restlessness, and drowsiness. Some of these effects may wear off within 1–2 weeks. Restlessness may include anxiety, nervousness, tremor, abnormal dreams, agitation, and confusion.

Symptom/effect	Frequency		Discuss with doctor		Stop taking drug now	Call doctor now
	Common	Rare	Only if severe	In all cases		
Nausea/constipation	●		●			
Restlessness/insomnia	●		●			
Weakness/blurred vision	●		●			
Drowsiness/dizziness	●		●			
Sexual dysfunction	●		●			
Hypertension/palpitations		●		●		
Suicidal thoughts or attempts		●		●	●	●

INTERACTIONS

Sedatives All drugs with a sedative action may increase sedative effect of venlafaxine.

Warfarin Venlafaxine may increase effect of warfarin; warfarin dose may need reduction.

Serotonergics including triptans, other SSRIs, tramadol, and St John's wort may interact dangerously with venlafaxine.

Antihypertensive drugs Venlafaxine may reduce the effectiveness of these drugs.

Monoamine oxidase inhibitors (MAOIs) Venlafaxine may interact with these drugs to produce a dangerous rise in blood pressure. At least 14 days should elapse between stopping MAOIs and starting venlafaxine.

PROLONGED USE

Withdrawal symptoms (e.g. dizziness, headache, anxiety, nausea, and insomnia) may occur if the drug is not stopped gradually over at least 4 weeks. There is also a small risk of suicidal thoughts and self-harm in children and adolescents, although the drug is rarely used for this age group.

Monitoring Blood pressure should be measured periodically if high doses are prescribed. Anyone experiencing confusion, drowsiness, muscle cramps, or seizures should be monitored for low sodium levels in the blood. Under-18s should be monitored for suicidal thoughts and self-harm.

VERAPAMIL

Brand names Cordilox, Securon, Univer, Verapress, Vera-Til, Vertab, Zolvera
Used in the following combined preparation Tarka

GENERAL INFORMATION

Verapamil belongs to a group of drugs known as calcium channel blockers, which interfere with the conduction of signals in the muscles of the heart and blood vessels. It is used in treating hypertension, abnormal heart rhythms, and angina. It reduces the frequency of angina attacks, although it does not help relieve pain while an attack is in progress. Verapamil increases the ability to tolerate physical exertion and can be used safely by people with asthma.

Verapamil is also prescribed for certain types of abnormal heart rhythm. It can be administered by injection as well as in tablet form for such disorders.

Verapamil is not generally prescribed for people with low blood pressure, slow heart beat, or heart failure because it may worsen these conditions.

INFORMATION FOR USERS

Your drug prescription is tailored for you. Do not alter dosage without checking with your doctor.

How taken/used

Tablets, SR tablets/capsules, liquid, injection.

Frequency and timing of doses
2–3 x daily (tablets, liquid); 1–2 x daily (SR tablets/capsules).

Adult dosage range
120–480mg daily.

Onset of effect
1–2 hours (tablets); 2–3 minutes (injection).

Duration of action
6–8 hours. During prolonged treatment some beneficial effects may last for up to 12 hours. SR tablets act for 12–24 hours.

Diet advice
Avoid grapefruit juice, which may increase blood levels of verapamil.

Storage
Keep in original container at room temperature out of the reach of children.

Missed dose
Take as soon as you remember. If your next dose is due within 3 hours (tablets, liquid) or 8 hours (SR tablets/capsules), take a single dose now and skip the next.

Stopping the drug
Do not stop the drug without consulting your doctor; symptoms may recur.

Exceeding the dose
An occasional unintentional extra dose is unlikely to be a cause for concern. Large overdoses may cause dizziness. Notify your doctor.

SPECIAL PRECAUTIONS

Be sure to tell your doctor if:
- You have a long-term liver problem.
- You have heart failure.
- You have myasthenia gravis.
- You have porphyria.
- You are taking other medicines.

Pregnancy
Not usually prescribed. May inhibit labour if taken during later stages of pregnancy. Discuss with your doctor.

Breast-feeding
The drug passes into the breast milk, but at normal doses adverse effects on the baby are unlikely. Discuss with your doctor.

Infants and children
Usually given on specialist advice only. Reduced dose necessary.

Over 60
No special problems.

Driving and hazardous work
Avoid until you have learned how verapamil affects you because the drug can cause dizziness.

Alcohol
Avoid. Alcohol may further reduce blood pressure, causing dizziness or other symptoms.

Surgery and general anaesthetics
Verapamil may need to be stopped before surgery. Consult your doctor or dentist.

POSSIBLE ADVERSE EFFECTS

The main adverse effect is constipation. The drug may also cause slowing of the heart rate, which may result in dizziness. Rare effects include gynaecomastia (breast enlargement in males) and an increase in gum tissue after prolonged use.

Symptom/effect	Frequency		Discuss with doctor		Stop taking drug now	Call doctor now
	Common	Rare	Only if severe	In all cases		
Constipation	●			●		
Headache	●			●		
Nausea/vomiting	●			●		
Ankle swelling	●			●		
Dizziness		●		●		
Rash		●		●		

PROLONGED USE

Rarely, gynaecomastia (breast enlargement in men) or enlargement of the gum tissues may occur with long-term use.

INTERACTIONS

Clarithromycin and erythromycin may increase the effects of verapamil.

Carbamazepine, ciclosporin, dabigatran, digoxin, theophylline, sirolimus, and ivabradine The effects of these drugs may be increased by verapamil; their doses may need to be reduced or the combination avoided.

Rifampicin and barbiturates may reduce the effects of verapamil.

Beta blockers When verapamil is taken with these drugs, there is a slight risk of abnormal heart beat and heart failure.

Simvastatin and atorvastatin There is an increased risk of muscle damage if these drugs are taken with verapamil.

Colchicine Verapamil may increase the effects of colchicine, and the combination should be avoided.

WARFARIN

Brand name None
Used in the following combined preparations None

GENERAL INFORMATION

Warfarin is an anticoagulant designed to prevent deep-vein thromboses: blood clots, particularly in the leg and pelvic veins, where blood flow is slowest. The clots could otherwise break off and travel to the lungs to cause pulmonary embolism. It is also used to reduce the risk of clots in the heart in people with atrial fibrillation (irregular heart rhythm) or artificial heart valves; these clots may travel to the brain and cause a stroke. Regular monitoring is needed to ensure proper maintenance, dosage, and safety with warfarin, using the International Normalized Ratio (INR) blood test. As the full benefits are not felt for two to three days, a faster-acting drug such as heparin (see p.275) is often used initially in people who have or who are at risk of developing a clot.

Due to its risk of excessive bleeding, and the advent of newer anticoagulants, the use of warfarin is in decline except in patients with artificial heart valves.

QUICK REFERENCE

Drug group Anticoagulant drug (p.62)

Overdose danger rating High

Dependence rating Low

Prescription needed Yes

Available as generic Yes

INFORMATION FOR USERS

Your drug prescription is tailored for you. Do not alter dosage without checking with your doctor.

How taken/used

Tablets.

Frequency and timing of doses
Once daily, taken at the same time each day.

Dosage range
Large variation in starting and maintenance dose, according to patient factors, but usually 10mg for 2 days (starting dose); 3–9mg daily at same time, determined by blood tests (maintenance dose).

Onset of effect
Within 24–48 hours; full effect after several days.

Duration of action
2–3 days.

Diet advice
Avoid cranberry juice and major diet changes (especially of salads and vegetables).

Storage
Keep in original container at room temperature out of the reach of children. Protect from light.

Missed dose
Take as soon as you remember. Take the following dose on your original schedule.

Stopping the drug
Do not stop taking the drug without consulting your doctor; stopping the drug may lead to worsening of the underlying condition.

OVERDOSE ACTION

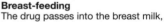

Seek immediate medical advice in all cases. Take emergency action if severe bleeding or loss of consciousness occur.

See Drug poisoning emergency guide (p.518).

SPECIAL PRECAUTIONS

Be sure to tell your doctor if:
- You have long-term liver or kidney problems.
- You have high blood pressure.
- You have a history of peptic ulcers.
- You have a bleeding disorder.
- You are taking other medicines.

Pregnancy
Not prescribed. Given in early pregnancy, the drug can cause malformations in the unborn child. Taken near the time of delivery, it may cause the mother to bleed excessively. Discuss with your doctor, who will prescribe alternative treatment.

Breast-feeding
The drug passes into the breast milk, but at normal doses adverse effects on the baby are unlikely. Discuss with your doctor.

Infants and children
Reduced dose necessary.

Over 60
No special problems.

Driving and hazardous work
Use caution. Even minor bumps can cause bad bruises and excessive bleeding.

Alcohol
Avoid major changes in alcohol consumption.

Surgery and general anaesthetics
Warfarin may need to be stopped before surgery. Discuss with your doctor or dentist.

POSSIBLE ADVERSE EFFECTS

Bleeding is the most common adverse effect. If you notice serious bruising, very prolonged bleeding from a minor wound, or blood in your urine or faeces, call your doctor immediately.

Symptom/effect	Frequency		Discuss with doctor		Stop taking drug now	Call doctor now
	Common	Rare	Only if severe	In all cases		
Bleeding/bruising	●			●	●	●
Nausea/vomiting		●		●		
Abdominal pain/diarrhoea		●		●		
Rash		●		●		
Hair loss		●		●		
Fever		●		●	●	●
Jaundice		●		●	●	●

INTERACTIONS

General note A wide range of drugs (e.g. aspirin and other non-steroidal anti-inflammatory drugs (NSAIDs), diuretics, chemotherapy, oral contraceptives, lipid-lowering drugs, amiodarone, barbiturates, cimetidine, steroids, certain laxatives, antidepressants, antibiotics and herbal medicines) interact with warfarin to affect the risk of bleeding. Consult your pharmacist before using over-the-counter medicines, and inform your warfarin clinic of any changes to your medicines.

PROLONGED USE

No special problems.

Monitoring Regular INR blood tests are carried out. Dose is adjusted accordingly and recorded in a treatment book, which should be carried with you at all times. More frequent testing may be needed if there is a significant change in your health.

ZIDOVUDINE/LAMIVUDINE

Brand names [zidovudine] Retrovir; [lamivudine] Epivir, Zeffix
Used in the following combined preparations Combivir, Trizivir

GENERAL INFORMATION

Zidovudine and lamivudine belong to the same class of drugs – nucleoside analogues – and are used in the treatment of HIV infection. The two drugs can be prescribed separately or combined in one tablet, which is usually prescribed with another class of drug (either a non-nucleoside reverse transcriptase inhibitor or a protease inhibitor) to treat HIV. This combination of three drugs is more effective at treating HIV than either a single or double regime of drugs.

Although it is not a cure for HIV, combination antiretroviral therapy (ART) slows the production of the virus and, therefore, reduces the viral load and consequent damage done to the immune system. The drugs need to be taken regularly and on a long-term basis to remain effective.

INFORMATION FOR USERS

Your drug prescription is tailored for you. Do not alter dosage without checking with your doctor.

How taken/used

Tablets, liquid, injection (zidovudine).

Frequency and timing of doses
1–2 x daily.

Adult dosage range
One tablet; 15–30ml liquid; dosage for injection calculated according to body weight.

Onset of effect
1 hour.

Duration of action
12–24 hours.

Diet advice
None.

Storage
Keep in original container at room temperature out of the reach of children.

Missed dose
Take as soon as you remember. If your next dose is due within 2 hours, take a single dose now and skip the next. It is very important not to miss doses on a regular basis as this can lead to the development of drug-resistant HIV.

Stopping the drug
Do not stop taking the drug without consulting your doctor.

Exceeding the dose
An occasional unintentional extra dose is unlikely to cause problems. But if you notice any unusual symptoms, or if a large overdose has been taken, notify your doctor.

SPECIAL PRECAUTIONS

Be sure to tell your doctor if:
• You have liver or kidney problems.
• You have other infections, such as hepatitis B or C.
• You are taking other medicines.

Pregnancy
Safety in pregnancy not established. If you are pregnant or planning pregnancy, discuss with your doctor.

Breast-feeding
Safety in breast-feeding not established. Breast-feeding is not recommended for HIV-positive mothers as the virus may be passed to the baby.

Infants and children
Reduced dose necessary under 12 years.

Over 60
Increased likelihood of adverse effects. Reduced dose may therefore be necessary.

Driving and hazardous work
No special problems.

Alcohol
No known problems.

POSSIBLE ADVERSE EFFECTS

The most common adverse effects of zidovudine/lamivudine are nausea, vomiting, and diarrhoea. Sometimes, anaemia may develop with prolonged use.

Symptom/effect	Frequency		Discuss with doctor		Stop taking drug now	Call doctor now
	Common	Rare	Only if severe	In all cases		
Nausea/vomiting	●			●		
Diarrhoea	●			●		
Fatigue	●			●		
Skin discoloration		●		●		
Anaemia		●		●		
Severe abdominal pain		●			●	●

INTERACTIONS

General note A wide range of drugs may interact with zidovudine and lamivudine, causing either an increase in adverse effects or a reduction in the effect of the antiretroviral drugs. Check with your doctor or pharmacist before taking any new drugs, including those acquired from your dentist or a supermarket, and herbal medicines.

PROLONGED USE

There is an increased risk of serious blood disorders, such as anaemia, with long-term use of zidovudine and lamivudine. There may also be a redistribution of fat from the limbs to the abdomen, back, and breasts. This may be accompanied by increases in blood levels of lipids and glucose.

Monitoring Regular blood checks will be carried out to monitor the viral load, blood count, and blood lipid and glucose levels.

ZOLEDRONIC ACID

Brand names Aclasta, Zerlinda, Zometa
Used in the following combined preparations None

GENERAL INFORMATION

Zoledronic acid is a bisphosphonate, one of a group of drugs used in the treatment of bone disorders. These drugs work directly on the bones, reducing the rate at which calcium is released from them and thereby making them less liable to fracture. The reduction of calcium release can cause blood calcium levels to fall, which is useful if the level is high (e.g. due to cancer). Zoledronic acid can only be given by infusion into a vein, and has a very long duration of action so that it can be used very infrequently.

It is used to treat various bone disorders, including Paget's disease of the bone, and osteoporosis in men and post-menopausal women – particularly those who have had a recent osteoporotic fracture or who are on long-term corticosteroids. Zoledronic acid is also used to prevent bone damage in patients with advanced cancer that has spread to bone.

QUICK REFERENCE

Drug group Drug for bone disorders (p.80) and anticancer drug (p.112)

Overdose danger rating Medium

Dependence rating Low

Prescription needed Yes

Available as generic No

INFORMATION FOR USERS

The drug is given only under medical supervision and is not for self-administration.

How taken/used

Intravenous infusion.

Frequency and timing of doses
Advanced cancer involving bone Every 3–4 weeks.
Paget's disease and high blood calcium associated with cancer One-off dose, can be repeated if required.
Osteoporosis Once yearly.

Adult dosage range
4–5mg.

Onset of effect
Up to 3 months.

Duration of action
Up to 1 year.

Diet advice
None. Calcium and/or vitamin D supplements may be prescribed before or after treatment with zoledronic acid.

Storage
Not applicable. The drug is not kept in the home.

Missed dose
The drug is administered in hospital under medical supervision. If you miss your dose, contact your doctor as soon as possible.

Stopping the drug
Discuss with your doctor. Stopping the drug may lead to worsening of the underlying condition.

Exceeding the dose
Overdosage is unlikely because the drug is given under close medical supervision. If you think you have received an overdose, tell your doctor as soon as possible.

POSSIBLE ADVERSE EFFECTS

The first dose of zoledronic acid may cause flu-like symptoms, including bone pain, fever, and fatigue; some people also experience gastrointestinal problems, such as sickness and vomiting. These symptoms tend to be milder if further doses are given.

Symptom/effect	Frequency		Discuss with doctor		Stop taking drug now	Call doctor now
	Common	Rare	Only if severe	In all cases		
Bone pain/fever/fatigue	●			●		
Sickness/vomiting	●			●		
Headache/dizziness		●		●		
Palpitations		●		●		
Rash/itching/facial swelling		●		●		●
Tingling/muscle spasms		●		●		●
Pain in the jaw		●		●		●

INTERACTIONS

None known

SPECIAL PRECAUTIONS

Be sure to tell your doctor if:
- You have had a recent hip fracture.
- You have kidney problems.
- You are or may be pregnant or are planning a pregnancy.
- You have had a previous allergic reaction to any bisphosphonate drug.
- You are taking other medicines.

 Pregnancy
Not recommended. Safety in pregnancy not established. Discuss with your doctor.

 Breast-feeding
Not recommended. Safety in breast-feeding not established. Discuss with your doctor.

 Infants and children
Not recommended.

 Over 60
No special problems.

 Driving and hazardous work
No special problems.

 Alcohol
No special problems.

PROLONGED USE

There have been rare reports of atypical femoral fractures and ulceration of jaw bones in patients taking bisphosphonates including zoledronic acid. Patients undergoing bisphosphonate treatment are advised to report any thigh, hip, or groin pain during to their doctor.

Monitoring Blood tests will be carried out to monitor your calcium levels. Your overall health will also be monitored.

ZOPICLONE

Brand names Zimovane, Zimovane LS
Used in the following combined preparations None

GENERAL INFORMATION

Zopiclone is a hypnotic (sleeping drug) used for the short-term treatment of insomnia. Sleep problems can take the form of difficulty in falling asleep, frequent night-time awakenings, and/or early morning awakenings. Hypnotic drugs are given only when non-drug measures – for example, avoidance of caffeine – have proved ineffective.

Unlike benzodiazepines, zopiclone has no anti-anxiety properties. Therefore, it may be suited for instances of insomnia that are not accompanied by anxiety, such as international travel or a change in shift-work routine.

Hypnotics are intended for occasional use only. Dependence can develop after as little as one week of continuous use.

QUICK REFERENCE

Drug group Sleeping drug (p.38)
Overdose danger rating Medium
Dependence rating Medium
Prescription needed Yes
Available as generic Yes

INFORMATION FOR USERS

Your drug prescription is tailored for you. Do not alter dosage without checking with your doctor.

How taken/used

Tablets.

Frequency and timing of doses
Once daily at bedtime when required. Tablets should be swallowed whole, without sucking or chewing.

Dosage range
3.75–7.5mg.

Onset of effect
Within 30 minutes.

Duration of action
4–6 hours.

Diet advice
None.

Storage
Keep in original container at room temperature out of the reach of children. Protect from light.

Missed dose
If you fall asleep without having taken a dose and wake some hours later, do not take the missed dose.

Stopping the drug
If you have been taking the drug continuously for less than 1 week, it can be safely stopped as soon as you feel you no longer need it. However, if you have been taking the drug for longer, consult your doctor.

Exceeding the dose
An occasional, unintentional extra dose is unlikely to cause problems. Large overdoses may cause prolonged sleep, drowsiness, lethargy, and poor muscle coordination and reflexes. Notify your doctor immediately.

SPECIAL PRECAUTIONS

Be sure to tell your doctor if:
- You have or have had any problems with alcohol or drug misuse.
- You have depression.
- You have myasthenia gravis.
- You have severe respiratory disease.
- You have liver or kidney problems.
- You are taking other medicines.

Pregnancy
Safety not established. Use in late pregnancy may affect the baby and cause withdrawal symptoms. Discuss with your doctor.

Breast-feeding
Safety not established. The drug is present in breast milk. Discuss with your doctor.

Infants and children
Not recommended.

Over 60
Increased risk of adverse effects. Reduced dose may be necessary.

Driving and hazardous work
Avoid such activities until you have learned how zopiclone affects you because the drug can cause drowsiness, reduced alertness, and slowed reactions.

Alcohol
Avoid. Alcohol increases the sedative effects of this drug.

POSSIBLE ADVERSE EFFECTS

The most common effects are daytime drowsiness, which normally diminishes after the first few days, and a bitter or metallic taste in the mouth. Persistent morning drowsiness or impaired coordination indicate excessive dose. The drug may cause depression and suicidal thoughts; if these symptoms occur, consult your doctor immediately.

Symptom/effect	Frequency		Discuss with doctor		Stop taking drug now	Call doctor now
	Common	Rare	Only if severe	In all cases		
Bitter or metallic taste	●		●			
Daytime drowsiness/headache	●			●		
Dizziness/weakness		●	●			
Nausea/vomiting/diarrhoea		●	●			
Amnesia/confusion		●		●	●	
Rash		●		●	●	●

INTERACTIONS

Sedatives All drugs, including alcohol, that have a sedative effect on the central nervous system are likely to increase the sedative effects of zopiclone. Such drugs include other sleeping and anti-anxiety drugs, antihistamines, antidepressants, opioid analgesics, and antipsychotics.

Erythromycin, clarithromycin, and ketoconazole may increase the levels and the effect of zopiclone, leading to adverse effects.

Carbamazepine, phenytoin, rifampicin, and St John's wort may reduce the effects of zopiclone.

PROLONGED USE

Intended for occasional use only. Continuous use of zopiclone, or any other sleeping drug, for as little as 1 or 2 weeks may cause dependence. Withdrawal symptoms may occur when the drug is stopped. These may include insomnia, anxiety, tremor, confusion, and panic attacks. Withdrawal symptoms are less likely when the drug is used for less than 4 weeks.

A–Z OF VITAMINS AND MINERALS

This section gives detailed information on 24 of the major vitamins and minerals that are required by the body for good health – chemicals that are essential, but which the body cannot make by itself. These include the main vitamins – A, C, D, E, K, H (biotin), and the B vitamins – together with 11 essential minerals.

The section on vitamins in Part 2 (p.107) gives in general terms the main sources of the major vitamins and minerals and their roles in the body, while the following profiles discuss each vitamin and mineral in detail.

The following pages may be particularly useful as a guide for those who think their diet lacks sufficient amounts of a certain vitamin or mineral, and for those with disorders of the digestive tract or liver, who may need larger amounts of certain vitamins. The table on p.108 gives the good dietary sources of each one.

The vitamin and mineral profiles

The profiles are arranged in alphabetical order and give information under standard headings. These include the different names by which each chemical is known; whether it is available over the counter or by prescription only; its role in body maintenance; specific foods in which it can be found; the recommended daily intake; how to detect a deficiency; how and when to supplement your diet; and the risks that are associated with excessive intake of a particular vitamin or mineral.

The Reference Nutrient Intake (RNI), sometimes just called the Reference Intake (RI), of vitamins and minerals appears on the packaging of many foods. It represents the amount of the nutrient that is enough to meet the needs of about 97 per cent of people in a particular group. The dosages for treating deficiency are usually considerably higher, but need to be determined by your doctor.

HOW TO UNDERSTAND THE PROFILES

Each vitamin and mineral profile contains information arranged under standard headings to enable you to find the information you need.

Availability
Tells you whether the vitamin or mineral is available over the counter or only by prescription.

Other names
Lists the chemical and non-chemical names by which the vitamin or mineral is also known.

Dietary and other natural sources
Tells you how the vitamin or mineral is obtained naturally.

When supplements are helpful
Suggests when your doctor may recommend that you take supplements.

Dosage range for treating deficiency
Gives a usual recommended dosage of vitamin or mineral supplements.

PANTOTHENIC ACID

Other names Calcium pantothenate, panthenol, pantothenol, vitamin B$_5$

Availability
Pantothenic acid, calcium pantothenate, and panthenol are available without prescription in a variety of multivitamin and mineral preparations.

Actions on the body
Pantothenic acid plays a vital role in the activities of many enzymes. It is essential for the production of energy from sugars and fats; for the manufacture of fats, corticosteroids, and sex hormones; for the utilization of other vitamins; for the proper function of the nervous system and the adrenal glands; and for normal growth and development.

Dietary and other natural sources
Pantothenic acid is present in almost all vegetables, cereals, and animal foods. Liver, kidney, heart, fish, and egg yolks are good dietary sources. Brewer's yeast, wheat germ, and royal jelly (the substance on which queen bees feed) are also rich in the vitamin.

Normal daily requirement
No Reference Nutrient Intake (RNI) for pantothenic acid has ever been established, but adult requirements are met by a 3–7mg intake daily.

When supplements are helpful
Most diets provide adequate amounts of pantothenic acid. Any deficiency is likely to occur in malnutrition together with other B vitamin deficiency diseases such as pellagra (see niacin), beriberi (see thiamine), or with alcoholism, and will be treated with B complex supplements. There is no firm evidence that large doses help, as some believe, in the prevention of greying hair, nerve disorders in diabetes, or psychiatric illness.

Symptoms of deficiency
Pantothenic acid deficiency is unlikely to occur unless a person is suffering from malnutrition. However, deficiency produced under experimental conditions can cause malaise, abdominal discomfort, and burning feet.

Dosage range for treating deficiency
Usually 5–20mg per day.

Symptoms and risks of excessive intake
In tests, doses of 1,000mg or more of pantothenic acid have not caused toxic effects. The risk of toxicity is considered to be very low, since pantothenic acid is a water-soluble vitamin that does not accumulate in the tissues. Any excess is eliminated rapidly in the urine. However, very high intakes of 10–20g can cause diarrhoea.

POTASSIUM

Other names Potassium acetate, potassium chloride, potassium citrate, potassium gluconate

Availability
Salts of potassium in small doses are available in a number of multivitamin and mineral supplements. They are available at higher doses in prescription-only drugs given as dietary supplements and in some diuretics given to offset the loss of potassium in the urine. Potassium salts are also widely available in sodium-free or low-sodium salt (used as a salt substitute). However, these salt substitutes should be avoided by people with impaired kidney function and those taking drugs that cause potassium retention, such as potassium-sparing diuretics (p.57).

Actions on the body
Potassium works together with sodium in controlling the body's water balance, and in the conduction of nerve impulses, contraction of muscle, and maintenance of a normal heart rhythm. Potassium is essential for maintenance of normal blood sugar levels.

Dietary and other natural sources
The best dietary sources of potassium are leafy green vegetables, tomatoes, oranges, potatoes, and bananas. Lean meat, pulses, chocolate, coffee, and milk are also rich in the mineral. Many methods of food processing may lower the potassium levels found in fresh food.

Normal daily requirement
The Reference Nutrient Intakes (RNIs) for potassium are: 0.8g (birth–3 months); 0.85g (4–6 months); 0.7g (7–12 months); 0.8g (1–3 years); 1.1g (4–6 years); 2.0g (7–10 years); 3.1g (11–14 years); 3.5g (15 years and over). There are no extra requirements in pregnancy or breast-feeding.

When supplements are helpful
Most diets contain adequate amounts of potassium, and supplements are rarely required in normal circumstances. However, people who drink large amounts of alcohol or eat lots of salty foods may become marginally deficient. People with a condition called diabetic ketoacidosis or with certain types of kidney disease may be deficient in potassium, but the most common cause is prolonged treatment with diuretics. Long-term use of corticosteroids may deplete the body's potassium. Prolonged vomiting and diarrhoea also cause potassium deficiency, so people who misuse laxatives may be affected. Supplements are usually advised only when symptoms suggest deficiency, or for people at particular risk.

Symptoms of deficiency
Early symptoms of potassium deficiency may include muscle weakness, fatigue, dizziness, and mental confusion. Impairment of nerve and muscle function may progress to cause disturbances of the heart rhythm and paralysis of the skeletal muscles as well as the muscles of the bowel, which leads to constipation.

Dosage range for treating deficiency
Depends on the preparation, the individual, and the cause and severity of deficiency. In general, daily doses equivalent to 2–4g of potassium chloride are given to prevent deficiency (for example, in people treated with diuretics that deplete potassium). Doses equivalent to 3.0–7.2g of potassium chloride daily are used to treat deficiency.

Symptoms and risks of excessive intake
Blood potassium levels are normally regulated by the kidneys, and any excess is rapidly eliminated in the urine. Massive doses cause serious disturbances of the heart rhythm and muscular paralysis. In people with impaired kidney function, excess potassium may build up and the risk of potassium poisoning is increased. People on haemodialysis treatment need to take a carefully controlled low-potassium diet.

439

Actions on the body
Explains the role played by each vitamin or mineral in maintaining healthy body function.

Normal daily requirement
Gives you a guide to the Reference Nutrient Intake (RNI) of each vitamin or mineral.

Symptoms of deficiency
Describes the common signs of deficiency.

Symptoms and risks of excessive intake
Explains the risks that may accompany excessive intake of each vitamin or mineral and warning signs to look out for.

BIOTIN

Other names Coenzyme R, vitamin H

Availability
Biotin is available without a prescription, alone and in a wide variety of multivitamin and mineral preparations.

Actions on the body
Biotin plays a vital role in the activities of several enzymes. It is essential for the breakdown of carbohydrates and fatty acids in the diet for conversion into energy, for the manufacture of fats, and for excretion of the products of protein breakdown. People with Type 2 diabetes often have low levels of biotin, and supplements may help to control blood sugar levels.

Dietary and other natural sources
Traces of biotin are present in a wide variety of foods. Dietary sources rich in this vitamin include liver, nuts, peas, beans, egg yolks, cauliflower, and mushrooms. A large proportion of the biotin we require is manufactured by bacteria in the intestine.

Normal daily requirement
A Reference Nutrient Intake (RNI) has not been established, but a daily dietary intake of 10–200mcg is safe.

When supplements are helpful
Adequate amounts of biotin are provided in most diets and by the bacteria living in the intestine, so supplements are rarely needed. However, deficiency can occur with prolonged, excessive consumption of raw egg whites (as in eggnogs), because these contain a protein – avidin – that prevents absorption of the vitamin in the intestine. The risk of deficiency is also increased during long-term treatment with antibiotics or sulfonamide antibacterial drugs, which may destroy the biotin-producing bacteria in the intestine. However, additional biotin is not usually necessary with a balanced diet.

Symptoms of deficiency
Deficiency symptoms include weakness, tiredness, dry skin, poor appetite, hair loss, and depression. Severe deficiency is rare but may cause eczema of the face and body, and inflammation of the tongue.

Dosage range for treating deficiency
Depends on the individual and on the nature and severity of the disorder. Dietary deficiency can be treated with doses of 150–300mcg of biotin daily. Deficiency of biotin resulting from a genetic defect that limits use of the vitamin by body cells can be treated with very large doses of 5mg given once or twice daily.

Symptoms and risks of excessive intake
None known.

CALCIUM

Other names Calcium carbonate, calcium chloride, calcium citrate, calcium glubionate, calcium gluceptate, calcium gluconate, calcium lactate, calcium phosphate

Availability
Oral forms are available without a prescription. Injectable forms of calcium are available only under medical supervision.

Actions on the body
The most abundant mineral in the body, calcium makes up more than 90 per cent of the hard matter in bones and teeth. It is essential for the formation and maintenance of strong bones and healthy teeth, as well as blood clotting, transmission of nerve impulses, and muscle contraction.

Dietary and other natural sources
The main dietary sources of calcium are milk and dairy products, sardines, dark green leafy vegetables, beans, peas, and nuts. Calcium is also present in drinking water in hard water areas.

Normal daily requirement
The Reference Nutrient Intakes (RNIs) for calcium are: 525mg (birth–1 year); 350mg (1–3 years); 450mg (4–6 years); 550mg (7–10 years); 1,000mg (males aged 11–18 years); 800mg (females aged 11–18 years); and 700mg (19 years and older). Daily requirements of calcium do not increase markedly during pregnancy, but rise to 1,250mg during breast-feeding.

When supplements are helpful
Unless a sufficient amount of dairy products is consumed (a pint of milk contains approximately 600mg) the diet may not contain enough calcium, and supplements may be needed. Breast-feeding women are especially vulnerable to calcium deficiency because breast-feeding demands large amounts of calcium, which may be extracted from the skeleton if intake is not adequate. Osteoporosis (fragile bones) has been linked to dietary calcium deficiency in some cases, but may not be helped by supplements in all women. Hormone replacement therapy or other treatment is usually necessary (see Drugs for bone disorders, p.80). People with coeliac disease may also need calcium supplements.

Symptoms of deficiency
When dietary intake is inadequate, the body obtains the calcium it needs from the skeleton. Long-term deficiency of calcium may lead to increased fragility of the bones. Low levels of calcium in the blood cause abnormal stimulation of the nervous system, resulting in cramp-like spasms in the hands, feet, and face. Vitamin D deficiency is the main cause of the bone-softening diseases rickets and osteomalacia.

Dosage range for treating deficiency
Vitamin D is needed for treatment of rickets and osteomalacia (p.80), but oral supplements of calcium of up to 800mg daily may be advised for children with rickets, and 1,000mg or more daily may be given for osteoporosis and osteomalacia. Low blood calcium levels are treated in hospital by intravenous injection of calcium.

Symptoms and risks of excessive intake
Excessive intake of calcium may reduce the amount of iron and zinc absorbed and may also cause constipation, confusion, and nausea. There is an increased risk of palpitations and, for susceptible people, of calcium deposits in the kidneys leading to kidney stones and kidney damage. These symptoms do not usually develop unless calcium is taken with large amounts of vitamin D.

CHROMIUM

Other names Chromium trichloride, chromium picolinate

Availability
Chromium supplements are available without prescription. However, only a very small proportion of chromium in the supplements is absorbed by the body (possibly 1–2 per cent).

Actions on the body
Chromium plays a vital role in the activities of several enzymes. It is involved in the breakdown of sugar for conversion into energy and in the manufacture of certain fats. The mineral works together with insulin and is thus essential to the body's ability to use sugar. Chromium may also be involved in the manufacture of proteins in the body.

Dietary and other natural sources
Traces of chromium are present in a wide variety of foods. Meat, dairy products, and wholemeal cereals are good sources of this mineral.

Normal daily requirement
Chromium is a trace element and only minute quantities are required. A Reference Nutrient Intake (RNI) has not been determined, but a safe intake for adults is about 25mcg.

When supplements are helpful
Most people who eat a healthy diet containing plenty of fresh or unprocessed foods receive adequate amounts of chromium. The use of chromium in diabetes is under investigation, but people with diabetes and those with diabetes-like symptoms may benefit from additional chromium. Supplements may also be helpful if symptoms suggest chromium deficiency.

Symptoms of deficiency
Chromium deficiency is very rare in Britain and typically occurs mainly in patients given long-term intravenous feeding. A diet of too many processed foods may contribute to chromium deficiency. Inadequate intake of chromium over a prolonged period may impair the body's ability to use sugar, leading to high blood sugar levels. However, in most cases, there are no symptoms. In some people, there may be diabetes-like symptoms such as tiredness, mental confusion, and numbness or tingling of the hands and feet. Deficiency may worsen pre-existing diabetes and may depress growth in children. It has also been suggested that chromium deficiency may contribute to the development of atherosclerosis (narrowing of the arteries).

Dosage range for treating deficiency
This depends on the individual and on the nature and severity of the disorder.

Symptoms and risks of excessive intake
Chromium is poisonous in excess. Levels that produce symptoms are usually obtained from occupational exposure or industrial waste in drinking water or the atmosphere, not from excessive dietary intake. Symptoms include inflammation of the skin and, if inhaled, damage to the nasal passages. People who are repeatedly exposed to chromium fumes have a higher-than-average risk of developing lung cancer. High levels may reduce kidney function.

COPPER

Other names Copper chloride, copper chloride dihydrate, copper gluconate, copper sulfate

Availability
Copper supplements are available in oral forms without a prescription. Copper chloride is an injectable form and is available only on prescription. Copper chloride dihydrate is part of a multiple-ingredient preparation for hospital use.

Actions on the body
Copper is an essential constituent of several proteins and enzymes. It plays an important role in the development of red blood cells, helps to form the dark pigment that colours hair and skin, and helps the body to use vitamin C. It is essential for the formation of collagen and elastin – proteins found in ligaments, blood vessel walls, and the lungs – and for the proper formation and maintenance of strong bones. It is also required for central nervous system activity.

Dietary and other natural sources
Most unprocessed foods contain copper. Liver, shellfish, nuts, mushrooms, wholemeal cereals, and dried pulses are particularly rich sources. Soft water may dissolve copper from pipes.

Normal daily requirement
The Reference Nutrient Intakes (RNIs) for copper are: 0.2mg (birth–3 months); 0.3mg (4 months–1 year); 0.4mg (1–3 years); 0.6mg (4–6 years); 0.7mg (7–10 years); 0.8mg (11–14 years); 1.0mg (15–18 years); and 1.2mg (19 years and over). Daily requirements do not change during pregnancy, but rise by 0.3mg when breast-feeding.

When supplements are helpful
A diet that regularly includes a selection of the foods mentioned above provides sufficient copper. Supplements are rarely necessary. However, doctors may advise additional copper for malnourished infants and children.

Symptoms of deficiency
Copper deficiency is very rare. The major change is anaemia due to failure of production of red blood cells, the main symptoms of which are pallor, fatigue, shortness of breath, and palpitations. In severe cases, abnormal bone changes may occur. An inherited copper deficiency disorder called Menke's syndrome (kinky hair disease) results in brain degeneration, retarded growth, sparse and brittle hair, and weak bones.

Dosage range for treating deficiency
This depends on the individual and on the nature and severity of the disorder.

Symptoms and risks of excessive intake
As little as 250mg of copper sulfate taken by mouth in a single dose can produce toxic effects. Symptoms of poisoning include nausea, vomiting, abdominal pain, diarrhoea, and general aches and pains. Large overdoses of copper may cause destruction of red blood cells (haemolytic anaemia), and liver and kidney damage. In Wilson's disease, an inherited disorder, the patient cannot excrete copper and suffers from long-term copper poisoning, and gradually develops liver and brain damage. The disease is treated with chelating agents such as penicillamine. Acute copper poisoning may occur in people who regularly drink home-made alcohol distilled through copper tubing.

FLUORIDE

Other names Calcium fluoride, sodium fluoride, sodium monofluorophosphate, stannous fluoride

Availability
Sodium fluoride may be added to drinking water and is available over the counter in single- or multiple-ingredient preparations. Mouth rinses, toothpastes, tablets, gels, and oral drops containing sodium fluoride, sodium monofluorophosphate, or stannous fluoride are available over the counter. Calcium fluoride is a naturally occurring form of the mineral.

Actions on the body
Fluoride helps to prevent tooth decay and contributes to the strength of bones. It is thought to work on the teeth by strengthening the mineral composition of the tooth enamel, making it more resistant to attack by acid in the mouth. Fluoride is most effective when taken during the formation of teeth in childhood, since it is then incorporated into the tooth itself. It may also strengthen developing bones.

Dietary and other natural sources
Fluoride has been added to drinking water in many areas, and water is therefore a prime source of this mineral (fluoride levels in water vary from area to area, and untreated water also contains a small amount of fluoride). Foods and beverages grown or prepared in areas with fluoride-treated water may also contribute fluoride. Tea and sea fish are also rich in fluoride.

Normal daily requirement
No Reference Nutrient Intake (RNI) has been established.

When supplements are helpful
Fluoride supplements are not usually necessary for adults, particularly those who use a fluoride toothpaste, although a dentist may recommend supplements for people who are especially prone to tooth decay. For children, supplements are not generally advised unless the drinking water contains a very low level of fluoride; infants less than 6 months old should not be given supplements even if the drinking water is low in fluoride. In all cases, supplements should only be used on the advice of a dentist. See below for more information about dosage ranges for supplements.

Symptoms of deficiency
Fluoride deficiency increases the risk of tooth decay, especially in children.

Dosage range for treating deficiency
Dietary supplements are not usually advised unless the drinking water contains less than 0.7 parts per million (ppm) of fluoride (0.7mg per litre). In such cases, the recommended dosage depends on the level of fluoride in the water and the age of the child; supplements are not recommended for infants under 6 months old. When the drinking water contains less than 0.3ppm, the recommended daily dose of fluoride is: 0.25mg (6 months–3 years); 0.5mg (3–6 years); and 1mg (over 6 years). When the drinking water contains 0.3–0.7ppm, supplements are not recommended for children under 3 years old; the recommended daily dose for older children is 0.25mg (3–6 years) and 0.5mg (over 6 years).

Symptoms and risks of excessive intake
Prolonged intake of water containing high concentrations of fluoride may lead to mottled or brown discoloration of the enamel in developing teeth, a condition known as fluorosis. Suggestions of a link between fluoridation of the water supply and cancer are without foundation. A child or adult who has taken a number of fluoride tablets may become seriously unwell and eventually lose consciousness. Give milk if the person is conscious, and seek immediate medical help (see p.518).

FOLIC ACID

Other names Folacin, folates, sodium folate, vitamin B_9, vitamin B_{11}

Availability
Folic acid is available without prescription, alone and in a variety of multivitamin and mineral preparations. Strengths of 500mcg and over are available only on prescription.

Actions on the body
Folic acid is essential for the activities of several enzymes. It is required for the manufacture of nucleic acids – the genetic material of cells – and thus for the processes of growth and reproduction. It is vital for the formation of red blood cells by the bone marrow and the development and proper function of the central nervous system. Taken before and during pregnancy, it can help prevent neural tube defects (abnormalities affecting development of the brain and spinal cord) in the unborn baby.

Dietary and other natural sources
The best sources are leafy green vegetables, yeast extract, and liver. Root vegetables, oranges, nuts, dried pulses, and egg yolks are also rich sources.

Normal daily requirement
The Reference Nutrient Intakes (RNIs) for folic acid, as folate, in micrograms (mcg) are: 50mcg (birth–1 year); 70mcg 1–3 years); 100mcg (4–6 years); 150mcg (7–10 years); 200mcg (11 years and over). For women planning pregnancy who are at low risk of having a baby with a neural tube defect: 400mcg per day before conception and during the first 12 weeks of pregnancy. Couples are considered to be at high risk of having a baby with a neural tube defect if either partner has a personal or family history of the condition (including a previous pregnancy); if the woman has a malabsorption disorder such as coeliac disease; if she has diabetes or sickle cell disease; or if she is taking anticonvulsant medication. Women at high risk should take 5mg per day before conception and during the first 12 weeks of pregnancy; women with sickle cell disease should continue taking 5mg daily throughout pregnancy. Daily requirements increase by 60mcg during breast-feeding.

When supplements are helpful
A varied diet containing fresh fruit and vegetables usually provides adequate amounts. However, minor deficiency is fairly common, and can be corrected by adding one uncooked fruit or vegetable or a glass of fruit juice daily. Supplements are recommended for women before and during pregnancy to prevent neural tube defects. They may also be needed in premature or low-birth-weight infants and those fed on goat's milk (breast and cow's milk contain adequate amounts of the vitamin). Doctors may recommend additional folic acid for people on haemodialysis or those with certain blood disorders, psoriasis, conditions in which absorption of nutrients from the intestine is impaired, severe alcoholism, or liver disease. Supplements may be helpful if you are a heavy drinker or if you are taking drugs that deplete folic acid, such as anticonvulsants, antimalarial drugs, oestrogen-containing contraceptives, certain analgesics, corticosteroids, and sulfonamides.

Symptoms of deficiency
Folic acid deficiency leads to abnormally low numbers of red blood cells (anaemia). The main symptoms include fatigue, loss of appetite, nausea, diarrhoea, and hair loss. Mouth sores are common and the tongue is often sore. Deficiency may also cause poor growth in infants and children.

Dosage range for treating deficiency
Symptoms of anaemia are usually treated with 5–15mg of folic acid daily, together with vitamin B_{12}. A lower maintenance dose may be substituted once the anaemia has responded.

Symptoms and risks of excessive intake
Excessive folic acid is not toxic. However, it may worsen the neurological symptoms of a coexisting vitamin B_{12} deficiency and should never be taken to treat anaemia without a full medical investigation of the cause of the anaemia.

IODINE

Other names Potassium iodate, potassium iodide, sodium iodide

Availability
Iodine supplements are available without prescription as kelp tablets and in several multivitamin and mineral preparations. Iodine skin preparations are also available without a prescription for antiseptic use. A small amount of iodine is routinely added to most table salts in order to prevent iodine deficiency from occurring. Treatments for thyroid suppression are available only on prescription.

Actions on the body
Iodine is essential for the formation of thyroid hormone, which regulates the body's energy production, promotes growth and development, and helps burn excess fat.

Dietary and other natural sources
Seafood is the best source of iodine, but bread and dairy products such as milk are the main sources of this mineral in most diets. Iodized table salt is also a good source. Iodine may be inhaled from the atmosphere in coastal regions.

Normal daily requirement
The Reference Nutrient Intakes (RNIs) for iodine in micrograms (mcg) are: 50mcg (birth–3 months); 60mcg (4–12 months); 70mcg (1–3 years); 100mcg (4–6 years); 110 mcg (7–10 years); 130mcg (11–14 years); and 140mcg (15 years and over).

When supplements are helpful
Most diets contain adequate amounts of iodine, and use of iodized table salt can usually make up for any deficiency. Supplements are rarely necessary except on medical advice. However, excessive intake of raw cabbage or nuts reduces uptake of iodine into the thyroid gland, and it may lead to deficiency if iodine intake is otherwise low. Kelp supplements may be helpful.

Adults exposed to radiation from radioactive iodine released into the environment may be given 100mg of iodine as a single dose (as potassium iodate 170mg) to prevent their thyroid gland absorbing the radioactive material; a lower dose is given to children according to age.

Iodine is used to treat people with thyrotoxicosis before surgery on the thyroid gland, and iodine-containing compounds are also used as X-ray contrast media.

Symptoms of deficiency
Deficiency may result in a goitre (enlargement of the thyroid gland) and hypothyroidism (deficiency of thyroid hormone). Symptoms of hypothyroidism include tiredness, physical and mental slowness, weight gain, facial puffiness, and constipation. Babies born to iodine-deficient mothers are lethargic and difficult to feed. Left untreated, many show poor growth and developmental delay.

Dosage range for treating deficiency
Iodine deficiency may be treated with doses of 150mcg of iodine daily, and then followed up by ensuring that iodized table salt is used.

Symptoms and risks of excessive intake
The amount of iodine that occurs naturally in food is non-toxic, but prolonged use of large amounts (6mg or more daily) may suppress the activity of the thyroid gland. Large overdoses of iodine compounds may cause abdominal pain, vomiting, bloody diarrhoea, and swelling of the thyroid and salivary glands.

IRON

Other names Ferrous fumarate, ferrous gluconate, ferrous sulfate, iron dextran, iron-polysaccharide complex, sodium feredelate

Availability
Ferrous sulfate, ferrous fumarate, ferrous gluconate, and iron-polysaccharide complex are all available without prescription, alone and in multivitamin and mineral preparations. Iron dextran, an injectable form, is available only on prescription.

Actions on the body
Iron has an important role in the formation of red blood cells (which contain two-thirds of the body's iron) and is a vital component of the oxygen-carrying pigment haemoglobin. It is involved in the formation of myoglobin, a pigment that stores oxygen in muscles for use during exercise. It is also an essential component of several enzymes, and is involved in the uptake of oxygen by the cells and the conversion of blood sugar to energy.

Dietary and other natural sources
Liver is the best dietary source of iron. Meat (especially organ offal), eggs, chicken, fish, leafy green vegetables, dried fruit, enriched or wholemeal cereals, breads and pastas, nuts, and dried pulses are also rich sources. Iron is better absorbed from meat, eggs, chicken, and fish than from vegetables. Foods containing vitamin C enhance iron absorption.

Normal daily requirement
The Reference Nutrient Intakes (RNIs) for iron are: 1.7mg (birth–3 months); 4.3mg (4–6 months); 7.8mg (7–12 months); 6.9mg (1–3 years); 6.1mg (4–6 years); 8.7mg (7–10 years); 11.3mg (males aged 11–18 years); 14.8mg (females aged 11–50 years); and 8.7mg (males aged 19 and over, and females aged 51 and over). Requirements may be increased during pregnancy and for 2 to 3 months after childbirth.

When supplements are helpful
Most average diets supply adequate amounts of iron. However, larger amounts are necessary during pregnancy. Supplements may be given throughout pregnancy and for 2 to 3 months after childbirth to maintain and replenish adequate iron stores in the mother. Premature babies may be prescribed supplements from a few weeks after birth to prevent deficiency. Supplements may be helpful in young vegetarians, women with heavy menstrual periods, and people with chronic blood loss due to disease (for example, peptic ulcer).

Symptoms of deficiency
Iron deficiency causes anaemia. Symptoms of anaemia include pallor, fatigue, shortness of breath, and palpitations. Apathy, irritability, and lowered resistance to infection may occur. Iron deficiency may also affect intellectual performance and behaviour.

Dosage range for treating deficiency
Depends on the individual and the nature and severity of the condition. In adults, iron-deficiency anaemia is usually treated with 100–200mg of elemental iron (usually as ferrous sulfate or gluconate) daily. In children, the dose is reduced according to age and weight. Iron supplements of 30–60mg daily may be given during pregnancy.

Symptoms and risks of excessive intake
An overdose of iron tablets is extremely dangerous. Pain in the abdomen, nausea, and vomiting may be followed by abdominal bloating, dehydration, and dangerously lowered blood pressure. Immediate medical attention must be sought (see p.518).

Excessive long-term intake, especially when iron is taken with large amounts of vitamin C, may in susceptible individuals cause iron to accumulate in organs, causing congestive heart failure, cirrhosis of the liver, and diabetes mellitus. This condition is known as haemochromatosis.

MAGNESIUM

Other names Magnesium carbonate, magnesium citrate, magnesium gluconate, magnesium glycerophosphate, magnesium hydroxide, magnesium sulfate

Availability
Magnesium is available without prescription in a variety of multivitamin and mineral preparations. Magnesium is also an ingredient of numerous over-the-counter antacid and laxative preparations, but it is not absorbed well from these sources.

Actions on the body
About 60 per cent of the body's magnesium is found in bones and teeth. Magnesium is essential for the formation of healthy bones and teeth, the transmission of nerve impulses, and the contraction of muscles. It activates several enzymes, and is important in the conversion of carbohydrates, fats, and proteins into energy.

Dietary and other natural sources
The best dietary sources of magnesium are leafy green vegetables. Nuts, wholemeal cereals, soya beans, cheese, and seafood are also rich in magnesium. Drinking water in hard water areas is a further source of this mineral.

Normal daily requirement
The Reference Nutrient Intakes (RNIs) for magnesium are: 55mg (birth–3 months); 60mg (4–6 months); 75mg (7–9 months); 80mg (10–12 months); 85mg (1–3 years); 120mg (4–6 years); 200mg (7–10 years); 280mg (11–14 years); 300mg (males aged 15 and over, and females aged 15–18 years); and 270mg (females aged 19 and over). Daily requirements do not increase during pregnancy but rise by 50mg during breast-feeding.

When supplements are helpful
A varied diet provides adequate amounts of magnesium, particularly in hard water areas. Supplements are usually necessary only on medical advice for deficiency of magnesium associated with certain conditions in which absorption from the intestine is impaired, which occurs in repeated vomiting or diarrhoea, advanced kidney disease, severe alcoholism, or prolonged treatment with certain diuretic drugs. Some anti-ulcer drugs (proton pump inhibitors) may also cause magnesium deficiency. Intravenous magnesium is used to treat eclampsia, cardiac arrhythmias, and myocardial infarction.

Oestrogens and oestrogen-containing oral contraceptives may reduce blood magnesium levels, but women who are on adequate diets do not need supplements.

Symptoms of deficiency
The symptoms of magnesium deficiency include anxiety, restlessness, tremors, confusion, palpitations, irritability, depression, and disorientation. Severe magnesium deficiency causes marked overstimulation of the nervous system, and results in seizures and cramp-like spasms of the hands and feet. Inadequate intake may be a factor in the development of coronary heart disease, and may also lead to calcium deposits in the kidneys, resulting in kidney stones.

Dosage range for treating deficiency
This depends on the individual and on the nature and severity of the disorder. Severe deficiency is usually treated in hospital by injection of magnesium sulfate.

Symptoms and risks of excessive intake
Magnesium toxicity (hypermagnesaemia) is rare, but can occur in people with impaired kidney function after prolonged intake of the large amounts that are found in antacid or laxative preparations. Symptoms include nausea, vomiting, dizziness (due to a drop in blood pressure), and muscle weakness. Very large increases in magnesium in the blood may cause fatal respiratory failure or heart arrest.

NIACIN

Other names Niacinamide, nicotinamide, nicotinic acid, vitamin B3, vitamin PP

Availability
Niacin is available without prescription in a wide variety of single-ingredient and multivitamin and mineral preparations. However, high doses of nicotinic acid are available only on prescription.

Actions on the body
Niacin plays a vital role in the activities of many enzymes. It is important in producing energy from blood sugar, and in the manufacture of fats. Niacin is also essential for the proper working of the nervous system, for a healthy skin and digestive system, and for the manufacture of steroid hormones.

Dietary and other natural sources
Liver, lean meat, poultry, fish, wholemeal cereals, nuts, and dried pulses are the best dietary sources of niacin.

Normal daily requirement
The Reference Nutrient Intakes (RNIs) for niacin are: 3mg (birth–6 months); 4mg (7–9 months); 5mg (10–12 months); 8mg (1–3 years); 11mg (4–6 years); 12mg (7–10 years and females aged 11–14 years); 15mg (males aged 11–14 years); 18mg (males aged 15–18 years); 14mg (females aged 15–18 years); 17mg (males aged 19–50 years); 13mg (females aged 19–50 years); 16mg (males aged 51 and over); and 12mg (females aged 51 and over). Daily requirements do not increase during pregnancy, but they rise by 2mg during breast-feeding.

When supplements are helpful
Most British diets provide adequate amounts of niacin, and dietary deficiency is rare. Supplements are required for niacin deficiency associated with bowel disorders in which absorption from the intestine is impaired, and for people with liver disease or severe alcoholism. They may also be required for older people on poor diets. Large doses of niacin (up to 6g daily) are sometimes used in the treatment of hyperlipidaemia (raised blood fat levels). There is no convincing medical evidence that niacin helps psychiatric disorders (except those associated with pellagra). Topical niacin (nicotinic acid) is used in mild to moderate acne and is being investigated for use in diabetes.

Symptoms of deficiency
Severe niacin deficiency causes pellagra (literally, rough skin). Symptoms include sore, red, cracked skin in areas exposed to sun, friction, or pressure, inflammation of the mouth and tongue, abdominal pain and distension, nausea, diarrhoea, and mental disturbances such as depression, anxiety, and dementia.

Dosage range for treating deficiency
For severe pellagra, adults are usually treated with 100–500mg nicotinamide daily by mouth, and children are usually given 100–300mg daily. For less severe deficiency, doses of 25–50mg are given. Nicotinyl alcohol tartrate is a drug with similar properties to nicotinamide, but it is not the same as niacin.

Symptoms and risks of excessive intake
At doses of over 50mg used to treat hyperlipidaemia, niacin (nicotinic acid) may cause transient itching, flushing, tingling, or headache. These symptoms diminish after a few weeks with repeated administration. Niacin in the form that occurs naturally in the body (nicotinamide) is free of these effects. Large doses of niacin may cause nausea and may aggravate a peptic ulcer. Side effects may be reduced by taking the drug on a full stomach. At doses of over 2g daily (which have been used to treat hyperlipidaemia), there is a risk of gout, liver damage, and high blood sugar levels, leading to extreme thirst.

PANTOTHENIC ACID

Other names Calcium pantothenate, panthenol, pantothenol, vitamin B_5

Availability
Pantothenic acid, calcium pantothenate, and panthenol are available without prescription in a variety of multivitamin and mineral preparations.

Actions on the body
Pantothenic acid plays a vital role in the activities of many enzymes. It is essential for the production of energy from sugars and fats; for the manufacture of fats, corticosteroids, and sex hormones; for the utilization of other vitamins; for the proper function of the nervous system and the adrenal glands; and for normal growth and development.

Dietary and other natural sources
Pantothenic acid is present in almost all vegetables, cereals, and animal foods. Liver, kidney, heart, fish, and egg yolks are good dietary sources. Brewer's yeast, wheat germ, and royal jelly (the substance on which queen bees feed) are also rich in the vitamin.

Normal daily requirement
No Reference Nutrient Intake (RNI) for pantothenic acid has ever been established, but adult requirements are met by a 3–7mg intake daily.

When supplements are helpful
Most diets provide adequate amounts of pantothenic acid. Any deficiency is likely to occur in malnutrition together with other B vitamin deficiency diseases such as pellagra (see niacin), beriberi (see thiamine), or with alcoholism, and will be treated with B complex supplements. There is no firm evidence that large doses help, as some believe, in the prevention of greying hair, nerve disorders in diabetes, or psychiatric illness.

Symptoms of deficiency
Pantothenic acid deficiency is unlikely to occur unless a person is suffering from malnutrition. However, deficiency produced under experimental conditions can cause malaise, abdominal discomfort, and burning feet.

Dosage range for treating deficiency
Usually 5–20mg per day.

Symptoms and risks of excessive intake
In tests, doses of 1,000mg or more of pantothenic acid have not caused toxic effects. The risk of toxicity is considered to be very low, since pantothenic acid is a water-soluble vitamin that does not accumulate in the tissues. Any excess is eliminated rapidly in the urine. However, very high intakes of 10–20g can cause diarrhoea.

POTASSIUM

Other names Potassium acetate, potassium chloride, potassium citrate, potassium gluconate

Availability
Salts of potassium in small doses are available in a number of multivitamin and mineral supplements. They are available at higher doses in prescription-only drugs given as dietary supplements and in some diuretics given to offset the loss of potassium in the urine. Potassium salts are also widely available in sodium-free or low-sodium salt (used as a salt substitute). However, these salt substitutes should be avoided by people with impaired kidney function and those taking drugs that cause potassium retention, such as potassium-sparing diuretics (p.57).

Actions on the body
Potassium works together with sodium in controlling the body's water balance, and in the conduction of nerve impulses, contraction of muscle, and maintenance of a normal heart rhythm. Potassium is essential for maintenance of normal blood sugar levels.

Dietary and other natural sources
The best dietary sources of potassium are leafy green vegetables, tomatoes, oranges, potatoes, and bananas. Lean meat, pulses, chocolate, coffee, and milk are also rich in the mineral. Many methods of food processing may lower the potassium levels found in fresh food.

Normal daily requirement
The Reference Nutrient Intakes (RNIs) for potassium are: 0.8g (birth–3 months); 0.85g (4–6 months); 0.7g (7–12 months); 0.8g (1–3 years); 1.1g (4–6 years); 2g (7–10 years); 3.1g (11–14 years); 3.5g (15 years and over). There are no extra requirements in pregnancy or breast-feeding.

When supplements are helpful
Most diets contain adequate amounts of potassium, and supplements are rarely required in normal circumstances. However, people who drink large amounts of alcohol or eat lots of salty foods may become marginally deficient. People with a condition called diabetic ketoacidosis or with certain types of kidney disease may be deficient in potassium, but the most common cause is prolonged treatment with diuretics. Long-term use of corticosteroids may deplete the body's potassium. Prolonged vomiting and diarrhoea also cause potassium deficiency, so people who misuse laxatives may be affected. Supplements are usually advised only when symptoms suggest deficiency, or for people at particular risk.

Symptoms of deficiency
Early symptoms of potassium deficiency may include muscle weakness, fatigue, dizziness, and mental confusion. Impairment of nerve and muscle function may progress to cause disturbances of the heart rhythm and paralysis of the skeletal muscles as well as the muscles of the bowel, which leads to constipation.

Dosage range for treating deficiency
Depends on the preparation, the individual, and the cause and severity of deficiency. In general, daily doses equivalent to 2–4g of potassium chloride are given to prevent deficiency (for example, in people treated with diuretics that deplete potassium). Doses equivalent to 3.0–7.2g of potassium chloride daily are used to treat deficiency.

Symptoms and risks of excessive intake
Blood potassium levels are normally regulated by the kidneys, and any excess is rapidly eliminated in the urine. Massive doses cause serious disturbances of the heart rhythm and muscular paralysis. In people with impaired kidney function, excess potassium may build up and the risk of potassium poisoning is increased. People on haemodialysis treatment need to take a carefully controlled low-potassium diet.

PYRIDOXINE

Other names Pyridoxine hydrochloride, vitamin B_6

Availability
Pyridoxine and pyridoxine hydrochloride are available without prescription in a variety of single-ingredient and multivitamin and mineral preparations.

Actions on the body
Pyridoxine plays a vital role in the activities of many enzymes. This B vitamin is essential for the release of carbohydrates stored in the liver and muscles for energy; for the breakdown and use of proteins, carbohydrates, and fats from food; and for the manufacture of niacin (vitamin B_3). It is needed for the production of red blood cells and antibodies, and for healthy skin. It is also important for normal function of the central nervous system.

Dietary and other natural sources
Liver, chicken, fish, wholemeal cereals, wheat germ, and eggs are rich in this vitamin. Bananas, avocados, and potatoes are also good sources.

Normal daily requirement
The Reference Nutrient Intakes (RNIs) for pyridoxine are: 0.2mg (birth–6 months); 0.3mg (7–9 months); 0.4mg (10 months–1 year); 0.7mg (1–3 years); 0.9mg (4–6 years); 1mg (7–10 years and females aged 11–14 years); 1.2mg (males aged 11–14 years); 1.5mg (males aged 15–18 years); 1.2mg (females aged 15 and over); and 1.4mg (males aged 19 and over). There are no extra requirements in pregnancy or breast-feeding.

When supplements are helpful
Most balanced diets contain adequate amounts of pyridoxine, and it is also manufactured in small amounts by bacteria that live in the intestine. However, breast-fed infants and older adults may require additional pyridoxine. Supplements may be given on medical advice together with other B vitamins to people with certain conditions in which absorption from the intestine is impaired. They may be used to treat one form of anaemia (sideroblastic) and certain rare genetic disorders termed pyridoxine dependency conditions. Supplements may also be recommended to prevent or treat deficiency caused by alcoholism, oral contraceptives, and treatment with drugs such as isoniazid, penicillamine, and hydralazine.

Symptoms of deficiency
Pyridoxine deficiency is rare unless it is due to drug treatment. Deficiency may cause weakness, nervousness, irritability, depression, skin disorders, inflammation of the mouth and tongue, and cracked lips. In adults, it may cause anaemia (abnormally low levels of red blood cells). Seizures may occur in infants.

Dosage range for treating deficiency
Depends on the individual and the nature and severity of the disorder. In general, deficiency is treated with 20–50mg up to 3 times per day for three weeks followed by 1.5–2.5mg daily in a multivitamin preparation for as long as necessary. Deficiency resulting from genetic defects that prevent use of the vitamin is treated with doses of 10–100mg daily in infants and 10–250mg daily in adults and children. Daily doses of 50–100mg (given with other B vitamins from day 10 of a menstrual cycle) to day 3 of the following cycle may help relieve premenstrual syndrome.

Symptoms and risks of excessive intake
The long-term safety of daily doses over 10mg has not been established. However, daily doses of over 200mg taken over a prolonged period may severely damage the nervous system, resulting in unsteadiness, numbness, and clumsiness of the hands.

RIBOFLAVIN

Other names Vitamin B_2, vitamin G

Availability
Riboflavin is available without a prescription, alone and in a wide variety of multivitamin and mineral preparations.

Actions on the body
Riboflavin plays a vital role in the activities of several enzymes. It is involved in the breakdown and utilization of carbohydrates, fats, and proteins and in the production of energy in cells using oxygen. It is needed for utilization of other B vitamins and for production of steroid hormones (by the adrenal glands).

Dietary and other natural sources
Riboflavin is found in most foods. Good dietary sources are liver, milk, cheese, eggs, leafy green vegetables, wholemeal cereals, and pulses. Brewer's yeast is also a rich source of the vitamin.

Normal daily requirement
The Reference Nutrient Intakes (RNIs) for riboflavin are: 0.4mg (birth–1 year); 0.6mg (1–3 years); 0.8mg (4–6 years); 1mg (7–10 years); 1.2mg (males aged 11–14 years); 1.1mg (females aged 11 and over); and 1.3mg (males aged 15 and over). Daily requirements rise by 0.3mg in pregnancy and by 0.5mg when breast-feeding.

When supplements are helpful
A balanced diet generally provides adequate amounts of riboflavin. Supplements may be beneficial in people on very low-calorie diets and older people on poor diets. Riboflavin requirements may also be increased by prolonged use of phenothiazine antipsychotics, tricyclic antidepressants, and oestrogen-containing oral contraceptives. Supplements are required for riboflavin deficiency associated with chronic diarrhoeal illnesses in which absorption of nutrients from the intestine is impaired. Riboflavin deficiency is also common among people with alcoholism. As with other B vitamins, the need for riboflavin is increased by injury, surgery, severe illness, and psychological stress. In all cases, treatment with supplements works best in a complete B-complex formulation.

Symptoms of deficiency
Prolonged deficiency may lead to chapped lips, cracks, and sores in the corners of the mouth; a red, sore tongue; and skin problems in the genital area. The eyes may itch, burn, and become unusually sensitive to light.

Dosage range for treating deficiency
Usually treated with doses of up to 30mg (in divided doses) in combination with other B vitamins.

Symptoms and risks of excessive intake
Excessive intake does not appear to have harmful effects.

SELENIUM

Other names Selenious acid, selenium sulfide, selenium yeast, selenomethionine, sodium selenite

Availability
Selenium is available without a prescription as 200mcg tablets and in a multivitamin and mineral preparation. Selenium sulfide is the active ingredient of several antidandruff shampoos.

Actions on the body
Selenium is a trace element, but it is an essential part of an enzyme system that protects cells against damage by oxygen "free radicals" (it is an antioxidant like vitamins A, C, and E).

Dietary and other natural sources
Meat, fish, wholemeal cereals, and dairy products are good dietary sources. The amount of selenium found in vegetables depends on the content of the mineral in the soil where they were grown. Selenium is found in foods combined in amino acids.

Normal daily requirement
The Reference Nutrient Intakes (RNIs) for selenium are: 10mcg (birth–3 months); 13mcg (4–6 months); 10mcg (7–12 months); 15mcg (1–3 years); 20mcg (4–6 years); 30mcg (7–10 years); 45mcg (11–14 years); 70mcg (males aged 15–18 years); 60mcg (females aged 15 and over); and 75mcg (males aged 19 and over). There is no extra requirement during pregnancy, but 15mcg extra daily are required when breast-feeding.

When supplements are helpful
Most normal diets provide adequate amounts of selenium, and supplements are, therefore, rarely necessary. At present, there is no conclusive medical evidence to support some claims that selenium may provide protection against cancer or that it prolongs life. A daily intake of more than 150mcg is not recommended, except on the advice of a doctor.

Symptoms of deficiency
Long-term lack of selenium may result in loss of stamina and degeneration of tissues, leading to premature ageing. Severe deficiency may cause muscle pain and tenderness, and can eventually lead to a fatal form of heart disease in children in areas where selenium levels in the diet are very low – for example, in one remote part of China.

Dosage range for treating deficiency
Depends on the individual and on the nature and severity of the disorder. Severe selenium deficiency may be treated with doses of up to 200mcg daily.

Symptoms and risks of excessive intake
Excessive intake may cause hair and nail loss, tooth decay and loss, fatigue, nausea, vomiting, and garlic breath. Total daily intake should not exceed 450mcg; large overdoses may be fatal.

SODIUM

Other names Sodium bicarbonate (baking soda), sodium chloride (table salt), sodium lactate, sodium phosphate

Availability
Sodium is widely available in the form of common table salt (sodium chloride). Sodium bicarbonate is used in many over-the-counter antacids. Sodium lactate is a prescription-only drug used in intravenous infusion fluid. Sodium phosphate is a laxative available only on prescription.

Actions on the body
Sodium works with potassium in control of the water balance in the body, conduction of nerve impulses, contraction of muscles, and maintenance of a normal heart rhythm.

Dietary and other natural sources
Sodium is present in almost all foods as a natural ingredient, or as an extra ingredient added during processing. The main sources are table salt, processed foods, cheese, breads and cereals, and smoked, pickled, or cured meats and fish. High concentrations are found in pickles and snack foods, including potato crisps and olives. Sodium is present in water that has been treated with water softeners. Manufactured foods may also contain sodium compounds such as monosodium glutamate.

Normal daily requirement
The Reference Nutrient Intakes (RNIs) for sodium are: 0.21g (birth–3 months); 0.28g (4–6 months); 0.32g (7–9 months); 0.35g (10–12 months); 0.5g (1–3 years); 0.7g (4–6 years); 1.2g (7–10 years); and 1.6g (11 years and over). Most British diets contain far more sodium than this: the average consumption of sodium is 3–7g daily. One teaspoon of table salt (6g) contains about 2g of sodium.

When supplements are helpful
The need for supplementation is rare in temperate climates, even with "low-salt" diets. In tropical climates, however, sodium supplements may help to prevent cramps and possibly heatstroke occurring as a result of sodium lost through excessive perspiration during heavy work. Sodium supplements may be given on medical advice to replace salt loss due to prolonged diarrhoea and vomiting, particularly in infants. They may also be given to prevent or treat deficiency due to certain kidney disorders, cystic fibrosis, adrenal gland insufficiency, or use of diuretics.

Symptoms of deficiency
Sodium deficiency caused by dietary insufficiency is rare. It is usually a result of conditions that increase loss of sodium from the body, such as diarrhoea, vomiting, and excessive perspiration. Early symptoms include lethargy, muscle cramps, and dizziness. In severe cases, there may be a marked drop in blood pressure leading to confusion, fainting, and palpitations.

Dosage range for treating deficiency
Depends on the individual and on the nature and severity of symptoms. In extreme cases, intravenous sodium chloride may be required.

Symptoms and risks of excessive intake
Excessive sodium intake is thought to contribute to the development of high blood pressure, which may increase the risk of heart disease, stroke, and kidney damage. Other adverse effects include abnormal fluid retention, which leads to swelling of the legs and face. Large overdoses, even of table salt, may cause seizures or coma and could be fatal. Table salt should never be used as an emetic (to trigger vomiting).

THIAMINE

Other names Aneurine hydrochloride, thiamin, thiamine hydrochloride, thiamine mononitrate, vitamin B_1

Availability
Thiamine is available without prescription in single-ingredient form and a variety of multivitamin and mineral preparations. It is also available on prescription, but as an injection only.

Actions on the body
Thiamine plays a vital role in the activities of many enzymes. It is essential for the breakdown and utilization of fats, alcohol, and carbohydrates. It is important for a healthy nervous system, healthy muscles, and normal heart function.

Dietary and other natural sources
Thiamine is present in all unrefined food. Good dietary sources include wholemeal or enriched cereals and breads, brown rice, pasta, liver, kidneys, meat, fish, beans, nuts, eggs, and most vegetables. Wheat germ and bran are excellent sources.

Normal daily requirement
The Reference Nutrient Intakes (RNIs) for thiamine are: 0.2mg (birth–9 months); 0.3mg (10–12 months); 0.5mg (1–3 years); 0.7mg (4–10 years and females aged 11–14 years); 0.9mg (males aged 11–14 years); 1.1mg (males aged 15–18 years); 0.8mg (females aged 15 and over); 1mg (males aged 19–50 years); and 0.9mg (males aged 51 and over). Daily requirements rise by 0.1mg in the last three months of pregnancy and by 0.2mg when breast-feeding.

When supplements are helpful
A balanced diet generally provides adequate amounts of thiamine. However, supplements may be helpful in older people on poor diets or those with high energy requirements caused, for example, by overactivity of the thyroid or heavy manual work. As with other B vitamins, requirements of thiamine are increased during severe illness, surgery, serious injury, and prolonged psychological stress. Additional thiamine is usually necessary on medical advice for deficiency associated with conditions in which absorption of nutrients from the intestine is impaired (such as excessive vomiting in pregnancy), and for prolonged liver disease or severe alcoholism.

Symptoms of deficiency
Deficiency may cause fatigue, irritability, loss of appetite, disturbed sleep, confusion, loss of memory, depression, abdominal pain, constipation, and beriberi, a disorder that affects the nervous system (so-called "dry" beriberi) and heart ("wet" beriberi). Symptoms of beriberi include tingling or burning sensations in the legs, cramps and tenderness in the calf muscles, incoordination, palpitations, seizures, and heart failure. In people with chronic alcoholism and those with malnutrition, thiamine deficiency may lead to a characteristic deterioration of central nervous system function known as Wernicke-Korsakoff's syndrome. The syndrome results in paralysis of the eye muscles, severe memory loss, and dementia, for which urgent treatment is needed.

Dosage range for treating deficiency
Depends on the nature and severity of the disorder but, in general, for mild chronic deficiency 10–25mg by mouth should be taken daily. Injections of the vitamin are sometimes given when deficiency is very severe or when symptoms have appeared suddenly. For severe deficiency, the dose is 200–300mg daily.

Symptoms and risks of excessive intake
The risk of adverse effects is very low because any excess is rapidly eliminated in the urine. However, prolonged use of large doses of thiamine may deplete other B vitamins, and thiamine should therefore be taken in a vitamin B complex formulation. There is a risk of allergic reactions with thiamine injections.

VITAMIN A

Other names Beta-carotene, carotenoids, retinoic acid, retinoids, retinol, retinol palmitate

Availability
Retinol, retinol palmitate, and beta-carotene are available without prescription in various single-ingredient and multivitamin and mineral preparations. Retinoids are used in prescription-only treatments for acne and psoriasis.

Actions on the body
Vitamin A is essential for normal growth and strong bones and teeth in children. It is necessary for normal vision and healthy cell structure. It helps to keep skin healthy and protect the linings of the mouth, nose, throat, lungs, and digestive and urinary tracts against infection. Vitamin A is also necessary for fertility in both sexes. Beta-carotene is an important antioxidant (i.e., it protects the body cells from damage).

Dietary and other natural sources
Liver (the richest source), fish liver oils, eggs, dairy products, orange and yellow vegetables and fruits (carrots, tomatoes, apricots, and peaches), and leafy green vegetables are good dietary sources. Vitamin A is also added to margarine.

Normal daily requirement
The Reference Nutrient Intakes (RNIs) for vitamin A are: 350mcg (up to 1 year); 400mcg (1–6 years); 500mcg (7–10 years); 600mcg (males aged 11–14 years, females aged 11 and over); 700mcg (males aged 15 and over, and pregnant women); 950mcg (breast-feeding).

When supplements are helpful
Most diets provide adequate amounts of vitamin A, but diets very low in fat or protein can lead to deficiency. Supplements are often given to young children in developing countries. They may also be needed by people with cystic fibrosis, obstruction of the bile ducts, overactivity of the thyroid gland, and certain intestinal disorders, and by people on long-term treatment with certain lipid-lowering drugs (e.g. colestyramine), which reduce absorption of the vitamin from the intestine. They are recommended with other vitamins for pregnant women, children under 5 years, and nursing mothers.

Symptoms of deficiency
Night blindness (difficulty in seeing in dim light) is the earliest symptom of deficiency; others include dry, rough skin, loss of appetite, and diarrhoea. Resistance to infection is decreased. Eyes may become dry and inflamed. Severe deficiency may lead to corneal ulcers.

Dosage range for treating deficiency
Deficiency is treated by intramuscular injection of 100,000 units every 2–4 months.

Symptoms and risks of excessive intake
Prolonged intake of more than 3mg a day in adults can cause loss of appetite, diarrhoea, dry or itchy skin, and hair loss. Fatigue and irregular menstruation are common. Headache, weakness, and vomiting may result from increased pressure of the fluid surrounding the brain. In extreme cases, bone pain and enlargement of the liver and spleen may occur. High doses of beta-carotene may turn the skin orange but are not dangerous. Excessive intake in pregnancy may lead to birth defects (see box, below).

VITAMIN A AND PREGNANCY

High doses of vitamin A in the early weeks of pregnancy can, rarely, cause defects in the baby, leading to damage of the central nervous system, face, eyes, ears, or palate. Pregnant women and those considering pregnancy should keep to the prescribed dose and not take extra vitamin A or eat liver products such as pâté (one serving of liver may contain 4–12 times the dose recommended for pregnancy). No other dietary restrictions are considered necessary.

VITAMIN B$_{12}$

Other names Cobalamin, cobalamins, cyanocobalamin, hydroxocobalamin

Availability
Vitamin B$_{12}$ is available without prescription in a wide variety of preparations. Hydroxocobalamin is given only by injection under medical supervision.

Actions on the body
Vitamin B$_{12}$ plays a vital role in the activities of several enzymes. It is essential for the manufacture of the genetic material of cells and thus for growth and development. The formation of red blood cells by the bone marrow is particularly dependent on this vitamin. It is also involved in the utilization of folic acid and carbohydrates in the diet, and is necessary for maintaining a healthy nervous system.

Dietary and other natural sources
Liver is the best dietary source of vitamin B$_{12}$. Almost all animal products, as well as seaweed, are also rich in the vitamin, but vegetables are not.

Normal daily requirement
Only minute quantities of vitamin B$_{12}$ are required. The Reference Nutrient Intakes (RNIs) are: 0.3mcg (birth–6 months); 0.4mcg (7–12 months); 0.5mcg (1–3 years); 0.8mcg (4–6 years); 1mcg (7–10 years); 1.2mcg (11–14 years); and 1.5mcg (15 years and over). Requirements of vitamin B$_{12}$ are unchanged during pregnancy but are increased by 0.5mcg per day during breast-feeding.

When supplements are helpful
A balanced diet usually provides more than adequate amounts of this vitamin, and deficiency is generally due to impaired absorption from the intestine rather than low dietary intake. However, a strict vegetarian or vegan diet lacking in eggs or dairy products is likely to be deficient in vitamin B$_{12}$, and supplements are usually needed. The most common cause of deficiency is pernicious anaemia, in which absorption of the vitamin is impaired due to inability of the stomach to secrete a particular substance – known as intrinsic factor – that normally combines with the vitamin so that it can be taken up in the intestine. Supplements are also prescribed on medical advice in certain bowel disorders, such as coeliac disease and various other causes of malabsorption, after surgery to the stomach or intestine, and in fish tapeworm infestation.

Symptoms of deficiency
Vitamin B$_{12}$ deficiency usually develops over months or years – the liver can store up to 6 years' supply. Deficiency leads to anaemia. The mouth and tongue often become sore. The brain and spinal cord may also be affected, leading to numbness and tingling of the limbs, memory loss, and depression.

Dosage range for treating deficiency
Depends on the individual and on the type and severity of deficiency. Pernicious anaemia (due to impaired absorption of vitamin B$_{12}$) is treated in adults with injections of 0.25mg–1mg (250–1,000mcg) on alternate days for 1–2 weeks, then 0.25mg per week until blood counts are normal, then 1mg every month (cobalamin) or every 2–3 months (hydroxocobalamin). Higher monthly doses of up to 1,000mcg of B$_{12}$ (on alternate days if there is neurological involvement), together with folic acid, may be given if the deficiency is severe. Children are treated with a total of 30–50mcg daily (cobalamin) or the same amounts as adults (hydroxocobalamin). Dietary deficiency is usually treated with oral supplements of 50–150mcg or more daily or 50–105mcg (cyanocobalamin) and 35–50mcg twice daily in infants. Deficiency that results from a genetic defect preventing use of the vitamin is treated with 250mcg every three weeks throughout life.

Symptoms and risks of excessive intake
Harmful effects from high doses of vitamin B$_{12}$ are rare. Allergic reactions may, rarely, occur with preparations given by injection.

VITAMIN C

Other names Ascorbic acid, calcium ascorbate, sodium ascorbate

Availability
Vitamin C is available without prescription in a wide variety of single-ingredient and multivitamin and mineral preparations. Ascorbic acid injection is given only under specialized medical supervision.

Actions on the body
Vitamin C plays an essential role in the activities of several enzymes. It is vital for the growth and maintenance of healthy bones, teeth, gums, ligaments, and blood vessels, and is an important component of all body organs. Vitamin C is also recognized as an important antioxidant (i.e., it protects the body cells against damage and may prevent fat deposits from building up in the blood vessels) and is important for the manufacture of certain neurotransmitters and adrenal hormones. It is required for the utilization of folic acid and absorption of iron. This vitamin is also necessary for normal immune responses to infection and for wound healing.

Dietary and other natural sources
Vitamin C is found in most fresh fruits and vegetables. Citrus fruits, tomatoes, potatoes, and leafy green vegetables are good dietary sources. This vitamin is easily destroyed by cooking; some fresh, uncooked fruit and vegetables should be eaten daily. Adding a daily source of vitamin C, such as a glass of orange juice, is also recommended.

Normal daily requirement
The Reference Nutrient Intakes (RNIs) for vitamin C are: 25mg (birth–1 year); 30mg (1–10 years); 35mg (11–14 years); 40mg (15 years and over); 50mg (pregnancy); and 70mg (breast-feeding).

When supplements are helpful
A healthy diet generally contains sufficient quantities of vitamin C. However, it is used up more rapidly after a serious injury, major surgery, burns, and in extremes of temperature. Supplements may be necessary to prevent or treat deficiency in older and chronically sick people, for smokers, and in severe alcoholism. They are recommended with other vitamins for pregnant women, children under 5 years, and nursing mothers. Women taking oestrogen-containing contraceptives may also require supplements. Although many people take larger doses (1g daily) for the prevention or treatment of colds, there is no convincing evidence that vitamin C in large doses prevents colds, although it may reduce the severity of symptoms.

Symptoms of deficiency
Mild deficiency may cause weakness and aches and pains. Severe deficiency results in scurvy, the symptoms of which include inflamed, bleeding gums, nosebleeds, excessive bruising, and internal bleeding. In adults, teeth become loose. In children, there is abnormal bone and tooth development. Wounds fail to heal and become infected. Deficiency of vitamin C often leads to anaemia (abnormally low levels of red blood cells), the symptoms of which are pallor, fatigue, shortness of breath, and palpitations. Untreated scurvy may cause seizures, coma, and death.

Dosage range for treating deficiency
For scurvy, at least 250mg of vitamin C is given daily for several weeks.

Symptoms and risks of excessive intake
The risk of harmful effects is low, since excess vitamin C is excreted in the urine. However, doses of over 2g daily may cause diarrhoea, nausea, and stomach cramps. Kidney stones may occasionally develop.

VITAMIN D

Other names Alfacalcidol, calcifediol, calciferol, calcitriol, colecalciferol, ergocalciferol, vitamin D$_2$, vitamin D$_3$

Availability
Vitamin D is available without prescription in a variety of multivitamin and mineral preparations. Injections and some oral preparations are given only under medical supervision.

Actions on the body
Vitamin D (together with parathyroid hormone) helps regulate the balance of calcium and phosphate in the body. It aids in the absorption of calcium from the intestinal tract, and is essential for strong bones and teeth.

Dietary and other natural sources
Margarine (to which vitamin D is added by law), oily fish (tuna, sardines, herring, and salmon), liver, dairy products, and egg yolks are usually good sources of this vitamin. It is also formed by the action of ultraviolet rays in sunlight on chemicals naturally present in the skin. Sunlight is a major source of vitamin D for most people.

Normal daily requirement
The Reference Nutrient Intakes (RNIs) for vitamin D are: 8.5–10mcg (birth–1 year); and 10mcg (all those over 1 year old, including women who are pregnant or breast-feeding). 1mcg of vitamin D equals 40 international units (IU).

When supplements are helpful
Vitamin D requirements are usually met by dietary sources and exposure to sunlight. However, a poor diet and inadequate sunlight may lead to deficiency; dark-skinned people and night-shift workers are more at risk. Premature infants, vegans, strict vegetarians, and older people may benefit from supplements. During winter months, the lack of sunlight may make it difficult for the body to make enough of the vitamin, and all adults may benefit from a daily supplement of 10mcg. Supplements are usually necessary on medical advice to prevent and treat vitamin D deficiency-related bone disorders, conditions in which absorption from the intestine is impaired, deficiency due to liver disease, certain kidney disorders, effects from prolonged use of certain drugs, and genetic defects. They are also used to treat hypoparathyroidism (inadequate secretion of parathyroid hormone). Supplements are recommended with other vitamins for pregnant women, children under 5 years, and nursing mothers, and with calcium to prevent or treat osteoporosis.

Symptoms of deficiency
Long-term deficiency leads to low blood levels of calcium (hypocalcaemia) and phosphate (hypophosphataemia), which results in softening of the bones. In children this causes abnormal bone development (rickets), and in adults, osteomalacia, leading to backache, muscle weakness, bone pain, and fractures.

Dosage range for treating deficiency
In general, rickets due to dietary deficiency is treated initially with 3,000–6,000 IU of vitamin D daily, depending on the age of the child, followed by a maintenance dose of 400 IU. Osteomalacia caused by deficiency of vitamin D is treated initially with 3,000–40,000 IU daily, followed by a daily maintenance dose of 400 IU. Deficiency due to impaired intestinal absorption or liver disease is treated with 40,000 IU daily (adults) and 10,000–25,000 IU daily (children). Hypocalcaemia due to hypoparathyroidism is treated with doses of up to 100,000 IU. Simple deficiency is usually treated with oral supplements of 400 IU.

Symptoms and risks of excessive intake
Doses of over 400 IU are not beneficial in most people (unless they have a poor diet or limited exposure to sunlight, when 800 IU per day may be needed) and may increase the risk of adverse effects. Prolonged excessive use disrupts the balance of calcium and phosphate and may lead to abnormal calcium deposits in the soft tissues, blood vessel walls, and kidneys, and retarded growth in children. Excess calcium may lead to symptoms such as weakness, increased urination, thirst, gastrointestinal disturbances, and depression.

VITAMIN E

Other names Alpha tocopherol, alpha tocopheryl acetate, tocopherol, tocopherols

Availability
Vitamin E is available without prescription in many single-ingredient and multivitamin and mineral preparations. It is also included in skin creams. Alpha tocopherol is the most powerful form.

Actions on the body
Vitamin E, a potent antioxidant, is vital for healthy cell structure, for slowing the effects of the ageing process on cells, and for maintaining the activities of certain enzymes. Vitamin E protects the lungs and other tissues from damage caused by pollutants, and protects red blood cells against destruction by poisons in the bloodstream. It also helps to maintain healthy red blood cells, and is involved in the production of energy in the heart and muscles.

Dietary and other natural sources
Some vegetable oils are good sources. Other sources rich in this vitamin include leafy green vegetables, wholemeal cereals, and wheat germ.

Normal daily requirement
Vitamin E is measured in milligrams of alpha-tocopherol equivalents (mg alpha-TE). Approximately 3–15mg daily are recommended. However, no UK recommendations have been made as vitamin E requirement depends on intake of polyunsaturated fatty acid, which varies widely. Recommended daily intakes in the USA are: 3mg alpha-TE (birth–6 months); 4mg alpha-TE (7–12 months); 6mg alpha-TE (1–3 years); 7mg alpha-TE (4–10 years); 10mg alpha-TE (males aged 11 and over); 8mg alpha-TE (females aged 11 and over); 10mg alpha-TE (pregnancy); 12mg alpha-TE (first 6 months of breast-feeding); and 11mg alpha-TE (second 6 months of breast-feeding).

When supplements are helpful
A normal diet supplies adequate amounts of vitamin E, and supplements are rarely necessary. However, people who consume large amounts of polyunsaturated fats in vegetable oils, especially if used in cooking at high temperatures, may need supplements. Supplements of vitamin E are also recommended for premature infants and people with impaired intestinal absorption or cystic fibrosis, as well as for liver disease in children.

Symptoms of deficiency
Vitamin E deficiency leads to destruction of red blood cells (haemolysis) and eventually anaemia (abnormally low levels of red blood cells), symptoms of which may include pallor, fatigue, shortness of breath, and palpitations. In infants, deficiency may cause irritability and fluid retention.

Dosage range for treating deficiency
Doses are generally four to five times the recommended intake in adults and children, for the relevant sex and age group.

Symptoms and risks of excessive intake
Harmful effects are rare, but there is a risk of diarrhoea and abdominal pain with doses of more than 1g per day. Prolonged use of over 250mg daily may lead to nausea, abdominal pain, vomiting, and diarrhoea. Long-term use of over 400mg daily has been linked to an increased risk of certain types of cancer.

VITAMIN K

Other names Menadiol, phytomenadione, vitamin K_1, vitamin K_2, vitamin K_3, vitamin K_4

Availability
Vitamin K is available without prescription as a dietary supplement in several multivitamin and mineral preparations. Injectable and oral preparations of vitamin K alone are used to treat bleeding disorders and are available only on prescription.

Actions on the body
Vitamin K is necessary for the formation in the liver of several substances that promote the formation of blood clots (blood clotting factors), including prothrombin (clotting factor II).

Dietary and other natural sources
The best dietary sources of vitamin K are leafy green vegetables and root vegetables, fruits, seeds, cow's milk, and yoghurt. Alfalfa is also an excellent source. In adults and children, the intestinal bacteria manufacture a large part of the vitamin K that is required.

Normal daily requirement
Newborn infants may be given 1mg of vitamin K (as phytomenadione) by single intramuscular injection. Alternatively, they may receive the vitamin orally; two doses of 2mg are given in the first week, and a third dose at 1 month for breast-fed babies (omitted in formula-fed babies due to the presence of vitamin K in formula feeds). In the UK, no recommended intake has been set for other age groups, but the US recommended daily intakes are: 15–100mcg (children and adolescents); 120mcg (adult males); and 90mcg (adult females).

When supplements are helpful
Vitamin K requirements are generally met adequately by dietary intake and by manufacture of the vitamin by bacteria that live in the intestine. Supplements are given routinely to newborn babies, since they lack intestinal bacteria capable of producing the vitamin and are therefore more at risk of deficiency than adults are. In adults and children, additional vitamin K is usually necessary only on medical advice for deficiency associated with prolonged use of antibiotics or sulfonamide antibacterials that destroy bacteria in the intestine, or when absorption of nutrients from the intestine is impaired. These conditions include liver disease, obstruction of the bile duct, and intestinal disorders causing chronic diarrhoea. Vitamin K may be given to reduce blood loss during labour or after surgery in people who have been taking oral anticoagulants. Vitamin K also reverses the effect of an overdose of oral anticoagulants.

Symptoms of deficiency
Vitamin K deficiency leads to low levels of prothrombin (hypoprothrombinaemia) and other clotting factors, resulting in delayed blood clotting and a tendency to bleed. This may cause easy bruising, oozing from wounds, nosebleeds, and bleeding from the gums, intestine, urinary tract, and, rarely, in the brain. (These effects are the same as those due to an overdose of warfarin, which counteracts vitamin K.)

Dosage range for treating deficiency
Depends on the individual and on the nature and severity of the disorder.

Symptoms and risks of excessive intake
Excess dietary intake of vitamin K has no known harmful effects, although it may increase the doses of oral anticoagulant medications needed. Synthetic vitamin K (menadione) may cause rupture of red blood cells (haemolysis) in people who have glucose-6-phosphate dehydrogenase (G6PD) deficiency. This may lead to reddish brown urine, jaundice, and, in extreme cases, anaemia. Adverse effects are extremely rare with vitamin K preparations taken by mouth.

ZINC

Other names Zinc acetate, zinc chloride, zinc gluconate, zinc oxide, zinc sulfate

Availability
Zinc supplements are available without prescription in single-ingredient and multivitamin and mineral preparations. Zinc chloride is used in ocular solutions and mouthwashes and as an injectable preparation given only under medical supervision during intravenous feeding. Zinc is also one ingredient included in a variety of topical formulations used for the treatment of minor skin irritations, dandruff, acne, haemorrhoids, and fungal infections.

Actions on the body
Zinc plays a vital role in the activities of over 100 enzymes. It is essential for the manufacture of proteins and nucleic acids (the genetic material of cells), and is involved in the function of the hormone insulin in utilizing carbohydrates. It is necessary for normal functioning of the immune system, a normal rate of growth, development of the reproductive organs, normal function of sperm, and healing of wounds and burns.

Dietary and other natural sources
Zinc is present in small amounts in a wide variety of foods. The mineral is better absorbed from animal sources than from plant sources. Protein-rich foods such as lean meat and seafood are the best sources of the mineral. Wholemeal breads and cereals, as well as dried pulses, are also good dietary sources.

Normal daily requirement
The Reference Nutrient Intakes (RNIs) for zinc are: 4mg (birth–6 months); 5mg (7 months–3 years); 6.5mg (4–6 years); 7mg (7–10 years); 9mg (11–14 years); 9.5mg (males aged 15 and over); and 7mg (females aged 15 and over). There is no extra requirement during pregnancy, but the RNI is 13mg in the first 4 months of breast-feeding and 9.5mg thereafter.

When supplements are helpful
A balanced diet containing natural, unprocessed foods usually provides adequate amounts of zinc. Dietary deficiency is rare in Britain, and is likely only in people who are generally malnourished, such as debilitated older people on poor diets. Supplements are usually recommended on medical advice for those with reduced absorption of the mineral due to certain intestinal disorders, such as cystic fibrosis; for those with increased zinc requirements due to sickle cell disease or major burns; and for those with liver damage occurring, for example, as a result of excessive alcohol intake. It has been suggested that zinc supplements may shorten the duration of the common cold but scientific studies suggest this is not the case.

Symptoms of deficiency
Deficiency may cause loss of appetite and impair the sense of taste. In children, it may also lead to poor growth and, in severe cases, to delayed sexual development and short stature. Severe, prolonged lack of zinc may result in a rare skin disorder involving hair loss, rash, inflamed areas of skin with pustules, and inflammation around the mouth, tongue, eyelids, and around the fingernails.

Dosage range for treating deficiency
Depends on the individual and on the cause and severity of the deficiency. In general, 50–150mg of elemental zinc daily is sufficient, usually in the form of zinc sulfate.

Symptoms and risks of excessive intake
Large overdoses of zinc salts in powder form are corrosive to tissues and may cause burns in the mouth and throat. Prolonged use of high doses may interfere with the absorption of copper, leading to deficiency, and may cause nausea, vomiting, headache, fever, malaise, and abdominal pain.

DRUGS OF ABUSE

The purpose of these pages is to clarify the medical facts concerning certain drugs (or classes of drugs) that are commonly misused in the UK. Their physical and mental effects, sometimes combined with a dangerous habit-forming potential, have led to their use outside a medical context. Some of the drugs listed in this section are illegal, while others have legitimate medical uses – such as anti-anxiety and sleeping drugs – and are also discussed in other parts of the book. Alcohol and volatile substances, although not medical drugs, are nevertheless drugs in a pharmacological sense and carry a substantial risk of misuse. These substances are not illegal, but the sale of alcohol products to young people is regulated by law, and the sale of volatile substances is restricted by voluntary agreement.

The individual profiles are designed to instruct and inform the reader, enabling readers to understand how these drugs affect the body, to become more aware of the hazards of drug misuse, and to be able to recognize signs of drug misuse in other people.

Since a large proportion of those who misuse drugs are young people, the following pages may serve as a useful source of reference for parents and teachers who are concerned that young people under their care may be taking drugs.

The drugs of abuse profiles

The profiles are arranged alphabetically under their medical or common names, with street names, drug categories, and cross-references to other parts of the book where appropriate. Each profile contains information on that drug under standard headings. Topics covered include the various ways it is taken, its habit-forming potential, its legitimate medical uses, its legal status, its effects and risks, the signs of misuse, and interactions with other drugs.

HOW TO UNDERSTAND THE PROFILES

Each drug of abuse profile contains standard headings under which you will find information covering important aspects of the drug.

Drug category
Categorizes the drug according to its principal effects on the body, with cross-references to other parts of the book where relevant.

Other common names
Lists the usual, alternative, and street names of each drug.

How taken
Tells you the various forms in which each substance is taken.

Short-term effects
Explains the immediate mental and physical effects of the drug.

Signs of misuse
Describes the outward effects of taking the drug, both short- and long-term, that concerned observers may notice.

Practical points
Gives tips on how to avoid abuse of the drug and suggests ways to stop or reduce intake.

Habit-forming potential
Explains to what extent the drug is likely to produce physical or psychological dependence.

Legitimate uses
Describes the accepted medical uses of the substance, if any.

Long-term effects and risks
Explains the serious long-term effects on health and the risks involved with regular use of the drug.

Interactions
Describes interactions that may occur with other drugs.

BENZODIAZEPINES

Other common names Tranquillizers, tranx, temmies
Drug category Central nervous system depressants (see Sleeping drugs, p.38, and Anti-anxiety drugs, p.39)

Habit-forming potential
The addictive potential of benzodiazepines is much lower than that of some other central nervous system depressants such as barbiturates. However, regular long-term use of these drugs can lead to physical and psychological dependence on their sedative effects.

How taken
By mouth as tablets or capsules, or by injection. Temazepam is the most widely abused benzodiazepine.

Legitimate uses
Benzodiazepines are commonly prescribed mainly for short-term treatment of anxiety and stress, as well as for relief of sleeplessness. They are also used in anaesthesia, both as premedication and for induction of general anaesthesia. Other medical uses include the management of alcohol withdrawal, control of epileptic seizures, and relief of muscle spasms. Most benzodiazepines are classified under Class C and Schedule IV of the Misuse of Drugs legislation (see p.13), although temazepam and flunitrazepam are under Schedule III.

Short-term effects
Benzodiazepines can reduce mental activity. In moderate doses, they may cause unsteadiness, reduce alertness, and slow the body's reactions, thus impairing driving ability as well as increasing the risk of accidents. Benzodiazepines may also cause amnesia (loss of memory regarding events that occurred while the person was under the influence of the drug). Any benzodiazepine in a high enough dose induces sleep. Large overdoses (especially by intravenous injection) may cause depression of the breathing mechanism and death.

Long-term effects and risks
Benzodiazepines tend to lose their sedative effect with long-term use (more than a few weeks). This may lead the user to increase the dose progressively, a manifestation of tolerance and physical dependence (see p.23). Older people may become apathetic or confused when taking these drugs. On stopping the drug, chronic users may develop withdrawal symptoms that may include anxiety, panic attacks, palpitations, shaking, insomnia, nightmares, nausea, dizziness, aches and pains, nausea, loss of appetite, and clumsiness. Symptoms can last for days or weeks. Babies born to women who take benzodiazepines regularly may suffer withdrawal symptoms during the first week of life.

Signs of misuse
Misuse can occur by injection in young people. Another type of misuse is a middle-aged or older person who may have been taking these drugs by prescription for months or years. He or she is usually unaware of the problem, and may admit to taking "nerve" or sleeping pills in normal or large quantities. Problems usually occur only if people attempt to cut down or stop taking the drugs without medical advice.

Interactions
Benzodiazepines increase the risk of sedation with any drug that has a sedative effect on the central nervous system. These include other anti-anxiety and sleeping drugs, alcohol, opioid analgesics, antipsychotics, tricyclic antidepressants, and antihistamines.

Practical points
Benzodiazepines should normally be used for courses of two weeks' duration or less. If these drugs have been taken for longer than two weeks, it is usually best to reduce the dose gradually in order to minimize the risk of withdrawal symptoms. If you have been taking benzodiazepines for many months or years, it is best to consult your doctor to work out a dose reduction programme. If possible, it will help to tell your family and friends and enlist their support.

450

CANNABIS

Other common names Marijuana, grass, pot, dope, reefers, weed, hash, ganja, skunk, skunkweed
Drug category Central nervous system depressant, hallucinogen, anti-emetic

Habit-forming potential
There is evidence that around one in ten users of cannabis become physically and psychologically dependent on its effects. Those who smoke cannabis mixed with tobacco may also become addicted to nicotine.

How taken
Usually smoked, either like tobacco or through a "bong" pipe. May be eaten, often in cakes or biscuits, or brewed like tea and drunk.

Legitimate uses
The leaves and resin of the plants Cannabis sativa and C. indica have been in use for over 2,000 years. Introduced into Western medicine in the mid-19th century, cannabis was taken for a variety of complaints, including anxiety, insomnia, rheumatic disorders, migraine, painful menstruation, strychnine poisoning, and opioid withdrawal. Today, derivatives (e.g. nabilone) can be prescribed with certain restrictions for relief of nausea and vomiting caused by treatment with anticancer drugs. Cannabis itself is listed under Class B and Schedule I of the Misuse of Drugs legislation (see p.13).

Short-term effects
Small doses promote a feeling of relaxation and well-being, enhance auditory and visual perception, and increase appetite talkativeness. In some people it may have little or no effect.
Under the drug's influence, short-term memory may be impaired and driving ability and coordination are disrupted for up to 24 hours. Confusion and emotional distress may result, and, rarely, hallucinations may occur. The effects last for one to three hours after smoking and for 12 hours or longer after it is eaten. Heavy use can lead to a schizophrenia-like illness, which subsides within days of stopping as blood levels go down.

Long-term effects and risks
Cannabis smoking increases the risk of bronchitis, emphysema, and lung cancer. Regular users may become apathetic and neglect work, studies, and personal appearance. In susceptible people, heavy use may trigger depression or psychotic illness such as schizophrenia. Cannabis is thought by some doctors to increase the likelihood of experimentation with other drugs.
Cannabis may increase heart rate and lower blood pressure, and people with heart disorders may be at risk from adverse effects. Regular use may reduce fertility in both men and women and, if used in pregnancy, may contribute to premature birth.

Signs of misuse
A cannabis user may appear unusually talkative or drunk. Appetite is increased, often resulting in eating binges known as the "munchies". The user may become defensive or aggressive when challenged about use of the drug. Cannabis smoke has a distinct herbal smell that may linger in the hair and clothes.

Interactions
Cannabis may increase the risk of sedation with any drug that have a sedative effect. These include anti-anxiety and sleeping drugs, general anaesthetics, opioid analgesics, antipsychotic, tricyclic antidepressants, antihistamines, and alcohol.

SYNTHETIC CANNABINOIDS

Since the early 2000s, increasing numbers of cannabis-like drugs have appeared. With names including K2, Spice, or simply herbal incense, these substances are often sprayed on to plant materials to mimic marijuana and they are used in the same way. However, they are more potent than natural cannabis and may have distinct and more dangerous adverse effects because of various adulterants.

ALCOHOL

Other common names Booze, drink (includes beer, wine, alcopops and spirits); also known as ethanol or ethyl alcohol
Drug category Central nervous system depressant; sedative

Habit-forming potential

It is difficult to measure the habit-forming potential of alcohol because individual responses vary so widely. Alcoholism is characterized by a person's inability to control intake. It involves psychological and physical dependence, evidenced by large daily consumption, heavy weekend drinking, or periodic binges. Regular drinking and heavy drinking do not cause alcoholism but, like alcoholism itself, carry significant health risks.

How taken

Orally, in the form of wines, beers and cider, and a wide range of spirits and liqueurs. Alcopops (lemonade- or fruit juice-based drinks) contain as much alcohol (3–5%) as beer or cider.

The alcohol content of drinks

Alcohol content is measured in units. To calculate the units in a drink, multiply the percentage of alcohol by volume (% ABV) x the amount (ml) in a serving, then divide the result by 1000. The units in some common drinks are shown below*:

1 unit	Small shot of spirits (25 ml @ 40% ABV)
1.5 units	Small glass of wine (125ml @ 12% ABV)
1.5 units	Serving of alcopop (275ml @ 5.5% ABV)
1.7 units	Bottle of beer, lager, or cider (330ml @ 5% ABV)
2.1 units	Standard glass of wine (175ml @ 12% ABV)
2.4 units	Can of beer, lager, or cider (440ml @ 5.5% ABV)

* Figures from NHS: www.nhs.uk/live-well/alcohol-support/calculating-alcohol-units/

Legitimate uses

The manufacture and sale of alcoholic drinks is closely regulated, both because it is a source of government revenue and to prevent the production of drinks containing methanol (methyl alcohol) – a toxin that can cause blindness. The sale of alcoholic beverages is restricted to those over the age of 18.

Medically, surgical spirit (concentrated alcohol that contains methanol, castor oil, methyl salicylate, and diethyl phthalate) is used as an antiseptic before injections to minimize the risk of infection. It is also used to harden the skin and thus prevent pressure sores in bedridden people, and foot sores in hikers and runners. Surgical spirit is extremely harmful if ingested.

Absorption of alcohol

Alcohol is rapidly absorbed from the stomach and particularly from the small intestine. Very strong drinks such as neat spirits are absorbed more slowly than weaker ones (as the alcohol reduces stomach movements that would push it into the intestine). Very dilute drinks are absorbed relatively slowly due to the large amount of water. In between these extremes, the stronger drinks will give higher blood levels. The presence of bubbles of carbon dioxide (in champagne, lemonade, and lager) may help to speed up absorption. So will mixing drinks; for example, drinking a glass of spirits after a beer will produce a higher concentration that is absorbed more quickly.

Food in the stomach slows the rate of absorption of alcohol. Full-cream milk seems particularly efficient for this purpose. Even the amount of carbohydrate in beer slows alcohol absorption a little, compared to a solution of alcohol in water at the same strength. Slowing the rate of absorption means that some of the alcohol can be broken down (metabolized, detoxified) before the rest is absorbed. This reduces the blood level and hence the effects of alcohol.

One unit of alcohol is the equivalent of about 15ml of pure alcohol, which is the amount that the average adult male can break down in 1 hour. If you drink at a faster rate, your blood alcohol level will continue to rise; most people, for example, will exceed the legal limit (80mg of alcohol per 100ml of blood in most of the UK, or 50mg/100ml in Scotland) after drinking only about 1–3 units of alcohol in 1 hour. It takes as many hours for your body to rid itself of all the alcohol as the number of units you have drunk. For example, if you had five pints of beer (10 units) in a few hours, it will, on average, take around 10 hours for the alcohol to be removed from your blood. However, there is considerable variation in these figures. Women achieve higher blood levels than men after drinking the same amount because women's bodies contain a lower percentage of water, into which the alcohol is distributed, and women break down alcohol more slowly than men of the same weight. A large-framed adult will have a lower blood level of alcohol than a smaller person after they have had the same amount to drink.

Short-term effects

Alcohol acts as a central nervous system depressant, reducing anxiety, tension, and inhibitions. In moderate quantities it gives a feeling of relaxation and confidence, and increases sociability and talkativeness, but does not improve mental performance. Moderate amounts also dilate small blood vessels, especially in the skin, leading to flushing and a feeling of warmth. Increasing amounts progressively impair concentration and judgement, and reactions are increasingly slowed. Accidents, particularly driving accidents, are more likely. As blood alcohol levels rise, violent or aggressive behaviour is possible. Speech is slurred, and the person becomes unsteady, staggers, and may experience double vision and loss of balance. Nausea and vomiting are frequent; incontinence may occur. Loss of consciousness may follow if blood alcohol levels continue to rise, and there is a risk of death from choking on vomit or cessation of breathing. Blood alcohol levels of only about 240–320mg of alcohol/100ml of blood are thus potentially fatal.

In addition to alcohol's effects on the central nervous system, it has a number of other effects. The most noticeable is its diuretic action. Dehydration after drinking is responsible for many of the symptoms of a hangover. The best means of prevention is to drink less, or at least to drink a glass of water for each unit of alcohol, during the same time period.

Alcoholic drinks are not the same as "alcohol". They contain other chemical ingredients that might have side effects; for example, the juniper oil in gin is also a diuretic. It is thought that many of the ingredients in drinks can add to the hangover experience. Congeners – complex organic molecules such as polyphenols, higher alcohols, and histamine, which occur in varying amounts in different alcoholic drinks – may also have toxic effects.

Long-term effects and risks

Heavy drinkers risk developing liver diseases, such as alcoholic hepatitis, liver cancer, cirrhosis, or fatty liver (excess fat deposits that may lead to cirrhosis). High blood pressure, strokes, and heart failure may also result from heavy drinking. Inflammation of the stomach (gastritis) and peptic ulcers are more common in people with alcoholism, who also have a higher than average risk of developing a dementia-like illness.

Long-term heavy drinking is generally associated with physical dependence. An alcoholic person may appear to be sober, even after heavy drinking, because of built-up tolerance. But a reverse tolerance effect is frequently seen in alcoholism, where relatively little alcohol can rapidly produce a state of intoxication. As well as health problems, alcohol dependence is associated with a range of personal and social problems. People with alcoholism may also have anxiety and depression, and because they often eat poorly, they are at risk of various nutritional deficiency diseases, particularly deficiency of thiamine (p.442). About 4 per cent of breast cancers in women may be related to alcohol intake. In developed countries, the risk of breast cancer rises with increased alcohol consumption.

Pregnancy and breast-feeding

Drinking during pregnancy, especially during the first three months, increases the risk of miscarriage, and can cause fetal abnormalities and poor physical and mental development in infants. Drinking heavily in pregnancy may lead to the baby developing fetal alcohol syndrome (FAS). Babies affected by FAS are abnormally small, develop poorly, and may have facial abnormalities, heart defects, and learning and behavioural problems. It is not known if there is a safe alcohol intake during pregnancy, but the more you drink, the greater the risk, and it is therefore recommended that women who are pregnant or trying to conceive should abstain from alcohol completely.

There is some evidence that regularly drinking more than 2 units of alcohol a day when breast-feeding may adversely affect your baby's development. However, an occasional drink is unlikely to be harmful, and it is advised that women who are breast-feeding should drink no more than 1 or 2 units of alcohol once or twice a week.

Signs of misuse
Alcohol consumption may be getting out of control if any or all of the following signs are noted:

- Changes in drinking pattern (for example, early morning drinking or a switch from beer to spirits);
- Changes in drinking habits (such as drinking alone or having a drink before an appointment or interview);
- Neglect of personal appearance;
- Personality changes or furtive behaviour;
- Poor eating habits;
- Increasingly frequent or prolonged bouts of intoxication with memory lapses (blackouts) about events that occurred during drinking episodes.

Physical symptoms may include nausea, vomiting, or shaking in the morning; abdominal pain; cramps; redness and enlarged blood vessels in the face; weakness in the legs and hands; unsteadiness; poor memory; and incontinence. The sudden stopping of heavy drinking, if not treated, can lead to delirium tremens (severe shaking, confusion, hallucinations, and occasionally fatal seizures) beginning after one to four days of abstinence and lasting for up to three days. Drugs such as clomethiazole, atenolol, and benzodiazepines, given short term under medical supervision, can control withdrawal symptoms.

Practical points
If you drink, know your limits. They vary from person to person, and your capacity depends on your weight, age, experience, and mental and emotional state. However, in general, the body can break down only about 1 unit of alcohol per hour. If you drink faster than this, your blood alcohol is likely to rise. But lower levels than this can affect judgement and reaction times, so the safest advice is not to drink at all if you plan to drive.

Men should not regularly drink more than 3–4 units of alcohol a day, and women should not regularly drink more than 2–3 units a day. The daily allowance of units should not be "saved up" in order to have a binge at the weekend.

If you are having trouble controlling your drinking, seek help and advice from your doctor or from an organization, such as Alcoholics Anonymous, dedicated to helping people with this problem. Even if you do not have a control problem you should avoid drinking heavily because alcohol can have harmful effects on many parts of your body.

INTERACTIONS WITH OTHER DRUGS

Alcohol interacts with a wide variety of drugs, and it is important to be aware of the interactions if you are on medication and want to have a drink. The main drug categories and their effects when taken with alcohol are shown below.

Type of drug	For example	Effects
Anti-anxiety drugs	Diazepam, lorazepam	Increased risk of sedation
Sleeping drugs	Temazepam, zopiclone	Increased risk of sedation
General anaesthetics	Propofol, thiopental	Increased risk of sedation
Antipsychotics	Chlorpromazine, haloperidol	Increased risk of sedation
Tricyclic antidepressants	Amitriptyline, dosulepin, lofepramine	Increased risk of sedation
Antihistamines	Chlorphenamine, promethazine	Increased risk of sedation
Antimuscarinics	Hyoscine	Increased risk of sedation
Muscle relaxants	Baclofen, tizanidine	Increased risk of sedation
Cannabis derivatives	Nabilone	Increased risk of sedation
Opioid analgesics	Morphine, dihydrocodeine, pethidine	Increased risk of sedation, fall in blood pressure, coma, death
Antidepressants, SSRIs	Citalopram, paroxetine	Possibly increased alcohol effects
Antihypertensives	Nifedipine, atenolol, losartan, lisinopril	Fall in blood pressure
	Clonidine, indoramin	Increased risk of sedation
Drugs of abuse	Barbiturates, heroin, volatile substances	Coma, death
Salicylates	Aspirin	Risk of stomach bleeding
Anti alcohol-dependence drugs	Disulfiram	Unpleasant reactions such as nausea, vomiting, throbbing headache, palpitations, flushing of face
Antibacterials	Metronidazole, tinidazole	Disulfiram-like reactions
Cytotoxics	Procarbazine	Disulfiram-like reactions
Drugs for diabetes	Insulin	Increased hypoglycaemia
	Sulfonylureas	Possibly increased effects
MAOIs	Phenelzine, isocarboxazid	Dangerous rise in blood pressure with tyramine in red wine; fall in blood pressure with other alcoholic drinks
Anticoagulants	Warfarin	Increased risk of bleeding
Antibiotics	Cycloserine	Risk of seizures
Anticonvulsants	Carbamazepine	CNS side effects increased
Dopamine-boosters	Bromocriptine	Reduced tolerance to drug

AMFETAMINE

Other common names Speed, uppers, whizz, blues (see also Ecstasy, p.451)
Drug category Central nervous system stimulant (see p.44)

Habit-forming potential
Regular use of amfetamine or methamfetamine rapidly leads to tolerance, requiring larger and larger doses to achieve the same effect. Users become psychologically dependent on the drug.

How taken
Usually swallowed as tablets or powder. Sometimes sniffed or mixed with water and injected.

Legitimate uses
During the 1950s and 1960s, amfetamine was widely given to reduce appetite for weight loss. Due to the risk of dependence and abuse, it is no longer used as an appetite suppressant. Amfetamine was also used to maintain wakefulness by drivers and pilots. It is still prescribed as dexamfetamine for attention deficit disorder (hyperactivity) and narcolepsy (see also Nervous system stimulants, p.44). Amfetamine is classified under Class B and Schedule II of the Misuse of Drugs legislation (p.13).

Short-term effects
Small doses of amfetamine reduce appetite and increase mental alertness and physical energy. Dry mouth, fast heart rate, rapid breathing, and dilated pupils are common. As these effects wear off, depression and fatigue may follow. At high doses, the drug may cause euphoria, tremor, sweating, anxiety, headache, palpitations, and chest pain. Large doses may cause confusion, hallucinations, delirium, collapse, seizures, coma, and death.

Long-term effects and risks
Regular use frequently leads to muscle damage, weight loss, and constipation. People who use amfetamine regularly may also become emotionally unstable; psychosis may develop. Severe depression and suicide are associated with withdrawal. Heavy long-term use reduces resistance to infection and also carries a risk of damage to the heart and blood vessels, leading to strokes and heart failure.

Use of amfetamine in early pregnancy increases the risk of birth defects, especially in the heart. Taken during pregnancy, amfetamine leads to premature birth and low birth weight.

Signs of misuse
A person under the influence of amfetamine may appear unusually energetic, cheerful, and talkative. Restlessness, agitation, and a lack of interest in food are typical symptoms; mood changes and paranoid delusions may also occur. Regular users may exhibit unusual sleeping patterns, staying awake for two or three nights at a stretch, then sleeping for up to 48 hours.

Interactions
Amfetamine counteracts the sedative effects of drugs that depress the central nervous system. It also increases blood pressure, opposing the effect of antihypertensives. Taken with monoamine oxidase inhibitors (MAOIs), it may lead to a dangerous rise in blood pressure. It also increases the risk of abnormal heart rhythms with digitalis drugs, levodopa, and certain anaesthetics given by inhalation.

METHAMFETAMINE

Methamfetamine, known as "crystal meth" or "ice", is about twenty times more potent than amfetamine, and is highly psychologically addictive. It is classified under Class A and Schedule II (p.13). It is usually sold as a colourless crystalline solid, which can be smoked or injected. It produces mental alertness, talkativeness, reduced appetite, increased energy, lack of fatigue, and insomnia. Other effects include restlessness, repetitive activity, twitching, jaw clenching, teeth grinding, and uninhibited sexual behaviour. Withdrawal leads to prolonged sleep, marked hunger, anxiety, and depression, with a craving for more of the drug. Excessive use can cause hallucinations and paranoia.

BARBITURATES

Other common names Barbs, downers
Drug category Central nervous system depressant (see also Sleeping drugs, p.38), sedative

Habit-forming potential
Long-term, regular use of barbiturates can be habit-forming. Both physical and psychological dependence may occur.

How taken
By mouth in the form of capsules or tablets. Occasionally mixed with water and injected.

Legitimate uses
In the past, barbiturates were widely prescribed as sleeping drugs. Since the 1960s, however, they have been almost completely replaced by a range of newer drugs, including benzodiazepines, which may also be addictive but are less likely to cause death from overdose. The widest use of barbiturates today is in anaesthesia (thiopental).

Most barbiturates are listed under Class B and Schedule III of the Misuse of Drugs Legislation (p.13).

Short-term effects
The short-term effects are similar to those of alcohol. A low dose produces relaxation, while larger amounts make the user more intoxicated and drowsy. Coordination is impaired and slurred speech, clumsiness, and confusion may occur. Increasingly large doses may produce loss of consciousness, coma, and death caused by depression of the person's breathing mechanism. In fact, the lethality of barbiturates in overdose is exploited in their use for euthanasia in animals and humans: deliberate pentobarbital overdose is used by organizations that offer assisted dying.

Long-term effects and risks
The greatest risk of long-term barbiturate use is physical dependence. In an addicted person, stopping the drug suddenly precipitates a withdrawal syndrome that varies in severity, depending partly on the type of barbiturate, its dose, and the duration of use. Symptoms may include irritability, disturbed sleep, nightmares, nausea, vomiting, weakness, tremors, and extreme anxiety. Abrupt withdrawal after several months of use may cause seizures, delirium, fever, and coma lasting for up to one week. Long-term, heavy use of barbiturates increases the risk of accidental overdose. The risk of chest infections is also increased because the cough reflex is suppressed by long-term, heavy use of these drugs.

Use of barbiturates during pregnancy may cause fetal abnormalities and, used regularly in the last three months, may lead to withdrawal symptoms in the newborn baby.

Signs of misuse
Long-term heavy use of barbiturates may cause prolonged bouts of intoxication with memory lapses (blackouts), neglect of personal appearance and responsibilities, personality changes, and episodes of severe depression.

Interactions
Barbiturates interact with a wide variety of drugs and increase the risk of sedation with any drug that has a sedative effect on the central nervous system. These include anti-anxiety drugs, opioid analgesics, antipsychotics, antihistamines, and tricyclic antidepressants. High doses taken with alcohol can lead to a fatal coma.

Barbiturates also increase the activity of certain enzymes in the liver, leading to an increase in the breakdown of certain drugs, thus reducing their effects. Tricyclic antidepressants, phenytoin, griseofulvin, and corticosteroids are affected in this way. However, the toxicity of a paracetamol overdose is likely to be greater in people taking barbiturates.

BENZODIAZEPINES

Other common names Tranquillizers, tranx, temmies
Drug category Central nervous system depressants (see Sleeping drugs, p.38, and Anti-anxiety drugs, p.39)

Habit-forming potential
The addictive potential of benzodiazepines is much lower than that of some other central nervous system depressants such as barbiturates. However, regular long-term use of these drugs can lead to physical and psychological dependence on their sedative effects.

How taken
By mouth as tablets or capsules, or by injection. Temazepam is the most widely abused benzodiazepine.

Legitimate uses
Benzodiazepines are commonly prescribed mainly for short-term treatment of anxiety and stress, as well as for relief of sleeplessness. They are also used in anaesthesia, both as premedication and for induction of general anaesthesia. Other medical uses include the management of alcohol withdrawal, control of epileptic seizures, and relief of muscle spasms. Most benzodiazepines are classified under Class C and Schedule IV of the Misuse of Drugs legislation (see p.13), although temazepam and flunitrazepam are under Schedule III.

Short-term effects
Benzodiazepines can reduce mental activity. In moderate doses, they may cause unsteadiness, reduce alertness, and slow the body's reactions, thus impairing driving ability as well as increasing the risk of accidents. Benzodiazepines may also cause amnesia (loss of memory regarding events that occurred while the person was under the influence of the drug). Any benzodiazepine in a high enough dose induces sleep. Large overdoses (especially by intravenous injection) may cause depression of the breathing mechanism and death.

Long-term effects and risks
Benzodiazepines tend to lose their sedative effect with long-term use (more than a few weeks). This may lead the user to increase the dose progressively, a manifestation of tolerance and physical dependence (see p.23). Older people may become apathetic or confused when taking these drugs. On stopping the drug, chronic users may develop withdrawal symptoms that may include anxiety, panic attacks, palpitations, shaking, insomnia, nightmares, headaches, dizziness, aches and pains, nausea, loss of appetite, and clumsiness. Symptoms can last for days or weeks. Babies born to women who take benzodiazepines regularly may suffer withdrawal symptoms during the first week of life.

Signs of misuse
Misuse can occur by injection in young people. Another type of misuser is a middle-aged or older person who may have been taking these drugs by prescription for months or years. He or she is usually unaware of the problem, and may freely admit to taking "nerve" or sleeping pills in normal or large quantities. Problems usually occur only if people attempt to cut down or stop taking the drugs without medical advice.

Interactions
Benzodiazepines increase the risk of sedation with any drug that has a sedative effect on the central nervous system. These include other anti-anxiety and sleeping drugs, alcohol, opioid analgesics, antipsychotics, tricyclic antidepressants, and antihistamines.

Practical points
Benzodiazepines should normally be used for courses of two weeks' duration or less. If these drugs have been taken for longer than two weeks, it is usually best to reduce the dose gradually in order to minimize the risk of withdrawal symptoms. If you have been taking benzodiazepines for many months or years, it is best to consult your doctor to work out a dose reduction programme. If possible, it will help to tell your family and friends and enlist their support.

CANNABIS

Other common names Marijuana, grass, pot, dope, reefers, weed, hash, ganja, skunk, skunkweed
Drug category Central nervous system depressant, hallucinogen, anti-emetic

Habit-forming potential
There is evidence that around one in ten users of cannabis become physically and psychologically dependent on its effects. Those who smoke cannabis mixed with tobacco may also become addicted to nicotine.

How taken
Usually smoked, either like tobacco or through a "bong" pipe. May be eaten, often in cakes or biscuits, or brewed like tea and drunk.

Legitimate uses
The leaves and resin of the plants *Cannabis sativa* and *C. indica* have been in use for over 2,000 years. Introduced into Western medicine in the mid-19th century, cannabis was taken for a variety of complaints, including anxiety, insomnia, rheumatic disorders, migraine, painful menstruation, strychnine poisoning, and opioid withdrawal. Today, derivatives (e.g. nabilone) can be prescribed with certain restrictions for relief of nausea and vomiting caused by treatment with anticancer drugs. Cannabis itself is listed under Class B and Schedule I of the Misuse of Drugs legislation (see p.13).

Short-term effects
Small doses promote a feeling of relaxation and well-being, enhance auditory and visual perception, and increase appetite and talkativeness. In some people it may have little effect.

Under the drug's influence, short-term memory may be impaired and driving ability and coordination are disrupted for up to 24 hours. Confusion and emotional distress may result, and, rarely, hallucinations may occur. The effects last for one to three hours after smoking and for 12 hours or longer after it is eaten. Heavy use can lead to a schizophrenia-like illness, which subsides within days of stopping as blood levels go down.

Long-term effects and risks
Cannabis smoking increases the risk of bronchitis, emphysema, and lung cancer. Regular users may become apathetic and neglect work, studies, and personal appearance. In susceptible people, heavy use may trigger depression or psychotic illness such as schizophrenia. Cannabis is thought by some doctors to increase the likelihood of experimentation with other drugs.

Cannabis may increase heart rate and lower blood pressure, and people with heart disorders may be at risk from adverse effects. Regular use may reduce fertility in both men and women and, if used in pregnancy, may contribute to premature birth.

Signs of misuse
A cannabis user may appear unusually talkative or drunk. Appetite is increased, often resulting in eating binges known as the "munchies". The user may become defensive or aggressive when challenged about use of the drug. Cannabis smoke has a distinct herbal smell that may linger in the hair and clothes.

Interactions
Cannabis may increase the risk of sedation with any drugs that have a sedative effect. These include anti-anxiety and sleeping drugs, general anaesthetics, opioid analgesics, antipsychotics, tricyclic antidepressants, antihistamines, and alcohol.

SYNTHETIC CANNABINOIDS

Since the early 2000s, increasing numbers of cannabis-like drugs have appeared. With names including K2, Spice, or simply herbal incense, these substances are often sprayed on to plant materials to mimic marijuana and they are used in the same way. However, they are more potent than natural cannabis and may have distinct and more dangerous adverse effects because of various adulterants.

COCAINE

Other common names Coke, crack, nose candy, snow
Drug category Central nervous system stimulant and local anaesthetic (p.36)

Habit-forming potential
Taken regularly, cocaine is habit-forming. Users may become psychologically dependent on its physical and psychological effects, and may step up their intake to maintain or increase these effects or to prevent the feelings of severe fatigue and depression that may occur after the drug is stopped. The risk of dependence is especially pronounced with the form of cocaine known as freebase or crack (see below).

How taken
Smoked, sniffed through a tube (snorted), or injected.

Legitimate uses
Cocaine was formerly widely used as a local anaesthetic. It is still sometimes given for topical anaesthesia in the eye, mouth, and throat prior to minor surgery or other procedures. However, because of its side effects and potential for abuse, cocaine has now been replaced in most cases by safer local anaesthetic drugs. Cocaine is classified under Class A and Schedule II of the Misuse of Drugs legislation (see p.13).

Short-term effects
Cocaine is a central nervous system stimulant. In moderate doses it overcomes fatigue and produces feelings of well-being. Appetite is reduced. Physical effects include an increase in heart rate and blood pressure, dilation of the pupils, tremor, and increased sweating. Large doses can lead to agitation, anxiety, paranoia, and hallucinations. Paranoia may cause violent behaviour. Very large doses cause seizures, heart failure, and rapid death. In some people, seizures and heart attack may occur after only moderate doses.

Long-term effects and risks
Heavy, regular use of cocaine can cause restlessness, anxiety, hyperexcitability, nausea, insomnia, and weight loss. Continued use may cause increasing paranoia and psychosis. Repeated sniffing also damages the membranes lining the nose and may eventually lead to the destruction of the septum (the structure separating the nostrils). Regular cocaine use leads to increased atheroma (fatty deposits in the arteries) and consequent risk of heart attacks.

Signs of misuse
A cocaine user may appear unusually energetic and exuberant under the influence of the drug and show little interest in food. Heavy, regular use may lead to disturbed eating and sleeping patterns. Agitation, mood swings, aggressive behaviour, and suspiciousness of other people may also be signs of heavy use.

Interactions
Cocaine can increase blood pressure, thus opposing the effect of antihypertensive drugs. Taken with monoamine oxidase inhibitors (MAOIs), it can cause a dangerous rise in blood pressure. It also increases the risk of adverse effects on the heart when taken with certain general anaesthetics.

CRACK

This potent form of cocaine occurs in the form of crystals that are smoked by vaporizing with a flame and inhaling the fumes; they may also be dissolved and injected. Highly addictive, crack appears to have more intense effects than other forms of cocaine, and it is associated with an increased risk of abnormal heart rhythms, high blood pressure, heart attacks, stroke, and death. Other consequences of crack abuse include coughing of black phlegm, wheezing, irreversible lung damage, hoarseness, and parched lips, tongue, and throat from inhaling the hot fumes. Mental deterioration, personality changes, social withdrawal, paranoia or violent behaviour, and suicide attempts may occur.

ECSTASY (MDMA)

Other common names E, XTC, methylenedioxymeth-amfetamine; other slang names vary from place to place
Drug category Central nervous system stimulant

Habit-forming potential
As with other amfetamines, regular use leads to tolerance, so that higher doses are required to achieve the same effect. Users may become psychologically dependent on the effects of the drug and the lifestyle that surrounds its use.

How taken
By mouth in tablet or capsule form.

Legitimate uses
MDMA was originally developed in 1912 as a drug to stop bleeding, but it was never used for this purpose. Today, although there have been claims that the drug may have a place in psychotherapy, it currently has no legitimate medical use. The drug is classified under Class A and Schedule I in the Misuse of Drugs legislation (see p.13).

Short-term effects
Ecstasy is most commonly used as a dance drug at raves or parties to increase the emotional effects of dancing to fast music and to enable users to dance for many hours. Adverse effects are more commonly due to recreational doses rather than to an overdose. Ecstasy stimulates the central nervous system, leading to increased wakefulness and energy and suppression of thirst, tiredness, and sleep. Because of its psychological effects (increasing a user's feelings of openness and emotional connection with others) it is often referred to as an empathogen.

Ecstasy can produce tight clenching of the jaw muscles (sometimes leading to involuntary tooth grinding, known as bruxism) and stiffness in other muscles. Various complications may occur: in particular, heatstroke due to prolonged dancing without replacing fluids lost by sweating. Heatstroke can lead to muscle breakdown, kidney failure, problems with the blood clotting mechanism, seizures, and death. In some cases there may be low sodium levels and brain swelling due to excessive intake of fluid in the absence of sufficient exertion to sweat it off. These patients may experience vomiting, headaches, and drowsiness. Liver damage and stroke have also occurred.

Long-term effects and risks
There is increasing evidence that ecstasy can impair both short- and long-term memory. In addition, some cases of psychiatric illness have been reported, such as schizophrenia and depression. Sleep disturbance and a craving for chocolate has also been reported. There may be an increased likelihood of developing depression even years after stopping the drug.

Signs of misuse
Ecstasy causes dilated pupils. Behaviour may be excitable or agitated. Ecstasy users may experience weight loss, tooth damage as a result of bruxism, and anxiety.

Interactions
Ecstasy interacts with a variety of drugs. If it is taken with monoamine oxidase inhibitors (MAOIs), it may lead to a dangerous rise in blood pressure. It also increases the risk of abnormal heart rhythms with digitalis drugs, levodopa, and certain anaesthetics given by inhalation. Ecstasy tends to counteract the sedative effects of drugs that depress the central nervous system, and its effect on the mind is reduced by these drugs. SSRI antidepressants (such as fluoxetine) appear to block the psychoactive effects of ecstasy, which often prompts users to take higher doses of ecstasy to overcome this blocking effect.

GHB

Other common names Liquid X, GBH, Liquid E, gamma hydroxybutyrate, sodium oxybate
Drug category Central nervous system depressant

Habit-forming potential
GHB is addictive if taken regularly in large doses.

How taken
By mouth. Often sold as liquid in bottles, but it may be presented as a capsule or as a powder that is commonly dissolved in water to produce a clear, colourless liquid that often has a salty taste. It may also be ingested as a number of other drugs that break down in the body to form GHB: for example, GBL (gamma-butyrolacone) and the industrial solvent 1,4BD (1,4 butanediol).

Legitimate uses
GHB is a naturally occurring chemical produced in the body in small amounts. It is also produced by fermentation, so appears in small amounts in beer and wine. Originally developed as an anaesthetic, it has been used to treat narcolepsy, insomnia, and alcohol and opioid withdrawal, but currently has no licensed medical use in the UK. It has also been misused as a date rape drug. Possession of GHB is illegal, and the drug is classified under Class C of the Misuse of Drugs legislation (see p.13).

Short-term effects
GHB is a central nervous system depressant. Its effects are somewhat similar to alcohol, with talkativeness, cheerfulness, and euphoria occurring soon after taking an average dose. Most people become drowsy but recover within 4–8 hours of ingestion. Some users may experience confusion, headache, or gastrointestinal symptoms such as vomiting or stomach pain. Excessive doses may cause unconsciousness, and seizures, slowed heart rate, low blood pressure, and respiratory arrest have been reported. Rapid recovery is the rule, but full recovery may take 96 hours, and hospital treatment may be necessary. Deaths have occurred after taking excessive doses of GHB, either from cardiorespiratory depression or from accidents while intoxicated by the drug.

Long-term effects and risks
Users may suffer a hung-over state for 2–3 days, and insomnia and dizziness may linger for up to 2 weeks. Longer-term effects of the drug have not been well studied. During prolonged regular use, a marked withdrawal syndrome may commence within hours of the last dose, and regular users even have to get up at night to take a further dose.

Signs of misuse
As the drug is taken in liquid form it is difficult to estimate the correct dose, and the response to a low dose varies widely. Many abusers simply consume it until they reach an adequate high. Sometimes this is achieved only shortly before becoming unconscious, so sudden unconsciousness, on the dance floor for example, may be caused by GHB intoxication. In such cases, the person may later wake up suddenly, after apparently having been in a deep coma. Abnormally long-lasting hangovers and dizziness may be signs of abuse.

Interactions
The effects will be increased by other central nervous system depressants – for example, alcohol, benzodiazepines, and antipsychotics. GHB may also add to the effects of opioid analgesic drugs and muscle relaxants. It is sometimes mixed with amfetamines in an attempt to prolong the high for several hours.

KETAMINE

Other common names Kit-Kat, Special K, Super K, vitamin K
Drug category General anaesthetic with analgesic properties (see p.36)

Habit-forming potential
Likely to lead to psychological addiction if taken regularly.

How taken
Usually swallowed as the liquid pharmaceutical preparation or as tablets/capsules, produced mainly by heating the liquid anaesthetic to evaporate the water, leaving ketamine crystals. Sometimes sniffed as a powder or smoked. The smoke has a characteristic bitter taste and produces a "high" very rapidly. Ketamine may also be injected into a muscle, and this is the preferred route of administration for heavy users. The drug is usually taken alone in a quiet place because the effects can be disturbing if it is taken in a noisy or crowded environment.

Legitimate uses
A general anaesthetic with analgesic properties, used both in human and veterinary medicine (it is on the WHO list of essential drugs for any healthcare system). It is related to phencyclidine and is classified under Class C and Schedule IV of the Misuse of Drugs legislation (see p.13).

Short-term effects
The effects may depend on mood and environment, but have a rapid onset. Ketamine stimulates the cardiovascular system, producing a racing heart. There are a number of psychological effects that may occur, including hallucinations and a feeling of paralysis in which the user cannot move or speak but is still fully conscious and can see and hear. This is sometimes called a "K-hole". Actions or words may be repeated persistently, or the user may have an out of body experience. Users may be unconcerned whether they live or die. Due to the analgesic effects, the user is unlikely to feel pain. Severe reactions, usually due to overdose, may include seizures, depression of the breathing mechanism, or heart failure.

Long-term effects and risks
The long-term use of ketamine may interfere with memory, learning, and attention span. Users may experience flashbacks. Psychosis may occur. There have also been reports that regular use of ketamine causes inflammation of the bladder and ureters, which can cause cystitis-like spasms ("K-cramps"), bladder pain, and blood in the urine. In some cases, it has necessitated surgical removal of the bladder.

Signs of misuse
Strange behaviour may suggest the psychological effects of ketamine. Painful injuries (such as cigarette burns) appear to go unnoticed.

Interactions
Barbiturates lengthen the duration of action that results from ketamine use, and in combination there is a risk of respiratory depression. Use of ketamine together with theophylline or aminophylline may increase the likelihood of seizures. People with alcoholism tend to be resistant to ketamine, although the psychological effects may be exaggerated during the recovery period.

KHAT

Other common names Cat, chaat, mriaa, quat
Drug category Central nervous system stimulant

Habit-forming potential
Dependence on khat is exclusively psychological. The main active constituent of khat is cathinone, an amfetamine-like substance that is responsible for the drug's potential to cause psychological dependence.

How taken
Khat is composed of the leaves and small twigs of a plant (Catha edulis) that grows on high ground in many tropical countries. A large amount of the leaves or stems are chewed, and the plant material is kept in the cheek while the juice is swallowed. Occasionally it is dried and drunk as a tea because cathinone is unstable in the fresh leaves.

Legitimate uses
Khat has no legitimate medical uses. The drug is widely used as a social stimulant in many Middle Eastern and African countries, especially in Yemen, Somalia, and Ethiopia, and is often taken at celebrations and gatherings. It has also been used as a traditional remedy to treat depression, fatigue, obesity, and gastric ulcers. However, the authorities in these countries are increasingly concerned about its adverse effects on health. Khat is not currently a controlled drug, but its active ingredient, cathinone, is listed under Class C and Schedule I of the Misuse of Drugs legislation (see p.13).

Short-term effects
Khat produces appetite suppression, dry mouth, euphoria, increased alertness, talkativeness, and hyperactivity. Gastrointestinal side effects are common, as well as a mild rise in the blood pressure, pulse, respiratory rate, and temperature. Insomnia, poor concentration, and malaise are also common side effects. Aggressive verbal outbursts and hallucinations may occur as a result of khat use, and psychosis has occurred. Depression and sedation may follow withdrawal after heavy or regular use.

Long-term effects and risks
Constipation is a very common side effect, and stomach ulcers are quite common in regular users of khat. Men may experience erectile dysfunction and reduced sex drive. Khat use may contribute to the risk of high blood pressure in young adults, and heart attacks are a known complication of khat use. Chronic use during pregnancy may lead to low birth weight, and the drug is excreted in breast milk.

Signs of misuse
The drug causes brownish-green staining of the teeth. Weight loss may occur as a result of appetite suppression.

Interactions
It causes additive effects with other phenylalkylamines, including amfetamine and phenylpropanolamine, to cause mental stimulation, a fast heart rate, and high blood pressure.

LSD

Other common names Lysergide, diethylamide, lysergic acid, acid, haze, microdots
Drug category Hallucinogen

Habit-forming potential
LSD may cause psychological dependence but it is not addictive, because of the speed with which tolerance (p.23) develops – within a few days. (This is the reason why other chemically related psychedelics, such as psilocybin in "magic mushrooms" and mescaline, are also not addictive.) Because of the rapid development of tolerance, a period of several days must elapse after taking LSD before another "dose" will produce the original effects.

How taken
By mouth, as tiny coloured tablets (known as microdots), or absorbed on to small squares of paper, gelatin sheets, or sugar cubes. It is unstable in tap water because the tiny amounts of chlorine present in the water break down the LSD molecule.

Legitimate uses
None. The early interest of the medical profession in LSD focused on its possible use in psychotherapy, but additional studies suggested that it could lead to psychosis in susceptible people. LSD is listed under Class A and Schedule I of the Misuse of Drugs legislation (see p.13).

Short-term effects
The effects of usual doses of LSD last for about 4–12 hours, beginning almost immediately after taking the drug. Initial effects include restlessness, dizziness, a feeling of coldness with shivering, and an uncontrollable desire to laugh. The subsequent effects include distortions in vision and, in some cases, in the perception of sound. Introspection is often increased and mystical, pseudoreligious experiences may occur. Loss of emotional control, unpleasant or terrifying hallucinations, and overwhelming feelings of anxiety, despair, or panic may occur (a "bad trip"), particularly if the user has underlying anxiety or depression. Suicide may be attempted. Driving and other hazardous tasks are extremely dangerous. Some people under the influence of this drug have fallen off high buildings, mistakenly believing they could fly.

Long-term effects and risks
The effects of long-term LSD use include an increase in the risk of mental disturbances, including severe depression. In those with existing psychological difficulties, it has been said to cause lasting mental problems (e.g. permanent psychosis). In addition, for months or even years after last taking the drug, some frequent users experience brief but vivid recurrences of LSD's effects (flashbacks), which cause anxiety and disorientation. However, there is no evidence of lasting physical ill-effects from LSD use.

Signs of misuse
A person under the influence of LSD may be behaving strangely but rarely shows any other outward signs of intoxication. Occasionally, a user who has taken LSD may seem overexcited and may become violent, or may appear withdrawn or confused.

Interactions
The acute agitation caused by LSD is managed with benzodiazepines, although occasionally antipsychotic drugs such as haloperidol may be needed. Interactions with other drugs acting on the brain, such as alcohol, may increase the likelihood of unpredictable or violent behaviour. LSD misusers who are given SSRI antidepressants (e.g. fluoxetine, paroxetine, or sertraline) may experience onset or worsening of flashbacks. When LSD is given to those taking lithium or tricyclic antidepressants, it may sometimes cause dissociative fugue states during which the users are unaware of their surroundings and may injure themselves.

MAGIC MUSHROOMS

Other common names *Psilocybe semilanceata*, mushies, liberty cap, shrooms
Drug category Hallucinogen

Habit-forming potential
Psilocybe mushrooms are not habit-forming or addictive, though those who get desirable experiences from them may wish to obtain the experience again. Tolerance is considerable, so that a person who takes the mushrooms repeatedly over a short space of time may obtain less and less of an effect from them. This rapid development of tolerance is similar to what happens with LSD. In addition, the active ingredient of magic mushrooms is a substance called psilocybin, and there is cross-tolerance between LSD and psilocybin.

How taken
Psilocybe mushrooms are usually eaten raw, but may be dried and used later when convenient. They can also be cooked into food or made into an infusion and drunk. A dose consists of about 20 or 30 of the small psilocybe mushrooms (*Psilocybe semilanceata*) that grow widely in the UK, or two or three of the larger psilocybe species, which do not normally grow in the UK.

Legitimate uses
There are no legitimate uses for any of the species of magic mushrooms that contain psilocybin, and they are listed under Class A of the Misuse of Drugs legislation (see p.13). Some researchers have suggested that there may be a medical use for psilocybin, but the evidence that this may be so is lacking at present. It is not a criminal offence if these mushrooms grow in a person's garden or field, but it is if they are picked for the purpose of consuming them. Other potentially hallucinogenic mushrooms (such as *Amanita muscaria*, fly agaric) are not covered by the Misuse of Drugs Act. However, they are potentially fatal if eaten.

Short-term effects
The short-term effects of psilocybe mushrooms commence within 15 to 20 minutes of taking them, build up over the next half an hour, and gradually fade over the next two or three hours. Shapes, colours, and meanings of things change, and the experience is usually enjoyable, although it may be disturbing. When the mushrooms are eaten by someone who has not taken them before, however, or when they are taken unknowingly, the effects may be very upsetting.

Long-term effects and risks
Magic mushrooms may pose a particular risk for a person who has a mental illness such as schizophrenia, since taking them may cause a relapse of their illness. There is also the risk of self-harm or accidents while under their influence. Flashbacks (a repeat of the hallucinogenic experience) can occur hours to weeks after taking these mushrooms.

Signs of misuse
A person under the influence of magic mushrooms may be behaving strangely, may be withdrawn or confused, or may be giggling. Occasionally they may seem excited or violent. The pupils may be dilated and the pulse rate fast, but there are usually no other signs of intoxication.

Interactions
The effects of magic mushrooms may be increased and made more unpredictable by alcohol or stimulant drugs such as cocaine and amfetamines. Sedative and hypnotic drugs may also make the effects of magic mushrooms more unpredictable.

MEPHEDRONE

Other common names MCAT, meow/miaow, meow-meow/miaow-miaow, meph, drone, 4-MMc
Drug category Central nervous system stimulant

Habit-forming potential
Mephedrone is closely related chemically to cathinone, an amfetamine-substance that is the main active ingredient of khat. From its similarity to amfetamine, mephedrone is likely to cause only psychological dependence. Also like amfetamine, tolerance to mephedrone develops rapidly so that, with repeated use, increasing doses are required to produce the same effect.

How taken
It is available as capsules, tablets, and a powder, which can be ingested, snorted, or injected. Street ecstasy and cocaine may also sometimes be cut with mephedrone.

Legitimate uses
Mephedrone has no legitimate clinical uses. In April 2010, it was classified as a Class B drug under the Misuse of Drugs legislation (see p.13), and sale and possession in the UK is illegal. This same classification also extends to all chemically related cathinone drugs (e.g. methylone and flephedrone).

Short-term effects
There are no scientific studies of mephedrone's effects under controlled conditions, but users report that it causes an elevated mood (even euphoria), improved mental performance, and feelings of empathy. Most users report that the effects are pleasant and closely resemble those of ecstasy or related amfetamine-like drugs, although mephedrone seems to produce more pronounced craving than these other drugs. Users cannot usually distinguish mephedrone from cocaine if snorted.

Mephedrone may also produce a number of adverse effects, including high blood pressure, palpitations, hallucinations, sweating, and seizures. The sweating may be accompanied by excessive thirst, but it is important not to overhydrate while taking mephedrone because of the risk of significantly lowering the sodium level in the blood. Disturbed sleep and hangover effects after its use are also likely.

Long-term effects and risks
Information about the long-term effects of mephedrone is very limited. There have been isolated cases of psychotic reactions with repeated use.

Signs of misuse
Like ecstasy, mephedrone causes dilated pupils and clenching or grinding of the teeth (bruxism). Users may appear agitated or elated. Snorting the drug may also cause nosebleeds, which may be severe.

Interactions
Mephedrone raises blood pressure to dangerously high levels if taken with a monoamine oxidase inhibitor (MAOI) antidepressant. It also increases the risk of heart rhythm disturbances if used concomitantly with digoxin, levodopa, or other sympathomimetic drugs (e.g. salbutamol and pseudoephedrine).

LEGAL HIGHS

The term "legal highs" originally referred to psychoactive drugs that were not illegal but are chemically very similar to (and mimic many of the effects of) ones that were, such as Ecstasy, cannabis, and cocaine. Mephedrone was in this category until it was made illegal in the UK in 2010. Others included naphyrone (NRG-1), butylone, MDPV, and flephedrone. All of these are now categorized as Class B drugs under UK law (p.13). Since 2016, under the Psychoactive Substances Act, all "legal highs" have been banned. It is now an offence with up to 7 years' imprisonment to produce, supply, distribute, or sell any psychoactive substance. The only permitted exclusions are alcohol, tobacco, nicotine, caffeine, and medical products.

NITRITES

Other common names Amyl nitrite, butyl nitrite, poppers, snappers
Drug category Vasodilators (see also p.56)

Habit-forming potential
Nitrites do not cause physical dependence; major withdrawal symptoms have never been reported. However, users may become psychologically dependent on the stimulant effect of these drugs.

How taken
By inhalation, usually from small bottles with screw or plug tops or from small glass ampoules that are broken open.

Legitimate uses
Amyl nitrite was originally introduced as a treatment for angina but has now largely been replaced by safer, longer-acting drugs. It is still available as an antidote for cyanide poisoning. Butyl and isobutyl nitrites are not used medically.

Short-term effects
Nitrites increase the flow of blood by relaxing blood vessel walls. They give the user a rapid high, felt as a strong rush of energy. Less pleasant effects include an increase in heart rate, intense flushing, dizziness, fainting, pounding headache, nausea, and coughing. High doses may cause fainting, and regular use or overdosage by swallowing nitrites may produce a blue discoloration of the skin due to alteration of haemoglobin in the red blood cells.

Long-term effects and risks
Nitrites are very fast-acting drugs. Their effects start within 30 seconds of inhalation and last for about 5 minutes. Regular users may become tolerant to these drugs, thus requiring higher doses to achieve the desired effects. Lasting physical damage, including cardiac problems, can result from chronic use of these drugs, and deaths have occurred.

The risk of toxic effects is increased in those with low blood pressure. Nitrites may also precipitate the onset of glaucoma in susceptible people, by increasing pressure inside the eye.

Signs of misuse
Nitrites have a pungent, fruity odour. They evaporate quickly; the contents of a small bottle left uncapped in a room usually disappear within 2 hours. Unless someone is actually taking the drug or is suffering from an overdose, the only sign of misuse may be a bluish skin discoloration, although this is rare. Overdose is usually through swallowing rather than inhaling, and can result in collapse, seizures, and coma.

Interactions
The blood-pressure-lowering effect of these drugs is greatly increased by sildenafil, tadalafil, and vardenafil (drugs for erectile dysfunction) and their concomitant use should be avoided. In susceptible individuals, the effect may be to precipitate a stroke or heart attack. Alcohol, beta blockers, calcium channel blockers, and tricyclic antidepressants also increase the blood-pressure-lowering effects of nitrites, thus increasing the risk of dizziness and fainting.

OPIOIDS (HEROIN)

Other common names Horse, junk, smack, scag, H, diamorphine, morphine, opium
Drug category Central nervous system depressant

Habit-forming potential
Opioid analgesics include not only those drugs derived from the opium poppy (opium and morphine) but also synthetic drugs whose medical actions are similar to those of morphine (pethidine and methadone). Frequent use of these drugs leads to tolerance, and all have a potential for dependence. Among them, heroin is the most potent, widely abused, and dangerous. It is also associated with criminal behaviour.

After only a few weeks of use, withdrawal symptoms may occur when the drug is stopped; fear of such withdrawal effects may be a strong inducement to go on using the drug. In heavy users, the drug habit is often coupled with a lifestyle that revolves around its use.

How taken
A white or speckled brown powder, heroin is smoked, sniffed, or injected, either intravenously or subcutaneously ("popping"). Other opioids may be taken by mouth.

Legitimate uses
Heroin is widely used both in the UK and in Belgium to treat acute severe pain, such as the pain following a heart attack or acute heart failure. It is not used medically in other countries. Heroin and morphine are powerful cough suppressants. Other opioids, such as morphine and methadone, are used as analgesics. Most opioids are listed under Class A and Schedule II of the Misuse of Drugs legislation (see p.13). Mild opioids such as codeine are also sometimes included in cough suppressant and antidiarrhoeal medications and are listed under Schedule V.

Short-term effects
Strong opioids induce a feeling of contentment and well-being. Pain is dulled and the activity of the nervous system is depressed; breathing and heart rate are slowed and the cough reflex is inhibited. First-time users often feel nauseated and vomit. With higher doses, there is increasing drowsiness, sometimes leading to coma and, in rare cases, death from respiratory arrest.

Long-term effects and risks
The long-term regular use of opioids leads to constipation, reduced sexual drive, disruption of menstrual periods, and poor eating habits. Poor nutrition and personal neglect may lead to general ill health.

Street drugs are often mixed (cut) with other substances, such as caffeine, quinine, talcum powder, and flour, that can damage blood vessels, affect the lungs, or lead to the formation of blood clots. There is also a risk of abscesses at the injection site. Dangerous infections, such as hepatitis, syphilis, and human immunodeficiency virus (HIV), may be transmitted via unclean or shared needles.

After several weeks of regular use, sudden withdrawal of opioids produces a flu-like withdrawal syndrome beginning 6–24 hours after the last dose. Symptoms may include runny nose and eyes, hot and cold sweats and goose flesh (hence "cold turkey"), sleeplessness, aches, tremor, anxiety, nausea, vomiting, diarrhoea, muscle spasms, and abdominal cramps. These effects are at their worst 48–72 hours after withdrawal and fade after 7–10 days.

Signs of misuse
An opioid misuser may exhibit such signs as apathy, neglect of personal appearance and hygiene, loss of appetite and weight, loss of interest in former hobbies and social activities, personality changes, and furtive behaviour. Users resort to crime to continue financing their habit. Signs of intoxication include pinpoint pupils and a drowsy or drunken appearance.

Interactions
Opioids dangerously increase the risk of sedation with any drug that has a sedative effect on the central nervous system, including benzodiazepines and alcohol.

PHENCYCLIDINE

Other common names PCP, angel dust, crystal, ozone

Drug category General anaesthetic (see p.36), hallucinogen

Habit-forming potential
There is little evidence that phencyclidine causes physical dependence. Some users become psychologically dependent on this drug and tolerant to its effects.

How taken
May be sniffed, used in smoking mixtures (in the form of angel dust), eaten (as tablets), or, in rare cases, injected.

Legitimate uses
Although it was once used as an anaesthetic (and was a forerunner of ketamine), it no longer has any medical use. Its use in veterinary medicine has also been discontinued. Phencyclidine is classified under Class A and Schedule II of the Misuse of Drugs legislation (p.13). Phencyclidine's effects on behaviour (see below) make it one of the most dangerous of all drugs of abuse. Fortunately, it is rarely misused in Europe.

Short-term effects
Phencyclidine taken in small amounts generally produces a high, but sometimes leads to anxiety or depression. Coordination of speech and movement deteriorates, and thinking and concentration are impaired. Hallucinations and violent behaviour may occur. Other possible effects include increases in blood pressure and heart rate, dilation of the pupils, dryness of the mouth, tremor, numbness, and greatly reduced sensitivity to pain, which may make it difficult to restrain a person who has become violent under the influence of the drug. Those under the influence often appear to have extraordinary strength. Shivering, vomiting, muscle weakness, and rigidity may also occur. Higher doses lead to coma or stupor and seizures. The recovery period is often prolonged, with alternate periods of sleep and waking, usually followed by memory blackout for the whole episode.

Long-term effects and risks
Repeated phencyclidine use may lead to paranoia, auditory hallucinations, violent behaviour, anxiety, severe depression, and schizophrenia. While depressed, the user may attempt suicide by overdosing on the drug. Heavy users may also develop brain damage, which may cause memory blackouts, disorientation, visual disturbances, and speech difficulties.

   Deaths due to prolonged seizures, cardiac or respiratory arrest, and ruptured blood vessels in the brain have been reported. After high doses or prolonged coma, there is also a risk of mental derangement, which may be permanent.

Signs of misuse
Phencyclidine users may appear drunk while under the influence of the drug. Hostile or violent behaviour and mood swings with bouts of depression may be more common with heavy use.

Interactions
Using phencyclidine may inhibit the effects of anticholinergic drugs, as well as beta blockers and antihypertensive drugs.

VOLATILE SUBSTANCES

Other common names Inhalants, glue, solvents, solvent abuse
Drug category Central nervous system depressant

Habit-forming potential
There is a low risk of physical dependence with volatile substance abuse, but regular users of these substances may become psychologically dependent. Young people with family and personality problems are at particular risk of becoming habitual users of volatile substances.

How taken
By breathing in the fumes, usually from a plastic bag placed over the nose and/or mouth or from a cloth or handkerchief soaked in the solvent, or directly from the container.

Legitimate uses
Volatile substances are used in a wide variety of industrial, domestic, and cosmetic products. They function as aerosol propellants for cosmetics and spray paints, hair lacquer, lighter fuel, glues, solvents, and deodorants. They are also used in adhesives, paints, paint stripper, lacquers, petrol, and cleaning fluids. Most products containing volatile substances may not be sold to people under the age of 18.

Short-term effects
The short-term effects include lightheadedness, dizziness, confusion, and progressive drowsiness; loss of coordination occurs with increasing doses. Accidents of all types are more likely. Heart rhythm might be disturbed, sometimes fatally. Large doses can lead to disorientation, hallucinations, and loss of consciousness. Nausea, vomiting, and headaches may also occur. There are about 30 deaths every year in the UK from volatile substance abuse.

Long-term effects and risks
One of the greatest risks of volatile substance abuse is accidental death or injury while intoxicated. Some products, especially aerosol gases, butane gas, and cleaning fluids, may seriously disrupt heart rhythm or cause heart failure and sometimes death. Aerosols and butane gas can also cause suffocation by sudden cooling of the airways, and these are particularly dangerous if squirted into the mouth. Butane gas has been known to ignite in the mouth. Aerosol products, such as deodorant and paint, may suffocate the user by coating the lungs. People have suffocated while sniffing volatile substances from plastic bags placed over their heads. There is also a risk of death from inhalation of vomit and depression of the breathing mechanism.

   Long-term misuse of solvent-based cleaning fluids can cause permanent liver or kidney damage, while long-term exposure to benzene (found in plastic cements, lacquers, paint remover, petrol, and cleaning fluid) may lead to blood and liver disorders. Hexane-based adhesives may cause nerve damage leading to numbness and tremor. Repeated sniffing of leaded petrol may cause lead poisoning.

   Regular daily use of volatile substances can lead to pallor, fatigue, and forgetfulness. Heavy use may affect the student's school performance and lead to weight loss, depression, and general deterioration of health.

Signs of misuse
Most misusers are adolescents between the ages of 10 and 17, although the average age for this type of drug abuse, 14–15, is thought to be falling.

   Obvious signs of solvent abuse include a chemical smell on the breath and traces of glue or volatile substances on the body or clothes. Other signs include furtive behaviour, uncharacteristic moodiness, unusual soreness or redness around the mouth, nose, or eyes, and a persistent cough.

Interactions
Sniffing volatile substances increases the risk of sedation with any drug that has a sedative effect on the central nervous system. Such drugs include anti-anxiety and sleeping drugs, opioids, tricyclic antidepressants, antipsychotics, and alcohol.

COMPLEMENTARY AND ALTERNATIVE MEDICINE

Complementary and alternative medicine (CAM) has become increasingly popular in recent years. However, there is little or no evidence that most alternative medicines work, and the safety and effectiveness of these remedies is largely unproven.

Equally, it cannot be assumed that they are necessarily safe. They are not regulated in the same way as conventional drugs, so there is no comprehensive mechanism for establishing their safety, toxicity, or even quality.

Buying alternative medicines

Only buy products from a reputable manufacturer, who will usually provide information leaflets and instructions for use with their products. Other medicines can only be dispensed by practitioners who are suitably trained and registered. Some alternative practitioners are also medically trained and qualified.

Using alternative medicines

You may be able to treat yourself for minor, short-lived conditions, such as a cold, but you should seek professional advice for more serious or persistent complaints. Always follow the instructions given when taking alternative medicines, and never exceed the recommended dose. Certain herbs and preparations contain natural drugs that can be harmful if not used with care.

Some alternative medicines can interact with other drugs or affect pre-existing disorders in an adverse way. You always should tell your practitioner about all the medications you are taking regardless of whether they are alternative remedies or conventional drugs. You should also not stop or reduce any conventional treatment without asking your doctor's advice.

HOMEOPATHY

Homeopathic treatment is based on the concept of "like cures like" and uses the principle that the body can be stimulated to overcome illness if a patient is given dilute doses of a substance that, at full strength, would produce symptoms of the illness. In practice, this means that homeopathic remedies are made by diluting plant and animal extracts so that the final level of active drug is extremely low – usually far below the level a pharmacologist would accept as having biological activity at a receptor.

Homeopathic remedies were previously available within the NHS, in order to provide patient choice rather than to signal endorsement of their proven effectiveness. The "gold standard" for testing the clinical effectiveness of any drug is a randomized, placebo-controlled trial (RCT). Tested in this way, homeopathic remedies have never consistently shown benefit over placebos. The only advantage of homeopathy is that the low level of drug present ensures these remedies are extremely safe. The real danger is that a homeopathic remedy is used without clinical effect, placing the patient at risk.

COMMON WESTERN HERBAL REMEDIES

African plum	Guar gum
Agnus castus	Hops
Andrographis	Lavender
Astragalus	Marigold
Borage oil	Motherwort
Chamomile	Nettle
Comfrey	Oat
Cramp bark	Passion flower
Dandelion	Peppermint
Dandelion root	Psyllium
Echinacea	Pumpkin seed
Evening primrose oil	Saw palmetto
Fennel	St John's wort
Feverfew	Thunder god vine
Garlic	Valerian
Ginger	Vervain
Ginseng	Yellow dock root
Goldenseal	

WESTERN HERBAL MEDICINE

Western herbal medicines are extracted from the leaves, roots, and other parts of whole plants. They usually contain a mixture of natural drugs, as distinct from a modern drug that has been isolated from a plant to provide a preparation of a single drug (e.g. digoxin). This mixture problem is compounded if several herbs are combined in a single herbal medicine. Furthermore, the natural drug content of herbal remedies is variable and unpredictable between batches. Hence under- or overdosing with the natural drugs they contain is a real possibility.

Using Western herbal remedies

Like all drugs, herbal remedies should be used with care, particularly as there are important interactions between some herbal medicines and conventional drugs. For example, liquorice (used to treat coughs and heal peptic ulcers) can raise blood pressure and interfere with antihypertensive medication. However, St John's wort (used for depression) should be singled out as causing the most important and occasionally fatal interactions with conventional drugs. You should never take this remedy if you are on prescription drugs unless you have first discussed this with your doctor.

CHINESE HERBAL MEDICINE

Chinese herbal medicine is part of the ancient system of healing known as Traditional Chinese Medicine (TCM). It differs from Western medicine in that symptoms are regarded as being due to disharmony in the body of the two complementary but opposing forces of yin and yang; its goal is to restore harmony of these forces. Western medicine, in contrast, focuses on the disease itself and its specific symptoms.

In China, TCM is taught alongside conventional Western medical practice and is used in all hospitals. However, research to demonstrate that Chinese herbal medicine is clinically effective has been complex, largely because of the way the herbs are used.

Using Chinese herbal remedies

Herbs are generally prescribed by the practitioner as a formula containing up to 15 ingredients. Each herb performs a particular function to restore yin and yang harmony. The herbs are usually boiled in water to make a tea but may also be available as tablets, pills, powders, pastes, ointments, creams, and lotions. The medicine is usually taken daily at the start of treatment, but this may be modified according to response.

A large range of Chinese herbal medicines for minor conditions can be bought over the counter from health shops, chemists, Chinese herbalists, or Chinese medicine centres. More complex remedies and formulas are prescribed by a practitioner.

Some Chinese medicinal plants are toxic, and some herbal remedies may be adulterated with conventional drugs that can be harmful if used inappropriately.

COMMON CHINESE HERBAL REMEDIES

Aconite	Ginger
Astragalus root	Ginseng
Balloon flower	Liquorice
Cassia	Magnolia bark
Chinese angelica	Peony
Chinese bitter melon	Peony root
Chinese gentian	Plantain
Chinese rhubarb	Poria
Chinese wormwood	Red sage
Chrysanthemum	Rehmannia
Cinnamon	Shiitake
Dandelion	Thorowax root
Fleeceflower	White peony
Fritillary	Wild jujube

MEDICINES AND TRAVEL

With increasing international travel to remote destinations, travellers are more likely to visit places with novel health hazards or poorly developed health services. Although few people have serious problems, it is advisable to consider the health aspects before travelling.

BEFORE YOU GO

If you take medicines regularly

Pack sufficient supplies to last for the entire trip. If any of your medicines are schedule II or III controlled drugs (see p.13), check with your doctor or pharmacist because these may be stopped by Customs. Take your repeat prescription record with you or ask your doctor to give you a letter with details of the drugs you have been prescribed to show to Customs' officials.

... and even if you don't

Take a few everyday medicines with you, including: a motion sickness remedy; simple painkillers (e.g. paracetamol or ibuprofen); an antidiarrhoeal; rehydration salts; a laxative; an antiseptic cream; a bite/sting relief spray or cream; a high-protection (SPF 25+) sunscreen; and an insect repellent.

If you are going to a high risk area for malaria, start taking the recommended antimalarials (p.95) before leaving.

If you are going to travel outside the usual tourist routes, you might need to carry an emergency sterile syringe and needle kit. If you will be away for a long time, see your dentist for a check-up first.

Vaccinations

Vaccinations are not normally necessary for travel to western Europe, North America, Australia, or New Zealand (although you should make sure that your tetanus and poliomyelitis boosters are up to date). However, you should consult your doctor if you are visiting other destinations. If you are taking children, make sure that they have had the full set of childhood vaccinations as well as any vaccinations needed for the areas in which you will be travelling.

If you are visiting an area where there is yellow fever, you will need an International Certificate of Vaccination. Many countries also require an International Certificate of Vaccination if you have already been to a country where yellow fever is present.

Other infectious diseases are a risk in many parts of the world, and appropriate vaccinations are a wise precaution. For example, visitors to Saudi Arabia, especially for the Hajj or Umrah pilgrimages, may be required to have the meningitis A, C, W135, and Y (now called the MenACWY) vaccine beforehand.

If you are planning to stay for a long time or you are backpacking, additional vaccinations may be advisable – for example, hepatitis A, hepatitis B, BCG (tuberculosis), and possibly rabies.

All immunizations should be completed well before departure as the vaccinations do not give instant protection, and some need more than one dose to be effective. The NHS has a website providing travel health advice (www.nhs.uk/conditions/travel-vaccinations/), including vaccination advice as well as information about specific health hazards such as malaria.

Outbreaks of disease

It is advisable to check beforehand if there is an outbreak of an infectious disease in the area you are planning to visit. You could ask your doctor or travel insurance company. Another good source of information about serious outbreaks of disease worldwide is the website of the US Centers for Disease Control and Prevention (wwwnc.cdc.gov/travel).

Insurance

Being taken ill when you are abroad can be expensive, especially in countries outside the European Union. You should always have travel insurance, and should make sure that it is valid for any activities that you may be undertaking (such as skiing).

WHILE YOU ARE TRAVELLING

Travel sickness

If you are prone to travel sickness, take a travel sickness medicine before you start your journey. Ask your doctor or pharmacist for advice on which drug to choose. Do not drink alcohol because it can interact with the drugs and may make you excessively sleepy.

Dehydration and other cabin problems

To prevent dehydration during a flight, drink plenty of non-alcoholic fluids and limit alcoholic drinks.

Sitting still during a long-haul flight may lead to deep vein thrombosis (a blood clot in the leg veins). However, the risk is very small for most people, and there is no evidence that taking aspirin before a long-haul flight prevents deep vein thrombosis. Once you are on the flight, get up and walk around the cabin now and again; also practise ankle- and knee-flexing exercises. Flight socks can help, too.

Taking medicines

Travelling across different time zones may make it difficult to determine when to take regular doses of medicines. The best advice is to take the doses at the correct intervals (e.g. every 8 hours for a drug normally taken 3 times a day) regardless of the clock time. People with diabetes who take insulin should consult their doctor or diabetes nurse for advice before travelling long distances.

Jet lag

Rapid travel across time zones can cause physical and psychological stress. This can be helped by having a quiet adjustment period of at least a day to settle into the new day/night timing. Those on regular medication should seek advice from their doctor about dosage adjustment before travelling. Melatonin is included in some jet-lag remedies, but its effectiveness is unproven and it is not licensed in the UK for treating jet-lag.

ON ARRIVAL

Insect bites

Many diseases are spread by insect bites. To reduce the chance of being bitten, wear long-sleeved shirts and trousers, apply insect repellent regularly, and sleep under an insecticide-impregnated mosquito net or in accommodation protected by screens and insecticide.

Malaria prevention

Travellers to malaria-affected areas should protect themselves by taking antimalarial tablets regularly (p.95) and taking steps to prevent mosquito bites (see above).

Traveller's diarrhoea

This type of diarrhoea is usually the result of different local bacteria. The condition is largely avoidable by drinking only bottled or sterilized liquids, and by avoiding ice in drinks, uncooked and unpeeled fruit and vegetables, salads, and meat that is not freshly and thoroughly cooked. Be cautious about shellfish, even if it seems to have been cooked. Avoid buying cooked food from street traders. When brushing teeth, rinse with bottled water, not tap water.

If you do get traveller's diarrhoea, it normally disappears quickly without medicines, so your primary concern should be on preventing dehydration by using rehydration salts. Although antidiarrhoeal drugs are of no value in reducing the overall duration of traveller's diarrhoea, they may be useful for reducing the frequency of bowel movements. Remember that severe diarrhoea can reduce the absorption and effectiveness of medicines taken by mouth.

Typhoid and cholera are two serious diseases spread by contaminated food and drink that may start like traveller's diarrhoea. If you are going to a country where these diseases are endemic, you should be immunized against them but it is still vital to maintain scrupulous food, water, and personal hygiene. Do not hesitate to call local medical help if diarrhoea seems to be getting out of control. Eating raw, salted, dried, or pickled fish may lead to liver fluke or tapeworm infestations.

Sun

Travellers, especially those with fair skins, should avoid exposure to the hottest sun (from 11 am to 3 pm), apply a high-protection factor (25+) sunscreen (p.141) protecting against both UVA and UVB, and use a wide-brimmed hat and clothing for additional sun protection.

There is no such thing as a healthy tan. People who are unaccustomed to hot climates may experience heat exhaustion and even sunstroke, causing weakness, dizziness, nausea, muscle cramps, and eventually unconsciousness. Rarely, severe sunstroke may be fatal. Drinking plenty of non-alcoholic fluids, limiting exposure to the sun, and avoiding exertion until you are acclimatized to the heat can often prevent this condition from developing.

Bites and stings

Seek expert advice if you are stung or bitten by any unfamiliar wildlife or by any mammal, and try to avoid such incidents by following local advice on where it is safe to walk or swim. Tropical and subtropical rivers and lakes may contain parasitic flukes that will infest people who drink, bathe, or swim in them. Walking outdoors with bare feet is inadvisable in many parts of the world, because of the possibility of becoming infected by parasitic worms in the soil that are able to penetrate the skin and enter the body. If out hiking, always wear good walking shoes or boots and long trousers. Keep to paths and avoid walking in long grass.

ON RETURN

If you have any unusual symptoms, such as persistent diarrhoea or unexplained fever, after you return, tell a doctor which country or countries you have visited. If you were taking antimalarial drugs while away, you may need to continue taking them for up to 4 weeks after your return, depending on the type of tablets taken.

TRAVEL IMMUNIZATION

The immunizations that you will need before travelling depend on the part of the world you plan to visit. Wherever you intend to go, make sure that you have been immunized against diphtheria, tetanus, and polio and have had booster doses if necessary. Advice on immunizations may change from time to time. Before you travel, ask your doctor or travel clinic for up-to-date information. The recommendations given here are for adults; consult your doctor about travel immunizations for children.

Disease	Number of doses	When effective	Period of protection	Who should be immunized
Cholera	2 oral doses, 1–6 weeks apart	1 week after 2nd dose	Up to 2 years	People travelling to areas where cholera is endemic or epidemic. Vaccination does not provide complete protection; it is also crucial to pay scrupulous attention to food, water, and personal hygiene.
Hepatitis A	2 injections, 6–12 months apart	2 weeks after 1st dose	1st dose protects for 1 year; 2nd dose for at least 20 years	Travellers to high-risk areas outside Northern and Western Europe, North America, Australia, New Zealand, and Japan.
Hepatitis B	3 injections, over a period of 3 weeks to 6 months	After 3rd dose	At least 5 years	People travelling to countries in which hepatitis B is prevalent and who might need medical or dental treatment and/or are likely to have unprotected sex.
Japanese encephalitis	2 injections, 28 days apart	About 1 week after 2nd dose	1–2 years	People staying for an extended period in rural areas where the disease is prevalent, including the Indian subcontinent, China, Southeast Asia, and the Far East.
Meningitis A, C, W135, and Y (MenACWY)	1 injection	After 2–3 weeks	About 5 years	People travelling to sub-Saharan Africa and parts of Saudi Arabia. Immunization certificate needed if travelling to Saudi Arabia for the Hajj and Umrah pilgrimages.
Rabies	3 injections: 1 week between 1st and 2nd doses, 2 or 3 weeks between 2nd and 3rd doses	After 3rd dose	Those at continued risk: 1 year; booster doses protect for 3–5 years. Travellers: about 10 years	Travellers to areas where rabies is endemic, particularly those at high risk (e.g. veterinary surgeons) and/or those travelling to areas with limited medical facilities. The vaccine may also be given after rabies exposure.
Typhoid	1 injection or 3 oral doses, each dose on an alternate day	2 weeks after injection, or 7–10 days after last oral dose	Injection: about 3 years. Oral vaccine: about 1 year	People travelling to areas with poor sanitation and hygiene, especially those at high risk of infection (e.g. aid workers in disaster areas). Scrupulous attention to personal hygiene is also important.
Yellow fever	1 injection	After 10 days	At least 10 years	Yellow fever vaccination is compulsory for entry to some countries and advisable for visits to others within yellow fever zones (which are mainly in Africa and South America). May also be needed when travelling from yellow fever zones.

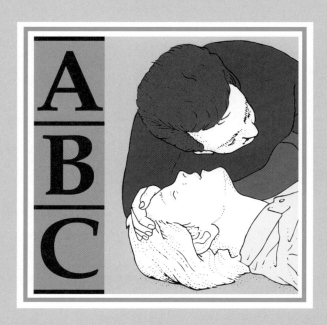

INFORMATION AND INDEX

USEFUL RESOURCES
GLOSSARY
DRUG FINDER
INDEX
DRUG POISONING EMERGENCY GUIDE

USEFUL RESOURCES

It is important to have as much information as possible about any medicines that you, or someone that you are caring for, are taking. All medicines, whether prescribed or bought over the counter, should come with a patient information leaflet. Always read these leaflets. If you are still in doubt about anything to do with a medicine, you should ask your doctor or pharmacist.

Organizations should be able to provide general information on medicines. Some of these societies are listed below. Further information is usually also available from your local hospital, as well as social services and local libraries. If you have access to the Internet you will also be able to find hundreds of websites that offer information.

Although much of the available advice on medicines and drugs is useful and reliable, some information may be misleading, oversimplified, or even wrong. Always be careful of following advice that does not appear to be from a qualified source, and discuss the matter with your doctor or pharmacist if you are unsure.

GENERAL INFORMATION

British Medical Association
Tel: 0300 123 1233
Online: www.bma.org.uk

Centers for Disease Control and Prevention (US)
Online: www.cdc.gov

Department of Health and Social Care
Online: www.gov.uk/government/organisations/department-of-health-and-social-care

Medicines and Healthcare products Regulatory Agency (MHRA)
Tel: 020 3080 6000
E-mail: info@mhra.gov.uk
Online: www.mhra.gov.uk

National Health Service
Online: www.nhs.uk

National Institute for Health and Clinical Excellence (NICE)
Tel: 0300 323 0140
E-mail: nice@nice.org.uk
Online: www.nice.org.uk

National Pharmacy Association
Tel: 01727 858687
Online: www.npa.co.uk

Patient UK
Online: patient.info

Public Health England
Online: www.gov.uk/government/organisations/public-health-england

Royal College of General Practitioners
Tel: 020 3188 7400
E-mail: info@rcgp.org.uk
Online: www.rcgp.org.uk

Royal Pharmaceutical Society
Tel: 020 7572 2737
Online: www.rpharms.com

US Office of Disease Prevention and Health Promotion
Online: health.gov

World Health Organization
Tel: 0041 22 791 2111
Online: www.who.int

DRUG DEPENDENCE

Alcoholics Anonymous
Tel: 0800 9177 650
E-mail: help@aamail.org
Online: www.alcoholics-anonymous.org.uk

DrugWise
Tel: 0330 123 6600
Online: www.drugwise.org.uk

Narcotics Anonymous
Helpline: 0300 999 1212
Online: ukna.org

DRUG REACTIONS

Allergy UK
Allergy Helpline: 01322 619898
E-mail: info@allergyuk.org
Online: www.allergyuk.org

MedicAlert
Tel: 01908 951045
E-mail: info@medicalert.org.uk
Online: www.medicalert.org.uk

SPECIFIC CONDITIONS

British Heart Foundation
Heartline: 0300 330 3311
E-mail: heretohelp@bhf.org.uk
Online: www.bhf.org.uk

British Lung Foundation
Helpline: 03000 030 555
E-mail: hello.blf.org.uk
Online: www.blf.org.uk

British Red Cross
Tel: 0344 871 1111
E-mail: contactus@redcross.org.uk
Online: www.redcross.org.uk

Cancer Research UK
Tel: 020 7242 0200
Online: www.cancerresearchuk.org

Guts UK (The Digestive Disorders Foundation)
Tel: 020 7486 0341
E-mail: info@gutscharity.org.uk
Online: gutscharity.org.uk

The Mental Health Foundation
Tel: 020 7803 1100
Online: www.mentalhealth.org.uk

MIND
Infoline: 0300 123 3393
Tel: 020 8519 2122
E-mail:supporterrelations@mind.org.uk
Online: www.mind.org.uk

The Pain Research Institute
Tel: 0151 529 5835 or 0151 529 5820
Online: www.liverpool.ac.uk/pain-research-institute/

Royal National Institute for the Blind
Tel: 0303 123 9999
E-mail: helpline@rnib.org.uk
Online: www.rnib.org.uk

RNID (Royal National Institute for Deaf People)
Tel: 0808 808 0123
Textphone: 0808 808 9000
E-mail: information@rnid.org.uk
Online: rnid.org.uk

Versus Arthritis (Arthritis Research UK)
Tel: 0300 790 0400
E-mail: enquiries@versusarthritis.org
Online: www.versusarthritis.org

DRUGS IN SPORT

Global Drug Reference Online
Online: www.globaldro.com

World Anti-Doping Agency
Online: www.wada-ama.org

MEDICINES AND TRAVEL

London School of Hygiene and Tropical Medicine
Tel: 020 7636 8636
Online: www.lshtm.ac.uk

MASTA (Medical Advisory Services for Travellers Abroad)
Tel: 0330 100 4200
E-mail: enquiries@masta.org
Online: www.masta-travel-health.com

National Travel Health Network and Centre
Online: www.nathnac.net

NHS: Travel vaccinations
Online: www.nhs.uk/conditions/travel-vaccinations

Tropical Medical Bureau (Ireland)
Tel: +353 1 2715 200
Online: www.tmb.ie

GLOSSARY

The following pages contain definitions of drug-related terms whose technical meanings are not explained in detail elsewhere in the book, or for which an easily located precise explanation may be helpful. These are words that may not be familiar to the general reader, or that have a slightly different meaning in a medical context from that in ordinary use. Some of the terms included refer to particular drug actions or effects; others describe methods of drug administration. A few medical conditions that may occur as a result of drug use are also defined.

The glossary is arranged in alphabetical order. To avoid repetition, where relevant, entries include cross-references to further information on that topic located in other sections of the book, or to another glossary term (indicated by italics).

A

Activator
See *Agonist*.

Addiction
A term referring to compulsive use of a drug that can cover anything from intense, habitual cravings for caffeine to physical and psychological dependence on drugs such as nicotine and *opioids*. See also *Dependence* and Drug dependence (p.23).

Adjuvant
A drug or chemical that enhances the therapeutic effect of another drug.

Adrenergic
See *Sympathomimetic*.

Adverse effect
Like "side effect" and "adverse reaction", this is a term for unwanted effects of a drug. Most adverse effects increase as the dose is increased. Other adverse effects appear not to be dose-related, such as an *idiosyncrasy* or an *allergic reaction*. See also Adverse effects (p.15).

Adverse reaction
See *Adverse effect*.

Agonist
A substance that has a stimulating effect on activities of body cells. An agonist drug (often called an activator) is one that binds to a *receptor* and activates it.

Allergic reaction
An intense or excessive reaction by the immune system to a trigger (allergen). An allergy (p.81) appears not on first exposure to the trigger but after repeated exposures. See also *Anaphylaxis*.

Amoebicide
A drug that kills single-celled microorganisms called amoebae. See Antiprotozoal drugs (p.94).

Anaemia
A condition in which the concentration of haemoglobin, the oxygen-carrying pigment in the blood, is below normal. Severe anaemia may cause fatigue, pallor, and occasionally, breathing difficulty.

Anaesthetic, general
A drug or drug combination given to produce unconsciousness before and during surgery or potentially painful investigative procedures. General anaesthesia is usually induced by injection of a drug such as propofol, and then maintained by inhalation of a mixture of anaesthetic gases. Intravenous maintenance of anaesthesia is also possible. See also *Premedication*.

Anaesthetic, local
A drug applied topically (see *Topical*) or injected to numb sensation in a small area. See also Local anaesthetics (p.36).

Analeptic
A drug that stimulates breathing. See also Respiratory stimulants (p.44).

Analgesia
Relief of pain, usually by drugs. See also Analgesics (p.36).

Anaphylaxis
A severe reaction to an allergen such as a bee sting or a drug (see Allergy, p.81). Symptoms may include swelling, breathing difficulty, and collapse. See also Anaphylactic shock (p.520).

Antagonist
A substance with an opposing effect on body cell activities. An antagonist drug (often called a blocker) binds to a *receptor* without activating it and prevents other substances (i.e. *agonists*) from occupying and activating that receptor.

Antibiotic
A substance that kills or arrests the growth of bacteria. See also Antibiotics (p.86) and Antibacterial drugs (p.89).

Antibody
A protein manufactured by lymphocytes (a type of white blood cell) to neutralize an antigen (foreign protein) in the body. The formation of antibodies is part of the body's defence against infection. *Immunization* to increase resistance to a specific disease involves either injection of specific antibodies or administration of a *vaccine* that stimulates antibody production. See also Vaccines and immunization (p.92).

Anticholinergic
A drug that blocks the action of acetylcholine, a neurotransmitter secreted by nerve cells. Anticholinergic drugs relax the bladder's squeezing muscles, tighten those of the sphincter, relax the muscles of the intestinal wall, and reduce saliva production. See also Autonomic nervous system (p.35).

Antidote
A substance used to neutralize or counteract the effects of a poison.

Antineoplastic
An anticancer drug (p.112).

Antioxidant
A substance that delays cell deterioration due to free radicals (unstable oxygen atoms), which are thought to play a role in aging and disease. Vitamins A, C, and E are antioxidants. See also Vitamins (p.107).

Antipyretic
A type of drug that reduces fever. Common antipyretic drugs are aspirin and paracetamol.

Antiseptic
A chemical that destroys bacteria and sometimes other microorganisms. See also Anti-infective skin preparations (p.135).

Antispasmodic
A drug that reduces spasm (abnormally strong or inappropriate contraction) of the digestive tract muscles.

Antitussive
A drug that prevents or relieves a cough. See also Drugs to treat coughs (p.52).

Aperient
A mild laxative. See Laxatives (p.69).

Astringent
A substance that causes tissue to dry and shrink by reducing its ability to absorb water. Astringents are used in various antiperspirants and skin tonics. They are also used in ear drops for inflammation of the outer ear because they promote healing of inflamed tissue.

B

Bactericidal
A term used to describe a drug that kills bacteria. See also Antibiotics (p.86) and Antibacterials (p.89).

Bacteriostatic
A term used to describe a drug that stops the growth or multiplication of bacteria. See also Antibiotics (p.86) and Antibacterials (p.89).

Balm
A soothing preparation applied to the skin.

Bioavailability

A term for the proportion of a drug dose that enters the bloodstream and so reaches body tissues; usually expressed as a percentage of the dose. Injection of a drug into a vein results in 100 per cent bioavailability. Drugs given by mouth generally have a lower bioavailability as some of the drug may not pass through the gut wall, and some may be broken down in the liver before reaching the rest of the body.

Blocker

See *Antagonist*.

Body mass index (BMI)

An indicator of healthy body weight. BMI is a number calculated by dividing a person's weight in kilograms by the square of their height in metres. The healthy range is 18.5–24.9.

Body salts

Also known as electrolytes, these are minerals present in body fluids such as blood, urine, and sweat, and within cells. These salts play an important role in regulating water balance, controlling acidity of the blood, conduction of nerve impulses, and muscle contraction. The balance of body salts can be upset by such conditions as diarrhoea and vomiting, and by the action of drugs such as diuretics (p.57).

Brand name

The name chosen by a manufacturer for its version of a product containing a generic drug. See also *Generic name* and How drugs are classified (p.13).

Bronchoconstrictor

A substance that narrows the airways in the lungs. An attack of asthma may be caused by the release of bronchoconstrictor substances such as histamine or certain prostaglandins.

Bronchodilator

A drug that widens the airways. See Bronchodilators (p.48).

C

Capsule

See p.19.

Cathartic

A drug that stimulates bowel action to soften bowel movements. See also Laxatives (p.69).

Chelating agent

A chemical used in the treatment of poisoning by metals such as iron, lead, arsenic, and mercury. It combines with the metal to form a less poisonous substance and in some cases increases excretion in the urine.

Chemotherapy

Drug treatment of cancer or infections. *Cytotoxic* drugs (p.112) and *antibiotics* (p.86) are examples of drugs used in chemotherapy.

Cholinergic

A drug, also called a *parasympathomimetic*, that acts by stimulating the parasympathetic nervous system. See also Autonomic nervous system (p.35).

Coma

A state of unconsciousness and unresponsiveness to external stimuli such as noise and pain. Coma results from damage to or disturbance of part of the brain.

Contraindication

A factor in a person's current condition, medical history, or genetic make-up that may increase the risks of an *adverse effect* from a drug, to the extent that the drug should not be prescribed (called an absolute contraindication), or should only be prescribed with caution (called a relative contraindication).

Counter-irritant

Another term for a *rubefacient*.

Cycloplegic

Refers to the action of paralysing the ciliary muscle in the eye. This muscle alters the shape of the lens when it contracts, enabling the eye to focus on objects. A cycloplegic drug prevents this action, thereby making both eye examination and eye surgery easier. See also Drugs affecting the pupil (p.130).

Cytotoxic

A drug that kills or damages cells. Drugs with this action are most commonly used to treat cancer. Although these drugs are primarily intended to affect abnormal cells, they may also kill or damage healthy ones. See also Anticancer drugs (p.112).

D

Dependence

A term that relates to psychological or physical dependence on a substance, or both. Psychological dependence involves intense mental cravings if a drug is unavailable or withdrawn. Physical dependence causes physical withdrawal symptoms (sweating, shaking, abdominal pain, and convulsions) if the substance is not taken. Dependence also implies loss of control over intake. See also Drug dependence (p.23).

Depot injection

Injection into a muscle of a drug that has been specially formulated to provide for a slow, steady absorption of its active ingredients by the surrounding blood vessels. Alternatively, some drugs may be injected under the skin using an applicator. This is known as an implant injection. The release period can be made to last up to several weeks. See also Methods of administration (p.17).

Designer drugs

A group of unlicensed substances whose only purpose is to duplicate the effects of certain illegal drugs of abuse or to provide even stronger effects. Designer drugs are very dangerous because their effects are unpredictable, they are often highly potent, and they may contain impurities.

Double-blind

A test used to determine the effectiveness of a new drug compared to an existing medicine or a *placebo*. Neither patients nor the doctors administering the drug know who is receiving which substance. Only after the test is completed is the identity of those who received the new drug revealed. Double-blind trials are performed for almost all new drugs. See Testing and approving new drugs (p.12).

Drip

A non-medical term for *intravenous infusion*.

E

Electrolytes

See *Body salts*.

Elixir

A clear, sweetened liquid, often containing alcohol, that forms the base for many liquid medicines such as those used to treat coughs.

Embrocation

An ointment or liniment rubbed on to the skin to relieve joint pain, muscle cramp, or muscle injury. An embrocation usually contains a *rubefacient*.

Emetic

Any substance that causes a person to vomit.

Emollient

A substance having a soothing, softening effect when applied to the skin. An emollient also has a moisturizing effect. See also Bases for skin preparations (p.135).

Empathogen

A drug that increases feelings of openness and emotional connection with other people. Term used for certain recreational drugs, e.g. Ecstasy.

Emulsion

A combination of two liquids that do not normally mix together but, on addition of a third substance (known as an emulsifying agent), can be mixed to give a complex liquid consisting of droplets of one liquid suspended in the other. An example of an emulsion is liquid paraffin.

Endorphins

A group of substances occurring naturally in the brain that bind to specialized receptors and reduce the perception of pain. *Opioid* analgesics such as morphine work by mimicking the action of endorphins. See also Analgesics (p.36).

Enteric coated

A term used for a drug that has been treated with a special coating so that, after being taken orally, it passes safely and unaltered through the stomach and acts on the intestine.

Enzyme

A protein that controls the rate of one or more chemical reactions in the body. There are thousands of enzymes active in the body. Each type of cell produces a specific range of enzymes. Cells in the liver contain enzymes that stimulate the breakdown of nutrients and drugs; cells in the digestive tract release enzymes that help digest food. Some drugs work by altering the activity of enzymes – for example, certain anticancer drugs halt tumour growth by altering enzyme function in cancer cells.

Epidural injection
An injection that resembles an *intrathecal injection* but delivers the drug into a more superficial space around the spine. Usually a local anaesthetic and analgesic are injected or infused together to provide regional anaesthesia.

Excitatory
A term meaning "having a stimulating or enhancing effect on cell activity". A chemical released from a nerve ending that causes muscle contraction is having an excitatory effect. See also *Inhibitory*.

Expectorant
A type of cough remedy that enhances sputum (phlegm) production and is used in treating a productive (sputum-producing) cough. See also Drugs to treat coughs (p.52).

F

Formula, chemical
A way of expressing the constituents of a chemical in symbols and numbers. There is a formula for every known chemical substance, including drugs and natural body chemicals. For example, water has the formula H_2O, indicating that it is composed of two hydrogen atoms (H_2) and one oxygen atom (O).

Formulary
A list of drugs produced as a guide to prescribers and other health professionals. The British National Formulary (BNF) is jointly produced by the British Medical Association and the Royal Pharmaceutical Society as a non-promotional guide to what is available and considered worth prescribing for most common conditions.

G

Gel
A viscous, usually translucent, jelly-like formulation of a drug for application to the skin.

Generic name
The official name for a substance that is therapeutically active. The term "generic" is distinct from a *brand name*, which is a term chosen by a manufacturer for its version of a product containing a generic drug. See also How drugs are classified (p.13).

GSL (General Sales List) medicines
Over-the-counter medicines considered suitable for sale by any retail outlet because of their safety record. Examples include aspirin and paracetamol. See also Managing your drug treatment (p.25).

H

Half-life
A term used in *pharmacology* for the time taken to reduce the blood level of a drug by half.

Hallucinogen
A drug that causes hallucinations. Common hallucinogens include the drugs of abuse LSD (p.453) and ketamine (p.452). Large amounts of alcohol may have a hallucinogenic effect, and hallucinations may also occur during withdrawal from alcohol (p.447). Certain prescribed drugs can cause hallucinations, e.g. opioids, some antidepressants, and dopamine agonists.

Hormone
A natural chemical produced by the body and released into the bloodstream by a gland or tissue. Each hormone has a specific range of functions, such as controlling the *metabolism* of cells, sexual development, and the response to stress or illness. Hormone-producing glands make up the endocrine system; the kidneys, gut, and brain also release hormones. See also Hormones and endocrine system (p.98).

I

Idiosyncrasy
A term for an *adverse effect* of a drug that happens on first use, but appears not to be dose related and is pharmacologically unexpected. Idiosyncratic reactions occur because people are different genetically and may react differently from usual to a drug.

Immunization
The process of inducing immunity (resistance to infection). See Vaccines and immunization (p.92).

Indication
The term used to describe a disorder, symptom, or condition for which a drug or treatment may be prescribed. For example, indications for the use of beta blockers include angina and high blood pressure (hypertension).

Infusion pump
A machine for administering a continuous, controlled amount of a drug or other fluid through a needle inserted into a vein or under the skin. See Methods of administration (p.17).

Inhalator
A mouthpiece similar to a cigarette holder into which a nicotine-impregnated plug is inserted. The inhalator and plug are a form of nicotine-replacement therapy used during attempts to give up smoking.

Inhaler
A device used for administering a drug in the form of powder or vapour. Inhalers are used principally in the treatment of respiratory disorders. See also Methods of administration (p.17) and Inhalers (p.49).

Inhibitory
A term meaning "with a blocking effect on cell activity". See also *Antagonist* and *Excitatory*.

Inoculation
A method of *immunization* in which a *vaccine* is scratched into the skin rather than injected. See also Vaccines and immunization (p.92).

Interaction
See Drug interactions, p.16.

Intramuscular injection
Injection of a drug into a muscle, usually in the upper arm or buttock. The drug is then absorbed into the bloodstream. See also Methods of administration (p.17).

Intrathecal injection
An injection of a drug into the space around the brain or spinal cord. This minimizes systemic effects of a drug while producing high levels in the enclosed nervous tissue. Local anaesthetic drugs are injected by this route to provide spinal anaesthesia. See also *Epidural injection*.

Intravenous infusion
Prolonged, slow introduction of fluid into a vein. The fluid flows at a controlled rate from a bag or bottle through a fine tube and a needle inserted into a vein. An intravenous infusion may also be administered via an *infusion pump*.

Intravenous injection
Direct injection of a drug into the bloodstream via a vein. Because it has a rapid effect, intravenous injection is useful in an emergency. See also Methods of administration (p.17).

JL

Jaundice
A condition in which the skin and whites of the eyes turn yellow due to a build-up in the blood of the yellow-brown bile pigment bilirubin. Jaundice is a sign of many liver disorders. Some drugs also cause jaundice as an *adverse effect*. See also Liver and kidney disease, p.22.

Liniment
A liquid medicine for application to the skin by being rubbed in. See also *Embrocation*.

Lotion
A liquid preparation that may be applied to large areas of skin. See also Bases for skin preparations (p.135).

M

Metabolism
The term for all chemical processes in the body that involve either the formation of new substances or the breakdown of substances to release energy or detoxify foreign substances.

MHRA
The Medicines and Healthcare products Regulatory Agency (MHRA) is the UK government licensing agency (part of the Department of Health) responsible for ensuring that medicines and medical devices work and are safe. No drug can be sold in the UK without a marketing authorization from the MHRA.

Miotic

A drug that constricts (narrows) the pupil. *Opioid* drugs such as morphine have a miotic effect. Certain miotic drugs are used deliberately to narrow the pupil, for example in the treatment of glaucoma. See also Drugs for glaucoma (p.128) and Drugs affecting the pupil (p.130).

Monoclonal antibody

An *antibody* generated by modified, genetically identical (monoclonal) human immune cells grown outside the body. The antibody acts in the same way as an antibody made in the body. These drugs are widely used in treating cancer (p.114) and immunotherapy (e.g. for rheumatoid arthritis and inflammatory bowel disease).

Mucolytic

A drug that liquefies mucus secretions in the airways. See also Drugs to treat coughs (p.52).

Mydriatic

A drug that dilates (widens) the pupil. Mydriatic drugs are used to facilitate examination of the retina in the eye. They may occasionally provoke the onset of glaucoma. See also Drugs affecting the pupil (p.130).

N

Narcotic

Once applied to drugs derived from the opium poppy, but no longer has a precise medical meaning; some American sources use the term to mean any potent abused drug. "Narcotic analgesic", a term largely replaced by *opioid* analgesic, refers to opium-derived and synthetic drugs that have pain-relieving properties and other effects similar to those of morphine (see Analgesics, p.36). See also Opioids (p.455).

Nebulizer

A method of administering a drug to the airways and lungs in aerosol form through a facemask. See also *Inhaler*.

Neuroleptic

Also called an antipsychotic, a drug used to treat psychotic illness. See Antipsychotic drugs (p.41).

Neurotransmitter

A body chemical that is released from a nerve ending in response to an electrical impulse. A neurotransmitter may carry a message from the nerve to another nerve so that the electrical impulse passes on, to a muscle to stimulate contraction, or to a gland to stimulate hormone secretion. Examples of neurotransmitters include acetylcholine and norepinephrine (noradrenaline). Many drugs either mimic or block the action of neurotransmitters. See also Brain and nervous system (p.34).

O

Opioid

One of a group of drugs (also called *narcotic* analgesics) that are prescribed to relieve pain, treat diarrhoea, and suppress coughs. See also Opioids (p.455).

Orphan drug

A drug that is effective for a rare medical condition, but that may not be marketed by a drug manufacturer due to the low profit potential. Such drugs may be given fast-track licensing by the authorities to compensate the manufacturer.

Over-the-counter (OTC) medicines

A term for drugs that can be bought from a pharmacy without a prescription. See also *GSL medicines, P medicines, POM*, and Managing your drug treatment (p.25).

P

Parasympathomimetic

A drug that is prescribed to stimulate the parasympathetic nervous system (see Autonomic nervous system, p.35). These drugs (also called *cholinergic* drugs) are used as *miotics* and to stimulate bladder contraction in urinary retention (see Drugs used in urinary disorders, p.126).

Parkinsonism

Neurological symptoms including tremor of the hands, muscle rigidity, and slowness of movement that resemble Parkinson's disease. Parkinsonism may be caused by prolonged treatment with an antipsychotic drug. See Drugs for parkinsonism (p.43).

Pharmacist

A registered health professional (or "chemist") concerned with the preparation, manufacture, and dispensing of drugs. Pharmacists can also advise users on the correct use of drugs.

Pharmacodynamics

The effects or actions that a drug produces in the body.

Pharmacokinetics

The term used to describe how the body deals with a drug from the point it enters the body to the point at which it acts. This includes how the drug is absorbed into the blood, distributed to different tissues, broken down, and excreted from the body.

Pharmacologist

A scientist concerned with the study of the *pharmacodynamics* and *pharmacokinetics* of drugs. Pharmacologists are one of the groups responsible for scientific research into new drugs and new uses for existing drugs. Clinical pharmacologists are usually qualified doctors.

Pharmacology

The science of the origin, appearance, chemistry, action, and use of drugs.

Pharmacopoeia

A publication that describes the drugs used in medicine. The term "pharmacopoeia" usually refers to an official national publication (such as the British Pharmacopoeia) that sets standards and describes the methods used to identify drugs and determine their purity.

Pharmacy

A term that is used to describe the science and technology involved in the study of drugs. The word is also used to refer to the place where the practice of preparing drugs, making up prescriptions, and dispensing the drugs is carried out.

Photophobia

Dislike of, or intolerance to, bright light.

Photosensitivity

An abnormal reaction of the skin to light, often causing reddening.

Placebo

A "medicine", often in tablet or capsule form, that contains no medically active ingredient. Placebos are frequently used in trials of new drugs (see *Double-blind*). See also Placebo response (p.15).

P medicines

These are *over-the-counter medicines* that may only be sold in a *pharmacy*. Most drugs that are not *POMs* are P (pharmacy) medicines. See also Managing your drug treatment (p.25).

POM

An abbreviation for Prescription Only Medicine. These drugs cannot be bought without a prescription from a doctor, dentist, prescribing nurse, or pharmacist. See also Prescription drugs (p.26).

Premedication

The term applied to drugs that are given to patients between one and two hours before an operation. The premedication usually contains an *opioid* analgesic to help relieve pain and anxiety and to reduce the dose of anaesthetic needed (see also *Anaesthetic, general*). In some cases, an *anticholinergic* drug is also included to reduce secretions in the airways.

Prescription

A written instruction from a doctor to a pharmacist, detailing the name of the drug to be dispensed, the dosage, how often it has to be taken, and other instructions as necessary. A prescription is written and signed by a prescriber and carries the name and address of the patient for whom the drug is prescribed. See also Managing your drug treatment (p.25).

Prophylactic

A drug, procedure, or piece of equipment used to prevent disease. The process of prevention is called prophylaxis.

Proprietary

A term now applied to a drug that is sold over the counter and having its name registered to a private manufacturer, i.e. a proprietor.

Prostaglandin

A fatty (organic) acid that acts in a similar way to a hormone. Prostaglandins occur in many different tissues and have various effects. These include causing inflammation in damaged tissue, lowering blood pressure, and stimulating contractions in labour.

Psychedelic
A drug that changes cognition and perception, often producing effects that include visual hallucinations. Most psychedelics are drugs of abuse, although some have legitimate therapeutic uses (e.g. ketamine).

Purgative
A drug that helps eliminate faeces from the body, to relieve constipation or to empty the bowel/intestine before surgery. See also *Cathartic* and Laxatives (p.69).

Pyrogen
A substance that causes a rise in temperature.

R

Receptor
A specific site on a cell with a characteristic chemical and physical structure that binds a body chemical or a drug. Receptors are usually located on the surface of a cell, although some are located inside the cell. Body chemicals such as *neurotransmitters* and *hormones* bind to their specific receptors to initiate a response in the cell. Most drugs have their effects by binding to receptors and either activating or blocking them. See also *Agonist* and *Antagonist*.

Replication
The duplication of genetic material (DNA or RNA) in a cell as part of the process of cell division that enables a tissue to grow or a virus to multiply.

Rubefacient
A preparation, also known as a counter-irritant, that, when applied to an area of skin, causes it to redden by increasing blood flow in vessels in that area. A rubefacient may be included in an *embrocation* or a *liniment*.

S

Sedative
A drug that dampens the activity of the central nervous system. Sleeping drugs (p.38) and anti-anxiety drugs (p.39) have a sedative effect, and many other drugs can produce sedation as a side effect.

Side effect
See *Adverse effect*.

Sterile
A term meaning free from live microorganisms. Drugs that are administered by certain methods, such as injection, must be sterile to avoid causing infection. See also *Pyrogen*.

Subcutaneous injection
A method of giving a drug by which the drug is injected under the skin and is then slowly absorbed into the surrounding blood vessels. See also Methods of administration (p.17).

Sublingual
A term meaning under the tongue. Some drugs are administered sublingually in tablet or spray form. The drug is rapidly absorbed through the lining of the mouth. See also Methods of administration (p.17).

Suppository
A bullet-shaped pellet usually containing a drug for insertion into the rectum. See also Methods of administration (p.17).

Sustained release
A term used to describe tablet formulations designed to release their drug contents slowly and over a prolonged period. These tablets often carry suffixes such as SR, MR, XL, or CR.

Sympatholytic
A term for a drug that blocks the effect of the sympathetic nervous system. Sympatholytic drugs work either by reducing the release of the *neurotransmitter* norepinephrine (noradrenaline), or by occupying the *receptors* to which the neurotransmitters epinephrine (adrenaline) and norepinephrine normally bind. Beta blockers are examples of sympatholytic drugs. See Autonomic nervous system (p.35).

Sympathomimetic
A term for a drug that has the same effect as stimulation of the sympathetic nervous system: for example, causing an increase in the heart rate and widening of the airways. A drug having a sympathomimetic action may work either by causing the release of the stimulatory *neurotransmitter* norepinephrine (noradrenaline) from the nerve endings or by mimicking neurotransmitter action (see Autonomic nervous system, p.35). The sympathomimetic drugs include certain bronchodilators (p.48) and decongestants (p.51).

Syrup
A solution of sucrose (sugar) in water. Syrup is used as a basis for some liquid medicines because it acts as an *antioxidant*; bacteria, fungi, and moulds do not grow in it; and its sweetness hides the taste of some drugs.

Systemic
Having a generalized effect, causing physical or chemical changes in tissues throughout the body. For a drug to have a systemic effect it must be absorbed into the bloodstream.

T

Tablet
See Drug forms, p.19.

Tardive dyskinesia
Abnormal, uncontrolled movements, mainly of the face, tongue, mouth, and neck, that may be caused by prolonged treatment with antipsychotic drugs (p.41).

Tolerance
The need to take a higher dosage of a drug in order to maintain the same physical or mental effect. See also Drug dependence (p.23).

Tonics
Remedies for relieving vague symptoms such as malaise, lethargy, and loss of appetite, for which no obvious cause can be found. Tonics may contain vitamins or minerals, but there is no scientific evidence that such ingredients have anything other than a *placebo* effect.

Topical
The term used to describe the application of a drug directly to the site where it is intended to have its effect, such as the skin.

Toxic reaction
Unpleasant and possibly dangerous symptoms caused by a drug, the result of an overdose. See also The effects of drugs (p.15).

Toxin
A poisonous substance such as a harmful chemical released by bacteria.

Tranquillizer, major
A drug used to treat psychotic illness such as schizophrenia. See Antipsychotic drugs (p.41).

Tranquillizer, minor
A sedative drug used to treat anxiety and emotional tension. See Anti-anxiety drugs (p.39).

Transdermal patch
An adhesive patch that is impregnated with a drug and placed on the skin, from where the drug is absorbed into underlying blood vessels. See also Methods of administration (p.17).

V

Vaccine
A substance containing a harmless form of a microorganism, administered to induce active immunity against a specific infectious disease (see Vaccines and immunization, p.92).

Vasoconstrictor
A drug that narrows blood vessels, sometimes prescribed to reduce nasal congestion (see Decongestants, p.51). Vasoconstrictors are also frequently given with injected local anaesthetics (p.36) (see also *Anaesthetic, local*).

Vasodilator
A drug that widens blood vessels. See Vasodilators (p.56).

W

Wafer
A sliver of material impregnated with a drug and placed on the tongue. As the wafer dissolves, the drug is absorbed through the lining of the mouth into the surrounding blood vessels.

Withdrawal symptom
Any symptom caused by abrupt stopping of a drug. These symptoms occur as a result of physical *dependence* on a drug. See also Drug dependence (p.23).

DRUG FINDER

This section contains the names of more than 3,000 individual drug products and substances. It provides a quick reference for information on specific drugs or other medications.

What it contains

The entries include all major generic drugs and many less widely used substances, a broad range of brand-named products, and many vitamins and minerals. Each gives the name, the generic name for branded drugs, the drug class (if relevant), and the use. Inclusion of a product does not imply the publisher's endorsement, nor does the exclusion of a particular product indicate disapproval.

How the references work

References are to the pages in Part 3, containing the drug profiles of each principal generic drug, and to the section in Part 2 that describes the relevant drug group, as appropriate. Some entries for drugs that do not have a full profile contain a brief description here.

Abbreviations

For brevity and ease of reading, names of the following drug types have been abbreviated:

Disease-modifying anti-rheumatic drug – DMARD
Non-steroidal anti-inflammatory drug – NSAID

A

abacavir antiretroviral drug for HIV/AIDS 116

abacavir with dolutegravir and lamivudine combined preparation of antiretroviral drugs for HIV/AIDS 116

abacavir with lamivudine combined preparation of antiretrovirals for HIV/AIDS 116

abacavir with lamivudine and zidovudine combined preparation of antiretroviral drugs for HIV/AIDS 116

abatacept cytokine modulator antirheumatic 75 for moderate to severe rheumatoid arthritis

abciximab antiplatelet drug 62

Abelcet brand name for amphotericin 160 (an antifungal 96)

Abidec brand-name multivitamin 107

Abilify brand name for aripiprazole (an antipsychotic 41)

abiretarone acetate anticancer drug 112 used for prostate cancer

Abraxane brand name for paclitaxel (an anticancer drug 112)

Abstral brand name for fentanyl (an opioid analgesic 36)

Abtard brand name for oxycodone, an opioid analgesic 36 to relieve post-operative pain

acamprosate drug for alcohol misuse 447 used in addition to counselling

acarbose oral drug for diabetes 100

Accolate brand name for zafirlukast (a leukotriene receptor antagonist for asthma 49 and bronchospasm 48)

Accrete D3 brand name for vitamin D 444 (a vitamin 107) with calcium carbonate, a calcium salt (a mineral 108)

Accupro brand name for quinapril (an ACE inhibitor 56)

Accuretic brand name for quinapril (an ACE inhibitor 56) with hydrochlorothiazide 270 (a diuretic 57)

Acea brand name topical gel preparation of metronidazole 325 (an antibiotic 86)

acebutolol beta blocker 55

aceclofenac NSAID 74

acemetacin NSAID 74

acenocoumarol (previously nicoumalone) anticoagulant drug 62

acetaminophen see paracetamol 352

acetazolamide carbonic anhydrase inhibitor diuretic 57 and drug for acute glaucoma 128

acetylcholine parasympathetic nervous system stimulant 44 used as a miotic 130

acetylcysteine mucolytic 52 (also used for paracetamol 352 overdose)

acetylsalicylic acid see aspirin 162

aciclovir 148, antiviral drug 91

Acidex preparations brand-name alginate oral suspension for heartburn and indigestion 66

acipimox lipid-lowering drug 61

acitretin drug for psoriasis 138

Aclasta brand name for zoledronic acid 431 (a drug for bone disorders 80)

aclidinium bromide antimuscarinic bronchodilator 48 used to treat chronic obstructive pulmonary disease

aclidinium with formeterol combined preparation of two bronchodilator drugs 48 for chronic obstructive pulmonary disease

Acnamino brand name for minocycline 327 (a tetracycline antibiotic 86 used for acne 137)

Acnocin brand name for co-cyprindiol, a combined preparation of cyproterone 218 and ethinylestradiol 252 used for acne 137

acrivastine antihistamine 82

Actelsar HCT brand-name antihypertensive 60 containing telmisartan (an angiotensin II blocker 56) with hydrochlorothiazide (a diuretic 57)

Actifed Chesty Coughs brand name for guaifenesin (an expectorant 52) with pseudoephedrine (a decongestant 51) and triprolidine (an antihistamine 82)

Actifed Dry Coughs brand name for dextromethorphan (a cough suppressant 52) with pseudoephedrine (a decongestant 51) and triprolidine (an antihistamine 82)

Actikerall brand name for 5-fluorouracil 261 with salicylic acid (drugs for actinic keratosis)

Actilyse brand name for alteplase 152 (a thrombolytic drug 63)

actinomycin D another name for dactinomycin (an anticancer drug 112)

Action Cold Sore Cream brand name cream containing aciclovir 148 used for cold sores

Actiq brand name for fentanyl (an opioid analgesic 36)

activated charcoal substance used in the emergency treatment of poisoning

Actonel brand name for risedronate 383 (a drug for bone disorders 80)

Actonel Combi brand name for calcium carbonate with calciferol and risedronate 383

Actonel Once a Week brand name for a once-weekly preparation of risedronate 383

Actos brand name for pioglitazone 361 (an oral drug for diabetes 100)

Actrapid brand name for short-acting insulin 284

Acular brand name for ketorolac (a NSAID 74)

Acumor brand name for galantamine (a drug for Alzheimer's disease 43)

ACWY Vax brand-name vaccine 92 to protect against meningococcal infections

Adalat brand name for nifedipine 340 (a calcium-channel blocker anti-angina drug 59 and antihypertensive 60)

Adalat Retard brand name for a modified-release preparation of nifedipine 340 (a calcium-channel blocker, anti-angina drug 59, and antihypertensive 60)

adalimumab DMARD 75

Adanif XL brand name for modified-release nifedipine 340, used for hypertension 60

adapalene retinoid for acne 137

Adartrel brand-name drug containing ropinirole 388 used to treat restless legs

Adasuve brand name for loxapine (an antipsychotic 41) used in treating schizophrenia

Adcal D3 brand name for calcium carbonate 434 (a mineral 107) with vitamin D 444 (a vitamin 107)

Adcetris brand name for brentuximab vedotin (a monoclonal antibody) used to treat cancer

Adcirca brand name for tadalafil 394, a drug used to treat erectile dysfunction 124

Adcortyl brand name for triamcinolone (a corticosteroid 99)

adefovir antiviral drug 91 for chronic hepatitis B

Adempas brand name for riociguat, a drug used for pulmonary hypertension

Adenocor brand name for adenosine (an anti-arrhythmic drug 58)

Adenoscan brand name for adenosine (an anti-arrhythmic drug 58)

adenosine anti-arrhythmic drug 58

Adenuric brand name for febuxostat (a drug for gout 77)

Adepend brand name for naltrexone (a drug for alcohol dependence 24, 447)

Adipine MR and **Adipine XL** brand names for modified-release preparations of nifedipine 340 (a calcium channel blocker 59)

Adizem-SR and **Adizem-XL** brand names for diltiazem 229 (a calcium channel blocker 59)

Adoport brand name for tacrolimus 405 (an immunosuppressant 115)

adrenaline see epinephrine 245, a bronchodilator 48 and drug for glaucoma 128 and cardiac resuscitation and anaphylaxis 512)

Advagraf brand name for tacrolimus 405 (an immunosuppressant 115)

Aerrane brand name for isoflurane (a gaseous general anaesthetic)

afatinib anticancer drug 112

Afinitor brand name for everolimus (an anticancer drug 112)

aflibercept treatment for macular degeneration

agalsidase alfa and beta drugs for metabolic disorders

Aggrastat brand name for tirofiban (antiplatelet drug 62 used to prevent heart attacks)

agomelatine an antidepressant drug 40

Agrippal brand-name influenza vaccine 92

Aidulan brand-name combined oral contraceptive 121 containing ethinylestradiol 252 and gestodene (female sex hormones 105)

Aindeem brand name for finasteride 258, a male sex hormone 104 for benign prostatic hyperplasia 126 and hair loss in men 140

Airomir brand name for salbutamol 391, a bronchodilator 48 used for asthma 49

AirSalb brand name for salbutamol 391, a bronchodilator 48 used for asthma 49

Aizea brand name for desogestrel 222, a progestogen-only oral contraceptive 121

Aknemin brand name for minocycline 327 (a tetracycline antibiotic 86)

Aknemycin Plus brand-name product containing tretinoin (a drug for acne 137) and erythromycin 243 (an antibiotic 86)

Akynzeo brand name for palonosetron with netupitant, a combined preparation used for nausea 46 and inner ear disorders

Alateris brand name for glucosamine

albendazole anthelmintic 97

albiglutide drug for diabetes 100

alclometasone topical corticosteroid 134

Aldactide brand name for co-flumactone (spironolactone 400 with hydroflumethiazide, both diuretics 57)

Aldactone brand name for spironolactone 400 (a potassium-sparing diuretic 57)

Aldara brand name for imiquimod (a drug for genital and perianal warts)

aldesleukin anticancer drug 112

Aldomet brand name for methyldopa (an antihypertensive 60)

Aldurazyme brand-name enzyme preparation used for metabolic disorders

Alecensa brand name for alectinib (an anticancer drug 112 used to treat lung cancer)

alectinib anticancer drug 112 for lung cancer

alemtuzumab monoclonal antibody anticancer drug 112

alendronic acid 149, drug for bone disorders 80

alfacalcidol vitamin D 444 (a vitamin 107)

alfentanil potent injectable analgesic related to fentanyl and used in general anesthesia 36

alfuzosin an alpha blocker 35 for prostate disorders 126

alginates 150 seaweed extracts used to neutralize stomach acids (antacids 66)

alginic acid ingredient combined with antacids 66 to help protect the stomach lining in gastro-oesophageal reflux disease

alimemazine (previously trimeprazine) antihistamine 82 and antipruritic 133

Alimta brand name for pemetrexed (anticancer drug 112)

alirocumab monoclonal antibody used to treat hyperlipidaemia

aliskiren drug used for hypertension 60

alitretinoin oral drug used for severe, chronic hand eczema 139

Alka-Seltzer Original brand-name analgesic 36 and antacid 66 containing aspirin 162, sodium bicarbonate, and citric acid

Allercalm brand name for chlorphenamine 194 (an antihistamine 82)

Aller-Eze brand name for azelastine (a topical antihistamine 82)

Allerief brand name for chlorphenamine 194 (an antihistamine 82) to relieve allergy symptoms

AllerTek brand name for cetirizine 191 (an antihistamine 82)

Alli brand name for orlistat 348 (anti-obesity drug)

allopurinol 151 (a drug for gout 77)

Almogran brand name for almotriptan (a drug for migraine 45)

almotriptan drug for migraine 45

Almuriva brand name for a transdermal patch containing rivastigmine 387 (treatment for Alzheimer's disease 43)

alogliptin drug for diabetes 100

Alomide brand name for lodoxamide (an anti-allergy drug 82)

Aloxi brand name for palonosetron (an anti-emetic 46)

alpha tocopheryl acetate vitamin E 444 (a vitamin 107)

Alphaderm brand name for hydrocortisone 277 (a corticosteroid 99) with urea (an emollient)

Alphagan brand name for brimonidine (a drug for glaucoma 128)

AlphaNine brand name for factor IX (a substance that affects blood clotting 62)

alprazolam benzodiazepine anti-anxiety drug 39

alprostadil prostaglandin used for erectile dysfunction 104, 124

Altacite Plus brand name for hydrotalcite (an antacid 66) with dimeticone (an antifoaming agent 66)

Altargo brand name for retapamulin (an antibacterial 89)

alteplase 152, tissue-type plasminogen activator thrombolytic drug 63

Alu-Cap brand name for aluminium hydroxide 153 (an antacid 66)

Aludrox brand name for aluminium hydroxide 153, magnesium carbonate, and magnesium hydroxide 309 (all antacids 66)

aluminium acetate astringent used for inflammation of the skin or outer ear canal 135; also used in rectal preparations 71

aluminium chloride antiperspirant

aluminium hydroxide 153 (an antacid 66)

Alvedon brand name for paracetamol 352 (a non-opioid analgesic 36)

Alventa XL brand name for venlafaxine 427 (an antidepressant 40)

alverine antispasmodic for irritable bowel syndrome 68

Alvesco brand name for ciclesonide (a corticosteroid for asthma 49)

Alzain brand name for pregabalin (an anticonvulsant 42 also used for neuropathic pain and anxiety disorders)

Alzest brand name for rivastigmine 387, used for Alzheimer's and Parkinson's disease

Alzhok brand name for memantine (a drug used to treat dementia 43)

amantadine antiviral 91 and drug used for parkinsonism 43

Amaryl brand name for glimepiride (an oral drug for diabetes 100)

Ambirix brand-name vaccine 92 against hepatitis A and B

AmBisome brand name for amphotericin 160 (an antifungal 96)

ambrisentan vasodilator 56 used for pulmonary hypertension

Ametop brand name for tetracaine (a local anaesthetic 36)

amfebutamone see bupropion 182 (an adjunct to smoking cessation used with counselling)

Amfexa brand name for dexamfetamine sulfate, a drug used for narcolepsy and attention deficit hyperactivity disorder

Amias brand name for candesartan 182, an angiotensin II blocker (a vasodilator 56 and antihypertensive 60)

amikacin aminoglycoside antibiotic 86

Amikin brand name for amikacin (an aminoglycoside antibiotic 86)

amiloride 154 (a potassium-sparing diuretic 57)

aminophylline a bronchodilator 48 related to theophylline 416

aminosalicylates drugs used for inflammatory bowel disease 70

aminosalicylic acid antibacterial drug used with other antituberculous drugs 90 to treat pulmonary tuberculosis

amiodarone 155, anti-arrhythmic 58

amisulpride 156, antipsychotic 41

Amitiza brand name for lubiprostone (laxative 69)

amitriptyline 157, tricyclic antidepressant 40

amlodipine 158, calcium channel blocker 59

Ammonaps brand name for sodium phenylbutyrate (drug for metabolic disorders)

amorolfine antifungal 96

amoxicillin 159, penicillin antibiotic 86

Amoxil brand name for amoxicillin 159

Amphero XL brand name for venlafaxine 427 (an antidepressant 40)

amphotericin 160, antifungal 96

ampicillin penicillin antibiotic 86

Ampres brand name for chloroprocaine (a local anaesthetic 36)

Amsidine brand name for amsacrine (an anticancer drug 112) used for lymphoma and leukaemia

Anabact brand name for metronidazole 325 (an antibacterial 89)

anagrelide drug for platelet disorders 62

anakinra DMARD 75

anastrozole 161, anticancer drug 112

Ancotil brand name for flucytosine (an antifungal 96)

Androcur brand name for cyproterone 218 (a synthetic anti-androgen 104)

Anectine brand name for suxamethonium (a muscle relaxant 78)

Angeliq brand-name preparation containing estradiol 249 and drospirenone for HRT 149

Angitil SR and **Angitil XL** brand names for diltiazem 229 (a calcium channel blocker 59)

Anhydrol Forte brand name for aluminium chloride (an antiperspirant)

anidulafungin antifungal drug 96 administered intravenously

Anoro Ellipta brand name for umeclidinium with vilanterol (both bronchodilators 48)

Anquil brand name for benperidol (an antipsychotic drug 41)

antazoline an antihistamine 82

anti-D immunoglobulin a drug used to prevent sensitization to Rhesus antigen

antihaemophilic fraction a blood protein used to promote blood clotting in haemophilia 62

Anugesic-HC brand-name preparation for haemorrhoids 71 containing hydrocortisone 277 (a corticosteroid 99)

Anusol branded haemorrhoid preparation 71 with zinc oxide, bismuth, and Peru balsam

APIDRA

Apidra brand name for insulin glulisine 284 (a drug for diabetes 100)

apixaban anti-clotting drug 62 used to prevent venous thromboembolism

apomorphine drug for Parkinson's disease 43

apraclonidine drug for glaucoma 128

apremilast drug that moderates inflammation, used for arthritis 75

aprepitant anti-emetic 46

Apresoline brand name for hydralazine (an antihypertensive 60)

Aprinox brand name for bendroflumethiazide 169 (a thiazide diuretic 57)

Aprokam brand name for cefuroxime (a cephalosporin antibiotic 86)

Aprovel brand name for irbesartan 287, an angiotensin II blocker (a vasodilator 56 and antihypertensive 60)

Aptivus brand name for tipranavir (an antiretroviral for HIV/AIDS 116)

Aquadrate brand name for urea (an emollient)

Aranesp brand name for darbepoetin alfa (a drug for anaemia)

Arava brand name for leflunomide (a DMARD 75)

Arcoxia brand name for etoricoxib (an analgesic 36 and NSAID 74)

Aricept brand name for donepezil 233 (a drug for Alzheimer's disease 43)

Arimidex brand name for anastrozole 161 (a drug for breast cancer 112)

aripiprazole antipsychotic drug 41

Arixtra brand name for fondaparinux (an anticoagulant 62)

Arjun brand name for ear drops containing olive oil

Arkolamyl brand name for olanzapine 344 (an antipsychotic 41) used for schizophrenia, bipolar disorder, and mania

Arlevert brand-name combined preparation containing cinnarizine 198 and dimenhydrinate (an antihistamine 82)

Aromasin brand name for exemestane (a drug for breast cancer 112)

Artelac SDU brand name for hypromellose (artificial tears 130)

artemether antimalarial drug 95

artemether with lumefantrine a combination antimalarial 95

artenimol with piperaquine phosphate a combination antimalarial 95

artesunate an antimalarial 95

Arthrotec branded antirheumatic 75 containing diclofenac 225 with misoprostol 330

articaine local anaesthetic 36

Arythmol brand name for propafenone (an anti-arrhythmic 58)

Arzerra brand name for ofatumumab (a monoclonal antibody anticancer drug 112)

AS Saliva Orthana brand-name artificial saliva

Asacol brand name for mesalazine 317 (a drug for ulcerative colitis 70)

Asasantin brand name for aspirin 162 with dipyridamole 230 (an antiplatelet drug 62)

ascorbic acid vitamin C 443 (a vitamin 107)

asenapine antipsychotic 41 used for manic episodes in bipolar disorder

Aserbine branded product for wound cleaning

Asilone brand name for aluminium hydroxide 153 and magnesium oxide (both antacids 66) with simeticone (an antifoaming agent 66)

Asmabec brand name for beclometasone 168

Asmanex brand name for mometasone 332 (a topical corticosteroid 134)

Asmavent brand name for salbutamol 391 (a bronchodilator 48) used for asthma

aspirin/aspirin dispersible 162, non-opioid analgesic 36 and antiplatelet drug 62

Aspro Clear brand name for soluble aspirin 162 (a non-opioid analgesic 36)

AT 10 brand name for dihydrotachysterol (vitamin D 444)

Atarax brand name for hydroxyzine (an antihistamine 82 and an anti-anxiety drug 39)

atazanavir antiretroviral for HIV/AIDS 116

atenolol 163, beta blocker 55

Atimos modulite brand name for formeterol fumarate (a bronchodilator 48) used for asthma

Ativan brand name for lorazepam 224 (a benzodiazepine, anti-anxiety drug 39, and sleeping drug 38)

atomoxetine drug for attention deficit hyperactivity disorder (ADHD) 44

atorvastatin 164, a lipid-lowering drug 61

atosiban drug to stop premature labour 125

atovaquone antiprotozoal 94 and antimalarial 95

atracurium drug used to relax the muscles in general anaesthesia

Atriance brand name for nelarabine (an anticancer drug 112)

Atripla brand-name drug containing efavirenz 241, emtricitabine 242, and tenofovir 409 used for HIV infection 116

Atrolak brand name for quetiapine 375 (an antipsychotic 41) used for schizophrenia, bipolar disorder, and depression

atropine 165, anticholinergic for irritable bowel syndrome 68 and a mydriatic 130

Atrovent brand name for ipratropium bromide 286 (a bronchodilator 48)

Aubagio brand name for teriflunomide (an immunosuppressant 115) for multiple sclerosis

Audavate brand name for betamethasone 172 (a corticosteroid 99)

Audmonal brand name for alverine (an antispasmodic used to treat irritable bowel syndrome 68)

Augmentin brand name for amoxicillin 159 (a penicillin antibiotic 86) with clavulanic acid (increases the effectiveness of amoxicillin)

Aureocort brand name for chlortetracycline (a tetracycline antibiotic 86) with triamcinolone (a corticosteroid 99)

Aurobeverine brand name for mebeverine 312 (an antispasmodic drug 68 used to treat irritable bowel syndrome)

Autopen preparations brand-name preparations of insulin 284 for injection pens

Avamys brand name for fluticasone 265

avanafil drug for erectile dysfunction 124

Avastin brand name for bevacizumab 173 (an anticancer drug 112)

Avaxim brand-name vaccine 92 to protect against viral hepatitis A

Avelox brand name for moxifloxacin (an antibiotic 86)

avelumab monoclonal antibody used to treat some cancers 112

Aviticol brand name for colecalciferol (vitamin D 444)

Avloclor brand name for chloroquine 193 (an antimalarial 95 and DMARD 75)

Avoca brand name for silver nitrate, used for warts and verrucas

Avodart brand name for dutasteride (a male sex hormone 104 for benign prostatic hypertrophy 126)

Avomine brand name for promethazine 370 (an antihistamine 82 and anti-emetic 46)

Avonex brand name for interferon beta 285 (a drug for multiple sclerosis)

Axalid brand name for pregabalin (anticonvulsant 42 also used for nerve pain 37 and anxiety 39)

axitinib anticancer drug 112 for kidney cancer

Axorid brand-name drug containing ketoprofen 292 and omeprazole 346 used for rheumatic disease and gout 77

Axsain brand name for capsaicin (a rubefacient)

azacitidine anticancer drug 112 used for some types of leukaemia

Azactam brand name for aztreonam (an antibiotic 86)

Azarga brand-name eye drops containing brinzolomide and timolol 417 for glaucoma 128

azathioprine 166, DMARD 75 and immunosuppressant 115

azelaic acid antibacterial 89 for acne 137

azelastine antihistamine 82

azidothymidine zidovudine 430 an antiretroviral for HIV/AIDS 116

Azilect brand name for rasagiline (a drug for parkinsonism 43)

azilsartan medoxomil angiotensin II blocker 56 used for hypertension 60

azithromycin antibiotic 86

Azocan brand name for fluconazole 260 (an antifungal drug 96)

Azopt brand name for brinzolamide 178 (a carbonic anhydrase inhibitor 129 drug used for glaucoma 128)

AZT zidovudine 430 (an antiretroviral for HIV/AIDS 116)

aztreonam antibiotic 86

Azyter brand name for azithromycin (an antibiotic 86)

Azzalure brand name for botulinum toxin 176

B

bacitracin antibiotic 86

baclofen 167, muscle relaxant 73

Bactroban brand name for mupirocin (an antibacterial for skin infections 135)

Balance Activ brand name for lactic acid gel, used to prevent bacterial vaginosis

Balneum products brand name for emollient bath and shower products containing soya

balsalazide drug for ulcerative colitis 70

Bambec brand name for bambuterol (a sympathomimetic bronchodilator 48)

bambuterol sympathomimetic bronchodilator 48

Baraclude brand name for entecavir (an antiviral 91 for hepatitis B)

baricitinib drug used for rheumatoid arthritis 75

basiliximab an immunosuppressant 115

Bavencio brand name for avelumab (a monoclonal antibody) used to treat some types of cancer 112

Beacita brand name for orlistat 348 (an anti-obesity drug 112)

beclometasone 168, corticosteroid 99

Beconase brand name for beclometasone 168 (a corticosteroid 99)

Bedol brand-name preparation for menopausal symptoms 105 containing estradiol 249

Bedranol SR brand name for propranolol 371 (a beta blocker 55)

Beechams Powders brand name for aspirin 162 (a non-opioid analgesic 36) and caffeine

Beechams Powders Capsules brand name for paracetamol 352 (a non-opioid analgesic 36) with phenylephrine (a decongestant 51) and caffeine (a stimulant 44)

belatacept monoclonal antibody used as an immunosuppressant 115 after transplants

belimumab monoclonal antibody used as an immunosuppressant 115 after transplants

Bemfola brand name for follitropin alfa (a drug for infertility 124)

Benadryl brand name for cetirizine 191 (an antihistamine 82)

bendamustine hydrochloride anticancer drug 112 for chronic lymphocytic leukaemia

bendroflumethiazide 169, (previously bendrofluazide) a thiazide diuretic 57

Benepali brand name for etanercept 250 in injectable form, used for severe rheumatoid arthritis and severe psoriasis

Benerva brand name for thiamine 442 used for thiamine deficiencies and related illnesses

Benlysta brand name for belimumab (a monoclonal antibody 114) in intravenous form used for systemic erythematosus lupus

benperidol an antipsychotic 41

benralizumab monoclonal antibody used to treat asthma 49

benserazide drug used to enhance the effect of levodopa 298 (a drug for parkinsonism 43)

Benylin Chesty Cough brand name for guaifenesin (expectorant 52) with levomenthol

benzalkonium chloride antiseptic 135

benzoic acid with salicylic acid combination antifungal product 96 used for ringworm 96

benzoyl peroxide 170, drug for acne 137 and fungal skin infections 96

benzydamine analgesic 46 used in mouthwashes and throat sprays

benzyl benzoate antiparasitic 136

benzylpenicillin also known as penicillin G, a penicillin antibiotic 86

Berlind retard brand name for modified-release indometacin (NSAID 74 used as analgesic 36)

Berocca branded multivitamin preparation 107

Besavar brand name for alfuzosin (an alpha blocker for prostate disorders 126)

Betacap brand name for betamethasone 172 (a corticosteroid 99)

Beta-Cardone brand name for sotalol 399 (a beta blocker 55)

beta carotene vitamin A 442 (a vitamin 107 and food additive)

Betadine brand name for povidone-iodine (an antiseptic 135)

Betaferon brand name for interferon beta 285 (a drug for multiple sclerosis 78)

Betagan brand name for levobunolol (a beta blocker 55 and drug for glaucoma 128)

betahistine 171, drug for Ménière's disease 46

Betaloc brand name for metoprolol 324 (a beta blocker 55)

betamethasone 172, corticosteroid 99

Beta-Prograne brand name for propranolol 371 (a beta blocker 55)

betaxolol beta blocker 55 also used in glaucoma 128

bethanechol parasympathomimetic for urinary retention 126 and paralytic ileus

Betmiga brand name for mirabegron, an antimuscarinic drug used to treat urinary frequency 126

Betnesol preparations branded ear, eye, and nose drops containing betamethasone 172

Betnovate brand name for betamethasone 172 (a corticosteroid 99)

Betoptic brand-name drug for glaucoma 128 containing betaxolol

Bettamousse brand name for betamethasone 172 (a corticosteroid 99)

bevacizumab 173, anticancer drug 112

bexarotene anticancer drug 112

Bexsero branded vaccine 92 for meningitis B

bezafibrate 174, lipid-lowering drug 61

Bezalip brand name for bezafibrate 174 (a lipid-lowering drug 61)

bicalutamide anticancer drug 112

bilastine antihistamine 82 used for allergic rhinitis and urticaria

Bilxona brand name for gliclazide 270 (a drug for diabetes 100)

bimatoprost drug for glaucoma 128

Bimizza brand-name combined oral contraceptive 121 containing ethinylestradiol 252 and desogestrel 222

Binosto brand name for alendronic acid 149 used for osteoporosis 80

Biotène Oralbalance brand name for artificial saliva

biotin 434, vitamin 107

BioXtra brand-name oral preparation for treating a dry mouth

Biquelle XL brand name for quetiapine 375 (an antipsychotic 41) used for psychoses and schizophrenia

bisacodyl stimulant laxative 69

bisoprolol 175, a beta blocker 55

bivalirudin anticlotting drug 62 used to prevent thromboembolism

Bleo-Kyowa brand name for bleomycin, a cytotoxic antibiotic for cancer 112

bleomycin cytotoxic antibiotic for cancer 112

Blephlagel brand-name eye gel containing carbomer (a lubricant) used for dry eyes

Blerone XL brand name for tolterodine 420 (an antimuscarinic used for urinary frequency 126)

Blincyto brand name for blinatumomab (an anticancer drug 112) used to treat leukaemia

boceprevir antiviral 91 for hepatitis C

Bocouture brand name for botulinum toxin 176 (a muscle relaxant 78)

Bolamyn SR brand name for modified-release metformin 318 (a drug for diabetes 100)

Bondronat brand name for ibandronic acid (a drug for bone disorders 80)

Bonefos brand name for sodium clodronate (a drug to control high blood calcium in cancer patients 112)

Bonjela brand name for choline salicylate (similar to aspirin 162) and cetalkonium chloride for cold sores, mouth ulcers, and teething pain

Bonjela Teething Gel brand-name preparation containing lidocaine (a local anaesthetic 36) and cetalkonium (an antiseptic 135)

Bonviva brand name for ibandronic acid (a drug for bone disorders 80)

Boostrix-IPV brand-name vaccine 92 for diphtheria, pertussis, poliomyelitis, and tetanus

Boots Allergy Relief brand name for chlorphenamine 194 (an antihistamine 82)

Boots Antibiotic Eye Drops brand name for eye drops containing chloramphenicol 192

Boots Anti-Dandruff Ketoconazole Shampoo brand-name shampoo containing ketoconazole 291 (an antifungal 96)

Boots Avert brand name for aciclovir 148 (an antiviral 91)

Boots Diareze brand name for loperamide 305 (an antidiarrhoeal 68)

Boots Hair Loss Treatment brand name for minoxidil 328 (a drug for hair loss 140)

Boots Hayfever and Allergy Relief All Day brand name for cetirizine 191 (an antihistamine 82)

Boots Heartburn Relief Tablets brand-name preparation for heartburn and indigestion containing ranitidine 380

Boots IBS Relief brand-name drug for irritable bowel syndrome 68 containing mebeverine 312

Boots Threadworm Tablets brand name for mebendazole 311 (an anthelmintic 97)

Boots Thrush Cream brand-name cream containing clotrimazole 209 (an antifungal 96)

boric acid with salicylic acid and tannic acid combined antifungal preparation 96 used for fungal nail infections

borneol with camphene, cineole, menthol, menthone, and pinene combined drug used for liver disorders

bortezomib anticancer drug 112

bosentan drug for pulmonary arterial hypertension

Bosulif brand name for bosutinib (an anticancer drug 112 used for certain types of leukaemia)

bosutinib anticancer drug 112 used for certain types of leukaemia

Botox brand name for botulinum toxin 176 (a muscle relaxant 78)

botulinum toxin 176, a muscle relaxant 78

Braltus brand name for tiotropium 418 (a bronchodilator drug used for asthma 49)

Bramitob brand name for tobramycin (an antibiotic 86)

Bramox brand name for midodrine, a vasoconstrictor used for hypotension (low blood pressure)

Brancico brand name for quetiapine 375 (an antipsychotic drug 41)

Brasivol branded abrasive paste for acne 137

Bravelle brand name for urofollitropin (a gonadotrophin drug for female infertility 124)

brentuximab a monoclonal antibody 113 used for cancer

Brevibloc brand name for esmolol (a beta blocker 55)

Brevinor brand-name oral contraceptive 121 containing ethinylestradiol 252 and norethisterone 342

Brevoxyl brand name for benzoyl peroxide (a drug for acne 137)

Brexidol brand name for piroxicam 362 (a NSAID 74)

Bricanyl brand name for terbutaline 411 (a bronchodilator 48 and drug used in premature labour 125)

Brilique brand name for ticagrelor (an antiplatelet drug 62) used for heart problems

brimonidine tartrate 177, drug for glaucoma 128

Brintellix brand name for vortioxetine (an antidepressant 40)

brinzolamide 178, drug for glaucoma 128

BritLofex brand name for lofexidine, a drug for opioid withdrawal symptoms 24

brivaracetam anticonvulsant 42

Briviact brand name for brivaracetam (an anticonvulsant 42)

Brochlor brand name for chloramphenicol 192

Brolene brand name for propamidine isethionate (an antibacterial 89) for eye infections

bromfenac NSAID 74 for eye inflammation

bromocriptine 179, pituitary agent 103 and drug for parkinsonism 43

brompheniramine antihistamine 82

Bronchitol brand name for mannitol in powder form, used for cystic fibrosis

Brufen and **Brufen Retard** brand names for ibuprofen 279 (a NSAID 74)

Brymont brand name for brimonidine tartrate 177 (a drug for glaucoma 128)

Buccastem brand name for prochlorperazine 366 (an anti-emetic 46)

BUCCOLAM

Buccolam brand name for midazolam (a benzodiazepine 38)

buclizine antihistamine 82 and anti-emetic 46 used for motion sickness

Budelin brand name for budesonide 180 (a corticosteroid 99)

Budenofalk brand name for budesonide 180 (a corticosteroid 99)

budesonide 180, corticosteroid 99

Bufyl brand name for bupivacaine (a local anaesthetic 36) with fentanyl (an opioid analgesic 36)

bumetanide 181, loop diuretic 57

Bupeaze brand name for buprenorphine (an opioid analgesic 36)

bupivacaine long-lasting local anaesthetic 36 used in labour 125

Buplast brand name for buprenorphine (an opioid analgesic 36)

Bupramyl brand name for a transdermal patch containing buprenorphine (opioid analgesic 36)

buprenorphine strong opioid analgesic 36

bupropion 182, an antidepressant used as an aid to smoking cessation with counselling

BurnEze brand name for benzocaine (a local anaesthetic 36)

Buscopan brand name for hyoscine butylbromide 278 (an antispasmodic for irritable bowel syndrome 68)

buserelin drug for menstrual disorders 120 and prostate cancer 112

Busilvex brand name for busulfan (an alkylating agent used for some leukaemias 112)

buspirone non-benzodiazepine anti-anxiety drug 39

busulfan alkylating agent used for certain leukaemias 112

Butec brand name for buprenorphine (an opioid analgesic 36)

BuTrans brand name for buprenorphine (an opioid analgesic 36)

butylcyanoacrylate a tissue and skin adhesive for closing wounds

Bydureon brand name for exenatide 254 (a drug for diabetes 100)

Byetta brand name for exenatide 254 (a drug for diabetes 100)

C

Cabaser brand name for cabergoline (a drug for parkinsonism 43)

cabazitaxel anticancer drug 112 used for prostate cancer

cabergoline drug for parkinsonism 43 and endocrine disorders 103

cabozantinib anticancer drug 112 used for thyroid cancer

cabzitaxel anticancer drug 112 used for prostate cancer

Cacit brand of calcium carbonate (a mineral 108)

Caelyx brand name for doxorubicin 237 (a cytotoxic anticancer drug 112)

caffeine stimulant 44 in coffee, tea, and cola drinks, added to some analgesics 36

Cala Soothe brand-name barrier cream

calamine substance containing zinc carbonate (an antipruritic 133) to soothe irritated skin

Calceos brand name for colecalciferol (vitamin D 444, a vitamin 107) and calcium carbonate (a mineral 108)

Calcichew preparations brand-name calcium carbonate products used for kidney failure, hyperphosphataemia, and calcium deficiency

calciferol vitamin D 444 (a vitamin 107)

calcipotriol 183, drug for psoriasis 138

calcitonin drug for bone disorders 80

calcitonin (salmon) (previously salcatonin) drug for bone disorders 80

calcitriol vitamin D 444 (a vitamin 107)

calcium 434, mineral 108

calcium acetate, chloride, and gluconate salts of calcium 434 (a mineral 108)

calcium carbonate calcium salt (a mineral 108) used as an antacid 66

calcium resonium drug to lower the amount of potassium in the blood

Calcort brand name for deflazacort (a corticosteroid 99, 134)

Calfovit D3 brand name for colecalciferol (vitamin D 444) with calcium phosphate 426 used for calcium and vitamin D deficiency

Calgel brand-name teething gel containing lidocaine (a local anaesthetic 36) and cetylpyridinium (an antibacterial 89)

Calmurid HC brand-name substance for eczema 139 containing hydrocortisone 277, lactic acid, and urea (an emollient)

Calpol brand name for paracetamol 352 (a non-opioid analgesic 36)

Calprofen brand name for ibuprofen 279

Camcolit brand name for lithium 303 (a drug for mania 41)

Campral EC brand name for acamprosate (a drug for alcohol abuse 447)

Campto brand name for irinotecan (an anticancer drug 112)

canagliflozin drug for diabetes 100

canagliflozin with metformin a combination of two drugs for diabetes 100

canakinumab monoclonal antibody immunosuppressant 115 used for gout 77 and certain immune system disorders

Cancidas brand name for caspofungin (an antifungal 96)

candesartan 184, angiotensin II blocker (a vasodilator 56 and antihypertensive 60)

Canesten brand name for clotrimazole 209 (an antifungal 96)

Canesten HC brand name for clotrimazole 209 (an antifungal 96) with hydrocortisone 277 (a corticosteroid 99)

Canesten Oral brand name for fluconazole 260 (an antifungal 96)

cangrelor an anticlotting drug 62 used with aspirin 162 to reduce the risk of blood clots

cannabidiol 185, phytocannabinoid used to treat epilepsy 42

cannabis drug of abuse 450

Capasal brand-name coal tar shampoo for dandruff 140 and psoriasis 138

Capastat brand name for capreomycin sulphate (an antituberculous drug 90)

capecitabine antimetabolite anticancer drug 112

Capexion brand name for tacrolimus 405 (an immunosuppressant 115)

Capimune brand name for ciclosporin 196 (an immunosuppressant 115)

Capoten brand name for captopril 186 (an ACE inhibitor 56)

Capozide brand name for captopril 186 (an ACE inhibitor 56) with hydrochlorothiazide 270 (a thiazide diuretic 57)

Caprelsa brand name for vandetanib (an anticancer drug 112) used for thyroid cancer

capreomycin antituberculous drug 90

capsaicin the active agent in chilli peppers used for topical pain relief

Capsorin brand name for ciclosporin 196 (an immunosuppressant 115)

captopril 186, an ACE inhibitor 56

Carac brand-name cream for fluorouracil 261 (an anti-cancer drug 112)

Carace Plus brand name for lisinopril 302 and hydrochlorothiazide 270 (a thiazide diuretic 57)

Caramet CR brand name for modified-release carbidopa, used for Parkinson's disease 43

Carbagen SR brand name for carbamazepine 187 (an anticonvulsant 42)

Carbaglu brand name for carglumic acid, a drug used for certain metabolic disorders

carbamazepine 187, anticonvulsant 42 and antipsychotic 41

carbetocin drug to control bleeding after childbirth 125

carbidopa substance that enhances the effect of levodopa 298 (a drug for parkinsonism 43)

carbimazole 188, antithyroid drug 102

carbocisteine mucolytic 52

Carbomix brand name for activated charcoal used to treat poisoning

carboplatin anticancer drug 112

carboprost drug to control bleeding after childbirth 125

Cardene brand name for nicardipine (a calcium channel blocker 59)

Cardicor brand name for bisoprolol 175 (a beta blocker 55)

Cardide SR brand name for modified-release indapamide 282 (a diuretic drug 57) used for hypertension 60

Cardioplen brand name for felodipine 256 (calcium channel blocker 59)

Cardioxane brand name for dexrazoxane, to treat side effects of cytotoxic anticancer drugs

Cardozin XL brand name for modified-release doxazosin 236 (an alpha-blocker antihypertensive 60)

Cardura brand name for doxazosin 236 (an antihypertensive 60, also used for prostate disorders 126)

Cardura XL brand-name modified-release preparation of doxazosin 236

Care Clotrimazole Cream brand name for clotrimazole 209 (an antifungal 96)

Care Fluconazole brand name for fluconazole 260 (an antifungal 96)

Carexil brand name for oxycodone (an opioid analgesic 36)

carglumic acid amino acid used for certain metabolic disorders

carisoprodol a muscle relaxant 78 related to meprobamate

Carmeleze brand name for carmellose sodium eye drops used for dry eyes

carmellose sodium lubricant drops for dry eyes

Carmil XL brand name for modified-release isosorbide mononitrate 289 (a nitrate vasodilator 56 and anti-angina drug 59)

Carmize brand name for carmellose sodium eye drops used for dry eyes

carmustine an alkylating agent for Hodgkin's disease and solid tumours 112

Carnitor brand name for carnitine (an amino acid used as a nutritional supplement 106)

carteolol beta blocker 55 for glaucoma 128

carvedilol beta blocker 55

Casodex brand name for bicalutamide (an anticancer drug 112)

caspofungin antifungal 96

castor oil stimulant laxative 69

Catacrom brand-name eye drops containing sodium cromoglicate 397

CLIOQUINOL

Catapres brand name for clonidine (an antihypertensive 60 and drug for migraine 45)

catumaxomab monoclonal antibody used for malignant ascites in cancer patients

Caverject brand name for alprostadil (a prostaglandin for erectile dysfunction 104, 124)

Cayston brand name for powder and solvent forms of aztreonam (an antibiotic 86) for use in nebulizers

Ceanel brand-name shampoo for dandruff 140 and psoriasis 138

cefaclor cephalosporin antibiotic 86

cefadroxil cephalosporin antibiotic 86

cefalexin 189, a cephalosporin antibiotic 86

cefixime cephalosporin antibiotic 86

cefotaxime cephalosporin antibiotic 86

cefradine cephalosporin antibiotic 86

ceftaroline fosamil cephalosporin antibiotic 86 used for pneumonia and skin infections

ceftazidime cephalosporin antibiotic 86

ceftobiprole cephalosporin antibiotic 86

ceftriaxone cephalosporin antibiotic 86

cefuroxime cephalosporin antibiotic 86

Celebrex brand name for celecoxib 190 (an NSAID 74)

celecoxib 190 NSAID 74

Celectol brand name for celiprolol (a beta blocker 55)

Celevac brand name for methylcellulose 321 (a laxative 69 and antidiarrhoeal 68)

celiprolol beta blocker 55

CellCept brand name for mycophenolate mofetil (an immunosuppressant 115)

Cellusan brand name for carmellose (artificial tears 130)

Celluvisc brand name for carmellose (artificial tears 130)

Celsentri brand name for maraviroc (a drug for HIV 116)

Ceporex brand name for cefalexin 189 (a cephalosporin antibiotic 86)

Ceprotin brand name for protein C concentrate (a blood product to promote blood clotting 62)

Ceptava brand name for mycophenolate (a drug used to prevent rejection in transplants)

Cepton brand name for chlorhexidine (an antiseptic 135) used for acne 137

Cerazette brand-name oral contraceptive 121 containing desogestrel 222 (a female sex hormone 105)

Cerelle brand-name oral contraceptive 121 containing desogestrel 222 (a female sex homone 105)

Cerezyme brand name for imiglucerase (an enzyme for replacement therapy)

ceritinib anticancer drug 112 for lung cancer

Certican brand name for everolimus (a protein kinase inhibitor anticancer drug 112) to help prevent organ rejection after liver transplant

certolizumab pegol antibody-drug for rheumatoid arthritis 75 and psoriatic arthritis

Cerumol brand-name preparation for ear wax removal 131

Cervarix brand-name human papillomavirus vaccine 92

cetirizine 191, an antihistamine 82

Cetraxal brand name for antibiotic eardrops containing ciprofloxacin 199 (a quinolone antibacterial 89)

Cetraben brand-name bath additive containing liquid paraffin for dry and scaling skin disorders

cetrimide antiseptic 135

cetrorelix drug for infertility 124

Cetrotide brand name for cetrorelix (a drug for infertility 124)

cetuximab anticancer drug 112

Champix brand name for varenicline 426 (a drug used as a smoking cessation aid)

Charcodote brand name for activated charcoal used to treat poisoning

Chemydur brand name for isosorbide mononitrate 289 (a nitrate vasodilator 56 anti-angina drug 59)

Chirocaine brand name for lignocaine (a local anaesthetic 36)

chloral hydrate sleeping drug 38

chlorambucil anticancer drug 112 used for chronic lymphocytic leukaemia and lymphatic and ovarian cancers, and immunosuppressant 115 for rheumatoid arthritis 75

chloramphenicol 192, antibiotic 86

chlordiazepoxide benzodiazepine anti-anxiety drug 39

chlorhexidine antiseptic 135

Chloromycetin brand name for chloramphenicol 192 (an antibiotic 86)

chloroquine 193, antimalarial 95 and DMARD 75

chlorphenamine (chlorpheniramine) 194, an antihistamine 82

chlorpromazine 195, phenothiazine antipsychotic 41 and anti-emetic 46

chlortalidone thiazide diuretic 57

chlortetracycline with triamcinolone topical preparation containing an antibiotic 86 and a corticosteroid 134 used to treat severe inflammatory skin disorders

Cholestagel brand name for colesevelam hydrochloride (a lipid-lowering drug 61) used for hyperlipidaemia

Cholib brand-name lipid-lowering drug 61 containing simvastatin 395 and fenofibrate (a fibrate drug) used for hyperlipidaemia

cholic acid bile acid used for biliary disorders

choline salicylate drug similar to aspirin 162 used in pain-relieving mouth gels 36 and ear drops 131

Cholurso brand name for ursodeoxycholic acid (used for cirrhosis of the liver and gallstones)

Choragon brand name for chorionic gonadotrophin (a drug for infertility 124)

choriogonadotropin alfa drug for infertility 124

chorionic gonadotrophin drug for infertility 124

chromium 435, mineral 108

Cialis brand name for tadalafil 394 (a drug for erectile dysfunction 124)

ciclesonide corticosteroid used for asthma 49

ciclosporin 196, immunosuppressant 115

Cidomycin brand name for gentamicin 268 (an aminoglycoside antibiotic 86)

cilastatin enzyme inhibitor used to make imipenem (an antibiotic 86) more effective

cilazapril ACE inhibitor 56

Cilest brand-name oral contraceptive 121 containing ethinylestradiol 252 and norgestimate (both female sex hormones 105)

Cilique brand-name oral contraceptive 121 containing ethinylestradiol 252 and norgestimate (both female sex hormones 105)

Cilodex brand name for ear drops containing ciprofloxacin 199 and dexamethasone 223 used for ear infections

cilostazol vasodilator 56

Ciloxan brand name for ciprofloxacin 199 (a quinolone antibacterial 89)

cimetidine 197, anti-ulcer drug 67

Cimizt brand-name combined oral contraceptive 121 containing ethinylestradiol 252 and desogestrel 222

Cimzia brand name for certolizumab pegol (an immunosuppressant 115) used for arthritis

cinacalcet calcium-regulating drug used to reduce calcium levels in overactivity of the parathyroid glands

cinchocaine local anaesthetic 36

cinnarizine 198, antihistamine anti-emetic 46

Cinqaero brand name for reslizumab (a monoclonal antibody) for severe asthma 49

cinryze drug for treating angioedema (a type of severe allergic reaction)

Cipralex brand name for escitalopram 201 (an antidepressant 40)

Cipramil brand name for citalopram 201 (an antidepressant 40)

ciprofibrate lipid-lowering drug 61

ciprofloxacin 199, quinolone antibacterial 89

Ciproxin brand name for ciprofloxacin 199 (a quinolone antibacterial 89)

Circadin brand name for melatonin (a hormone) used as a sleeping drug 38 to treat insomnia

cisatracurium drug used to relax the muscles in general anaesthesia

cisplatin 200, anticancer drug 112

citalopram 201, antidepressant 40

Citanest brand name for prilocaine (a local anaesthetic 36)

CitraFleet brand-name stimulant laxative 69

Citramag brand name for magnesium citrate (an osmotic laxative 69)

citric acid simple linctus used for coughs 52

cladribine anticancer drug 112

Clairette brand-name combined preparation containing ethinylestradiol 252 and cyproterone 218 used for acne 137

Clarelux brand name for clobetasol 204 (a topical corticosteroid 134)

Clarie XL brand name for modified-release clarithromycin 202 (a macrolide antibiotic 86)

clarithromycin 202, a macrolide antibiotic 86

Clarityn brand name for loratadine 307 (an antihistamine 82)

Clarityn Allergy brand name for loratadine 307 (an antihistamine 82)

Clasteon brand name for sodium clodronate (a bisphosphonate used for bone disorders 80)

clavulanic acid substance to enhance the effect of amoxicillin 159 (a penicillin antibiotic 86)

clemastine antihistamine 82

Clenil Modulite brand name for beclometasone (a corticosteroid 99)

clevidipine calcium channel blocker 59 used for hypertension 60

Cleviprex brand name for clevidipine (a calcium channel blocker) used for hypertension 60

Clexane brand name for enoxaparin (a low-molecular-weight heparin 275, an anticoagulant 62)

Climagest brand-name preparation for menopausal symptoms 105 containing estradiol 249 and norethisterone 342

Climanor brand name for medroxypro-gesterone 306 (a female sex hormone 105)

Climaval brand-name preparation for menopausal symptoms 105 containing estradiol 249

clindamycin 203, lincosamide antibiotic 86

Clinitar brand name for coal tar (a substance used to treat psoriasis 138 and dandruff 140)

Clinitas brand name for sodium hyaluronate eye drops used for dry eyes

Clinitas Carbomer brand name for carbomer eye drops used for dry eyes

Clinorette brand-name preparation containing estradiol 249 with norethisterone 342 (both female sex hormones 105)

clioquinol antibacterial 89 and antifungal 96 for outer ear infections 131

CLIPPER

Clipper brand name for beclometasone 168 (a corticosteroid 99)

Clivarine brand name for reviparin (a type of heparin 275, an anticoagulant 62)

ClobaDerm brand name for clobetasol 204 (a topical corticosteroid 134)

Clobavate brand name for clobetasone (a topical corticosteroid 134) used for psoriasis 138 and eczema 139

clobazam benzodiazepine anti-anxiety drug 39 and anticonvulsant 42

clobetasol 204, topical corticosteroid 134

clobetasone topical corticosteroid 134

clofarabine anticancer drug 112

clofazimine drug for leprosy 89

clomethiazole non-benzodiazepine, non-barbiturate sleeping drug 38

Clomid brand name for clomifene 205 (a drug for infertility 124)

clomifene 205, drug for infertility 124

clomipramine 206, tricyclic antidepressant 40

clonazepam 207, benzodiazepine anticonvulsant 42

clonidine antihypertensive 60 and drug for migraine 45

clopamide thiazide diuretic 57

clopidogrel 208, antiplatelet drug 62

Clopixol brand name for zuclopenthixol (an antipsychotic 41)

Clotam brand name for tolfenamic acid (a drug for migraine 45)

clotrimazole 209, antifungal 96

clozapine 210, antipsychotic 41

Clozaril brand name for clozapine 210 (an antipsychotic 41)

coal tar substance for psoriasis 138 and eczema 139

co-amilofruse generic product containing amiloride 154 with furosemide 266 (both diuretics 57)

co-amilozide generic product containing amiloride 154 with hydrochlorothiazide 270 (both diuretics 57)

co-amoxiclav generic product containing amoxicillin 159 (a penicillin antibiotic 86) with clavulanic acid (a substance that increases the effectiveness of amoxicillin)

CoAprovel brand name for irbesartan 287 (an antihypertensive 60) with hydrochlorothiazide (a thiazide diuretic 57)

Cobalin-H brand name for hydroxocobalamin (a vitamin 107)

co-beneldopa generic product containing levodopa 298 (a drug for parkinsonism 43) with benserazide (a drug that enhances the effect of levodopa)

cobicistat drug for HIV/AIDS 116

cobimetinib anticancer drug 112

cocaine local anaesthetic 36 and drug of abuse 451

co-careldopa generic product containing levodopa 298 (a drug for parkinsonism 43) with carbidopa (a drug that enhances the effect of levodopa)

co-codamol generic product containing codeine 211 with paracetamol 352 (both analgesics 36)

co-cyprindiol generic product containing cyproterone 218 (an anti-androgen 104) with ethinylestradiol 252 (female sex hormone 105)

co-danthramer generic product containing dantron with poloxamer (both stimulant laxatives 69)

co-danthrusate generic product containing dantron with docusate (both stimulant laxatives 69)

codeine 211, opioid analgesic 36, cough suppressant 52, and antidiarrhoeal 68

Co-Diovan brand name for hydrochlorothiazide 270 with valsartan 390 used to control hypertension 60

Codipar brand name for codeine 211 with paracetamol 352 (both analgesics 36)

Codis brand-name product containing aspirin 162 and codeine 211 (both analgesics 36)

co-dydramol generic product containing paracetamol 352 with dihydrocodeine 228 (both analgesics 36)

co-fluampicil generic product containing flucloxacillin 259 with ampicillin (both penicillin antibiotics 86)

co-flumactone generic product containing hydroflumethiazide with spironolactone 400 (both diuretics 57)

Colazide brand name for balsalazide (a drug for ulcerative colitis 70)

colchicine 212, drug for gout 77

cold cream antipruritic 133

colecalciferol vitamin D 444 (a vitamin 107)

Colestid brand name for colestipol (a lipid-lowering drug 61)

colestipol lipid-lowering drug 61

colestyramine 213, lipid-lowering drug 61

Colief brand name for lactase, used to relieve symptoms of lactose intolerance in infants

Colifoam brand name for hydrocortisone 277 (a corticosteroid 99)

colistimethate injection form of colistin (an antibiotic 86)

colistin antibiotic 86

collodion substance that dries to form a sticky film, protecting broken skin 132

Colofac brand name for mebeverine 312 (an antispasmodic drug for irritable bowel syndrome 68)

Colofac IBS brand name for mebeverine 312 (an antispasmodic drug for irritable bowel syndrome 68)

Colofac MR brand name for mebeverine 312 (an antispasmodic drug for irritable bowel syndrome 68)

Colomycin brand name for colistin (an antibiotic 86)

Colpermin brand name for peppermint oil (a substance for indigestion 66 and spasm of the bowel 68)

co-magaldrox generic product containing aluminium hydroxide 153 with magnesium hydroxide 309 (both antacids 66)

Combigan brand-name preparation for glaucoma 128 containing brimonidine 177 with timolol 417 (a beta blocker 55)

Combivent brand-name inhaler containing salbutamol 391 and ipratropium bromide 286 (both bronchodilators 48)

Combivir brand-name preparation containing zidovudine/lamivudine 430 (antiretrovirals used for HIV/AIDS 116)

Combodart brand-name preparation containing tamsulosin 407 (a male sex hormone 104) and dutasteride (a male sex hormone 104) used to treat urinary retention 126

Competact brand-name preparation containing metformin 318 and pioglitazone 361 (both oral drugs for diabetes 100)

Compound W brand-name keratolytic 140 for warts, containing salicylic acid

Comtess brand name for entacapone (a drug for parkinsonism 43)

Concerta XL brand name for methylphenidate 322 (a nervous system stimulant 44)

Condyline brand name for podophyllotoxin (a drug for genital warts)

Congescor brand name for bisoprolol 175 (a beta-blocker 55)

conjugated oestrogens 214, female sex hormone 105 and drug for bone disorders 80

Conotrane brand name for benzalkonium chloride (an antiseptic 135) with dimeticone (a base for skin preparations 135)

Consion XL brand name for galantamine for attention deficit hyperactivity disorder (ADHD)

Constella brand name for linaclotide (a laxative 69)

Contiflo XL brand name for tamsulosin 407 (a drug for urinary retention 126)

Convulex brand name for sodium valproate 398 (an anticonvulsant 42)

Copaxone brand name for glatiramer (a drug for multiple sclerosis)

Copegus brand name for ribavirin (an antiviral 91)

co-phenotrope 215, generic antidiarrhoeal drug 68 containing diphenoxylate with atropine 165

copper 435, mineral 108

Coracten brand name for nifedipine 340 (an anti-angina drug 59 and antihypertensive 60)

Cordarone X brand name for amiodarone 155 (an anti-arrhythmic 58)

Corgard brand name for nadolol (a beta blocker 55)

Coro-Nitro brand name for glyceryl trinitrate 272 (an anti-angina drug 59)

Corsodyl brand-name mouthwash and oral gel containing chlorhexidine (an antiseptic 135)

corticotrophin a pituitary hormone 103

Cortiment brand name for budesonide 180 (a corticosteroid 99)

cortisol previous name for hydrocortisone 277

cortisone corticosteroid 99

Cosentyx brand name for secukinumab (a monoclonal antibody antirheumatic drug 75)

co-simalcite generic product containing hydrotalcite (an antacid 66) with dimeticone (an antifoaming agent 66)

Cositam XL brand name for tamsulosin 407 (an alpha-blocker drug used to treat benign prostatic hyperplasia 104)

CosmoCol brand name for macrogol 69 (a laxative 69)

CosmoFer brand name for iron dextran (iron 437, a mineral 108)

Cosopt brand-name preparation containing dorzolamide 234 and timolol 417 (drugs for glaucoma 128)

Cotellic brand name for cobimetinib (an anticancer drug 112) used for skin cancer

co-tenidone generic product containing atenolol 163 (a beta blocker 55) with chlortalidone (a thiazide diuretic 57)

co-triamterzide generic product containing hydrochlorothiazide 276 with triamterene 423 (both diuretics 57)

co-trimoxazole 216, generic product containing trimethoprim 424 with sulfamethoxazole (an antibacterial 89 and antiprotozoal 94)

Covermark brand name for a masking cream for skin disfigurement

Coversyl brand name for perindopril 354 (an ACE inhibitor 56)

Covonia brand-name medicine for coughs

Cozaar brand name for losartan 308 (an antihypertensive 60)

Cozaar-Comp brand-name preparation containing losartan 308 and hydrochlorothiazide 269 (a thiazide diuretic 57)

DEQUALINIUM

Co-zidocapt brand-name preparation containing captopril 186 (an ACE inhibitor vasodilator 56) and hydrochlorthiazide 269 (a thiazide diuretic 57)

Creon brand name for pancreatin (a preparation of pancreatic enzymes 72)

Cresemba brand name for isavuconazole (an antifungal drug 96)

Crestor brand name for rosuvastatin 389 (a lipid-lowering drug 61)

Crinone brand name for progesterone (a female sex hormone 105)

crisantaspase anticancer drug 112

Crixivan brand name for indinavir (antiretroviral for HIV/AIDS 116)

crizotinib tyrosine kinase inhibitor anticancer drug 112

cromoglicate 389, anti-allergy drug 82

Cromolux brand name for eye drops containing sodium cromoglicate 397

crotamiton antipruritic 133 and antiparasitic 136 for scabies

Crystacide brand name for hydrogen peroxide cream (an antiseptic 135)

Cubicin brand name for daptomycin (an antibiotic 86)

Cuplex brand-name wart preparation that contains copper acetate, lactic acid, and salicylic acid

Cuprofen Plus brand-name preparation containing ibuprofen 279 (an NSAID 74) and codeine 211 (an opioid analgesic 36)

Curasept brand-name mouthwash containing chlorhexidine (an antiseptic 135)

Curatoderm brand name for tacalcitol (a drug for psoriasis 138)

Curosurf brand name for poractant alfa (used to mature the lungs of premature babies)

Cutivate brand-name ointment containing fluticasone 265 (a corticosteroid 99)

cyanocobalamin vitamin B12 443 (a vitamin 107)

Cyclimorph brand name for morphine 334 (an opioid analgesic 36) with cyclizine (an anti-emetic 46)

cyclizine antihistamine 82 used as an anti-emetic 46

Cyclogest brand name for progesterone (a female sex hormone 105)

cyclopenthiazide thiazide diuretic 57

cyclopentolate anticholinergic mydriatic 130

cyclophosphamide 217, an anticancer drug 112

Cyclo-Progynova brand name for estradiol 249 with levonorgestrel 300 (both female sex hormones 105)

cycloserine antibiotic 86 used to treat tuberculosis 90

Cyklokapron brand name for tranexamic acid (an antifibrinolytic to promote blood clotting 62)

Cymalon brand-name preparation for cystitis 126 containing sodium bicarbonate, citric acid, sodium citrate, and sodium carbonate

Cymbalta brand name for duloxetine (an antidepressant 40 and drug for diabetic neuropathy)

Cymevene brand name for ganciclovir (an antiviral 91)

cyproheptadine antihistamine 82 and drug for migraine 45

Cyprostat brand name for cyproterone 218 (an anti-androgen 104)

cyproterone 218, synthetic anti-androgen 104

Cyramza brand name for ramucirumab (a monoclonal antibody anticancer drug 112)

Cystagon brand name for mercaptamine (a drug used for a metabolic disorder)

Cysticide brand name for praziquantel (an anthelmintic 97)

Cystopurin brand name for potassium citrate (used for cystitis 126)

Cystrin brand name for oxybutynin 351 (a drug for urinary disorders 126)

Cytacon brand name for cyanocobalamin (vitamin B12 443)

Cytamen brand name for cyanocobalamin (vitamin B12 443)

cytarabine drug for leukaemia 112

Cytotec brand name for misoprostol 330 (an anti-ulcer drug 67)

Cytoxan brand name for cyclophosphamide 217 (an anticancer drug 112)

D

dabigatran 219, anticoagulant 62

dabrafenib anticancer drug 112 for skin cancer

Dacadis MR brand name for modified-release gliclazide 270 (a drug for diabetes 100)

dacarbazine drug for malignant melanoma and cancer of soft tissues 112

daclatasvir antiviral 91 for chronic hepatitis C

Dacogen brand name for decitabine (a cytotoxic anticancer drug 112) used for leukaemia

Daklinza brand name for daclatasvir (an antiviral 91) used for chronic hepatitis C

Daktacort brand name for hydrocortisone 277 (a corticosteroid 99) with miconazole 326 (an antifungal 96)

Daktarin brand name for miconazole 326 (an antifungal 96)

Dalacin brand name for clindamycin 203 (a lincosamide antibiotic 86)

Dalacin C brand name for clindamycin 203 (a lincosamide antibiotic 86)

Dalacin T brand name for clindamycin 203 (a lincosamide antibiotic 86)

dalfopristin an antibiotic 86

Dalmane brand name for flurazepam (a benzodiazepine sleeping drug 38)

dalteparin a type of heparin 275 (an anticoagulant 62)

dalvabancin glycopeptide antibacterial 89 used to treat skin infections

danaparoid anticoagulant 62

danazol drug for menstrual disorders 120

Dandrazol brand name for ketoconazole 291 (an antifungal 96)

Danol brand name for danazol (a drug for menstrual disorders 120)

Dantrium brand name for dantrolene (a muscle relaxant 78)

dantrolene muscle relaxant 78

dantron stimulant laxative 69

dapagliflozin 220, drug for diabetes 100

dapoxetine serotonin re-uptake inhibitor used to treat premature ejaculation

dapsone antibacterial 89 and antiprotozoal 94

daptomycin lipopeptide antibiotic 86

Daraprim brand name for pyrimethamine 374 (an antimalarial 95)

daratumumab monoclonal antibody and anticancer drug 112 used to treat myeloma (a type of cancer of the bone marrow)

darbepoetin alfa drug used for anaemia

darifenacin antimuscarinic drug used for urinary disorders 126

darunavir drug used for HIV infection 116

Darzalex brand name for daratumumab (a monoclonal antibody and anticancer drug 112) used to treat myeloma

dasabuvir antiviral drug 91

dasatinib anticancer drug 112 for leukaemia

daunorubicin cytotoxic antibiotic (an anticancer drug 112)

DaunoXome brand name for daunorubicin (an anticancer drug 112)

Daxas brand name for roflumilast, an anti-inflammatory drug used for obstructive airways disease

Day Nurse brand-name preparation containing paracetamol 352 (a non-opioid analgesic 36), pseudoephedrine (a decongestant) and pholcodine (a cough suppressant)

Daylett brand name for a combined oral contraceptive 121 containing ethinylestradiol 252 and drospirenone

DDAVP brand name for desmopressin 221 (a pituitary hormone 103)

DDI see didanosine

Deca-Durabolin brand name for nandrolone (an anabolic steroid 104)

Decapeptyl SR brand name for triptorelin (an anticancer drug 112)

decitabine anticancer drug 112 used for leukaemia

Deep Relief branded preparation containing ibuprofen 279 (a NSAID 74) with levomenthol

DEET another name for diethyltoluamide (a mosquito repellent)

deferasirox drug used to remove excess iron from the blood

deferiprone drug used to remove excess iron from the blood in thalassaemia

deflazacort a corticosteroid 99, 134

degarelix a drug for advanced prostate cancer

delamanid an antituberculous drug 90

Delmosart brand name for methylphenidate 322, used to treat attention deficit hyperactivity disorder (ADHD)

Deltacortril Enteric brand name for prednisolone 365 (a corticosteroid 99)

Deltastab brand name for prednisolone 365 (a corticosteroid 99)

Deltyba brand name for delamanid (an antituberculous drug 90)

demeclocycline a tetracycline antibiotic 86

Demorem brand-name oral solution containing ondansetron 347 used for nausea 46

denosumab a drug for bone disorders 80

Dentinox infant brand name for simethicone drops used for infant colic

Denzapine brand name for clozapine (an antipsychotic 41)

Depakote brand name for valproic acid (a drug for mania 41)

Depalta brand name for duloxetine (an antidepressant 40 and analgesic 36 for neuropathic pain)

Depefex XL brand name for venlafaxine 427 (an antidepressant 40)

Depixol brand name for flupentixol 263 (an antipsychotic 41 and antidepressant 40)

DepoCyte brand name for cytarabine (an anticancer drug 112)

Depo-Medrone brand name for methylprednisolone (a corticosteroid 99)

Deponit brand name for glyceryl trinitrate 272 (an anti-angina drug 59)

Depo-Provera brand name for medroxyprogesterone 313 (a female sex hormone 105)

Dequacaine brand name for benzocaine (a local anaesthetic 36) with dequalinium (an antibacterial 89)

dequalinium antibacterial 89 for mouth infections

DERBAC-M

Derbac-M brand-name shampoo containing malathion 310 (an antiparasitic 136)

Dermabond brand name for octylcyanoacrylate (a skin adhesive)

Dermacolor brand name for a masking cream for skin disfigurement

Dermacort brand-name preparation for hydrocortisone cream 277

Dermovate brand name for clobetasol 204 (a topical corticosteroid 134)

Desferal brand name for desferrioxamine (an antidote for an iron overdose)

desferrioxamine antidote for an iron overdose

desflurane gaseous general anaesthetic

Desitrend brand name for levetiracetam 297 (an anticonvulsant 42)

desloratadine 307, antihistamine 82

DesmoMelt brand name for desmopressin 221, a pituitary hormone 103 used for diabetes insipidus 103

desmopressin 221, pituitary hormone 103 used for diabetes insipidus 103

Desmospray brand-name nasal spray containing desmopressin 221, a pituitary hormone 103 for diabetes insipidus 103

Desmotabs brand name for desmopressin 221, a pituitary hormone 103 used for diabetes insipidus 103

desogestrel 222, female sex hormone 105 and oral contraceptive 121

Desomono brand-name progesterone-only oral contraceptive 121 containing desogestrel 222

Desorex brand-name progesterone-only oral contraceptive 121 containing desogestrel 222

Destolit brand name for ursodeoxycholic acid (a drug for gallstones 72)

Desunin brand name for colecalciferol (vitamin D 444)

Detrunorm brand name for propiverine (a drug used to treat urinary frequency 126)

Detrusitol brand name for tolterodine 420 (an anticholinergic and antispasmodic drug used to treat urinary disorders 126)

Detrusitol XL brand name for tolterodine 420 (an anticholinergic and antispasmodic drug used to treat urinary disorders 126)

Dettol brand-name liquid skin antiseptic 135 containing chloroxylenol

Dexafree brand name for dexamethasone 223 (a corticosteroid 99)

dexamethasone 223, corticosteroid 99

dexamfetamine amfetamine 449, used for narcolepsy and hyperactivity in children 44

Dexedrine brand name for dexamfetamine (an amfetamine 449)

dexibuprofen NSAID 74

Deximune brand name for ciclosporin 196, an immunosuppressant 115

dexketoprofen NSAID 74

dexrazoxane an iron chelator used to prevent cardiotoxicity in patients receiving anticancer drugs

Dexsol brand name for dexamethasone 223 (a corticosteroid 99)

DF 118 brand name for dihydrocodeine 228 (an opioid analgesic 36)

DHC Continus brand name for dihydrocodeine 225 (an opioid analgesic 36)

Diabiom brand name for pioglitazone 361 (a drug for diabetes 100)

Diafer brand name for iron 437 (a mineral 108) used to treat iron-deficiency anaemia

Diagemet XL brand name for modified-release metformin 318 (a drug for diabetes 100)

Dialar brand of diazepam 224 (a benzodiazepine anti-anxiety drug 39, muscle relaxant 78, and anticonvulsant 42)

Diamicron brand name for gliclazide 270 (an oral drug for diabetes 100)

diamorphine 334, opioid analgesic 36

Diamox brand name for acetazolamide (a carbonic anhydrase inhibitor diuretic 57 and drug for glaucoma 128)

Dianette brand name for cyproterone 218 (an anti-androgen 104) with ethinylestradiol 252 (a female sex hormone 105)

Diazemuls brand name for diazepam 224 (a benzodiazepine anti-anxiety drug 39, muscle relaxant 78, and anticonvulsant 42)

diazepam 224, benzodiazepine anti-anxiety drug 39, muscle relaxant 78, and anticonvulsant 42

diazoxide antihypertensive 60 also used for hypoglycaemia 100

diclofenac 225, NSAID 74

Dicloflex brand name for diclofenac 225 (a NSAID 74)

Diclomax Retard brand name for diclofenac 225 (a NSAID 74)

dicobalt edetate antidote for cyanide poisoning

Diconal brand name for dipipanone (an opioid analgesic drug 36) with cyclizine (an anti-emetic drug 46)

dicycloverine 226 (previously dicyclomine) drug for irritable bowel syndrome 68

didanosine antiretroviral for HIV/AIDS 116

dienogest female sex hormone 105 used with estradiol 249 for contraception 121

diethylamine salicylate rubefacient

diethylstilbestrol (previously stilboestrol) a female sex hormone 105

diethyltoluamide (DEET) a mosquito repellent

Differin brand name for adapalene (a retinoid for acne 137)

Difflam brand name for benzydamine (an analgesic 36)

Diffundox XL brand name for tamsulosin 407 (an alpha blocker for urinary retention 126)

Diflucan brand name for fluconazole 260 (an antifungal 96)

diflucortolone topical corticosteroid 134

digifab drug used for overdose of digoxin 227

digitoxin digitalis drug 54

digoxin 227, digitalis drug 54

dihydrocodeine 228, opioid analgesic 36

dihydrotachysterol vitamin D 444 (a vitamin 107)

Dilacort brand name for prednisolone 365

Dilcardia SR brand name for diltiazem 229 (a calcium channel blocker 59)

diloxanide furoate antiprotozoal 94 for amoebic dysentery

diltiazem 229, calcium channel blocker 59 and antihypertensive 60

Dilzem SR brand name for diltiazem 229 (an antihypertensive and calcium channel blocker 59)

Dilzem XL brand name for diltiazem 229 (an antihypertensive and calcium channel blocker 59)

dimethyl fumarate drug for multiple sclerosis

dimethyl sulfoxide drug used to treat bladder inflammation

dimeticone silicone-based substance used in barrier creams 135 and antifoaming agent 66

dinoprostone prostaglandin used to terminate pregnancy 125

dinutuximab beta monoclonal antibody used to treat certain cancers 112

Diocalm brand-name antidiarrhoeal 68 containing attapulgite and morphine 334

Diocalm Ultra brand name for loperamide 305 (an antidiarrhoeal 68)

Dioctyl brand name for docusate (a stimulant laxative 69)

Dioderm brand name for hydrocortisone 277 (a corticosteroid 99)

Dioralyte brand name for rehydration salts containing sodium bicarbonate, glucose, potassium chloride, and sodium chloride 434

Diovan brand name for valsartan 390 (an antihypertensive drug 60)

diphenhydramine antihistamine 82, anti-emetic 46, and antipruritic 133

diphenoxylate opioid antidiarrhoeal 68

dipipanone opioid analgesic 36

Diprivan brand name for propofol (a general anesthetic 36)

Diprobase brand-name emollient preparation

Diprosalic branded skin preparation containing betamethasone 172 (a corticosteroid 99) and salicylic acid (a keratolytic 137)

Diprosone brand name for betamethasone 172 (a corticosteroid 99)

dipyridamole 230, an antiplatelet drug 62

disopyramide an anti-arrhythmic 58

Disprin brand name for soluble aspirin 162 (a non-opioid analgesic 36)

Disprin Extra brand-name soluble analgesic 36 containing aspirin 162 and paracetamol 352

Disprol brand name for paracetamol 352 (a non-opioid analgesic 36)

Distaclor brand name for cefaclor (a cephalosporin antibiotic 86)

Distamine brand name for penicillamine (a DMARD 75)

disulfiram 231, alcohol misuse deterrent 24, 447

dithranol drug for psoriasis 138

Dithrocream brand name for dithranol (a drug for psoriasis 138)

Ditropan brand name for oxybutynin 351 (an anticholinergic and antispasmodic drug for urinary disorders 126)

Diumide-K Continus brand name for furosemide 266 (a loop diuretic 57) with potassium (a mineral 108)

Diuresal brand name for furosemide 266 (a loop diuretic 57)

Diurexan brand name for xipamide (a diuretic 57) used to treat hypertension

Dixarit brand name for clonidine (a drug for migraine 45)

dobutamine drug for heart failure and shock

docetaxel anticancer drug 112

docusate faecal softener, stimulant laxative 69, and ear wax softener 131

Docusol brand name for oral solution containing docusate used as a laxative 69

Dolenio brand name for glucosamine, used for osteoarthritis

Dolmatil brand name for sulpiride 156 (an antipsychotic 41)

dolutegravir antiviral 91 used with other medications to treat HIV 116

domperidone 232, anti-emetic 46

donepezil 233, drug for Alzheimer's disease 43

Dopacard brand name for dopexamine (a drug for heart failure)

dopamine drug for heart failure, kidney failure, and shock

dopexamine drug for heart failure

Doralese brand name for indoramin (a drug for prostate disorders 126 and an antihypertensive 60)

ELUDEN

Doralese Tiltab brand name for indoramin (an antihypertensive 60 also used for prostate enlargement 126)

Dorisin XL brand name for modified-release fluvastatin (a lipid-lowering drug 61)

dornase alfa drug for cystic fibrosis 72

dorzolamide 234, a carbonic anhydrase inhibitor for glaucoma 128

Dostinex brand name for cabergoline (a drug for parkinsonism 43 and endocrine disorders 103)

dosulepin 235, (previously dothiepin) a tricyclic antidepressant 40

Doublebase brand-name paraffin-containing gel used for dry and scaling skin disorders

Dovobet brand name for betamethasone 172 (a corticosteroid 99) with calcipotriol 183 (a drug for psoriasis 138)

Dovonex brand name for calcipotriol 183 (a drug for psoriasis 138)

Doxadura brand name for doxazosin 236 (an antihypertensive 60 and drug for prostate disorders 126)

doxapram respiratory stimulant 44

doxazosin 236, alpha blocker antihypertensive 60 and drug for prostate disorders 126

doxepin tricyclic antidepressant 40 and drug for pruritus in eczema 139

doxorubicin 237, cytotoxic anticancer drug 112

Doxorubin brand name for doxorubicin 237 (a cytotoxic anticancer drug 112)

doxycycline 238, a tetracycline antibiotic 86

Doxylar brand name for doxycycline 238 (a tetracycline antibiotic 86)

Doxzogen XL brand name for modified-release doxazosin 236 (an alpha blocker antihypertensive 60 and drug for prostate disorders 126)

doylamine drug given with pyridoxine 440 to treat nausea in pregnancy

Drapolene branded barrier cream containing benzalkonium chloride and cetrimide (skin antiseptics 135) for dry and scaling skin

Dretine brand-name combined oral contraceptive 121 containing ethinylestradiol 252 and drospirenone

Driclor brand name for aluminium chloride (an antiperspirant)

dronaderone anti-arrhythmic 58

droperidol antipsychotic 41

Dropodex brand name for dexamethasone 223 (a corticosteroid 99)

drospirenone a progestogen female sex hormone 105

Droxia brand name for hydroxycarbamide (an anticancer drug 112)

Duac brand-name gel for acne 137 containing benzoyl peroxide 170 and clindamycin 203 (a lincosamide antibiotic 86)

Duac Once Daily brand-name preparation for acne 137 containing benzoyl peroxide 170 and clindamycin 203 (a lincosamide antibiotic 86)

Duaklir brand name for aclidinium bromide with formoterol (both bronchodilator drugs 48) used for chronic obstructive pulmonary disease

Dualtis brand-name capsule containing docosahexaenoic acid and eicosapentaenoic acid (lipid-lowering substances 61)

Duavive brand name form of HRT 105 containing oestrogen

Duciltia brand name for duloxetine (an antidepressant 40)

Dukoral brand-name cholera vaccine 451

dulaglutide 239, drug for diabetes 100

Dulco-lax brand name for sodium picosulfate (a stimulant laxative 69)

duloxetine antidepressant 40 and drug for diabetic neuropathy and urinary disorders 126

Duodopa brand name for co-careldopa (a generic product containing levodopa 298, a drug for parkinsonism 43, with carbidopa, a drug that enhances the effect of levodopa)

Duofilm brand-name wart preparation containing lactic acid, salicylic acid, and collodion 135

DuoResp Spiromax brand name for budenoside 178 with formoterol (a bronchodilator 48) used for obstructive airways disease

DuoTrav brand-name preparation for glaucoma 128 containing travoprost with timolol 417 (a beta blocker 55)

Duphalac brand name for lactulose 293 (a laxative 69)

dupilumab monoclonal antibody used for allergic diseases

Durogesic brand name for fentanyl (an opioid analgesic 36)

durvalumab monoclonal antibody for cancer 112 of the lungs, bladder, or urinary tract

Dutasteride male sex hormone 104 for benign prostatic hyperplasia 126

Dyazide brand name for hydrochlorothiazide 270 with triamterene 423 (both diuretics 57)

dydrogesterone 240, female sex hormone 105

Dyloject brand-name injectable form of diclofenac 225 (a NSAID 74)

Dymista brand-name spray containing fluticasone 265 (a corticosteroid 99) with azelastine (an antihistamine 82) used to treat allergic rhinitis

Dynastat brand name for parecoxib (an analgesic 36 and NSAID 74)

Dysport brand name for botulinum toxin 176 used as a muscle relaxant 78

E

E45 cream brand-name emollient 139

EarCalm brand-name preparation for treatment of superficial ear infections 131 containing acetic acid

Earex brand-name preparation for ear wax removal 131

Earol brand-name olive oil ear spray to remove earwax

Easyhaler brand name for salbutamol 391 (a bronchodilator 48) used to treat asthma 49

Ebesque XL brand name for quetiapine 375 (an antipsychotic 41)

Ebixa brand name for memantidine, used for Alzheimer's disease 43

Ecalta brand name for anidalafungin (an antifungal 96)

Eciferol brand name for ergocalciferol (vitamin D 444)

Econacort brand name for econazole (an antifungal 96) with hydrocortisone 277 (a corticosteroid 99)

econazole antifungal drug 96

Ecopace brand name for captopril 186 (an ACE inhibitor 56)

Ecstasy 451, street name for methylenedioxy-methamfetamine (MDMA), an amfetamine 449

eculizumab monoclonal antibody used to treat certain blood disorders

Eczmol brand-name emollient containing chlorhexidine for eczema and dermatitis 139

Edarbi brand name for azilsartan medoxomil (an antihypertensive 60)

Edicil MR brand name for modified-release gliclazide 270 (a drug for diabetes 100)

edoxaban anticlotting drug 62 used to prevent stroke in patients with atrial fibrillation and deep vein thrombosis

Edronax brand name for reboxetine (an antidepressant 40)

edrophonium drug for diagnosis of myasthenia gravis 79

Edurant brand name for rilpivirine (an antiretroviral for HIV/AIDS 116)

efavirenz 241, antiretroviral for HIV/AIDS 116

Efexor XL brand name for venlafaxine 427 (an antidepressant drug 40)

Effentora brand name for fentanyl (an opioid analgesic 36)

Efflosomyl brand name for tolterodine 420 (an anticholinergic 126)

Efient brand name for prasugrel (an anticlotting drug 62) used for acute coronary syndrome

eflornithine drug to treat facial hair in women

eformoterol see formoterol (a sympathomimetic bronchodilator 48)

Efracea brand name for doxycycline 238 (a tetracycline antibiotic 86)

Efudix brand-name cream containing fluorouracil 261 (an anticancer drug 112)

Eklira brand name for aclidinium bromide (a bronchodilator 48) used for obstructive airways disease

Elantan brand name for isosorbide mononitrate 289 (a nitrate vasodilator 56 and anti-angina drug 59)

elbasvir antiviral 91 used to treat hepatitis C

Eldepryl brand name for selegiline (a drug for parkinsonism 43)

Eldisine brand name for vindesine (an anticancer drug 112)

eletriptan drug for migraine 45

Elevin brand-name combined oral contraceptive 121 containing ethinylestradiol 252 and levonorgestrel 300

Elidel cream brand name for pimecrolimus (an anti-inflammatory used to treat eczema 139)

Eliquis brand name for apixaban (an anticoagulant 62)

EllaOne brand name for ulipristal 425 (a drug used for emergency contraception 121)

Elleste brand name for estradiol 249 (an oestrogen 105 for treatment of menopausal symptoms 105)

Elleste Duet brand-name preparation for menopausal symptoms 105 containing estradiol 249 and norethisterone 342

Elleste Solo brand name for estradiol 249 (an oestrogen 105 for treatment of menopausal symptoms 105)

Elmino brand name for modified-release galantamine (a drug used to treat Alzheimer's disease 43)

Elocon brand name for mometasone 332 (a topical corticosteroid 134)

Eloine brand-name combined oral contraceptive 121 containing ethinylestradiol 252 and drospirenone

Elonva brand name for corifollitropin alfa (a gonadotrophin used for female infertility 124)

elotuzumab monoclonal antibody used to treat myeloma

eltrombopag drug used to treat platelet disorders

Eltroxin brand name for levothyroxine 301 (a thyroid hormone 102)

Eluden brand name for a skin patch containing rivastigmine 387 (a drug for Alzheimer's disease 43)

ELUXADOLINE

eluxadoline drug for irritable bowel syndrome 68

Elvanse brand name for lisdexamfetamine mesilate (a nervous system stimulant 44) used for attention deficit hyperactivity disorder

elvitegravir antiviral used for HIV/AIDS 116

Emadine brand name for emedastine (an antihistamine 82)

emedastine antihistamine 82

Emelpin branded ointment containing wax and soft paraffin for dry and scaling skin disorders

Emend brand name for aprepitant (an anti-emetic 46)

Emerade brand name for epinephrine 245 injection used for anaphylaxis

Emeside brand name for ethosuximide (an anticonvulsant 42)

Emflex brand name for acemetacin (a NSAID 74)

emicizumab monoconal antibody used to treat haemophilia 62

Emla brand-name local anaesthetic 36 containing lignocaine and prilocaine

Emmerres brand name for levonorgestrel 300 used for emergency contraception 123

Emollin an aerosol spray containing paraffin used for dry and scaling skin disorders

Emozul brand name for esomeprazole 67 (an anti-ulcer drug 67)

empagliflozin drug for diabetes 100

Empliciti brand name for elotuzumab (a monoclonal antibody anticancer drug 112) used for myeloma

Emselex brand name for darifenacin (a drug used for urinary disorders 126)

emtricitabine 242, antiretroviral for HIV/AIDS 116

Emtriva brand name for emtricitabine 242 (an antiretroviral for HIV/AIDS 116)

Emulsiderm brand-name emollient used for dry skin conditions

Emustil brand name for artificial tears containing soybean oil

enalapril 243, ACE inhibitor vasodilator 56 and antihypertensive 60

Enbrel brand name for etanercept 250 (an immunosuppressant 115, DMARD 75, and drug for psoriasis 138)

En-De-Kay brand name for fluoride 436 (a mineral 108)

enfuvirtide antiretroviral for HIV/AIDS 116

Engerix B brand-name vaccine 92 to protect against viral hepatitis B

ENO's brand-name antacid 66 containing sodium bicarbonate, sodium carbonate, and citric acid

enoxaparin type of heparin 275 (an anticoagulant 62)

enoximone drug for heart failure 53

Enstilar brand-name topical medication containing calcipotriene (vitamin D 444) and betamethasone 172 for psoriasis 138

entacapone drug for parkinsonism 43

entecavir antiviral 91 for hepatitis B

Entocort brand name for budesonide 180 (a corticosteroid 99)

Entonox brand name for a mixture of nitrous oxide and oxygen used as an analgesic 36

Entresto brand name for a fixed-dose combination of sacubitril and valsartan 390 (an antihypertensive drug 60) used to treat heart failure

Entyvio brand name for vedolizumab (a monoclonal antibody) for Crohn's disease 70

Envarsus brand name for tacrolimus 405 used to prevent rejection after transplants

Enyglid brand name for repaglinide 381 (a drug for diabetes 100)

enzalutamide anti-androgen drug 104 used for prostate cancer

Enzira brand-name influenza vaccine 92

Epaderm brand-name ointment containing emulsifying wax and paraffin used for dry and scaling skin disorders

Epanutin brand name for phenytoin 359 (an anticonvulsant 42)

Epaxal brand-name hepatitis A vaccine 92

Epclusa brand name for sofosbuvir with velpatasvir (antivirals 91) used for hepatitis C

Eperzan brand name for albiglutide (a drug for diabetes 100)

ephedrine 244, bronchodilator 48 and decongestant 51

Epiduo brand-name preparation containing aldapalene (a retinoid) and benzoyl peroxide used for acne 137

Epidyolex brand name for cannabidiol 185 (an anticonvulsant 42)

Epilim brand name for sodium valproate 398 (an anticonvulsant 42)

Epilim Chronosphere brand name for prolonged-release sodium valproate 398 (an anticonvulsant 42)

epinastine antihistamine 82

epinephrine 245, a bronchodilator 48 and drug for glaucoma 128; also known as adrenaline

EpiPen brand name for epinephrine 245 (an anti-allergy drug 82)

epirubicin cytotoxic anticancer drug 112

Episenta brand name for sodium valproate 398 (an anticonvulsant 42)

Epistatus brand name for midazolam (an anticonvulsant 42) used to treat epilepsy in children and adolescents

Epival brand name for prolonged-release sodium valproate 398 (an anticonvulsant 42)

Epivir brand name for lamivudine 430 (an antiretroviral for HIV/AIDS 116)

eplerenone drug for heart failure following a heart attack 53

epoetin also called erythropoietin 248 (a kidney hormone 98 for anaemia due to kidney failure)

epoprostenol prostaglandin used for its vasodilator effects 56

Eposin brand name for etoposide (an anticancer drug 112)

Eppinix XL brand name for modified-release ropinirole 388 (a drug used to treat Parkinson's disease 43)

Eprex brand name for erythropoietin 248 (a kidney hormone 98 used for anaemia due to kidney failure)

eprosartan angiotensin II blocker (a vasodilator 56 and antihypertensive 60)

Eptadone brand name for methadone 319 (an opioid 455 used as an analgesic 36 and to ease heroin withdrawal)

eptifibatide antiplatelet drug 62 for prevention of heart attacks

Equasym brand name for methylphenidate 322 (a nervous system stimulant 44)

Equasym XL brand name for methylphenidate 322 (a nervous system stimulant 44)

Erbitux brand name for cetuximab (an anticancer drug 112)

erdosteine mucolytic drug used for bronchitis

Erdotin brand name for erdosteine (a mucolytic drug used for bronchitis)

erenumab monoclonal antibody used to prevent migraines 45

Ergamisol brand name for levamisole (an anthelmintic 97) for roundworm infestation

ergocalciferol vitamin D 444 (a vitamin 107)

ergometrine uterine stimulant 125

Ergoral brand name for ergocalciferol (vitamin D 444)

ergotamine 246, drug for migraine 45

eribulin anticancer drug 112 for breast cancer

Erivedge brand name for vismodegib (an anticancer drug 112) used to treat skin cancer

Erlibelle brand-name combined oral contraceptive 121 containing ethinylestradiol 252 and levonorgestrel 300

erlotinib anticancer drug 112

Eroset brand name for a combination analgesic 36 containing paracetamol 352 and dihydrocodeine 228

ertapenem antibiotic 86

Erwinase brand name for crisantaspase (an anticancer drug 112)

Erymax brand name for erythromycin 247 (an antibiotic 86)

Erythrocin brand name for erythromycin 247 (an antibiotic 86)

Erythrolar brand name for erythromycin 247 (an antibiotic 86)

erythromycin 247, antibiotic 86

Erythroped brand name for erythromycin 247 (an antibiotic 86)

erythropoietin 248, kidney hormone 98 used for anaemia due to kidney failure; also known as epoetin

Esbriet brand name for perfenidone (an antifibrotic drug) used for pulmonary fibrosis

escitalopram 201, antidepressant 40

eslicarbazepine acetate anticonvulsant 42 used for epilepsy

esmolol beta blocker 55

Esmya brand name for ulipristal 425 (an oral contraceptive 121)

esomeprazole anti-ulcer drug 67

Espranol brand name for buprenorphine (an opioid analgesic 36)

Estracyt brand name for estramustine (an anticancer drug 112)

Estraderm MX brand-name skin patch containing estradiol 249 used for menopausal symptoms

estradiol 249, an oestrogen 105

Estradot brand-name skin patch containing estradiol 249 used for menopausal symptoms 105

estramustine alkylating agent for cancer of the prostate 112

Estring brand-name vaginal ring containing estradiol 249 for menopausal symptoms 105

estriol oestrogen 105

estrone oestrogen 105

E-tabs brand name for tocopherol (vitamin E 444)

etamsylate antifibrinolytic used to promote blood clotting 62

etanercept 250, immunosuppressant 115, DMARD 75, and drug for psoriasis 138

ethambutol 251, antituberculous drug 90

ethinylestradiol 252, female sex hormone 105 and oral contraceptive 121

ethosuximide anticonvulsant 42

etodolac NSAID 74

etomidate drug to induce general anaesthesia

etonorgestrel a progestogen 121

Etopan XL brand name for modified-release etodolac (an NSAID 74)

Etopophos brand name for etoposide (an anticancer drug 112)

etoposide drug for cancers of the lung, lymphatic system, and testes 112

etoricoxib analgesic 36 and NSAID 74

FLECAINIDE

etravirine drug used for HIV 116

Etrivex brand name for clobetasol 204 (a topical corticosteroid 134)

Eucerin brand-name cream containing urea used for dry and scaling skin disorders

Eucreas brand-name preparation containing vildagliptin and metformin 318 (both drugs for diabetes100)

Eudemine brand name for diazoxide (used for hypoglycaemia 100 and as antihypertensive 60)

Eumovate brand name for clobetasone (a topical corticosteroid 134)

Eurartesim brand name for artenimol with piperaquinephosphate used for falciparum malaria 95

Eurax brand name for crotamiton (antipruritic 133)

Eurax-Hydrocortisone brand name for hydrocortisone 277 (a corticosteroid 99) with crotamiton (an antipruritic 133)

Evacal D3 brand name for colecalciferol (vitamin D 444) with calcium carbonate (calcium 434)

everolimus protein kinase inhibitor anticancer drug 112

Eviplera brand-name preparation containing rilpivirine, emtricitabine 242, and tenofovir 409 (drugs for HIV/AIDS 116)

Evirex brand name for raloxifene 378 (an anti-oestrogen sex hormone antagonist 105 for osteoporosis 80)

Evista brand name for raloxifene 378 (an anti-oestrogen sex hormone antagonist 105 for osteoporosis 80)

evolocumab 253, monoclonal antibody for the treatment of hyperlipidaemia 61

Evoltra brand name for clofarabine (an anticancer drug 112) used for leukaemia

Evolve HA brand name for eye drops containing sodium hyaluronate, a lubricant used for dry eyes

Evorel brand name for estradiol 249 (a female sex hormone 105)

Evotaz brand-name combined preparation of atazanavir and cobicistat used for HIV 116

Evoxil brand name for levofloxacin 299 (an antibacterial 89)

Evra brand-name contraceptive patch containing ethinylestradiol 252 with norelgestromin (both female sex hormones 105)

Exelon brand name for rivastigmine 387 (a drug for Alzheimer's disease 43)

Exembol brand name for argatroban monohydrate (an anticlotting drug 62)

exemestane anti-breast-cancer drug 112

exenatide 254, injectable drug for diabetes 100

Exforge brand name for amlodipine 158 (a calcium channel blocker 59) with valsartan 390 (an antihypertensive 60)

Exjade brand name for desferasirox, a drug to reduce excess iron in the body

Ex-Lax brand name for senna (a laxative 69)

Exocin brand name for ofloxacin (an antibiotic 86)

Exorex brand name for coal tar lotion (for psoriasis 138 and eczema 139)

Extavia brand name for interferon 285 (an antiviral 91 and anticancer drug 112)

Exterol brand-name ear drops for wax removal 131 containing urea (an emollient) and hydrogen peroxide (an antiseptic 135)

Exviera brand name for dasabuvir (an antiviral drug 91)

Eydelto brand name for dorzolamide 234 eye drops used to treat glaucoma 128

Eykappo brand name for chloramphenicol 192 (an antibiotic 68) used to treat eye infections

Eylamdo brand name for dorzolamide 234 eye drops used to treat glaucoma 128

Eylea brand name for aflibercept (an anti-VEGF drug) used for macular degeneration

Eyreida brand name for bitamaprost (a drug used to treat glaucoma 128)

Eysano brand name for timolol 417 (a drug used to treat glaucoma 128)

Eytazox brand name for acetazolamide (a diuretic 57) for glaucoma 128 and epilepsy 42

ezetimibe 255, lipid-lowering drug 61

Ezetrol brand name for ezetimibe 255 (a lipid-lowering drug 61)

Ezinelle brand name for levonorgestrel 300 (an oral contraceptive 121)

F

factor VIIa blood extract to promote blood clotting 62

factor VIII blood extract to promote blood clotting 62

factor IX blood extract to promote blood clotting 62

factor XIII blood extract to promote blood clotting 62

famciclovir antiviral drug 91

famotidine anti-ulcer drug 67

fampridine drug for multiple sclerosis 78

Fampyra brand name for fampridine (a drug for multiple sclerosis 78)

Famvir brand name for famciclovir (an antiviral drug 91)

Faramsil brand name for modified-release tamsulosin 407, for prostate disorders 126

Fareston brand name for toremifene (an anticancer drug 112)

Farydak brand name for panobinostat (an anticancer drug 112 used for myeloma)

fasenra monoclonal antibody for asthma 49

Fasigyn brand name for tinidazole (an antibacterial 89)

Faslodex brand name for fluvestrant (an anti-breast cancer drug 112)

Faverin brand name for fluvoxamine (an antidepressant 40)

Feanolla brand-name oral contraceptive 121 containing desogestrel 222

febuxostat drug used to treat gout 77

Fefol brand name for folic acid 436 (a vitamin 107) with iron 437 (a mineral 108)

felbinac NSAID 74 for joint and muscle pain

Feldene brand name for piroxicam 362 (an NSAID 74 and drug for gout 77)

Felendil XL brand name for felodipine 256 (a calcium channel blocker 59)

felodipine 256, calcium channel blocker 59

Felogen XL brand name for felodipine 256 (a calcium channel blocker 59)

Felotens XL brand name for felodipine 256 (a calcium channel blocker 59)

Femara brand name for letrozole (an anticancer drug 112)

Femodene brand-name oral contraceptive 121 containing ethinylestradiol 252 and gestodene

Femodette brand-name oral contraceptive 121 containing gestodene and ethinylestradiol 252

Femoston 1/10 & 2/10 brand-name preparations for menopausal symptoms 105 containing estradiol 249 and dydrogesterone 240

Femoston-conti brand-name preparation for menopausal symptoms 105 containing estradiol 249 and dydrogesterone 240

FemSeven brand name for estradiol 249 (an oestrogen 105)

FemSeven Conti brand name for estradiol 249 with levonorgestrel 300 for hormone replacement therapy 105

Fenacto preparations brand name for preparations of gastro-resistant diclofenac 225 (a NSAID 74)

Fenbid brand name for ibuprofen 279 (an NSAID 74)

Fencino brand name for fentanyl (an opioid analgesic 36)

Fendrix brand-name hepatitis B vaccine 92

fenofibrate lipid-lowering drug 61

fenoprofen NSAID 74

Fenopron brand name for fenoprofen (an NSAID 74)

Fentalis brand-name skin patch containing fentanyl (an opioid analgesic 36)

fentanyl an opioid analgesic 36 used in general anaesthesia and labour 125

fenticonazole nitrate an antifungal 96 used for vaginal and vulval infections

Feospan brand name for iron 437 (a mineral 108)

Feraccru brand name for iron 437 (a mineral 108)

Ferinject brand name for ferric carboxymaltose (an injectable form of iron 437 for anaemia)

ferric carboxymaltose injectable form of iron 437 for anaemia

Ferriprox brand name for deferiprone (used to treat iron overload)

Ferrograd brand name for iron 437 (a mineral 108)

Ferrograd C brand name for iron 437 (a mineral 108) with vitamin C 443 (a vitamin 107)

Ferrograd Folic brand name for folic acid 436 (a vitamin 107) with iron 437 (a mineral 108)

ferrous fumarate iron 437 (a mineral 108)

ferrous gluconate iron 437 (a mineral 108)

ferrous sulfate iron 437 (a mineral 108)

Fersaday brand name for iron 437 (a mineral 108)

fesoterodine fumarate antimuscarinic drug used for urinary frequency 126

fexofenadine antihistamine 82

Fibrazate (bezatard) XL brand name for bezafibrate 174 (a lipid-lowering drug 61)

Fibrogammin P brand name for factor XIII (a blood extract to promote blood clotting 62)

Fibro-vein brand name for sodium tetradecyl sulfate (a drug for varicose veins)

fidaxomicin macrocyclic antibacterial 89

Fifty:50 aemollient ointment containing liquid paraffin and white soft paraffin

filgrastim 257, blood growth stimulant

Finacea brand name for azelaic acid (an antibacterial 89 used for acne 137)

finasteride 258, male sex hormone 104 for benign prostatic hypertrophy 126

fingolimod immunomodulating drug used for multiple sclerosis 78

Firazyr brand name for icatibant, a drug used for angioedema

Firmagon brand name for degarelix (an anticancer drug 112 used for prostate cancer)

Flagyl brand name for metronidazole 325 (an antibacterial 89 and antiprotozoal 94)

Flamazine brand name for silver sulfadiazine (a topical antibacterial 89)

flavoxate urinary antispasmodic 126

Flebogammadif brand name for human immunoglobulin (a preparation injected to prevent infectious diseases 92)

flecainide anti-arrhythmic drug 58

FLECTONE XL

Flectone XL brand name for tamsulosin 407 (an alpha blocker to treat prostate disorders 126)

Fleet preparations brand-name sodium acid phosphate products used to treat constipation 69 and to empty the bowel before medical procedures

Flexitol brand-name balm containing urea used for dry and scaling skin conditions

Flixonase brand name for fluticasone 265 (a corticosteroid 99)

Flixotide brand name for fluticasone 265 (a corticosteroid 99)

Flolan brand name for epoprostenol (an anticoagulant 62 and vasodilator 56)

Flomax MR brand name for modified-release tamsulosin 407 (an alpha blocker for prostate disorders 126)

Flomaxtra XL brand name for tamsulosin 407 (an alpha blocker for prostate disorders 126)

Flotros brand name for trospium chloride (an antimuscarinic to treat urinary frequency 126)

Fluanxol brand name for flupentixol 263 (an antipsychotic drug 41)

Fluarix brand-name vaccine 92 to protect against influenza

Fluarix Tetra brand-name vaccine 92 to protect against influenza

flucloxacillin 259, penicillin antibiotic 86

fluconazole 260, antifungal 96

flucytosine antifungal 96

Fludara brand name for fludarabine (an anticancer drug 112)

fludarabine anticancer drug 112

fludrocortisone corticosteroid 99

fludroxycortide (previously flurandrenolone) a topical corticosteroid 134

Fluenz Tetra brand-name nasal spray vaccine 92 to protect against influenza

flumazenil antidote for benzodiazepine overdose 450

flumetasone corticosteroid 99

FluMist Quadrivalent brand-name nasal spray vaccine 92 to protect against influenza

fluocinolone topical corticosteroid 134

fluocinonide topical corticosteroid 134

fluocortolone topical corticosteroid 134

Fluomozin brand name for dequalinium (an antibacterial 89) used for bacterial vaginosis

Fluor-a-day brand name for fluoride 436 (a mineral 108)

fluorescein drug used to stain the eye before examination

fluoride 436, mineral 108

Fluorigard brand name for fluoride 436 (a mineral 108)

fluorometholone corticosteroid 99 for eye disorders

fluorouracil 261, anticancer drug 112

fluoxetine 262, antidepressant 40

flupentixol 263, antipsychotic 41 used in depression 40

fluphenazine antipsychotic drug 41

flurazepam benzodiazepine sleeping drug 38

flurbiprofen NSAID 74

flutamide 264, anticancer drug 112

fluticasone 265, corticosteroid 99

Flutiform brand name for combined formoterol (a sympathomimetic bronchodilator 48) and fluticasone 265 (a corticosteroid 99)

fluvastatin lipid-lowering drug 61

fluvoxamine antidepressant 40

FML brand name for fluorometholone (a corticosteroid 99)

folic acid 436, vitamin 107

folinic acid vitamin 107

follicle-stimulating hormone (FSH) natural hormone for infertility 124

follitropin alfa drug for infertility 124

follitropin beta drug for infertility 124

fomepizole antidote for ethylene glycol and methanol poisoning

Fomicyt brand name for fosfomycin (an antibacterial 89)

fondaparinux anticoagulant 62

Foradil brand name for formoterol (a bronchodilator 48)

Forceval brand-name multivitamin 107

Formagin brand name for degarelix (an anticancer drug 112 used for advanced prostate cancer)

formoterol (previously eformoterol) a sympathomimetic bronchodilator 48

Forsteo brand name for teriparatide (a drug for bone disorders 80)

Fortipine LA brand name for modified-release nifedipine 340 (a calcium channel blocker 59)

Fortum brand name for ceftazidime (a cephalosporin antibiotic 86)

Forxiga brand name for dapagliflozin 220 (a drug for diabetes 100)

Fosamax brand name for alendronic acid 149 (a drug for bone disorders 80)

fosamprenavir antiretroviral for HIV/AIDS 116

fosaprepitant pro-drug of aprepitant (an anti-emetic 46)

Fosavance brand name for alendronic acid 149 (a drug for bone disorders 80) with colecalciferol (vitamin D 444)

Foscan brand name for temoprofin (an anticancer drug 112)

foscarnet antiviral drug 91

Foscavir brand name for foscarnet (an antiviral drug 91)

fosfomycin antibacterial drug 89

fosinopril ACE inhibitor 56

fosphenytoin 359, a pro-drug of phenytoin (an anticonvulsant 42)

Fostair brand name for beclometasone 168 (a corticosteroid 99) with formoterol (a sympathomimetic brochodilator 48)

Fostiman Freederm brand name for nicotinamide gel (used to treat acne 137)

Fotivda brand name for tivozinab (an anti-cancer drug 112) used to treat kidney cancers

Fragmin brand name for dalteparin (a low-molecular-weight heparin 275 used as an anticoagulant 62)

framycetin topical aminoglycoside antibiotic 86 for ear, eye, and skin infections

frangula mild stimulant laxative 69

Frisium brand name for clobazam (a benzodiazepine anti-anxiety drug 39)

frovatriptan drug for migraine 45

Frumil brand name for amiloride 154 with furosemide 266 (both diuretics 57)

Frusene brand name for furosemide 266 with triamterene 423 (both diuretics 57)

Frusol brand name for furosemide 266 (a loop diuretic 57)

FSH follicle-stimulating hormone (a natural hormone for infertility 124)

Fucibet brand name for betamethasone 172 (a corticosteroid 99) with fusidic acid (an antibiotic 86)

Fucidin brand name for fusidic acid (an antibiotic 86)

Fultium-D3 brand name for colecalciferol 437 (vitamin D 444)

Fulvestrant anticancer drug 112 used for treatment of breast cancer

Fungizone brand name for amphotericin 160 (an antifungal 96)

furosemide (previously frusemide) 266, a loop diuretic 57

fusidic acid antibiotic 86

Fuzatal XL brand name for alfuzosin hydrochloride (an alpha blocker used to treat prostate disorders 126)

Fuzeon brand name for enfuvirtide (an antiretroviral for HIV/AIDS 116)

Fybogel brand name for ispaghula (a bulk-forming agent used as a laxative 69 and antidiarrhoeal 68)

Fycompa brand name for perampanel (an anticonvulsant 42)

Fyramadel brand name for ganirelix (a drug used to treat infertility 124)

G

gabapentin 267, anticonvulsant 42

Gabitril brand name for tiagabine (an anticonvulsant 42)

Gabup brand name for sublingual buprenorphine (an opioid analgesic 36)

galantamine drug for Alzheimer's disease 43

Galantex brand name for galantamine (a drug used to treat Alzheimer's disease 43)

Galcodine brand name for codeine 211 (a cough suppressant 52)

Galebon brand name for modified-release tamsulosin 407 (an alpha blocker used to treat prostate disorders 126)

Galenphol brand name for pholcodine (a cough suppressant 52)

Galfer brand name for iron 437 (a mineral 108)

Galfer FA brand name for folic acid 436 (a vitamin 107) with iron 437 (a mineral 108)

Galpseud brand name for pseudoephedrine (a sympathomimetic decongestant 51)

Galsya XL brand name for galantamine (a drug used to treat Alzheimer's disease 43)

Galvus brand name for vildagliptin (a drug for diabetes 100)

gamma globulin immunoglobulin 92

gamolenic acid extract of evening primrose

ganciclovir antiviral 91

Ganfort brand-name preparation containing bimatoprost (a drug for glaucoma 128) with timolol 417 (a beta blocker 55)

ganirelix drug used to treat infertility 124

Gardasil brand-name vaccine 92 against human papillomavirus

Gatalin XL brand name for galantamine (a drug used to treat Alzheimer's disease 43)

Gaviscon Advance brand-name antacid 66 containing potassium bicarbonate with alginate

Gaviscon Extra Strength brand-name antacid 66 containing aluminium hydroxide 153, sodium bicarbonate, magnesium trisilicate, and alginic acid

Gaviscon Infant Oral brand-name antacid 66 containing alginates 150

Gazylan XL brand name for galantamine (a drug used to treat Alzheimer's disease 43)

Gazyvaro brand name for obinutuzumab (a monoclonal antibody anticancer drug 112)

Gedarel brand-name combined oral contraceptive 121 containing ethinylestradiol 252 and desogestrel 222

Gefitinib anticancer drug 112

GelTears brand of artificial tears 130

gemcitabine anticancer drug 112

gemeprost drug used in labour 125

HUMAN MIXTARD

gemfibrozil lipid-lowering drug 61

gemtuzumab monoclonal antibody 113 used to treat acute myeloid leukaemia

Gemzar brand name for gemcitabine (an anticancer drug 112)

Genfura brand name for nitrofurantoin (an antibacterial 89) used for urinary tract infections

Genotropin brand name for somatropin (a synthetic pituitary hormone 103)

gentamicin 268, aminoglycoside antibiotic 86

Germolene brand-name preparation containing phenol with chlorhexidine (both antiseptics 135)

Germoloids HC brand name for hydrocortisone 277 (a corticosteroid 134) with lidocaine (a local anaesthetic 36) for haemorrhoids 71

gestodene progestogen 105 and oral contraceptive 121

Gestone brand name for progesterone (a female sex hormone 105)

Gielism brand name for alverine citrate (an antispasmodic drug 68) for menstrual pain

Gilenya brand name for fingolimod (an immunomodulator for multiple sclerosis 78)

Giotrif brand name for afatinib (an anticancer drug 112)

Glandosane brand name for artificial saliva

glatiramer drug for multiple sclerosis

Glensoludex brand name for dexamethasone 223 (a corticosteroid 99)

Gliadel brand name for carmustine (an anticancer drug 112) used for malignant glioma brain tumours

glibenclamide 269, oral drug for diabetes 100

gliclazide 270, oral drug for diabetes 100

Glidipion brand name for pioglitazone 361 (a drug for diabetes 100)

glimepiride oral drug for diabetes 100

glipizide oral drug for diabetes 100

Glivec brand name for imatinib 280 (an anticancer drug 112)

GlucaGen brand name for glucagon 271 (a drug for hypoglycaemia 100)

glucagon 271, a drug for hypoglycaemia 100

Glucient SR brand name for modified-release metformin 318 (an oral drug for diabetes 100)

Glucobay brand name for acarbose (an oral drug for diabetes 100)

Glucophage brand name for metformin 318 (an oral drug for diabetes 100)

Glucophage SR brand name for modified-release metformin 318 (an oral drug for diabetes 100)

glucosamine substance used for osteoarthritis of the knee

Glusartel brand name for glucosamine (a substance used for osteoarthritis of the knee)

glutaraldehyde topical wart treatment

Glutarol brand name for glutaraldehyde (a topical wart preparation)

glycerol drug used to reduce pressure inside the eye 127; an ingredient in cough mixtures 52, skin preparations 135, laxative suppositories 69, and ear-wax softening drops 131

glyceryl trinitrate 272, anti-angina drug 59

glycopyrronium bromide anticholinergic used in general anaesthesia

Glypressin brand name for terlipressin (a drug similar to vasopressin, a pituitary hormone 103, used to stop bleeding)

Glytrin brand name for a spray form of glyceryl trinitrate 267 (an anti-angina drug 59)

gold metal used medically as a DMARD 75

Golden Eye brand name for propamidine isethionate (an antibacterial used topically on the eye 89)

golimumab monoclonal antibody for severe ulcerative colitis 70 and rheumatoid arthritis 75

gonadorelin a drug for infertility 124

gonadotrophin chorionic drug used to treat infertility 124

Gonal-f brand name for follitropin alfa (a gonadotrophin for female infertility 124)

Gonapeptyl brand name for triptorelin (a drug used to treat infertility 124)

goserelin 273, female sex hormone 105 and anticancer drug 112, also used for menstrual disorders 120 and infertility 124

granisetron anti-emetic 46

Granocyte brand name for lenograstim (a blood growth stimulant)

granpidam a generic drug similar to sildenafil 394 (a drug used to treat pulmonary hypertension and erectile dysfunction)

Granupas brand name for aminosalicylic acid (an antibacterial drug used to treat tuberculosis 90)

Grazax brand name for grass pollen extract used to treat hay fever

Grepid brand name for clopidogrel 208 (an antiplatelet drug 62)

griseofulvin antifungal drug 96

Grisol AF brand-name spray containing griseofulvin (an antifungal 96) used for athlete's foot

growth hormone also called somatropin, a pituitary hormone 103

GTN 300mcg brand name for glyceryl trinitrate 272 (an anti-angina drug 59)

guanethidine antihypertensive drug 60

guanfacine non-stimulant drug used to treat attention deficit hyperactivity disorder (ADHD)

guselkumab monoclonal antibody used to treat psoriasis 138

Gygel brand-name gel containing nonoxinol (a spermicidal contraceptive)

Gyno-Daktarin brand name for miconazole 326 (an antifungal 96)

Gyno-Pevaryl brand name for econazole (an antifungal 96)

Gynoxin brand name for fenticonazole nitrate (an antifungal drug 96) used for vaginal and vulval candidiasis

H

Haelan brand name for fludroxycortide (a topical corticosteroid 134)

haem arginate drug used to treat porphyria

Haemoctin brand name for factor VIII (a substance used to promote blood clotting 62)

Haemonine brand name for factor X (a substance used to promote blood clotting 62)

Halaven brand name for eribulin (an anticancer drug 112)

Haldol brand name for a syrup preparation of haloperidol 274 (an antipsychotic 41)

Haldol decanoate brand name for an injectable form of haloperidol 274 (an antipsychotic 41)

Half Securon brand name for modified-release verapamil 428 used to treat hypertension 60

Half Sinemet CR brand name for modified-release co-careldopa 298 (a drug for Parkinson's disease 43)

haloperidol 274, antipsychotic 41

Hapoctasin brand-name skin patch containing buprenorphine (an opioid analgesic 36)

Harvoni brand name for sofosbuvir with ledipasvir (both antiviral drugs 91) used for chronic hepatitis C

Havrix brand-name vaccine 92 against hepatitis A

Hayfever and Allergy Relief/Hayfever Relief brand names for cetirizine 191 (an antihistamine 82)

Hayleve brand name for chlorphenamine 194 (an antihistamine 82) used for allergies

Haymine brand name for chlorphenamine 194 (an antihistamine 82) used for allergies

HBvaxPRO brand-name vaccine 92 against viral hepatitis B

Hc45 brand name for a cream containing hydrocortisone 277 (a corticosteroid 134)

hCG human chorionic gonadotrophin (a drug for infertility 124)

Hedex brand name for paracetamol 352 (a non-opioid analgesic 36)

Hedex Extra brand name for paracetamol 352 (a non-opioid analgesic 36) with caffeine

Hedrin brand name for dimeticone (a drug used for head lice 136)

Hedrin Once brand name for dimeticone (a drug used for head lice 136)

Helixate NexGen brand name for factor VIII (a substance to promote blood clotting 62)

Hemabate brand name for carboprost (a drug to control bleeding after childbirth 125)

Hemlibra brand name for emicizumab (a monoclonal antibody) used for haemophilia

heparin 275, an anticoagulant 62

heparinoid a drug applied topically to reduce inflammation of the skin 132

Hepatect CP brand-name immunoglobulin 92 used for hepatitis B

Hepatyrix brand-name vaccine 92 to protect against viral hepatitis A/typhoid

Hepsera brand name for adefovir (an antiviral 91 for chronic hepatitis B)

Herceptin brand name for trastuzumab 422 (an anticancer drug 112)

heroin diamorphine 334 (an opioid 455 and analgesic 36)

Herzuma brand name for trastuzumab 422 (a monoclonal antibody) used for breast cancer

hexamine another name for methenamine, a drug for urinary tract infections 126

hexetidine antiseptic 135

Hexopal brand name for inositol nicotinate (a vasodilator 56)

Hibisol brand name for chlorhexidine (an antiseptic 135)

Hibitane brand name for chlorhexidine (an antiseptic 135)

Hidrasec brand name for racecadotril (an antidiarrhoeal drug 68)

Hiprex brand name for hexamine/methenamine (a drug for urinary tract infections 126)

Hirudoid brand name for heparinoid (a topical anti-inflammatory 134)

histamine hydrochloride drug used for acute myeloid leukaemia

Histoacryl brand name for enbucrilate (a tissue adhesive)

Hormonin brand name for estradiol 249 (a female sex hormone 105)

Humalog brand name for insulin lispro 284 (a drug for diabetes 100)

Human Actrapid brand name for insulin 284 (a drug for diabetes 100)

Human Insulatard brand name for insulin 284 (a drug for diabetes 100)

human menopausal gonadotrophins (also called menotrophin) a drug for infertility 124

Human Mixtard brand name for insulin 284 (a drug for diabetes 100)

HUMATROPE

Humatrope brand name for somatropin, a pituitary hormone 103 (a synthetic pituitary hormone 103)

Humira brand name for adalimumab (DMARD 75)

Humulin preparations brand name for insulin 284 (a drug for diabetes 100)

Hyabak brand name for eye drops containing sodium hyaluronate (a lubricant)

hyaluronidase substance that helps injections penetrate tissues

Hycamtin brand name for topotecan (an anticancer drug 112)

Hycoscan brand name for eye drops containing sodium hyaluronate (a lubricant)

hydralazine antihypertensive drug 60

Hydrea brand name for hydroxycarbamide (an anticancer drug 112)

hydrochlorothiazide 276, thiazide diuretic 57

hydrocortisone 277, corticosteroid 99 and antipruritic 133

Hydrocortistab brand name for hydrocortisone 277 (a corticosteroid 99)

hydroflumethiazide thiazide diuretic 57

hydrogen peroxide antiseptic mouthwash 135

Hydromol Ointment preparation for eczema, psoriasis, and other dry skin conditions

Hydromoor brand name for hypromellose eye drops 130

hydromorphone opioid analgesic 36

hydrotalcite antacid 66

hydroxocobalamin vitamin B12 443 (a vitamin 107)

hydroxycarbamide (previously hydroxyurea) a drug for chronic myeloid leukaemia 112

hydroxychloroquine antimalarial 95 and DMARD 75

hydroxyzine antihistamine 82 and anti-anxiety drug 39

Hygroton brand name for chlortalidone (a thiazide diuretic 57)

hyoscine 278, drug for irritable bowel syndrome 68, affecting the pupil 130, and to prevent motion sickness 46

Hypnovel brand name for midazolam (a benzodiazepine 38 used as premedication)

Hypovase brand name for prazosin (an alpha blocker 56 antihypertensive 60 and drug for prostate disorders 126)

hypromellose substance in artificial tear preparations 130

Hypurin brand name for insulin 284 (a drug for diabetes 100)

Hytrin brand name for terazosin (an alpha blocker 56 antihypertensive 60 and drug for prostate disorders 126)

I

Iasibon brand name for ibandronic acid (a bisphosphonate for bone disorders 80)

ibandronic acid bisphosphonate drug for bone disorders 80

Ibrance brand name for palbociclib (an anticancer drug 112) used for breast cancer

Ibrutinib a tyrosine kinase inhibitor anticancer drug 112

Ibugel brand name for ibuprofen 279 (NSAID 74)

Ibuleve brand-name gel for muscular pain relief containing ibuprofen 279 (a NSAID 74)

Ibumousse brand-name foam for muscle pain relief containing ibuprofen 279 (a NSAID 74)

ibuprofen 279, non-opioid analgesic 36 and NSAID 74

icatibant drug to treat angioedema

ichthammol substance in skin preparations for eczema 139

Iclusig brand name for ponatinib (a tyrosine kinase inhibitor anticancer drug 112)

idarubicin cytotoxic antibiotic (an anticancer drug 112)

idarucizumab monoclonal antibody used to reverse the bleeding effects of dabigatran 219 (an anticoagulant 62)

idelalisib tyrosine kinase inhibitor anticancer drug 112

idoxuridine antiviral drug 91

Ifirmasta brand name for irbesartan 287 (an antihypertensive 60)

ifosfamide anticancer drug 112

Ikervis brand name for ciclosporin 196 (an immunosuppressant 115) for eye inflammation

Ikorel brand name for nicorandil 338 (an anti-angina drug 59)

Ilaris brand name for canakinumab (a monoclonal antibody used for gout 77)

Ilaxten brand name for bilastine (an antihistamine 82)

iloprost vasodilator 56 used for pulmonary hypertension

Ilube brand name for acetylcysteine (a mucolytic 52) with hypromellose (a substance in artificial tear preparations 130)

imatinib 280, an anticancer drug 112

Imbruvica brand name for ibrutinib (a tyrosine kinase anticancer drug 112)

Imdur brand name for isosorbide mononitrate 289 (a nitrate vasodilator 56 and anti-angina drug 59)

imidapril ACE inhibitor 56

imiglucerase enzyme used for replacement therapy

Imigran brand name for sumatriptan 404 (a drug for migraine 45)

imipenem antibiotic 86

imipramine 281, tricyclic antidepressant 40 and drug for urinary disorders 126

imiquimod drug to treat genital warts

Immukin brand name for interferon gamma 285 (an antiviral 91)

immunoglobulin preparation injected to prevent infectious diseases 92

Imnovid brand name for pomalidomide (a drug similar to thalidomide 415 used for cancer)

Imodium brand name for loperamide 305 (an antidiarrhoeal 68)

Implanon brand name for etonorgestrel (a progestogen 105)

Imunovir brand name for inosine pranobex (an antiviral 91)

Imuran brand name for azathioprine 166 (a DMARD 75 and immunosuppressant drug 115)

Incivo brand name for telaprevir (an antiviral for HIV/AIDS 116)

Inconex XL brand name for modified-release tolterodine 420 (a drug used to treat urinary frequency 126)

Incruse Ellipta brand name for an inhaled form of umeclidinium (a bronchodilator 48) used for obstructive airways disease

indacaterol long-acting bronchodilator 48 used for obstructive airways disease

indapamide 282, thiazide-like diuretic 57

Indermil brand name for enbucrilate (a tissue adhesive)

indinavir antiretroviral for HIV/AIDS 116

Indipam XL brand name for modified-release indapamide 282 (a thiazide-like diuretic 57) used for hypertension 60

Indivina brand-name preparation for menopausal symptoms 105 containing estradiol 249 with medroxyprogesterone 313

Indocid brand name for indometacin (a NSAID 74 and drug for gout 77)

indometacin NSAID 74 and drug for gout 77

indoramin antihypertensive 60 and drug for urinary disorders 126

Inegy brand-name preparation containing simvastatin 395 with ezetimibe 255 (both lipid-lowering drugs 61)

Infacol brand name for dimeticone (an antifoaming agent 66)

Inflectra brand name for infliximab 283 (a drug for inflammatory bowel disease 70 and DMARD 75)

infliximab 283, drug for inflammatory bowel disease 70 and DMARD 75

Influvac Sub-unit branded influenza vaccine 92

ingenol mebutate a protein kinase activator used for actinic keratosis

Inhalvent brand name for ipratropium bromide 286 (a bronchodilator 48)

Inhixa biosimilar drug to enoxaparin (an anticoagulant 62)

Inlyta brand name for axitinib (a protein kinase anticancer drug 112)

Innohep brand name for tinzaparin (a low-molecular-weight heparin 275 used as an anticoagulant 62)

Innovace brand name for enalapril 243 (a vasodilator 56 and antihypertensive 60)

Innozide brand name for enalapril 243 (a vasodilator 56 and antihypertensive 60)

inosine pranobex antiviral drug 91

inositol drug related to nicotinic acid

inotuzumab ozogamicin monoclonal antibody used to treat cancer 112

Inovelon brand name for rufinamide (an anticonvulsant drug 42)

Inspra brand name for eplerenone (a drug for heart failure following a heart attack 53)

Instanyl brand name for a spray containing fentanyl (an opioid analgesic 36)

Insulatard brand name for insulin 284 (a drug for diabetes 100)

insulin 284, drug for diabetes 100

insulin aspart type of insulin 284 (a drug for diabetes 100)

insulin detemir type of insulin 284 (a drug for diabetes 100)

insulin glargine type of insulin 284 (a drug for diabetes 100)

insulin glulisine type of insulin 284 (a drug for diabetes 100)

insulin isphane type of insulin 284 (a drug for diabetes 100)

insulin lispro type of insulin 284 (a drug for diabetes 100)

Insuman brand name for insulin (human) 284 (a drug for diabetes 100)

Intal brand name for sodium cromoglicate 397 (an anti-allergy drug 82)

Intelence brand name for etravirine (an antiviral 91) used to treat HIV 116

interferon 285, antiviral drug 91 and anticancer drug 112

Intron-A brand name for interferon 285 (an antiviral 91 and anticancer drug 112)

Intuniv brand name for modified-release guanfacine (a non-stimulant drug used for attention deficit hyperactivity disorder)

Invanz brand name for ertapenem (an antibiotic 86)

Invega brand name for modified-release paliperidone (an antipsychotic drug 41)

LABETALOL

Invirase brand name for saquinavir (an antiretroviral for HIV/AIDS 116)

Invita D3 brand name for colecalciferol (vitamin D 444)

Invivac brand name for influenza vaccine 92

Invodol SR brand name for modified-release tramadol 421 (an opioid analgesic 36)

Invokana brand name for canagliflozin (a drug for diabetes 100)

iodine 437, mineral 108

Iopidine brand name for apraclonidine (a drug for glaucoma 128)

ipilimumab monoclonal antibody anticancer drug 112

Ipocol brand name for mesalazine 317 (a drug for ulcerative colitis 70)

Ipramol brand name for ipratropium 286 with salbutamol 391 (both bronchodilators 48) used for obstructive airways disease

ipratropium bromide 286, bronchodilator 48

irbesartan 287, angiotensin II blocker (a vasodilator 56 and antihypertensive 60)

Iressa brand name for gefitinib (an anticancer drug 112)

irinotecan anticancer drug 112

iron 437, mineral 108

Ironorm brand name for oral drops containing iron 437 used for anaemia

isavuconazole triazole antifungal drug 96

Isentress brand name for raltegravir (an antiviral 91) used to treat HIV 116

Isib brand name for isosorbide mononitrate 289 (a vasodilator 56 and anti-angina drug 59)

Ismo brand name for isosorbide mononitrate 289 (a vasodilator 56 and anti-angina drug 59)

isocarboxazid monoamine oxidase inhibitor (MAOI) antidepressant 40

Isodur brand name for isosorbide mononitrate 289 (a vasodilator 56 and anti-angina drug 59)

isoflurane volatile liquid inhaled as a general anaesthetic

Isoket brand name for isosorbide dinitrate 289 (a vasodilator 56 and anti-angina drug 59)

isometheptene mucate a drug for migraine 45

isoniazid 288, antituberculous drug 90

isophane insulin type of insulin 284 (a drug for diabetes 100)

isoprenaline bronchodilator 48

Isopto Alkaline brand name for hypromellose (a substance in artificial tear preparations 130)

Isopto Plain brand-name eye drops containing phenylephrine (a decongestant 51) and hypromellose (a substance in artificial tear preparations 130)

isosorbide dinitrate 289, nitrate vasodilator 56 and anti-angina drug 59

isosorbide mononitrate 289, nitrate vasodilator 56 and anti-angina drug 59

Isotard brand name for isosorbide mononitrate 289 (a vasodilator 56 and anti-angina drug 59)

isotretinoin 290, drug for acne 137

Isotrex brand name for isotretinoin 290 (a drug for acne 137)

Isotrexin brand name for isotretinoin 290 with erythromycin 247 (a drug for acne 137)

Isovorin brand name for levofolinate, used to reduce the toxicity of methotrexate 320 during chemotherapy

Ispagel brand name for ispaghula (a bulk-forming agent) for constipation 69 and diarrhoea 68

ispaghula bulk-forming agent for constipation 69 and diarrhoea 68

isradipine calcium channel blocker used for hypertension 60

Isteranda brand-name contraceptive 121 containing levonorgestrel 300

Istin brand name for amlodipine 158 (a calcium channel blocker 59 and antihypertensive 60)

itraconazole an antifungal 96

ivabradine anti-angina drug 59

ivacaftor 414, drug used for cystic fibrosis

Ivemend brand name for fosaprepitant (an anti-emetic 46)

ivermectin anthelmintic 97

ixazomib proteasome inhibitor drug used to treat (blood) cancer 112

ixekizumab monoclonal antibody used to treat psoriasis 138

J

Jakavi brand name for ruxolitinib (a tyrosine kinase inhibitor anticancer drug 112)

Janumet brand-name preparation of sitagliptin 396 with metformin 318 (both drugs for diabetes 100)

Januvia brand name for sitagliptin 396 (a drug for diabetes 100)

Jardiance brand name for empagliflozin (a drug for diabetes 100)

Javlor brand name for vinflunine (an anticancer drug 112)

Jaydess brand-name intrauterine contraceptive device containing levonorgestrel 300

Jentadueto brand name for linagliptin with metformin 318 (both drugs for diabetes 100)

Jevtana brand name for cabazitaxel (a taxane anticancer drug 112) used for prostate cancer

Jext brand name for epinephrine 245

Jinarc brand name for tolvaptan (a diuretic drug 57) used for polycystic kidney disease and low blood sodium

Joy-rides brand name for hyoscine hydrobromide 278 (used to prevent motion sickness 46)

Juliperla brand-name combined oral contraceptive 121 containing ethinylestradiol 252 and gestodene

Jylamvo brand name for methotrexate 320 (an immunosuppressant drug 115)

K

Kadcyla brand name for trastuzumab 422 (an anticancer drug 112)

Kaftrio brand name for a fixed-dose combination of elexacaftor/ivacaftor/tezacaftor 414 (a treatment for cystic fibrosis)

Kalcipos-D brand name for colecalciferol (vitamin D 444) with calcium carbonate (calcium 427)

Kaletra brand name for lopinavir 306 with ritonavir (both antiretrovirals for HIV/AIDS 116)

Kalspare brand name for triamterene 423 with chlortalidone (both diuretics 57)

Kalydeco brand name for ivacaftor 414 (a drug used for cystic fibrosis)

kaolin absorbent used as an antidiarrhoeal 68

Kapake brand name for codeine 211 and paracetamol 352 (both analgesics 36)

Katya branded combined oral contraceptive 121 containing ethinylestradiol 252 and gestodene

Kay-Cee-L brand name for a potassium supplement 431 (a mineral 108)

Keflex brand name for cefalexin 189 (a cephalosporin antibiotic 86)

Keftid brand name for cefaclor (a cephalosporin antibiotic 86)

Kemadrin brand name for procyclidine 367 (a drug for parkinsonism 43)

Kemicetine brand name for chloramphenicol 192 (an antibiotic 86)

Kenalog brand name for triamcinolone (a corticosteroid 99)

Kengrexal brand name for cangrelor (an antiplatelet drug 62)

Kentera brand name for oxybutynin 351 (a drug for urinary disorders 126)

Keppra brand name for levetiracetam 297 (an anticonvulsant 42)

Keral brand name for dexketoprofen (an NSAID 74)

Kerstipon brand name for rivastigmine 387 (a drug used for Alzheimer's disease 43)

Ketalar brand name for ketamine (used as general anaesthetic; also a drug of abuse 452)

ketamine drug used to induce general anaesthesia; also a drug of abuse 452

ketoconazole 291, an antifungal 96

ketoprofen 292, a NSAID 74

ketorolac a NSAID 74 used as an analgesic 36

ketotifen an antihistamine 82 similar to sodium cromoglicate 397 for allergies and asthma 49

Ketovite brand-name vitamin supplement 107

Kevzara brand name for sarilumab (a monoclonal antibody) used to treat rheumatoid arthritis 75

Keytruda brand name for pembrolizumab (a monoclonal antibody)

Kineret brand name for anakinra (a DMARD 75)

Kisplyx brand name for lenvatinib (an anticancer drug 112) used for kidney cancer

Kisqali brand name for ribociclib (an anticancer drug 112) to treat breast cancer

Kivexa brand name for abacavir with lamivudine 430 (both antiretrovirals for HIV/AIDS 116)

Klaricid brand name for clarithromycin 202 (an antibiotic 86)

Klean-prep brand-name osmotic laxative 69

Kliofem brand-name product for menopausal symptoms 105 containing estradiol 249 and norethisterone 342

Kliovance brand-name product for menopausal symptoms 105 containing estradiol 249 and norethisterone 342

Kogenate brand name for factor VIII (a substance to promote blood clotting 62)

Kolanticon brand name for aluminium hydroxide 153 and magnesium oxide (both antacids 66) with dicycloverine 226 (an anticholinergic antispasmodic 68) and simeticone (an antifoaming agent 66)

Kolbam brand name for cholic acid used for biliary disorders

Komboglyze brand name for metformin 318 with saxagliptin (both drugs for diabetes 100)

Konakion brand name for phytomenadione (vitamin K 445)

Kwells/Kwells Adult brand name for hyoscine hydrobromide 278 used to prevent motion sickness 46

Kyprolis brand name for carfilzomib (an anticancer drug 112) used for myeloma (a type of cancer of the bone marrow)

Kytril brand name for granisetron (an anti-emetic 46)

L

Laaglyda MR brand name for modified-release gliclazide 270 (a drug for diabetes 100)

labetalol beta blocker 55

LACIDIPINE

lacidipine calcium channel blocker 59

lacosamide anticonvulsant drug 42 used to control epilepsy

Lacri-Lube brand-name ointment used for dry eyes 130

lactic acid ingredient in wart preparations, emollients, and pessaries

Lactugal brand name for lactulose 293 (an osmotic laxative 69)

lactulose 293, osmotic laxative 69

Lamictal brand name for lamotrigine 294 (an anticonvulsant 42)

Lamisil AT 1% Cream/Gel/Spray brand name for terbinafine 410 (an antifungal 96)

Lamisil Cream brand name for terbinafine 410 (an antifungal 96)

Lamisil Once brand name for terbinafine 410 (an antifungal 96)

Lamisil Tablets brand name for terbinafine 410 (an antifungal 96)

lamivudine 430, antiretroviral for HIV/AIDS 116 and hepatitis B

lamotrigine 294, anticonvulsant 42

Lanoxin brand name for digoxin 227 (a digitalis drug 54)

lanreotide anticancer drug 112, also used for endocrine disorders 103

lansoprazole 295, anti-ulcer drug 67

Lantus brand name for insulin glargine (a type of insulin 284, a drug for diabetes 100)

lapatinib anticancer drug 112

Larafen brand name for ketoprofen 292 (a NSAID 74)

Larbex XL brand name for modified-release doxazosin 236 (an alpha blocker antihypertensive 60 and drug for prostate disorders 126)

Largactil brand name for chlorpromazine 195 (a phenothiazine antipsychotic 41 and anti-emetic 46)

Lariam brand name for mefloquine 315 (an antimalarial 95)

Lasilactone brand name for furosemide 266 with spironolactone 400 (both diuretics 57)

Lasix brand name for furosemide 260 (a loop diuretic 57)

Lasoride brand name for amiloride 154 (a potassium-sparing diuretic 57)

latanoprost 296, drug for glaucoma 128

Latuda brand name for lurasidone hydrochloride (an antipsychotic drug 41)

Laxido brand name for macrogol (a laxative 69) used to treat chronic constipation

Laxoberal brand name for sodium picosulfate (a laxative 69)

Leandra brand name for a combination contraceptive 121 containing levonorgestrel 300 and ethinylestradiol 252

Lecaent brand name for pregabalin (an anticonvulsant 42) used for seizures and pain

ledipasvir antiviral 91 used to treat hepatitis C

leflunomide DMARD 75

Lemsip Max brand name for paracetamol 352 (a non-opioid analgesic 36) with phenylephrine (a decongestant 51) and caffeine

Lemtrada brand name for alemtuzumab (an anticancer drug 112)

lenalidomide immunomodulating anticancer drug 112

lenograstim blood growth stimulant

lenvatinib protein kinase inhibitor used to treat cancer 112

Lenvima brand name for lenvatinib (an anticancer drug 112) used for thyroid cancer

lercanidipine calcium channel blocker 59

Lescol brand name for fluvastatin (a lipid-lowering drug 61)

Lestramyl brand-name combined oral contraceptive 121 containing ethinylestradiol 252 and desogestrel 222

letrozole anticancer drug 112

leuprorelin a drug for menstrual disorders 120 and prostate cancer 112

Leustat brand name for cladribine (a cyotoxic anticancer drug 112) used for leukaemia

Levact brand name for bendamustine hydrochloride (a cytotoxic anticancer drug 112) used for leukaemia, non-Hodgkin's lymphoma, and multiple myeloma

levamisole anthelmintic 97

Levemir brand name for insulin 284 (a drug for diabetes 100)

Levest brand name for a combined oral contraceptive 121 containing ethinylestradiol 252 and levonorgestrel 300

levetiracetam 297, anticonvulsant 42

Levinan brand name for levomepromazine (an antipsychotic drug 41) used in palliative care and for schizophrenia

Levitra brand name for vardenafil (a drug for erectile dysfunction 124)

levobunolol beta blocker 55 and drug for glaucoma 128

levobupivacaine local anaesthetic 36

levocetirizine 191, antihistamine 82

levodopa 298, drug for parkinsonism 43

levofloxacin 299, an antibacterial 89

levomenthol an alcohol from mint oils used as an inhalation and topical antipruritic 133

levomepromazine (previously methotrimeprazine) an antpsychotic 41

Levonelle 1500 brand name for levonorgestrel 300 (a female sex hormone 105 and oral contraceptive 121)

Levonelle One Step brand name for levonorgestrel 300 (a female sex hormone 105 and oral contraceptive 121)

levonorgestrel 300, female sex hormone 105 and oral contraceptive 121

Levosert intravaginal form of levonorgestrel 300 for contraception or heavy periods 120

levothyroxine 301 (previously thyroxine) a thyroid hormone 102

Lexpec brand name for folic acid 436

Librium brand name for chlordiazepoxide (a benzodiazepine anti-anxiety drug 39)

lidocaine (previously lignocaine) local anaesthetic 36, anti-arrhythmic 58, and antipruritic 133

Li-liquid brand name for lithium 303 (a drug for mania 41)

linaclotide drug for irritable bowel syndrome 68

linagliptin drug for diabetes 100

linezolid antibiotic 86

Lioresal brand name for baclofen 167 (a muscle relaxant 78)

liothyronine (also called tri-iodothyronine) thyroid hormone 102

Lipantil brand name for fenofibrate (a lipid-lowering drug 61)

lipegfilgrastim drug used with chemotherapy drugs to stimulate white blood cell production

Lipitor brand name for atorvastatin 164 (a lipid-lowering drug 61)

Lipostat brand name for pravastatin 364 (a cholesterol-lowering agent 61)

liquid paraffin lubricating agent used as a laxative 69 and also in artificial tears 130

Liquifilm Tears brand-name eye drops containing polyvinyl acetate (artificial tears 130)

liquorice substance for peptic ulcers 67

liraglutide drug for diabetes 100

lisdexamfetamine drug used to treat attention deficit hyperactivity disorder (ADHD)

lisinopril 302, ACE inhibitor 56

Liskonum brand name for lithium 303 (a drug for mania 41)

Litak brand name for cladribine (a cytotoxic anticancer drug 112) for hairy cell leukaemia

lithium 303, drug for mania 41

Livial brand name for tibolone (a female sex hormone 105)

Lixiana brand name for edoxaban (an anticlotting drug 62)

lixisenatide drug for diabetes 100

Lizinna brand-name combined oral contraceptive 121 containing ethinylestradiol 252 and norgestimate

Loceryl brand name for amorolfine (an antifungal 96)

Locoid brand name for hydrocortisone 277 (a corticosteroid 99)

Lodine SR brand name for etodolac (a NSAID 74)

Lodotra brand name for modified-release prednisolone 365 (a corticosteroid 99) used for rheumatoid arthritis 75

lodoxamide anti-allergy drug 82

Loestrin 20 and **Loestrin 30** brand-name oral contraceptives 121 containing ethinylestradiol 252 and norethisterone 342

lofepramine 304, tricyclic antidepressant 40

lofexidine drug to treat opioid withdrawal symptoms 24

Lojuxta brand name for lomitapide (a lipid-lowering drug 61)

lomitapide lipid-lowering drug 61

Lomont brand name for lofepramine 304 (a tricyclic antidepressant 40)

lomustine alkylating agent for Hodgkin's disease 112

Longtec brand name for oxycodone (an opioid analgesic 36)

Loniten brand name for minoxidil 328 (an antihypertensive 60)

Lonsurf brand name for a combination of trifluridine and tipiracil (both anticancer drugs 112) used for bowel cancer

loperamide 305, antidiarrhoeal 68

Lopid brand name for gemfibrozil (a lipid-lowering drug 61)

lopinavir 306, antiretroviral for HIV/AIDS 116

loprazolam benzodiazepine sleeping drug 38

Lopresor brand name for metoprolol 324 (a cardioselective beta blocker 55)

loratadine 307, antihistamine 82

lorazepam 224, benzodiazepine anti-anxiety drug 39 and sleeping drug 38

lormetazepam benzodiazepine sleeping drug 38

Loron brand name for sodium clodronate (a drug for bone disorders 80 in some types of cancer 112)

losartan 308, angiotensin II blocker (a vasodilator 56 and antihypertensive 60)

Losec brand name for omeprazole 346 (an anti-ulcer drug 67)

Losinate MR brand name for modified-release tamsulosin 407 used for benign prostatic hyperplasia 126

Lotprosin XL brand name for modified-release galantamine (a drug for dementia 43)

Lotriderm brand-name product containing betamethasone 172 (a corticosteroid 99) and clotrimazole 209 (an antifungal 96)

Lubion brand name for progesterone 105 used to treat female infertility 124

METFORMIN

lubiprostone laxative 69

Lubristil brand name for hyaluronate (artificial tears 130)

Lucentis brand name for ranibizumab (a drug for wet age-related macular degeneration)

Lucette brand-name combined oral contraceptive 121 containing ethinylestradiol 252 and drospirenone

lumacaftor drug used to treat cystic fibrosis

Lumecare carbomer, hypromellose, sodium hyaluronate brands of artificial tears 130

lumefantrine antimalarial drug 95

Lumigan brand name for bimatoprost (a drug for glaucoma 128)

lurasidone hydrochloride antipsychotic 41

Lustral brand name for sertraline 393 (an antidepressant 40)

luteinizing hormone (LH) drug for infertility 124

Lutigest brand name for progesterone 105 used to treat female infertility 124

lutropin alfa drug for infertility 124

Luventa XL brand name for modified-release galantamine (a drug for dementia 43)

Luveris brand name for lutropin alfa used to treat female infertility 124

Luvinsta XL brand name for modified-release fluvastatin (a lipid-lowering drug 61)

Lyclear brand name for permethrin 355 (a topical antiparasitic 136)

Lyflex brand name for baclofen 167 (a muscle relaxant 78)

lymecycline 413, tetracycline antibiotic 86

Lynlor brand name for oxycodone (an opioid analgesic 36)

Lynparza brand name for olaparib 345 (an anticancer drug 112)

Lypsyl Aciclovir 5% Cold Sore Cream branded preparation of aciclovir 148 (an antiviral 91)

Lyrica brand name for pregabalin (an anticonvulsant 42 also used to relieve neuropathic pain)

Lyrinel XL brand name for oxybutynin 351 (a drug for urinary disorders 126)

Lysodren brand name for mitotane (an anticancer drug 112)

Lyxumia brand name for lixisenatide (a drug for diabetes 100)

M

Maalox branded antacid containing aluminium hydroxide 153 and magnesium hydroxide 309

Maalox Plus brand-name antacid containing aluminium hydroxide 153, magnesium hydroxide 309, and simeticone (an antifoaming agent 66)

Mabron brand name for tramadol 421 (an opioid analgesic 36)

MabThera brand name for rituximab 385 (an anticancer drug 112)

Macrobid brand name for nitrofurantoin (an antibacterial 89)

macrogol drug used to treat constipation 69

Macugen brand name for pegaptanib (a drug for age-related macular degeneration)

Madopar brand name for levodopa 298 (a drug for parkinsonism 43) with benserazide (a drug to enhance the effect of levodopa)

Madopar CR brand name for levodopa 298 (a drug for parkinsonism 43) combined with benserazide (enhances effects of levodopa)

Maexeni brand name for a combination contraceptive 121 containing ethinylestradiol 252 and levonorgestrel 300

magnesium 438, mineral 108

magnesium alginate antifoaming agent 66

magnesium aspartate magnesium supplement 438 (a mineral 108)

magnesium carbonate antacid 66

magnesium citrate osmotic laxative 69

magnesium glycerol phosphate magnesium supplement 438 (a mineral 108)

magnesium hydroxide 309, antacid 66 and laxative 69

magnesium oxide antacid 66

magnesium sulfate osmotic laxative 69

magnesium trisilicate antacid 66

Malarivon brand-name antimalarial 95 containing chloroquine 193

Malarone brand-name antimalarial 95 containing proguanil 368 with atovaquone

malathion 310, antiparasitic 136 for head lice and scabies

Mandanol brand of hypromellose eye drops

Maneo brand name for tramadol 421 (an opioid analgesic 36)

Manerix brand name for moclobemide (a reversible MAOI antidepressant 40)

Manevac brand name for ispaghula (a bulk-forming agent 66) with senna (a stimulant laxative 69)

mannitol osmotic diuretic 57

maraviroc drug to treat HIV infection 116

Marcain brand name for bupivacaine (a local anaesthetic 36 used in labour 125)

Marevan brand name for warfarin 429 (an anticoagulant 62)

Mariosea XL brand name for tolterodine 420 (an anticholinergic 126)

Marixeno brand name for memantine (a drug used to treat dementia 43)

Marol brand name for tramadol 421 (an opioid analgesic 36)

Martapan brand name for dexamethasone 223 (a corticosteroid 99)

Marvelon brand-name oral contraceptive 121 containing ethinylestradiol 252 and desogestrel 222 (both female sex hormones 105)

Matrifen brand name for fentanyl (an opioid analgesic 36)

Maxalt brand name for rizatriptan (a drug for migraine 45)

Maxidex brand name for dexamethasone 223 (a corticosteroid 99) with hypromellose (a substance in artificial tear preparations 130)

Maxitram SR brand name for tramadol 421 (an opioid analgesic 36)

Maxitrol brand name for dexamethasone 223 (a corticosteroid 99) with hypromellose (used in artificial tear preparations 130), and neomycin and polymyxin B (both antibiotics 86)

Maxolon brand name for metoclopramide 323 (a gastrointestinal motility regulator and anti-emetic 46)

Maxolon High Dose brand of metoclopramide 323 (a gastrointestinal motility regulator and anti-emetic 46) used with chemotherapy only

Maxolon SR brand name for modified-release metoclopramide 323 (a gastrointestinal motility regulator and anti-emetic 46)

Maxtrex brand name for methotrexate 320 (an antimetabolite anticancer drug 112)

MCT oil substance used for cystic fibrosis

mebendazole 311, anthelmintic 97

mebeverine 312, antispasmodic drug for irritable bowel syndrome 68

Medijel brand name for a pain-relieving mouth gel containing lidocaine (a local anaesthetic 36) and aminacrine (an antiseptic 135)

Medikinet XL brand name for methylphenidate 322 (a nervous system stimulant 44)

Medrone brand name for methylprednisolone (a corticosteroid 99)

medroxyprogesterone 313, female sex hormone 105 and anticancer drug 112

mefenamic acid 314, NSAID 74

mefloquine 315, antimalarial 95

Megace brand name for megestrol (a female sex hormone 105 and anticancer drug 112)

megestrol female sex hormone 105 and anticancer drug 112

Meijumet brand name for metformin 318 (a drug used to treat diabetes 100)

Mekinist brand name for trametinib (an anticancer drug 112) used for skin cancer

melatonin hormone 98

meloxicam NSAID 74 and non-opioid analgesic 36

melphalan alkylating agent for multiple myeloma 112

memantidine NMDA receptor antagonist used to treat Alzheimer's disease 43

menadiol vitamin K 445 (a vitamin 107)

Menitorix brand-name vaccine 92 against Haemophilus influenzae/Neisseria meningitidis

Menopur brand name for menotrophin (a drug for infertility 124; also known as human menopausal gonadotrophins)

menotrophin drug for infertility 124; also known as human menopausal gonadotrophins

menthol alcohol from mint oils used as an inhalation and topical antipruritic 133

Menveo brand-name vaccine 92 to protect against meningococcal A, C, W135, and Y

mepacrine antiprotozoal 94 for giardiasis

Mepact brand name for mifamurtide (an anticancer drug 112)

mepivacaine local anaesthetic 36

mepolizumab monoclonal antibody used to treat asthma 49

Mepradec brand name for omeprazole 346 (an anti-ulcer drug 67)

meprobamate anti-anxiety drug 39

meptazinol opioid analgesic 36

Meptid brand name for meptazinol (an opioid analgesic 36)

mercaptamine drug for metabolic disorders

mercaptopurine 316, anticancer drug 112

Mercilon brand-name oral contraceptive 121 containing ethinylestradiol 252 and desogestrel 222 (female sex hormones 105)

Merocaine Lozenges brand-name preparation for sore throat and minor mouth infections, containing benzocaine (a local anaesthetic 36) and cetylpyridinium (a topical antiseptic 135)

Meronem brand name for meropenem (an antibiotic 86)

meropenem antibiotic 86

mesalazine 317, drug for ulcerative colitis 70

mesna drug used to protect the urinary tract from damage by some anticancer drugs 112

mesterolone a male sex hormone 104

Mestinon brand name for pyridostigmine 373 (a drug for myasthenia gravis 79)

mestranol female sex hormone 105 and oral contraceptive 121

Metabet brand name for metformin 318 (a drug used to treat diabetes 100)

Metanium brand-name barrier ointment 135 containing titanium dioxide, titanium peroxide, and titanium salicylate

metaraminol drug used to treat hypotension (low blood pressure)

metformin 318, drug for diabetes 100

METHADONE

methadone 319, opioid drug 455 used as an analgesic 36 and to treat heroin dependence

Methadose brand name for methadone 319 (an opioid 455 used as an analgesic 36 and to ease heroin withdrawal)

Metharose brand name for methadone 319 (an opioid 455 used as an analgesic 36 and to ease heroin withdrawal)

methenamine antibacterial drug 89 for urinary tract infections 126

methocarbamol muscle relaxant 78

Methofill brand name for methotrexate 320 (a DMARD 75)

methotrexate 320, an anticancer drug 112 and a DMARD 75

methyl salicylate topical analgesic 36 for muscle and joint pain

methylcellulose 321, laxative 69, antidiarrhoeal 68, and artificial tear preparation 130

methyldopa an antihypertensive 60

methylnaltrexone bromide drug used to relieve constipation 69 in patients taking opioids 37

methylphenidate 322, nervous system stimulant 44 used for attention deficit hyperactivity disorder (ADHD) and narcolepsy

methylprednisolone corticosteroid 99

methysergide drug to prevent migraine 45

metipranolol beta blocker 55 for glaucoma 128

metirosine drug for phaeochromocytoma (tumour of the adrenal glands 112)

metoclopramide 323, gastrointestinal motility regulator and anti-emetic 46

Metoject branded preparation of methotrexate 320 (an anticancer drug 112 and DMARD 75)

metolazone thiazide-like diuretic 57

Metopirone brand name for metyrapone (a diuretic 57)

metoprolol 324, beta blocker 55

Metosyn brand name for fluocinonide (a topical corticosteroid 134)

Metrogel brand name for topical metronidazole 325 (an antibacterial 89)

Metrolyl brand name for metronidazole 325 (an antibacterial 89 and antiprotozoal 94)

metronidazole 325, antibacterial 89 and antiprotozoal 94

mexiletine anti-arrhythmic drug 58

Mezavant XL brand-name modified release preparation of mesalazine 317 (a drug for ulcerative colitis 70)

Mezolar brand name for fentanyl (an opioid analgesic 36)

Mezzopram brand name for omeprazole 346 (an anti-ulcer drug 67)

mianserin antidepressant 40

micafungin antifungal drug 96

Micardis brand name for telmisartan (an angiotensin II blocker vasodilator 56 and antihypertensive drug 60)

Micardis Plus brand-name antihypertensive 60 containing telmisartan (an angiotensin II blocker vasodilator 56) with hydrochlorothiazide 276 (a thiazide diuretic 57)

miconazole 326, antifungal 96

Microgynon 30 brand-name oral contraceptive 121 containing ethinylestradiol 252 and levonorgestrel 300

Micronor brand-name oral contraceptive 121 containing norethisterone 342

Micropirin brand name for aspirin 162 (a non-opioid analgesic 36 and antiplatelet drug 62)

Microval brand-name oral contraceptive 121 containing levonorgestrel 300

midazolam benzodiazepine 38 premedication

Midrid brand-name drug for migraine 45 containing paracetamol 352 and isometheptene mucate

mifamurtide anticancer drug 112 used to treat some bone cancers

Mifegyne brand name for mifepristone (a drug used during labour 125)

mifepristone drug used during labour 125

Migard brand name for frovatriptan (a drug used to treat migraines)

Migraleve brand-name drug for migraine 45 containing codeine 211, paracetamol 352, and buclizine

Migraleve Ultra drug for migraine 45

MigraMax brand-name drug for migraine 45 containing aspirin (a non-opioid analgesic 36) with metoclopramide 323 (a gastrointestinal motility regulator and anti-emetic 46)

Migril branded drug for migraine 45 containing ergotamine 246, caffeine, and cyclizine

Mildison brand name for hydrocortisone 277 (a corticosteroid 99)

Milk of Magnesia brand name for magnesium hydroxide 309 (an antacid 66 and laxative 69)

Millinette 20/75 & 30/75 brand-name combined oral contraceptive 121 containing ethinylestradiol 252 and gestodene (a progestogen 105)

Milpar brand-name laxative 69 containing magnesium hydroxide 309 and liquid paraffin

milrinone drug used for its vasodilator effects 56 and for heart failure

Minijet Adrenaline brand name for epinephrine 245 (a drug for anaphylaxis 512)

Minims Atropine brand name for atropine 165 (a mydriatic 130)

Minims Chloramphenicol brand name for chloramphenicol 192 (an antibiotic 86)

Minims Cyclopentolate brand name for cyclopentolate (an anticholinergic mydriatic 130)

Minims Dexamethasone brand name for dexamethasone 223 (a corticosteroid 99)

Minims Gentamicin brand name for gentamicin 268 (an aminoglycoside antibiotic 86)

Minims Phenylephrine brand name for phenylephrine (a decongestant 51)

Minims Pilocarpine brand name for pilocarpine 360 (a miotic for glaucoma 128)

Minims Prednisolone brand name for prednisolone 365 (a corticosteroid 99)

Minitran brand name for glyceryl trinitrate 272 (an anti-angina drug 59)

Minocin brand name for minocycline 327 (a tetracycline antibiotic 86)

minocycline 327, tetracycline antibiotic 86

Minodiab brand name for glipizide (an oral drug for diabetes 100)

minoxidil 328, antihypertensive 60 and treatment for male pattern baldness 140

Mintec brand name for peppermint oil (a substance for irritable bowel syndrome 68)

Mintreleq XL brand name for a modified-release preparation of quetiapine 375 (an antipsychotic 41)

mirabegron smooth muscle relaxant used for urinary disorders 126

Mirapexin brand name for pramipexole (a drug for parkinsonism 43)

Mircera brand name for erythropoietin 248

Mirena intrauterine contraceptive device 121 containing levonorgestrel 300 (a female sex hormone 105)

mirtazapine 329, antidepressant 40

Mirvaso brand name for brimonidine 177 (a treatment for rosacea)

Misofen brand name for misoprostol 330 (an anti-ulcer drug 67) with diclofenac 225 (a NSAID 36)

misoprostol 330, anti-ulcer drug 67

mitomycin cytotoxic antibiotic for breast, stomach, and bladder cancer 112

mitotane anticancer drug 112 used for adrenocortical cancer

mitoxantrone (previously mitozantrone) an anticancer drug 112)

mivacurium drug used to relax muscles during general anaesthesia

Mixtard preparations brand names for insulin 284 (a drug for diabetes 100)

mizolastine antihistamine 82

Mizollen brand name for mizolastine (an antihistamine 82)

Mobiflex brand name for tenoxicam (NSAID 74)

moclobemide monoamine oxidase inhibitor (MAOI) antidepressant 40

modafinil 331, a nervous system stimulant 44 used for narcolepsy and excessive sleepiness

Modecate brand name for fluphenazine (an antipsychotic 41)

Modigraf brand name for tacrolimus 405 (an immunosuppressant 115)

Modisal brand name for isosorbide mononitrate 289 (a nitrate vasodilator 56 and anti-angina drug 59)

Modrasone brand name for alclometasone (a topical corticosteroid 134)

Moduret-25 brand name for amiloride 154 with hydrochlorothiazide 276 (both diuretics 57)

Moduretic brand name for amilcride 154 with hydrochlorothiazide 276 (both diuretics 57)

moexipril an ACE inhibitor 56

Mogadon brand name for nitrazepam 341 (a benzodiazepine sleeping drug 38)

Molap brand name for lacidipine (a calcium channel blocker used for hypertension 60)

Molative brand-name laxative 69 to relieve persistent constipation

Molaxole brand name laxative 69 containing macrogol (an osmotic laxative), bicarbonate, chloride, potassium, and sodium

Molipaxin brand name for trazodone (an antidepressant 40)

Molita branded preparation containing aspirin 162 and dipyridamole 230 to prevent stroke

mometasone 332, topical corticosteroid 134

Monofer brand name for iron isomaltoside (an injectable form of iron 437) used for anaemia

Monomax brand name for isosorbide mononitrate 289 (a vasodilator 56 and anti-angina drug 59)

Monomil XL brand name for isosorbide mononitrate 289 (a vasodilator 56 and anti-angina drug 59)

Mononine brand name for factor IX (a substance to promote blood clotting 62)

Monopost brand name for latanoprost 296 (a drug for glaucoma 128)

Monosorb XL brand name for isosorbide mononitrate 289 (nitrate vasodilator 56 and anti-angina drug 59)

Monotrim brand name for trimethoprim 424 (an antibacterial 89)

montelukast 333, leukotriene antagonist for asthma 49 and bronchospasm 48

Monuril brand name for fosfomycin (an antibiotic 86) used to treat urinary tract infections

Morphgesic SR brand name for morphine 334 (an opioid analgesic 36)

morphine 334, opioid analgesic 36

Motens brand name for lacidipine (a calcium channel blocker 59)

Motifene brand name for diclofenac 225 (an NSAID 74)

Motilium brand name for domperidone 232 (an anti-emetic 46)

Moventig brand name for naloxegol (a laxative 69) for constipation in patients taking opioids 36

Movicol brand-name osmotic laxative 69

moxifloxacin an antibiotic 86

moxisylyte (previously thymoxamine) a drug used in eye examinations 130 and a vasodilator 56 used to improve blood supply to the limbs

moxonidine 335, a centrally acting antihypertensive 60

Mozobil brand name for plerixafor, a drug used to mobilize stem cells in patients with multiple myeloma or lymphoma

MST Continus brand name for morphine 334 (an opioid analgesic 36)

MucoClear brand-name nebulizer solution containing sodium chloride

Mucodyne brand name for carbocisteine (a mucolytic decongestant 52)

Mucogel brand-name antacid 66 containing aluminium hydroxide 153 and magnesium hydroxide 309

Multaq brand name for dronaderone (an anti-arrhythmic 58)

Munalea brand-name combined oral contraceptive 121 containing ethinylestradiol 252 and desogestrel 222

mupirocin antibacterial for skin infections 135

Murine Eye Drops branded drops containing naphazoline a sympathomimetic 35

Muse brand name for alprostadil (a drug used for erectile dysfunction 104, 124)

MXL brand name for morphine sulphate 334 (an opioid analgesic 36)

Mycamine brand name for micafungin (an antifungal 96 used for candidiasis

Mycobutin brand name for rifabutin (an antituberculous drug 90)

mycophenolate mofetil immunosuppressant drug 115

Mydriacyl brand name for tropicamide (a mydriatic 130)

Mydriasert brand name for eye drops containing tropicamide (a mydriatic 130) used in eye investigations and surgery

Mydrilate brand name for cyclopentolate (an anticholinergic mydriatic 130)

Myelobromol brand name for mitobronitol (an anticancer drug 112)

Myfenax brand name for mycophenalate (an immunosuppressant 115)

Myfortic brand name for mycophenolic acid (an immunosuppressant 115)

Mylafent brand name skin patch containing fentanyl (an opioid analgesic 36)

Mylan brand name for cinnarizine 198 (an antihistamine anti-emetic drug 46)

Mylatrip brand name for frovatriptan (a drug used to treat migraine 45)

Mylotarg brand name for gemtuzumab (a monoclonal antibody used to treat leukaemia)

Myocet brand name for doxorubicin 237 (a cytotoxic anticancer drug 112)

Myocrisin brand name for sodium aurothiomalate (a DMARD 75)

Myotonine brand name for bethanechol (a parasympathomimetic drug used to treat urinary retention 126)

Mysimba brand name for naltrexone and bupropion combination used to control obesity

N

nabilone anti-emetic 46 used to treat nausea and vomiting induced by anticancer drugs 112

nabumetone NSAID 74

Nacrez brand-name oral contraceptive 121 containing desogestrel 222

nadolol beta blocker 55

nafarelin drug for menstrual disorders 120

naftidrofuryl 336, vasodilator 56

Nalcrom brand name for sodium cromoglicate 397 (an anti-allergy drug 82)

nalidixic acid antibacterial 89

nalmefene (nalmetrene) drug used to treat alcohol dependence 447

Nalorex brand name for naltrexone (a drug for opioid withdrawal 24)

naloxegol drug used to treat constipation 69 in patients taking opioid analgesics 36

naloxone an antidote for opioid 455 poisoning

naltrexone a drug for opioid withdrawal 24

Nandover XL brand name for fluvastatin (a lipid-lowering drug 61)

nandrolone anabolic steroid 104

Napratec branded antirheumatic drug containing naproxen 337 (a NSAID 74 and drug for gout 77) and misoprostol 330 (an anti-ulcer drug 67)

naproxen 337, NSAID 74 and drug for gout 77

Naramig brand name for naratriptan (a drug for migraine 45)

naratriptan drug for migraine 45

Nardil brand name for phenelzine 356 (an MAOI antidepressant 40)

Naropin brand name for ropivacaine (a local anaesthetic 36)

Nasacort brand name for triamcinolone (a corticosteroid 99)

Naseptin brand name for chlorhexidine (an antiseptic 135) with neomycin (an aminoglycoside antibiotic 86)

Nasobec brand-name nasal spray containing beclometasone 168 (a corticosteroid 99) used for allergic rhinitis

Nasofan branded nasal spray containing fluticasone 265 (a corticosteroid 99) used for allergic rhinitis

Nasonex brand name for mometasone 332 (a topical corticosteroid 134)

natalizumab monoclonal antibody used to treat multiple sclerosis

Natecal brand name for calcium carbonate (calcium 434) with colecalciferol (vitamin D 444) used to prevent or treat vitamin D and calcium deficiency

nateglinide drug for diabetes 100

Natrilix brand name for indapamide 282 (a thiazide-like diuretic 57)

Natzon branded sublingual tablet containing buprenorphine (an opioid analgesic 36)

Navelbine brand name for vinorelbine (an anticancer drug 112)

Navidrex brand name for cyclopenthiazide (a thiazide diuretic 57)

Navispare brand name for cyclopenthiazide with amiloride 154 (both diuretics 57)

Nazdol MR brand name for gliclazide 270 (a drug used to treat diabetes 100)

Nebbaro brand name for omega-3 acid ethyl esters (a lipid-lowering drug 61)

Nebcin brand name for tobramycin (an aminoglycoside antibiotic 86)

Nebido brand name for testosterone 412 (a male sex hormone 104)

Nebilet brand name for nebivolol (a beta blocker 55 antihypertensive 60)

nebivolol beta blocker drug 55

necitumumab monoclonal antibody used to treat lung cancer

Neditol XL brand name for modified-release tolterodine 420 (a drug used to treat urinary disorders 126)

nedocromil drug similar to sodium cromoglicate 397 used to prevent asthma attacks 49

nefopam non-opioid analgesic 36

Negaban brand name for temocillin (an antibiotic 86)

nelarabine antimetabolite and anticancer drug 112

nelfinavir antiretroviral for HIV/AIDS 116

Nemdatine brand name for memantine (a drug for dementia 43)

Neoclarityn brand name for desloratadine 307 (an anithistamine 82)

Neo-Cytamen brand name for hydroxocobalamin (vitamin B12 443) used for vitamin B deficiencies and pernicious anaemia

Neofel XL brand name for modified-release felodipine 256 (a calcium channel blocker used for hypertension 60)

Neofordex brand name for dexamethasone 223 (a corticosteroid 99)

neomycin aminoglycoside antibiotic 86 used in ear drops 131

Neo-Naclex brand name for bendroflumethiazide 169 (a thiazide diuretic 57)

Neoral brand name for ciclosporin 196 (an immunosuppressant 115)

NeoRecormon brand name for erythropoietin 248 (a kidney hormone 98)

neostigmine drug for myasthenia gravis 79

Neotigason brand name for acitretin (a drug for psoriasis 138)

Neovent brand name for a salmeterol 392 inhaler used for obstructive airways disease

Neozipine XL brand name for prolonged-release nifedipine 340 (a calcium channel blocker used for hypertension 60)

nepafenac non-steroidal anti-inflammatory eye drops 74 used for pain relief after eye surgery

Nerisone brand name for diflucortolone (a topical corticosteroid 134)

Netillin brand name for netilmicin (an aminoglycoside antibiotic 86)

Neulasta brand name for pegfilgrastim (a blood growth stimulant)

Neupogen brand name for filgrastim 257 (a blood growth stimulant)

Neupro brand name for rotigotine (a drug for parkinsonism 43)

Neurontin brand name for gabapentin 267 (an anticonvulsant 42 also used to relieve neuropathic pain)

Nevanac brand name for nepafenac eye drops (an NSAID 74) for pain relief after eye surgery

nevirapine antiretroviral for HIV/AIDS 116

Nexavar brand name for sorafenib (an anticancer drug 112)

Nexium brand name for esomeprazole (an anti-ulcer drug 67)

Nexplanon brand name for a contraceptive implant containing etonogestrel (a progestogen female sex hormone 105)

niacin 438, a vitamin 107

Nicam brand name for nicotamide (vitamin B 107) used for acne 137

nicardipine calcium channel blocker 59

Nicef brand name for cefradine (a cephalosporin antibiotic 86)

NICOPASS

Nicopass brand name of nicotine 339 used as a smoking cessation aid

nicorandil 338, anti-angina drug 59

Nicorette brand of nicotine 339 used as a smoking cessation aid

nicotinamide B vitamin 436 (a vitamin 107)

nicotine 339, nervous system stimulant 44, smoking cessation aid, drug of abuse, and insecticide

Nicotinell brand name for nicotine 339 used as a smoking cessation aid

nicotinic acid vasodilator 56, lipid-lowering drug 61, and vitamin 107

Nidef brand name for nifedipine 340 (a calcium channel blocker 59)

nifedipine 340, a calcium channel blocker 59

Nifedipress MR brand name for nifedipine 340 (a calcium channel blocker 59)

Niferex brand name for iron 437 (a mineral 108)

Night Nurse brand-name preparation for cold symptoms containing paracetamol 352 (a non-opioid analgesic 36) with promethazine 370 (an antihistamine 82 and anti-emetic 46) and dextromethorphan (a cough suppressant 52)

nilotinib anticancer drug 112

nimodipine calcium channel blocker 59

Nimotop brand name for nimodipine (a calcium channel blocker 59)

Nimvastid brand name for rivastigmine 387 (a drug for dementia 43)

Ninlaro brand name for iazomib (a protein kinase inhibitor anticancer drug 112) used to treat myeloma (a type of bone marrow cancer)

nintedanib protein kinase inhibitor anticancer drug 112

Nipatra brand name for sildenafil 394 (a drug for pulmonary hypertension 60)

Nipent brand name for pentostatin (an anticancer drug 112)

NiQuitin CQ brand name of nicotine 339 used as a smoking cessation aid

niraparib anticancer drug 112 used to treat ovarian cancer

nisoldipine calcium channel blocker 59

nitrazepam 341, benzodiazepine sleeping drug 38

Nitrocine brand name for glyceryl trinitrate 272 (an anti-angina drug 59)

Nitro-Dur brand name for glyceryl trinitrate 272 (an anti-angina drug 59)

nitrofurantoin antibacterial 89

Nitrolingual brand name for glyceryl trinitrate 272 (an anti-angina drug 59)

Nitromin brand name for glyceryl trinitrate 272 (an anti-angina drug 59)

Nitronal brand name for glyceryl trinitrate 272 (an anti-angina drug 59)

nitroprusside antihypertensive 60

nitrous oxide anaesthetic gas

Nivestim brand name for filgrastim 257, a blood growth stimulant used to treat neutropenia (low levels of white blood cells)

nivolumab a monoclonal antibody 112 used to treat skin cancer and kidney cancer

nizatidine anti-ulcer drug 67

Nizoral brand name for ketoconazole 291 (an antifungal 96)

Nocutil brand name for desmopressin 221 (a pituitary hormone for diabetes insipidus 103)

nomegestrol progestogen (female sex hormone 105) for used in contraceptives 121

Non-Drowsy Sudafed brand name for phenylephrine (a decongestant 51)

nonoxinol-9 spermicidal agent

Nootropil brand name for piracetam (an anticonvulsant 42)

Noqdirna brand name for desmopressin 221 (a drug for urinary disorders 126)

noradrenaline see norepinephrine

Nordimet brand name for methotrexate 320 (a DMARD 75)

Norditropin brand name for somatropin (a synthetic pituitary hormone 103)

norepinephrine (previously noradrenaline) a drug similar to epinephrine 245 used to treat shock

norethisterone 342, a female sex hormone 105 and oral contraceptive 121

norfloxacin antibacterial 89

Norgalax brand name for docusate (a stimulant laxative 69)

norgestimate progestogen (female sex hormone 105) used in oral contraceptives 121

Norgeston brand-name oral contraceptive 121 containing levonorgestrel 300

norgestrel progestogen (female sex hormone 105)

Noriday brand-name oral contraceptive 121 containing norethisterone 342

Norimin brand-name oral contraceptive 121 containing ethinylestradiol 252 and norethisterone 342

Norimode brand name for loperamide 305 (an antidiarrhoeal 68)

Norinyl-1 brand-name oral contraceptive 121 containing norethisterone 342 and mestranol

Noristerat brand-name injectable contraceptive 121 containing norethisterone 342 (a female sex hormone 105)

Normacol Plus brand name for frangula with sterculia (both laxatives 69)

Normaloe brand name for loperamide 305 (an antidiarrhoeal 68)

Normosang brand name for haem arginate (a drug to treat porphyria)

Norphyllin SR brand name for aminophylline 416 (a bronchodilator 48)

Norprolac brand name for quinagolide (a drug for infertility 124 and hyperprolactinaemia 103)

nortriptyline tricyclic antidepressant 40

Norvir brand name for ritonavir (an antiretroviral for HIV/AIDS 116)

Novofem brand-name preparation containing estradiol 249 with norethisterone 342 (both female sex hormones 105)

NovoMix brand name for insulin 284 (a drug for diabetes 100)

NovoRapid brand name for insulin 284 (a drug for diabetes 100)

NovoSeven brand of factor VIIa (a blood extract to promote blood clotting 62)

Noxafil brand name for posaconazole (an antifungal 96)

Noyada brand name for captopril 186 (an ACE inhibitor 56)

Nozinan brand name for levomepromazine (an antipsychotic 41)

Nucala brand name for mepolizumab (a monoclonal antibody for severe asthma 49)

Nuelin brand name for theophylline 416 (a bronchodilator 48)

Nulojix brand name for belatercept (an immunosuppressant 115)

Nurofen brand name for ibuprofen 279 (a non-opioid analgesic 36 and NSAID 74)

Nurofen Plus brand name for ibuprofen 279 (a NSAID 74) with codeine 211 (an opioid analgesic 36)

Nu-Seals Aspirin brand of aspirin 162 (a non-opioid analgesic 36 and antiplatelet drug 62)

Nutraplus brand name for urea (an emollient)

Nutrizym GR brand name for pancreatin (a preparation of pancreatic enzymes 72)

Nuvelle Continuous brand-name preparation for menopausal symptoms 105 containing estradiol 249 and levonorgestrel 300 (both female sex hormones 105)

Nuwiq brand name for factor VIII (a substance to promote blood clotting 62)

Nystaform brand name for nystatin 343 (an antifungal 96) with chlorhexidine (an antiseptic 135)

Nystaform-HC brand name for hydrocortisone 277 (a corticosteroid 99) with nystatin 343 (an antifungal 96) and chlorhexidine (an antiseptic 135)

Nystan brand name for nystatin 343 (an antifungal 96)

nystatin 343, antifungal 96

Nytol brand-name preparation for sleep disturbance containing diphenhydramine (an antihistamine 82)

O

Oasis brand-name preparation for cystitis containing sodium citrate and sucrose

obinutuzumab a monoclonal antibody anticancer drug 112

Occlusal brand name for salicylic acid (a wart remover)

Octasa brand name for mesalazine 317 (a drug for ulcerative colitis 70)

Octim brand name for desmopressin 221 (a pituitary hormone 103 used for diabetes insipidus 103)

octreotide a synthetic pituitary hormone 103 used to relieve symptoms of pancreatic cancer

Ocufen brand name for flurbiprofen (a NSAID 74)

Ocu-Lube brand name for eye drops containing hypromellose (a lubricant) used for dry eyes 130

Ocusan brand-name drops containing sodium hyaluronate (a lubricant) for dry eyes 130

Odefsey brand name for a combination of emtricitabine 242, tenofovir 409, and rilpivirine (antiviral drugs 91) used to treat HIV/AIDS 116

ODM5 brand name for eye drops containing sodium chloride used for dry eyes 130

Oestrogel brand name for estradiol 249 (a female sex hormone 105)

oestrogen female sex hormone 105

ofatumumab monoclonal antibody anticancer drug 112

Ofcram PR brand name for modified-release dipyridamole 230 (an antiplatelet drug 62)

Ofev brand name for nintedanib (a tyrosine protein kinase inhibitor anticancer drug 112)

ofloxacin antibacterial 89

Oftaquix brand-name topical preparation of levofloxacin 299 (an antibacterial 89)

Oilatum Emollient brand-name bath additive containing liquid paraffin for dry skin 132

Oilatum Gel brand name for a shower gel containing liquid paraffin for dry skin 132

olanzapine 344, antipsychotic 41

olaparib 345, anticancer drug 112

olaratumab a monoclonal antibody used to treat solid tumours

Olbetam brand name for acipimox (a lipid-lowering drug 61)

Oldaram brand name for modified-release tramadol 421 (an opioid analgesic 36)

PANADOL ULTRA

Oleax brand name for olive oil ear drops

Olena brand name for fluoxetine 262 (an antidepressant 40)

olmesartan angiotensin II blocker (a vasodilator 56 and antihypertensive 60)

Olmetec brand name for olmesartan (an angiotensin II blocker vasodilator 56 and antihypertensive 60)

olodaterol bronchodilator 48

olopatadine antihistamine 82

olsalazine drug for ulcerative colitis 70

Olumiant brand name for baricitinib (an antirheumatic drug 75)

Olysio brand name for simeprevir (a drug for HIV/AIDS 116)

Omacor brand name for omega 3 acid ethyl esters (a lipid-lowering drug 61)

omalizumab monoclonal antibody for asthma 49

ombitsavir with paritaprevir and ritonavir combination of antiviral drugs 91 used for chronic hepatitis C

omega-3-acid ethyl esters lipid-lowering drugs 61

omega-3-marine triglycerides lipid-lowering drugs 61

omeprazole 346, anti-ulcer drug 67

Omicur brand name for amorolfine (an antifungal drug 96)

Omnitrope preparations brand name for somatropin (a growth hormone 103)

Onbrez Breezhaler brand name for indacaterol (a bronchodilator 48) used for obstructive airways disease

Oncaspar brand name for pegaspargase (an anticancer drug 112) used for leukaemia

ondansetron 347, anti-emetic 46

Ondemet brand name for ondansetron 347 (an anti-emetic 46)

One-Alpha brand name for alfacalcidol (a vitamin 107)

Onexila XL brand name for oxycodone (an opioid analgesic 36)

Ongentys brand name for opicapone (a drug for Parkinson's disease 43)

Onglyza brand name for saxagliptin (a drug for diabetes 100)

Onivyde brand name for irinotecan (an anticancer drug 112)

Onkotrone brand name for pixantrone (an anticancer drug 112)

Ontruzant brand name for trastuzumab 422 (a monoclonal antibody) used for breast cancer

Opatanol brand name for olopatadine (an antihistamine 82)

Opdivo brand name for nivolumab (an anticancer drug 112)

Opilon brand name for moxisylyte (a vasodilator 56)

Opiodur brand name for a skin patch containing fentanyl (an opioid analgesic 36)

opium morphine 334 (an opioid analgesic 36)

Opizone brand name for naltrexone, used for opioid 455 and alcohol 447 dependence

Oprymea brand name for pramipexole (a drug for Parkinson's disease 43)

Opsumit brand name for macitentan used for pulmonary hypertension

Opticrom brand name for sodium cromoglicate 397 (an anti-allergy drug 82)

Optilast branded drops containing azelastine (an antihistamine 82) for allergic conjunctivitis

Optimax brand name for tryptophan (a drug used to treat anxiety 39 and depression 40)

Optive preparations branded drops containing carmellose sodium (a lubricant) for dry eyes

Optrex Allergy brand name for sodium cromoglicate 397 (an anti-allergy drug 82)

Optrex Infected Eyes brand-name preparation containing chloramphenicol 192 (an antibiotic 86)

Optrex Red Eyes brand-name drops containing naphazoline (a topical sympathomimetic)

Optrex Sore Eyes brand-name preparation containing witch hazel (an astringent)

Orabase branded ointment containing carmellose to protect the skin or mouth from damage

Oraldene brand-name antiseptic mouthwash containing hexetidine

Oramorph brand name for morphine 334 (an opioid analgesic 36)

Orap brand name for pimozide (an antipsychotic 41)

Orbifen brand name for ibuprofen 279 (an NSAID 74)

orciprenaline sympathomimetic used as a bronchodilator 48

Orencia brand name for abatacept (a cytokine modulator antirheumatic drug 75 for moderate to severe rheumatoid arthritis)

Orgalutran brand name for ganirelix used for female infertility 124

Orgaran brand name for danaparoid (an anticoagulant 62)

orlistat 348, anti-obesity drug

Orovite brand-name multivitamin 107

Orphacol brand name for cholic acid used for biliary disorders

orphenadrine 349, anticholinergic muscle relaxant 78 and drug for parkinsonism 43

Ortho-Creme brand name for nonoxinol-9 (a spermicidal agent)

Orthoforms brand name for nonoxinol-9 (a spermicidal agent)

Ortho-Gynest brand name for estriol (a female sex hormone 105)

Oruvail brand name for ketoprofen 292 (an NSAID 74)

oseltamivir 350, antiviral drug 91 for influenza

Osmanil brand name for a skin patch containing fentanyl (an opioid analgesic 36)

ospemifene drug used to relieve vulvar and vaginal atrophy

Ostiral brand name for raloxifene 378 used to prevent/treat postmenopausal osteoporosis 80

Otex brand-name preparation for removal of ear wax containing urea (an emollient) and hydrogen peroxide (an antiseptic 135)

Otezla brand name for apremilast used for psoriatic arthritis

Otomize brand name for dexamethasone 223 (a corticosteroid 99) and neomycin (an aminoglycoside antibiotic 86)

Otrivine brand name for xylometazoline (a decongestant 51)

Otrivine-Antistin brand name for antazoline (an antihistamine 82) with xylometazoline (a decongestant 51)

Ovaleap brand name for follitropin alfa (a drug for female infertility 124)

Ovestin brand name for estriol (a female sex hormone 105)

Ovex brand name for mebendazole 311 (an anthelmintic 97)

Ovitrelle brand name for choriogonadotropin alfa (a drug for female infertility 124)

Ovranette brand-name oral contraceptive 121 containing ethinylestradiol 252 and levonorgestrel 300

Oxactin brand name for fluoxetine 262 (an antidepressant 40)

oxaliplatin an anticancer drug 112

oxazepam a benzodiazepine anti-anxiety drug 39

oxcarbazepine an anticonvulsant 42

Oxeltra brand name for modified-release oxycodone (an opioid analgesic 36)

oxerutins drugs used to relieve oedema especially in the lower limbs

Oxis brand name for formoterol (a bronchodilator 48)

oxpentifylline see pentoxifylline (a vasodilator 56 used for peripheral vascular disease)

oxprenolol a beta blocker 55

Oxyal brand name for eye drops containing sodium hyaluronate (a lubricant) for dry eyes

oxybuprocaine local anaesthetic 36

oxybutynin 351, anticholinergic and antispasmodic for urinary disorders 126

oxycodone opioid analgesic 36

OxyContin brand name for oxycodone (an opioid analgesic 36)

Oxylan brand name for modified-release oxycodone (an opioid analgesic 36)

oxymetholone anabolic steroid for aplastic anaemia

OxyNorm brand name for oxycodone (an opioid analgesic 36)

Oxy On-The-Spot brand-name topical preparation of benzoyl peroxide 170 (a drug for acne 137)

oxytetracycline tetracycline antibiotic 86

oxytocin uterine stimulant 125

Ozurdex brand name for dexamethasone 223 (a corticosteroid 99)

P

Pabal brand name for carbetocin (a uterine stimulant 125)

Pabrinex preparations brand name for preparations containing B and C vitamins 107

paclitaxel an anticancer drug 112

Palexia preparations brand name for preparations containing tapentadol (an opioid analgesic 36)

palbociclib protein kinase inhibitor used to treat breast cancer

palifermin drug used to treat side effects of cancer treatment

paliperidone antipsychotic drug 41

palivizumab antiviral drug 91

Palladone brand name for hydromorphone (an opioid analgesic 36)

palonosetron anti-emetic 46

Paludrine brand name for proguanil 368 (an antimalarial 95)

Paludrine/Avloclor brand name for chloroquine 193 with proguanil 368 (both antimalarials 95)

pamidronate drug for bone disorders 80

Pamsvax XL brand name for modified-release tamsulosin 407 (a drug for benign prostatic hyperplasia 126)

Panadeine brand name for paracetamol 352 (a non-opioid analgesic 36) with codeine 211

Panadol brand name for paracetamol 352 (a non-opioid analgesic 36)

Panadol Extra brand name for paracetamol 352 (a non-opioid analgesic 36) with caffeine

Panadol NightPain brand name for paracetamol 352 (a non-opioid analgesic 36) with diphenhydramine (an antihistamine 82)

Panadol OA brand name for paracetamol 352 (a non-opioid analgesic 36)

Panadol Ultra brand name for paracetamol 352 with codeine 211 (both analgesics 36)

PANCREASE

Pancrease brand name for pancreatin (a preparation of pancreatic enzymes 72)
pancreatin preparation of pancreatic enzymes 72
Pancrex brand name for pancreatin (a preparation of pancreatic enzymes 72)
pancuronium muscle relaxant 78 used during general anaesthesia
Panitaz brand name for buprenorphine (an opioid analgesic 36)
panitumumab anticancer drug 112
PanOxyl brand name for benzoyl peroxide 170 (a drug for acne 137)
panthenol pantothenic acid 439 (a vitamin 107)
pantoprazole ulcer-healing drug 67
pantothenic acid 439, vitamin 107
papaveretum opioid analgesic 36 containing morphine 334, codeine 211, and papaverine (a muscle relaxant 78)
papaveretum and hyoscine injection preparation used in general anaesthesia containing papaveretum (an opioid analgesic 36) and hyoscine 278 (an anticholinergic)
papaverine muscle relaxant 78
paracetamol 352, non-opioid analgesic 36
Paracodol brand-name analgesic 36 containing codeine 211 and paracetamol 352
Paramax brand-name migraine drug 45 containing paracetamol 352 and metoclopramide 323 (a gastrointestinal motility regulator and anti-emetic 46)
Paramol brand name for paracetamol 352 with dihydrocodeine 228 (both analgesics 36)
Paravict brand name for paracetamol 352 (a non-opioid analgesic 36)
parecoxib analgesic 36 and NSAID 74
paricalcitol synthetic form of vitamin D 444
Pariet brand name for rabeprazole 377 (an anti-ulcer drug 67)
Parlodel brand name for bromocriptine 179 (a pituitary agent 103 and drug for parkinsonism 43)
Parmid brand name for felodipine 256 (a calcium channel blocker 59)
Paroven brand name for oxerutin (a drug used to treat peripheral vascular disease 56)
paroxetine 353, antidepressant 40
Parvolex brand name for acetylcysteine (a mucolytic 52) and antidote for paracetamol 352 poisoning
pasireotide drug for Cushing's disease (abnormally high levels of corticosteroid hormones)
Pavacol-D brand name for pholcodine (a cough suppressant 52)
pazopanib tyrosine kinase inhibitor anticancer drug 112
PecFent brand name for a spray containing fentanyl (an opioid analgesic 36)
pegaptanib drug for age-related macular degeneration
Pegasys brand name for peginterferon alfa (an antiviral 91 for hepatitis C)
pegfilgrastim blood growth stimulant
peginterferon alfa antiviral 91 for hepatitis C
pegvisomant drug used to control excess growth hormone production in acromegaly
pembrolizumab monoclonal antibody anticancer drug 112
pemetrexed anticancer drug 112
Penbritin brand name for ampicillin (a penicillin antibiotic 86)
penciclovir antiviral drug 91
penicillamine DMARD 75
penicillins class of antibiotics 86
penicillin G see benzylpenicillin

penicillin V see phenoxymethylpenicillin 358
Pentacarinat brand name for pentamidine (an antiprotozoal 94)
pentamidine antiprotozoal drug 94
Pentasa brand name for mesalazine 317 (a drug for ulcerative colitis 70)
pentazocine opioid analgesic 36
Pentostam brand name for sodium stibogluconate (an antiprotozoal 94)
pentostatin anticancer drug 112
pentoxifylline (previously oxpentifylline) a vasodilator 56 for peripheral vascular disease
peppermint oil substance to relieve indigestion and bowel spasm 68
perampanel anticonvulsant 42
Percutol brand name for glyceryl trinitrate 272 (an anti-angina drug 59)
Perfan brand name for enoximone (a drug for heart failure 53)
pergolide drug for parkinsonism 43
Pergoveris brand name for lutropin alfa (a drug for female infertility 124)
Periactin brand name for cyproheptadine (an antihistamine 82)
pericyazine antipsychotic 41
Perinal brand name for hydrocortisone 277 (a corticosteroid 99) with lignocaine (a local anaesthetic)
perindopril 354, ACE inhibitor 56
Periostat brand name for doxycycline 238 (a tetracycline antibiotic 86)
Perizam brand name for clobazam (a benzodiazepine anti-anxiety drug 39 and anticonvulsant 42)
Perjeta brand name for pertuzumab (a monoclonal antibody anticancer drug 112)
permethrin 355, a topical antiparasitic 136
perphenazine antipsychotic drug 41 and anti-emetic 46
Persantin brand name for dipyridamole 230 (an antiplatelet drug 62)
Persantin Retard brand-name modified-release dipyridamole 230 (an antiplatelet drug 62)
pertuzumab monoclonal antibody anticancer drug 112
pethidine opioid analgesic 36 and drug used in labour 125
Petyme brand name for tamsulosin 407 (an alpha blocker for prostate disease 126)
Pevanti brand name for prednisolone 365 (a corticosteroid 99)
Pevaryl brand name for econazole (an antifungal drug 96)
Pharmorubicin brand name for epirubicin hydrochloride (a cytotoxic anticancer drug 112) used for breast cancer
phenelzine 356, monoamine oxidase inhibitor (MAOI) antidepressant 40
Phenergan brand name for promethazine 370 (an antihistamine 82 and anti-emetic 46)
phenindione an oral anticoagulant 62
phenobarbital 357, barbiturate anticonvulsant 42
phenol antiseptic used in throat lozenges and sprays 135
phenoxybenzamine drug for phaeochromo-cytoma (a tumour of the adrenal glands 112)
phenoxymethylpenicillin 358, penicillin antibiotic 86
phentolamine antihypertensive 60
phenylephrine decongestant 51
phenytoin 359, anticonvulsant 42
pholcodine cough suppressant 52
Phorpain branded gel containing ibuprofen 279
Phosex brand name for calcium acetate (removes excess phosphate from blood)

Phosphate-Sandoz brand name for phosphate supplement (a mineral 108)
phosphorus mineral 108
Phyllocontin Continus brand name for aminophylline 416 (a bronchodilator 48)
Physeptone brand name for methadone 319 (an opioid 455 used as an analgesic 36 and to ease heroin withdrawal)
Physiotens brand name for moxonidine 335 (a centrally acting antihypertensive 60)
phytomenadione vitamin K 445 (a vitamin 107)
Picato brand name for ingenol mebutate (a drug used for light-induced skin damage)
Picolax brand name for sodium picosulfate and magnesium citrate (both laxatives 69)
pilocarpine 360, miotic for glaucoma 128
pimecrolimus anti-inflammatory drug used for eczema 139
pimozide antipsychotic 41
pindolol beta blocker 55
Pinefeld XL brand name for modified-release felodipine 256 used for hypertension 60
Pinexel PR brand name for modified-release tamsulosin 407 (a drug used for urinary disorders 126)
Pinmactil brand name for fluvastatin (a lipid-lowering drug 61)
pioglitazone 361, oral drug for diabetes 100
piperacillin penicillin antibiotic 86
Pipexus brand name for pramipexole (a drug used to treat Parkinson's disease 43)
piracetam anticonvulsant 42
pirfenidone drug to treat pulmonary fibrosis
Piriton brand name for chlorphenamine 194 (an antihistamine 82)
piroxicam 362, NSAID 74 and drug for gout 77
pivmecillinam antibiotic 86
pixantrone anticancer drug 112 used for non-Hodgkin's lymphoma
Pixuvri brand name for pixantrone (an anticancer drug 112 used for non-Hodgkin's lymphoma)
pizotifen 363, drug for migraine 45
Plaquenil brand name for hydroxychloroquine (an antimalarial 95 and DMARD 75)
Platinex brand name for cisplatin 200, an anticancer drug 112
Plavix brand name for clopidogrel 208 (an antiplatelet drug 62)
Plegridy brand name for peginterferon beta-1a (a drug used for multiple sclerosis)
Plenachol brand name for colecalciferol (vitamin D 444)
Plenadren brand name for hydrocortisone 277
Plendil brand name for felodipine 256 (a calcium channel blocker 59)
Plenvu brand-name osmotic laxative for cleansing the bowel
plerixafor drug used to mobilize stem cells in patients with multiple myeloma or lymphoma
Pletal brand name for cilostazol (a vasodilator 56)
podophyllin topical treatment for genital warts
podophyllotoxin topical treatment for genital warts
Politid XL brand name for venlafaxine 427 (an antidepressant 40)
Pollenase brand name for chlorphenamine 194 (an antihistamine 82) for allergies and hayfever
Pollinex brand name for tree pollen extract for seasonal allergic hay fever due to tree pollen
poloxamer stimulant laxative 69
Polyfax brand name for bacitracin with polymyxin B (both antibiotics 86)
polymyxin B antibiotic 86

QUESTRAN LIGHT

polystyrene sulphonate drug to remove excess potassium from the blood

Polytar brand name for coal tar (used for eczema 139, psoriasis 138, and dandruff 140)

polyvinyl alcohol ingredient of artificial tear preparations 130

pomalidomide drug similar to thalidomide 415 used for multiple myeloma

ponatinib tyrosine kinase inhibitor anticancer drug 112

Ponstan brand name for mefenamic acid 314 (an NSAID 74)

porfimer anticancer drug 112

Portrazza brand name for necitumumab (an anticancer drug 112) used for lung cancer

posaconazole antifungal 96

Potaba brand name for potassium aminobenzoate used for Peyronie's disease (thickening of penile tissue)

Potactasol brand name for topotecan (an anticancer drug 112) used for ovarian, cervical, and lung cancer

potassium 439, mineral 108

potassium bicarbonate antacid 66

potassium chloride potassium 439 (a mineral 108)

potassium citrate drug for cystitis that reduces the acidity of urine 126

potassium permanganate antiseptic 135

povidone-iodine antiseptic 135

Pradaxa brand name for dabigatran 219 (an anticoagulant 62)

Praluent brand name for alirocumab (a lipid-lowering drug 61)

pramipexole drug for parkinsonism 43

pramocaine local anaesthetic 36

Prandin brand name for repaglinide 381 (an oral drug for diabetes 100)

prasugrel anticoagulant 63

pravastatin 364, cholesterol-lowering drug 61

Praxbind brand name for idarucizumab used to reverse the anticoagulant effect of dabigatran 219

Praxilene brand name for naftidrofuryl 336 (a vasodilator 56)

praziquantel anthelmintic 97 for tapeworm infestations

prazosin alpha blocker used for hypertension 60 and benign prostatic hyperplasia 126

Preblacon XL brand name for tolterodine 420 (a drug for urinary disorders 126)

Pred Forte brand name for prednisolone 365 (a corticosteroid 99) for ophthalmic use

Predenema brand name for prednisolone 365 (a corticosteroid 99)

Predfoam brand name for prednisolone 365 (a corticosteroid 99)

prednisolone 365 (a corticosteroid 99)

prednisone alternative name for prednisolone 365 (a corticosteroid 99)

Predsol brand name for prednisolone 365 (a corticosteroid 99)

Predsol-N brand name for prednisolone 365 (a corticosteroid 99) with neomycin (an aminoglycoside antibiotic 86)

Prefibin brand name for sublingual buprenorphine (an opioid analgesic 36)

pregabalin anticonvulsant 42 and drug for treatment of neuropathic pain

Pregaday brand name for folic acid 436 (a vitamin 107) with iron 437 (a mineral 108)

Pregnyl brand name for chorionic gonadotrophin (a drug for infertility 124)

Premarin brand name for conjugated oestrogens 214 (a female sex hormone 105)

Premique branded preparation for menopausal symptoms 105 containing conjugated oestrogens 214 and medroxyprogesterone 313

Prempak-C brand-name drug for menopausal symptoms 105 containing conjugated oestrogens 214 and norgestrel

Prenotrix brand name for buprenorphine (an opioid analgesic 36)

Prestylon brand name for omega-3-acid ethyl ester (a lipid-lowering drug 61)

Prevenar 13 brand-name vaccine 92 against pneumococcal infections

Prezista brand name for darunavir (a drug for HIV 116)

Priadel brand name for lithium 303 (a drug for mania 41)

Priligy brand name for dapoxetine used for premature ejaculation

prilocaine local anaesthetic 36

Prilotekal brand name for prilocaine (a local anaesthetic 36)

Primacor brand name for milrinone (a vasodilator drug 56) for heart failure

primaquine antimalarial 95 and antiprotozoal 94

Primaxin brand name for imipenem (an antibiotic 86) with cilastatin

primidone anticonvulsant 42

Primolut N brand name for norethisterone 342 (a female sex hormone 105)

Prioderm brand name for malathion 310 (a topical antiparasitic 136)

Pro-Banthine brand name for propantheline (an anticholinergic antispasmodic for irritable bowel syndrome 68 and urinary incontinence 126)

probenecid uricosuric for gout 77

procarbazine drug for lymphatic cancers and small-cell cancer of the lung 112

prochlorperazine 366, phenothiazine anti-emetic 46 and antipsychotic 41

Procoralan brand name for ivabradine (an anti-angina drug 59)

Proctofoam HC brand name for hydrocortisone 277 (a corticosteroid 99) with pramocaine (a local anaesthetic 36)

Proctosedyl brand name for hydrocortisone 277 (a corticosteroid 99) with cinchocaine (a local anaesthetic 36)

procyclidine 367, anticholinergic for parkinsonism 43

Pro-Epanutin brand name for fosphenytoin sodium 359 used for epilepsy 42

progesterone a female sex hormone 105

Prograf brand name for tacrolimus 405 (an immunosuppressant 115)

proguanil with atovaquone 368, an antimalarial drug 95

Progynova brand name for estradiol 249 (a female sex hormone 105)

Progynova TS brand name for estradiol 249 (a female sex hormone 105)

Proleukin brand name for aldesleukin (an anticancer drug 112) used for kidney cancer

Prolia brand name for denosumab (a monoclonal antibody for bone disorders 80)

promazine 369, phenothiazine antipsychotic 41

Prometax brand name for rivastigmine 387 (a drug for Alzheimer's disease 43)

promethazine 370, antihistamine 82 and anti-emetic 46

Propaderm brand name for beclometasone 168 (a corticosteroid 99)

propamidine isetionate antibacterial 89 for eye infections

propantheline anticholinergic anti-spasmodic for irritable bowel syndrome 68 and urinary incontinence 126

Propecia brand name for finasteride 258 (a male sex hormone 104 for benign prostatic hypertrophy 126)

propiverine drug for urinary frequency 126

propofol anaesthetic agent 36

propranolol 371, beta blocker 55 and anti-anxiety drug 39

propylthiouracil 372, antithyroid drug 102

Proscar brand name for finasteride 258 (a drug for benign prostatic hyperplasia 126)

Prostap SR brand name for leuprorelin (a drug for menstrual disorders 120)

Prosurin XL brand name for tamsulosin 407 used for benign prostatic hyperplasia 126

protamine an antidote for heparin 275

Protelos brand name for strontium ranelate 401 (a drug for bone disorders 80)

Prothiaden brand name for dosulepin 235 (a tricyclic antidepressant 40)

Protium brand name for pantoprazole (an ulcer healing drug 67)

Protopic brand name for tacrolimus 405 (an immunosuppressant 115)

Provera brand name for medroxyprogesterone 313 (a female sex hormone 105)

Provigil brand name for modafinil 331 (a nervous system stimulant 44 used for narcolepsy and excessive sleepiness)

Pro-Viron brand name for mesterolone (a male sex hormone 104)

proxymetacaine local anaesthetic 36

Prozac (and Prozep) brand names for fluoxetine 262 (an antidepressant 40)

prucalopride drug used for chronic constipation in women

pseudoephedrine sympathomimetic decongestant 51

Psoriderm brand-name bath product containing tar used for psoriasis 138

Psyquet XL brand name for modified-release quetiapine 375 (an antipsychotic 41)

Psytixol brand name for flupentixol 263 (an antipsychotic 41)

Pulmicort brand name for budesonide 180 (a corticosteroid 99)

Pulmozyme brand name for dornase alfa (a drug for cystic fibrosis 52)

Pulvinal brand name for salbutamol 391 (a bronchodilator 48)

Puregon brand name for follitropin alfa with lutropin alfa used to treat female infertility 124

Pyralvex brand-name preparation for mouth ulcers containing salicylic acid

pyrazinamide antituberculous drug 90

pyridostigmine 373, drug for myasthenia gravis 79

pyridoxine 440, vitamin 107

pyrimethamine 374, antimalarial 95

Q

Qlaira brand-name combined oral contraceptive 121 containing estradiol 249 and dienogest (a synthetic progestogen 105)

Qtern brand-name preparation of saxagliptin and dapagliflozin 220 (both drugs for diabetes 100)

Questran brand name for colestyramine 213 (a lipid-lowering drug 61)

Questran Light brand name for colestyramine 213 (a lipid-lowering drug 61)

QUETIAPINE

quetiapine 375, antipsychotic 41
quinagolide drug for hyperprolactinaemia 103
quinapril ACE inhibitor 56
quinidine anti-arrhythmic drug 58
quinine 376, antimalarial drug 95
Quinoric brand name for hydroxychloroquine (a DMARD 75)
Quinsair brand name for levofloxacin 299 (an antibiotic 86) used for lung infections
quinupristin antibiotic 86
Quodixor brand name for ibandronic acid (a bisphosphonate drug for bone disorders 80)
Qutenza brand-name preparation of capsaicin used to treat rheumatic and neuropathic pain
Qvar brand name for beclometasone (a corticosteroid 99)

R

rabeprazole 377, an anti-ulcer drug 67
Rabipur brand-name rabies vaccine 454
racecadotril antidiarrhoeal drug 68
Ralnea XL brand name for modified-release ropinirole 382 (drug for Parkinson's disease 43)
raloxifene 378, anti-oestrogen sex hormone antagonist 105 used for osteoporosis 80
raltegravir drug for HIV 116
raltitrexed anticancer drug 112
ramipril 379, ACE inhibitor 56
ramucirumab monoclonal antibody anticancer drug 112
Ranexa brand name for ranolazine (a drug for angina 59)
ranibizumab drug used for wet age-related macular degeneration
ranitidine 380, anti-ulcer drug 67
Ranitil brand name for ranitidine 380 (an anti-ulcer drug 67)
ranolazine drug for angina 59
Rapamune brand name for sirolimus (an immunosuppressant 115)
Rapitil brand name for nedocromilan (an anti-allergy drug 82)
Raponer XL brand name for modified-release ropinirole 388 (drug for Parkinson's disease 43)
Raporsin XL brand name for modified-release doxazosin 236 (an alpha-blocker antihypertensive 60 and drug for prostate disorders 126)
rasagiline drug for parkinsonism 43
rasburicase drug used to reduce high uric acid blood levels
Rasilez brand name for aliskiren (an antihypertensive 60)
Rawel XL brand name for modified-release indapamide 282 (a thiazide-like diuretic 57 used for hypertension 60)
Raxone brand name for idebenone (a drug for Alzheimer's disease 43)
Razylan brand name for modified-release raloxifene 378 (a drug for postmenopausal osteoporosis 80)
Rebetol brand name for ribavirin (antiviral 91)
Rebif brand name for interferon 285 (an antiviral 91 and anticancer drug 112)
reboxetine antidepressant 40
Recivit brand name for fentanyl (an opioid analgesic 36)
Rectogesic rectal preparation 71 containing glyceryl trinitrate 272 (an anti-angina drug 59)
Redoxon brand name for vitamin C 443 (a vitamin 107)
Refolinon brand name for calcium folinate (used to reduce toxicity of methotrexate 320)

Regaine brand name for minoxidil 328 (for treatment of male pattern baldness 140)
regorafenib protein kinase inhibitor anticancer drug 112
regulose osmotic laxative 69
Regurin preparations brand-name preparations containing trospium (an anticholinergic drug for urinary disorders 126)
Relactagel brand name for lactic acid gel used for vaginal and vulval conditions
Relaxit brand-name lubricant laxative 69
Relenza brand name for zanamivir, an antiviral 91
Reletrans brand name for buprenorphine (an opioid analgesic 36)
Relevtec brand name for buprenorphine (an opioid analgesic 36)
Relifex brand name for nabumetone (NSAID 74)
Relistor brand name for methylnaltrexone bromide, used to prevent constipation in patients taking opioids
Relpax brand name for eletriptan (a drug for migraine 45)
Reltebon brand name for oxycodone (an opioid analgesic 36)
Relvar brand name for fluticasone 265 (a corticosteroid 99) with vilanterol (a bronchodilator 48)
Remicade brand of infliximab 283 (a drug for Crohn's disease 70 and DMARD 75)
remifentanil drug used in anaesthesia
Reminyl brand name for galantamine (a drug for dementia 43)
Remsima brand name for infliximab 283 (a DMARD 75)
Renacet brand name for tablets containing calcium acetate (calcium 434) used for high blood phosphate levels
Renagel brand name for sevelamer (a drug used for high blood phosphate levels)
RenehaVis brand name for sodium hyaluronate (artificial tears 130)
Rennie brand name for calcium carbonate with magnesium carbonate (both antacids 66)
Rennie Deflatine brand-name antacid 66 containing calcium carbonate with magnesium carbonate and simeticone (antifoaming agent)
Rennie Duo brand-name antacid 66 containing calcium carbonate with magnesium carbonate and alginate (an antifoaming agent)
Renvela brand name for sevelamer (a drug used for high blood phosphate levels)
ReoPro brand name for abciximab (an anti-platelet drug 62 to prevent heart attacks)
repaglinide 381, oral drug for diabetes 100
Repatha brand name for evolocumab 253 used for high blood lipid levels 61
Rephoren brand name for calcium acetate (calcium 434) with magnesium carbonate (magnesium 438) used for high blood phosphate levels
Repinex XL brand name for ropinirole 388 (a drug for parkinsonism 43)
Replenine-VF brand name for factor IX (a substance to promote blood clotting 62)
Requip brand name for ropinirole 388 (a drug for parkinsonism 43)
Requip XL brand name for ropinirole 388 (a drug for parkinsonism 43)
reslizumab monoclonal antibody used to treat asthma 49
Resolor brand name for prucalopride (a laxative 69)
Resonium A brand name for polystyrene sulphonate (a drug to remove excess potassium from the blood)

Respontin brand name for ipratropium bromide 286 (a bronchodilator 48)
Restandol brand name for testosterone 412 (a male sex hormone 104)
Retacrit brand name for epoetin zeta (an erythropoietin 248)
Retalzem brand name for modified-release diltiazem 229 (a calcium channel blocker 59)
retapamulin antibacterial 89 used for superficial bacterial skin infections
reteplase thrombolytic 63
retigabine anticonvulsant drug 42
retinoic acid vitamin A 442 (a vitamin 107)
retinoids vitamin A 442 (a vitamin 107)
retinol vitamin A 442 (a vitamin 107)
Retrovir brand name for zidovudine 430 (an antiretroviral for HIV/AIDS 116)
Revatio brand name for sildenafil 394 (a drug for pulmonary hypertension)
Revaxis brand-name vaccine 92 to protect against diphtheria/tetanus/poliomyelitis
Revestive brand name for teduglutide (used to improve intestinal absorption of nutrients)
Revocon brand name for tetrabenazine (a drug for tremor)
Revolade brand name for eltrombopag (a drug used to treat platelet disorders)
Rewisca brand name for pregabalin (an anticonvulsant 42 and drug for neuropathic pain)
Reyataz brand name for atazanavir (an antiretroviral for HIV/AIDS 116)
Rezolsta brand name for a combination of darunavir and clobicistat (both drugs for HIV 116)
Rhinocort brand name for budesonide 180 (a corticosteroid 99)
Rhinolast brand name for azelastine (an antihistamine 82)
Riamet brand name for artemether with lumefantrine (both antimalarials 95)
ribavirin antiviral 91 used for certain lung infections in infants and children
ribociclib protein kinase inhibitor used to treat breast cancer
rifabutin antituberculous drug 90
Rifadin brand name for rifampicin 382 (an antituberculous drug 90)
rifampicin 382, an antituberculous drug 90
Rifater brand name for isoniazid 288 with rifampicin 382 and pyrazinamide (all antituberculous drugs 90)
rifaximin antibacterial 89
Rifinah brand name for isoniazid 288 with rifampicin 382 (both antituberculous drugs 90)
Rigevidon brand name combined oral contraceptive 121 containing ethinylestradiol 252 and levonorgestrel 300
rilpivirine antiretroviral for treating HIV/AIDS 116
Rilutek brand name for riluzole (a glutamate inhibitor used to help patients with sclerosis)
riluzole glutamate inhibitor to relieve sclerosis
Rimactane brand name for rifampicin 382 (an antituberculous drug 90)
rimexolone corticosteroid 99
Rinatec brand name for ipratropium bromide 286 (a bronchodilator 48)
Rinstead pastilles brand-name preparation for mouth ulcers and denture sores containing cetylpyridinium (a topical antiseptic 135) and menthol
riociguat drug for pulmonary hypertension
risedronate 383, a drug for bone disorders 80
Risperdal brand name for risperidone 384 (an antipsychotic drug 41)

SILVER SULFADIAZINE

risperidone 384, an antipsychotic 41

Ritalin brand name for methylphenidate 322 (a nervous system stimulant 44)

ritonavir antiretroviral for HIV/AIDS 116

rituximab 385, anticancer drug 112

rivaroxaban 386, anticoagulant 62

rivastigmine 387, drug for Alzheimer's disease 43

Rixathon brand name for rituximab 385 (a monoclonal antibody anticancer drug 112)

rizatriptan drug for migraine 45

Roaccutane brand name for isotretinoin 290 (a drug for acne 137)

RoActemra brand name for tocilizumab (an immunosuppressant 115 and antirheumatic drug 75)

Robaxin brand name for methocarbamol (a muscle relaxant 78)

Robinul-Neostigmine brand name for neostigmine (a drug for myasthenia gravis 79)

Robitussin Chesty Cough brand name for guaifenesin (an expectorant 52)

Robitussin Dry Cough brand name for dextromethorphan (a cough suppressant 52)

Rocaltrol brand name for calcitriol (a vitamin 107)

Rocephin brand name for ceftriaxone (an antibiotic 86)

rocuronium drug to relax the muscles during general anaesthesia

Rodomel XL brand name for modified-release venlafaxine 427 (an antidepressant 40)

Roferon-A brand name for interferon 285 (an antiviral 91 and anticancer drug 112)

roflumilast drug for obstructive airways disease

rolapitant drug used to prevent nausea and vomiting in patients receiving chemotherapy

romiplostim drug for thrombocytopenia (low levels of platelets in the blood)

Ropilynz brand name for ropinirole 388 (a drug for parkinsonism 43)

ropinirole 388, drug for parkinsonism 43

Ropiqual brand name for ropinirole 388 (a drug for parkinsonism 43)

ropivacaine local anaesthetic 36

Rosiced brand name for metronidazole 325 (an antibacterial 89 and antiprotozoal 94)

rosuvastatin 389, a lipid-lowering drug 61

Rotarix brand-name vaccine 92 to protect against gastroenteritis caused by rotavirus

rotigotine drug for parkinsonism 43

Rowachol brand-name preparation of essential oils for gallstones 72

Rowatinex brand-name preparation to dissolve kidney stones 77 and treat kidney infections

Rozex brand name for metronidazole 325 (an antibacterial 89)

rucaparib antineoplastic drug used to treat ovarian cancer

rufinamide anticonvulsant drug 42 used to control epilepsy

rupatadine antihistamine 82

ruxolitinib tyrosine kinase inhibitor anticancer drug 112

Rythmodan brand name for disopyramide (an anti-arrhythmic 58)

S

Sabril brand name for vigabatrin (an anticonvulsant 42)

sacubitril with valsartan 390, combination drug used for heart failure

Saflutan brand name for tafluprost used for glaucoma 128

Saizen brand name for somatropin (a synthetic pituitary hormone 103)

Salactol brand-name wart preparation containing salicylic acid, lactic acid, and collodion 135

Salagen brand name for pilocarpine 360 (a miotic for glaucoma 128)

Salamol brand name for salbutamol 391 (a bronchodilator 48)

Salatac brand-name wart preparation containing salicylic acid, lactic acid, and collodion 135

Salazopyrin brand name for sulfasalazine 403 (a drug for inflammatory bowel disease 70 and DMARD 75)

Salbulin brand name for salbutamol 391 (a bronchodilator 48 and drug used in labour 125)

salbutamol 391, bronchodilator 48 and drug used in labour 125

salcatonin see calcitonin (salmon)

salicylic acid keratolytic for acne 137, dandruff 140, psoriasis 138, and warts

Saliveze brand name for artificial saliva

salmeterol 392, bronchodilator 48

Salofalk brand name for mesalazine 317 (a drug for ulcerative colitis 70)

Samsca brand name for tolvaptan (a diuretic 57) used for syndrome of inappropriate antidiuretic hormone secretion (in which water builds up in the body)

Sanatogen preparations brand-name multivitamin preparations 107

Sancuso brand name for a skin patch containing granisetron (an anti-emetic 46)

Sandimmun brand name for ciclosporin 196 (an immunosuppressant 115)

Sandocal brand name for calcium 434 (a mineral 108)

Sando-K brand name for potassium 439 (a mineral 108)

Sandostatin brand name for octreotide (a synthetic pituitary hormone 103 used to relieve symptoms of cancer of the pancreas 112)

Sandrena brand-name preparation for menopausal symptoms 105 containing estradiol 249

Santizor brand name for tolterodine 420 (an anticholinergic 126)

Santizor XL brand name for tolterodine 420 (a drug for urinary disorders 126)

sapropterin dihydrochloride drug for phenylketonuria, a metabolic disorder

saquinavir antiretroviral for HIV/AIDS 116

sarilumab monoclonal antibody used to treat rheumatoid arthritis 75

Sativex brand name for cannabidiol 185 used for spasticity

Savlon brand name for chlorhexidine with cetrimide (both skin antiseptics 135)

saxagliptin drug for diabetes 100

Saxenda brand name for liraglutide (a drug used to treat diabetes 100)

Sayana Press brand name for progesterone (a female sex hormone 105)

Scheriproct brand name for prednisolone 365 (a corticosteroid 99) with cinchocaine (a local anaesthetic 36)

Scopoderm brand name for a skin patch containing hyoscine 278 (an anti-emetic 46)

Scopoderm TTS brand name for an anti-emetic 46 containing hyoscine 278

Sea-Legs brand name for meclozine (an antihistamine 82 to prevent motion sickness 46)

Sebco brand-name preparation containing coal tar, salicylic acid, and sulphur used for scaly scalp disorders

Sebivo brand name for telbivudine (an antiviral drug 91) used for hepatitis B

Sectral brand name for acebutolol (a beta blocker 55)

secukinumab monoclonal antibody antirheumatic drug 75

Securon SR brand name for verapamil 428 (an anti-arrhythmic 58 and anti-angina drug 59)

selegiline drug for severe parkinsonism 43

Selenase brand name for selenium 441 (a mineral 108)

selenium 441, mineral 108

SelenoPrecise brand name for selenium 441 (a mineral 108)

Selexid brand name for pivmecillinam (a penicillin antibiotic 86)

Selexipag drug for pulmonary hypertension

Selincro brand name for nalmefene used to treat alcohol dependence 447

Selsun brand-name dandruff shampoo 140 containing selenium sulphide

senna stimulant laxative 69

Senokot brand name for senna (a stimulant laxative 69)

Septanest brand name for articaine (a local anaesthetic 36) with epinephrine 245

Septrin brand name for co-trimoxazole 216 (an antibacterial 89 and anti-protozoal 94)

Seractil brand name for dexibuprofen (NSAID 74)

Serc brand name for betahistine 171 (a drug for Ménière's disease 46)

Sereflo brand name for fluticasone (a corticosteroid 99) with salmeterol (a bronchodilator 48)

Serenace brand name for haloperidol 274 (a butyrophenone antipsychotic 41)

Seretide brand name for salmeterol 392 (a bronchodilator 48) with fluticasone 265 (a corticosteroid 99)

Serevent brand name for salmeterol 392 (a bronchodilator 48)

Seroquel brand name for quetiapine 375 (an antipsychotic 41)

Seroxat brand name for paroxetine 353 (an antidepressant 40)

sertraline 393, antidepressant 40

Setlers brand-name antacid 66 containing calcium carbonate

Setofilm brand name for ondansetron 347 (an anti-emetic 46)

sevelamer drug for removing excess phosphate from the blood

Sevikar brand name for olmesartan (an angiotensin II blocker, vasodilator 56, and antihypertensive 60)

Sevodyne brand name for buprenorphine (an opioid analgesic 36)

sevoflurane general anaesthetic

Sevredol brand name for morphine 334 (an opioid analgesic 36)

Shortec brand name for modified-release oxycodone (an opioid analgesic 36)

Signifor brand name for pasireotide used for Cushing's disease (high levels of corticosteroid hormones)

Siklos brand name for hydroxycarbamide (an anticancer drug 112) used for leukaemia and sickle-cell disease

sildenafil 394, drug for erectile dysfunction 104, 124 and pulmonary hypertension

siltuximab monoclonal antibody anticancer drug 112

silver nitrate skin disinfectant 135

silver sulfadiazine topical antibacterial 89 used to prevent infection in burns 135

SIMBRINZA

Simbrinza brand name for eye drops containing brimodine 177 and brinzolamide 178 (drugs for glaucoma 128)

simeprevir antiviral drug 91 used for hepatitis C

simeticone antifoaming agent 66

Simple linctus brand-name preparation for dry coughs containing citric acid (a soothing agent)

Simponi brand name for golimumab (a monoclonal antibody antirheumatic drug 75)

Simulect brand name for basiliximab (an immunosuppressant 115)

Simvador brand name for simvastatin 395 (a lipid-lowering drug 61)

simvastatin 395, a lipid-lowering drug 61

Sinemet brand name for levodopa 298 with carbidopa (both drugs for parkinsonism 43)

Sinemet CR brand name for modified-release levodopa 298 with carbidopa (both drugs for parkinsonism 43)

Singulair brand name for montelukast 333 (a leukotriene antagonist) for asthma 49 and bronchospasm 48

Sinthrome brand name for acenocoumarol (an anticoagulant 62)

Siopel brand-name barrier cream containing cetrimide and dimeticone

sirolimus immunosuppressant 115

Sirturo brand name for bedaquiline (an antituberculous drug 90)

sitagliptin 396, oral drug for diabetes 100

Sivextro brand name for tedizolid (an antibiotic for skin infections 135)

Skinoren brand name for azelaic acid (an antibacterial 89 drug for acne 137)

Slocinx XL brand name for modified–release doxazosin 236 (an antihypertensive 60 used for heart failure)

Slo-Phyllin brand name for theophylline 416 (a bronchodilator 48)

Slow-Sodium brand name for sodium chloride 441 (a mineral 108)

Slow-Trasicor brand name for slow-release oxprenolol (a beta blocker 55)

Slozem brand name for diltiazem 229 (a calcium channel blocker 56)

Sno Tears brand name for polyvinyl alcohol (used in artificial tear preparations 130)

Sodiofolin brand of folinic acid (a vitamin 107)

sodium 441, mineral 108

sodium acid phosphate phosphate supplement

sodium aurothiomalate substance containing gold, a DMARD 75

sodium bicarbonate antacid 66

sodium chloride common salt; contains sodium 441 (a mineral 108)

sodium citrate drug for urinary tract infections 126

sodium clodronate agent used for high blood calcium in cancer patients 112

sodium cromoglicate 397, anti-allergy drug 82

sodium feredetate iron 437, a mineral 108

sodium fluoride 436, a mineral 108

sodium nitroprusside vasodilator 56

sodium oxybate drug used for narcolepsy

sodium picosulfate stimulant laxative 69

sodium valproate 398, anticonvulsant drug 42

Soffen brand name for liquid paraffin used for dry and scaling skin conditions

Sofiperla brand-name combined oral contraceptive 121 containing ethinylestradiol 252 and gestodene

sofosbuvir antiviral drug 91 used for hepatitis C

Sofradex brand name for dexamethasone 223 (a corticosteroid 99) with framycetin and gramicidin (both antibiotics 86)

SoftDrops brand name for eye drops containing hypermellose (a lubricant) used for dry eyes

Solaraze brand name for a gel containing diclofenac 225 used for sunburn

Solarcaine brand name for benzocaine (a local anaesthetic 36) with triclosan (an antimicrobial drug 133)

Solian brand name for amisulpride 156, an antipsychotic 41

solifenacin drug for urinary disorders 126

Soliris brand name for eculizumab (a monoclonal antibody used for certain blood disorders)

Solpadeine Migraine brand-name analgesic 36 containing codeine 211 and ibuprofen 279

Solpadeine Plus brand-name analgesic 36 containing codeine 211, paracetamol 352, and caffeine

Solpadol brand-name analgesic containing codeine 211 and paracetamol 352

Soltamox brand name for tamoxifen 406, an anti-oestrogen anticancer drug 112

Solu-Cortef brand name for hydrocortisone 277 (a corticosteroid 99)

Solu-Medrone brand name for methylprednisolone (a corticosteroid 99)

Solvazinc brand name for zinc 445 (a mineral 108)

somatropin synthetic pituitary hormone 103

Somatuline brand name for lanreotide (an anticancer drug 112 and drug for endocrine disorders 103)

Somavert brand name for pegvisomant used for growth hormone disorders 103

Sominex brand name for promethazine 370 (a sedating antihistamine 82)

Sondate brand name for quetiapine 375 (an antipsychotic 41 and antidepressant 40)

Soolantra brand name for ivermectin (an antiparasitic drug 136)

Soothelip brand name cold-sore cream containing aciclovir 148 (an antiviral 91)

sorafenib anticancer drug 112

Sotacor brand name for sotalol 399 (a beta blocker 55)

sotalol 399, a beta blocker 55

Sovaldi brand name for sofosbuvir (an antiviral drug 91) used for hepatitis C

Spasmonal brand name for alverine citrate (an antispasmodic for irritable bowel syndrome 68)

Spectrila brand name for asparignase (an anticancer drug 112) used for childhood leukaemia

Spedra brand name for avanafil (a drug for erectile dysfunction 124)

Spiriva brand name for tiotropium 418 (a bronchodilator 48)

Spiriva Resprimat brand name for tiotropium 418 (a bronchodilator 48)

Spiroco XL brand name for modified-release ropinirole 388 (a drug for Parkinson's disease 43 and restless legs)

spironolactone 400, potassium-sparing diuretic 57

Sporanox brand name for itraconazole (an antifungal 96)

Sprilon brand-name skin preparation 135 containing dimeticone and zinc oxide

Sprycel brand name for dasatinib (an anticancer drug 112 used to treat leukaemia)

Stalevo brand-name product containing levodopa 298 with carbidopa (a drug that enhances the effect of levodopa) and entacapone (drugs for parkinsonism 43)

Starlix brand name for netaglenide (an oral drug for diabetes 100)

stavudine antiretroviral used for HIV/AIDS 116

Stayveer brand name for bosentan (a drug used to treat pulmonary hypertension)

Stelara brand name for ustekinumab (an immunosuppressant 115)

Stemetil brand name for prochlorperazine 366 (a phenothiazine anti-emetic 46 and antipsychotic 41)

sterculia bulk-forming agent used as an antidiarrhoeal 68 and laxative 69

Ster-Zac brand name for triclosan (an antimicrobial 133)

Stesolid brand name for diazepam 224 (a benzodiazepine anti-anxiety drug 39, muscle relaxant 78, and anticonvulsant 42)

Stiemycin brand name for erythromycin 247 (an antibiotic 86)

stilboestrol see diethylstilbestrol

Stilnoct brand name for zolpidem (a sleeping drug 38)

Stirlescent brand name for an effervescent form of naproxen 337 (a NSAID 74)

Stivarga brand name for regorafenib (a protein kinase inhibitor anticancer drug 112)

St John's wort herbal antidepressant that interacts with many other drugs

Strattera brand name for atomoxetine (a drug for attention deficit hyperactivity disorder (ADHD) 44)

Strefen brand-name preparation for sore throats containing flurbiprofen (a NSAID 74)

Strepsils branded preparation for mouth and throat infections containing amylmetacresol and dichlorobenzyl alcohol (both antiseptics 135)

Streptase brand name for streptokinase (a thrombolytic 63)

streptokinase thrombolytic 63

streptomycin antituberculous drug 90 and aminoglycoside antibiotic 86

Stribild brand name for a combined preparation containing cobicistat, elvitegravir, emtricitabine 242, and tenofovir 409 (antiretrovirals for HIV/AIDS 116)

Striverdi Respimat brand name for olodaterol (a bronchodilator 48)

Strivit-D3 brand name for colecalciferol (vitamin D 444)

strontium ranelate 401, drug for bone disorders 80

Stugeron brand name for cinnarizine 198 (an antihistamine anti-emetic 46)

Sublimaze brand name for fentanyl (an opioid analgesic 36)

Suboxone brand name for buprenorphine (an opioid analgesic 36) with naloxone used to treat opioid dependence

Subutex brand name for buprenorphine (an opioid analgesic 36)

sucralfate 402, ulcer-healing drug 67

sucroferric oxyhydroxide drug used for high phosphate levels in the blood

Sudafed brand name for pseudoephedrine (a decongestant 51)

Sudafed-Congestion Cold and Flu brand name for paracetamol 352 (a non-opioid analgesic 36) and pseudoephedrine (a decongestant 51)

Sudocrem brand-name skin preparation containing benzyl benzoate and zinc oxide

Sukkarto SR brand name for modified-release metformin 318 (a drug for diabetes 100)

Sulazine EC brand name for sulfasalazine 403 used for inflammatory bowel disease 70

sulfadiazine sulfonamide antibacterial 89

sulfadoxine drug used with pyrimethamine 374 for malaria 95

TENSIPINE MR

sulfamethoxazole sulfonamide antibacterial 89 combined with trimethoprim 424 in co-trimoxazole 216

sulfasalazine 403, drug for inflammatory bowel disease 70 and a DMARD 75

sulfinpyrazone drug for gout 77

sulfur topical antibacterial 89 and antifungal 96 for acne 137 and dandruff 140

sulindac NSAID 74

sulpiride 156, antipsychotic 41

Sulpor brand name for sulpiride 156 (an antipsychotic 41)

sumatriptan 404, drug for migraine 45

sunitinib anticancer drug 112

Sunveniz XL brand name for modified-release venlafaxine 427 (an antidepressant 40)

Sunya brand-name combined oral contraceptive 121 containing ethinylastradiol 248 and gestodene

Supralip brand name for a fenofibrate (a lipid-lowering drug 61)

Suprane brand name for desflurane (a general anaesthetic)

Suprax brand name for cefixime (a cephalosporin antibiotic 86)

Suprecur brand name for buserelin (a drug for menstrual disorders 120 and prostate cancer 112)

Suprefact brand name for buserelin (a drug for menstrual disorders 120 and prostate cancer 112)

Surgam brand name for tiaprofenic acid (a NSAID 74)

Sustanon brand name for testosterone 412 (a male sex hormone 104)

Sustiva brand name for efavirenz 241 (an antiretroviral for HIV/AIDS 116)

Sutent brand name for sunitinib (an anticancer drug 112)

suxamethonium a muscle relaxant used during general anaesthesia

Sycrest brand name for asenapine (an antipsychotic drug 41) used for bipolar disorder

Sylvant brand name for siltuximab (an anticancer drug 112)

Symbicort brand name for formoterol (a bronchodilator 48) with budesonide 180 (a corticosteroid 99)

Symdeko brand name for a fixed-dose combination of tezacaftor/ivacaftor 414 (a treatment for cystic fibrosis)

Symkevi brand name for a fixed-dose combination of tezacaftor/ivacaftor 414 (a treatment for cystic fibrosis)

Symtuza brand name for darunavir, cobicistat, emtricitabine 242, and tenofovir 409 (antiviral drugs) used to treat HIV

Synacthen brand name for tetracosactide (used to assess adrenal gland function 103)

Synalar brand name for fluocinolone (a topical corticosteroid 134)

Synalar C brand name for fluocinolone (a topical corticosteroid 134) with clioquinol (an antiseptic 135)

Synalar N brand name for fluocinolone (a topical corticosteroid 134) with neomycin (an aminoglycoside antibiotic 86)

Synarel brand name for nafarelin (a drug for menstrual disorders 120)

Syner-KINASE brand-name anticoagulant drug 62

Synjardy brand name for empagliflozin with metformin 313 (both drugs for diabetes 100)

Syntocinon brand name for oxytocin (a uterine stimulant 125)

Syntometrine brand name for ergometrine with oxytocin (both uterine stimulants 125)

Sytron brand name for sodium feredetate (iron 437, a mineral 108)

T

Tabphyn MR brand name for tamsulosin 407 (an alpha blocker for prostate disorders 126)

tacalcitol a drug for psoriasis 138

Tacni brand name for tacrolimus 405 (an immunosuppressant drug 115)

tacrolimus 405, an immunosuppressant 115

tadalafil 394, a drug for erectile dysfunction 124

tafamidis drug used to inhibit neurological impairment in nervous system disorders

Tafinlar brand name for dabrafenib (a protein kinase anticancer drug 112)

tafluprost drug for glaucoma 128

Tagamet brand name for cimetidine 197 (an anti-ulcer drug 67)

Tagrisso brand name for osimertinib (a protein kinase inhibitor)

Talidex brand name for thalidomide, used to treat a number of cancers

Talmanco a brand name for tadalafil 394 (a drug used for erectile dysfunction 124 and pulmonary hypertension)

Taltz brand name for ixekizumab used for psoriasis 138

Tambocor brand name for flecainide (an anti-arrhythmic 58)

Tamfrex XL brand name for tamsulosin 407 (an alpha blocker used to treat prostate disorders 126)

Tamiflu brand name for oseltamivir 350 (an antiviral drug 91 to protect against influenza)

tamoxifen 406, anticancer drug 112

tamsulosin 407, alpha blocker used to treat prostate disorders 126

Tamurex brand name for tamsulosin 407 (an alpha blocker used for prostate disorders 126)

Tanatril brand name for imidapril (an ACE inhibitor 56)

Tapclob brand name for clobazam (a benzodiazepine anti-anxiety drug 39 and anticonvulsant 42)

tapentadol opioid analgesic drug 36

Taptiqom brand name for tafluprost (a drug for glaucoma 128)

Tarceva brand name for erlotinib (an anticancer drug 112)

Tardiben brand name for tetrabenazine (a drug used to treat movement disorders)

Targaxan brand name for rifaximin (an antibacterial 89)

Targinact brand name for modified-release naloxone with oxycodone (an opioid analgesic drug 36) used to treat severe pain and restless legs

Targocid brand name for teicoplanin (an antibiotic 86)

Targretin brand name for bexarotene (an anticancer drug 112)

Tarivid brand name for ofloxacin (an antibiotic 86)

Tasigna brand name for nilotinib (an anticancer drug 112)

Tasmar brand name for tolcapone (a drug for parkinsonism 43)

Tavanic brand name for levofloxacin 299 (an antibacterial 89)

Tavegil brand name for clemastine (an antihistamine 82)

Taxceus brand name for docetaxel (an anticancer drug 112)

Taxotere brand name for docetaxel (an anticancer drug 112)

tazarotene retinoid (see vitamin A 442) for psoriasis 138

tazobactam an antibiotic 86

Tazocin brand name for piperacillin (an antibiotic 86) with tazobactam (a substance that increases the effectiveness of piperacillin)

TCP brand-name antiseptic 135 containing phenol, chlorinated and halogenated phenols, sodium salicylate and glycerol

Tear-Lac brand-name artificial tear preparation 130 containing hypromellose

Tears Naturale brand-name artificial tear preparation 130 containing hypromellose

Tecentriq brand name for atezolizumab (a monoclonal antibody)

Tecfidera brand name for dimethyl fumarate used for multiple sclerosis

tedizolid antibacterial drug 89

tegafur anticancer drug 112

Teglutik brand name for riluzole (a drug used to help patients with amyotrophic lateral sclerosis)

Tegretol brand name for carbamazepine 187 (an anticonvulsant 42)

Tegretol Retard brand name for modified-release carbamazepine 187 (an anticonvulsant 42)

teicoplanin antibiotic 86

telaprevir antiviral drug 91

telavancin antibacterial drug 89

telbivudine antiviral drug 91

Telfast brand name for fexofenadine (an antihistamine 82)

telithromycin antibiotic 86

telmisartan vasodilator 56 and antihypertensive drug 60

Telzir brand name for fosamprenavir (an antiretroviral for HIV/AIDS 116)

temazepam 408, benzodiazepine sleeping drug 38

Temgesic brand name for buprenorphine (an opioid analgesic 36)

temocillin antibiotic 86

Temodal brand name for temozolomide (an anticancer drug 112)

Temomedac brand name for temozolomide (an anticancer drug 112)

temozolomide anticancer drug 112

temsirolimus protein kinase inhibitor anticancer drug 112

tenecteplase thrombolytic 63

Tenif brand name for atenolol 163 (a beta blocker 55) with nifedipine 340 (an anti-angina drug 59 and antihypertensive 60)

tenofovir 409, antiviral 91 and drug for HIV/AIDS 116

Tenoret-50 brand name for atenolol 163 (a beta blocker 55) with chlortalidone (a thiazide diuretic 57)

Tenoretic brand name for atenolol 163 (a beta blocker 55) with chlortalidone (a thiazide diuretic 57)

Tenormin brand name for atenolol 163 (a beta blocker 55)

tenoxicam NSAID 74

Tenprolide XL brand name for quetiapine 375 (an antipsychotic 41)

Tensaid XL brand name for indapamide 282 (a thiazide-like diuretic 57)

Tensipine MR brand name for nifedipine 340 (a calcium channel blocker 59)

TEOPTIC

Teoptic brand name for carteolol (a beta blocker 55 used for glaucoma 128)

Tepadina brand name for thiotepa (an anticancer drug 112) used in stem cell treatment

Tephine brand name for sublingual buprenorphine (an opioid analgesic drug 36)

terazosin sympatholytic antihypertensive 60, also used for prostate disorders 126

terbinafine 410, antifungal 96

terbutaline 411, sympathomimetic bronchodilator 48 and uterine muscle relaxant 125

teriflunomide immunosuppressant drug 115 used for multiple sclerosis

teriparatide drug for bone disorders 80

terlipressin drug similar to vasopressin (a pituitary hormone 103) used to stop bleeding

Teromeg brand name for omega-3-acid ethyl esters (used to treat elevated triglycerides 61)

Tertroxin brand name for liothyronine (a thyroid hormone 102)

Testim brand name for testosterone 412 (a male sex hormone 104)

Testogel brand name for testosterone 412 (a male sex hormone 104)

testosterone 412, male sex hormone 104

Tetmodis brand name for tetrabenazine (a drug for tremor)

tetrabenazine drug for tremor

tetracaine (previously amethocaine) a local anaesthetic 36

tetracosactide drug similar to corticotropin, used to assess adrenal gland function 103

tetracycline 413, antibiotic 86 and antimalarial drug 95

Tetralysal 300 brand name for lymecycline 413 (a tetracycline antibiotic 86)

Teveten brand name for eposartan (an angiotensin II blocker antihypertensive drug 60)

Teysuno brand name for tegafur with gimeracil and oteracil (all anticancer drugs 112)

tezacaftor with ivacaftor fixed-dose combination drug used for cystic fibrosis

T-Gel brand name for coal tar (a substance used in treating dandruff 140 and psoriasis 138)

thalidomide 415, drug for leprosy 89 and multiple myeloma (a type of bone marrow cancer)

theophylline/aminophylline 416, bronchodilator drug 48

thiamine 442, vitamin 107

thiopental fast-acting barbiturate used to induce general anaesthesia

thiotepa anticancer drug 112

Thorens brand name for colecalciferol (vitamin D 444)

Thyrogen brand name for thyrotropin alfa (a thyroid-stimulating hormone) used for thyroid cancer 102

thyroid hormones synthetic thyroid hormones used for hypothyroidism 102

tiagabine anti-epileptic 42

tiaprofenic acid NSAID 74

tibolone female sex hormone 105

ticagrelor antiplatelet drug 62

ticarcillin penicillin antibiotic 86

tigecycline antibiotic 86 and antibacterial 89 used for soft-tissue and skin infections 135

Tilade brand name for nedocromil (a bronchodilator 48)

Tildiem brand name for diltiazem 229 (an anti-angina drug 59)

Tilodol SR brand name for modified-release tramadol 421 (an opioid analgesic 36)

Tilofyl brand name for a skin patch containing fentanyl (an opioid analgesic 36)

Tiloryth brand name for erythromycin 247 (an antibiotic 86)

Timentin brand name for ticarcillin (a penicillin antibiotic 86) with clavulanic acid (a substance that increases the effectiveness of ticarcillin)

Timodine brand name for hydrocortisone 277 (a corticosteroid 99) with nystatin 343 (an antifungal 96), benzalkonium chloride (an antiseptic 135), and dimeticone (a base for skin preparations 135)

timolol 417, beta blocker 55 and drug for glaucoma 128

Timoptol brand name for timolol 417 (a beta blocker 55 and drug for glaucoma 128)

Timoptol LA brand-name long-acting preparation of timolol 417

tinidazole antibacterial 89 and antiprotozoal 94

tinzaparin type of heparin 275 (an anticoagulant drug 62)

tioconazole antifungal 96

tioguanine antimetabolite for acute leukaemia 112

Tiopex brand name for timolol 417 (a beta blocker 55 and drug for glaucoma 128)

tiotropium 418, bronchodilator 48

tipranavir antiretroviral for HIV/AIDS 116

tirofiban antiplatelet drug 62 for the prevention of heart attacks

tissue-type plasminogen activator see alteplase

Tivicay brand name for dolutegravir (a drug for HIV 116)

tivozanib protein kinase inhibitor used to treat kidney cancer

tizanidine a muscle relaxant 78

Tobi brand name for tobramycin (an antibiotic 86)

Tobradex brand name for dexamethasone 223 (a corticosteroid 99) with tobramycin (an antibiotic 86)

tobramycin aminoglycoside antibiotic 86

Tobravisc brand name for a topical preparation of tobramycin (an aminoglycoside antibiotic 86) used for eye infections

tocilizumab immunosuppressant 115 and antirheumatic drug 75

tocopherol vitamin E 444 (a vitamin 107)

tocopheryl vitamin E 444 (a vitamin 107)

tofacitinib drug for rheumatoid arthritis 75

tolbutamide 419, drug for diabetes 100

tolcapone drug for parkinsonism 43

tolfenamic acid drug for migraine 45

tolterodine 420, anticholinergic and antispasmodic for urinary disorders 126

Tolucombi brand name for telmisartan (a vasodilator 56) with hydrochlorothiazide (276, a diuretic drug 57) used for hypertension 60

Tolura brand name for telmisartan (a vasodilator 56) used to treat hypertension 60

tolvaptan drug similar to vasopressin (a pituitary hormone 103)

Tomudex brand name for raltitrexed (an anticancer drug 112) used for bowel cancer

Tonpular XL brand name for a modified-release preparation of venlafaxine 427 (an antidepressant 40)

Topamax brand name for topiramate (an anticonvulsant 42)

Topogyne brand name for misoprostol 330 used in the termination of pregnancy

topotecan anticancer drug 112

torasemide loop diuretic 57

Torem brand name for torasemide (a loop diuretic 57)

toremifene anticancer drug 112

Torisel brand name for temsirolimus (a protein kinase inhibitor anticancer drug 112)

Tostran brand name for testosterone 412 (a male hormone 104)

Toujeo brand name for insulin glargine 284 (a drug for diabetes 100)

Toviaz brand name for fesoterodine (a drug used for urinary frequency 126)

Tracleer brand name for bosentan (a drug for pulmonary hypertension)

Tractocile brand name for atosiban (a drug used to stop premature labour 125)

Tradorec XL brand-name modified-release preparation of tramadol 421 (an opioid analgesic 36)

Trajenta brand name for linagliptin (a drug for diabetes 100)

Tramacet brand-name product containing tramadol 421 and paracetamol 352 (both analgesics 36)

tramadol 421, opioid analgesic 36

Tramquel SR brand-name modified-release preparation of tramadol 421 (an opioid analgesic 36)

Tramulief SR brand-name modified-release preparation of tramadol 421 (an opioid analgesic 36)

Trandate brand name for labetalol (a beta blocker 55)

trandolapril ACE inhibitor 56

tranexamic acid antifibrinolytic used to promote blood clotting 62

Tranquilyn brand name for methylphenidate 322 (a nervous system stimulant 316) used to treat attention deficit hyperactivity disorder (ADHD)

Transiderm-Nitro brand name for glyceryl trinitrate 272 (an anti-angina drug 59)

Transtec brand name for buprenorphine (an opioid analgesic 36)

Transvasin brand-name topical treatment for muscle aches and sprains 78

tranylcypromine monoamine oxidase inhibitor (MAOI) antidepressant 40

trastuzumab 422, anticancer drug 112

Travatan brand name for travoprost (a drug for glaucoma 128)

travoprost drug for glaucoma 128

Traxam brand name for felbinac (an NSAID 74)

trazodone antidepressant 40

Treclin brand name for clindamycin 203 (an antibiotic 86) with tretinoin (a drug used for acne 137)

Trental brand name for pentoxifylline (a vasodilator 56)

treosulfan drug for ovarian cancer 112

Tresiba preparations brand name for preparations of insulin 284 (a drug for diabetes 100)

tretinoin drug for acne 137

Trevicta brand name for paliperidone (an antipsychotic drug 41)

triamcinolone corticosteroid 99 also used for ear disorders 131

triamterene 423, potassium-sparing diuretic 57

Triapin brand-name preparation containing felodipine 256 (a calcium channel blocker 59) and ramipril 379 (an ACE inhibitor 56)

tribavirin see ribavirin

triclosan topical antimicrobial 133

Tridestra brand-name preparation for menopausal symptoms 105 containing estradiol 249 and medroxyprogesterone acetate 313

trientine drug used for Wilson's disease (a metabolic disorder in which copper builds up in the body)

Triesence brand name for triamcinolone (a corticosteroid 99) used to treat allergy 81

trifluoperazine a phenothiazine antipsychotic 41 and an anti-emetic 46

trihexyphenidyl (previously benzhexol) a drug for parkinsonism 43)

tri-iodothyronine see liothyronine

Trileptal brand name for oxcarbazepine (an anticonvulsant 42)

Trimbow brand-name combination inhaler containing beclometasone 168 (a corticosteroid 99), formoterol, and glycopyrronium (both bronchodilators 48)

trimethoprim 424, an antibacterial 89

trimipramine a tricyclic antidepressant 40

Trimovate brand name for clobetasone (a topical corticosteroid 134) with nystatin 343 (an antifungal 96) and oxytetracycline (a tetracycline antibiotic 86)

tripotassium dicitratobismuthate bismuth compound used in treating peptic ulcers 67

triprolidine an antihistamine 82

Triptafen brand name for amitriptyline 157 with perphenazine (an antipsychotic 41 and anti-emetic 46) used to treat depression 40

triptorelin anticancer drug 112 and drug for menstrual disorders 120

Trisenox brand name for arsenic (a chemical used as an anticancer drug 112 to treat leukaemia)

Trisequens brand name for estradiol 249 and norethisterone 342 (female sex hormones 105)

Tritace brand name for ramipril 379 (an ACE inhibitor 56)

Triumeq brand name for abacavir with dolutegravir and lamivudine 430 (all antiretrovirals for HIV/AIDS 116)

Trizivir brand name for abacavir with zidovudine/lamivudine 430 (all antiretrovirals for HIV/AIDS 116)

Trobalt brand name for retigabine (an anticonvulsant 42)

Trolactin brand name for dipyridamole 230 (an antithrombotic drug 62)

tropicamide mydriatic 130

trospium anticholinergic for urinary disorders 126

Trosyl brand name for tioconazole (an antifungal 96)

Trulicity brand name for dulaglutide 239 (a drug for diabetes 100)

Trusopt brand name for dorzolamide 234 (a drug for glaucoma 128)

Truvada brand name for tenofovir 409 with emtricitabine 242 (both drugs for HIV/AIDS 116)

Truxima brand name for rituximab 385 (a monoclonal antibody)

TUMS brand name for an antacid 66 containing calcium carbonate

Twinrix brand-name vaccine 92 to protect against hepatitis A/hepatitis B

Tybost brand name for cobicistat (a drug for HIV/AIDS 116)

Tygacil brand name for tigecycline (an antibiotic 86)

Tylex brand name for paracetamol 352 (a non-opioid analgesic 36) and codeine phosphate (an opioid analgesic 36)

Tymbrineb brand name for an injectable preparation of tobramycin (an aminoglycoside antibiotic 86)

Tysabri brand name for natalizumab (a monoclonal antibody)

Tyvera brand name for thiamine (vitamin B1 442)

Tyverb brand name for lapatinib (an anticancer drug 112)

U

Uard brand name for diltiazem 229 (a calcium channel blocker 59) used for hypertension 60

** ulipristal** 425, drug used for emergency contraception 121

Ultibro Breezhaler brand-name inhaler containing glycopyrronium and indacaterol (both bronchodilators 48)

Ultralanum Plain brand name for fluocortolone (a topical corticosteroid 134)

Ultraproct brand name for fluocortolone (a topical corticosteroid 134) with cinchocaine (a local anaesthetic 36)

umeclidinium bronchodilator drug 48 used to treat chronic obstructive pulmonary disease

umeclidinium with vilanterol a combination bronchodilator preparation 48 used to treat chronic obstructive pulmonary disease

undecenoic acid antifungal 96 for athlete's foot

Unguentum M brand-name preparation for dry skin conditions 132

Uniphyllin Continus brand name for theophylline 416 (a bronchodilator 48)

Uniroid HC brand name for hydrocortisone 277 (a corticosteroid 99) with cinchocaine (a local anaesthetic 36)

Univer brand name for verapamil 428 (an anti-arrhythmic 58 and anti-angina drug 59)

Upostelle brand-name progesterone-only oral contraceptive 121 containing levonorgestrel 300

Uptravi brand name for selexipag (a drug that lowers blood pressure in the lungs) used for pulmonary hypertension

Uraplex brand name for trospium chloride (a drug for urinary frequency 126)

urea topical treatment to moisturize dry skin 132 and soften ear wax 131

Uricto brand name for allopurinol 151 (a drug for gout 77)

Urispas-199 brand name for flavoxate (a urinary antispasmodic 126)

urofollitropin drug for pituitary disorders 103

urokinase anticlotting drug 62

ursodeoxycholic acid drug for gallstones 72

Ursofalk brand name for ursodeoxycholic acid (a drug used for treating gallstones 72)

ustekinumab immunosuppressant 115

Utovlan brand name for norethisterone 342 (a female sex hormone 105)

Utrogestan brand name for progesterone (a female sex hormone 105)

Uvistat brand-name sunscreen preparation 141

V

Vagifem brand name for estradiol 249 (a female sex hormone 105)

valaciclovir antiviral 91

Valcade brand name for bortezomib (an anticancer drug 112)

Valcyte brand name for valganciclovir (an antiviral 91)

Valdoxan brand name for agomelatine (an antidepressant 40)

valganciclovir antiviral 91 for cytomegalovirus

Valios brand name for memantine (a drug for Alzheimer's disease 43)

Valket Retard brand name for ketoprofen 292 (an NSAID 74)

Valni XL brand name for modified-release nifedipine 340 (a calcium-channel blocker 59)

Valpeda brand-name topical preparation containing halquinol (an antiseptic)

valproate 398, anticonvulsant 42

valproic acid anticonvulsant 42

valsartan 390, antihypertensive 60

Valtrex brand name for valaciclovir, an antiviral drug 91

Vamju brand name for modified-release gliclazide 270 (a drug for diabetes 100)

Vancocin brand name for vancomycin, an antibiotic 86 for serious infections

vancomycin antibiotic 86 for serious infections

vandetanib protein kinase inhibitor anticancer drug 112

Vaniqa brand name for eflornithine (a drug to control facial hair in women)

Vanquoral brand name for ciclosporin 196 (an immunosuppressant 115)

Vantobra brand-name nebulizer solution of tobramycin (an aminoglycoside antibiotic 86) used for lung infections

VAQTA brand-name vaccine 92 to protect against viral hepatitis

vardenafil drug for erectile dysfunction 124

varenicline 426, drug used as a smoking cessation aid

Vargatef brand name for nintedanib (an anticancer drug 112)

Varilrix brand name for varicella-zoster vaccine (chickenpox/shingles) 92

Vascalpha brand name for modified-release felodipine 256 (a calcium channel blocker 59)

Vaseline Petroleum Jelly brand-name ointment used for dry skin 132

Vasogen brand-name barrier cream 135 containing calamine, dimeticone, and zinc oxide

vasopressin a pituitary hormone 103 used for diabetes insipidus 103

Vasran brand name for alfuzosin (an alpha blocker for prostate disorders 126)

Vectibix brand name for panitumumab (an anticancer drug 112)

vecuronium muscle relaxant 78 used in general anaesthesia

vedolizumab monoclonal antibody used for inflammatory gastrointestinal disorders

Vedrop brand name for D-alpha tocopherol (vitamin E 444)

Veil brand-name skin preparation 135 to camouflage scars

Veletri brand name for epoprostenol (an anticlotting drug 62)

Velosef brand name for cefradine, a cephalosporin antibiotic 86

Velphoro brand name for iron 437 for patients with kidney failure

Vemlidy brand name for tenofovir 409 (a drug used to treat hepatitis)

vemurafinib anticancer drug 112

Venaxx XL brand name for a modified-release preparation of venlafaxine 427 (an antidepressant 40)

Vencarm XL brand name for a modified-release preparation of venlafaxine 427 (an antidepressant 40)

Venclyxto brand name for venetoclax (an anticancer drug 112) used to treat leukaemia

Venlablue XL brand name for a modified-release preparation of venlafaxine 427 (an antidepressant 40)

VENLADEX XL

Venladex XL brand name for a modified-release preparation of venlafaxine 427 (an antidepressant 40)

venlafaxine 427, antidepressant 40

Venlalic XL brand name for a modified-release preparation of venlafaxine 427 (an antidepressant 40)

Venlaneo XL brand name for a modified-release preparation of venlafaxine 427 (an antidepressant 40)

Venlasov XL brand name for a modified-release preparation of venlafaxine 427 (an antidepressant 40)

Venofer brand-name iron supplement 437

Vensir XL brand name for a modified-release preparation of venlafaxine 427 (an antidepressant 40)

Ventavis brand name for iloprost (a vasodilator drug 56 used to treat pulmonary hypertension)

Ventolin brand name for salbutamol 391 (a bronchodilator 48 and drug used in labour 125)

Ventra brand name for esomeprazole (an ulcer-healing drug 67)

Vepesid brand name for etoposide (an anticancer drug 112)

Veracur brand name for formaldehyde (a substance for warts)

verapamil 428, calcium channel blocker for angina 59, arrhythmias 58, and hypertension 60

Verapress MR brand name for a modified-release preparation of verapamil 428 (a calcium channel blocker for angina 59, arrhythmias 58, and hypertension 60)

Vermox brand name for mebendazole 311 (an anthelmintic 97)

Verrugon brand name for salicylic acid (a keratolytic for warts)

Vertab SR brand name for a modified-release preparation of verapamil 428 (a calcium channel blocker for angina 59, arrhythmias 58, and hypertension 60)

verteporfin drug used for age-related macular degeneration

Vertine brand name for salmeterol 392 (a bronchodilator 48) used for asthma 49

Vesicare brand name for solifenacin (a drug for urinary disorders 126)

Vesomni brand name for tamsulosin 407 (an alpha blocker for prostate disorders 126)

Vexarin XL brand name for a modified-release preparation of venlafaxine 427 (an antidepressant 40)

VFEND brand name for voriconazole (an antifungal 96)

Viagra brand name for sildenafil 394 (a drug for erectile dysfunction 104, 124)

Viazem XL brand name for diltiazem 229 (a calcium channel blocker 59 and antihypertensive 60)

Vibativ brand name for an intravenous preparation of telavancin (an antibacterial drug 89) used to treat pneumonia

Vibramycin and Vibramycin-D brand names for doxycycline 238 (a tetracycline antibiotic 86)

Vibrox brand name for doxycycline 238 (a tetracycline antibiotic 86)

Vicks Sinex brand-name decongestant containing oxymethazoline (a decongestant)

Victanyl brand name for a skin patch containing fentanyl (an opioid analgesic drug 36)

Victoza brand name for liraglutide (a drug for diabetes 100)

Victrelis brand name for boceprivir (an antiviral 91 for hepatitis B and C)

Vidaza brand name for azacitidine (an anticancer drug 112 for some leukaemias)

Videne brand name for povidone-iodine (an antiseptic 135)

Videx brand name for didanosine (an antiretroviral for HIV/AIDS 116)

Viekirax brand-name preparation containing ombitasvir, paritaprevir, and ritonavir (all antivirals 91) used for hepatitis C

ViePax Winfex XL brand name for a preparation containing venlafaxine 427 (an antidepressant drug 40)

vigabatrin anticonvulsant 42

Vigam brand name for human normal immunoglobulin (a preparation injected to prevent infectious diseases 92)

vilanterol bronchodilator 48

vildagliptin drug used to treat diabetes 100

Vimovo brand name for naproxen 337 (a NSAID 74 and drug for gout 77) with esomeprazole (an anti-ulcer drug 67)

Vimpat brand name drug for lacosamide (an anticonvulsant drug 42 used to control epilepsy)

vinblastine anticancer drug 112

vincristine anticancer drug 112

vindesine anticancer drug 112

vinflunine anticancer drug 112

vinorelbine anticancer drug 112

Vipdomet brand-name preparation containing metformin 318 with alogliptin (both drugs for diabetes 100)

Vipidia brand name for alogliptin (a drug for diabetes 100)

Viraferon brand name for interferon alfa 285 (an antiviral drug 91 used to treat viral hepatitis)

Viramune brand name for nevirapine (an antiretroviral used to treat HIV/AIDS 116)

Viread brand name for tenofovir 409 (an antiviral drug 91 and drug for HIV/AIDS 116)

Viridal Duo brand name for alprostadil (a prostaglandin used to treat erectile dysfunction 104, 124)

Viscotears brand of artificial tears 130

Viskaldix brand name for pindolol (a beta blocker 55) and clopamide (a thiazide diuretic 57)

Visken brand name for pindolol (a beta blocker drug 55)

vismodegib anticancer drug 112

Vistamethasone brand name for betamethasone 172 (a corticosteroid 99)

Vistaprep bowel cleansing preparation used prior to colonoscopy

Visudyne brand name for verteporfin (a drug used for age-related muscular degeneration)

Vita-E brand name for alpha tocopherol (vitamin E 444)

vitamin A 442 (a vitamin 107)

vitamin B1 thiamine 442 (a vitamin 107)

vitamin B2 riboflavin 440 (a vitamin 107)

vitamin B6 pyridoxine 440 (a vitamin 107)

vitamin B12 hydroxocobalamin 443 (a vitamin 107)

vitamin B complex see vitamins 107

vitamin C ascorbic acid 443 (a vitamin 107)

vitamin D 444 (a vitamin 107)

vitamin E 444 (a vitamin 107)

vitamin K 445 (a vitamin 107)

Vitaros brand name for alprostadil (a prostaglandin for erectile dysfunction 104, 124)

Vitekta brand name for elvitegravir (an antiretroviral drug for HIV/AIDS 116)

Vivadex brand name for tacrolimus 405 (an immunosuppressant 115)

Vivotif brand-name vaccine 92 to protect against typhoid fever

Vizarsin brand name for sildenafil 394 (a drug for erectile dysfunction 124)

Vokanamet brand name for a combined preparation containing canagliflozin and metformin 318 (both drugs for diabetes 100)

Voleze brand name for rivastigmine 387 (a drug for Alzheimer's disease 43)

Volibris brand name for ambrisentan (a vasodilator 56) for pulmonary hypertension

Volsaid Retard brand name for diclofenac 225 (an NSAID 74)

Voltarol brand name for diclofenac 225 (an NSAID 74)

Voractiv brand name for rifampicin 382 (an antituberculous drug 90)

voriconazole antifungal 96

vortioxetine antidepressant 40

Vosevi brand-name drug containing sofosbuvir, velpatasvir, and oxilaprevir (antiviral drugs 91) used to treat hepatitis C

Votrient brand name for pazopanib (a protein kinase inhibitor) used to treat kidney cancer

Votubia brand name for everolimus (an immunosuppressant 115)

W

warfarin 429, anticoagulant 62

Warticon brand name for podophyllotoxin (a drug for genital warts)

Wellvone brand name for atovaquone (an antiprotozoal 94 and an antimalarial 95)

witch hazel astringent used in topical 134 and rectal preparations 71

X

Xadago brand name for safinamide (a drug for Parkinson's disease 43)

Xaggitin XL brand name for methylphenidate 322 (a drug used to treat attention deficit hyperactivity disorder (ADHD))

Xalacom brand name for latanoprost 296 with timolol 417 (both drugs for glaucoma 128)

Xalatan brand name for latanoprost 296 (a drug for glaucoma 128)

Xalkori brand name for crizotinib (an anticancer drug 112)

Xaluprine brand name for mercaptopurine 316 (an anticancer drug 112)

Xanax brand name for alprazolam (a benzodiazepine anti-anxiety drug 39)

Xarelto brand name for rivaroxaban 386 (an anticoagulant 62)

Xatral XL brand name for alfuzosin (a drug for prostate disorders 104)

Xeljanz brand name for tofacitinib (a drug for rheumatoid arthritis 75)

Xeloda brand name for capecitabine (an anticancer drug 112)

Xenazine a brand name for tetrabenazine (a drug used to treat movement disorders)

Xenical brand name for orlistat 348 (an anti-obesity drug 106)

Xeomin brand name for botulinum toxin 176

Xeplion brand name for paliperidone (an antipsychotic drug 41)

Xetinin brand name for clarithromycin 202 (a macrolide antibiotic 86)

Xgeva brand name for denosumab (a monoclonal antibody) used to treat bone metastases and osteoporosis

ZYVOX

Xifaxanta brand name for rifaximin (an antibacterial 89)

Xigduo brand name for metformin 318 with dapagliflozin 220 (both drugs used for diabetes 100)

Xigris brand name for drotrecogin alfa (an anti-thrombotic drug 63)

xipamide thiazide-like diuretic 57

Xolair brand name for omalizumab, used for severe asthma

Xultophy brand name for insulin 284 and liraglutide (both drugs used to treat diabetes 100)

Xydalba brand name for dalbavancin (an antibiotic 86) used for MRSA infections

xylometazoline a decongestant 51

Xyloproct brand-name anal preparation 71 containing hydrocortisone 277, aluminium acetate, lidocaine, and zinc oxide

Xyzal brand name for levocetirizine (an antihistamine 82)

Y

Yacella brand-name oral contraceptive 121 containing ethinylestradiol 252 with drospirenone (a progestogen 105)

Yasmin brand-name oral contraceptive containing ethinylestradiol 252 with drospirenone (a progestogen 105)

Yemex brand name for fentanyl (an opioid painkiller 36)

Yentreve brand name for duloxetine (a drug for stress incontinence 126)

Yervoy brand name for ipilimumab (an anticancer drug 112)

Yiznell brand-name oral contraceptive 121 containing ethinylestradiol 252 with drospirenone (a progestogen 105)

Yondelis brand name for trabectedine (an anticancer drug 112)

Z

Zacco brand name for clobazam (a benzodiazepine 39)

Zacin brand name for topical capsaicin (a plant alkaloid) used to treat pain

Zaditen brand name for ketotifen (a drug used to prevent asthma 49)

zafirlukast leukotriene antagonist for asthma 49 and bronchospasm 48

Zalasta brand name for olanzapine 344 (a second-generation antipsychotic 41)

zaleplon sleeping drug 38

Zaltrap brand name for aflibercept (used to treat eye conditions affecting vision)

Zaluron brand name for quetiapine 375 (a second-generation antipsychotic 41)

Zalviso brand name for sufentanil (an opioid analgesic 36)

Zamadol brand name for tramadol 421 (an opioid analgesic 36)

Zanaflex brand name for tizanidine (a muscle relaxant 78)

zanamivir antiviral drug 91

Zanidip brand name for lercanidipine (a calcium channel blocker 59)

Zantac brand name for ranitidine 380 (an anti-ulcer drug 67)

Zapain brand name for codeine phosphate 211 (an opioid analgesic 36) and paracetamol 352 (a non-opioid analgesic 36)

Zaponex brand name for clozapine 210 (an antipsychotic 41)

Zarontin brand name for ethosuximide (an anticonvulsant 42)

Zaroxolyn brand name for metolazone (a diuretic 57)

Zarzio brand name for filgastrim 257 (a blood growth stimulant)

Zebinix brand name for eslicarbazepine (an anticonvulsant 42)

Zedbac brand name for azithromycin (an antibiotic 86)

Zeffix brand name for lamivudine 430 (an antiretroviral for hepatitis B)

Zelapar brand name for selegiline (a drug used in treating Parkinson's disease 43)

Zelboraf brand name for vemurafinib (an anticancer drug 112)

Zelleta brand name for desogestrel 222 (a progestogen 105)

Zemplar brand name for paricalcitol (synthetic form of vitamin D 444)

Zemret brand name for diltiazem 229 (a calcium channel blocker 58)

Zemtard brand name for diltiazem 229 (a calcium channel blocker 58)

Zepatier brand-name combination of elbasvir and grazoprevir (both antivirals 91) for hepatitis C

Zeridame SR brand-name modified-release preparation of tramadol 421 (an opioid analgesic 36)

Zerit brand name for stavudine (an antiretroviral for HIV/AIDS 116)

Zerocream brand-name cream for dry skin

Zeroguent brand-name cream for dry skin

Zerolatum Plus brand-name bath oil for dry skin

Zeroneum brand-name bath oil for dry skin

Zestoretic brand name for lisinopril 302 (an ACE inhibitor 56) and hydrochlorothiazide 276 (a diuretic 57)

Zestril brand name for lisinopril 302 (an ACE inhibitor 56)

Ziagen brand name for abacavir (an antiretroviral drug for HIV/AIDS 116)

Ziclaseg brand name for gliclazide (a drug used to treat diabetes 100)

Zicron brand name for gliclazide (a drug used to treat diabetes 100)

Zidoval brand name for topical metronidazole 325 (an antibacterial 89 and antiprotozoal 94)

zidovudine (AZT) 430, antiretroviral used to treat HIV/AIDS 116

Zimovane and **Zimovane LS** brand names for zopiclone 432 (a sleeping drug 38)

Zinacef brand name for cefuroxime (a cephalosporin antibiotic 86)

Zinamide brand name for pyrazinamide (an antimycobacterial) for tuberculosis 90

Zinbryta brand name for daclizumab (a drug for multiple sclerosis)

zinc 445, mineral 108

zinc oxide soothing agent 135

zinc sulfate zinc 445 (a mineral 108)

Zindaclin brand-name topical gel for acne 137 containing clindamycin 200 (an antibiotic 86)

Zineryt brand-name acne preparation 137 containing erythromycin 247 (an antibiotic 86) and zinc 437 (a mineral 108)

Zinforo brand name for cetaroline (an antibacterial 89)

Zinnat brand name for cefuroxime (a cephalosporin antibiotic 86)

Zirtek brand name for cetirizine 188 (an antihistamine 82)

Zispin brand name for mirtazapine 329 (an antidepressant 40)

Zithromax brand name for azithromycin (an antibiotic 86)

Zlatal brand name for methotrexate 320 (a DMARD)

Zochek brand name for alfuzosin (an alpha blocker for urinary disorders 126)

Zocor brand name for simvastatin 395 (a lipid-lowering drug 61)

Zoely brand name for estradiol 249 and nomegestrol (both female sex hormones 105)

Zofran brand name for ondansetron 347 (an anti-emetic 46)

Zoladex brand name for goserelin 273 (a female sex hormone 105 and anticancer drug 112)

zoledronic acid 431, drug for bone disorders 80

zolmitriptan drug for migraine 45

zolpidem sleeping drug 38

Zolvera brand name for verapamil 428 (a calcium channel blocker for angina 59 and arrhythmias 58)

Zomacton brand name for somatropin (a synthetic pituitary hormone 103)

Zomestine brand name for oxycodone (an opioid analgesic 36)

Zometa brand name for zoledronic acid 423 (a drug for bone disorders 80)

Zomig brand name for zolmitriptan (a drug for migraine 45)

Zomorph brand name for morphine 334 (an opioid analgesic 36) with cyclizine (an anti-emetic 46)

Zonegran brand name for zonisamide (an anticonvulsant 42)

zonisamide anticonvulsant 42

zopiclone 432, sleeping drug 38

Zorac brand-name topical preparation for psoriasis 138 containing tazarotene (a retinoid)

Zoton brand name for lansoprazole 295 (an anti-ulcer drug 67)

Zovirax brand name for aciclovir 148 (an antiviral 91)

zuclopenthixol an antipsychotic 41

Zumenon brand name for estradiol 249 (a female sex hormone 105)

Zyban brand name for bupropion 180 (a drug used as an adjunct to smoking cessation)

Zyclara brand name for imiquimod (a drug used in treating genital and perianal warts)

Zydol brand name for tramadol 412 (an opioid analgesic 36)

Zykadia brand name for ceritinib (an anticancer drug 112) used to treat lung cancer

Zyloric brand name for allopurinol 151 (a drug for gout 77)

Zyomet brand name for metronidazole 319 (an antibacterial 89 and antiprotozoal 94)

ZypAdhera brand-name depot injection containing olanzapine 344 (an antipsychotic 41)

Zyprexa and **Zyprexa Velotab** brand names for olanzapine 344 (an antipsychotic 41)

Zytiga brand name for abiraterone (an anticancer drug 112)

Zytram brand name for tramadol 421 (an opioid analgesic 36)

Zyvox brand name for linezolid (an antibiotic 86)

INDEX

This general index contains references to the information in all sections of the book. It can be used to look up topics such as groups of drugs, diseases, and conditions. References for generic and brand-name drugs are also listed, with references to

the appropriate drug profile or the listing in the Drug Finder (pp.468–499). Entries that contain a page reference followed by the letter "g" indicate that the entry is defined in the Glossary (pp.463–467) on the page specified.

DRUG POISONING EMERGENCY GUIDE

The information on the following pages is intended to give practical advice for dealing with a known or suspected drug poisoning emergency. Although many of the first-aid techniques described can be used in a number of different types of emergency, these instructions apply specifically to drug overdose or poisoning.

Emergency action is necessary in any of the following circumstances:

- If a person has taken an overdose of any of the high-danger drugs listed in the box on p.520.
- If a person has taken an overdose of a less dangerous drug, but has one or more of the danger symptoms listed (right).
- If a person has taken, or is suspected of having taken, an overdose of an unknown drug.
- If an infant or child has swallowed, or is suspected of having swallowed, any medicines or any drug of abuse.

What to do

If you are faced with a drug poisoning emergency, it is important to carry out first aid and arrange immediate medical help in the correct order. The Priority Action Decision Chart (below left) will help you to assess the situation and to determine your priorities. The following information should help you to remain calm in an emergency if you ever need to deal with a case of drug poisoning.

DANGER SYMPTOMS

Take emergency action if the person has one or more of the following symptoms:

- Vomiting
- Seizures
- Shallow or irregular breathing
- Unresponsive or impaired level of response

PRIORITY ACTION DECISION CHART

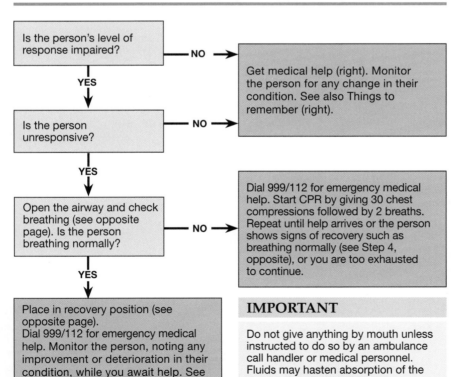

Is the person's level of response impaired? — NO → Get medical help (right). Monitor the person for any change in their condition. See also Things to remember (right).

YES ↓

Is the person unresponsive? — NO →

YES ↓

Open the airway and check breathing (see opposite page). Is the person breathing normally? — NO → Dial 999/112 for emergency medical help. Start CPR by giving 30 chest compressions followed by 2 breaths. Repeat until help arrives or the person shows signs of recovery such as breathing normally (see Step 4, opposite), or you are too exhausted to continue.

YES ↓

Place in recovery position (see opposite page). Dial 999/112 for emergency medical help. Monitor the person, noting any improvement or deterioration in their condition, while you await help. See also Things to remember (right).

IMPORTANT

Do not give anything by mouth unless instructed to do so by an ambulance call handler or medical personnel. Fluids may hasten absorption of the drug, increasing the danger.

GETTING MEDICAL HELP

In an emergency, one person competent in first aid should stay with the casualty, while others summon help. Clear the area of any hazards, then start first aid (see the Priority Action Decision Chart, left). Ask someone else to call for help as soon as you have checked breathing. If you are on your own, call for help before you start CPR. Any syringes (see below) should be handled only when wearing gloves and placed in a jar with a lid or in a sharps box.

Calling an ambulance may be the fastest method of transport to hospital. The call handler will advise you what first aid to give. If possible, tell the call handler or ambulance personnel what drug was taken, how much, and the person's age.

THINGS TO REMEMBER

Effective treatment of drug poisoning depends on medical personnel making a rapid assessment of the type and amount of drug taken. Collecting evidence that will assist this will help. After you have carried out first aid, look for empty or opened medicine containers. Keep any of the drug that is left, together with its container (or syringe), and take these with the casualty. Save any vomit for analysis by the hospital.

ESSENTIAL FIRST AID

UNRESPONSIVE CASUALTY

CHECKING BREATHING

If a casualty is unresponsive, open their airway and check the person's breathing (below). If the person is breathing normally, place them in the recovery position (right). If they are not breathing normally, start cardiopulmonary resuscitation (CPR) as shown below.

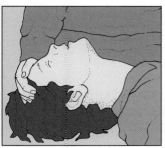 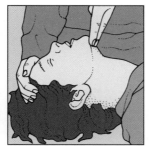

1 Lay the casualty on their back on a firm surface. Place one hand on the forehead and gently tilt the head back. Clear any obvious obstructions from the mouth.

2 Place two fingers under the point of the casualty's chin, and lift the jaw. Then look, listen, and feel for breathing for no more than 10 seconds.

3 Place your ear over the person's mouth and look along the chest. Look for chest movements that indicate breathing, feel for breaths on your cheek, and listen for sounds of breathing. If the person is not breathing normally, call for emergency help.

RECOVERY POSITION

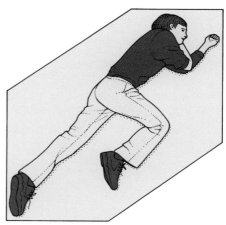

The recovery position is the safest position for an unresponsive person who is breathing normally. It will help maintain an open airway and allow fluids or vomit to drain from the mouth, to prevent choking. Place the casualty on their side with the upper leg and lower arm bent to stop them rolling forward. Tilt the head back to keep the airway open. Support it by placing the hand of the uppermost arm, palm down, under the cheek. Monitor breathing and pulse while awaiting help. If the person stops breathing, turn them on their back and start CPR (below).

CARDIOPULMONARY RESUSCITATION (CPR)

In an adult, blood oxygen levels remain the same for a couple of minutes after the heart has stopped, so start with chest compressions. After 2–4 minutes oxygen levels fall, so rescue breaths are needed. This sequence is called cardiopulmonary resuscitation (CPR). If you are alone, call for help before starting CPR.

> If unable or unwilling to give rescue breaths, just give chest compressions. The emergency services will instruct callers on chest compressions only.

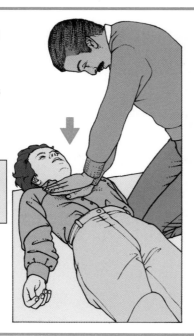

1 Place the heel of your hand on the centre of the chest and place your other hand on top. Press down about one third the depth of the chest, then release the pressure but do not remove your hands. Give 30 compressions at a rate of 100 per minute.

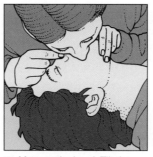 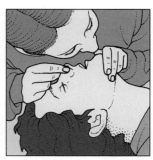

2 Move to the head. Tilt the casualty's head back and pinch the nose shut with one hand, while lifting the casualty's chin with your other one. Take a breath and breathe into the casualty's mouth until you see their chest rise.

3 Remove your mouth and look along the chest to see the casualty's chest fall. Repeat to give two breaths.

4 Continue a sequence of 30 compressions followed by 2 rescue breaths until emergency help arrives, the casualty shows signs of becoming responsive, such as coughing, moving purposefully, and opening their eyes, the person starts to breathe normally, or you are too exhausted to continue.

DEALING WITH A SEIZURE

Certain types of drug poisoning may provoke seizures. These may occur in people who are initially responsive as well as in unresponsive casualties. The person usually falls to the ground twitching or making uncontrolled movements of the limbs and body. If you witness a seizure:

● Try to ensure that the person does not suffer injury by moving away furniture or any dangerous objects.
● Loosen clothing around neck if possible.
● Do not attempt to put anything into the person's mouth.
● Do not try to hold the person down.
● Once the seizure is over, the person may fall into a deep sleep, so place them in the recovery position (see p.519).

HIGH-DANGER DRUGS

Below is a list of drugs with a high overdose rating in the drug profiles or included in the drugs of abuse. If you suspect that someone has taken an overdose of any of these drugs, seek immediate medical attention.

Amiodarone
Amitriptyline
Aspirin
Atenolol
Atropine
Betahistine
Bisoprolol
Bupropion
Chloroquine
Clomipramine
Codeine
Colchicine
Dabigatran
Digoxin
Dihydrocodeine
Dosulepin
   (dothiepin)
Epinephrine
   (adrenaline)
Exenatide
Glibenclamide
Gliclazide
Heparin
Imipramine
Insulin
Isoniazid
Lithium
Mefloquine
Metformin
Methadone
Methotrexate
Methylphenidate
Metoprolol
Modafinil
Morphine/
   diamorphine
Nicotine
Orphenadrine
Oxybutynin
Paracetamol

Phenelzine
Phenobarbital
Phenytoin/
   fosphenytoin
Pioglitazone
Procyclidine
Propranolol
Pyridostigmine
Quinine
Rivaroxaban
Sitagliptin
Sotalol
Theophylline/
   aminophylline
Timolol
Tolbutamide
Tolterodine
Tramadol
Venlafaxine
Warfarin

Drugs of abuse
Alcohol
Amfetamines
Barbiturates
Benzodiazepines
Cannabis (marijuana)
Cocaine (including crack)
Ecstasy (MDMA)
GHB
Ketamine
Khat
LSD
Magic mushrooms
Mephedrone
Nitrites
Opioids (including
   heroin)
Phencyclidine
Volatile substances

DEALING WITH ANAPHYLACTIC SHOCK

Anaphylactic shock can occur as the result of a severe allergic reaction to a drug (such as penicillin). Blood pressure drops dramatically and the airways may become narrowed. The reaction usually occurs within minutes. The main symptoms are:

● Breathing difficulty
● Pallor
● Blotchy red rash
● Anxiety
● Swelling of tongue or throat

A person known to be at risk of anaphylaxis may be carrying a pre-filled epinephrine/adrenaline syringe, called an autoinjector, for immediate self-injection.

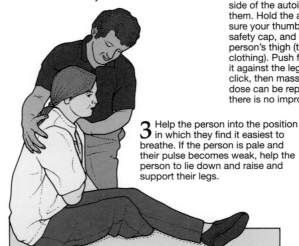

1 Dial 999/112 for emergency help, telling them you think the person has had a severe allergic reaction.

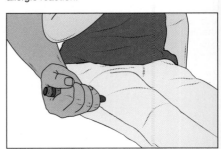

2 If the person has an epinephrine/adrenaline autoinjector, help them to use it. If they are unable to do this, follow the instructions on the side of the autoinjector and administer it for them. Hold the autoinjector in your fist (make sure your thumb is not on the top), remove the safety cap, and press the needle against the person's thigh (the dose can be given through clothing). Push firmly until you hear a click, hold it against the leg for 10 seconds until you hear it click, then massage the leg for 10 seconds. The dose can be repeated at 5-minute intervals if there is no improvement or if symptoms recur.

3 Help the person into the position in which they find it easiest to breathe. If the person is pale and their pulse becomes weak, help the person to lie down and raise and support their legs.

4 Monitor the person's breathing and level of responsiveness while waiting for medical help to arrive. If they become unresponsive, treat as described on p.519.

DEALING WITH VOMITING

Vomiting is the body's response to many potentially harmful things, including contaminated food, viral infections, and severe pain. It also occurs as an adverse effect of some drugs and as a result of drug overdose.

Do not attempt to induce vomiting by pushing fingers down the casualty's throat. When vomiting does occur, remember the following:

● Vomiting can be a result of poisoning.
● Vomiting due to drugs is usually a result of an overdose rather than a side effect. Check in the relevant drug profile whether vomiting is a possible adverse effect of the suspected drug. If vomiting appears to be due to an overdose, get medical help urgently.

● Even if vomiting has stopped, monitor the person's breathing and level of reponse; they may have a seizure or become unresponsive.
● If the person is unresponsive, check their breathing and place them in the recovery position (see p.519).

1 Ensure that the casualty leans well forward to avoid either choking or inhaling vomit. If the casualty appears to be choking, encourage coughing.

2 Keep a sample of vomit for analysis (see Things to remember p.518).

3 Give water to rinse the mouth. Advise the person to spit out the water rather than swallow it.